Lecture Notes in Co

Commenced Publication in 1973
Founding and Former Series Editors:
Gerhard Goos, Juris Hartmanis, and Jan van Leeuwen

Editorial Board

David Hutchison
  Lancaster University, UK
Takeo Kanade
  Carnegie Mellon University, Pittsburgh, PA, USA
Josef Kittler
  University of Surrey, Guildford, UK
Jon M. Kleinberg
  Cornell University, Ithaca, NY, USA
Alfred Kobsa
  University of California, Irvine, CA, USA
Friedemann Mattern
  ETH Zurich, Switzerland
John C. Mitchell
  Stanford University, CA, USA
Moni Naor
  Weizmann Institute of Science, Rehovot, Israel
Oscar Nierstrasz
  University of Bern, Switzerland
C. Pandu Rangan
  Indian Institute of Technology, Madras, India
Bernhard Steffen
  University of Dortmund, Germany
Madhu Sudan
  Microsoft Research, Cambridge, MA, USA
Demetri Terzopoulos
  University of California, Los Angeles, CA, USA
Doug Tygar
  University of California, Berkeley, CA, USA
Gerhard Weikum
  Max-Planck Institute of Computer Science, Saarbruecken, Germany

Guang-Zhong Yang   David Hawkes
Daniel Rueckert   Alison Noble
Chris Taylor (Eds.)

Medical Image Computing and Computer-Assisted Intervention – MICCAI 2009

12th International Conference
London, UK, September 20-24, 2009
Proceedings, Part II

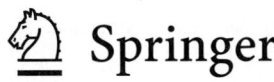
Springer

Volume Editors

Guang-Zhong Yang
Imperial College London, Institute of Biomedical Engineering
London, UK
E-mail: g.z.yang@imperial.ac.uk

David Hawkes
University College London, Centre for Medical Image Computing
London, UK
E-mail: d.hawkes@ucl.ac.uk

Daniel Rueckert
Imperial College London, Department of Computing
London, UK
E-mail: d.rueckert@imperial.ac.uk

Alison Noble
University of Oxford, Institute of Biomedical Engineering
Oxford, UK
E-mail: noble@robots.ox.ac.uk

Chris Taylor
University of Manchester, School of Computer Science
Manchester, UK
E-mail: chris.taylor@manchester.ac.uk

Library of Congress Control Number: 2009934167

CR Subject Classification (1998): I.5, I.2.10, I.2.9, J.3, J.6, I.4, K.4.1

LNCS Sublibrary: SL 6 – Image Processing, Computer Vision, Pattern Recognition, and Graphics

ISSN   0302-9743
ISBN-10   3-642-04270-8 Springer Berlin Heidelberg New York
ISBN-13   978-3-642-04270-6 Springer Berlin Heidelberg New York

This work is subject to copyright. All rights are reserved, whether the whole or part of the material is concerned, specifically the rights of translation, reprinting, re-use of illustrations, recitation, broadcasting, reproduction on microfilms or in any other way, and storage in data banks. Duplication of this publication or parts thereof is permitted only under the provisions of the German Copyright Law of September 9, 1965, in its current version, and permission for use must always be obtained from Springer. Violations are liable to prosecution under the German Copyright Law.

springer.com

© Springer-Verlag Berlin Heidelberg 2009
Printed in Germany

Typesetting: Camera-ready by author, data conversion by Scientific Publishing Services, Chennai, India
Printed on acid-free paper   SPIN: 12757428   06/3180   5 4 3 2 1 0

Preface

The 12th International Conference on Medical Image Computing and Computer-Assisted Intervention, MICCAI 2009, was held in London, England at Imperial College during September 20–24, 2009. The venue was situated in one of London's finest locations, adjacent to landmarks such as The Royal Albert Hall and the Science, Natural History and Victoria and Albert Museums, with Hyde Park just a short walk away.

Over the last decade, the MICCAI conferences have become a premier international event, with papers of very high standard addressing the multidisciplinary fields of biomedical image computing, computer-assisted intervention and medical robotics. The conference has attracted annually leading scientists, engineers and clinicians from a wide range of disciplines.

This year, we received a record submission of 804 papers from 36 different countries worldwide. These covered medical image computing (functional and diffusion image analysis, segmentation, physical and functional modelling, shape analysis, atlases and statistical models, registration, data fusion and multiscale analysis), computer-assisted interventions and robotics (planning and image guidance of interventions, simulation and training systems, clinical platforms, visualization and feedback, robotics and human–robot interaction), and clinical imaging and biomarkers (computer-aided diagnosis, organ/system specific applications, molecular and optical imaging and imaging biomarkers).

A careful, systematic review process was put in place to ensure the best possible program for MICCAI 2009. The Program Committee (PC) of the conference was composed of 39 members, each with recognized international reputation in the main topics covered by the conference. Each one of the 804 submitted papers was assigned to two PC members (a Primary and a Secondary). At least three external reviewers (outside the PC) were assigned to each paper according to their expertise. These external reviewers provided double-blind reviews of the papers, including those submitted by the conference organizers. All reviewers, except a handful who provided last minute "emergency" reviews, refereed between 8 and 10 papers each, giving each reviewer a reasonable sample for ranking the relative quality of the papers. Authors were given the opportunity to rebut the anonymous reviews.

Then, each PC member graded (typically 20) papers as primary based on the external reviews, the rebuttal and his/her own reading of the papers. In addition he/she provided input, as Secondary PC, to typically 20 more papers assigned to various Primary PCs. In summary, each paper was graded by two PC members and three external reviewers (i.e., by five assessors). During a two-day PC meeting involving the PC members held during May 17–18, 2009, papers were selected in a three-stage process:

- First stage: initial acceptance of those papers ranked very high and rejection of those papers ranked very low. Eight groups were formed, each comprising four or five PC members. The groups considered acceptance of the top three papers from each PC member and rejection of the bottom eight. Any papers in doubt were transferred to the second stage.
- Second stage: the same groups of PC members ranked the remaining papers and accepted between 9 and 18 of the highest ranking papers per group and rejected between 18 and 32 of the lowest ranking papers.
- Third stage: a different set of groups were formed and assigned the remaining undecided papers to the "accept" or "reject" category through an iterative process.

In all, we accepted 259 papers (32%) to be included in the proceedings of MICCAI 2009. Of these, 43 were selected for podium presentation (5%) and 216 for poster presentation at the conference (27%).

The review process was developed from that used in previous MICCAI conferences. In particular we are grateful to Rasmus Larsen for his input on the statistical basis for the protocol. Each step of the process ensured that, for random selections of papers to PC members, the probability of correctly assigning rejections and acceptances was at least 95%. With the combined skill and expertise of the PC, we are confident that it exceeded this figure and that we ran a robust system. Acceptance of papers at MICCAI is a competitive process and with such a strong submission rate it is inevitable that many good papers were not able to be included in the final program and we understand the frustration of authors. We too have had many papers rejected. We congratulate those who had papers accepted and encourage those who did not to persevere and submit again next year.

We wish to thank the reviewers and the PC for giving up their precious time ensuring the high quality of reviews and paper selection. These tasks are time consuming and require skill and good judgment, representing a significant effort by all. The continued improvement in the quality of the conference is entirely dependent on this tremendous effort.

We particularly wish to thank James Stewart of *precisionconference.com* for the efficient organization of the website and rapid response to any queries and requests for changes, many of them totally unreasonable and at a very short notice.

One highlight of MICCAI 2009 was the workshops and tutorials organized before and after the main conference. We had a record number of submissions which resulted in a very exciting, diverse and high-quality program. The workshops provided a comprehensive coverage on topics that were not fully explored during the main conference, including "grand challenges," and some emerging areas of MICCAI, whereas the tutorials provided educational material for training new professionals in the field including students, clinicians and new researchers. We are grateful to all workshop and tutorial organizers for making these events a great success.

We would also like to thank our two invited keynote speakers, Sir Michael Brady, University of Oxford, UK, and Koji Ikuta, Nagoya University, Japan. Their presentations on "Oncological Image Analysis" and "Nano and Micro Robotics for Future Biomedicine" were both inspiring and entertaining.

The conference would not be possible without the commitment and hard work of the local organizing team. In particular, we thank our Associate Editors Adrian Chung and Su-Lin Lee for their help in working with all authors in improving the final manuscript, and Dominique Drai, Ron Gaston, Thomy Merzanidou, Christiana Christodoulou, Karim Lekadir, Felipe Orihuela-Espina, Lichao Wang, Fani Deligianni, and Dong Ping Zhang for checking the original submissions and for assisting in the compilation of the proceedings.

We are grateful to Ferdinando Rodriguez y Baena for coordinating the corporate sponsorship and industrial/academic exhibitions, Dan Elson and Fernando Bello for coordinating MICCAI workshops and tutorials, Eddie Edwards for managing the conference registration and social events, and Raphaele Raupp for assisting with all the conference logistics. We also thank Robert Merrifield for his kind help in graphics design and George Mylonas for his huge effort in designing and implementing the hardware/software platforms for the conference e-Teaser sessions.

We are extremely grateful to Betty Yue, Ulrika Wernmark and their team for their tireless effort in managing all aspects of the conference organization—it is through their effort that we managed to have a seamless event on a busy campus where many dedicated facilities including the fully equipped poster hall had to be installed specially for the conference. We also thank all the session Chairs and Co-chairs in managing and coordinating the presentations during the conference.

We would also like to thank the MICCAI Society for providing valuable input and support to the conference, especially Guido Gerig for coordinating the MICCAI Young Scientist Awards and Richard Robb for coordinating the Best Paper Awards.

Last but not least, we would like to thank all our sponsors for their kind support, particularly in this most difficult economic climate. Their generosity ensured the highest quality of the conference and essential support to students and young researchers.

It was our pleasure to welcome the MICCAI 2009 attendees to London. In addition to attending the workshop, we trust that the attendees also took the opportunity to explore the rich culture and history of the city. We look forward to meeting you again at MICCAI 2010 in Beijing, China.

September 2009

Guang-Zhong Yang
David Hawkes
Daniel Rueckert
Alison Noble
Chris Taylor

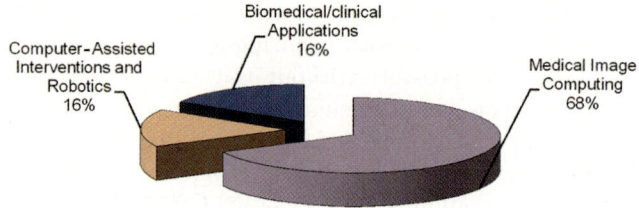
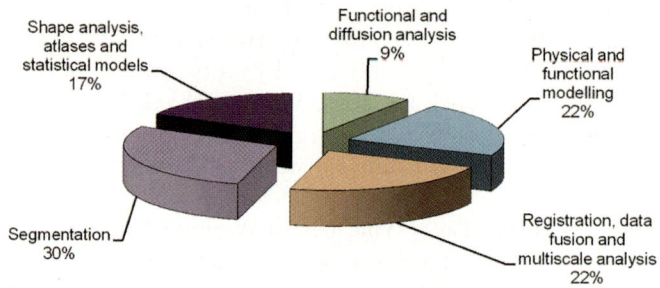
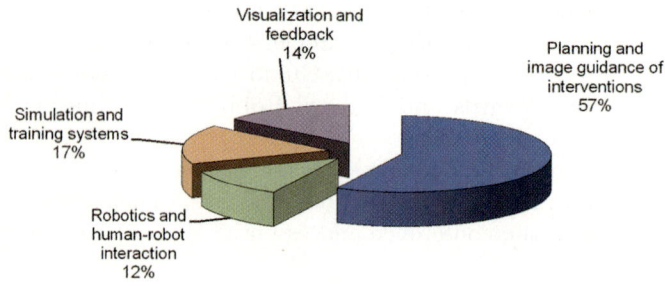
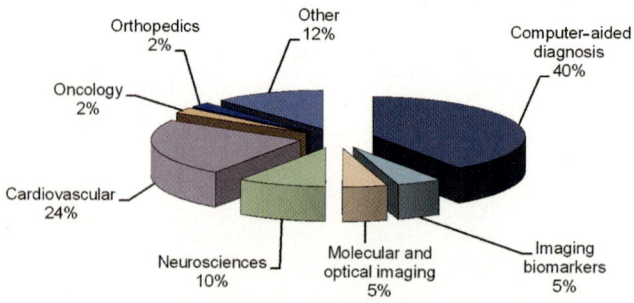

Organization

General Chairs

Guang-Zhong Yang   Imperial College London, UK

Program Co-chairs

David Hawkes   University College London, UK
Daniel Rueckert   Imperial College London, UK
Guang-Zhong Yang   Imperial College London, UK

Workshop Chair and Co-chairs

Alison Noble (Chair)   University of Oxford, UK
Nobuhiko Hata   Harvard University, USA
Xavier Pennec   INRIA, France

Tutorial Chair and Co-chairs

Chris Taylor (Chair)   University of Manchester, UK
Hongen Liao   University of Tokyo, Japan
Frederik Maes   KU Leuven, Belgium

Associate Editors

Adrian Chung   Imperial College London, UK
Su-Lin Lee   Imperial College London, UK

Coordinator for MICCAI Young Scientist Awards

Guido Gerig   University of Utah, USA

Coordinator for Best Paper Awards

Richard Robb   Mayo Clinic College of Medicine
Rochester, Minnesota, USA

Program Committee

Christian Barillot	IRISA, France
Wolfgang Birkfellner	University of Vienna, Austria
Ela Claridge	University of Birmingham, UK
Tim Cootes	University of Manchester, UK
Randy Ellis	Queen's University, Canada
Gabor Fichtinger	Queen's University, Canada
Jim Gee	University of Pennsylvania, Philadelphia, USA
Guido Gerig	University of Utah, USA
Polina Golland	Massachusetts Institute of Technology, USA
Tianzi Jiang	Chinese Academy of Sciences, China
Leo Joskowicz	Hebrew University of Jerusalem, Israel
Rasmus Larsen	Technical University of Denmark, Denmark
Cristian Lorenz	Philips Research Labs, Germany
Frederik Maes	University of Leuven, Belgium
Kensaku Mori	Nagoya University, Japan
Nassir Navab	Technical University of Munich, Germany
Mads Nielsen	University of Copenhagen, Denmark
Poul Nielsen	University of Auckland, New Zealand
Wiro Niessen	Erasmus Medical Center, The Netherlands
Sebastien Ourselin	University College London, UK
Xavier Pennec	INRIA, France
Graeme Penney	King's College London, UK
Franjo Pernus	University of Ljubljana, Slovenia
Terry Peters	Robarts Research Institute, Canada
Ichiro Sakuma	University of Tokyo, Japan
Tim Salcudean	University of British Columbia, Canada
Yoshinobu Sato	University of Osaka, Japan
Julia Schnabel	University of Oxford, UK
Dinggang Shen	University of North Carolina, USA
Gabor Szekely	ETH Zurich, Switzerland
Russell Taylor	John Hopkins University, USA
Jocelyne Troccaz	CNRS, France
Max Viergever	University of Utrecht, The Netherlands
Simon Warfield	Harvard University, USA
Sandy Wells	Harvard University, USA
Carl-Frederik Westin	Harvard University, USA
Chenyang Xu	Siemens Corporate Research, USA

Local Organizing Committee

Ferdinando Rodriguez y Baena	Imperial College London, UK
Fernando Bello	Imperial College London, UK
Brian Davies	Imperial College London, UK
Eddie Edwards	Imperial College London, UK
Daniel Elson	Imperial College London, UK
David Firmin	Imperial College London, UK
Andrew Todd-Pokropek	University College London, UK
Ulrika Wernmark	Imperial College London, UK
Betty Yue	Imperial College London, UK

Reviewers

Abolmaesumi, Purang
Abugharbieh, Rafeef
Alexander, Daniel
Aljabar, Paul
Alvino, Christopher
Amini, Amir
An, Jungha
Angelini, Elsa
Arridge, Simon R.
Ashburner, John
Astley, Sue
Atkinson, David
Awate, Suyash
Axel, Leon
Aylward, Stephen

Babalola, Kolawole
Barratt, Dean
Batchelor, Philip
Baumann, Michael
Bazin, Pierre-Louis
Beckmann, Christian
Beichel, Reinhard
Bello, Fernando
Berger, Marie-Odile
Betke, Margrit
Bhalerao, Abhir
Bhotika, Rahul
Bischof, Horst
Blezek, Daniel
Bloch, Isabelle

Boctor, Emad
Bouix, Sylvain
Boukerroui, Djamal
Bourgeat, Pierrick
Brady, Mike
Bromiley, Paul
Buelow, Thomas
Bullitt, Elizabeth

Camara, Oscar
Camp, Jon
Cattin, Philippe C.
Chakravarty, M. Mallar
Chou, Yiyu
Christensen, Gary
Chung, Adrian
Chung, Albert C. S.
Cinquin, Philippe
Clark, Chris
Colchester, Alan
Collins, D. Louis
Colliot, Olivier
Comaniciu, Dorin
Commowick, Olivier
Cook, Philip
Coulon, Olivier
Crozier, Stuart
Crum, William

Dam, Erik
Darvann, Tron

Dauguet, Julien
Davatzikos, Christos
Dawant, Benoit
de Bruijne, Marleen
Deligianni, Fani
Delingette, Hervé
Deriche, Rachid
Descoteaux, Maxime
Desvignes, Michel
Douiri, Abdel
Duan, Qi
Duchesne, Simon
Duncan, James S
Dupont, Pierre

Ecabert, Olivier
Edwards, Philip
El-Baz, Ayman

Fan, Yong
Farag, Aly
Fenster, Aaron
Feuerstein, Marco
Figl, Michael
Fillard, Pierre
Fischer, Bernd
Fitzpatrick, J Michael
Fleig, Oliver
Fletcher, P. Thomas
Florack, Luc
Frangi, Alejandro
Freysinger, Wolfgang
Funka-Lea, Gareth

Gibaud, Bernard
Gilson, Wesley
Glocker, Ben
Gonzalez Ballester, Miguel Angel
Gooding, Mark
Graham, Jim
Grau, Vicente
Grimson, Eric
Groher, Martin
Guetter, Christoph
Guimond, Alexandre

Hager, Gregory D
Hahn, Horst
Hamarneh, Ghassan
Hanson, Dennis
Harders, Matthias
Hartley, Richard
Hastreiter, Peter
Hata, Nobuhiko
Haynor, David
Heimann, Tobias
Hellier, Pierre
Heng, Pheng Ann
Hipwell, John
Holmes, David
Hornegger, Joachim
Howe, Robert
Hu, Mingxing
Huang, Heng
Huang, Xiaolei
Hunter, Peter

Jain, Ameet
Janke, Andrew
Jannin, Pierre
Jenkinson, Mark
Jolly, Marie-Pierre
Jomier, Julien
Joshi, Sarang

Kabus, Sven
Kakadiaris, Ioannis
Karamalis, Athanasios
Karssemeijer, Nico
Kaus, Michael
Kazanzides, Peter
Keeve, Erwin
Keil, Andreas
Khamene, Ali
Khurd, Parmeshwar
Kikinis, Ron
Kindlmann, Gordon
King, Andrew
Kirchberg, Klaus
Klein, Stefan
Klinder, Tobias

Kruggel, Frithjof
Kurtcuoglu, Vartan
Kutter, Oliver

Laine, Andrew
Langs, Georg
Lapeer, Rudy
Lee, Su-Lin
Lelieveldt, Boudewijn
Lenglet, Christophe
Lepore, Natasha
Li, Chunming
Li, Shuo
Li, Yonghui
Liang, Jianming
Liao, Rui
Likar, Bostjan
Linguraru, Marius George
Liu, Alan
Liu, Tianming
Liu, Yong
Loeckx, Dirk
Loew, Murray
Lohmann, Gabriele
Lötjönen, Jyrki
Lu, Le
Luboz, Vincent

Ma, Burton
Madabhushi, Anant
Makram-Ebeid, Sherif
Malandain, Gregoire
Manduca, Armando
Mangin, Jean-Francois
Manniesing, Rashindra
Marsland, Stephen
Martel, Anne
Martí, Robert
Martin-Fernandez, Marcos
Mattes, Julian
Mazza, Edoardo
McClelland, Jamie
McGraw, Tim
Meijering, Erik
Metaxas, Dimitris
Meyer, Chuck

Miller, James
Milles, Julien
Modersitzki, Jan
Mohamed, Ashraf
Morel, Guillaume
Murgasova, Maria
Mylonas, George

Nain, Delphine
Nash, Martyn
Nicolau, Stephane
Niethammer, Marc
Nishikawa, Atsushi

O'Donnell, Lauren
O'Donnell, Thomas
Ogier, Arnaud
Olivo-Marin, Jean-Christophe
Olszewski, Mark

Pang, Wai-Man
Papademetris, Xenios
Paragios, Nikos
Patriciu, Alexandru
Paul, Perrine
Paulsen, Rasmus
Pauly, Olivier
Peitgen, Heinz-Otto
Peyrat, Jean-Marc
Pham, Dzung
Pichon, Eric
Pitiot, Alain
Pluim, Josien
Pohl, Kilian Maria
Poignet, Philippe
Prager, Richard
Prastawa, Marcel
Prause, Guido
Prima, Sylvain

Qian, Xiaoning

Radeva, Petia
Rajagopal, Vijayaraghavan
Rajagopalan, Srinivasan
Ramamurthi, Krishnakumar

Reinhardt, Joseph
Rexilius, Jan
Reyes, Mauricio
Rhode, Kawal
Ridgway, Gerard
Rittscher, Jens
Riviere, Cameron
Robb, Richard A
Robinson, Emma
Rodriguez y Baena, Ferdinando
Rohde, Gustavo
Rohlfing, Torsten
Rohling, Robert
Rohr, Karl
Rousseau, François
Russakoff, Daniel

Sabuncu, Mert Rory
Salvado, Olivier
Schweikard, Achim
Sermesant, Maxime
Shechter, Guy
Shen, Xilin
Shi, Pengcheng
Shimizu, Akinobu
Shu, Ni
Siddiqi, Kaleem
Siewerdsen, Jeffrey
Sjöstrand, Karl
Sled, John G.
Smith, Stephen
Sporring, Jon
Staib, Lawrence
Stewart, James
Stoyanov, Danail
Studholme, Colin
Styner, Martin
Subramanian, Navneeth
Suetens, Paul
Summers, Ronald
Sundar, Hari
Szczerba, Dominik
Szilagyi, Laszlo

Tanner, Christine
Tao, Xiaodong

Tasdizen, Tolga
Taylor, Zeike
ter Haar Romeny, Bart M.
Thévenaz, Philippe
Thiran, Jean-Philippe
Thiriet, Marc
Thirion, Bertrand
Todd Pokropek, Andrew
Toews, Matthew
Tosun, Duygu
Tristán-Vega, Antonio
Tsechpenakis, Gavriil
Twining, Carole

Unal, Gozde

van Assen, Hans
van Ginneken, Bram
Van Leemput, Koen
van Walsum, Theo
Vandermeulen, Dirk
Vannier, Michael
Vercauteren, Tom
Vik, Torbjörn
Villard, Pierre-Frederic
Vrooman, Henri

Wachinger, Christian
Wahle, Andreas
Wang, Defeng
Weber, Stefan
Weese, Jürgen
Wein, Wolfgang
West, Jay
Whitaker, Ross
Whitcher, Brandon
Wiemker, Rafael
Wolf, Ivo
Wong, Stephen
Woolrich, Mark

Xue, Zhong

Yan, Pingkun
Yang, Hua
Yaniv, Ziv

Yendiki, Anastasia
Yeo, Boon Thye
Yoo, Terry
Young, Alistair
Yushkevich, Paul

Zhang, Hui
Zhang, Yong

Zheng, Guoyan
Zheng, Yefeng
Zhou, S. Kevin
Zhou, Xiang (Sean)
Zhu, Hongtu
Zikic, Darko
Zollei, Lilla
Zwiggelaar, Reyer

MICCAI Society, Board of Directors

Nicholas Ayache — INRIA, Sophia Antipolis, France
Kevin Cleary — Georgetown University, Washington DC, USA
James Duncan — Yale University, New Haven, Connecticut, USA
Gabor Fichtinger — Queen's University, Kingston, Ontario, Canada
Guido Gerig — University of Utah, Salt Lake City Utah, USA
Polina Golland — Massachusetts Institute of Technology, USA
Tianzi Jiang — Chinese Academy of Sciences, China
Dimitris Metaxas — Rutgers University, Piscataway, New Jersey, USA
Nassir Navab — Technical University of Munich, Germany
Alison Noble — University of Oxford, Oxford, UK
Sebastien Ourselin — University College London UK
Terry Peters — Robarts Research Institute, London, Ontario, Canada
Richard Robb — Mayo Clinic College of Medicine, Minnesota, USA
Ichiro Sakuma — University of Tokyo, Japan
Guang-Zhong Yang — Imperial College London, UK

MICCAI Society, Executive Officers

President, James Duncan
Executive Director, Richard Robb
Secretary, Nicholas Ayache
Treasurer, Terry Peters
Elections Officer, Karl Heinz Hoehne
Awards Officer, Guido Gerig

MICCAI Society, Staff

Society Secretariat, Janette Wallace, Canada
Membership Coordinator, Gabor Szekely, Switzerland
Publication Coordinator, Nobuhiko Hata, USA
Communications Coordinator, Kirby Vosburgh, USA
Industry Relations Coordinator, Tina Kapur, USA

MICCAI Young Scientist Awards, New York City, 2008

Each year MICCAI awards outstanding work written and presented by students. Both oral and poster presentations are eligible for the awards, and the awards are presented to the winners in a public ceremony at the end of the conference. Six MICCAI Young Scientist Awards were presented by the MICCAI Society at MICCAI 2008:

- *The Effect of Automated Marker Detection on In Vivo Volumetric Stent Reconstruction*: Gert Schoonenberg, Pierre Lelong, Raoul Florent, Onno Wink, Bart ter Haar Romeny, Technische Universiteit Eindhoven, The Netherlands, Philips Healthcare Best NL, Philips France, Paris, France.
- *Passive Ventricular Mechanics Modelling Using Cardiac MR Imaging of Structure and Function*: Vicky Y. Wang, Hoi Leng Lam, Daniel B. Ennis, Alistair A. Young, Martyn P. Nash, University of Auckland New Zealand, UCLA, USA.
- *On-the-Fly Motion-Compensated Cone-Beam CT Using an A Priori Motion Model*: Simon Rit, Jochem Wolthaus, Marcel von Herk, Jan-Jakob Sonke, The Netherlands Cancer Institute, The Netherlands.
- *A Constrained Non-Rigid Registration Algorithm for use in Prostate Image-Guided Radiotherapy*: William Greene, Sudhakar Chelikani, Kailas Purushothaman, Zhe Chen, Jonathan Krisely, Lawrence Staib, Xenophon Papademetris, Jim Duncan, Yale University, USA.
- *Fully Bayesian Joint Model for MR Brain Scan Tissue and Subcortical Structure Segmentation*: Benoit Scherrer, Florence Forbes, Catherine Garbay, Michel Dojat, INSERN, CNRS, INRIA, Université Joseph Fourier, Grenoble France.
- *Sparse Approximation of Currents for Statistics on Curves and Surfaces*: Stanley Durrleman, Xavier Pennec, Alain Trouve, Nicholas Ayache, INRIA Sophia-Antipolis, ENS-Cachan, France.

Elsevier MedIA-MICCAI Prize 2008

Two prizes were awarded by Elsevier during MICCAI 2008 to the first authors of two outstanding articles of the special issue of the *Medical Image Analysis* journal (volume 12, issue 5, October 2008) dedicated to the previous MICCAI 2007 conference.

- First prize awarded to Cyril Poupon for the article: *Real-time MR diffusion tensor and Q-ball imaging using Kalman filtering*, Cyril Poupon, Alexis Roche, Jessica Dubois, Jean-François Mangin, Fabrice Poupon, Medical Image Analysis 12(5) (2008), pages 527-534.
- Second prize awarded to Gabor Fichtinger for the article: *Robotic assistance for ultrasound-guided prostate brachytherapy*, Gabor Fichtinger, Jonathan P. Fiene, Christopher W. Kennedy, Gernot Kronreif, Iulian Iordachita, Danny Y. Song, Everette C. Burdette, Peter Kazanzides, Medical Image Analysis 12(5) (2008), pages 535-545.

Table of Contents – Part II

Shape Modelling and Analysis

Building Shape Models from Lousy Data 1
Marcel Lüthi, Thomas Albrecht, and Thomas Vetter

Statistical Location Model for Abdominal Organ Localization 9
Jianhua Yao and Ronald M. Summers

Volumetric Shape Model for Oriented Tubular Structure from DTI Data 18
Hon Pong Ho, Xenophon Papademetris, Fei Wang, Hilary P. Blumberg, and Lawrence H. Staib

A Generic Probabilistic Active Shape Model for Organ Segmentation ... 26
Andreas Wimmer, Grzegorz Soza, and Joachim Hornegger

Organ Segmentation with Level Sets Using Local Shape and Appearance Priors 34
Timo Kohlberger, M. Gökhan Uzunbaş, Christopher Alvino, Timor Kadir, Daniel O. Slosman, and Gareth Funka-Lea

Liver Segmentation Using Automatically Defined Patient Specific B-Spline Surface Models 43
Yi Song, Andy J. Bulpitt, and Ken W. Brodlie

Airway Tree Extraction with Locally Optimal Paths 51
Pechin Lo, Jon Sporring, Jesper Johannes Holst Pedersen, and Marleen de Bruijne

A Deformable Surface Model for Vascular Segmentation 59
Max W.K. Law and Albert C.S. Chung

A Deformation Tracking Approach to 4D Coronary Artery Tree Reconstruction 68
Yanghai Tsin, Klaus J. Kirchberg, Guenter Lauritsch, and Chenyang Xu

Automatic Extraction of Mandibular Nerve and Bone from Cone-Beam CT Data 76
Dagmar Kainmueller, Hans Lamecker, Heiko Seim, Max Zinser, and Stefan Zachow

Conditional Variability of Statistical Shape Models Based on Surrogate Variables 84
Rémi Blanc, Mauricio Reyes, Christof Seiler, and Gábor Székely

Surface/Volume-Based Articulated 3D Spine Inference through Markov
Random Fields 92
  Samuel Kadoury and Nikos Paragios

A Shape Relationship Descriptor for Radiation Therapy Planning 100
  *Michael Kazhdan, Patricio Simari, Todd McNutt, Binbin Wu,
  Robert Jacques, Ming Chuang, and Russell Taylor*

Feature-Based Morphometry 109
  *Matthew Toews, William M. Wells III, D. Louis Collins, and
  Tal Arbel*

Constructing a Dictionary of Human Brain Folding Patterns 117
  *Zhong Yi Sun, Matthieu Perrot, Alan Tucholka, Denis Rivière, and
  Jean-François Mangin*

Topological Correction of Brain Surface Meshes Using Spherical
Harmonics 125
  Rachel Aine Yotter, Robert Dahnke, and Christian Gaser

Teichmüller Shape Space Theory and Its Application to Brain
Morphometry 133
  *Yalin Wang, Wei Dai, Xianfeng Gu, Tony F. Chan, Shing-Tung Yau,
  Arthur W. Toga, and Paul M. Thompson*

A Tract-Specific Framework for White Matter Morphometry Combining
Macroscopic and Microscopic Tract Features 141
  *Hui Zhang, Suyash P. Awate, Sandhitsu R. Das, John H. Woo,
  Elias R. Melhem, James C. Gee, and Paul A. Yushkevich*

Shape Modelling for Tract Selection 150
  Jonathan D. Clayden, Martin D. King, and Chris A. Clark

Topological Characterization of Signal in Brain Images Using Min-Max
Diagrams 158
  *Moo K. Chung, Vikas Singh, Peter T. Kim, Kim M. Dalton, and
  Richard J. Davidson*

Particle Based Shape Regression of Open Surfaces with Applications to
Developmental Neuroimaging 167
  *Manasi Datar, Joshua Cates, P. Thomas Fletcher, Sylvain Gouttard,
  Guido Gerig, and Ross Whitaker*

Setting Priors and Enforcing Constraints on Matches for Nonlinear
Registration of Meshes 175
  Benoît Combès and Sylvain Prima

Parametric Representation of Cortical Surface Folding Based on
Polynomials 184
  Tuo Zhang, Lei Guo, Gang Li, Jingxin Nie, and Tianming Liu

Intrinsic Regression Models for Manifold-Valued Data 192
   *Xiaoyan Shi, Martin Styner, Jeffrey Lieberman, Joseph G. Ibrahim,
Weili Lin, and Hongtu Zhu*

Gender Differences in Cerebral Cortical Folding: Multivariate
Complexity-Shape Analysis with Insights into Handling Brain-Volume
Differences 200
   Suyash P. Awate, Paul Yushkevich, Daniel Licht, and James C. Gee

Cortical Shape Analysis in the Laplace-Beltrami Feature Space 208
   Yonggang Shi, Ivo Dinov, and Arthur W. Toga

Shape Analysis of Human Brain Interhemispheric Fissure Bending in
MRI 216
   Lu Zhao, Jarmo Hietala, and Jussi Tohka

Subject-Matched Templates for Spatial Normalization 224
   Torsten Rohlfing, Edith V. Sullivan, and Adolf Pfefferbaum

Mapping Growth Patterns and Genetic Influences on Early Brain
Development in Twins 232
   *Yasheng Chen, Hongtu Zhu, Dinggang Shen, Hongyu An,
John Gilmore, and Weili Lin*

Tensor-Based Morphometry with Mappings Parameterized by
Stationary Velocity Fields in Alzheimer's Disease Neuroimaging
Initiative.. 240
   Matías Nicolás Bossa, Ernesto Zacur, and Salvador Olmos

Motion Analysis, Physical Based Modelling and Image Reconstruction

High-Quality Model Generation for Finite Element Simulation of
Tissue Deformation 248
   Orcun Goksel and Septimiu E. Salcudean

Biomechanically-Constrained 4D Estimation of Myocardial Motion 257
   Hari Sundar, Christos Davatzikos, and George Biros

Predictive Simulation of Bidirectional Glenn Shunt Using a Hybrid
Blood Vessel Model 266
   Hao Li, Wee Kheng Leow, and Ing-Sh Chiu

Surgical Planning and Patient-Specific Biomechanical Simulation for
Tracheal Endoprostheses Interventions 275
   *Miguel A. González Ballester, Amaya Pérez del Palomar,
José Luís López Villalobos, Laura Lara Rodríguez, Olfa Trabelsi,
Frederic Pérez, Ángel Ginel Cañamaque, Emilia Barrot Cortés,
Francisco Rodríguez Panadero, Manuel Doblaré Castellano, and
Javier Herrero Jover*

Mesh Generation from 3D Multi-material Images 283
  Dobrina Boltcheva, Mariette Yvinec, and Jean-Daniel Boissonnat

Interactive Simulation of Flexible Needle Insertions Based on Constraint
Models 291
  *Christian Duriez, Christophe Guébert, Maud Marchal,
  Stephane Cotin, and Laurent Grisoni*

Real-Time Prediction of Brain Shift Using Nonlinear Finite Element
Algorithms 300
  *Grand Roman Joldes, Adam Wittek, Mathieu Couton,
  Simon K. Warfield, and Karol Miller*

Model-Based Estimation of Ventricular Deformation in the Cat
Brain 308
  *Fenghong Liu, S. Scott Lollis, Songbai Ji, Keith D. Paulsen,
  Alexander Hartov, and David W. Roberts*

Contact Studies between Total Knee Replacement Components
Developed Using Explicit Finite Elements Analysis 316
  *Lucian Gheorghe Gruionu, Gabriel Gruionu, Stefan Pastrama,
  Nicolae Iliescu, and Taina Avramescu*

A Hybrid 1D and 3D Approach to Hemodynamics Modelling for a
Patient-Specific Cerebral Vasculature and Aneurysm 323
  *Harvey Ho, Gregory Sands, Holger Schmid, Kumar Mithraratne,
  Gordon Mallinson, and Peter Hunter*

Incompressible Cardiac Motion Estimation of the Left Ventricle Using
Tagged MR Images 331
  Xiaofeng Liu, Khaled Z. Abd-Elmoniem, and Jerry L. Prince

Vibro-Elastography for Visualization of the Prostate Region: Method
Evaluation 339
  *Seyedeh Sara Mahdavi, Mehdi Moradi, Xu Wen,
  William J. Morris, and Septimiu E. Salcudean*

Modeling Respiratory Motion for Cancer Radiation Therapy Based on
Patient-Specific 4DCT Data 348
  Jaesung Eom, Chengyu Shi, Xie George Xu, and Suvranu De

Correlating Chest Surface Motion to Motion of the Liver Using
ε-SVR – A Porcine Study 356
  *Floris Ernst, Volker Martens, Stefan Schlichting, Armin Beširević,
  Markus Kleemann, Christoph Koch, Dirk Petersen, and
  Achim Schweikard*

Respiratory Motion Estimation from Cone-Beam Projections Using a
Prior Model 365
    *Jef Vandemeulebroucke, Jan Kybic, Patrick Clarysse, and
David Sarrut*

Heart Motion Abnormality Detection via an Information Measure and
Bayesian Filtering 373
    *Kumaradevan Punithakumar, Shuo Li, Ismail Ben Ayed, Ian Ross,
Ali Islam, and Jaron Chong*

Automatic Image-Based Cardiac and Respiratory Cycle Synchronization
and Gating of Image Sequences 381
    Hari Sundar, Ali Khamene, Liron Yatziv, and Chenyang Xu

Dynamic Cone Beam Reconstruction Using a New Level Set
Formulation 389
    Andreas Keil, Jakob Vogel, Günter Lauritsch, and Nassir Navab

Spatio-temporal Reconstruction of dPET Data Using Complex Wavelet
Regularisation 398
    Andrew McLennan and Michael Brady

Evaluation of q-Space Sampling Strategies for the Diffusion Magnetic
Resonance Imaging 406
    Haz-Edine Assemlal, David Tschumperlé, and Luc Brun

On the Blurring of the Funk–Radon Transform in Q–Ball Imaging 415
    *Antonio Tristán-Vega, Santiago Aja-Fernández, and
Carl-Fredrik Westin*

Multiple Q-Shell ODF Reconstruction in Q-Ball Imaging 423
    *Iman Aganj, Christophe Lenglet, Guillermo Sapiro, Essa Yacoub,
Kamil Ugurbil, and Noam Harel*

Neuro, Cell and Multiscale Image Analysis

Lossless Online Ensemble Learning (LOEL) and Its Application to
Subcortical Segmentation 432
    *Jonathan H. Morra, Zhuowen Tu, Arthur W. Toga, and
Paul M. Thompson*

Improved Maximum a Posteriori Cortical Segmentation by Iterative
Relaxation of Priors 441
    *Manuel Jorge Cardoso, Matthew J. Clarkson, Gerard R. Ridgway,
Marc Modat, Nick C. Fox, and Sebastien Ourselin*

Anatomically Informed Bayesian Model Selection for fMRI Group Data
Analysis 450
    Merlin Keller, Marc Lavielle, Matthieu Perrot, and Alexis Roche

A Computational Model of Cerebral Cortex Folding 458
    Jingxin Nie, Gang Li, Lei Guo, and Tianming Liu

Tensor-Based Morphometry of Fibrous Structures with Application to
Human Brain White Matter 466
    Hui Zhang, Paul A. Yushkevich, Daniel Rueckert, and James C. Gee

A Fuzzy Region-Based Hidden Markov Model for Partial-Volume
Classification in Brain MRI 474
    Albert Huang, Rafeef Abugharbieh, and Roger Tam

Brain Connectivity Using Geodesics in HARDI 482
    Mickaël Péchaud, Maxime Descoteaux, and Renaud Keriven

Functional Segmentation of fMRI Data Using Adaptive Non-negative
Sparse PCA (ANSPCA) 490
    Bernard Ng, Rafeef Abugharbieh, and Martin J. McKeown

Genetics of Anisotropy Asymmetry: Registration and Sample Size
Effects 498
    Neda Jahanshad, Agatha D. Lee, Natasha Leporé, Yi-Yu Chou,
    Caroline C. Brun, Marina Barysheva, Arthur W. Toga,
    Katie L. McMahon, Greig I. de Zubicaray, Margaret J. Wright, and
    Paul M. Thompson

Extending Genetic Linkage Analysis to Diffusion Tensor Images to Map
Single Gene Effects on Brain Fiber Architecture 506
    Ming-Chang Chiang, Christina Avedissian, Marina Barysheva,
    Arthur W. Toga, Katie L. McMahon, Greig I. de Zubicaray,
    Margaret J. Wright, and Paul M. Thompson

Vascular Territory Image Analysis Using Vessel Encoded Arterial Spin
Labeling 514
    Michael A. Chappell, Thomas W. Okell, Peter Jezzard, and
    Mark W. Woolrich

Predicting MGMT Methylation Status of Glioblastomas from MRI
Texture 522
    Ilya Levner, Sylvia Drabycz, Gloria Roldan, Paula De Robles,
    J. Gregory Cairncross, and Ross Mitchell

Tumor Invasion Margin on the Riemannian Space of Brain Fibers 531
    Dana Cobzas, Parisa Mosayebi, Albert Murtha, and
    Martin Jagersand

A Conditional Random Field Approach for Coupling Local Registration
with Robust Tissue and Structure Segmentation 540
    Benoit Scherrer, Florence Forbes, and Michel Dojat

Robust Atlas-Based Brain Segmentation Using Multi-structure
Confidence-Weighted Registration 549
  Ali R. Khan, Moo K. Chung, and Mirza Faisal Beg

Discriminative, Semantic Segmentation of Brain Tissue in MR
Images 558
  Zhao Yi, Antonio Criminisi, Jamie Shotton, and Andrew Blake

Use of Simulated Atrophy for Performance Analysis of Brain Atrophy
Estimation Approaches 566
  *Swati Sharma, Vincent Noblet, François Rousseau, Fabrice Heitz,
  Lucien Rumbach, and Jean-Paul Armspach*

Fast and Robust 3-D MRI Brain Structure Segmentation 575
  *Michael Wels, Yefeng Zheng, Gustavo Carneiro, Martin Huber,
  Joachim Hornegger, and Dorin Comaniciu*

Multiple Sclerosis Lesion Segmentation Using an Automatic Multimodal
Graph Cuts 584
  *Daniel García-Lorenzo, Jeremy Lecoeur, Douglas L. Arnold,
  D. Louis Collins, and Christian Barillot*

Towards Accurate, Automatic Segmentation of the Hippocampus and
Amygdala from MRI 592
  D. Louis Collins and Jens C. Pruessner

An Object-Based Method for Rician Noise Estimation in MR Images ... 601
  *Pierrick Coupé, José V. Manjón, Elias Gedamu, Douglas Arnold,
  Montserrat Robles, and D. Louis Collins*

Cell Segmentation Using Front Vector Flow Guided Active Contours .. 609
  Fuhai Li, Xiaobo Zhou, Hong Zhao, and Stephen T.C. Wong

Segmentation and Classification of Cell Cycle Phases in Fluorescence
Imaging 617
  *Ilker Ersoy, Filiz Bunyak, Vadim Chagin,
  M. Christina Cardoso, and Kannappan Palaniappan*

Steerable Features for Statistical 3D Dendrite Detection 625
  *Germán González, François Aguet, François Fleuret,
  Michael Unser, and Pascal Fua*

Graph-Based Pancreatic Islet Segmentation for Early Type 2 Diabetes
Mellitus on Histopathological Tissue 633
  *Xenofon Floros, Thomas J. Fuchs, Markus P. Rechsteiner,
  Giatgen Spinas, Holger Moch, and Joachim M. Buhmann*

Detection of Spatially Correlated Objects in 3D Images Using
Appearance Models and Coupled Active Contours.................... 641
   Kishore Mosaliganti, Arnaud Gelas, Alexandre Gouaillard,
   Ramil Noche, Nikolaus Obholzer, and Sean Megason

Intra-retinal Layer Segmentation in Optical Coherence Tomography
Using an Active Contour Approach................................. 649
   Azadeh Yazdanpanah, Ghassan Hamarneh, Benjamin Smith, and
   Marinko Sarunic

Mapping Tissue Optical Attenuation to Identify Cancer Using Optical
Coherence Tomography... 657
   Robert A. McLaughlin, Loretta Scolaro, Peter Robbins,
   Christobel Saunders, Steven L. Jacques, and David D. Sampson

Analysis of MR Images of Mice in Preclinical Treatment Monitoring of
Polycystic Kidney Disease.. 665
   Stathis Hadjidemetriou, Wilfried Reichardt, Martin Buechert,
   Juergen Hennig, and Dominik von Elverfeldt

Actin Filament Tracking Based on Particle Filters and Stretching Open
Active Contour Models.. 673
   Hongsheng Li, Tian Shen, Dimitrios Vavylonis, and Xiaolei Huang

Image Analysis and Computer Aided Diagnosis

Toward Early Diagnosis of Lung Cancer 682
   Ayman El-Baz, Georgy Gimel'farb, Robert Falk,
   Mohamed Abou El-Ghar, Sabrina Rainey,
   David Heredia, and Teresa Shaffer

Lung Extraction, Lobe Segmentation and Hierarchical Region
Assessment for Quantitative Analysis on High Resolution Computed
Tomography Images.. 690
   James C. Ross, Raúl San José Estépar, Alejandro Díaz,
   Carl-Fredrik Westin, Ron Kikinis, Edwin K. Silverman, and
   George R. Washko

Learning COPD Sensitive Filters in Pulmonary CT 699
   Lauge Sørensen, Pechin Lo, Haseem Ashraf, Jon Sporring,
   Mads Nielsen, and Marleen de Bruijne

Automated Anatomical Labeling of Bronchial Branches Extracted
from CT Datasets Based on Machine Learning and Combination
Optimization and Its Application to Bronchoscope Guidance 707
   Kensaku Mori, Shunsuke Ota, Daisuke Deguchi, Takayuki Kitasaka,
   Yasuhito Suenaga, Shingo Iwano, Yosihnori Hasegawa,
   Hirotsugu Takabatake, Masaki Mori, and Hiroshi Natori

Multi-level Ground Glass Nodule Detection and Segmentation in CT
Lung Images 715
  Yimo Tao, Le Lu, Maneesh Dewan, Albert Y. Chen, Jason Corso,
  Jianhua Xuan, Marcos Salganicoff, and Arun Krishnan

Global and Local Multi-valued Dissimilarity-Based Classification:
Application to Computer-Aided Detection of Tuberculosis 724
  Yulia Arzhaeva, Laurens Hogeweg, Pim A. de Jong,
  Max A. Viergever, and Bram van Ginneken

Noninvasive Imaging of Electrophysiological Substrates in Post
Myocardial Infarction 732
  Linwei Wang, Heye Zhang, Ken C.L. Wong, Huafeng Liu, and
  Pengcheng Shi

Unsupervised Inline Analysis of Cardiac Perfusion MRI 741
  Hui Xue, Sven Zuehlsdorff, Peter Kellman, Andrew Arai,
  Sonia Nielles-Vallespin, Christophe Chefdhotel,
  Christine H. Lorenz, and Jens Guehring

Pattern Recognition of Abnormal Left Ventricle Wall Motion in Cardiac
MR 750
  Yingli Lu, Perry Radau, Kim Connelly, Alexander Dick, and
  Graham Wright

Septal Flash Assessment on CRT Candidates Based on Statistical
Atlases of Motion 759
  Nicolas Duchateau, Mathieu De Craene, Etel Silva, Marta Sitges,
  Bart H. Bijnens, and Alejandro F. Frangi

Personalized Modeling and Assessment of the Aortic-Mitral Coupling
from 4D TEE and CT 767
  Razvan Ioan Ionasec, Ingmar Voigt, Bogdan Georgescu,
  Yang Wang, Helene Houle, Joachim Hornegger, Nassir Navab, and
  Dorin Comaniciu

A New 3-D Automated Computational Method to Evaluate In-Stent
Neointimal Hyperplasia in In-Vivo Intravascular Optical Coherence
Tomography Pullbacks... 776
  Serhan Gurmeric, Gozde Gul Isguder, Stéphane Carlier, and
  Gozde Unal

MKL for Robust Multi-modality AD Classification 786
  Chris Hinrichs, Vikas Singh, Guofan Xu, and Sterling Johnson

A New Approach for Creating Customizable Cytoarchitectonic
Probabilistic Maps without a Template 795
  Amir M. Tahmasebi, Purang Abolmaesumi, Xiujuan Geng,
  Patricia Morosan, Katrin Amunts, Gary E. Christensen, and
  Ingrid S. Johnsrude

A Computer-Aided Diagnosis System of Nuclear Cataract via
Ranking 803
   Wei Huang, Huiqi Li, Kap Luk Chan, Joo Hwee Lim,
   Jiang Liu, and Tien Yin Wong

Automated Segmentation of the Femur and Pelvis from 3D CT Data
of Diseased Hip Using Hierarchical Statistical Shape Model of Joint
Structure 811
   Futoshi Yokota, Toshiyuki Okada, Masaki Takao, Nobuhiko Sugano,
   Yukio Tada, and Yoshinobu Sato

Computer-Aided Assessment of Anomalies in the Scoliotic Spine in 3-D
MRI Images 819
   Florian Jäger, Joachim Hornegger, Siegfried Schwab, and Rolf Janka

Optimal Graph Search Segmentation Using Arc-Weighted Graph for
Simultaneous Surface Detection of Bladder and Prostate 827
   Qi Song, Xiaodong Wu, Yunlong Liu, Mark Smith,
   John Buatti, and Milan Sonka

Automated Calibration for Computerized Analysis of Prostate Lesions
Using Pharmacokinetic Magnetic Resonance Images 836
   Pieter C. Vos, Thomas Hambrock, Jelle O. Barenstz, and
   Henkjan J. Huisman

Spectral Embedding Based Probabilistic Boosting Tree (ScEPTre):
Classifying High Dimensional Heterogeneous Biomedical Data 844
   Pallavi Tiwari, Mark Rosen, Galen Reed, John Kurhanewicz, and
   Anant Madabhushi

Automatic Correction of Intensity Nonuniformity from Sparseness of
Gradient Distribution in Medical Images 852
   Yuanjie Zheng, Murray Grossman, Suyash P. Awate, and
   James C. Gee

Weakly Supervised Group-Wise Model Learning Based on Discrete
Optimization 860
   René Donner, Horst Wildenauer, Horst Bischof, and Georg Langs

Image Segmentation and Analysis

ECOC Random Fields for Lumen Segmentation in Radial Artery IVUS
Sequences 869
   Francesco Ciompi, Oriol Pujol, Eduard Fernández-Nofrerías,
   Josepa Mauri, and Petia Radeva

Dynamic Layer Separation for Coronary DSA and Enhancement in
Fluoroscopic Sequences 877
   *Ying Zhu, Simone Prummer, Peng Wang, Terrence Chen,
   Dorin Comaniciu, and Martin Ostermeier*

An Inverse Scattering Algorithm for the Segmentation of the Luminal
Border on Intravascular Ultrasound Data 885
   *E. Gerardo Mendizabal-Ruiz, George Biros, and
   Ioannis A. Kakadiaris*

Image-Driven Cardiac Left Ventricle Segmentation for the Evaluation
of Multiview Fused Real-Time 3-Dimensional Echocardiography
Images 893
   *Kashif Rajpoot, J. Alison Noble, Vicente Grau,
   Cezary Szmigielski, and Harald Becher*

Left Ventricle Segmentation via Graph Cut Distribution Matching 901
   *Ismail Ben Ayed, Kumaradevan Punithakumar, Shuo Li,
   Ali Islam, and Jaron Chong*

Combining Registration and Minimum Surfaces for the Segmentation
of the Left Ventricle in Cardiac Cine MR Images..................... 910
   Marie-Pierre Jolly, Hui Xue, Leo Grady, and Jens Guehring

Left Ventricle Segmentation Using Diffusion Wavelets and Boosting 919
   Salma Essafi, Georg Langs, and Nikos Paragios

3D Cardiac Segmentation Using Temporal Correlation of Radio
Frequency Ultrasound Data 927
   *Maartje M. Nillesen, Richard G.P. Lopata, Henkjan J. Huisman,
   Johan M. Thijssen, Livia Kapusta, and Chris L. de Korte*

Improved Modelling of Ultrasound Contrast Agent Diminution for
Blood Perfusion Analysis 935
   *Christian Kier, Karsten Meyer-Wiethe, Günter Seidel, and
   Alfred Mertins*

A Novel 3D Joint Markov-Gibbs Model for Extracting Blood Vessels
from PC–MRA Images 943
   *Ayman El-Baz, Georgy Gimel'farb, Robert Falk,
   Mohamed Abou El-Ghar, Vedant Kumar, and David Heredia*

Atlas-Based Improved Prediction of Magnetic Field Inhomogeneity for
Distortion Correction of EPI Data 951
   Clare Poynton, Mark Jenkinson, and William Wells III

3D Prostate Segmentation in Ultrasound Images Based on Tapered and
Deformed Ellipsoids 960
   *Seyedeh Sara Mahdavi, William J. Morris, Ingrid Spadinger,
   Nick Chng, Orcun Goksel, and Septimiu E. Salcudean*

An Interactive Geometric Technique for Upper and Lower Teeth
Segmentation 968
  Binh Huy Le, Zhigang Deng, James Xia, Yu-Bing Chang, and
  Xiaobo Zhou

Enforcing Monotonic Temporal Evolution in Dry Eye Images 976
  Tamir Yedidya, Peter Carr, Richard Hartley, and
  Jean-Pierre Guillon

Ultrafast Localization of the Optic Disc Using Dimensionality
Reduction of the Search Space 985
  Ahmed Essam Mahfouz and Ahmed S. Fahmy

Using Frankenstein's Creature Paradigm to Build a Patient Specific
Atlas 993
  Olivier Commowick, Simon K. Warfield, and Grégoire Malandain

Atlas-Based Automated Segmentation of Spleen and Liver Using
Adaptive Enhancement Estimation 1001
  Marius George Linguraru, Jesse K. Sandberg, Zhixi Li,
  John A. Pura, and Ronald M. Summers

A Two-Level Approach towards Semantic Colon Segmentation:
Removing Extra-Colonic Findings 1009
  Le Lu, Matthias Wolf, Jianming Liang, Murat Dundar,
  Jinbo Bi, and Marcos Salganicoff

Segmentation of Lumbar Vertebrae Using Part-Based Graphs and
Active Appearance Models 1017
  Martin G. Roberts, Tim F. Cootes, Elisa Pacheco, Teik Oh, and
  Judith E. Adams

Utero-Fetal Unit and Pregnant Woman Modeling Using a Computer
Graphics Approach for Dosimetry Studies 1025
  Jérémie Anquez, Tamy Boubekeur, Lazar Bibin, Elsa Angelini, and
  Isabelle Bloch

Cross Modality Deformable Segmentation Using Hierarchical Clustering
and Learning 1033
  Yiqiang Zhan, Maneesh Dewan, and Xiang Sean Zhou

3D Multi-branch Tubular Surface and Centerline Extraction with 4D
Iterative Key Points 1042
  Hua Li, Anthony Yezzi, and Laurent Cohen

Multimodal Prior Appearance Models Based on Regional Clustering of
Intensity Profiles 1051
  François Chung and Hervé Delingette

3D Medical Image Segmentation by Multiple-Surface Active Volume
Models 1059
    Tian Shen and Xiaolei Huang

Model Completion via Deformation Cloning Based on an Explicit
Global Deformation Model 1067
    Qiong Han, Stephen E. Strup, Melody C. Carswell,
    Duncan Clarke, and Williams B. Seales

Supervised Nonparametric Image Parcellation 1075
    Mert R. Sabuncu, B.T. Thomas Yeo, Koen Van Leemput,
    Bruce Fischl, and Polina Golland

Thermal Vision for Sleep Apnea Monitoring 1084
    Jin Fei, Ioannis Pavlidis, and Jayasimha Murthy

Tissue Tracking in Thermo-physiological Imagery through
Spatio-temporal Smoothing 1092
    Yan Zhou, Panagiotis Tsiamyrtzis, and Ioannis T. Pavlidis

Depth Data Improves Skin Lesion Segmentation 1100
    Xiang Li, Ben Aldridge, Lucia Ballerini, Robert Fisher, and
    Jonathan Rees

A Fully Automatic Random Walker Segmentation for Skin Lesions in a
Supervised Setting 1108
    Paul Wighton, Maryam Sadeghi, Tim K. Lee, and M. Stella Atkins

Author Index 1117

Table of Contents – Part I

Cardiovascular Image Guided Intervention and Robotics

Optimal Transseptal Puncture Location for Robot-Assisted Left Atrial Catheter Ablation 1
  Jagadeesan Jayender, Rajni V. Patel, Gregory F. Michaud, and Nobuhiko Hata

Towards Guidance of Electrophysiological Procedures with Real-Time 3D Intracardiac Echocardiography Fusion to C-arm CT 9
  Wolfgang Wein, Estelle Camus, Matthias John, Mamadou Diallo, Christophe Duong, Amin Al-Ahmad, Rebecca Fahrig, Ali Khamene, and Chenyang Xu

Personalized Pulmonary Trunk Modeling for Intervention Planning and Valve Assessment Estimated from CT Data 17
  Dime Vitanovski, Razvan Ioan Ionasec, Bogdan Georgescu, Martin Huber, Andrew Mayall Taylor, Joachim Hornegger, and Dorin Comaniciu

Robotic Force Stabilization for Beating Heart Intracardiac Surgery 26
  Shelten G. Yuen, Michael C. Yip, Nikolay V. Vasilyev, Douglas P. Perrin, Pedro J. del Nido, and Robert D. Howe

Non-rigid Reconstruction of the Beating Heart Surface for Minimally Invasive Cardiac Surgery 34
  Mingxing Hu, Graeme P. Penney, Daniel Rueckert, Philip J. Edwards, Fernando Bello, Roberto Casula, Michael Figl, and David J. Hawkes

Surgical Navigation and Tissue Interaction

3D Meshless Prostate Segmentation and Registration in Image Guided Radiotherapy 43
  Ting Chen, Sung Kim, Jinghao Zhou, Dimitris Metaxas, Gunaretnam Rajagopal, and Ning Yue

A Computer Model of Soft Tissue Interaction with a Surgical Aspirator 51
  Vincent Mora, Di Jiang, Rupert Brooks, and Sébastien Delorme

Optimal Matching for Prostate Brachytherapy Seed Localization with Dimension Reduction 59
  Junghoon Lee, Christian Labat, Ameet K. Jain, Danny Y. Song, Everette C. Burdette, Gabor Fichtinger, and Jerry L. Prince

Prostate Biopsy Assistance System with Gland Deformation Estimation for Enhanced Precision 67
  Michael Baumann, Pierre Mozer, Vincent Daanen, and Jocelyne Troccaz

Prediction of the Repair Surface over Cartilage Defects: A Comparison of Three Methods in a Sheep Model 75
  Manuela Kunz, Steven Devlin, Ren Hui Gong, Jiro Inoue, Stephen D. Waldman, Mark Hurtig, Purang Abolmaesumi, and James Stewart

Intra-operative Optical Imaging and Endoscopic Navigation

A Coaxial Laser Endoscope with Arbitrary Spots in Endoscopic View for Fetal Surgery... 83
  Noriaki Yamanaka, Hiromasa Yamashita, Ken Masamune, Hongen Liao, Toshio Chiba, and Takeyoshi Dohi

Toward Video-Based Navigation for Endoscopic Endonasal Skull Base Surgery 91
  Daniel Mirota, Hanzi Wang, Russell H. Taylor, Masaru Ishii, and Gregory D. Hager

Correcting Motion Artifacts in Retinal Spectral Domain Optical Coherence Tomography via Image Registration 100
  Susanna Ricco, Mei Chen, Hiroshi Ishikawa, Gadi Wollstein, and Joel Schuman

Single Fiber Optical Coherence Tomography Microsurgical Instruments for Computer and Robot-Assisted Retinal Surgery 108
  Marcin Balicki, Jae-Ho Han, Iulian Iordachita, Peter Gehlbach, James Handa, Russell Taylor, and Jin Kang

Motion Modelling and Image Formation

Coronary Tree Extraction Using Motion Layer Separation 116
  Wei Zhang, Haibin Ling, Simone Prummer, Kevin Shaohua Zhou, Martin Ostermeier, and Dorin Comaniciu

A Fast Alternative to Computational Fluid Dynamics for High Quality Imaging of Blood Flow 124
  Robert H.P. McGregor, Dominik Szczerba, Krishnamurthy Muralidhar, and Gábor Székely

Interventional 4-D Motion Estimation and Reconstruction of Cardiac Vasculature without Motion Periodicity Assumption 132
  Christopher Rohkohl, Günter Lauritsch, Marcus Prümmer, and Joachim Hornegger

Estimating Continuous 4D Wall Motion of Cerebral Aneurysms from
3D Rotational Angiography 140
  Chong Zhang, Mathieu De Craene, Maria-Cruz Villa-Uriol,
  Jose M. Pozo, Bart H. Bijnens, and Alejandro F. Frangi

NIBART: A New Interval Based Algebraic Reconstruction Technique
for Error Quantification of Emission Tomography Images 148
  Olivier Strauss, Abdelkabir Lahrech, Agnès Rico,
  Denis Mariano-Goulart, and Benoît Telle

Image Registration

A Log-Euclidean Polyaffine Registration for Articulated Structures in
Medical Images 156
  Miguel Ángel Martín-Fernández, Marcos Martín-Fernández, and
  Carlos Alberola-López

Nonrigid Registration of Myocardial Perfusion MRI Using Pseudo
Ground Truth 165
  Chao Li and Ying Sun

Parallax-Free Long Bone X-ray Image Stitching 173
  Lejing Wang, Joerg Traub, Simon Weidert, Sandro Michael Heining,
  Ekkehard Euler, and Nassir Navab

Diffusion Tensor Field Registration in the Presence of Uncertainty 181
  Mustafa Okan Irfanoglu, Cheng Guan Koay, Sinisa Pajevic,
  Raghu Machiraju, and Peter J. Basser

Non-rigid Registration of High Angular Resolution Diffusion Images
Represented by Gaussian Mixture Fields 190
  Guang Cheng, Baba C. Vemuri, Paul R. Carney, and
  Thomas H. Mareci

Modelling and Segmentation

Toward Real-Time Simulation of Blood-Coil Interaction during
Aneurysm Embolization 198
  Yiyi Wei, Stéphane Cotin, Le Fang, Jérémie Allard,
  Chunhong Pan, and Songde Ma

A Dynamical Shape Prior for LV Segmentation from RT3D
Echocardiography 206
  Yun Zhu, Xenophon Papademetris, Albert J. Sinusas, and
  James S. Duncan

A Statistical Model of Right Ventricle in Tetralogy of Fallot for
Prediction of Remodelling and Therapy Planning 214
    *Tommaso Mansi, Stanley Durrleman, Boris Bernhardt,
Maxime Sermesant, Hervé Delingette, Ingmar Voigt, Philipp Lurz,
Andrew M. Taylor, Julie Blanc, Younes Boudjemline,
Xavier Pennec, and Nicholas Ayache*

Bayesian Maximal Paths for Coronary Artery Segmentation from 3D
CT Angiograms.. 222
    *David Lesage, Elsa D. Angelini, Isabelle Bloch, and
Gareth Funka-Lea*

Image Segmentation and Classification

Hierarchical Normalized Cuts: Unsupervised Segmentation of Vascular
Biomarkers from Ovarian Cancer Tissue Microarrays 230
    *Andrew Janowczyk, Sharat Chandran, Rajendra Singh,
Dimitra Sasaroli, George Coukos, Michael D. Feldman, and
Anant Madabhushi*

Nonparametric Intensity Priors for Level Set Segmentation of Low
Contrast Structures 239
    *Sokratis Makrogiannis, Rahul Bhotika, James V. Miller,
John Skinner Jr., and Melissa Vass*

Improving Pit–Pattern Classification of Endoscopy Images by a
Combination of Experts 247
    *Michael Häfner, Alfred Gangl, Roland Kwitt, Andreas Uhl,
Andreas Vécsei, and Friedrich Wrba*

Fast Automatic Segmentation of the Esophagus from 3D CT Data
Using a Probabilistic Model 255
    *Johannes Feulner, S. Kevin Zhou, Alexander Cavallaro,
Sascha Seifert, Joachim Hornegger, and Dorin Comaniciu*

Automatic Segmentation of the Pulmonary Lobes from Fissures,
Airways, and Lung Borders: Evaluation of Robustness against Missing
Data 263
    *Eva M. van Rikxoort, Mathias Prokop, Bartjan de Hoop,
Max A. Viergever, Josien P.W. Pluim, and Bram van Ginneken*

Segmentation and Atlas Based Techniques

Joint Segmentation of Image Ensembles via Latent Atlases 272
    *Tammy Riklin Raviv, Koen Van Leemput,
William M. Wells III, and Polina Golland*

Robust Medical Images Segmentation Using Learned Shape and
Appearance Models 281
  Ayman El-Baz and Georgy Gimel'farb

A Spatio-temporal Atlas of the Human Fetal Brain with Application to
Tissue Segmentation 289
  Piotr A. Habas, Kio Kim, Francois Rousseau, Orit A. Glenn,
  A. James Barkovich, and Colin Studholme

Spatiotemporal Atlas Estimation for Developmental Delay Detection in
Longitudinal Datasets 297
  Stanley Durrleman, Xavier Pennec, Alain Trouvé, Guido Gerig, and
  Nicholas Ayache

On the Manifold Structure of the Space of Brain Images 305
  Samuel Gerber, Tolga Tasdizen, Sarang Joshi, and Ross Whitaker

Neuroimage Analysis

Gyral Folding Pattern Analysis via Surface Profiling................. 313
  Kaiming Li, Lei Guo, Gang Li, Jingxin Nie, Carlos Faraco,
  Qun Zhao, Stephen Miller, and Tianming Liu

Constrained Data Decomposition and Regression for Analyzing Healthy
Aging from Fiber Tract Diffusion Properties......................... 321
  Sylvain Gouttard, Marcel Prastawa, Elizabeth Bullitt, Weili Lin,
  Casey Goodlett, and Guido Gerig

Two-Compartment Models of the Diffusion MR Signal in Brain White
Matter 329
  Eleftheria Panagiotaki, Hubert Fonteijn, Bernard Siow, Matt G. Hall,
  Anthony Price, Mark F. Lythgoe, and Daniel C. Alexander

Multivariate Tensor-Based Brain Anatomical Surface Morphometry via
Holomorphic One-Forms 337
  Yalin Wang, Tony F. Chan, Arthur W. Toga, and Paul M. Thompson

Local White Matter Geometry Indices from Diffusion Tensor
Gradients 345
  Peter Savadjiev, Gordon Kindlmann, Sylvain Bouix,
  Martha E. Shenton, and Carl-Fredrik Westin

Surgical Navigation and Robotics

i-BRUSH: A Gaze-Contingent Virtual Paintbrush for Dense 3D
Reconstruction in Robotic Assisted Surgery 353
  Marco Visentini-Scarzanella, George P. Mylonas,
  Danail Stoyanov, and Guang-Zhong Yang

Targeting Accuracy under Model-to-Subject Misalignments in
Model-Guided Cardiac Surgery 361
   Cristian A. Linte, John Moore, Andrew D. Wiles,
   Chris Wedlake, and Terry M. Peters

Patient Specific 4D Coronary Models from ECG-gated CTA Data for
Intra-operative Dynamic Alignment of CTA with X-ray Images 369
   Coert T. Metz, Michiel Schaap, Stefan Klein, Lisan A. Neefjes,
   Ermanno Capuano, Carl Schultz, Robert Jan van Geuns,
   Patrick W. Serruys, Theo van Walsum, and Wiro J. Niessen

Towards Interactive Planning of Coil Embolization in Brain
Aneurysms 377
   Jeremie Dequidt, Christian Duriez, Stephane Cotin, and
   Erwan Kerrien

Temporal Estimation of the 3d Guide-Wire Position Using 2d X-ray
Images 386
   Marcel Brückner, Frank Deinzer, and Joachim Denzler

3-D Respiratory Motion Compensation during EP Procedures by
Image-Based 3-D Lasso Catheter Model Generation and Tracking 394
   Alexander Brost, Rui Liao, Joachim Hornegger, and Norbert Strobel

System Design of a Hand-Held Mobile Robot for Craniotomy 402
   Gavin Kane, Georg Eggers, Robert Boesecke, Jörg Raczkowsky,
   Heinz Wörn, Rüdiger Marmulla, and Joachim Mühling

Dynamic Active Constraints for Hyper-Redundant Flexible Robots 410
   Ka-Wai Kwok, George P. Mylonas, Loi Wah Sun,
   Mirna Lerotic, James Clark, Thanos Athanasiou, Ara Darzi, and
   Guang-Zhong Yang

Nonmagnetic Rigid and Flexible Outer Sheath with Pneumatic
Interlocking Mechanism for Minimally Invasive Surgical Approach ... 418
   Hiromasa Yamashita, Siyang Zuo, Ken Masamune,
   Hongen Liao, and Takeyoshi Dohi

Data-Derived Models for Segmentation with Application to Surgical
Assessment and Training 426
   Balakrishnan Varadarajan, Carol Reiley, Henry Lin,
   Sanjeev Khudanpur, and Gregory Hager

Task versus Subtask Surgical Skill Evaluation of Robotic Minimally
Invasive Surgery 435
   Carol E. Reiley and Gregory D. Hager

Development of the Ultra-Miniaturized Inertial Measurement Unit
WB3 for Objective Skill Analysis and Assessment in Neurosurgery:
Preliminary Results 443
    Massimiliano Zecca, Salvatore Sessa, Zhuohua Lin, Takashi Suzuki,
    Tomoya Sasaki, Kazuko Itoh, Hiroshi Iseki, and Atsuo Takanishi

Novel Endoscope System with Plasma Flushing for Off-Pump Cardiac
Surgery 451
    Ken Masamune, Tetsuya Horiuchi, Masahiro Mizutani,
    Hiromasa Yamashita, Hiroyuki Tsukihara, Noboru Motomura,
    Shinichi Takamoto, Hongen Liao, and Takeyoshi Dohi

Endoscopic Orientation Correction 459
    Kurt Höller, Jochen Penne, Armin Schneider,
    Jasper Jahn, Javier Gutiérrez Boronat, Thomas Wittenberg,
    Hubertus Feußner, and Joachim Hornegger

Time-of-Flight 3-D Endoscopy 467
    Jochen Penne, Kurt Höller, Michael Stürmer, Thomas Schrauder,
    Armin Schneider, Rainer Engelbrecht, Hubertus Feußner,
    Bernhard Schmauss, and Joachim Hornegger

In Vivo OCT Coronary Imaging Augmented with Stent
Reendothelialization Score 475
    Florian Dubuisson, Claude Kauffmann, Pascal Motreff, and
    Laurent Sarry

Optical Biopsy Mapping for Minimally Invasive Cancer Screening 483
    Peter Mountney, Stamatia Giannarou, Daniel Elson, and
    Guang-Zhong Yang

Biopsy Site Re-localisation Based on the Computation of Epipolar
Lines from Two Previous Endoscopic Images 491
    Baptiste Allain, Mingxing Hu, Laurence B. Lovat, Richard Cook,
    Sebastien Ourselin, and David Hawkes

Probabilistic Region Matching in Narrow-Band Endoscopy for Targeted
Optical Biopsy 499
    Selen Atasoy, Ben Glocker, Stamatia Giannarou, Diana Mateus,
    Alexander Meining, Guang-Zhong Yang, and Nassir Navab

Tracked Regularized Ultrasound Elastography for Targeting Breast
Radiotherapy 507
    Hassan Rivaz, Pezhman Foroughi, Ioana Fleming, Richard Zellars,
    Emad Boctor, and Gregory Hager

Image Guidance for Spinal Facet Injections Using Tracked
Ultrasound 516
    John Moore, Colin Clarke, Daniel Bainbridge, Chris Wedlake,
    Andrew Wiles, Danielle Pace, and Terry Peters

Cervical Vertebrae Tracking in Video-Fluoroscopy Using the Normalized
Gradient Field 524
   Rianne Reinartz, Bram Platel, Toon Boselie, Henk van Mameren,
   Henk van Santbrink, and Bart ter Haar Romeny

Expertise Modeling for Automated Planning of Acetabular Cup in
Total Hip Arthroplasty Using Combined Bone and Implant Statistical
Atlases 532
   Itaru Otomaru, Kazuto Kobayashi, Toshiyuki Okada,
   Masahiko Nakamoto, Yoshiyuki Kagiyama, Masaki Takao,
   Nobuhiko Sugano, Yukio Tada, and Yoshinobu Sato

Wide-Angle Intraocular Imaging and Localization 540
   Christos Bergeles, Kamran Shamaei, Jake J. Abbott, and
   Bradley J. Nelson

Inverse C-arm Positioning for Interventional Procedures Using
Real-Time Body Part Detection 549
   Christian Schaller, Christopher Rohkohl, Jochen Penne,
   Michael Stürmer, and Joachim Hornegger

A Method to Correct for Brain Shift When Building Electrophysiological
Atlases for Deep Brain Stimulation (DBS) Surgery 557
   Srivatsan Pallavaram, Benoit M. Dawant, Rui Li, Joseph S. Neimat,
   Michael S. Remple, Chris Kao, Peter E. Konrad, and
   Pierre-François D'Haese

Image Registration

Asymmetric Image-Template Registration 565
   Mert R. Sabuncu, B.T. Thomas Yeo, Koen Van Leemput,
   Tom Vercauteren, and Polina Golland

A Demons Algorithm for Image Registration with Locally Adaptive
Regularization 574
   Nathan D. Cahill, J. Alison Noble, and David J. Hawkes

A Meta Registration Framework for Lesion Matching 582
   Sharmishtaa Seshamani, Purnima Rajan, Rajesh Kumar,
   Hani Girgis, Themos Dassopoulos, Gerard Mullin, and
   Gregory Hager

Automatic Robust Medical Image Registration Using a New Democratic
Vector Optimization Approach with Multiple Measures 590
   Matthias Wacker and Frank Deinzer

Task-Optimal Registration Cost Functions 598
   B.T. Thomas Yeo, Mert Sabuncu, Polina Golland, and Bruce Fischl

Hybrid Spline-Based Multimodal Registration Using Local Measures
for Joint Entropy and Mutual Information 607
   Andreas Biesdorf, Stefan Wörz, Hans-Jürgen Kaiser,
   Christoph Stippich, and Karl Rohr

A Robust Solution to Multi-modal Image Registration by Combining
Mutual Information with Multi-scale Derivatives 616
   Philip A. Legg, Paul L. Rosin, David Marshall, and James E. Morgan

Multimodal Image Registration by Information Fusion at Feature
Level 624
   Yang Li and Ragini Verma

Accelerating Feature Based Registration Using the
Johnson-Lindenstrauss Lemma 632
   Ayelet Akselrod-Ballin, Davi Bock, R. Clay Reid, and
   Simon K. Warfield

Groupwise Registration and Atlas Construction of 4th-Order Tensor
Fields Using the $\mathbb{R}^+$ Riemannian Metric 640
   Angelos Barmpoutis and Baba C. Vemuri

Closed-Form Jensen-Renyi Divergence for Mixture of Gaussians and
Applications to Group-Wise Shape Registration 648
   Fei Wang, Tanveer Syeda-Mahmood, Baba C. Vemuri,
   David Beymer, and Anand Rangarajan

Attribute Vector Guided Groupwise Registration 656
   Qian Wang, Pew-Thian Yap, Guorong Wu, and Dinggang Shen

Statistical Regularization of Deformation Fields for Atlas-Based
Segmentation of Bone Scintigraphy Images 664
   Karl Sjöstrand, Mattias Ohlsson, and Lars Edenbrandt

Graphical Models and Deformable Diffeomorphic Population
Registration Using Global and Local Metrics 672
   Aristeidis Sotiras, Nikos Komodakis, Ben Glocker,
   Jean-François Deux, and Nikos Paragios

Efficient Large Deformation Registration via Geodesics on a Learned
Manifold of Images 680
   Jihun Hamm, Christos Davatzikos, and Ragini Verma

A Non-rigid Registration Method for Serial microCT Mouse Hindlimb
Images 688
   Jung W. Suh, Dustin Scheinost, Donald P. Dione,
   Lawrence W. Dobrucki, Albert J. Sinusas, and
   Xenophon Papademetris

Non-rigid Image Registration with Uniform Gradient Spherical Patterns 696
  Shu Liao and Albert C.S. Chung

Methods for Tractography-Driven Surface Registration of Brain Structures 705
  Aleksandar Petrović, Stephen M. Smith, Ricarda A. Menke, and Mark Jenkinson

A Combined Surface And VOlumetric Registration (SAVOR) Framework to Study Cortical Biomarkers and Volumetric Imaging Data 713
  Eli Gibson, Ali R. Khan, and Mirza Faisal Beg

Fast Tensor Image Morphing for Elastic Registration 721
  Pew-Thian Yap, Guorong Wu, Hongtu Zhu, Weili Lin, and Dinggang Shen

DISCO: A Coherent Diffeomorphic Framework for Brain Registration under Exhaustive Sulcal Constraints............................... 730
  Guillaume Auzias, Joan Glaunès, Olivier Colliot, Matthieu Perrot, Jean-François Mangin, Alain Trouvé, and Sylvain Baillet

Evaluation of Lobar Biomechanics during Respiration Using Image Registration 739
  Kai Ding, Youbing Yin, Kunlin Cao, Gary E. Christensen, Ching-Long Lin, Eric A. Hoffman, and Joseph M. Reinhardt

Evaluation of 4D-CT Lung Registration............................. 747
  Sven Kabus, Tobias Klinder, Keelin Murphy, Bram van Ginneken, Cristian Lorenz, and Josien P.W. Pluim

Slipping Objects in Image Registration: Improved Motion Field Estimation with Direction-Dependent Regularization 755
  Alexander Schmidt-Richberg, Jan Ehrhardt, Rene Werner, and Heinz Handels

Multi-modal Registration Based Ultrasound Mosaicing................ 763
  Oliver Kutter, Wolfgang Wein, and Nassir Navab

A Novel Method for Registration of US/MR of the Liver Based on the Analysis of US Dynamics 771
  Sergiy Milko, Eivind Lyche Melvær, Eigil Samset, and Timor Kadir

Alignment of Viewing-Angle Dependent Ultrasound Images 779
  Christian Wachinger and Nassir Navab

MR to Ultrasound Image Registration for Guiding Prostate Biopsy and
Interventions 787
  Yipeng Hu, Hashim Uddin Ahmed, Clare Allen, Doug Pendsé,
  Mahua Sahu, Mark Emberton, David Hawkes, and Dean Barratt

Combining Multiple True 3D Ultrasound Image Volumes through
Re-registration and Rasterization 795
  Songbai Ji, David W. Roberts, Alex Hartov, and Keith D. Paulsen

Biomechanically Constrained Groupwise US to CT Registration of the
Lumbar Spine 803
  Sean Gill, Parvin Mousavi, Gabor Fichtinger, Elvis Chen,
  Jonathan Boisvert, David Pichora, and Purang Abolmaesumi

A General PDE-Framework for Registration of Contrast Enhanced
Images 811
  Mehran Ebrahimi and Anne L. Martel

Statistically Deformable 2D/3D Registration for Accurate
Determination of Post-operative Cup Orientation from Single Standard
X-ray Radiograph 820
  Guoyan Zheng

A Novel Intensity Similarity Metric with Soft Spatial Constraint for a
Deformable Image Registration Problem in Radiation Therapy 828
  Ali Khamene, Darko Zikic, Mamadou Diallo, Thomas Boettger, and
  Eike Rietzel

Intra-operative Multimodal Non-rigid Registration of the Liver for
Navigated Tumor Ablation 837
  Haytham Elhawary, Sota Oguro, Kemal Tuncali, Paul R. Morrison,
  Paul B. Shyn, Servet Tatli, Stuart G. Silverman, and Nobuhiko Hata

Neuroimage Analysis: Structure and Function

A Novel Measure of Fractional Anisotropy Based on the Tensor
Distribution Function 845
  Liang Zhan, Alex D. Leow, Siwei Zhu, Marina Barysheva,
  Arthur W. Toga, Katie L. McMahon, Greig I. De Zubicaray,
  Margaret J. Wright, and Paul M. Thompson

Iterative Co-linearity Filtering and Parameterization of Fiber Tracts in
the Entire Cingulum 853
  Marius de Groot, Meike W. Vernooij, Stefan Klein,
  Alexander Leemans, Renske de Boer, Aad van der Lugt,
  Monique M.B. Breteler, and Wiro J. Niessen

Think Global, Act Local; Projectome Estimation with BlueMatter 861
  Anthony J. Sherbondy, Robert F. Dougherty,
  Rajagopal Ananthanarayanan, Dharmendra S. Modha, and
  Brian A. Wandell

Dual Tensor Atlas Generation Based on a Cohort of Coregistered
non-HARDI Datasets... 869
  Matthan Caan, Caroline Sage, Maaike van der Graaf,
  Cornelis Grimbergen, Stefan Sunaert, Lucas van Vliet, and Frans Vos

Estimating Orientation Distribution Functions with Probability
Density Constraints and Spatial Regularity......................... 877
  Alvina Goh, Christophe Lenglet, Paul M. Thompson, and René Vidal

Quantifying Brain Connectivity: A Comparative Tractography Study ... 886
  Ting-Shuo Yo, Alfred Anwander, Maxime Descoteaux, Pierre Fillard,
  Cyril Poupon, and T.R. Knösche

Two-Tensor Tractography Using a Constrained Filter 894
  James G. Malcolm, Martha E. Shenton, and Yogesh Rathi

Characterization of Anatomic Fiber Bundles for Diffusion Tensor Image
Analysis 903
  Rubén Cárdenes, Daniel Argibay-Quiñones,
  Emma Muñoz-Moreno, and Marcos Martin-Fernandez

A Riemannian Framework for Orientation Distribution Function
Computing.. 911
  Jian Cheng, Aurobrata Ghosh, Tianzi Jiang, and Rachid Deriche

Bias of Least Squares Approaches for Diffusion Tensor Estimation from
Array Coils in DT–MRI 919
  Antonio Tristán-Vega, Carl-Fredrik Westin, and
  Santiago Aja-Fernández

A Novel Global Tractography Algorithm Based on an Adaptive Spin
Glass Model.. 927
  Pierre Fillard, Cyril Poupon, and Jean-François Mangin

Tractography-Based Parcellation of the Cortex Using a
Spatially-Informed Dimension Reduction of the Connectivity
Matrix 935
  Pauline Roca, Denis Rivière, Pamela Guevara, Cyril Poupon, and
  Jean-François Mangin

Belief Propagation Based Segmentation of White Matter Tracts in
DTI.. 943
  Pierre-Louis Bazin, John Bogovic, Daniel Reich,
  Jerry L. Prince, and Dzung L. Pham

Design and Construction of a Realistic DWI Phantom for Filtering
Performance Assessment 951
 Antonio Tristán-Vega and Santiago Aja-Fernández

Statistical Detection of Longitudinal Changes between Apparent
Diffusion Coefficient Images: Application to Multiple Sclerosis 959
 *Hervé Boisgontier, Vincent Noblet, Félix Renard, Fabrice Heitz,
 Lucien Rumbach, and Jean-Paul Armspach*

Tensor-Based Analysis of Genetic Influences on Brain Integrity Using
DTI in 100 Twins 967
 *Agatha D. Lee, Natasha Leporé, Caroline Brun, Yi-Yu Chou,
 Marina Barysheva, Ming-Chang Chiang, Sarah K. Madsen,
 Greig I. de Zubicaray, Katie L. McMahon, Margaret J. Wright,
 Arthur W. Toga, and Paul M. Thompson*

Robust Extrapolation Scheme for Fast Estimation of 3D Ising Field
Partition Functions: Application to Within-Subject fMRI Data
Analysis 975
 Laurent Risser, Thomas Vincent, Philippe Ciuciu, and Jérôme Idier

Parcellation of fMRI Datasets with ICA and PLS-A Data Driven
Approach 984
 Yongnan Ji, Pierre-Yves Hervé, Uwe Aickelin, and Alain Pitiot

Adjusting the Neuroimaging Statistical Inferences for
Nonstationarity 992
 *Gholamreza Salimi-Khorshidi, Stephen M. Smith, and
 Thomas E. Nichols*

Using Real-Time fMRI to Control a Dynamical System by Brain
Activity Classification 1000
 *Anders Eklund, Henrik Ohlsson, Mats Andersson, Joakim Rydell,
 Anders Ynnerman, and Hans Knutsson*

Modeling Adaptation Effects in fMRI Analysis 1009
 *Wanmei Ou, Tommi Raij, Fa-Hsuan Lin, Polina Golland, and
 Matti Hämäläinen*

A Cluster Overlap Measure for Comparison of Activations in fMRI
Studies 1018
 Guillermo A. Cecchi, Rahul Garg, and A. Ravishankar Rao

Author Index 1027

Building Shape Models from Lousy Data

Marcel Lüthi, Thomas Albrecht, and Thomas Vetter

Computer Science Department, University of Basel, Switzerland
{marcel.luethi,thomas.albrecht,thomas.vetter}@unibas.ch

Abstract. Statistical shape models have gained widespread use in medical image analysis. In order for such models to be statistically meaningful, a large number of data sets have to be included. The number of available data sets is usually limited and often the data is corrupted by imaging artifacts or missing information. We propose a method for building a statistical shape model from such "lousy" data sets. The method works by identifying the corrupted parts of a shape as statistical outliers and excluding these parts from the model. Only the parts of a shape that were identified as outliers are discarded, while all the intact parts are included in the model. The model building is then performed using the EM algorithm for probabilistic principal component analysis, which allows for a principled way to handle missing data. Our experiments on 2D synthetic and real 3D medical data sets confirm the feasibility of the approach. We show that it yields superior models compared to approaches using robust statistics, which only downweight the influence of outliers.

1 Introduction

Statistical shape models have become a widely used tool in medical image analysis, computer vision, and computer graphics. From a technical point of view, the methods for model building are well established. The first and most challenging step is to establish correspondence among the examples. Once the shapes are in correspondence, each shape is regarded as a random observation, and standard methods from statistics can be applied. In practice, however, building statistically representative models is much more difficult. Often, acquiring a large enough data set of sufficient quality constitutes the most difficult step. This is especially true in the medical domain, where the image acquisition process is tailored to the physician's needs and to minimize harm for the patient. The data available to the researcher is therefore often noisy, incomplete, and contains artifacts.

In this paper we propose a method for building statistical shape models from data sets which can include incomplete and corrupted shapes. The main motivation for our work comes from a project involving the construction of a statistical model of the human skull from CT data. In many scans, teeth are missing completely or contain dental fillings resulting in severe metal artifacts. Others show only the region of the skull that was used to diagnose a certain pathology. As is often the case with medical data, some skulls show severe pathologies which should not be included in a model representing the normal anatomy.

To be able to build statistically representative models, we need to make sure that the corrupted parts do not distort the space of possible shapes the model can represent. Our approach identifies the corrupted parts as statistical outliers and excludes them from the model building. This is done by dividing the shapes into parts and checking for each part individually whether it is corrupted. During model building, the best reconstruction of the corrupted parts is estimated from the remaining data sets. This is achieved in a statistically sound way using the EM algorithm for Probabilistic PCA. Performing the outlier analysis part-wise has two advantages: In statistical shape modeling, the observations are usually high-dimensional objects which can naturally be decomposed into smaller structures. Rather than throwing away all the information, we still use the parts that are intact to learn the shape variability of these substructures. More importantly, however, looking for outliers on individual parts makes it possible to detect small, local outliers, which would remain unrecognized if the shape was analyzed as a whole.

In our approach missing data and artifacts are just different instances of statistical outliers. There are two main approaches for dealing with outliers. *Outlier identification* can be performed to identify corrupted samples and exclude them from the data set. Methods for identifying outliers are well known in statistics [1]. Most of the traditional methods, however, consider only the case in which the number of examples is much larger than the dimensionality of the data. Such methods are not applicable to shape statistics. In recent years, outlier detection in high-dimensional data has been greatly advanced in the field of bioinformatics, where outlier-ridden data is the rule and not the exception [2,3]. The second approach for dealing with outliers is to *robustify* the procedure, i.e. to adapt it such that outliers have less influence on the results. This can be achieved by using robust statistics [4] or by incorporating prior information [5,6]. All steps of the workflow leading to a statistical shape model, from image denoising, segmentation, and registration to principal component analysis could benefit from being robustified [4]. In our method, however, we want corrupted parts to remain visible until the registration process has been performed. This makes it possible to detect and eliminate them completely. Therefore, we do not robustify any of these preprocessing steps. Knowing that a part of a shape is an outlier allows us to choose an adequate strategy to deal with it.

2 Method

We first give a brief overview of our approach. Let a set of surfaces be given. We single out one surface as the reference shape, which we know to be complete and free of artifacts. This reference is segmented into parts as illustrated in Figure 1(a). While the method would work with arbitrary patches of reasonable size, we usually use anatomically significant parts for ease of interpretation. Before attempting any statistical analysis, we need to identify corresponding points in all the shapes. We assume that every target shape can be obtained by deforming the reference surface with a smooth vector field, which we find using a non-rigid registration algorithm. Figure 1(b) shows the result of warping the reference surface with such a vector field. We observe that both artifacts and missing data result in (locally) unnatural deformations. We aim at identifying these as statistical outliers. To do so, we rigidly align the individual parts of each shape to the corresponding part of the reference and apply an outlier identification algorithm to the locally aligned shapes. The parts that were identified as outliers are marked

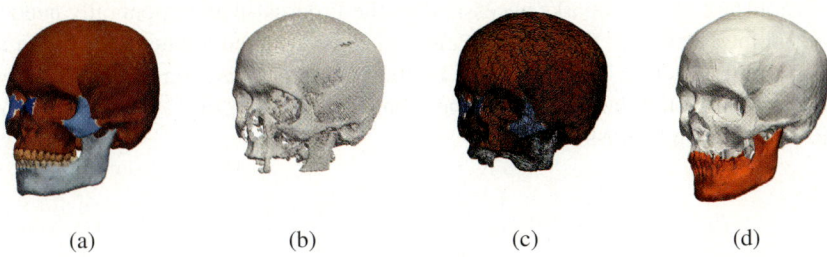

(a) (b) (c) (d)

Fig. 1. Workflow of the outlier detection: 1(a) A reference surface is segmented into parts. 1(b) Some shape used for model building are incomplete or noisy. 1(c) The reference is warped to match the shape of the target. The missing parts lead to an unnatural deformation and can thus be identified as outliers. 1(d) The outlier parts are reconstructed from the remaining data.

as missing in the surface. The statistical model is built from these partial data sets using a PCA method that can handle missing data. We propose the use of the EM algorithm for probabilistic PCA (PPCA) [7,8]. Figure 1(d) shows a reconstruction obtained by the PPCA algorithm.

In the following we provide the details of the methods we use in the individual steps of the workflow. However, the approach is general and does not depend on the particular registration or outlier identification algorithm used.

Registration. To establish correspondence among the examples we use a registration algorithm based on Thirion's Demons algorithm [9]. Similar to the approach of Paragios et al. [10], we do not register the surfaces directly, but rather their distance images. After registration, each shape $\Gamma_i \subset \mathbb{R}^3$ ($i = 1, \ldots, n$) can be represented as a warp of a reference surface Γ_1 with a vector field $\phi_i : \Gamma_1 \to \mathbb{R}^3$:

$$\Gamma_i = \{x + \phi_i(x) \mid x \in \Gamma_1\}. \tag{1}$$

The vector field ϕ_i can be used to transfer any discretisation of the reference Γ_1 to the shape Γ_i and thus allows us to treat the surfaces as discrete random observations (i.e. the surfaces become random vectors).

The parameter in the registration algorithm which controls the smoothness of the vector field is deliberately chosen to be small, in order to make the outliers visible and limit their influence on neighboring regions. In the case that smoother registration results are required for the final shape model, the registration can be run again after the outliers have been identified.

Procrustes Alignment. The reference shape Γ_1 is partitioned into m parts, which we denote by Γ_1^j, $j = 1, \ldots, m$. Since the surfaces are in correspondence, the same partitioning is induced on all shapes. To perform outlier identification, we first align the individual parts of each shape to the corresponding part of the reference by Procrustes alignment. In this way only the shape of the part and not its position in space is considered in the outlier identification. As correspondence among the shapes has already been established, the landmarks necessary for the Procrustes alignment only need to be labeled on the reference. These points can either be selected manually or by an automatic procedure. Let $x_k^j, k = 1, \ldots, N$ be the landmark points on the j-th part of the reference. To align the shapes, we find the rotation matrix $R \in \mathrm{I\!R}^{3 \times 3}$, translation vector $t \in \mathrm{I\!R}^3$ and scaling factor $s \in \mathrm{I\!R}$ as:

$$(s, R, t) = \arg\min_{s,R,t} \frac{1}{N} \sum_{k=1}^{N} \|x_k^j - (sR(x_k^j + \phi_i(x_k^j)) + t)\|^2. \tag{2}$$

The minimum of (2) admits a closed form solution and can be found efficiently (see Umeyama [11]).

Outlier Identification in High Dimensional Data. The place in this workflow to identify and remove outliers is after the alignment step, before they have a chance to corrupt the statistics, but after they have been brought into correspondence. We use the algorithm *PCOut*, proposed by Filzmoser et al. [2], which is especially designed for detecting outliers in high-dimensional spaces. As the method is quite intricate and its details are not critical for understanding our method, we only give a broad overview and refer the interested reader to the original paper [2].

The main idea of *PCOut* is to *robustly* build a PCA model and then identify those samples that do not fit well into this model. In order to build the robust PCA model, it suffices to robustly estimate the mean and covariance matrix. *PCOut* uses the robust estimators median and MAD (mean absolute deviation) to rescale the data, and performs a principal components analysis of this rescaled data. A weighting scheme using a robust kurtosis measure is used to identify the data sets that do not fit the PCA model well enough, according to a user-specified threshold. This value is referred to as the "outlier boundary".

Probabilistic Principal Component Analysis. In the last step, the parts that were identified as outliers are marked as missing in the surface. There exist several methods for PCA that can deal with incomplete data [12]. One such algorithm, which is based on a sound probabilistic framework, is probabilistic PCA (PPCA) [7,8]. Formulated in terms of the EM algorithm, PPCA can be seen as an iterative method, which simultaneously provides an estimation of the principal subspace and a reconstruction of the missing data given this subspace. It corresponds to the following generative model for an observation s:

$$s = Wx + \mu + \varepsilon. \tag{3}$$

That is, s is given as a linear mapping W of the latent variable $x \sim \mathcal{N}(0, \mathcal{I})$ plus the mean of the observation μ and some additive Gaussian noise $\varepsilon \sim \mathcal{N}(0, \sigma\mathcal{I})$. The mapping W can be found using an EM algorithm, which consists of the following steps:

E-Step: $X = W^T W^{-1} W^T S$ **M-Step:** $W^{\text{new}} = S^T X^T (XX^T)^{-1}$.

Here, S is a matrix of all the observed data and X is the matrix of the latent variables x. Of most relevance for our work is that this EM algorithm enables us to extend the E-Step such that missing data can be handled. To reconstruct the complete vector s from the incomplete data s^*, PPCA finds the unique pair (x, s^*) such that $\|Wx - s^*\|^2$ is minimized. The completed observation can be obtained explicitly by computing $s = Wx$ (i.e. s is the maximum a-posteriori reconstruction of $p(s|x)$). In each iteration of the algorithm the reconstruction is improved, as the current estimation of the subspace given by W becomes more accurate.

3 Results

We performed experiments on a synthetic data set of 2D hand contours and a 3D data set of human skull surfaces. Our implementation is solely based on freely available software packages. The registration algorithm is a variant of the Demons algorithm, as implemented in the Insight Toolkit [13]. The algorithms for outlier detection and PPCA are readily available as R packages [14,2,15]. The same parameter settings were used for all our experiments. To align the parts, we automatically determined 20 evenly distributed landmarks for each part. In all experiments we computed the first 10 principal components. While the individual algorithms have many parameters that could be tuned, our experiments showed that the given default values yield good results. Only the parameter of the *outlier boundary* for the algorithm *PCOut* critically influences the result (cf. Section 2). We found a value of 0.45 to work well with all our data sets.

For the first experiment we considered the case in which only the outlier framed in Figure 2 is present. Our algorithm successfully identifies the outlier and removes it from the analysis. The reconstruction computed by the PPCA algorithm is shown in Figure 3(c). Figure 3 clearly shows that in the presence of such outliers, standard PCA will fail. For comparison, we computed a robust PCA using the *PCAproj* algorithm as provided in the R package *pcapp* [16]. While the effect of the outlier is reduced, it still influences the model as illustrated in Figure 3(d). We performed a further experiment, now including all artifacts shown in Figure 2. Figure 4 shows the variation represented by the first two principal components. The variation in the data is captured well, without being influenced by the outliers. We observe that a cusp appears in the model. This may happen at the borders of a segment, when an outlier part is reconstructed using PPCA, but the model is not expressive enough to fit the remaining shape exactly. Table 1 shows a quantitative comparison of the different methods to a ground truth model, which is built from the complete data sets from Figure 2. We evaluated the Hausdorff distance

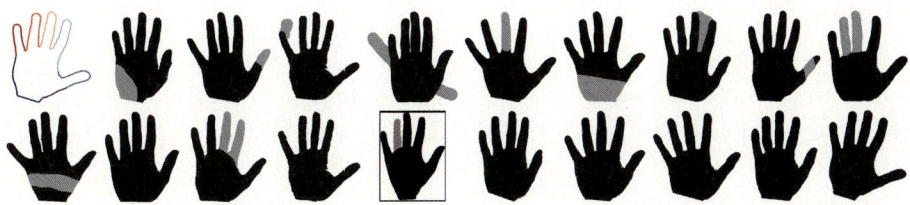

Fig. 2. The hand data set consisting of 19 hands. The hand is divided into 6 parts, as shown by the colors in the first shape. The grey area in the shape images shows manually introduced defects. The framed data-set marks the corrupted shape used in the first experiment.

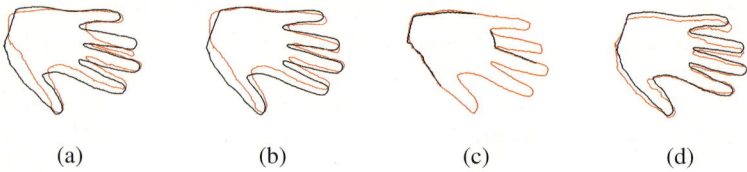

(a) (b) (c) (d)

Fig. 3. Different methods for building shape models from noisy data: 3(a) The mean (black) and 2nd variation using standard PCA. 3(b) The mean and 2nd variation with our method. 3(c) The reconstruction from the PPCA algorithm (red) together with the corrupted shape. 3(d) A result from robust PCA: The outlier is still visible and leads to the thinning of the ring finger.

Table 1. Hausdorff distance (in mm) between the ground truth model and the models computed from data with outliers (σ_i stands for 1σ in the direction of the i−th principal component)

	mean μ	$\mu + \sigma_1$	$\mu - \sigma_1$	$\mu + \sigma_2$	$\mu - \sigma_2$	$\mu + \sigma_3$	$\mu - \sigma_3$
PCA	5.77	13.31	12.61	15.90	16.07	15.60	14.19
robust PCA (PCAproj)	5.45	7.12	8.05	6.45	7.91	8.37	8.54
outlier PPCA	1.90	6.09	4.62	6.72	6.30	5.88	5.96

between the mean and first three principal components of the ground truth to the models computed with regular PCA, robust PCA, and our proposed method. Our method clearly gives the best approximation to the ground truth model.

We finally applied the algorithm to a data set of 23 human skulls. Some of the skull shapes in the data set are shown in Figure 5. As before, the artifacts are detected as outliers and automatically reconstructed, as shown in the same figure. In this test, the method reaches its breaking point. As a common problem in skull data is that some or all of the teeth are missing, the reconstruction of the teeth looks slightly unnatural. This is due to the small number of examples in which the teeth are intact. However, in the final statistical model, this effect is only visible in the last few principle components. Further, as the parts are still identified as outliers, a different reconstruction strategy could be used, such as using a statistical model of the teeth. The comparison with robust PCA

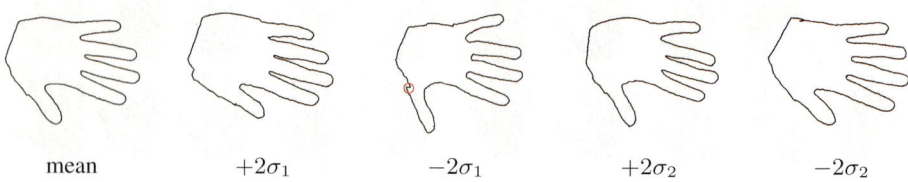

mean $+2\sigma_1$ $-2\sigma_1$ $+2\sigma_2$ $-2\sigma_2$

Fig. 4. The first two principal components of the model. No artifacts are visible, despite the large number of artifacts in the data set. At segment boundaries, small discontinuities can appear (red circle), when the segment is reconstructed from limited data.

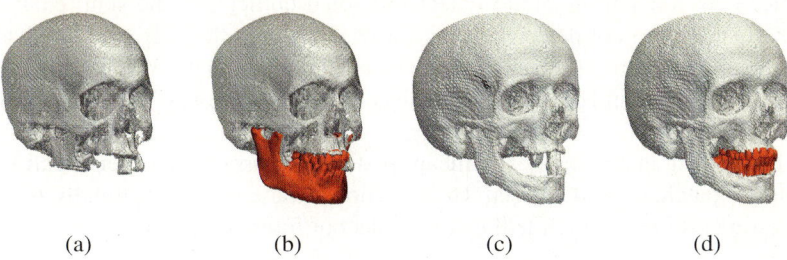

(a)   (b)   (c)   (d)

Fig. 5. 3D Reconstruction 5(a) and 5(c) show two example surfaces from a skull data set. Their reconstruction is shown in 5(b) and 5(d) respectively.

given in Figure 6 leads again to the conclusion, that in the presence of large outliers, explicit outlier removal yields superior results than applying robust PCA.

4 Discussion

We presented an approach for building a statistical shape model in the presence of artifacts and missing data. The main idea is to divide the shapes into parts, and to perform outlier detection on each part individually. Once a part is identified as an outlier, it is removed from the data set. The remaining shape is still used to build the model. In this way, it becomes possible to build shape models from data sets in which almost every shape has some defect. Compared to robust approaches for model building, our method has the advantage that it does not only downweight the influence of an outlier but eliminates it completely. Further, explicit identification of corrupted parts is useful, as it enables us to choose an adequate strategy to replace it. The strategy we presented here is to complete these parts implicitly during model building. Depending on the application, a different approach could be to either remove the parts completely from the analysis, or to perform a reconstruction using a dedicated shape model for this specific part. In general, some of the methods used in our workflow might not be suitable for some applications. For instance, the rigid alignment removes the rotational component,

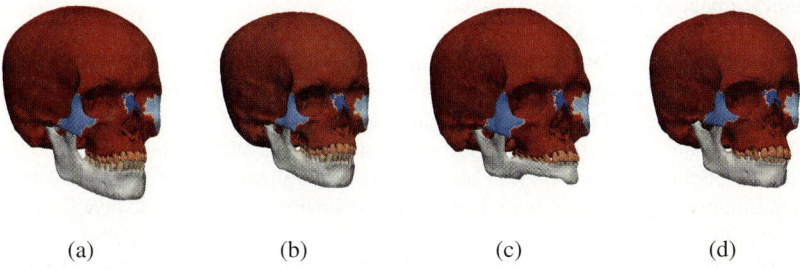

(a)   (b)   (c)   (d)

Fig. 6. Models from real data. 6(a) and 6(b) show the mean and the first principal variation using our method. The outliers are clearly visible when using standard PCA (Figure 6(c)) and still influence the results of robust PCA (Figure 6(d)).

and hence makes it impossible to detect rotational outliers. In the skull example, an open jaw is therefore not detected as an outlier. However, the only step that has to be changed in order to detect such cases is the local alignment. In this respect, the approach we presented here should be seen as a strategy to deal with "lousy" data sets rather than a ready-made method.

While we used anatomically significant parts to perform outlier identification, arbitrary surface patches could be used. How to choose these patches optimally is by itself an interesting problem, which will be the subject of future research.

Acknowledgments. We thank Dr. Zdzislaw Krol and Dr. Stefan Zimmerer, University Hospital Basel, for their support and for providing us with the radiological data. This work was funded by the Swiss National Science Foundation in the scope of the NCCR CO-ME project 5005-66380.

References

1. Rousseeuw, P., Leroy, A., Wiley, J., InterScience, W.: Robust regression and outlier detection. Wiley, New York (1987)
2. Filzmoser, P., Maronna, R., Werner, M.: Outlier identification in high dimensions. Computational Statistics and Data Analysis 52(3), 1694–1711 (2008)
3. Becker, C., Gather, U.: The largest nonidentifiable outlier: A comparison of multivariate simultaneous outlier identification rules. Computational Statistics and Data Analysis 36(1), 119–127 (2001)
4. De la Torre, F., Black, M.: Robust principal component analysis for computer vision. In: Intl. Conf. on Computer Vision (ICCV), vol. 1, pp. 362–369 (2001)
5. Cremers, D., Kohlberger, T., Schnorr, C.: Nonlinear shape statistics in mumford-shah based segmentation. LNCS, pp. 93–108. Springer, Heidelberg (2002)
6. Albrecht, T., Lüthi, M., Vetter, T.: A statistical deformation prior for non-rigid image and shape registration. In: IEEE Conference on Computer Vision and Pattern Recognition (2008)
7. Tipping, M.E., Bishop, C.M.: Probabilistic principal component analysis. Journal of the Royal Statistical Society 61, 611–622 (1999)
8. Roweis, S.: EM Algorithms for PCA and SPCA. In: Advances in neural information processing systems (NIPS), pp. 626–632 (1998)
9. Thirion, J.P.: Image matching as a diffusion process: an analogy with maxwell's demons. Medical Image Analysis 2(3), 243–260 (1998)
10. Paragios, N., Rousson, M., Ramesh, V.: Non-rigid registration using distance functions. Computer Vision and Image Understanding 89(2-3), 142–165 (2003)
11. Umeyama, S.: Least-squares estimation of transformation parameters between two point patterns. IEEE Trans. on Pattern Analysis and Machine Intelligence 13, 376–380 (1991)
12. Little, R., Rubin, D.: Statistical analysis with missing data. Wiley, Chichester (2002)
13. Ibanez, L., Schroeder, W., Ng, L., Cates, J.: The ITK Software Guide. Kitware, Inc. (2005)
14. R Development Core Team: R: A Language and Environment for Statistical Computing. R Foundation for Statistical Computing, Vienna, Austria (2008) (ISBN 3-900051-07-0)
15. Stacklies, W., Redestig, H., Scholz, M., Walther, D., Selbig, J.: pcaMethods - a Bioconductor package providing PCA methods for incomplete data. Bioinformatics (March 2007)
16. Croux, C., Filzmoser, P., Oliveira, M.: Algorithms for Projection–Pursuit robust principal component analysis. Chemometrics and Intelligent Laboratory Systems 87(2) (2007)

Statistical Location Model for Abdominal Organ Localization

Jianhua Yao and Ronald M. Summers

Imaging Biomarkers and Computer Aided Diagnosis Lab, Clinical Center,
The National Institutes of Health, Bethesda, MD 20892, USA

Abstract. Initial placement of the models is an essential pre-processing step for model-based organ segmentation. Based on the observation that organs move along with the spine and their relative locations remain relatively stable, we built a statistical location model (SLM) and applied it to abdominal organ localization. The model is a point distribution model which learns the pattern of variability of organ locations relative to the spinal column from a training set of normal individuals. The localization is achieved in three stages: spine alignment, model optimization and location refinement. The SLM is optimized through maximum a posteriori estimation of a probabilistic density model constructed for each organ. Our model includes five organs: liver, left kidney, right kidney, spleen and pancreas. We validated our method on 12 abdominal CTs using leave-one-out experiments. The SLM enabled reduction in the overall localization error from 62.0±28.5 mm to 5.8±1.5 mm. Experiments showed that the SLM was robust to the reference model selection.

1 Introduction

Segmentation of anatomical structures is often the first step in computer-aided diagnosis using medical images. In recent years there has been considerable interest in methods that use deformable models or atlases to segment anatomical structures. One category of deformable models, such as active contour models [1] and geodesic level sets [2], is based on the optimization of objective functions. Another category of models, including active shape models (ASM) [3], probabilistic atlases [4], and statistical shape models [5], is constructed based on prior information extracted from samples. The motivation is to achieve robust segmentation by constraining solutions to be valid examples of the structure modeled in a population.

Abdominal organ segmentation on CT scans is a challenging task due to the following reasons. First, different organs have similar Hounsfield number, which limits the use of thresholding methods. Second, organs have irregular shapes and often demonstrate large anatomical variations amongst individuals. Third, image artifacts, such as beam-hardening, partial-volume and motion, raise more difficulties.

Instead of segmenting each organ separately, multi-organ segmentation has attracted investigations in recent years [4-6]. Park et al. [4] constructed a probabilistic atlas of three organs (liver, both kidneys) and the spinal cord. The atlas was optimized in a Bayesian framework using mutual information as the similarity measure. Okada

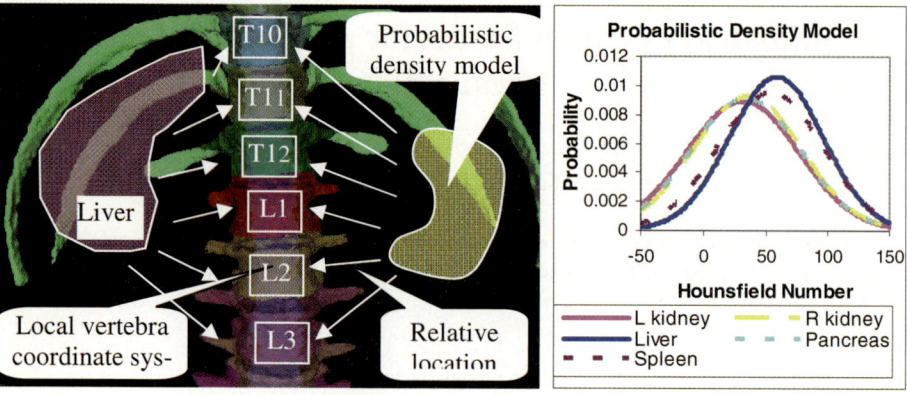

Fig. 1. Organ location model. Left: relative location model; right: probabilistic density model.

et al. [5] proposed a hierarchical statistical atlas to embed the constraints on inter-relations amongst organs in an orga`nization of probabilistic atlases and statistical shape models. Shimizu [6] et al. proposed a simultaneous extraction method for 12 abdominal organs based on abdominal cavity standardization and the EM algorithm.

Initial placement of the models is essential to the success of model-based methods, and this is especially important for organ segmentation due to the large variability. Most methods [4] [7] require the models be placed in close proximity of the targets. Some methods relied on human experts for manual initialization and guidance [4]. Fujimoto et al. [7] set up a coordinate system centered at the T12 vertebra and employed normalized distance for model initialization.

In this paper, we propose a novel method to initialize the model location for multi-organ segmentation. We observed that the spinal column supports the human upper body. When the spine moves, the organs move along with it and the relative location between the organs and the spine remains relatively stable. Furthermore, the organ location configurations amongst normal individuals are similar. Therefore, we model the statistics of the organ location relative to the spinal column using a point distribution model. The organs are also equipped with probabilistic density models. Our model includes five abdominal organs: liver, spleen, pancreas and both kidneys.

2 Methods

Our method is summarized as follows. In the modeling phase, we first segment the spinal column and partition it into vertebrae. The vertebrae are used as anchor points, and the relative locations between organs and vertebrae are recorded. We then build a statistical location model (SLM) to learn all possible configurations of organ relative locations from a training set of normal individuals. We also build a probabilistic density model for each organ. In the application phase, the SLM is applied to a new data set to obtain the initial organ location through maximum a posteriori (MAP) estimation of the probabilistic density model.

2.1 Automated Spinal Column Extraction and Partitioning

The details of the automated spinal column extraction and partitioning can be found in [8]. A threshold of 200 HU is applied to mask out the bone pixels. Then a connected component analysis is conducted to obtain the initial spine segmentation. The spinal cord is then extracted using a watershed algorithm and a directed acyclic graph search. Then curved planar reformation is computed along the centerline to partition the spinal column into vertebrae. After that, the ribs are detected using features such as size, location, shape, orientation and density. Finally the vertebrae are labeled on the basis of two pieces of anatomical knowledge: 1) one vertebra has at most two attached ribs; 2) ribs are attached only to thoracic vertebrae. Figure 1 illustrated one example of partitioned spinal column. In our model, only six vertebrae, T10, T11, T12, L1, L2 and L3, are included since they are present in most abdominal CT scans.

2.2 Organ Location Model

We build an organ location model based on the spinal column. We fit a B-Spline curve for the centerline of the spinal cord. A local frame $\{c(V_i), \vec{t}(V_i), \vec{f}_1(V_i), \vec{f}_2(V_i)\}$ is established for each vertebra V_i. Here $c(V_i)$ is the center point of V_i at the spinal cord, $\vec{t}(V_i)$ is the tangent of the spinal cord, $\vec{f}_1(V_i)$ and $\vec{f}_2(V_i)$ are two orthogonal vectors on the plane perpendicular to $\vec{t}(V_i)$. Given the local frame at V_i, the relative location and orientation of each organ can be computed.

In the modeling phase, we manually segment each organ and compute its 3D surface. For an organ O_j, we use the center of mass of the 3D surface as its center. The relative location between an organ O_j and a vertebra V_i is defined as,

$$rl(O_j, V_i) = c(O_j) - c(V_i) \quad (1)$$

here $c(O_j)$ is the center of organ O_j and $c(V_i)$ is the center of vertebra V_i. The location vector of organ O_j is then defined as,

$$L(O_j) = \{rl(O_j, V_1), rl(O_j, V_2), \ldots, rl(O_j, V_n)\} \quad (2)$$

here n is the number of vertebrae in the model ($n=6$ for vertebra T10 to L3). The location vector for multiple organs is the concatenation of the location vector of each organ in the model, i.e.,

$$L = \{L(O_1), L(O_2), \ldots, L(O_m)\} = \{rl(O_1, V_1), rl(O_1, V_2), \ldots, rl(O_m, V_n)\} \quad (3)$$

here m is the total number of organs in the model ($m=5$). The location vector is a 90 dimensional vector (5*6*3=90). The organ location model is illustrated in Figure 1.

2.3 Probabilistic Density Model

We build a probabilistic density model for each organ. The model is a conditional Gaussian model using sample mean and variance over the manually segmented organ region. The density model of an organ O_j is represented as,

$$G(O_j) = (\mu(O_j), \sigma(O_j)) \quad (4)$$

where $\mu(O_j)$ is the mean tissue density and $\sigma^2(O_j)$ is the variance. Given this model, the conditional probability of a tissue y_i belonging to organ O_j is,

$$p(y_i \mid O_j) = \frac{1}{\sqrt{2\pi\sigma^2(O_j)}} \exp\left(\frac{-(y_i - \mu(O_j))^2}{2\sigma^2(O_j)}\right) \qquad (5)$$

Figure 1 (right) shows the probabilistic density models of five organs.

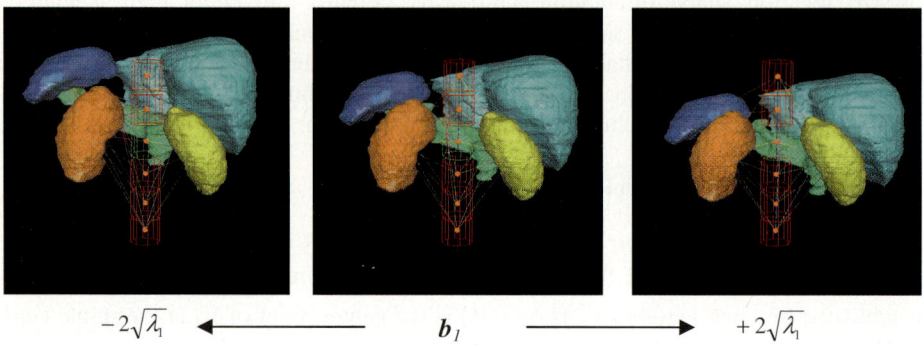

Fig. 2. Statistical location model (SLM). Cylinders are vertebra models. Note variations in the relative locations of liver (cyan), left kidney (yellow), right kidney (orange), spleen (blue) and pancreas (green) as the largest mode b_1 is varied.

2.4 Statistical Location Model

Our aim is to build a statistical location model (SLM) for abdominal organs. The SLM describes both the typical location and variability of the organs from a training set of normal individuals. This is achieved by a point distribution model (PDM).

In order to compute the statistics, all training models must first be aligned. We randomly select a reference model from the training set and align other models to it. The technique is described in detail in Section 2.5.1. The alignment is through the spinal column and the aligned location models form an "allowable location domain", which can be modeled using a PDM.

A principal component analysis (PCA) method is employed to extract the "modes of variation" from the training set. Given a set of N aligned location models $\{L_i\}$ (Eq. 3), the mean location model $\overline{L}$ is computed,

$$\overline{L} = \frac{1}{N} \sum_{i=1}^{N} L_i \qquad (6)$$

A covariance matrix S is constructed using the deviation from the mean model,

$$S = \frac{1}{N} \sum_{i=1}^{N} (L_i - \overline{L})(L_i - \overline{L})^T \qquad (7)$$

The eigenvectors $\{e_1, e_2, .. e_N\}$ and their corresponding eigenvalues $\{\lambda_1, \lambda_2, ..., \lambda_N\}$ are computed. The variance explained by each eigenvector is equal to its corresponding eigenvalue. The first t ($t<N$) eigenvectors are often sufficient to define the "allowable location domain". Any location model in the domain can be represented by taking the mean and adding a linear combination of the eigenvectors, i.e.,

$$L(b) = \overline{L} + Eb \tag{8}$$

where $E=\{e_1, e_2, .. e_t\}$ is the matrix of first t eigenvectors, and $b=(b_1, b_2, ..., b_t)^T$ is the model parameter vector. By varying b, we can generate new location instances within the "allowable location domain". Given an instantiated location model $L(b)$, the relative location $rl(O_j, V_i)$ can be extracted from the vector (Eq. 3), and the location of an organ can be computed as,

$$l(O_j) = \frac{1}{n}\sum_{i=1}^{n}\left(c(V_i) + rl(O_j, V_i)\right) \tag{9}$$

Figure 2 shows examples of instantiated location models by varying the largest mode b_1 of the SLM.

2.5 Organ Localization Using SLM

Given the SLM, the organ localization is treated as an optimization problem in which we maximize the similarity between one instantiated model and an image. After the spinal column is extracted and partitioned from the image (section 2.1), the organ localization is conducted in three steps: first, the spinal column in the SLM is aligned with the spinal column in the image (2.5.1); second, the model parameter is optimized through MAP estimation of the probabilistic density model (2.5.2); and third, the location of each organ is locally refined (2.5.3).

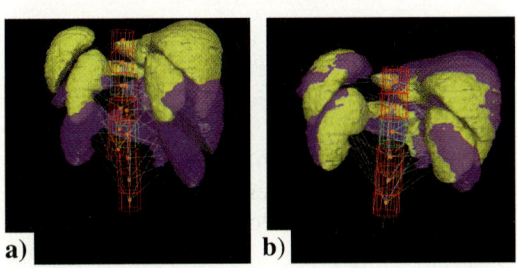

Fig. 3. Model alignment. a) Before alignment, b) after alignment

2.5.1 Model Alignment

The location models are aligned using the spinal column. That is, the vertebrae in one model are aligned to their corresponding vertebrae in another model. The organs are then relocated according to the spine alignment. Assuming the translation of vertebra V_i from the moving model to the fixed model is $\Delta t(V_i)$, the new location of organ O_j is,

$$l(O_j) = \frac{1}{n}\sum_{i=1}^{n}\left(c(V_i) + \Delta t(V_i) + rl(O_j, V_i)\right) \tag{10}$$

Currently only the positions of the vertebrae are aligned, not the orientation. Figure 3 shows two models before and after the alignment.

2.5.2 Model Optimization

The optimization of the SLM is through MAP estimation of the probabilistic density model. Given a location model $L(b)$, we can extract the organ location $l(O_j)$ using

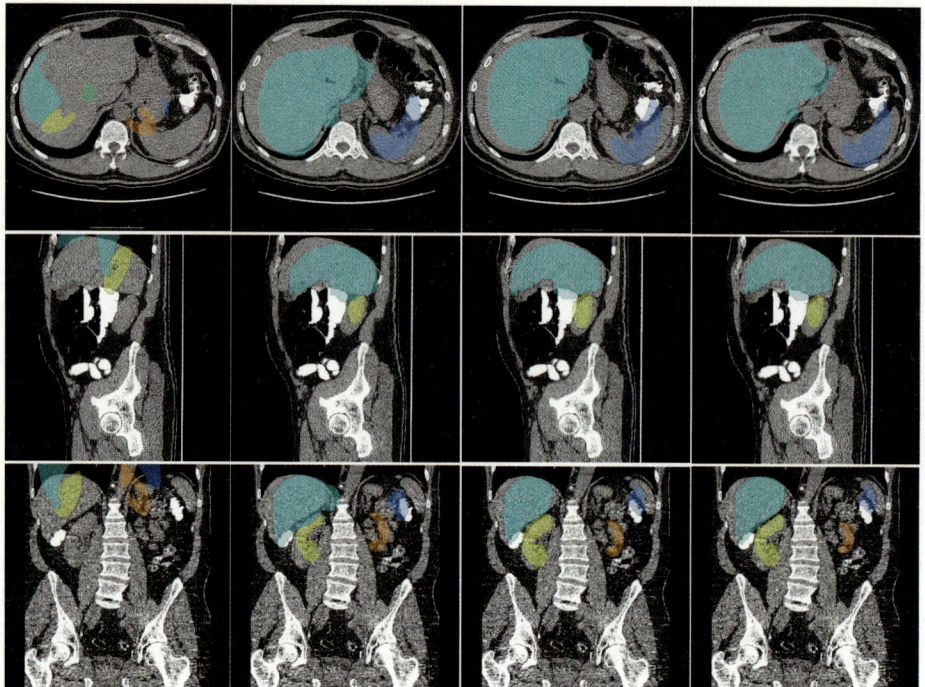

Fig. 4. Organ localization example. Reference models are superimposed on the image data, orientation not optimized. Liver (cyan), left kidney (yellow), right kidney (orange), spleen (blue) and pancreas (green).
1st row: axial view; 2nd row: sagittal view; 3rd row: coronal view
1st column: initial state; 2nd column: after spine alignment; 3rd column: after model optimization; 4th column: after local refinement.

Eq. 3 and 9. The manually segmented organ region in the reference model is moved to location $l(O_j)$, and the set of voxels inside the region are generated, denoted as $\Omega(O_j, L(b))$. The average probability that $\Omega(O_j, L(b))$ coincides with organ O_j is,

$$P(\Omega(O_j, L(b)) \mid O_j) = \frac{1}{\|\Omega(O_j, L(b))\|} \sum_{y_i \in \Omega(O_j, L(b))} p(y_i \mid O_j) \quad (11)$$

here $p(y_i|O_j)$ is defined in the probabilistic density model (Eq. 5). To obtain the optimal location model, we maximize the a posteriori probability for all organs. That is, the optimal model parameter b is,

$$b^{opt} = \arg\max_b \left(\sum_{j=1}^{m} P(\Omega(O_j, L(b)) \mid O_j) \right) \quad (12)$$

The optimization algorithm is Powell's method.

2.5.3 Location Refinement

Since the SLM can only model the variability present in the training set, we conduct a location refinement for each organ independently. The refinement is conducted in a small neighborhood of $L(b^{opt})$ and through MAP estimation of the probabilistic density model, i.e.,

$$\Delta l(O_j)^{opt} = \arg\max_{\Delta l}\left(P(\Omega(O_j, L(b^{opt}) + \Delta l) \mid O_j)\right) \quad (13)$$

here $\Delta l(O_j)^{opt}$ is the optimal location adjustment.

Figure 4 shows an example of organ localization using the statistical location model. The reference model is superimposed on the image data.

2.6 Validation Dataset and Analysis

Our method was validated on 12 (6 males and 6 females) abdominal CT scans. The CT reconstruction interval is 1 mm. We manually segmented the five organs from all cases. The center of mass is treated as the location of an organ. The localization error is computed as the distance between the manually determined organ location and the computed organ location,

$$\Delta d(O_j) = \| l(O_j)^{cp} - l(O_j)^{gt} \|$$
$$\Delta d = \frac{1}{5}\sum_{j=1}^{5}\Delta d(O_j) \quad (14)$$

here $l(O_j)^{cp}$ is the computed organ location (Eq. 10), $l(O_j)^{gt}$ is the location determined by manual segmentation (used as ground truth), Δd is the overall localization error.

In our validation, we adopted a leave-one-out strategy. That is, we used 11 data sets to build a SLM, and applied the SLM on the left-out data to compute the organ locations.

3 Results

The eigenvalues of the SLM built from 12 data sets are shown in Table 1. It shows that the first 6 modes of the SLM cover more than 95% of the variability.

Table 1. Eigenvalues of the SLM

λ_1'	λ_2'	λ_3'	λ_4'	λ_5'	λ_6'	λ_7'	λ_8'	λ_9'	λ_{10}'	λ_{11}'	λ_{12}'
42.6%	27.1%	10.0%	7.5%	5.9%	2.5%	1.9%	1.1%	0.7%	0.3%	0.1%	0%

$\lambda_i' = \lambda_i/\lambda_t$, λ_t is the sum of all λs.

Figure 5 shows the statistics (mean and standard deviation of all leave-one-out experiments) of the localization error in each stage of the organ localization. The localization error was reduced dramatically (91%) from the initial stage to after the final refinement. Figure 6 shows the localization error of each organ. It shows that the liver is most accurately located, but the differences of localization errors amongst organs are small.

To evaluate the sensitivity to the reference model selection, we build different SLMs using different data sets for the reference models. The leave-one-out strategy was again adopted in the validation. Table 2 shows the results with different reference models. It indicates that our model is robust to the reference model selection.

Table 2. Localization error (mm) of different reference models

model	1	2	3	4	5	6	7	8	9	10	11	12
mean (mm)	5.9	5.8	6.3	6.2	5.9	5.5	5.8	5.7	5.6	5.9	5.6	5.9
stdev (mm)	1.4	1.0	1.7	1.6	1.9	1.3	1.2	1.6	1.4	1.5	1.5	1.5

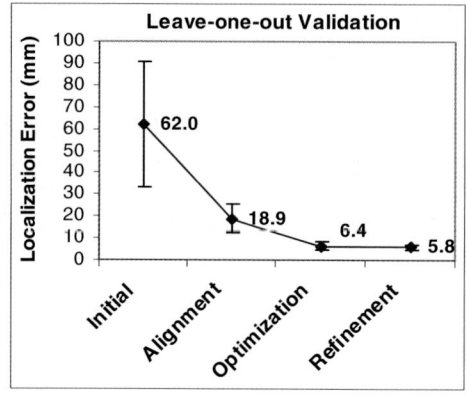
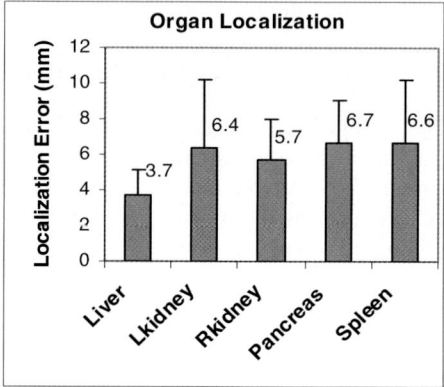

Fig. 5. Localization error in each stage of organ localization

Fig. 6. Localization error for each organ

4 Discussion

The SLM is similar to the active shape model (ASM) [3] in the way that the model is constructed. Instead of modeling the variability of labeled landmark positions as in the ASM, we model the variability of the abdominal organ locations relative to the spinal column. Our model ensures that the instantiated organ locations are consistent with the ones in the training set. The organ localization is only the first step towards a fully automated organ segmentation method. The final segmentation can be achieved using techniques such as level sets [2], ASMs [3], and statistical atlases [5].

More work is still needed to improve the SLM. For instance, variability of organ orientation and scale can be incorporated so that the SLM can bring the model even closer to the target during the initialization. Furthermore, the constraint of relative locations amongst organs can be incorporated to prevent organs from intersecting each other. The model will be trained on a larger training set to provide better estimation of the variability being modeled. Currently the model only works when vertebrae T10-L3 are present in the dataset. Although this requirement is met for most abdominal CTs, we could improve the spine alignment to accommodate data sets with fewer vertebrae.

In conclusion, we have developed a novel SLM that provides accurate and fast initialization of multiple organs in abdominal CT segmentation.

References

1. Kass, M., Witkin, A., Terzopoulos, D.: Snakes: Active Contour Models. International Journal of Computer Vision, 321–331 (1988)
2. Caselles, V., Kimmel, R., Sapiro, G.: Geodesic active contours. In: IEEE International Conference on Computer Vision, Cambridge, MA USA (1995)
3. Cootes, T.F., Taylor, C., Cooper, D., Graham, J.: Active shape models - their training and application. Computer Vision and Image Understanding 61, 38–59 (1995)
4. Park, H., Bland, P.H., Meyer, C.R.: Construction of an Abdominal Probabilistic Atlas and its Application in Segmentation. IEEE Trans. Med. Imag. 22(4), 483–492 (2003)
5. Okada, T., Yokota, K., Masatoshi, H., et al.: Construction of Hierarchical Multi-Organ Statistical Atlases and Their Application to Multi-Organ Segmentation from CT Images. In: Metaxas, D., Axel, L., Fichtinger, G., Székely, G. (eds.) MICCAI 2008, Part I. LNCS, vol. 5241, pp. 502–509. Springer, Heidelberg (2008)
6. Shimizu, A., Ohno, R., Ikegami, T., Kobatake, H., et al.: Segmentation of multiple organs in non-contrast 3D abdominal CT images. Int. J. CARS (2), 135–142 (2007)
7. Kaneko, T., Gu, L., Fujimoto, H.: Abdominal organ recognition using 3D mathematical morphology. In: Proc. of 15th Int Conf. on Pattern Recognition, Barcelona (2000)
8. Yao, J., O'Connor, S.D., Summers, R.M.: Automated Spinal Column Extraction and Partitioning. In: IEEE ISBI, Arlington, VA (2006)

Volumetric Shape Model for Oriented Tubular Structure from DTI Data

Hon Pong Ho[1], Xenophon Papademetris[1,2], Fei Wang[3], Hilary P. Blumberg[3], and Lawrence H. Staib[1,2]

Departments of [1]Biomedical Engineering, [2]Diagnostic Radiology and [3]Psychiatry, Yale University, New Haven, CT, USA

Abstract. In this paper, we describe methods for constructing shape priors using orientation information to model white matter tracts from magnetic resonance diffusion tensor images (DTI). Shape Normalization is needed for the construction of a shape prior using statistical methods. Moving beyond shape normalization using boundary-only or orientation-only information, our method combines the idea of sweeping and inverse-skeletonization to parameterize 3D volumetric shape, which provides point correspondence and orientations over the whole volume in a continuous fashion. Tangents from this continuous model can be treated as a de-noised reconstruction of the original structural orientation inside a shape. We demonstrate the accuracy of this technique by reconstructing synthetic data and the 3D cingulum tract from brain DTI data and manually drawn 2D contours for each tract. Our output can also serve as the input for subsequent boundary finding or shape analysis.

1 Introduction

Shape priors are powerful tools for image analysis [1,2,3,4,5,6,7,8]. In cases where the signal-to-noise ratio is low, using a prior model, typically generated by manual delineation, can substantially improve the accuracy of the end result. With Magnetic Resonance Diffusion Tensor Imaging (MR-DTI) [9,10,11], see Fig. 1 (left), one can now evaluate directional structural information within a volume in addition to the boundary of a shape. There is a natural demand for incorporating volumetric structural information into prior models for DTI data [12,13,14]. Such models are useful for quantifying and comparing white matter structure in neurologic and psychiatric disorders.

1.1 Shape Representation

Common shape representations include the boundary mesh [3,8], the distance map [1,4,5,7], and coefficients of harmonic functions [6]. In the context of shape sampling, we can manually specify boundary points and use straight lines in 2D or triangles in 3D to represents the actual boundary of a shape. A distance map can be computed based on the shortest distance from each point to the boundary.

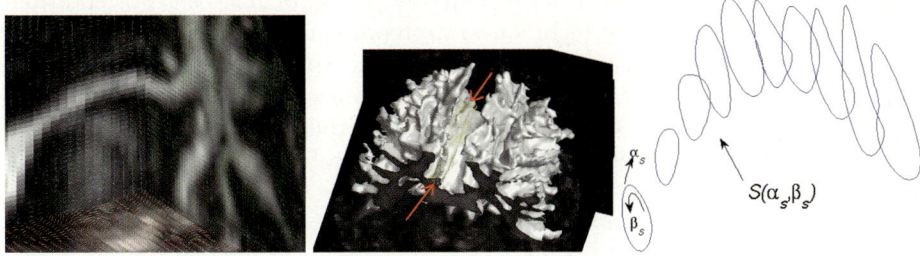

Fig. 1. (Left) Diffusion Tensor Image showing fractional anisotropy (FA) and main diffusion orientations. (Middle) Position and orientation around the cingulum tract within the white matter. (Right) One of the manual segmentations of the cingulum tract.

Such implicit representations have the advantage of representing complex shapes using a single map. On the other hand, a projection from boundary points to harmonic functions transforms the representation from the spatial to a frequency domain. A frequency representation is generally shift and rotation invariant as well as continuous in the spatial domain and therefore easy to resample.

1.2 Point Correspondence in a Volume

Shape normalization [15] establishes a common ground for comparing shapes. Boundary samples on one training shape need to be at the same relative locations on all the others in order to provide a meaningful comparison. If point correspondence cannot be established manually, this could be a point-based registration problem. When using a labeled map, for example the FA map in Fig. 1 (left), instead of boundary points, this could be an intensity-based registration [16]. However, accurate non-rigid intensity-based inter-subject registration can be very difficult for small structures. Assuming intensity maps can be registered reasonably well, if no interior landmark points or features [3] are given, internal point correspondence established over these homogeneous regions through registration is purely controlled by the interpolation between boundaries and smoothing constraints, which are unrelated to the internal structure of the training shape. In cm-reps [17], a shape is parameterized based on an object map and a manual skeleton, which provides interior landmarks, using the idea of inverse-skeletonization. Sun et al. [15] further analyze the cm-rep approach targeted at the corpus callosum from 2D brain DTI.

1.3 Training Shape with Orientation Data

Our goal is to create a set of normalized 3D training shapes with meaningful interior point correspondence. In most cases, specifying internal landmark points over all shapes would be impractical. So, we restrict our input to a limited number of 2D contours, see Fig. 1 (right), which are drawn on several slices of an image volume. Unlike previous surface-driven [15,17] or line-based orientation-driven [12,14] normalization techniques, we represent the training shapes using combinations of continuous basis functions and incorporate orientation data into our normalization process. The analysis of normalized shapes and their underlying orientation patterns can be performed on either the frequency domain or at freely selected spatial locations without the problem of under-sampling or re-meshing.

2 Fourier Surface and Volume in 3D

We begin with a set of 2D manual contours drawn on z-planes, see Fig. 1 (right). We represent each individual contour as a closed curve, with $x(\beta_s), y(\beta_s)$ expressed in terms of the arc-length parameter $\beta_s \in [0, 2\pi]$ and decompose as Fourier series. The Fourier coefficients of the contour at each z level are themselves decomposed as Fourier series over the range $\alpha_s \in [0, \pi]$. We construct the Fourier surface [6]: $S(\alpha_s, \beta_s) =$

$$\begin{bmatrix} x(\alpha_s, \beta_s) \\ y(\alpha_s, \beta_s) \\ z(\alpha_s, \beta_s) \end{bmatrix} = \sum_{k_1=0}^{K_1} \sum_{k_2=0}^{K_2} \begin{bmatrix} a_{11}(k_1,k_2) \cdots a_{14}(k_1,k_2) \\ a_{21}(k_1,k_2) \cdots a_{24}(k_1,k_2) \\ a_{31}(k_1,k_2) \cdots a_{34}(k_1,k_2) \end{bmatrix} \begin{bmatrix} \cos(k_1,\alpha_s)\cos(k_2,\beta_s) \\ \cos(k_1,\alpha_s)\sin(k_2,\beta_s) \\ \sin(k_1,\alpha_s)\cos(k_2,\beta_s) \\ \sin(k_1,\alpha_s)\sin(k_2,\beta_s) \end{bmatrix} \quad (1)$$

K_1, K_2 are the number of harmonics used to represent the long-axis and circumferential variations. To compute the coefficients a_{ij} for all frequencies, we perform Fourier Transforms:

$$a_{11}(k_1, k_2) = \int_{\alpha_s=0}^{2\pi} \int_{\beta_s=0}^{2\pi} x(\alpha_s, \beta_s) \cos(k_1, \alpha_s) \cos(k_2, \beta_s) d\alpha_s d\beta_s \quad (2)$$

Although we define the contours' α_s parameter up to π, the $x(\alpha_s, \beta_s)$ are repeated in reverse z-direction such that we have a full period of samples, see [6] for details. The other a_{ij} can be computed similarly. To perform integration in (2) by discrete summations, $S(\alpha_s, \beta_s)$ is preprocessed to be equally spaced.

After computing the surface coefficients $a_{ij}(k_1, k_2)$ from the input contours, our goal is to solve for the unknown coefficients $a_{ij}(k_1, k_2, k_3)$, defined in Eq. (3), which also carry orientation information from the image data $D(x, y, z) \in \Re^6$. D is the symmetric diffusion tensor computed at each voxel from the DTI data. This computation can be performed by inverse Fourier Transform of $V(\alpha, \beta, \gamma)$:

$$\begin{bmatrix} x(\alpha, \beta, \gamma) \\ y(\alpha, \beta, \gamma) \\ z(\alpha, \beta, \gamma) \end{bmatrix} = \sum_{k_1=0}^{K_1} \sum_{k_2=0}^{K_2} \sum_{k_3=0}^{K_3} \begin{bmatrix} a_{11}(k_1,k_2,k_3) \cdots a_{18} \\ a_{21}(k_1,k_2,k_3) \cdots a_{28} \\ a_{31}(k_1,k_2,k_3) \cdots a_{38} \end{bmatrix} \begin{bmatrix} \cos(k_1\alpha)\cos(k_2\beta)\cos(k_3\gamma) \\ \cos(k_1\alpha)\sin(k_2\beta)\cos(k_3\gamma) \\ \sin(k_1\alpha)\cos(k_2\beta)\cos(k_3\gamma) \\ \sin(k_1\alpha)\sin(k_2\beta)\cos(k_3\gamma) \\ \cos(k_1\alpha)\cos(k_2\beta)\sin(k_3\gamma) \\ \cos(k_1\alpha)\sin(k_2\beta)\sin(k_3\gamma) \\ \sin(k_1\alpha)\cos(k_2\beta)\sin(k_3\gamma) \\ \sin(k_1\alpha)\sin(k_2\beta)\sin(k_3\gamma) \end{bmatrix} \quad (3)$$

$$\text{where } V(\alpha, \beta, 0) = S(\alpha_s, \beta_s) \text{ are the boundary conditions} \quad (4)$$

which is an extension of the Fourier surface with an additional parameter γ representing the boundary-to-axis variation of the volume. K_3 defines the number

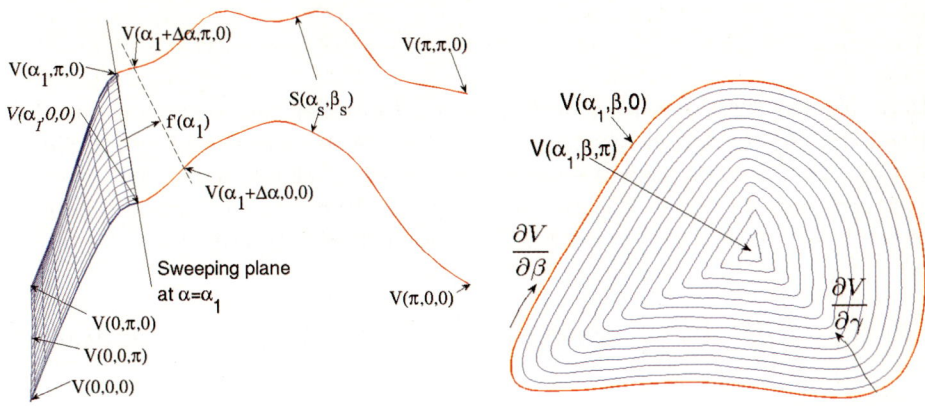

Fig. 2. (Left) A cross section of the parameterized shape with the sweeping plane. (Right) An example of minimum energy 2D front propagation on the sweeping plane.

of harmonics used for this variation. Generally, parameter $\alpha \neq \alpha_s$ and $\beta \neq \beta_s$. Also, we do not have interior samples of V. In the next section, we will discuss our method of generating ordered samples of $V(\alpha, \beta, \gamma)$ from $S(\alpha_s, \beta_s)$. The input structural orientation data is given by the eigen-decomposition of D and taking the main eigenvector $\mathbf{v}$ denoting the orientations of the underlying tissue. We will represent the orientations by the partial derivative of $V(\alpha, \beta, \gamma)$ w.r.t. α:

$$\frac{\partial}{\partial \alpha} V(\alpha, \beta, \gamma) = \mathbf{v}(D), \quad \mathbf{v}: \Re^6 \to \Re^3 \qquad (5)$$

3 Volumetric Parameterization through the Sweeping Plane

Similar to the challenge in white matter fiber tracking [11,12,13], $\mathbf{v}(D)$ contains noise and irrelevant orientations belonging to other structures and thus we cannot normalize the shape solely depending on the data orientations. Our method combines the idea of sweeping [18,13] and inverse-skeletonization [15] to generate ordered samples of $V(\alpha, \beta, \gamma)$ which satisfies (4) as well as (5). Without specifying a skeleton, we iteratively track the tract's axis $V(\alpha, \beta, \pi)$ from the orientation data. We use a sweeping plane to assist the estimation to reduce local tracking error by taking boundary information into account. With the estimated axis position and a 2D boundary extracted from the input surface $S(\alpha, \beta)$, we find the inverse-skeleton on the sweeping plane by solving a minimum energy front propagation equation using a 2D level set method [19], see Fig. 2 (right), as described below:

Assume the first manual contour is the same in our final volume, i.e. $V(0, \beta, 0)$ = $S(0, \beta_s)$. Let $N(\alpha_0, \beta, \gamma)$ be the inward normal of the contour. We solve for $V(\alpha_0, \beta, \gamma)$, the area enclosed by $V(0, \beta, 0)$, according to:

$$\frac{\partial}{\partial \gamma} V(\alpha_0, \beta, \gamma) = (1 - \varepsilon K(\beta, \gamma)) N(\alpha_0, \beta, \gamma), \quad \beta \in [0, 2\pi], \gamma \in [0, \pi] \quad (6)$$

Here, $K(\beta, \gamma)$ is the curvature of the evolving front and ε is a small constant. Let $V(\alpha_0, \beta, \gamma)$ be the first sweeping plane, see Fig. 2 (left). Let $(\bar{x}(\alpha_0), \bar{y}(\alpha_0), \bar{z}(\alpha_0))$ $= V(\alpha_0, \beta, \pi)$ be the estimated tract's axis location relative to the first contour. We then compute the average orientation $f'(\alpha_0)$ from D over a neighborhood Ω of the most recent axis point defined by the maximum inscribed disc from that point:

$$f'(\alpha_0) = \iiint_{(x,y,z) \in \Omega} W_\alpha\left(x - \bar{x}(\alpha_0), y - \bar{y}(\alpha_0), z - \bar{z}(\alpha_0)\right) \mathbf{v}(D(x,y,z)) dx dy dz \quad (7)$$

with weighting function and maximum axis point-to-boundary distance:

$$W_\alpha(d_1, d_2, d_3) = e^{-\sqrt{(d_1)^2 + (d_2)^2 + (d_3)^2}/d(\alpha)} \quad (8)$$

$$d(\alpha) = \max_\alpha dist\bigl(V(\alpha, \beta, 0), (\bar{x}(\alpha), \bar{y}(\alpha), \bar{z}(\alpha))\bigr) \quad (9)$$

Now we move to the next α value by advancing $\Delta \alpha$ step in the parametric space and Δs step in the image space along the average orientation:

$$\alpha_1 = \alpha_0 + \Delta \alpha \quad (10)$$

$$V(\alpha_1, \beta, \pi) = V(\alpha_0, \beta, \pi) + \Delta s f'(\alpha_0) / |f'(\alpha_0)| \quad (11)$$

Before going back to (6), we need $V(\alpha_1, \beta, 0)$ which is not $S(\alpha_1, \beta_s)$ in general except when $\alpha = \alpha_0$. However, we know that $V(\alpha_1, \beta, 0)$ must be on $S(\alpha_s, \beta_s)$. So we reconstruct $V(\alpha_1, \beta, 0)$, which will later become part of the reconstructed surface, from parameterized data points by the intersection between the sweeping plane passing through $V(\alpha_1, \beta, \pi)$ with the normal $f'(\alpha_1)$ and the input surface $S(\alpha_s, \beta_s)$. That is, we solve by gradient descent on a set of surface parameters $\{(\alpha_s, \beta_s)\}$ for:

$$V(\alpha_1, \beta, 0) = \{S(\alpha_s, \beta_s) | \bigl(S(\alpha_s, \beta_s) - V(\alpha_1, \beta, \pi)\bigr) \cdot f'(\alpha_1) = 0\} \quad (12)$$

After looping through Equations (6)-(12) for all $\alpha \in [0, \pi]$, we obtain a set of P sweeping planes with nested level contours on each plane. P will increase if Δs decreases. From the nested contours on each plane, we sample K_3 number of contours with uniform separation. The first contour on each plane must be the boundary and the last one must be the tract axis. Each level contour is also equally sampled, having $2K_2$ number of points, with the first point defined as the closest point to the previous contour. The first boundary point is defined to be the closest point to the first boundary point on the previous plane. In order to measure the distance of points between two sweeping planes, we apply a rigid transformation to align their tract centers and plane orientations. At the end, we have $P \times 2K_2 \times K_3$ number of ordered points of $V(\alpha, \beta, \gamma)$. We then project our sampling points $V(\alpha, \beta, \gamma)$ into Fourier space defined by (3) and take derivatives to obtain the orientation vectors.

Table 1. Reconstruction errors for the synthetic tract orientations. Example artificial contours shown on the right. Errors are the angles in degrees between the reconstructed tangents and ground truth orientations. Four methods compared: (1) our method, (2) fit input contours to volumetric basis functions without sweeping, (3) linearly interpolate input contours and use central differences to compute tangents, and (4) forward difference for tangents. The last three methods do not depend on orientation data, and thus are not affected by orientation noise.

Method \ Error (degree)	Basis fcn w sweep	Basis fcn w/o sweep	Mesh & Central diff.	Mesh & Forward diff.
Min	0.083-0.170	0.036-0.041	0.017-0.030	0.029-0.118
(w noise)	0.0234-0.15			
Max	5.61-14.0	31.8-37.9	20.4-63.5	26.0-89.5
(w noise)	11.98-15.55			
Mean	2.62-2.96	3.52-3.97	3.06-3.47	2.97-3.57
(w noise)	2.93-4.23			
Variance	1.50-1.95	3.37-5.49	3.39-5.59	3.72-8.04
(w noise)	1.93-2.84			

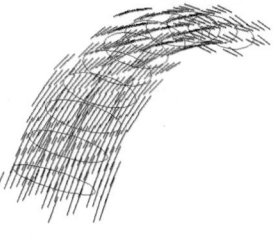

4 Experimental Results

As a validation, we synthesize a tract with orientations by sampling the tangents of a portion of a parametric conical spiral [20]. $K_1 = 10$ is the number of input contours. $K_2 = 41$ and $K_3 = 6$ are user-defined. K_1 and K_2 are the same in $S(\alpha_s, \beta_s)$ so that $V(\alpha, \beta, \gamma)$ reconstructs $S(\alpha_s, \beta_s)$ with very small numerical errors. Table 1 compares results on a synthetic image. Input contours are obtained from numerical intersections of vertical planes and the spirals at different locations. The table shows the range of results from 5 sets of contours, and there are 10 contours in each set. Synthetic tensors are formed from the spiral tangents with additional gaussian noise variance from 0.01 to 0.2. With orientation noise variance below 0.1, the basis function approach with sweeping performs the best in terms of average and maximum error as well as error variance. Using basis functions has a smoothing effect which slightly increases the minimum error. However, finite differences are sensitive to individual inaccurate input contours. When orientation data becomes unreliable, the average error of the first method will be similar to the finite difference schemes; however, it is still better in terms of maximum error and error variance. We also applied this method to a set of 18 normal human MR-DTI images with manually traced cingula. Fig. 3 shows our reconstructed orientations of the cingulum tract from real DTI data and visually compares to the original main diffusion direction. Our process filtered out unaligned diffusion vectors, mostly near the tract boundary, which are likely due to partial volume effects or were corrupted by noise. Additional reconstructed surfaces and orientations are given in Fig. 4. Our method does not change the input surface $S(\alpha_s, \beta_s)$, but modifies its parameterization to become $V(\alpha, \beta, 0)$.

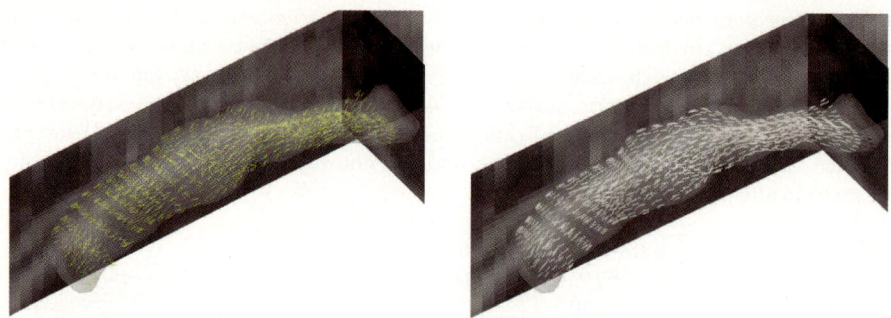

Fig. 3. Unaligned orientations (lines in the left figure) in a cingulum tract from DTI data and the reconstructed shape (transparent gray volume) and orientations (lines in the right figure)

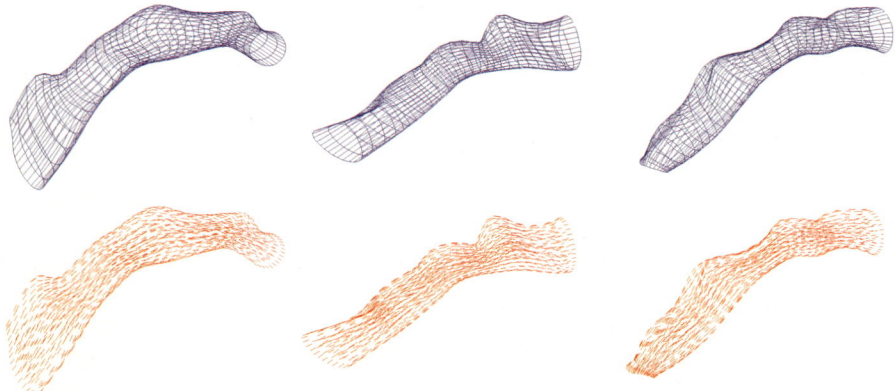

Fig. 4. Examples of reconstructed tract surfaces $V(\alpha, \beta, 0)$ (top row) and the corresponding orientations $\frac{\partial}{\partial \alpha} V(\alpha, \beta, \gamma)$ (bottom row)

5 Conclusion

We demonstrated a technique to parameterize tracts with boundary and volumetric orientations. Using volumetric basis functions makes the computation of the derivative simple, flexible and precise, which is important for brain tractography [18] based on a prior model derived from these training shapes. Future work includes improving the manual tract surface $S(\alpha_s, \beta_s)$ by simultaneously sweeping the FA data.

References

1. Chan, T., Zhu, W.: Level set based shape prior segmentation. In: IEEE Computer Society Conference on Computer Vision and Pattern Recognition (CVPR), vol. 2, pp. 1164–1170 (2005)
2. Cootes, T.F., Edwards, G.J., Taylor, C.J.: Active appearance models. IEEE Transactions on Pattern Analysis and Machine Intelligence 23(6), 681–685 (2001)

3. Cootes, T.F., Taylor, C.J., Cooper, D.H., Graham, J.: Active shape models-their training and application. Computer Vision and Image Understanding 61(1), 38–59 (1995)
4. Huang, X., Metaxas, D.N.: Metamorphs: Deformable shape and appearance models. IEEE Transactions on Pattern Analysis and Machine Intelligence 30(8), 1444–1459 (2008)
5. Leventon, M.E., Grimson, W.E.L., Faugeras, O.: Statistical shape influence in geodesic active contours. In: IEEE Conference on Computer Vision and Pattern Recognition, Proceedings, vol. 1, pp. 316–323 (2000)
6. Staib, L.H., Duncan, J.S.: Model-based deformable surface finding for medical images. IEEE Transactions on Medical Imaging 15(5), 720–731 (1996)
7. Tsai, A., Yezzi, A., Wells, W., Tempany, C., Tucker, D., Fan, A., Grimson, W.E., Willsky, A.: A shape-based approach to the segmentation of medical imagery using level sets. IEEE Transactions on Medical Imaging 22(2), 137–154 (2003)
8. Wang, Y., Staib, L.: Boundary finding with prior shape and smoothness models. IEEE Transactions on Pattern Analysis and Machine Intelligence 22(7), 738–743 (2000)
9. Basser, P.J., Jones, D.K.: Diffusion-tensor MRI: theory, experimental design and data analysis - a technical review. NMR Biomed. 15(7-8), 456–467 (2002)
10. Jellison, B.J., Field, A.S., Medow, J., Lazar, M., Salamat, S.M., Alexander, A.L.: Diffusion tensor imaging of cerebral white matter: A pictorial review of physics, fiber tract anatomy, and tumor imaging patterns. AJNR Am. J. Neuroradiol. 25(3), 356–369 (2004)
11. Mori, S., van Zijl, P.C.: Fiber tracking: principles and strategies - a technical review. NMR Biomed. 15(7-8), 468–480 (2002)
12. O'Donnell, L., Westin, C.L.: White matter tract clustering and correspondence in populations. Med. Image Comput. Comput. Assist. Interv. MICCAI (October 2005)
13. Parker, G.J.M., Wheeler-Kingshott, C.A.M., Barker, G.J.: Estimating distributed anatomical connectivity using fast marching methods and diffusion tensor imaging. IEEE Transactions on Medical Imaging 21(5), 505–512 (2002)
14. Wakana, S., Jiang, H., Nagae-Poetscher, L.M., van Zijl, P.C., Mori, S.: Fiber tract-based atlas of human white matter anatomy. Radiology 230(1), 77–87 (2004)
15. Sun, H., Yushkevich, P., Zhang, H., Cook, P., Duda, J., Simon, T., Gee, J.: Shape-based normalization of the corpus callosum for DTI connectivity analysis. IEEE Transactions on Medical Imaging 26(9), 1166–1178 (2007)
16. Rueckert, D., Sonoda, L.I., Hayes, C., Hill, D.L., Leach, M.O., Hawkes, D.J.: Non-rigid registration using free-form deformations: application to breast mr images. IEEE Trans. Med. Imaging 18(8), 712–721 (1999)
17. Yushkevich, P., Zhang, H., Gee, J.: Continuous medial representation for anatomical structures. IEEE Trans. on Medical Imaging 25(12), 1547–1564 (2006)
18. Jackowski, M., Kao, C.Y., Qiu, M., Constable, T.R., Staib, L.H.: White matter tractography by anisotropic wavefront evolution and diffusion tensor imaging. Medical Image Analysis 9(5), 427–440 (2005)
19. Osher, S., Sethian, J.A.: Fronts propagating with curvature-dependent speed: Algorithms based on hamilton-jacobi formulations. J. of Comp. Physics 79, 12–49 (1988)
20. von Seggern, D.H.: CRC Standard Curves and Surfaces: A Mathematica Notebook. CRC Press, Boca Raton

A Generic Probabilistic Active Shape Model for Organ Segmentation

Andreas Wimmer[1,2], Grzegorz Soza[2], and Joachim Hornegger[1]

[1] Chair of Pattern Recognition, Department of Computer Science,
Friedrich-Alexander University Erlangen-Nuremberg
andreas.wimmer@informatik.uni-erlangen.de
[2] Siemens Healthcare Sector, Computed Tomography, Forchheim, Germany

Abstract. Probabilistic models are extensively used in medical image segmentation. Most of them employ parametric representations of densities and make idealizing assumptions, e.g. normal distribution of data. Often, such assumptions are inadequate and limit a broader application. We propose here a novel probabilistic active shape model for organ segmentation, which is entirely built upon non-parametric density estimates. In particular, a nearest neighbor boundary appearance model is complemented by a cascade of boosted classifiers for region information and combined with a shape model based on Parzen density estimation. Image and shape terms are integrated into a single level set equation. Our approach has been evaluated for 3-D liver segmentation using a public data base originating from a competition (http://sliver07.org). With an average surface distance of 1.0 mm and an average volume overlap error of 6.5 %, it outperforms other automatic methods and provides accuracy close to interactive ones. Since no adaptions specific to liver segmentation have been made, our probabilistic active shape model can be applied to other segmentation tasks easily.

1 Introduction

Probabilistic modeling plays an important role in medical image segmentation. When dealing with images of complex anatomical structures, often impaired with noise or low contrast, it is convincing to search for the most likely boundary, region, or shape. In a related fashion, active shape models [1,2] use statistical knowledge about an object's shape and local gray level appearance for segmentation, traditionally assuming normal distribution of both. Deciding for a certain parametric distribution may be necessary because the model is not manageable without, or because little knowledge is available about the true nature of data. Often, a model works under the given assumptions for a specific problem, but a generalization to other fields of application is not possible.

In order to overcome such limitations, we propose a novel active shape model, which is entirely built upon non-parametric estimates of probabilities. In particular, we use a nearest neighbor appearance model of the organ boundary, a cascade of boosted classifiers to detect the object region, and Parzen density estimation to deduce a shape model. No assumptions about the underlying distribution of data are made, and no specific training, such as establishing correspondences between landmark points, is required. All image and shape terms are combined in a single equation within the level set framework [3]. Employing an implicit shape representation moreover avoids a parameterization of the target shape. While the proposed model is highly generic, it can nevertheless compete with or even outperform methods tailored to a specific problem, which is demonstrated for liver segmentation using a public data base [4].

The remainder of this paper is organized as follows. In the next section, related work is reviewed. The proposed boundary and region models are described in Sect. 3, along with the shape model. In Sect. 4, the application of the active shape model to liver segmentation is detailed, and evaluation results are presented. The paper concludes with a discussion of the obtained results and directions for further research.

2 Related Work

At the 2007 MICCAI conference, a competition for liver segmentation was held at a conference workshop [4,5]. The majority of automatic methods ranking in the highest quantile incorporated shape knowledge. They were mostly based on active shape models (ASM) [1], such as the approach proposed in [6], where a heuristic intensity model is used for incorporating image information.

In order to increase flexibility, a recursive subdivision of the liver shape into smaller patches was proposed in [7]. Individual models are trained, and during segmentation, an adhesiveness constraint ensures that patches overlap smoothly.

The ASM principle has been widely extended in [8] with marginal space learning and steerable features for rapidly detecting the liver pose and initializing the first modes of the shape model. Segmentation is then performed in a hierarchical manner from coarse to fine scales, with image information being inferred from a probabilistic boosting tree.

3 Probabilistic Active Shape Model

We segment an organ by evolving an active surface, which is implicitly described through the zero level set of a level set function $\phi(\boldsymbol{x})$, with $\boldsymbol{x} \in \mathbb{R}^3$ [3]. In contrast to explicit shape representations, e.g. through meshes, the implicit representation is parameter free and consequently does not depend on the target shape. Furthermore, when deforming the surface through the level set framework, self intersections do not pose a problem.

A popular edge based level set segmentation method is geodesic active contours [9], which is associated with the following partial differential equation to track the evolving boundary over time.

$$\frac{\partial}{\partial t}\phi = g\,|\nabla\phi|\,\mathrm{div}\left(\frac{\nabla\phi}{|\nabla\phi|}\right) + \nabla g \cdot \nabla\phi \qquad (1)$$

The first term accounts for the smoothness of the boundary, while the second part constitutes an advection term. The stopping function g is the reciprocal of an edge detector, which in turn depends on the image I. A common choice for g is $1/\left(1+|\nabla I|^2\right)$.

3.1 Boundary Model

In most cases, a simple edge detector based on the image gradient is not sufficient to deal with poorly discriminable tissues or noise. In contrast, the information contained in an intensity profile sampled at the organ boundary is much richer and more specific. An appearance model may be obtained by sampling profile vectors perpendicular to the boundary in a training stage. Traditionally [2], profiles were assumed to be normally distributed. In that case, the appearance model is given by the mean vector and covariance matrix. However, a normal distribution of profiles often is not present. In Fig. 1(a), profiles sampled from the liver boundary in computed tomography (CT) images are shown. The mean vector is not characteristic for the sample set.

As a non-parametric alternative, we instead build a nearest neighbor appearance model of the organ boundary. This approach, originally proposed in [10], allows capturing arbitrary distributions of profile vectors. During the training stage, additional false profiles are sampled off the true organ boundary. In order to evaluate the boundary probability, the k nearest neighbors found in the training set are determined using the L_2 norm. Amongst these, the number of true boundary profiles divided by k yields the desired probability. How to incorporate this procedure into a level set evolution has been described in [11]. For each point which is part of the narrow band around the active surface, an intensity profile is sampled. The profile orientation is given by the gradient of the level set function $\nabla \phi$, which is collinear to the normal. The boundary probability is then determined by finding the nearest neighbors in the training set and calculating the ratio mentioned before. The result is a probability image, from which a stopping function is calculated, as described for (1).

3.2 Region Model

Since the capture range of the boundary model is limited, an inaccurate initialization can result in slow convergence to the targeted boundary. In the worst case, the algorithm will stop at a local extremum. We therefore complement the boundary model with a region model, which leads to a global optimization.

Organs may have inhomogeneous intensities and contain tumors and vessels filled with contrast agent. Hence, a region model should be able to represent complex intensity distributions. Since distributions of different tissues may overlap, it is also advantageous to incorporate contextual information. As an example, high intensity values may be observed for voxels within vessels and for voxels within bones. While in the former case, the voxel shall be included in the segmentation if surrounded by organ tissue, in the latter case it shall be excluded.

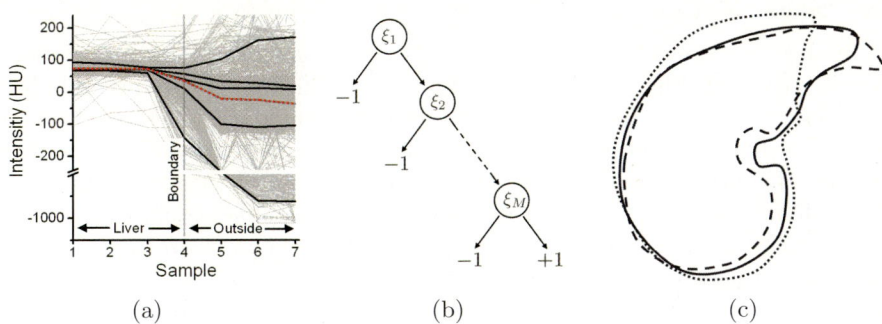

Fig. 1. (a) Profiles sampled from the liver boundary in CT images. The intensity scale is given in Hounsfield units (HU). Characteristic modes are highlighted (solid lines). The mean profile (dotted line) is not representative. (b) Cascade of boosted classifiers. At each stage ξ_i, a sample is either rejected (-1) or passed on to the next stage. Samples accepted at the final stage ($+1$) are considered to be part of the organ. (c) Principle of the kernel density shape model depicted for the 2-D case. Evolving active contour (solid line) and reference shapes (dashed lines) are rigidly aligned. The active contour is moved towards each reference shape, weighted according to their similarity.

How to define meaningful features and train a classifier to meet these requirements is not evident in advance. We therefore build a cascade χ of M boosted classifiers, as illustrated in Fig. 1(b). At each stage $i = 1, 2, \ldots, M$, a strong classifier ξ_i either rejects a sample or passes it on to the next stage. Only when the sample is accepted at the final stage, it is considered to be part of the organ. A strong classifier ξ_i is a weighted combination of weak classifiers and is determined by the AdaBoost [12] algorithm. Classification and regression trees (CART) [13] are used here as weak classifiers in order to further increase flexibility and handle complex region statistics. Within a CART, the decision which branch to take is based on Haar-like features [14]. They resolve to simple intensity differences, which are defined in large combinatorial numbers for a neighborhood around the sample voxel. Thereby, contextual information is integrated in the region model. While training a cascade of boosted classifiers may take several days, the application is extremely fast through the use of integral images. Further details can be found in [14]. Our implementation is based on OpenCV[1].

The result $\chi(\boldsymbol{x})$ of the cascade is $+1$, if the sample voxel $\boldsymbol{x}$ is accepted and -1, if it is rejected. This region information is incorporated as a dilatation or erosion of the surface into the level set equation (1), which leads to

$$\frac{\partial}{\partial t}\phi = g\left|\nabla\phi\right|\operatorname{div}\left(\frac{\nabla\phi}{\left|\nabla\phi\right|}\right) + \nabla g \cdot \nabla\phi + \chi g\left|\nabla\phi\right|. \tag{2}$$

---

[1] http://opencvlibrary.sourceforge.net

3.3 Shape Model

We further increase the robustness of the proposed active surface by incorporating a shape model. Shape knowledge is highly valuable in regions with ambiguous or missing image information. For example, the boundaries between liver and stomach or liver and muscle tissue may be virtually non-existent, depending on the level of contrast enhancement. When the surface is about to leak into other tissue, shape knowledge allows constraining such an unlikely deformation.

Most ASMs assume a normal distribution of shapes. The according shape space captured by the model is spanned by the mean shape and a linear combination of Eigen modes, which are obtained through principal component analysis performed on a training set [1]. We pursue the more generic non-parametric approach of [15], which is to determine the probability of observing a shape through Parzen density estimation [16]. The employed distance metric for shapes represented through level set functions is

$$\Delta(\phi_1, \phi_2) = \int_x (H(\phi_1) - H(\phi_2))^2 \, d\boldsymbol{x}. \quad (3)$$

$H(.)$ denotes the Heaviside function, which is 1 if the argument is non-negative and 0 otherwise. When evaluating the distance, both shapes have to be aligned. This is achieved intrinsically by normalizing the center of gravity, scaling, and principal axes of both shapes, i.e. of $H(\phi_1)$ and $H(\phi_2)$.

Given a set of N reference shapes $\{\phi_i\}_{i=1}^N$, a Parzen estimate of the probability of a shape ϕ is given by

$$P(\phi) \propto \frac{1}{N} \sum_{i=1}^{N} K_\sigma(\Delta(\phi, \phi_i)), \quad (4)$$

where K_σ is a Gaussian kernel, whose standard deviation σ is chosen according to the nearest neighbor distances: $\sigma^2 = \frac{1}{N} \sum_{i=1}^{N} \min_{j \neq i} \Delta^2(\phi_i, \phi_j)$. By optimizing this shape probability with respect to ϕ, a constraint is derived for the level set equation which evolves the surface towards similar shapes. The principle is illustrated in Fig. 1(c). Instead of maximizing (4), a minimization problem is obtained by taking the negative logarithm. Calculating the functional derivative of $-\log P(\phi)$ with respect to ϕ leads to a shape constraint term, which extends the active surface of (2) to a probabilistic active shape model.

$$\frac{\partial}{\partial t}\phi = g|\nabla\phi| \operatorname{div}\left(\frac{\nabla\phi}{|\nabla\phi|}\right) + \nabla g \cdot \nabla\phi + \chi g |\nabla\phi| + \frac{\sum_{i=1}^{N} K_\sigma(\Delta(\phi, \phi_i)) \frac{\partial}{\partial \phi} \Delta^2(\phi, \phi_i)}{2\sigma^2 \sum_{i=1}^{N} K_\sigma(\Delta(\phi, \phi_i))} \quad (5)$$

We refer to [15] for further details on the derivation of the shape constraint.

4 Evaluation

The proposed algorithm has been evaluated for liver segmentation from CT scans. Both training and test images were taken from a public data base, which had been assembled for a segmentation competition held at a workshop of the 2007 MICCAI conference [4,5]. Since ground truth segmentations are not provided for test images and the evaluation is conducted by the organizers, results are meaningful and comparable. The 20 training and 10 test images have a slice resolution of 512 × 512 voxel and 64 to 502 slices. Intra slice spacing varies between 0.56 mm × 0.56 mm and 0.86 mm × 0.86 mm, inter slice spacing varies between 0.7 mm and 5 mm. The data base comprises both normal and abnormal liver shapes with tumors and varying levels of contrast enhancement.

The boundary appearance model was built by sampling intensity profiles of length 7 with 1 mm spacing. In addition to true boundary profiles, negative examples were obtained with offsets of ±1 mm and ±3 mm. During segmentation, the $k = 10$ nearest neighbors were used to estimate the boundary probabilities. A cascade with $M = 5$ stages was trained for the region model. With the inter slice spacing being large compared to the intra slice spacing, we decided for 2−D Haar-like features. In order to train with a large context while at the same time preventing the classifier from over fitting, we conducted training and application for slices down sampled to a resolution of 128 × 128 voxel. Using a window of 12 × 12 voxel, the Haar feature pool consisted of about 16000 features. In contrast to PCA based approaches, no training of the shape model is required here.

For segmentation, the initial pose of the shape model was determined by extracting the largest object detected by the region model. In order to accelerate convergence, segmentation was performed in a multi-scale manner, starting with an image down sampled by a factor of 4. The whole process ran without user interaction and took about 3 min. per image on a 3 GHz CPU.

The obtained segmentation results were submitted to the organizers of the competition and evaluated with respect to volume overlap and difference as

Table 1. Results of the evaluation metrics and scores for all test cases. The maximum score, corresponding to a segmentation identical with the reference, would be 100. While interactive systems have reached scores in the range of 73 to 82, the majority of automatic systems falls within the range of 52 to 69. See http://sliver07.org for all results and [4,5] for details on the metrics and the score scale.

Case	Ovrl. Error [%]	Score	Vol. Diff. [%]	Score	Avg. Dist. [mm]	Score	RMS Dist. [mm]	Score	Max. Dist. [mm]	Score	Total Score
1	6.41	74.98	1.16	93.82	1.02	74.51	1.99	72.32	18.61	75.51	78.23
2	6.41	74.95	-0.64	96.59	0.98	75.62	2.31	67.93	22.29	70.68	77.15
3	5.10	80.08	0.54	97.11	1.00	75.10	1.83	74.65	15.82	79.19	81.23
4	7.27	71.62	4.31	77.09	1.20	70.05	2.49	65.47	28.99	61.86	69.22
5	5.61	78.10	1.86	90.13	0.96	76.04	2.12	70.55	21.91	71.17	77.20
6	7.99	68.77	-3.02	83.94	1.27	68.25	2.37	67.14	18.28	75.95	72.81
7	5.04	80.33	2.79	85.17	0.73	81.71	1.42	80.25	13.00	82.89	82.07
8	7.06	72.42	3.45	81.65	1.18	70.59	2.17	69.90	14.16	81.37	75.19
9	6.79	73.49	3.85	79.55	0.84	78.97	1.47	79.64	16.01	78.94	78.12
10	7.04	72.52	-3.92	79.17	1.01	74.76	1.80	75.01	14.15	81.38	76.57
Avg.	6.47	74.72	2.55	86.42	1.02	74.56	2.00	72.29	18.32	75.89	76.78

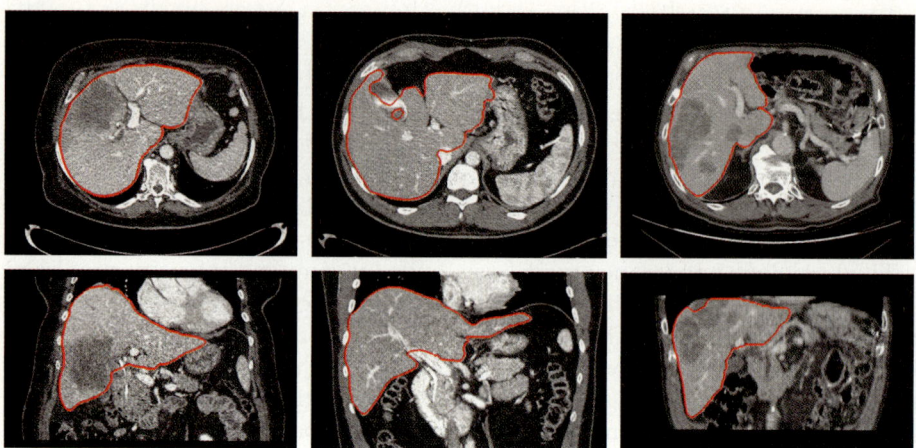

Fig. 2. From left to right, segmentation results for cases 3, 6, and 10 in transversal (top) and coronal (bottom) views. The large tumor in case 3 and the majority of tumors in case 10 were correctly included in the segmentation. For case 6, the shape model was too restrictive in the region of the gall bladder, which therefore was not completely excluded. What appears as a circle in the transversal view is actually a bulge in 3-D.

well as symmetric average, root mean squared, and maximum surface distance. Results are listed in Table 1 and displayed in Fig. 2 for several data sets.

5 Discussion and Conclusion

We have presented a novel probabilistic active shape model for organ segmentation, which combines boundary, region, and shape information in a single level set equation. Non-parametric estimates are used for all involved densities, which leads to a generic approach that can be applied to various segmentation tasks.

The proposed algorithm has been evaluated for liver segmentation from CT images using a public data base (cf. Sect. 4). As shown in Table 1, our method achieved constantly high scores for all test cases. On average, the surface distance is 1.0 mm and the overlap error is 6.5 %, which is close to interactive methods [4,5] and meets clinical requirements.

Failure to exclude the portal vein resulted in a higher overlap error and surface distance in case 4. For some cases where heart and liver share similar levels of contrast enhancement, the region term was not able to discriminate between both of them, leading to slight over segmentation indicated by positive volume differences in Table 1.

The advantages of our non-parametric approach are most evident when dealing with images that differ from the ordinary. For example, case 6 was accurately segmented except for a small part of the gall bladder, although the liver is unlike most training shapes. In contrast, ASM approaches perform considerably worse for organs significantly different from the mean, since the underlying PCA inherently assumes a normal distribution of shapes. This can be observed also for the top ranking method of the competition [6], even though it was trained with an extensive data base of 112 images [5], much more than the 20 images we used.

For the future, we are confident that results can be further improved by increasing the training set, from which all three terms will benefit. In addition, we plan to apply the proposed approach to the segmentation of other structures. Preliminary results show a high accuracy also for the segmentation of the nucleus caudate. No changes to the core system were made, which emphasizes the broad applicability of our method.

References

1. Cootes, T.F., Taylor, C.J., Cooper, D.H., Graham, J.: Active shape models – their training and application. CVIU 61(1), 38–59 (1995)
2. Cootes, T.F., Taylor, C.J.: Statistical models of appearance for medical image analysis and computer vision. In: SPIE Medical Imaging, vol. 4322, pp. 236–248 (2001)
3. Sethian, J.A.: Level Set Methods and Fast Marching Methods, 2nd edn. Cambridge University Press, New York (1999)
4. Heimann, T., Styner, M., van Ginneken, B.: 3D Segmentation in the Clinic – A Grand Challenge. In: MICCAI Workshop Proceedings (2007)
5. Heimann, T., van Ginneken, B., Styner, M., et al.: Comparison and evaluation of methods for liver segmentation from CT datasets. In: IEEE TMI (2009)
6. Kainmüller, D., Lange, T., Lamecker, H.: Shape constrained automatic segmentation of the liver based on a heuristic intensity model. In: 3D Segmentation in the Clinic – A Grand Challenge, pp. 109–116 (2007)
7. Okada, T., Shimada, R., Sato, Y., Hori, M., Yokota, K., Nakamoto, M., et al.: Automated segmentation of the liver from 3D CT images using probabilistic atlas and multi-level statistical shape model. In: Ayache, N., Ourselin, S., Maeder, A. (eds.) MICCAI 2007, Part I. LNCS, vol. 4791, pp. 86–93. Springer, Heidelberg (2007)
8. Ling, H., Zhou, S.K., Zheng, Y., Georgescu, B., Suehling, M., Comaniciu, D.: Hierarchical, learning-based automatic liver segmentation. In: CVPR (2008)
9. Caselles, V., Kimmel, R., Sapiro, G.: Geodesic active contours. International Journal of Computer Vision 22(1), 61–79 (1997)
10. van Ginnecken, B., Frangi, A.F., Staal, J.J., ter Haar Romeny, B.M., Viergever, M.A.: Active shape model segmentation with optimal features. IEEE Transactions on Medical Imaging 21(8), 924–933 (2002)
11. Wimmer, A., Soza, G., Hornegger, J.: Implicit active shape model employing boundary classifier. In: ICPR (2008)
12. Freund, Y., Schapire, R.E.: A decision-theoretic generalization of on-line learning and an application to boosting. JCSS 55(1), 119–139 (1997)
13. Breiman, L., Friedman, J.H., Olshen, R.A., Stone, C.J.: Classification and Regression Trees. Chapman & Hall, New York (1984)
14. Viola, P., Jones, M.: Robust real-time face detection. International Journal of Computer Vision 57(2), 137–154 (2004)
15. Cremers, D., Osher, S.J., Soatto, S.: Kernel density estimation and intrinsic alignment for shape priors in level set segmentation. IJCV 69(3), 335–351 (2006)
16. Parzen, E.: On the estimation of a probability density function and the mode. Annals of Mathematical Statistics 33, 1065–1076 (1962)

Organ Segmentation with Level Sets Using Local Shape and Appearance Priors

Timo Kohlberger[1], M. Gökhan Uzunbaş[1], Christopher Alvino[1], Timor Kadir[2], Daniel O. Slosman[3], and Gareth Funka-Lea[1]

[1] Siemens Corporate Research, Imaging and Visualization Dept., Princeton, USA
[2] Siemens Healthcare Molecular Imaging, Oxford, UK
[3] Clinic Generale-Beaulieu, Geneva, Switzerland

Abstract. Organ segmentation is a challenging problem on which recent progress has been made by incorporation of local image statistics that model the heterogeneity of structures outside of an organ of interest. However, most of these methods rely on landmark based segmentation, which has certain drawbacks. We propose to perform organ segmentation with a novel level set algorithm that incorporates local statistics via a highly efficient point tracking mechanism. Specifically, we compile statistics on these tracked points to allow for a local intensity profile outside of the contour and to allow for a local surface area penalty, which allows us to capture fine detail where it is expected. The local intensity and curvature models are learned through landmarks automatically embedded on the surface of the training shapes. We use Parzen windows to model the internal organ intensities as one distribution since this is sufficient for most organs. In addition, since the method is based on level sets, we are able to naturally take advantage of recent work on global shape regularization. We show state-of-the-art results on the challenging problems of liver and kidney segmentation.

1 Introduction

Level set methods have many strengths that make them suitable for general organ segmentation, which include the ability to naturally represent complex shapes non-parametrically, and the ability to incorporate powerful shape models [4,10,15,5]. Until recently, most level set-based segmentation methods have focused on global data likelihood models [16] and global priors on contours such as surface area penalty [9]. Unfortunately, such global models do not fully exploit the fact that surrounding image intensities and local organ curvatures vary in a predictably local fashion, e.g., in the segmentation of livers in computed tomography (CT) images in which the outside intensities and contour curvatures are naturally heterogeneous.

Thus many mechanisms to allow for local evolution have been introduced both in the computer vision literature [13], and in the medical imaging literature [11,6,12]. Some methods allow for local intensity models in a level set framework, but not in a way that allows position dependent knowledge to be accounted for [13]. Other methods use landmarks to represent the organ boundary [8,6,12,11], and allow incorporation of shape through active shape models [3]. While these methods have achieved significant progress on difficult organ segmentation problems such as the liver, no completely satisfactory solution exists due to high variability in anatomical shape, from disease, and in acquisition protocol. Additionally, segmenting only within the space of shapes allowable by ASM's is a limiting factor since ASM's tend to naturally produce shapes that smooth out naturally high curvature structures. Furthermore, determining segmentation boundaries in between points requires, as a final step, choosing some method of interpolating between landmarks [11].

In this paper, we introduce a novel efficient point tracking mechanism into standard level set evolution, which allows us to formulate the problem as a maximum a posteriori estimation problem with both a local likelihood model for the data term as well as a local prior model for the surface area penalty term. In doing this, we extend the work of [14], where point tracking is used to define correspondence during level set evolution, by simplifying the tracking for greater efficiency at the cost of maintaining an approximate correspondence that is still sufficient for segmentation. In addition, we show how introducing shape-guidance into this level set framework is natural and we can take advantage of recent work on shape-guided level set methods (see [5] and references therein.) We validate the efficacy of this point tracking method on complex organ segmentation problems such as liver and kidney segmentation, while also showing that it is very efficient. We show that the method produces segmentations with state of the art overlap and surface error statistics, as made popular in the MICCAI 2007 Liver challenge.

2 Key Point Tracking on Evolving Zero Level Sets

To facilitate the application of local prior statistics and constraints it is necessary to track explicit points on the evolving surface. This is done as follows.

Consider a set of discrete points $\{x_i(t)\}_{i=1,\ldots,N}$ defined on the initial zero level set of a signed distance function $\phi(\mathbf{x}, t), \mathbf{x} \in \Omega \subset \mathbb{R}^3$ at $t = 0$. As explained in [14] and the references therein, those can be tracked along with the evolution of the zero level set by mapping them along its outer normal $\mathbf{n}(\mathbf{x}_i(t), t) = -\nabla \phi(\mathbf{x}_i(t), t) / |\nabla \phi(\mathbf{x}_i(t), t)|$ by the amount of the level set speed $\Delta\phi(\cdot, t+1)$:

$$\mathbf{x}_i(t+1) \leftarrow \mathbf{x}_i(t) + \Delta\phi(\mathbf{x}_i(t), t+1)\,\mathbf{n}(\mathbf{x}_i(t), t). \tag{1}$$

This is to be carried out for each level set update, see Fig. 1 for an example.

However, in the case of a narrow-band implementation, especially when the speed of the level set is high, the update of the key point $\mathbf{x}_i(t)$ might locate the new position $\mathbf{x}_i(t+1)$ such that it lies outside of the band of $\phi(\cdot, t+1)$. In order to handle such cases, we linearly search along the normal of $\phi(\cdot, t)$ to a pre-defined extent, i.e. along the line $\mathbf{x}_i(t) + \tau\,\mathbf{n_0}(\mathbf{x}_i(t), t)$, with $\tau > 0$. (We found sampling τ at intervals of one voxel length to be a reasonable value.) By this we bring down the fraction of "lost" key points typically below 0.1%.

Furthermore, due to numerical inaccuracies in the update scheme (1), the key points may deviate from the zero levelset after some iterations. For such points, we apply an additional correction scheme:

$$\mathbf{x}_i(t) \leftarrow \mathbf{x}_i(t) + \phi(\mathbf{x}_i(t), t)\, \mathbf{n_0}(\mathbf{x}_i(t), t), \tag{2}$$

which guarantees that the updated key points are always on the zero level.

In the following, we use the described algorithm to establish shape correspondences between the initial shape $\phi(\cdot, 0)$, which we will refer to as reference shape, and the segmenting shape $\phi(\cdot, t)$. Obviously, because of neglecting the tangential evolution of similarity features, such a correspondence is only approximate, but will be sufficient in the following if the reference and the target shape are not too dissimilar and are roughly rigidly aligned. Compared to Poisson-equation-based methods, cf. [14], this method has the advantage of being computationally much more efficient. For example, tracking 3126 key points in the case shown in Fig. 1 along with a narrow-band consisting of 35000 voxels added only 2.3% to the average computation time of a level set update.

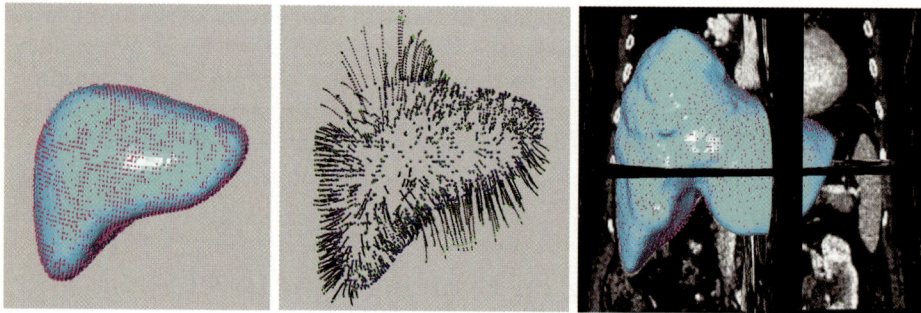

Fig. 1. (a) Example of initial key points on an initial zero level being rigidly aligned to the organ to segment. (b) Evolution of each key point along the normals of the zero level sets while carrying out a standard data-driven segmentation iteration. (c) Result after 200 level set/key point tracking iterations. Given a sufficient similarity of the initial shape as well as an initial alignment, tracking points along the normal at each iteration is sufficient to retrieve an approximate shape correspondence.

3 Levelset Segmentation Driven by Local Feature Models

Given a set of explicit points that have correspondences to the initial shape, we can assign locally measured features of different level set evolutions to one common reference shape. Such measurements from the segmentation of a set of training samples are accumulated on the reference shape to deduce localized feature models and it is these models which then are introduced as priors in the segmentation approach.

3.1 Local Intensity Statistics

To build a localized intensity prior, we carried out a standard data-driven segmentation approach [2] on expert-generated binary annotation masks of the intended organs, while employing the scheme presented in section 2 to track the key points in parallel. Thereby the initial/reference shape was a typical shape of the organ and rigidly aligned to each of those masks.

Once the zero level set had converged at or near the binary edge, at each key point, we sampled the local intensity outside the contour from the intensity volume being aligned with the annotation mask. Specifically, we convolved with small Gaussian windows which were centered at each point separately for inside and outside voxels, which in the latter case reads:

$$I_{j,\rho}^{out}(\mathbf{x}_i) = \frac{\int_{\Omega_i} g_\rho(\mathbf{x}_i - \mathbf{y}) \left(1 - H(\phi_i(\mathbf{y}))\right) I_j(\mathbf{y}) \, d\mathbf{y}}{\int_{\Omega_i} g_\rho(\mathbf{x}_i - \mathbf{y}) \left(1 - H(\phi_i(\mathbf{y}))\right) d\mathbf{y}} \quad (3)$$

with $g_\rho(\mathbf{x}) = \exp(-\mathbf{x}^\top \mathbf{x}/(2\rho^2))$, $I_j(\mathbf{x})$ referring to the value of the intensity volume (not the segmentation mask) at $\mathbf{x}$, and H denoting the Heaviside function.

In a next step, for each key point on the reference shape, we accumulated these samples across the training cases by fitting Gaussian distributions, whose spatially dependent parameters were determined according to:

$$\mu_{out}(\mathbf{x}_i) = \frac{1}{L} \sum_{j=1}^{L} I_{j,\rho}^{out}(\mathbf{x}_i), \quad \sigma_{out}^2(\mathbf{x}_i) = \frac{1}{L-1} \sum_{j=1}^{L} \left(\mu_{out}(\mathbf{x}_i) - I_{j,\rho}^{out}(\mathbf{x}_i)\right)^2.$$

See Fig. 2(a)-(b) for an example on the liver.

Subsequently, during the course of the level set evolution, the such inferred Gaussian likelihoods are not only available at tracked key point locations, but can be interpolated to any voxel in the narrow-band. In case of a simple nearest-neighbor interpolation, the prior probability of observing an intensity $I(\mathbf{x})$ at a location $\mathbf{x}$ near or at the zero level can thus be approximated by

$$p_{out}(I(\mathbf{x})|\mathbf{x}) := \frac{1}{\sqrt{2\pi\sigma_{out}^2(\mathbf{x}_{l(x)})}} \exp\left(-\frac{(I(\mathbf{x}) - \mu_{out}(\mathbf{x}_{l(x)}))^2}{2\sigma_{out}^2(\mathbf{x}_{l(x)})}\right), \quad (4)$$

with $l(x) = \arg\min_{i=1,\ldots,N} \|\mathbf{x} - \mathbf{x}_i\|_{L_2}^2$ being the closest key point with regards to the Euclidean distance. With respect to implementing the latter, we found [1] to provide a very efficient solution.

3.2 Local Mean Curvature Constraint

Local correspondences between the evolving and a reference shape not only enable spatially dependent intensity priors, but also allow for a spatially dependent weighting of feature measurements, such as the mean curvature.

Given the tracked key points at the boundaries of ground truth annotation masks, as described in the previous section, one can similarly sample local mean curvatures and average them over the set of training cases, which yields an average mean curvature for each key point (see Fig. 2(c) for an example):

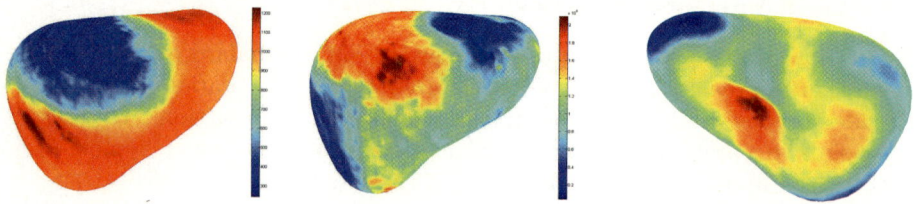

Fig. 2. Means (a) and variances (b) of the outward-bound local intensities across 100 liver shapes, which were traced back to the shown reference shape. (c) Average measured mean curvatures. Despite high shape variability, sharp correspondences are retrieved by the proposed key point tracking method, which is visible especially at the rib region in (a)+(b), and at the liver tips in (c).

$$\kappa_P(\mathbf{x}_i) = \frac{1}{L} \sum_{j=1}^{L} \operatorname{div} \frac{\nabla \phi_j(\mathbf{x}_i)}{|\nabla \phi_j(\mathbf{x}_i)|} \, . \tag{5}$$

Instead of inferring prior densities, which would involve second-order derivates of ϕ in the energy and thus numerically problematic fourth-order derivatives in the Euler-Lagrange equations, here we propose to introduce the spatially-dependent prior by modulating the weight of the area term, cf. [2], in the energy:

$$E_C(\phi) = \int_\Omega \omega_C(\mathbf{x}) \, |\nabla H(\phi)| \, d\mathbf{x}, \quad \text{with} \quad \omega_C(\mathbf{x}) = \frac{\xi}{1 + \nu \kappa_P^2(\mathbf{x})} \, , \tag{6}$$

with a parameter ν controlling the amount of weight variation and ξ denoting a global weigth.

Thus, we penalize surface area of the segmenting contour more strongly at locations when low curvatures were observed on the training contours, and viceversa for high curvatures. For example, by this the curvature term can be weak at the tip regions of a liver shape, while enforcing low curvatures everywhere at relatively straight regions. See Fig. 3 for examples on the CT liver.

4 Organ Segmentation Approach

In the following we combine the localized feature priors with established ideas in order to obtain a highly accurate, robust and generic organ segmentation approach. Thereby our objects of study are the segmentation of the liver and the right kidney in 3D CT images.

4.1 Local Models for the Liver and the Kidney

We applied the technique described in Sec. 3.1 on 100 liver and 20 right kidney ground truth segmentations, in order to estimate the local mean and variance of the intensities inside and outside the segmentation boundary. For the outside intensities, we obtained maps which clearly reflect heterogeneous intensity regions of the neighboring tissue classes, see Fig. 2(a)-(b).

By contrast, the accumulated inside measurements turned out to be very homogeneous per training case, but to vary in a range of about 150 Hounsfield units across all training cases. Both observations are in line with the fact that the tissues of both organs exhibit relatively homogeneous CT intensities, while their mean fluctuates with the concentration of contrast agent. In order to account for these effects, we chose an adaptive region-based Parzen density model, cf. e.g. [4], for the observed intensities inside the organ:

$$p_{in}(I(\mathbf{x})|\phi) := \sum_{l=I_{min}}^{I_{max}} \frac{h(l)}{H} g_\sigma(I(\mathbf{x}) - l) , \quad \text{where} \quad H = \sum_{l=I_{min}}^{I_{max}} h(l) , \quad (7)$$

with $h(I)$ denoting the histogram of observed (discrete) intensities $I \in [I_{min}, I_{max}]$.

Combining the new local intensity term for the outside and the region-based term for the inside yields the energy:

$$E_I(\phi) = -\int_\Omega \alpha H(\phi) \log p_{in}(I(\mathbf{x})|\phi) + (1-\alpha)(1-H(\phi)) \log p_{out}(I(\mathbf{x})|\mathbf{x}) \, d\mathbf{x} ,$$

while the role of the weights α and $(1-\alpha)$ are to balance those opposing forces which typically occur in slightly different value ranges.

With regards to the local curvature models, we determined the local mean curvatures as described in Sec. 3.2 for each organ. By this we obtained curvature maps which reflect the different convex and concave region of each organ, see Fig. 2(c).

4.2 Global Shape Prior and Final Approach

Although the spatially modulated curvature term imposes local constraints on the shape, in order to increase robustness of the overall segmentation approach, we also add prior information based on a *global* statistical shape model. Specifically, we follow a similar approach as recently reported in [5], where projections $\hat\phi$ of the current level set map ϕ into a linear subspace of learned shape variations are used to guide the shape evolution, by adding a term of the form $E_S(\phi) := \int_\Omega (\phi - \hat\phi)^2 d\mathbf{x}$ to the overall energy. In our experiments, we used a liver model which was built on a training set of 100 liver and 20 right kidney shapes, respectively.

Finally, the overall segmentation algorithm amounts to minimize the weighted sum of intensity-dependent E_I, the curvature-dependent E_C and the shape-prior-based energy E_S, by iteratively descending along the negative energy gradient, which is represented by the partial differential equation:

$$\frac{\partial E}{\partial \phi} = \delta_\epsilon(\phi) \left(\omega_I \Big(\alpha \log p_{in}(I|\mathbf{x}) - \beta \log p_{out}(I|\phi)\Big) + \omega_C(\mathbf{x}) \text{div} \frac{\nabla \phi}{|\nabla \phi|} + \omega_S(\phi - \hat\phi) \right).$$

Thereby, the key points $\{\mathbf{x}_i\}$ are updated according to (1) in every iteration in parallel.

In our experiments, ϕ was initialized by the reference shape of the local features models, which were manually aligned with the organ in question with regards to translation and rotation. The latter can easily be automatized by an atlas registration technique, or a Pictorial structure based approach, for example.

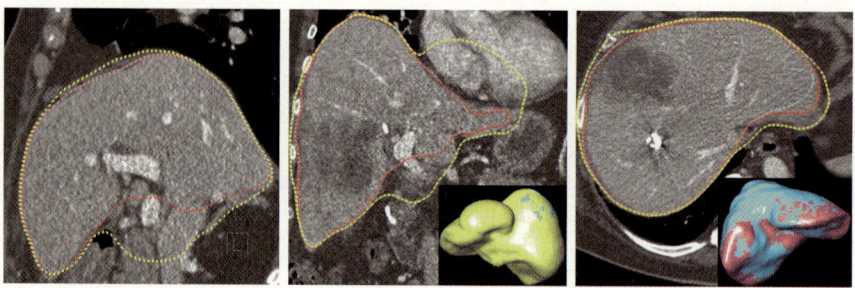

Fig. 3. Qualitative comparison of a standard approach with adaptive Parzen density estimation of the background intensities, cf. [4], and a global mean curvature force, cf. [2], (yellow) against the proposed local intensity prior (blue) and the locally modulated area penalization term in addition (red).

5 Experiments

Besides qualitative comparisons of the new local feature priors versus existing global approaches (see Fig. 3), we evaluated our algorithm on the 20 (mostly pathological) CT liver cases from the MICCAI '07 Liver challenge [7], and for the right kidney on 13 other CT cases which were annotated by own experts. None of them were included in the training sets. The reference shape of the local feature models served as initial shapes, which were manually aligned to each organ. The iteration were let run until convergence. All parameter values were the very same for all cases, except for a slightly weaker global curvature weight ξ in the kidney cases. The obtained volumetric and surface-based errors in Table 1 show that our proposed method produces state-of-the-art results, especially w.r.t. the average surface distance error of only 1.46mm/0.88mm for the liver/kidney, respectively. In addition, the fact that these results were gained without adjusting none of the involved parameter to any individual data set clearly shows the high degree of generalization and, given the strong variability of liver shapes and appearances in the test set, the high robustness of the presented algorithm.

Table 1. Volumetric and surface errors, cf. [7], as well as scores for the 20 training data sets of the Liver 2007 Challenge, as well as for 13 other CT right kidney data sets

Mean/std.dev.	Overlap. Err. [%]	Volume Diff. [%]	Avg. Surf. Dist. [mm]	RMS Surf. Dist. [mm]	Maximum Dist. [mm]	Challenge Score
20 liver cases	8.44±1.7	3.94±2.72	1.46±0.38	2.91±0.95	24.18±8.34	66.67±8.5
13 r.kidney cases	10.6 ± 1.9	4.82 ± 3.44	0.88 ± 0.23	1.92±0.52	15.31±4.51	72.8±7.3

6 Conclusion

In conclusion, we have developed a new method for general organ segmentation with level sets that incorporates local intensity statistics and local curvature by means of an efficient point-based tracking mechanism. We have shown that using level set methods enables us to incorporate recent advances in shape regularized segmentation. We have achieved results that are both qualitatively and quantitatively strong on some of the most challenging problems in organ segmentation.

In practice, we have not found point correspondence problems to effect the performance of the algorithm, however for future work we wish to investigate the effect of the tangential component of the tracked points. Proper treatment of this task would require ensuring correct correspondence, which is not explicitly guaranteed even by the method of [14].

In addition, we wish to investigate limitations of uni-modal statistical models employed by the tracked points, and whether using multi-modal or more sophisticated methods would yield improved segmentation.

Acknowledgments. We would like to thank Haibin Ling for helpful discussions and Bogdan Georgescu for providing some of the annotations we used.

References

1. Arya, S., Mount, D.M., Netanyahu, N.S., Silverman, R., Wu, A.Y.: An optimal algorithm for approximate nearest neighbor searching fixed dimensions. J. ACM 45(6), 891–923 (1998)
2. Chan, T., Vese, L.: Active contours without edges. T-IP 10(2), 266–277 (2001)
3. Cootes, T.F., Taylor, C.J., Cooper, D.H., Graham, J.: Active shape models—their training and applications. CVIU 61(1), 38–59 (1995)
4. Cremers, D., Rousson, M., Deriche, R.: A review of statistical approaches to level set segmentation: integrating color, texture, motion and shape. IJCV 72(2), 195–215 (2007)
5. Farzinfar, M., Xue, X., Teoh, E.K.: Joint parametric and non-parametric curve evolution for medical image segmentation. In: Forsyth, D., Torr, P., Zisserman, A. (eds.) ECCV 2008, Part I. LNCS, vol. 5302, pp. 167–178. Springer, Heidelberg (2008)
6. Heimann, T., Münzing, S., Meinzer, H., Wolf, I.: A shape-guided deformable model with evolutionary algorithm initialization for 3D soft tissue segmentation. In: Karssemeijer, N., Lelieveldt, B. (eds.) IPMI 2007. LNCS, vol. 4584, pp. 1–12. Springer, Heidelberg (2007)
7. Heimann, T., van Ginneken, B., Styner, M., et al.: Comparison and evaluation of methods for liver segmentation from ct datasets. In: T-MI (in press, 2009)
8. Kainmueller, D., Lange, T., Lamecker, H.: Shape constrained automatic segmentation of the liver based on a heuristic intensity model. In: Proc. MICCAI Workshop on 3D Segmentation in the Clinic: A Grand Challenge (2007)
9. Lee, J., Kim, N., Lee, H., Seo, J.B., Won, H.J., Shin, Y.M., Shin, Y.G.: Efficient liver segmentation exploiting level-set speed images with 2.5D shape propagation. In: MICCAI Workshop on 3D Segmentation in the Clinic (2007)
10. Leventon, M.E., Grimson, W.E., Faugeras, O.: Statistical shape influence in geodesic active contours. In: CVPR 2000, vol. 1, pp. 1316–1323. IEEE, Los Alamitos (2000)
11. Ling, H., Zhou, S.K., Zheng, Y., Georgescu, B., Sühling, M., Comaniciu, D.: Hierarchical, learning-based automatic liver segmentation. In: CVPR (2008)

12. Okada, T., Shimada, R., Sato, Y., Hori, M., Yokota, K., Nakamoto, M., Chen, Y., Nakamura, H., Tamura, S.: Automated segmentation of the liver from 3d ct images using probabilistic atlas and multi-level statistical shape model. In: Ayache, N., Ourselin, S., Maeder, A. (eds.) MICCAI 2007, Part I. LNCS, vol. 4791, pp. 86–93. Springer, Heidelberg (2007)
13. Piovano, J., Papadopoulo, T.: Local statistic based region segmentation with automatic scale selection. In: Forsyth, D., Torr, P., Zisserman, A. (eds.) ECCV 2008, Part II. LNCS, vol. 5303, pp. 486–499. Springer, Heidelberg (2008)
14. Pons, J.-P., Hermosillo, G., Keriven, R., Faugeras, O.: How to deal with point correspondences and tangential velocities in the level set framework. In: ICCV, pp. 894–899. IEEE, Los Alamitos (2003)
15. Tsai, A., Yezzi, A., Wells, W., Tempany, C., Tucker, D., Fan, A., Grimson, W.E., Willsky, A.: A shape-based approach to the segmentation of medical imagery using level sets. IEEE Trans. Medical Imaging 22(2), 137–154 (2003)
16. Wimmer, A., Soza, G., Hornegger, J.: Two-stage semi-automatic organ segmentation framework using radial basis functions and level sets. In: Proc. MICCAI Workshop on 3D Segmentation in the Clinic: A Grand Challenge (2007)

Liver Segmentation Using Automatically Defined Patient Specific B-Spline Surface Models

Yi Song, Andy J. Bulpitt, and Ken W. Brodlie

School of Computing, University of Leeds, UK
{scsys,A.J.Bulpitt,K.W.Brodlie}@leeds.ac.uk

Abstract. This paper presents a novel liver segmentation algorithm. This is a model-driven approach; however, unlike previous techniques which use a statistical model obtained from a training set, we initialize patient-specific models directly from their own pre-segmentation. As a result, the non-trivial problems such as landmark correspondences, model registration etc. can be avoided. Moreover, by dividing the liver region into three sub-regions, we convert the problem of building one complex shape model into constructing three much simpler models, which can be fitted independently, greatly improving the computation efficiency. A robust graph-based narrow band optimal surface fitting scheme is also presented. The proposed approach is evaluated on 35 CT images. Compared to contemporary approaches, our approach has no training requirement and requires significantly less processing time, with an RMS error of 2.44±0.53mm against manual segmentation.

1 Introduction

This work forms part of a project to develop virtual environments for training in interventional radiological procedures. It requires major abdominal structures, e.g. liver, kidney and blood vessels etc, to be segmented with particular interest in those cases where typical pathology is presented. The data for liver segmentation in this study therefore comes from patients with various pathologies and is obtained from different sources using different protocols which vary in quality and resolution and include both contrast enhanced and non-enhanced data. These diversities increase the variability of the liver data in both shape and texture.

Many techniques for liver segmentation have been proposed and implemented in recent years, see [1] for a recent review. These can be classified as texture-based and model-driven approaches. Due to the similar intensity values of some surrounding structures in CT data, approaches which are mainly based on local intensity or intensity gradient features are usually not sufficient to differentiate liver tissue. Therefore, model-based approaches have been widely explored where prior knowledge about the typical shape of a liver is used to constrain the segmentation process. Despite a number of different representations [2,3,4], many of these approaches rely on principal component analysis of corresponding landmark points marked on a training set to calculate allowed modes of variation of the shape model which may result in limited deformations impeding the exact adaptation to the structure of interest. Although techniques [5,6] have been developed to overcome this, these approaches still require the shape model to be roughly aligned and oriented to the structure of interest so that the iterative search procedure can lock onto the target.

In this paper, a novel shape model construction method is presented. Unlike previous work utilizing training datasets to capture the mean modes of shape variations, our patient-specific shape model is directly derived from each image dataset. Our previous work [7] has shown how a target region can be captured through applying morphological erosion on an edge enhanced image followed by a region growing algorithm (Fig. 1a); this pre-segmentation is then automatically embedded into a curvature-driven level set to evolve a smooth surface toward the real boundary. Due to the similarity of intensity values with surrounding structures, the liver pre-segmentation is likely to include some non-liver tissues (Fig. 1b). Hence in this paper, we construct a three-patch surface model (Fig. 1c) to eliminate such unwanted parts from the pre-segmentation. Only the most reliable information from the pre-segmentation is used to initialize our three-patch shape model, representing upper, right lobe and lower liver boundaries. A graph-based optimal surface fitting scheme is then applied independently on each patch (Fig. 1e), from which we obtain a refined pre-segmentation result having non-liver tissues removed (Fig. 1d).

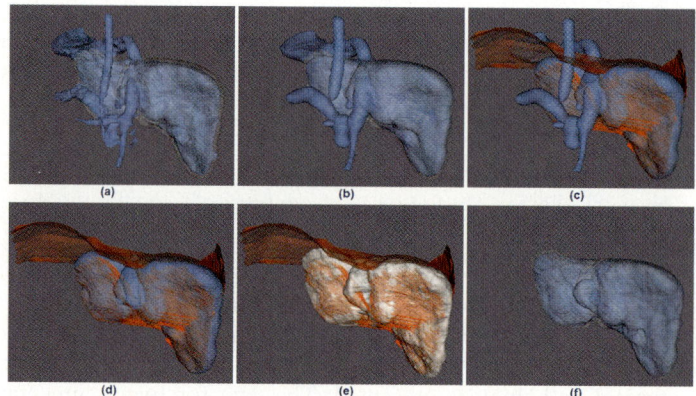

Fig. 1. Model construction[1]. (a) Initial liver estimation (blue) with manual segmentation (white). (b) Pre-segmentation (blue) with manual segmentation (white). (c) Deformed surface patches (orange) on the pre-segmentation (blue). (d) Refined pre-segmentation after non-liver tissues are removed. (e) Manual segmentation with surface patches (orange), for comparison with (d). (f) Final result of liver segmentation (blue) with the manual segmentation (white).

2 Method

The method consists of the following three main steps:

1) Liver pre-segmentation. This is obtained by applying our previous work [7] followed by a smoothness operation using a curvature-driven level set approach. The liver pre-segmentation serves as a basis for the subsequent segmentation.

---

[1] All the cases illustrated in this paper are from the datasets provided by [8].

2) Model initialization and deformation. This is a fully automatic process to remove unwanted tissues from the pre-segmentation. Firstly a three-patch surface model is initialized, representing the upper, right lobe and lower liver surfaces, separately (section 2.1). Next a graph-based optimal surface fitting scheme (section 2.2) is applied to recover the "real" liver boundaries (Fig. 1c,1e), from which we can obtain a refined pre-segmentation result with non-liver tissues removed (Fig. 1d).

3) Liver pre-segmentation refinement and precise liver region recovery by level set evolution (section 2.3). To recover some missing parts, such as some tips or small perturbations of the liver edges, due to morphological and smoothness operations in step one, we re-implement the level set evolution but driven by both image force and inner force, to obtain a more accurate liver contour (Fig. 1f).

2.1 Model Initialization

The feature points for the three-patch surface construction are identified on each coronal slice of the pre-segmentation images. Due to the property of B-Splines, the sensitivity of the surface to some poorly located feature points is reduced when it is initialized from a large number of points.

2.1.1 Upper Liver Surface Construction
The upper liver surface aims to separate liver and heart regions by using a curved surface approximating the base of the right and left lungs.

Initially, the lungs are segmented using region growing, seeded automatically by finding points with the lowest HU value directly above the highest part of the liver right lobe found from the pre-segmentation. From the segmentations the corner points on the bottom of each lung (Fig. 2a) are detected automatically on every coronal slice and a number of points sampled between the left and right corners of right/left lung along large gradient values. The number of sampled points is determined by the distance between the left and right bottom corners of the right and left lung. The B-Spline reconstruction technique [9] is applied to create the curved surface approximating the set of sample points (Fig. 2).

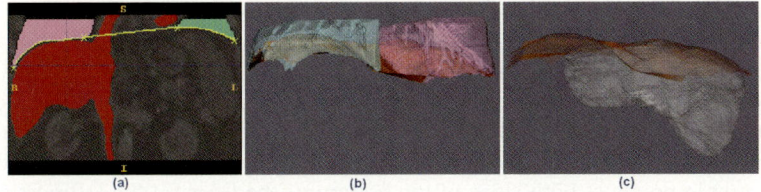

Fig. 2. Upper liver surface construction. (a) Feature points of lungs and B-Spline reconstruction (2D). (b) Constructed upper liver surface (orange) fitting to the bottom of the lungs (3D). (c) Upper liver surface is overlapped on the manual segmentation result (white).

2.1.2 Liver Right Lobe Boundary Construction
The liver right lobe boundary is created to delineate the abdominal cavity wall even when it is only partially detectable on the image. The initialized curved surface

encapsulates the right lung wall[2] and the right lobe of the liver pre-segmentation (Fig. 3b, 4b). A point set for B-Spline interpolation is created by sampling points in each coronal slice. For the lung wall, three evenly spaced points are selected. For feature points on the liver right lobe wall, to avoid noise introduced to the pre-segmentation, only two points located close to the bottom of the lung and one point located at the inferior segment of the right lobe (Fig. 3a) are used.

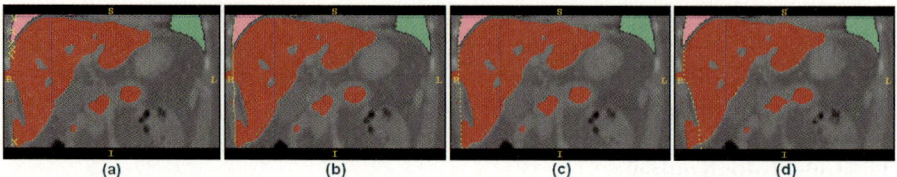

Fig. 3. Liver right lobe boundary (yellow) initialization and deformation (2D). (a) Feature points (yellow). (b) B-Spline reconstruction. (c) Discretization. (d) Deformation.

The initialization and deformation result (3D) of the liver right lobe wall is also shown in Fig. 4. For comparison, we overlay the fitted boundary onto the manual segmentation result in Fig. 4d. More detailed discussion on the deformation procedure is given in section 2.2.

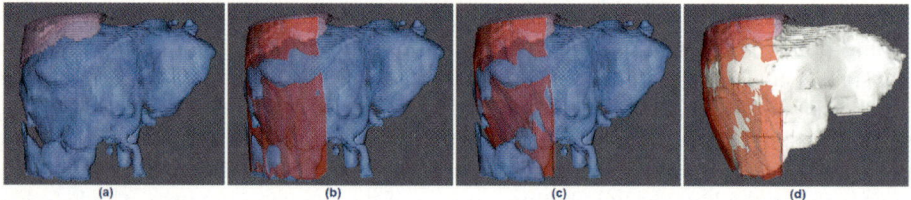

Fig. 4. Liver right lobe boundary initialization and deformation (3D). (a) Liver pre-segmentation (blue) and right lung detection (pink). (b) Liver right lobe boundary initialization (red). (c) Liver right lobe boundary deformation (fitting). (d) Deformed liver right lobe boundary (red) overlays on the manual segmentation result (white).

2.1.3 Lower Liver Surface Construction

The objective of approximating the lower liver surface is to exclude any non-liver tissues under the liver. The main problematic area in our pre-segmentation result is the portal vein, which is located near the centre of the liver. Therefore, we choose two pairs of sample points at both sides of the bottom of the liver, 1) the leftmost point on the left lobe boundary and a second point on the left lobe boundary but 7mm under the first, 2) the lowest point on the inferior segment of the right lobe and a point which is 7 mm above (Fig. 5a). The distance is only used as a reference to obtain the second point in each pair. This distance is small enough to ensure the initialized liver lower patch excludes the portal vein. In a similar manner to the other surfaces, the lower liver surface is created from the sample points by using B-Spline reconstruction (Fig. 5b).

---

[2] The right lung always exists for liver segmentation where the top of the liver right lobe is included in image sources.

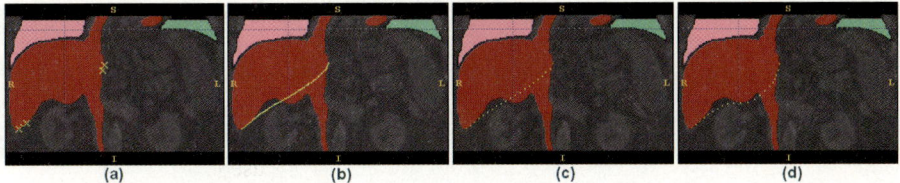

Fig. 5. Lower liver surface (yellow) initialization and deformation (2D). (a) Feature points (yellow). (b) B-Spline reconstruction. (c) Discretisation. (d) Deformation.

2.2 Deformable Model

Similar to the work presented in [5,10], the initial liver model (Fig. 6a) is deformed to create the "real" liver boundary (Fig. 6d) by applying a graph based fitting scheme. The details of constructing the directed graph can be found in [10]. A simplified visualization of this graph structure is given in Fig. 6c. To increase computation efficiency and robustness to outliers, we introduce the narrow band concept of the level set method. The lower liver surface is used to illustrate our approach.

According to the property of the B-Spline, the continuous lower liver surface can be discretised at any desired resolution [9]. In practice, to increase robustness to the local minimum, we adopt a sampling scheme where an average distance between adjacent vertices is about 3 times the voxel size of the original image (Fig. 3c,5c). We denote the discretised lower liver surface as $S_{t=0} = (V_0, E)$ with vertices set V_0 and edges set E. The graph search determines the optimal position v_i^* for each vertex $v_i \in V_0$. The final optimized surface is denoted as $S^* = (V^*, E)$. The vertex at any location can then be derived using B-Spline interpolation.

The external force is computed from the edge map of the pre-segmentation image, which serves as a template eliminating any region outside the liver region (Fig. 6b). The region inside the liver pre-segmentation is denoted by R_{ps}. Defining an infinite line $L(v_i)$ starting at vertex v_i with the direction $N(v_i, t)$, $L(v_i)$ intersects with an edge on the edge map at point p_i^*. A spring force drives the vertex v_i in the corresponding direction:

$$F_{ext}(v_i) = \begin{cases} \delta & if \left| p_i^* - v_i \right| > \delta \\ \left| p_i^* - v_i \right| & if \left| p_i^* - v_i \right| \leq \delta \\ 0 & v_i \notin R_{ps} \end{cases} \quad (1)$$

δ is the width of the narrow band around S_t. A smoothness constraint, denoted by Δ, is imposed on the geometric relations of the nodes in the graph. That is, a shift between any pair of neighbouring points on each sought surface cannot be bigger than Δ. A smaller value of Δ forces the sought surface to be smoother.

The surface fitting scheme is implemented in an iterative way. The process is stopped when either the predefined number of iterations has been achieved or the average vertex movement falls below a given threshold. More example results of deformation have been depicted in Fig. 3(5)d (2D) and Fig. 4c (3D).

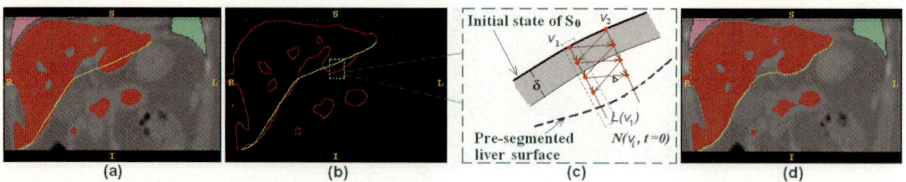

Fig. 6. Deformable model (patient-2). (a) Model initialization. (b) Edge map. (c) Graph. (d) Model deformation.

2.3 Pre-segmentation Refinement and Precise Liver Segmentation

Using the three optimized surface patches, the tissues outside the boundary (indicated by the surface normal direction) can be removed from the pre-segmentation (Fig. 1d). The result is a refined liver pre-segmentation which is the input of the level set evolution for accurate liver shape recovery (automatically).

The level set evolution in this section is driven by a joint force, i.e. image based force (external force) and curvature force (internal force), where the image based force is dominant. The external force is computed from a probabilistic map [11].

As the refined estimation is close to the real boundary, only a few iterations are required and thus the final result is not sensitive to the choice of parameters. We use 0.2 and 0.8, corresponding to the weights of curvature and image force respectively, for all experiments.

3 Evaluation and Experimental Results

In our project, it is desirable to segment liver inner structures, e.g. tumors and vessels, as separate objects. For comparison, we automatically integrate the explicitly segmented inner structures into the liver segmentation (Fig. 7b). The surface patches constructed in section 2 are used to trim vessels outside the liver region (Fig. 7a).

3.1 Evaluation of Accuracy

Our approach has been evaluated on 20 patient CT datasets[3] provided by the organizers of the MICCAI Workshop on 3D Segmentation in the Clinic [8] and 5 further patient CT data from the CRaIVE[4] project. Both volume-based and mesh-based evaluations are conducted. Manual segmentations are taken as references.

1) Volume comparison.
This is measured based on three criteria defined by [12], which are all expressed as a fraction of the volume of reference models; 1) True positive volume fraction (TPVF): the fraction of voxels in the intersection of our segmentation and the reference model; 2) False negative volume fraction (FNVF): the fraction of voxels defined in manual segmentation but missed by our method; 3) False positive volume fraction (FPVF): the fraction of voxels falsely identified by our method. The average TPVF is

---

[3] Since there is no training process required by our method, we use their 20 training datasets for testing as well. The results of 10 test datasets have been submitted to [8] for evaluation.
[4] Collaborators in Radiological Interventional Virtual Environments, http://www.craive.org.uk

95.77(±2.07)%. FNVF and FPVF are 4.23(±2.07)% and 4.31(±2.49)%, respectively.. To be comparable with other liver segmentation experiments, we also calculate the overlap error and volume difference (Table 1).

2) Mesh comparison

This experiment is based on the distance measurement between vertices of the reference model and our result. The mesh is created by using the marching cubes algorithm from the VTK library, using the same parameters for all datasets. The average RMS error is 2.44±0.53mm. The average maximum distance 16.84±4.35mm and the average mean distance is -0.15±0.22mm.

3.2 Evaluation of Efficiency

Our method was performed on an Intel Core2 2.66GHz processor. The average segmentation time is about 1 minute (step1: 15sec.; step2: 25-30sec.; step3: 10sec.). The comparison to recent liver segmentation experiments is given in Table 1.

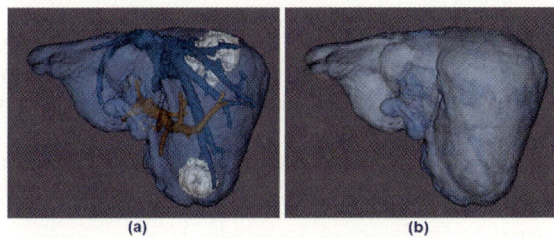

Fig. 7. (a) Liver Segmentation (light blue), tumor (white) and vessels (dark blue and brown). (b) Segmentation after merging (in blue), overlapped with the manual segmentation (white).

Table 1. Comparison to recent liver segmentation experiments. They are listed in the order of the best automatic, fastest automatic and best semi-automatic methods.

Method	Overlap Error [%]	Volume Diff. [%]	Avg. Dist. [mm]	RMS Dist. [mm]	Max. Dist. [mm]	Run time	Datasets tested	contrast
Kainmueller [13]	7.0	-3.6	1.1	2.3	20.9	15 mins	10	yes
Rusko [14]	10.7	-4.3	1.8	3.8	28.3	56 sec.	10	yes
Lee et al. [15]	6.9	-1.3	1.1	2.1	21.3	7.4 mins	10	yes
Our approach	8.15	0.079	-0.15	2.44	16.84	1 min	25	mixed

4 Conclusions and Future Work

Despite a large body of literature, (semi-) automatic liver segmentation from a 3D volume remains a challenge. Due to the large variations in shape and intensity pattern, the success of the classic statistical model-based approaches is often compromised by the limited number of training datasets. To overcome this, we propose a novel model-driven approach which creates a deformable model from each patient dataset directly. Moreover, by converting the problem of building one complex shape model into constructing three much simpler models that can be fitted independently, we greatly improve the computation efficiency.

Acknowledgments. This work is funded by the UK EPSRC (EP/E002749). The authors would like to thank Dr F. Bello and Dr P. Villard from Imperial College for help with evaluation. We would also like to thank Dr D. Gould at University of Liverpool for data acquisition and valuable clinical advice.

References

1. Campadelli, P., Casiraghi, E.: Liver Segmentation from CT Scans: A Survey. In: Masulli, F., Mitra, S., Pasi, G. (eds.) WILF 2007. LNCS (LNAI), vol. 4578, pp. 520–528. Springer, Heidelberg (2007)
2. Florin, C., Paragios, N., Funka-Lea, G., Williams, J.: Liver Segmentation Using Sparse 3D Prior Models with Optimal Data Support. In: Karssemeijer, N., Lelieveldt, B. (eds.) IPMI 2007. LNCS, vol. 4584, pp. 38–49. Springer, Heidelberg (2007)
3. Ling, H., Zhou, S.K., Zheng, Y., et al.: Hierarchical, Learning-based Automatic Liver Segmentation. In: IEEE conf. on Computer Vision and Pattern Recognition, pp. 1–8 (2008)
4. Wimmer, A., Soza, G., Hornegger, J.: Two-stage Semi-automatic Organ Segmentation Framework Using Radial Basis Functions and Level Set. In: Heimann, T., Styner, M., van Ginneken, B. (eds.) MICCAI workshop on 3D Segmentation in the Clinic, pp. 179–188 (2007)
5. Heimann, T., Meinzer, H., Wolf, I.: A Statistical Deformable model for the Segmentation of Liver CT Volumes. In: MICCAI workshop on 3D Segmentation in the Clinic (SLIVER 2007), pp. 161–166 (2007)
6. Lamecker, H., Lange, T., Seebass, M.: A Statistical Shape Model for the Liver. In: Dohi, T., Kikinis, R. (eds.) MICCAI 2002. LNCS, vol. 2489, pp. 421–427. Springer, Heidelberg (2002)
7. Song, Y., Bulpitt, A., Brodlie, K.: Efficient Semi-automatic Segmentation for Creating Patient Specific Models for Virtual Environments. In: MICCAI workshop CVII, pp. 22–34 (2008)
8. Heimann, T., van Ginneken, B., Styner, M., et al.: Comparison and Evaluation of Methods for Liver Segmentation from CT datasets. J. IEEE Trans. on Medical Imaging (2009) (in press) doi:10.1109/TMI.2009.2013851
9. Song, Y., Bai, L.: 3D Modeling for Deformable Objects. In: Perales, F.J., Fisher, R.B. (eds.) AMDO 2008. LNCS, vol. 5098, pp. 175–187. Springer, Heidelberg (2008)
10. Li, K., Millington, S., Wu, X., Chen, D., Sonka, M.: Simultaneous segmentation of multiple closed surfaces using optimal graph searching. In: Christensen, G.E., Sonka, M. (eds.) IPMI 2005. LNCS, vol. 3565, pp. 406–417. Springer, Heidelberg (2005)
11. Zhu, S.C., Yuille, A.: Region Competition: Unifying Snakes, Region Growing, and Bayes/MDL for Multiband Image Segmentation. J. IEEE Trans. PAMI 18, 884–900 (1996)
12. Udupa, J.K., Leblanc, V.R., Schmidt, H., et al.: A Methodology for Evaluating Image Segmentation Algorithm. In: SPIE, vol. 4684, pp. 266–277 (2002)
13. Kainmueller, D., Lange, T., Lamecker, H.: Shape Constrained Automatic Segmentation of the Liver based on a Heuristic Intensity Model. In: Heimann, T., Styner, M., van Ginneken, B. (eds.) MICCAI workshop on 3D Segmentation in the Clinic, pp. 109–116 (2007)
14. Rusko, L., Bekes, G., Nemeth, G., Fidrich, M.: Fully Automatic Liver Segmentation for Contrast-enhanced CT images. In: Heimann, T., Styner, M., van Ginneken, B. (eds.) MICCAI workshop on 3D Segmentation in the Clinic, pp. 143–150 (2007)
15. Lee, J., Kim, N., Lee, H., et al.: Efficient Liver Segmentation Exploiting Level-set Speed Images with 2.5D Shape Porpagation. In: Heimann, T., Styner, M., van Ginneken, B. (eds.) MICCAI workshop on 3D Segmentation in the Clinic, pp. 189–196 (2007)

Airway Tree Extraction with Locally Optimal Paths

Pechin Lo[1], Jon Sporring[1], Jesper Johannes Holst Pedersen[2], and Marleen de Bruijne[1,3]

[1] Image Group, Department of Computer Science,
University of Copenhagen, Denmark
pechin@diku.dk
[2] Department of Cardio Thoracic Surgery, Rigshospitalet - Copenhagen University Hospital, Denmark
[3] Biomedical Imaging Group Rotterdam, Departments of Radiology & Medical Informatics, Erasmus MC, Rotterdam, The Netherlands

Abstract. This paper proposes a method to extract the airway tree from CT images by continually extending the tree with locally optimal paths. This is in contrast to commonly used region growing based approaches that only search the space of the immediate neighbors. The result is a much more robust method for tree extraction that can overcome local occlusions. The cost function for obtaining the optimal paths takes into account of an airway probability map as well as measures of airway shape and orientation derived from multi-scale Hessian eigen analysis on the airway probability. Significant improvements were achieved compared to a region growing based method, with up to 36% longer trees at a slight increase of false positive rate.

1 Introduction

Analysis of the airways in computed tomography (CT) is crucial for the understanding of various lung diseases [1]. However due to the difficulties of the extraction process, the airways remain among the least understood structures in the lungs.

Most methods used for segmenting the airway tree from CT images are based on the concept of region growing [2,3,4,5]. The main problem with the standard region growing approach is that the segmentation may "leak" to surrounding lung parenchyma, if the contrast with the airway wall is low due to e.g. noise or pathology. Various strategies have been used to solve this problem, e.g. using geometric criteria to detect and remove leakage [2,3,4], or using improved appearance models to avoid leakage [5].

In this paper, we propose a new method for airway tree extraction method that continually extends the tree with locally optimal paths. The advantage of using such a path search approach is that the algorithm is able to look further ahead and can therefore overcome local occlusions. Occlusions may be caused for instance by noise or pathologies such as mucus plugging. Using the trained appearance model described in [5] as the basis for our cost function, the Dijkstra algorithm is applied within a sphere centered at a seed point to obtain candidate airway paths. Candidate paths that satisfy various criteria based on airway probability, shape, and orientation are retained, and potential bifurcation points and new end points are stored and subsequently used as new seed points. This process is repeated until no more valid candidate paths can be found.

The work is inspired by minimal path based approaches in vessel segmentation and diffusion tensor imaging (DTI) tractography (see e.g. [6,7]). These approaches are however typically either limited to extracting a single optimal path or require a user to specify the end points in advance. Another example is [8], where a complete vessel tree is extracted as a collection of optimal paths from a converged fast marching algorithm. In contrast to [8], we may be able to extract also less salient branches and thus find a more complete tree by searching for optimal paths locally and recursively. The notion of performing optimal path extraction locally was recently also proposed in [9], where various examples are shown in which a local approach outperforms the global approach. However, the focus of that paper was on extracting single paths or contours and the method is not capable of handling bifurcations.

Our work is similar in spirit to [10], which aims at reaching a more global solution for airway segmentation by detecting potential airway branches throughout the lungs with a tube detection scheme, and subsequently connecting these using a graph search method. However, our method is more flexible and can be customized to other tree segmentation tasks by simply modifying the cost function and the confidence measure.

2 Tracking Locally Optimal Paths

This section explains how the Dijkstra algorithm is applied locally and how the optimal paths are selected. We assume that a cost function F, a confidence measure D, and a list of initial candidate points are provided. A candidate point is a point that belongs to a previously extracted airway branch, and for which the departing paths are not yet extracted. Each candidate point is associated with the orientation and the average radius of the airway branch it belongs to.

At every iteration, a candidate point is taken from the list and evaluated. New paths extending from the candidate points are generated through a process of candidate path extraction and selection. Additional new candidate points from these new paths will then be added into the list. The iterative process ends once no more candidate points are available for evaluation.

2.1 Extracting Candidate Paths

Given a candidate point $\boldsymbol{x}_0$, with the branch orientation $\boldsymbol{d}_0$, optimal paths are computed from $\boldsymbol{x}_0$ to every point within a sphere of radius r_s using the Dijkstra algorithm. We refer to these optimal paths as the candidate path from $\boldsymbol{x}_0$ to $\boldsymbol{x}$. The traveling cost between two neighboring voxels is computed using cost function F.

Candidate paths are extracted for all points on the surface of the sphere that satisfy the following conditions:

1) Local minima: End points should form a local minimum, in terms of minimal cost from x_0, on the surface of the sphere.

2) Departing angle: To limit the search to branches that do not deviate too much from the initial direction, end points should satisfy $\angle(x - x_0), d_0 \leq \alpha$, as shown in Fig. 1(c).

2.2 Evaluating the Candidate Paths

The most likely airway branches are selected from the extracted candidate paths by the following three selection criteria in a low to high cost order:

1) Confidence: The majority of points on a path must have high confidence measure D. Hence, we require the Nth percentile of the confidence measure of a path to be greater than β in order to be selected.

2) Straightness: As airway branches are relatively straight in general, we require a path C to satisfy $l_{path}(C) < \gamma l(x_0, x)$, where $l_{path}(C)$ is the length of the path C and $l(x_0, x)$ is the distance from x_0 to x.

3) Non-overlap: Selected paths are not allowed to overlap each other and should be at least δ mm apart. The distance between a candidate path and the previously selected paths is measured as the minimum distance between the end point of the candidate path and the points in the selected paths. We also ensure that a selected candidate path will not intersect with other paths obtained from previously evaluated candidate points. Prior to applying this criterion, an additional trimming process is added to remove low confidence points at the end of the path, which exist because of the used of fixed end points. The trimmed path is stored if the path is selected.

A maximum of N_{max} paths is retained.

2.3 Updating the List of Candidate Points

The end points of the newly selected paths are added to the list of candidate points. All potential bifurcation points, defined as points where candidate paths depart from a selected path, are also added to the list. The direction for each of the new candidate points is the direction of the selected path it belongs to.

3 Cost Function

Unlike most current airway segmentation methods [2,3,4,10] that use only image intensity, our proposed method operates on the soft classification resulting from a voxel classification based appearance model [5].

The appearance model uses a K nearest neighbor (KNN) classifier that is trained to differentiate between voxels from airway and non-airway classes using various local image descriptors at different scales. To circumvent the requirement for high-quality ground truth segmentations of the complete airway tree, we follow the interactive training procedure described in [5]. A moderated KNN [11] output is used, where the posterior probability of a feature vector $\boldsymbol{f}(\boldsymbol{x})$, obtained at voxel position $\boldsymbol{x}$, to belong to the airway class is defined as

$$P_A(\boldsymbol{f}(\boldsymbol{x})) = \frac{K_A(\boldsymbol{f}(\boldsymbol{x})) + 1}{K + 2},$$

where $K_A(\boldsymbol{f}(\boldsymbol{x}))$ is the number of nearest neighbors around $\boldsymbol{f}(\boldsymbol{x})$ that belong to the airway class obtained from a total of K nearest neighbors.

The airway probability $P_A(\boldsymbol{f}(\boldsymbol{x}))$ is used directly as the confidence measure D in Section 2 to discard unlikely paths. The cost function F is designed such that local paths are searched in the direction of probable airways, which appear as bright, cylindrical structures in P_A. The local orientation of the airways is derived through multi-scale Hessian eigen analysis on the airway probability map. The scale is selected for each voxel independently using the scale normalized [12] Frobenius norm of the Hessian matrix $\omega(\sigma_i) = \sigma_i^2 \sqrt{\lambda_1(\sigma_i)^2 + \lambda_2(\sigma_i)^2 + \lambda_3(\sigma_i)^2}$, where $|\lambda_1| \geq |\lambda_2| \geq |\lambda_3|$ are the eigenvalues of the Hessian matrix. The local scale, σ_l, is then obtained as the smallest scale that corresponds to a local maximum of $\omega(\sigma_i)$ across a list of scales $\{\sigma_{min}, \ldots, \sigma_{max}\}$, where σ_{max} is chosen slightly larger than the current airway radius. A measure M_{tube}, indicating how well the surrounding image structure fits the model of a solid bright tube, can then be defined as

$$M_{tube}(\boldsymbol{x}) = \begin{cases} 0, & \lambda_1(\sigma_l) \geq 0 \text{ or } \lambda_2(\sigma_l) \geq 0, \\ \frac{|\lambda_2(\sigma_l)| - |\lambda_3(\sigma_l)|}{|\lambda_2(\sigma_l)|}, & \text{otherwise,} \end{cases}$$

The orientation of the tube at $\boldsymbol{x}$ is given by $\boldsymbol{v}_3(\boldsymbol{x})$, which is the eigenvector corresponding to $\lambda_3(\sigma_l)$.

The cost function F combines the airway probability, tubeness measure, and airway direction estimates as:

$$F(\boldsymbol{x}_s, \boldsymbol{x}_t) = \frac{\|\boldsymbol{x}_s - \boldsymbol{x}_t\|_2}{|<\frac{\boldsymbol{x}_s - \boldsymbol{x}_t}{\|\boldsymbol{x}_s - \boldsymbol{x}_t\|_2}, \boldsymbol{v}_3(\boldsymbol{x}_t)>|P_A(\boldsymbol{f}(\boldsymbol{x}_t)(1 + M_{tube}(\boldsymbol{x}_t))},$$

where $\boldsymbol{x}_s$ and $\boldsymbol{x}_t$ is the source and target location. The cost $F(\boldsymbol{x}_s, \boldsymbol{x}_t)$ is low, when both the local airway probability is high and the propagation direction is parallel with the estimated airway orientation. The term with M_{tube} is used to lower the cost further, when the local structure at $\boldsymbol{x}_t$ resembles a solid bright tube.

4 Experiment and Results

Experiments were conducted on low-dose CT images from the Danish Lung Cancer Screening Trial (DLCST) [13], where participants were current or former smokers at an age between 50-70 years. All images had a slice thickness of 1 mm and in-plane voxel size ranging from 0.72 to 0.78 mm. A total of 32

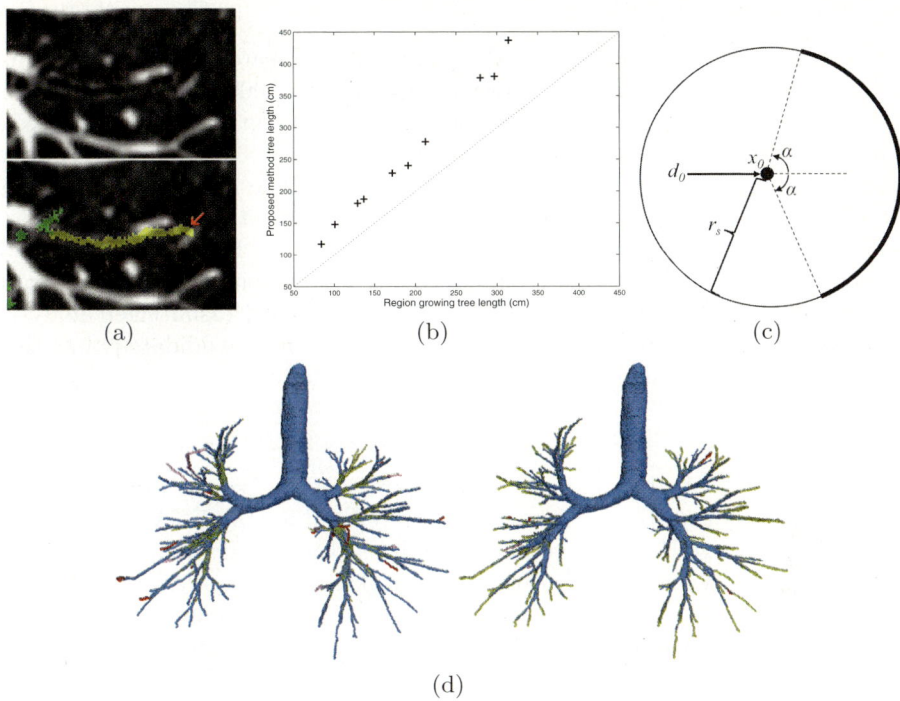

Fig. 1. (a) Example of a case where it is not possible to segment the correct part (the largest part of the branch) from the leakage, with the branch segment highlighted in yellow and an arrow indicating the leakage. (b) A scatter plot of the tree length obtained by both methods for the 10 test cases. (c) A schematic of the search sphere. (d) Surface rendering of the results from proposed method (left) and region growing based method (right), with correct regions in blue, missing regions in yellow, partly wrong regions in purple and false positives in red.

randomly selected images were used for the training of the voxel classification based appearance model. The method was tested on an additional 10 randomly selected CT scans from different subjects.

Results were compared to a region growing based method that uses a trained airway appearance model and exploits the fact that orientation of airways and vessels are similar [5]. Airways branches from the second up to and including the third generation obtained by this method were used to initialize the proposed method. Since extraction of these first few branches is relatively easy, simpler methods such as intensity based region growing could be used for initialization instead.

The centerlines of the initial segmentation were used as the initial set of candidate points needed for the proposed method. A simplified version of the segmentation algorithm presented in [2], without any leakage detection, were used to extract the centerlines. The direction and radius associated to each candidate point is derived from the branch they belong to. For newly added candidate points, the radius is simply propagated directly from their parents.

4.1 Parameter and Settings

For extracting the optimal paths, the radius of the search sphere was set to $r_s = 20$ mm and the maximum allowed angle to $\alpha = 100$ degrees. In selection of the optimal paths, at most $N = 30$ percent of points on the path may have a confidence below $\beta = 0.5$, the straightness measure $\gamma = 1.05$, minimum required distance between selected optimal paths $\delta = 3$ mm. The maximum number of selected paths from a single candidate point N_{max} was set to 2.

For the appearance model, $K = 21$ was used for the KNN classifier and 7 scales distributed exponentially from 0.5 to 3.5 mm were used both to generate the features (refer to [5] for details) and for the multi-scale Hessian eigen analysis.

To prevent paths from growing into border of the lungs, candidate points that were within 3 mm of the lung surface were not evaluated.

4.2 Results

All results were evaluated manually by an experienced observer using the dedicated airway segmentation evaluation tool developed for the EXACT'09 airway extraction challenge [14]. The results were divided into individual branches using the simplified version of [2], without any leakage detection. Airway branches are subsequently visually inspected and classified into the categories 'correct', 'wrong', or 'partly wrong' based on several views obtained from different cut planes at different angles and positions. Branches are said to be correct, if there is no leakage visible at all. A branch is said to be wrong, if the majority (more than 50%) of it is leakage, and partly wrong, if the majority is correct.

As the evaluation tool was designed for evaluating segmentation and not centerlines, results from the proposed method were dilated in order to make them compatible with the evaluation tool.

As the evaluation process only separates branches at bifurcations, we are unable to isolate leakage from a branch, if it extends from the endpoints and does not bifurcate. This usually occurred at the end segments, where a whole branch is classified as 'partly wrong' due to a small amount of leakage at the end. Figure 1(a) shows an example of this situation. All partly wrong regions were excluded from further evaluation.

Compared to the results from the region growing approach, we observe a significant ($p < 0.01$) increase of 36% in total tree length for the results of the proposed method, from an average of 192 cm tree length to 258 cm. The tree length is defined as the sum of the lengths of all branches obtained, excluding the trachea and main bronchi. The average false positive rate, computed as a percentage of the total tree with the trachea and main bronchi excluded, was 3.79% for the proposed method, slightly larger than for the region growing based method (1.35%). The total number of branches extracted was similar for both methods, around 174 branches on average. A plot showing the tree length for the 10 cases from the two methods are given in Fig. 1(b). Surface renderings of a randomly selected case are given in Fig. 1(d).

Finally, a third segmentation was constructed as the union of the airway trees extracted from the two methods. A comparison of the union against the result from the region growing based method shows a significant ($p < 0.01$) increase of 9% in branch count. Results from the proposed method cover 96% of the tree length in the union, while results from the region growing based method only have 71% coverage.

5 Discussion and Conclusions

The proposed method improves results significantly, especially in terms of tree length, where an average improvement of 36% was observed. The branches missed by the proposed method that were extracted correctly using the region growing based method were very short, with an average length of 5 mm. Despite having similar branch count when comparing the proposed method and the region growing based method, significant increase (9%) in branch count was observed when comparing the results from the region growing based method against the union. This indicates that the proposed method is capable of obtaining new branches, and not only merely extending branches obtainable by the region growing based method. It should be noted that the multi-scale version of the work from [5], used for comparison, is a method that gives results comparable to other recent state of the art methods such as [4].

In the current work, the estimate of the airway radius is propagated from old to new candidate points unaltered. Although this estimate is only used to determine the upper bound in the scale selection of Section 3, more reliable estimates of local tubeness and tube orientation may be found if the radius is updated with each bifurcation to reflect the overall decrease in airway diameter towards the higher generations. Alternatively, an airway wall segmentation algorithm such as [15] could be used to obtain the radius, with the additional advantage that the result can be directly used for airway dimension analysis.

Another potential improvement would be to introduce a "multi-radius" scheme, which involves searching paths within multiple search spheres of different radii. This might increase the number of new branches found, as shorter branches may then be extracted using a smaller radius, while occlusions can still be overcome using the larger radii.

In conclusion, an airway tree extraction method that is based on a recursive search for locally optimal paths is presented. In contrast to common airway tree segmentation methods that only consider the immediate neighbors of seed points, our method considers both the appearance and structure of a whole path. This enables the method to extend past local occlusions caused by noise or pathologies such as mucus plugging. The proposed method handles bifurcations automatically, which is a topic rarely touched upon by optimal path tracking methods.

Acknowledgments. This work is partly funded by the Danish Council for Strategic Research (NABIIT), the Netherlands Organization for Scientific Research (NWO), and AstraZeneca, Lund, Sweden.

References

1. Berger, P., Perot, V., Desbarats, P., de Lara, J.M.T., Marthan, R., Laurent, F.: Airway wall thickness in cigarette smokers: quantitative thin-section CT assessment. Radiology 235(3), 1055–1064 (2005)
2. Schlathölter, T., Lorenz, C., Carlsen, I.C., Renisch, S., Deschamps, T.: Simultaneous segmentation and tree reconstruction of the airways for virtual bronchoscopy. In: Sonka, M., Fitzpatrick, J.M. (eds.) SPIE Medical Imaging, vol. 4684, pp. 103–113. SPIE, San Jose (2002)
3. Tschirren, J., Hoffman, E., McLennan, G., Sonka, M.: Intrathoracic airway trees: segmentation and airway morphology analysis from low-dose CT scans. IEEE T. Med. Imaging 24(12), 1529–1539 (2005)
4. van Ginneken, B., Baggerman, W., van Rikxoort, E.: Robust segmentation and anatomical labeling of the airway tree from thoracic CT scans. In: Metaxas, D., Axel, L., Fichtinger, G., Székely, G. (eds.) MICCAI 2008, Part I. LNCS, vol. 5241, pp. 219–226. Springer, Heidelberg (2008)
5. Lo, P., Sporring, J., Ashraf, H., Pedersen, J., de Bruijne, M.: Vessel-guided airway segmentation based on voxel classification. In: Brown, M., de Bruijne, M., van Ginneken, B., Kiraly, A., Kuhnigk, J., Lorenz, C., Mori, K., Reinhardt, J. (eds.) Proc. of First International Workshop on Pulmonary Image Analysis (2008)
6. Jbabdi, S., Bellec, P., Toro, R., Daunizeau, J., Pélégrini-Issac, M., Benali, H.: Accurate anisotropic fast marching for diffusion-based geodesic tractography. Journal of Biomedical Imaging 2008(1), 1–12 (2008)
7. Jackowski, M., Papademetris, X., Dobrucki, L.W., Sinusas, A.J., Staib, L.H.: Characterizing vascular connectivity from microCT images. In: Duncan, J.S., Gerig, G. (eds.) MICCAI 2005. LNCS, vol. 3750, pp. 701–708. Springer, Heidelberg (2005)
8. Gülsün, M.A., Tek, H.: Robust vessel tree modeling. In: Metaxas, D., Axel, L., Fichtinger, G., Székely, G. (eds.) MICCAI 2008, Part I. LNCS, vol. 5241, pp. 602–611. Springer, Heidelberg (2008)
9. Benmansour, F., Cohen, L.: Fast object segmentation by growing minimal paths from a single point on 2D or 3D images. Journal of Mathematical Imaging and Vision 33(2), 209–221 (2009)
10. Graham, M.W., Gibbs, J.D., Higgins, W.E.: Robust system for human airway-tree segmentation. In: SPIE Medical Imaging. SPIE, vol. 6914, 69141J (2008)
11. Kittler, J., Alkoot, F.M.: Moderating k-NN classifiers. Pattern Analysis & Applications 5(3), 326–332 (2002)
12. Lindeberg, T.: Feature detection with automatic scale selection. Int. J. Comput. Vision 30(2), 79–116 (1998)
13. Pedersen, J., Ashraf, H., Dirksen, A., Bach, K., Hansen, H., Toennesen, P., Thorsen, H., Brodersen, J., Skov, B., Døssing, M., Mortensen, J., Richter, K., Clementsen, P., Seersholm, N.: The Danish randomized lung cancer CT screening trial - overall design and results of the prevalence round. Journal of Thoracic Oncology (April 2009)
14. Lo, P., van Ginneken, B., Reinhardt, J., de Bruijne., M.: Extraction of airways from CT 2009 (EXACT 2009). In: Proc. of Second International Workshop on Pulmonary Image Analysis (under preparation 2009)
15. Kiraly, A.P., Odry, B.L., Naidich, D.P., Novak, C.L.: Boundary-specific cost functions for quantitative airway analysis. In: Ayache, N., Ourselin, S., Maeder, A. (eds.) MICCAI 2007, Part I. LNCS, vol. 4791, pp. 784–791. Springer, Heidelberg (2007)

A Deformable Surface Model for Vascular Segmentation

Max W.K. Law and Albert C.S. Chung

Lo Kwee-Seong Medical Image Analysis Laboratory,
Department of Computer Science and Engineering,
The Hong Kong University of Science and Technology, Hong Kong
{maxlawwk,achung}@cse.ust.hk

Abstract. Inspired by the motion of a solid surface under liquid pressure, this paper proposes a novel deformable surface model to segment blood vessels in medical images. In the proposed model, the segmented region and the background region are respectively considered as liquid and an elastic solid. The surface of the elastic solid experiences various forces derived from the second order intensity statistics and the surface geometry. These forces cause the solid surface to deform in order to segment vascular structures in an image. The proposed model has been studied in the experiments on synthetic data and clinical data acquired by different imaging modalities. It is experimentally shown that the new model is robust to intensity contrast changes inside blood vessels and thus very suitable to perform vascular segmentation.

1 Introduction

Vascular segmentation is essential to the clinical assessment of blood vessels. To extract vasculatures from medical images, the deformable surface models have been actively studied in the past decade. Lorigo et al. have proposed the CURVES algorithm in [1]. CURVES makes use of the minimal curvature to aid the detection of thin vessels. Vasilevskiy and Siddiqi [2] have introduced the image gradient-flux to deform surfaces for the segmentation of vascular structures. The image gradient-flux encapsulates both the image gradient magnitude and direction. It is capable of detecting small and low contrast vasculatures. Rochery et al. have devised the higher order active contour model in [3]. The higher order active contour model factors in the image intensity, the geometry of target structures and the contour smoothness to extract tubular structures. Klein et al. [4] have presented the use of a B-Spline based deformable surface model to segment vessels. Yan and Kissim have elaborated the capillary action [5] for segmentation of vessels. The capillary force aims at pulling the evolving surface into thin and low contrast vessels. Nain et al. devised the shape driven flow [6] to reduce the chance of false positive detection when segmenting vessels.

In this paper, a novel deformable surface model is proposed. The deformable surface can be viewed as the surface of an elastic solid (the background region) that is in contact with the liquid (the segmented region). The surface is represented as a level set function. It experiences forces derived from the second order intensity statistics and the surface geometry. These forces are related by the force equilibrium equation of a solid-liquid interface [7]. The dynamics of the surface are governed by the net force acting on the surface. The surface deformation equation can inspect the second order intensity change along the surface tangential plane as well as the surface normal direction. It helps deform the surface to propagate through the position where changes of object intensity contrast happen.

The proposed model is studied using a synthetic and numerical image volume. It is also compared against a well founded vascular segmentation approach, the CURVES algorithm [1], by using the clinical datasets consisting of three different imaging modalities. It is experimentally shown that the proposed model is suitable to perform segmentation of vascular structures.

2 Methodology

2.1 The Proposed Model

In the proposed model, the segmented region and the background region are respectively regarded as liquid and an elastic solid (Fig. 1). As such, the solid surface is the boundary that separates the segmented region and the background region. There are three kinds of forces acting on the solid surface. First, the liquid exerts pressure on the solid surface. Second, the surface of the elastic solid has surface stress which opposes the change of the surface area of the solid. Third, an external bulk stress is acted on the surface of the solid. These forces are derived based on the second order intensity variation and the geometry of the solid surface. Given P is the pressure exerted by the liquid, $\mathbf{s}$ and $\mathbf{B}$ are symmetric tensors which represent the surface stress force and the bulk stress force at the solid surface respectively, at the force equilibrium position, these forces are related as [7],

$$(P - \text{div}_S \mathbf{s})\boldsymbol{n} + \mathbf{B}\boldsymbol{n} = \mathbf{0}, \tag{1}$$

where div_S is surface divergence and $\boldsymbol{n}$ is the inward surface normal of the solid.

By placing an initial surface inside the target vessels, the proposed model allows the solid surface to deform according to the net force acting on it. This aims at seeking the force equilibrium position of the surface. Denote $\mathcal{C}$ be the solid surface, the change of the surface with respect to time t is determined by the net force acting on the surface,

$$\mathcal{C}_\mathbf{t} = (P - \text{div}_S \mathbf{s})\boldsymbol{n} + \mathbf{B}\boldsymbol{n}. \tag{2}$$

The liquid pressure and the bulk stress experienced by the solid surface are devised based on the second order intensity statistics, which are widely used for the detection of vasculatures [8] [9] [10]. The pressure exerted by the liquid is defined as $P = -\Delta I$. Inside tubular structures, the Laplacian responses are negative and with large magnitudes. A large negative Laplacian response results in a high liquid pressure inside tubular structures to push the solid surface. On the other hand, the bulk stress acting on the solid surface $\mathbf{B}$ is defined as the negative second order intensity change along the surface normal, i.e. $\mathbf{B} = -\alpha I_{nn} \mathbf{n}\mathbf{n}^T$, where α determines the strength of the stress force. Since the second order intensity changes are large along the vessel cross-sectional planes, and small along the vessel direction, this bulk stress force intends to pull the solid along the vessel cross-sectional planes.

The second order intensity change magnitudes decrease at the positions away from the vessel centers and thus, the stress force as well as the liquid pressure decline accordingly. The bulk stress and the liquid pressure finally become small or vanish at the vessel boundaries. The surface receives very small or no force at the vessel boundaries where the deformation of the surface is therefore stopped at the vessel boundaries. Besides, the surface stress of the solid which opposes to the change of the solid surface area is designed to be constant and isotropic. As discussed in Section 2.3, such a constant and isotropic surface stress leads to a smooth resultant surface. Given $\mathbf{u}$ and $\mathbf{v}$ are two arbitrary orthogonal tangential directions of the surface, the tensor of the constant and isotropic surface stress can be written as, $\mathbf{s} = \gamma[\mathbf{u}\ \mathbf{v}][\mathbf{u}\ \mathbf{v}]^T$, where γ controls the surface stress strength.

Assigning the aforementioned forces to Eqn. 2, we have $\mathcal{C}_{\mathbf{t}} = (-\Delta I - \text{div}_s(\gamma[\mathbf{u}\ \mathbf{v}][\mathbf{u}\ \mathbf{v}]^T))\mathbf{n} - \alpha I_{nn}\mathbf{n}\mathbf{n}^T$. Since $\Delta I = \text{Tr}(\mathbf{H})$ and $\text{div}_S([\mathbf{u}\ \mathbf{v}][\mathbf{u}\ \mathbf{v}]^T) = -2\kappa \mathbf{n}$ [11] for the Euclidean mean curvature of the surface κ,

$$\mathcal{C}_{\mathbf{t}} = (-\text{Tr}([\mathbf{u}\ \mathbf{v}]^T \mathbf{H}[\mathbf{u}\ \mathbf{v}]) + 2\gamma\kappa)\mathbf{n} - (1+\alpha)(I_{nn}\mathbf{n}\mathbf{n}^T)\mathbf{n}. \qquad (3)$$

For the simplicity of discussion, denote $\gamma' = 2\gamma$, $\alpha' = 1 + \alpha$, $\mathbf{G}(\mathbf{H};\mathbf{n}) = (\mathbf{n}^T\mathbf{H}\mathbf{n})(\mathbf{n}\mathbf{n}^T) = I_{nn}\mathbf{n}\mathbf{n}^T$, $\mathbf{M} = \begin{bmatrix} I_{uu} & I_{uv} \\ I_{uv} & I_{vv} \end{bmatrix} = \begin{bmatrix} \mathbf{u}^T\mathbf{H}\mathbf{u} & \mathbf{u}^T\mathbf{H}\mathbf{v} \\ \mathbf{u}^T\mathbf{H}\mathbf{v} & \mathbf{v}^T\mathbf{H}\mathbf{v} \end{bmatrix} = [\mathbf{u}\ \mathbf{v}]^T\mathbf{H}[\mathbf{u}\ \mathbf{v}]$,

$$\mathcal{C}_{\mathbf{t}} = (-\text{Tr}(\mathbf{M}) + \gamma'\kappa)\mathbf{n} - \alpha'\mathbf{G}(\mathbf{H};\mathbf{n})\mathbf{n}. \qquad (4)$$

2.2 Vessel Specific Image Features and Multiscale Detection

If the surface is deforming along a vessel, the surface tangential plane is equivalent to the cross-sectional plane of the vessel. The eigenvalues of $\mathbf{M}$ would be negative and with large magnitudes. Furthermore, vessels are mainly in tubular shape with roughly circular cross-sections. Therefore, the ratio and the signs of these two eigenvalues are exploited to suppress the surface deformation speed in the structures producing non-negative eigenvalues or large difference between the two eigenvalues. The surface deformation equation (Eqn. 4) is refined as $\mathcal{C}_{\mathbf{t}} = (-f(\mathbf{H};\mathbf{u},\mathbf{v}) + \gamma'\kappa)\mathbf{n} - \alpha'\mathbf{G}(\mathbf{H};\mathbf{n})\mathbf{n}$, and

$$f(\mathbf{H};\mathbf{u},\mathbf{v}) = \begin{cases} \text{Tr}(\mathbf{M}) \exp\left(1 - \frac{\xi_2}{\xi_1}\right) & \text{if } \xi_1 < 0 \text{ and } \xi_2 < 0, \\ 0 & \text{otherwise}, \end{cases} \qquad (5)$$

where ξ_1 and ξ_2 are the eigenvalues of $\mathbf{M}$ and $|\xi_1| \leq |\xi_2|$.

Since vessel sizes vary in practice, the second order intensity statistics are computed on the images smoothed by Gaussian kernels with various scales (defined by the value of σ as shown in Fig. 2a) for multiscale detection. The scales are sampled logarithmically as discussed by Sato et al. in [10]. Suppose the Hessian matrix obtained at the scale σ is $\mathbf{H}^\sigma$ and the associated Hessian matrix along the surface is $\mathbf{M}^\sigma$, the surface deformation equation becomes,

$$\mathcal{C}_{\mathbf{t}} = -f(\mathbf{H}^{\arg\max_\sigma |\text{Tr}(\mathbf{M}^\sigma)|}; \boldsymbol{u}, \boldsymbol{v})\boldsymbol{n} - \alpha' \mathbf{G}(\mathbf{H}^{\arg\max_\sigma |\boldsymbol{n}^T \mathbf{H}^\sigma \boldsymbol{n}|}; \boldsymbol{n})\boldsymbol{n} + \gamma' \kappa \boldsymbol{n}, \quad (6)$$

where the terms $\arg\max_\sigma |\text{Tr}(\mathbf{M}^\sigma)|$ and $\arg\max_\sigma |\boldsymbol{n}^T \mathbf{H}^\sigma \boldsymbol{n}|$ select the scales that exhibit the largest second order intensity changes along the surface tangential plane and along the surface normal, among a set of pre-defined scales.

The solid surface is represented as the zero boundaries of the level set function [12]. The evolution of the level set function was implemented according to the description by Whitaker [13] and based on the Insight-Toolkits [14]. The level set function evolution was stopped when the change of the level set function was less than 0.0001 per segmented voxel over 40 evolution iterations. When the level set function is evolving, $\mathbf{H}$ in one scale is obtained in a 3∗3∗3 local window by taking central difference on one buffered image, which is Gaussian-smoothed before the evolution begins. $\mathbf{M}$ is retrieved from $\mathbf{H}$ and the surface tangents $\boldsymbol{u}$ and $\boldsymbol{v}$. Bilinear interpolation is used at the positions with non-integer coordinates. This procedure is repeated for each scale. The complexity of evaluating Eqn. 6 for one voxel is linear with respect to the number of scales used.

2.3 Properties of the Proposed Model

The function $f(\cdot)$ (Eqn. 5) has a large magnitude when the eigenvalues are negative, with large and similar magnitudes. This corresponds to the scenario that the surface is deforming along the vessel, as illustrated in Case 1 of Figs. 2b-d. In Cases 2 and 3 of Figs. 2b-d, the magnitudes of either one of or both of the eigenvalues of $\mathbf{M}^\sigma$ are small. In such cases, the resultant values of $f(\cdot)$ are suppressed by the exponential term. The surface is deformed according to the second and the third terms in the right hand side of Eqn. 6. The surface beyond vessel boundaries in Case 2 and the solid surface approaching the vessel boundary in Case 3 are expanded and shrunk respectively, according to the value of $\boldsymbol{n}^T \mathbf{H} \boldsymbol{n}$. The surface is in turn converged to the vessel boundary. Besides, Case 4 of Fig. 2 corresponds to the situation that the surface reaches the vessel boundary and the second order intensity variations along all directions are small. The deforming surface is therefore halted at the vessel boundary.

Regarding the parameters of the proposed model, the solid stress strength α' is used to specify how much the second order intensity change along the surface normal influences the speed of surface deformation. A small value of α' reduces the surface deformation speed induced by the second order intensity change along the surface normal. It causes the surface deforming aggressively along tubular structures. Enlarging the value of α' increases the chance of detecting non-tubular structures, such as, high curvature vessels or junctions. On the other

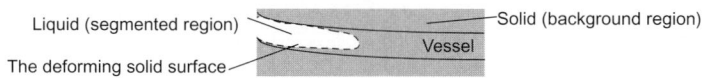

Fig. 1. The proposed deformable surface model

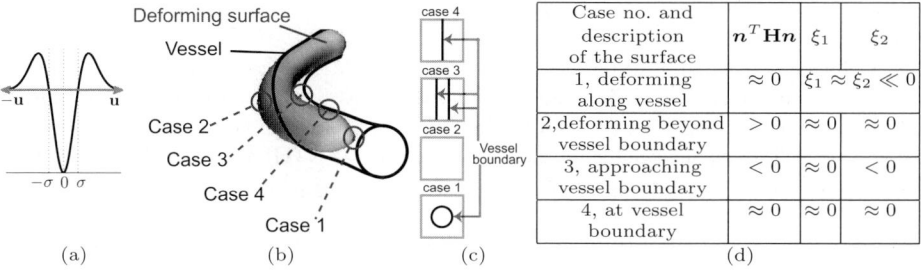

Fig. 2. (a) A plot of the second derivative of a Gaussian function along $\boldsymbol{u}$. (b) An example showing various situations when the surface is deforming to segment a vessel. (c) The surface tangential planes in different cases in (b). The black lines show the positions where the vessel boundary crosses the tangential planes. (d) The descriptions of various terms appeared in the definitions of $f(\cdot)$ and $\mathbf{G}(\cdot)$. σ is assumed to be the same as the vessel radius.

hand, the surface stress term of the solid (the third term in the right hand side of Eqn. 6) is analogous to the curvature regularization term which is commonly utilized in active contour methods. The value of γ' determines the smoothness of the resultant surface.

As the proposed model makes use of a 2D-circular-constraint (Eqn. 5), it exhibits extra flexibility on handling branches as compared to Hessian based methods which have a more restrictive 3D-tubular-constraint. Meanwhile, the proposed method inspects the second order intensity changes along the surface tangential plane and the surface normal direction separately. This makes our method more robust when the vessel intensity contrast varies rapidly along the vessel. The rapid change of vessel contrast can be caused by image noise or closely located objects with intensity similar to the vessels. A rapid change of vessel intensity contrast can significantly alter the directions of the image gradient and the principle directions of the Hessian matrix. It can undesirably terminate the deformation of the moving surface inside vessels in some deformable surface models, which are grounded on the image gradient [1][5] or the Hessian matrix [15]. For the proposed model, the intensity variations are measured along the directions defined by the deforming surface. When the surface is deforming along and inside vessels, the surface tangential plane at the evolving tip of the surface is equivalent to the vessel cross-sectional plane. Inspecting the intensity changes along the surface tangential plane is therefore able to capture the second order intensity changes along vessel cross-sectional plane. It consequently keeps the surface deforming along vessel despite of the rapid change of intensity contrast.

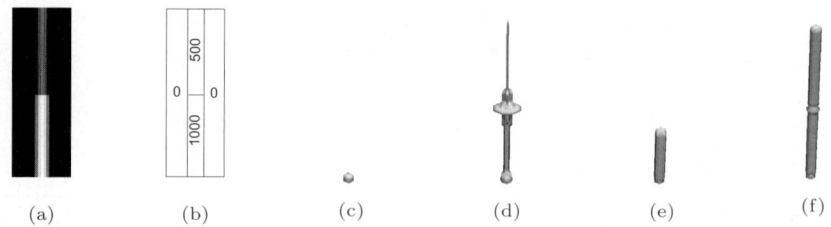

Fig. 3. The synthetic and numerical image volume with the size of $20 \times 20 \times 60$ voxels, consists of a vertical tube with a radius of 2 voxels. (a) The $x = 10$ slice of the image volume. (b) The intensity values in different parts of the image volume. (c) The initial surface. (d-f) The surface deformation results of $\mathcal{C}_t = -f(\mathbf{H}^{\arg\max_\sigma |\text{Tr}(\mathbf{M}^\sigma)|}; \boldsymbol{u}, \boldsymbol{v})\boldsymbol{n}$; $\mathcal{C}_t = -\mathbf{G}(\mathbf{H}^{\arg\max_\sigma |\boldsymbol{n}^T \mathbf{H}^\sigma \boldsymbol{n}|}; \boldsymbol{n})\boldsymbol{n}$; the proposed model using $\alpha' = 1$ and $\gamma' = 0$.

3 Experimental Results

The proposed method is validated by using four volumetric images: a numerical image volume consisting of a synthetic tube (Fig. 3a), an intracranial phase contrast magnetic resonance angiographic (PCMRA) image[1](Fig. 4a), an intracranial time-of-flight magnetic resonance angiographic (TOFMRA) image [1] (Fig. 4d) and a cardiac computed tomographic angiographic (CTA) image [2](Fig. 4g).

3.1 Synthetic Data

In this section, we employ a synthetic tube (Figs. 3a and b) which exaggerates a rapid change of intensity contrast along a vessel. With this rapid change of vessel intensity contrast, we demonstrate the behavior of the term involving the second order intensity change along the surface tangential plane, and the term involving the second order intensity change along surface normal in the surface deformation equation. These two terms are $f(\cdot)\boldsymbol{n}$ and $\mathbf{G}(\cdot)\boldsymbol{n}$ in Eqn. 6 respectively.

In this experiment, an initial surface is placed at the bottom of the tube (Fig. 3c). Two resultant surfaces are obtained by deforming this initial surface according to $\mathcal{C}_t = -f(\mathbf{H}^{\arg\max_\sigma |\text{Tr}(\mathbf{M}^\sigma)|}; \boldsymbol{u}, \boldsymbol{v})\boldsymbol{n}$ and $\mathcal{C}_t = -\mathbf{G}(\mathbf{H}^{\arg\max_\sigma |\boldsymbol{n}^T \mathbf{H}^\sigma \boldsymbol{n}|}; \boldsymbol{n})\boldsymbol{n}$. Five logarithmic scale samples are taken from the range of 1 to 5 voxel length. The resultant surfaces are shown in Figs. 3d and e respectively. Since the surface tangential plane at the evolving tip corresponds to the vessel cross-sectional plane, the deforming surface can propagate through the position where the tube intensity contrast changes. However, it cannot segment the entire tube as $f(\cdot)$ is small or zero when the surface tangential plane does not correspond to the vessel cross-sectional plane, where ξ_1 and ξ_2 are not both negative and with similar magnitudes (see Eqn. 5).

---

[1] Acquired using a Philips 3T ACS Gyroscan MR scanner without the use of contrast agent, at the University Hospital of Zurich, Switzerland.
[2] Rotterdam Coronary Artery Algorithm Evaluation Framework, "http://coronary.bigr.nl/"

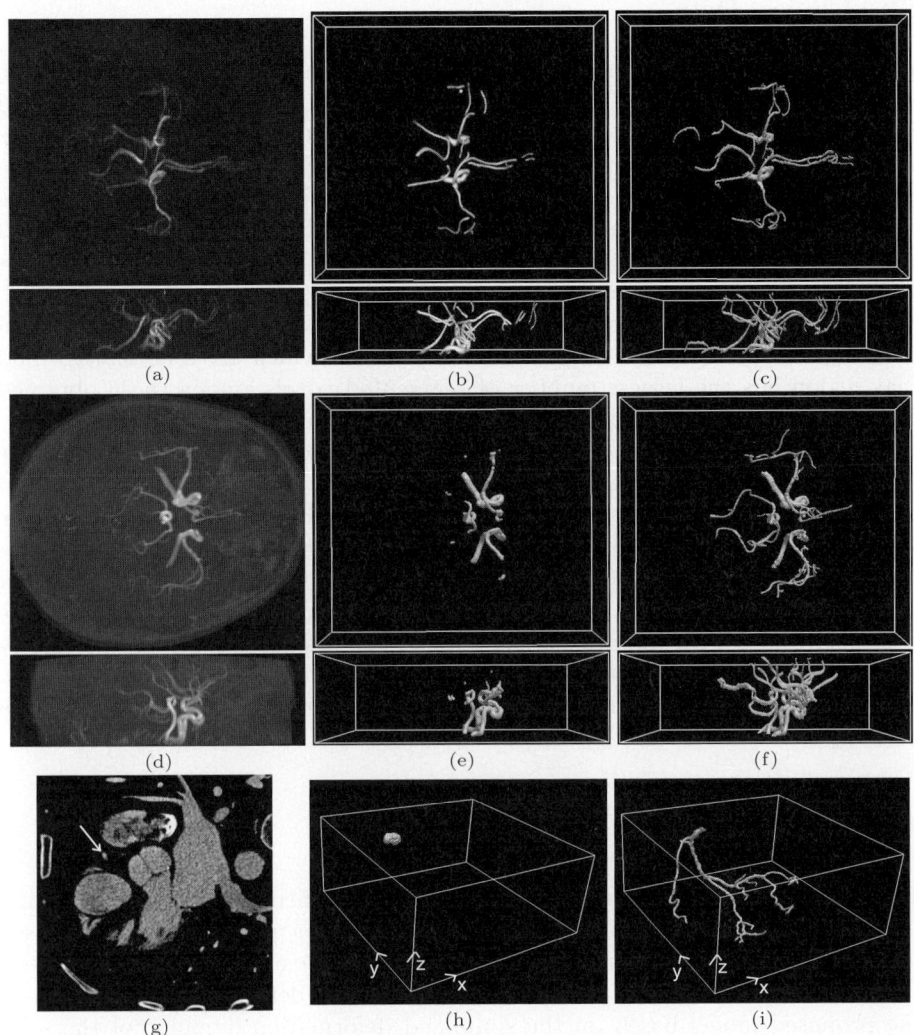

Fig. 4. (a, d, g) The three clinical datasets used in the experiments, an intracranial PCMRA image with $512 \times 512 \times 46$ voxels and voxel size of 0.39mm×0.39mm×0.8mm; an intracranial TOFMRA image with $512 \times 512 \times 60$ voxels and voxel size of 0.39mm×0.39mm×0.95mm; and the $z = 190$ slice of a cardiac CTA image with $512 \times 512 \times 190$ voxels and voxel size of 0.34mm×0.34mm×0.4mm, the white arrow points at the position where the initial surface/contour is placed. (b, e, h) The segmentation results using the CURVES algorithm. (c, f, i) The segmentation results using the proposed method.

Besides, in Fig. 3e, the deforming surface is halted by the rapid change of intensity contrast. Finally, by making use of both $f(\cdot)\boldsymbol{n}$ and $\mathbf{G}(\cdot)\boldsymbol{n}$, deforming the surface based on Eqn. 6 can segment the entire tube Fig. 3f, despite of the large change of tube intensity contrast.

3.2 Clinical Data

We have applied both our method and the CURVES algorithm [1] to segment the vasculatures in the three clinical datasets (Figs. 4a, d, g). The initial surface and contour of the proposed method and CURVES in the first and the second cases are obtained by thresholding the regions with 0.5% of the highest intensity in the entire image. In the CTA dataset, a single-voxel region manually placed in the right coronary artery is employed as the initial surface for the proposed method and the initial contour for CURVES. Five scale samples are obtained analogous to the synthetic experiment for the multiscale detection of the proposed model. The values of the parameters α' and γ' are 0.75 in all cases. For CURVES, in each dataset, we only show the segmented region which gives no leakage and that region has the largest number of segmented voxels among those obtained using various parameter values in the evolution equation of CURVES.

Comparing Figs. 4b and c, the proposed method is capable of segmenting more vessels in the PCMRA image. The main reason is that the analysis of the second order intensity variation along the surface tangential plane helps the surface deform along vessels, despite the present of intensity contrast variations along vascular structures. In the TOFMRA image and the CTA image, we have found that the evolving contours of CURVES leak frequently at the boundaries where adjacent tissues with intensity similar to vessels present. CURVES could only segment a small portion of the vessels (see Figs. 4e and h) before leakages happen. Besides, the proposed method has no problem to extract the vasculatures from the TOFMRA and the CTA images (Figs. 4f and i).

4 Discussion and Conclusion

The surface dynamics described in Eqn. 2 is a simplified case of the motion of a solid surface under liquid pressure in practice [16]. For instance, in the proposed model, the solid surface is assumed to be purely elastic and the bonding between the atoms on the solid surface does not break during deformation. Nevertheless, the proposed model based on the simplified deformation dynamic of the solid surface well serves the purpose of segmentation of vessels. Meanwhile, handling stenoses or aneurysms, and quantitative evaluation for a specific applications will be the future research directions of this work.

In summary, this paper proposes a novel physics-based deformable surface model for segmenting blood vessels in medical images. By considering the second order intensity statistics as various forces acting on the deforming surface, the proposed method allows the surface to propagate along vessels despite the presence of undesired intensity contrast fluctuations along vessels. The proposed method has been studied in the experiments using synthetic data, and compared with a classic deformable surface model, the CURVES algorithm [1], in the experiments using medical images acquired by various imaging modalities. It is demonstrated that the proposed method is well suited to segment vasculatures from medical images.

References

1. Lorigo, L., Faugeras, O., Grimson, W., Keriven, R., Kikinis, R., Nabavi, A., Westin, C.: Curves: Curve evolution for vessel segmentation. MedIA 5(3), 195–206 (2001)
2. Vasilevskiy, A., Siddiqi, K.: Flux maximizing geometric flows. PAMI 24(12), 1565–1578 (2002)
3. Rochery, M., Jermyn, I., Zerubia, J.: Higher order active contours. IJCV 69(1), 27–42 (2006)
4. Klein, A., Lee, F., Amini, A.: Quantitative coronary angiography with deformable spline models. TMI 16(5), 468–482 (1997)
5. Yan, P., Kassim, A.: Segmentation of volumetric mra images by using capillary active contour. MedIA 10(3), 317–329 (2006)
6. Nain, D., Yezzi, A., Turk, G.: Vessel segmentation using a shape driven flow. In: Barillot, C., Haynor, D.R., Hellier, P. (eds.) MICCAI 2004. LNCS, vol. 3216, pp. 51–59. Springer, Heidelberg (2004)
7. Weissmuller, J., Kramer, D.: Balance of force at curved solid metal - liquid electrolyte interfaces. Langmuir 21(10), 4592–4603 (2005)
8. Frangi, A., Niessen, W., Viergever, M.: Multiscale vessel enhancement filtering. In: Wells, W.M., Colchester, A.C.F., Delp, S.L. (eds.) MICCAI 1998. LNCS, vol. 1496, pp. 130–137. Springer, Heidelberg (1998)
9. Koller, T., Gerig, G., Szekely, G., Dettwiler, D.: Multiscale detection of curvilinear structures in 2-d and 3-d image data. In: IEEE International Conference on Computer Vision, pp. 864–869 (1995)
10. Sato, Y., Nakajima, S., Shiraga, N., Atsumi1, H., Yoshida, S., Koller, T., Gerig, G., Kikinis, R.: Three-dimensional multi-scale line filter for segmentation and visualization of curvilinear structures in medical images. MedIA 2(2), 143–168 (1998)
11. Gurtin, M., Weissmuller, J., Larche, F.: A general theory of curved deformable interfaces in solids at equilibrium. Philosophical Magazine 78(5), 1093–1109 (1998)
12. Malladi, R., Sethian, J., Vemuri, B.: Shape modeling with front propagation: A level set approach. PAMI 17(2), 158–175 (1995)
13. Whitaker, R.: A level-set approach to 3d reconstruction from range data. IJCV 29(33), 203–231 (1998)
14. Ibanez, L., Schroeder, W., Ng, L., Cates, J.: The ITK Software ToolKit
15. Descoteaux, M., Collins, L., Siddiqi, K.: Geometric flows for segmenting vasculature in MRI: Theory and validation. In: Barillot, C., Haynor, D.R., Hellier, P. (eds.) MICCAI 2004. LNCS, vol. 3216, pp. 500–507. Springer, Heidelberg (2004)
16. Kramer, D., Weissmuller, J.: Note on surface stress and surface tension and their interrelation via shuttleworth's equation and the lippmann equation. Surf. Sci. 601(14), 3042–3051 (2007)

A Deformation Tracking Approach to 4D Coronary Artery Tree Reconstruction

Yanghai Tsin[1], Klaus J. Kirchberg[1], Guenter Lauritsch[2], and Chenyang Xu[1]

[1] Siemens Corporate Research, Princeton, NJ, USA
[2] Siemens Healthcare, Forchheim, Germany
first_name.last_name@siemens.com

Abstract. This paper addresses reconstruction of a temporally deforming 3D coronary vessel tree, *i.e.*, 4D reconstruction from a sequence of angiographic X-ray images acquired by a rotating C-arm. Our algorithm starts from a 3D coronary tree that was reconstructed from images of one cardiac phase. Driven by gradient vector flow (GVF) fields, the method then estimates deformation such that projections of deformed models align with X-ray images of corresponding cardiac phases. To allow robust tracking of the coronary tree, the deformation estimation is regularized by smoothness and cyclic deformation constraints. Extensive qualitative and quantitative tests on clinical data sets suggest that our algorithm reconstructs accurate 4D coronary trees and regularized estimation significantly improves robustness. Our experiments also suggest that a hierarchy of deformation models with increasing complexities are desirable when input data are noisy or when the quality of the 3D model is low.

1 Introduction

A four dimensional (4D) representation of the coronary artery tree – *i.e.*, a temporally deforming 3D coronary artery model, would have many interesting applications, *e.g.*, motion compensated tomographic reconstruction, stenosis detection [1], foreshortening-free visualization, accurate measurement of cardiac motion parameters, and motion-based heart disease diagnosis. Automatic 4D reconstruction is challenging using traditional 2D cardiac monoplane or biplane angiograms due to difficulties with calibration and limited baselines, as shown by several prior studies [2,3,4]. This paper introduces a 4D reconstruction method using intra-operative rotational C-arm systems. Compared to biplane X-ray, rotational X-ray on a C-arm is clinically more prevalent, less costly, and it enables tomographic reconstruction.

4D reconstruction seems to have a straightforward solution: by repeating 3D reconstruction for every cardiac phase. However, this is not a viable solution in practice for several reasons. First, independent 3D reconstruction results in the loss of vessel branch correspondences, which are necessary for a diagnostically useful time-dynamic model. The second reason is related to the rotational acquisition protocol. As opposed to biplane X-ray, no two images are acquired at exactly the same heart phase. A small temporal offset can cause a significant spatial error for fast motion cardiac phases (e.g. in early systole [5]), rendering 3D reconstruction impractical. This is less of an issue for slowly moving cardiac phases. Indeed, there is research aimed at finding the optimal cardiac phase that are best for 3D coronary tree reconstruction [6].

In this work, starting from a successfully reconstructed 3D model [7] for a relatively static cardiac phase, we explicitly estimate coronary tree deformations from one cardiac phase to the next. Since we *track* deformations of the 3D coronary tree, this is a *4D reconstruction by deformation tracking* approach.

State-of-the-art work in coronary artery tree reconstruction was done by Blondel et al. [1]. The authors use 4D B-solids to model coronary motion with reported computation times of 15 to 30 minutes. Our approach is distinct in the following important ways. First, we derive the external force from *gradient vector flow (GVF)* [8] computed from the vessel enhancement filter responses (*"vesselness"*) [9]. GVF was proven to have superior capture range and convergence behavior over a regular gradient. It is also known that GVF is robust to noise perturbations, while 2D centerline extraction is extremely sensitive to noise, rendering centerline-based methods unstable in noisy sequences. Second, we adopted more robust motion models (rigid and affine), involving $90 \sim 180$ parameters, compared to the B-solid motion model used in [1] involving 30,000 parameters. Complex models have two known disadvantages, 1) costly to optimize; and more importantly 2) prone to over-fit noise. We show in our experiments that simpler 4D reconstruction algorithm is able to handle structural perturbations (due to missing branches) and heavy image noise perturbations more stably.

A biplane 4D reconstruction method is reported in [10]. Besides differences in the image acquisition procedures (thus different problems), the external driving forces (GVF versus gradient-based potential field) and data representations are different. In our work, we work directly on 3D point sets while the method in [10] requires a B-spline fitting preprocessing step that brings additional challenges such as selection of control points for B-spline and detecting bifurcation points. In the approach presented by Jandt et al. [11], the 4D motion vector field of the coronary tree is recovered by correspondence matching of multi-phase 3D centerline models. In contrast, our method circumvents the aforementioned inherent inaccuracy of 3D models reconstructed for high-velocity cardiac phases (see above) by requiring only one baseline 3D reconstruction. Furthermore, our approach solves the challenging correspondence problem implicitly.

Motion estimation is a well-studied topic in the computer vision community, *e.g.* [12] and [13]. Our problem differs from the traditional tracking problem in that image plane motions are induced by two major sources: the rotation of the projection plane around the patient, and nonrigid cardiac deformation. In our problem, the former is known given the calibrated C-arm rotation. What is left to be estimated is the cardiac deformation. In addition, a X-ray image is in its projective nature different from a photometric image, as it can be seen as a superposition of multiple transparent layers. 2D motion field estimation thus requires different techniques.

2 Method

In the following we denote vectors and matrices as boldface letters, e.g., $\mathbf{R}$. A letter with a tilde means that it is in a homogeneous coordinate, $\widetilde{\mathbf{X}}_n^{(p)} = \left[\mathbf{X}_n^{(p)T}, 1 \right]^T$. A letter with a prime, e.g., $\mathbf{u}', \mathbf{X}'$ represents deformation updated version of the same point (in 2D and 3D), $\mathbf{u}, \mathbf{X}$.

Problem Formulation. We are given a sequence of F X-ray images, $\mathcal{I} = \{\mathbf{I}_f\}$ and their corresponding projection matrices $\{\mathbf{P}_f\}$, $f = 1, 2, \ldots, F$, taken by an X-ray C-arm. Recorded ECG signals allow us to map each frame f into one of P discrete cardiac phases, $p = 0, 1, \ldots, P-1$. A 3D model of the coronary artery tree is reconstructed from a heart phase involving a low amount of motion. Without loss of generality, we term the optimal phase the *base phase* and denote it as phase 0. The model is in the form of a set of N 3D points, $\mathcal{X}^{(0)} = \left\{ \mathbf{X}_n^{(0)} \right\}$, $n = 1, 2, \ldots, N$. The problem is to infer a temporally deforming coronary artery tree, $\mathcal{X}^{(p)}$ for all cardiac phases, from the images, such that projections of $\mathcal{X}^{(p)}$ align with observations in all image frames corresponding to the cardiac phase.

Deformation Models. In this study, we model deformation of a coronary tree by two 3D parametric deformation models, i.e., *rigid* and *affine*. The affine model can capture the majority of the beating motion associated with the cardiac cycle. Both transformations can be represented by a compact 4×4 matrix $\mathbf{T}(\boldsymbol{\theta})$, where $\boldsymbol{\theta}$ is the vector of motion parameters. Forward and inverse mappings between $\mathbf{T}$ and $\boldsymbol{\theta}$ are assumed understood [14, Ch. 1.4 pp. 16].

A 4D Coronary Tree Model. Then deformation from phase $p-1$ to p is

$$\widetilde{\mathbf{X}}_n^{(p)} = \mathbf{T}\left(\boldsymbol{\theta}^{(p-1)} \right) \cdot \widetilde{\mathbf{X}}_n^{(p-1)} \qquad (1)$$

Note that all points in a 3D model $\mathbf{X}^{(p-1)}$ are deformed to the next phase by the same $\mathbf{T}$. By applying (1) recursively, we have

$$\widetilde{\mathbf{X}}_n^{(p)} = \left(\prod_{i=p-1}^{0} \mathbf{T}\left(\boldsymbol{\theta}^{(i)} \right) \right) \cdot \widetilde{\mathbf{X}}_n^{(0)} \doteq \mathcal{T}^{(p)}(\boldsymbol{\theta}) \cdot \widetilde{\mathbf{X}}_n^{(0)}, \qquad (2)$$

where $\mathcal{T}^{(p)}(\boldsymbol{\theta}) \doteq \prod_{i=p-1}^{0} \mathbf{T}\left(\boldsymbol{\theta}^{(i)} \right)$ is the *accumulative deformation* from frame 0 to p and $\boldsymbol{\theta} = (\boldsymbol{\theta}^{(0)T}, \ldots, \boldsymbol{\theta}^{(P-1)T})^T \in \mathcal{R}^{mP \times 1}$ is a concatenation of $\boldsymbol{\theta}^{(p)}$, and m is the parameter length (6 for rigid and 12 for affine).

Deformation Update. We adopt an iterative deformation update approach. Initially, the 4D coronary tree is trivial, i.e., $\mathcal{X}^{(p)} = \mathcal{X}^{(0)}, \forall p$. Due to cardiac deformations, projections of this trivial 4D coronary reconstruction will not align with the observed X-ray images except for the base phase. The iterative update approach then seeks to find updates to $\mathbf{T}^{(p)}, \forall p$, such that the projections progressively match towards the image observations. In the following, we will use a *compositional* update rule:

$$\mathbf{T}(\boldsymbol{\theta}^{(p)}) \leftarrow \mathbf{T}(\delta\boldsymbol{\theta}^{(p)}) \cdot \mathbf{T}(\boldsymbol{\theta}^{(p)}). \quad (3)$$

Put all the update parameters in a vector $\delta\boldsymbol{\theta} \doteq (\delta\boldsymbol{\theta}^{(0)T}, \ldots, \delta\boldsymbol{\theta}^{(P-1)T})^T \in \mathcal{R}^{mP \times 1}$ and by slight abuse of notation, denote

$$\mathcal{T}^{(p)}(\boldsymbol{\theta}, \delta\boldsymbol{\theta}) \doteq \prod_{i=p-1}^{0} \left(\mathbf{T}\left(\delta\boldsymbol{\theta}^{(i)}\right) \cdot \mathbf{T}\left(\boldsymbol{\theta}^{(i)}\right) \right) \quad (4)$$

as the *updated accumulative deformation*. An updated 2D projection $\widetilde{\mathbf{u}}'$ (in homogeneous coordinate) is derived by

$$\widetilde{\mathbf{u}}'_{nf}(\boldsymbol{\theta}, \delta\boldsymbol{\theta}) \doteq [x'_{nf}, y'_{nf}, z'_{nf}]^T \cong \mathbf{P}_f^{(p)} \cdot \mathcal{T}^{(p)}(\boldsymbol{\theta}, \delta\boldsymbol{\theta}) \cdot \widetilde{\mathbf{X}}_n^{(0)}. \quad (5)$$

where $\cong$ means equal up to a scale. Note that the phase-frame correspondence $p \leftrightarrow f$ is known given the recorded ECG signal. Next, the updated 2D projection in nonhomogeneous coordinate is

$$\mathbf{u}'_{nf} = \left[\frac{x'_{nf}}{z'_{nf}}, \frac{y'_{nf}}{z'_{nf}} \right]^T \approx \mathbf{u}_{nf} + \begin{bmatrix} \mathbf{d}_{1nf} \\ \mathbf{d}_{2nf} \end{bmatrix} \cdot \delta\boldsymbol{\theta} \quad (6)$$

where in the second (approximate) equality we used first order approximations and $\mathbf{d}_{knf}, k = 1, 2$ are *data term* related Jacobian for point n in frame f. Denote

$$\mathbf{v}_{nf} \doteq [v_{1nf}, v_{2nf}]^T \doteq \mathbf{u}'_{nf} - \mathbf{u}_{nf} \quad (7)$$

as the *desired vector flow* in a 2D image. Thus for each point n and a frame f, we have derived two linear constraints on the deformation update parameters,

$$\mathbf{d}_{knf}^T \cdot \delta\boldsymbol{\theta} \approx v_{knf}, \quad k = 1, 2. \quad (8)$$

In this study, we choose the gradient vector flow (GVF) field to provide v_{knf} due to many known advantages as stated previously in this paper.

Cyclic Deformation Constraints. Cardiac motions are cyclic, which implies that after a complete cycle, a point should end up at the same starting point,

$$\mathcal{T}^{(P)}(\boldsymbol{\theta}, \delta\boldsymbol{\theta}) \widetilde{\mathbf{X}}_n^{(0)} = \widetilde{\mathbf{X}}_n^{(0)}. \quad (9)$$

A first order approximation can be derive for each point $\mathbf{X}_n^{(0)}$

$$\mathbf{c}_{kn}^T \cdot \delta\boldsymbol{\theta} \approx c_{kn}, \quad k = 1, 2, 3 \quad (10)$$

each for a coordinate X, Y, Z. The right hand side has an intuitive explanation of *cyclic residues*, i.e., cyclic motion residue due to currently estimated deformation model $\boldsymbol{\theta}$. The above constraints express the requirement to make up for these residues using the deformation update $\delta\boldsymbol{\theta}$.

Smooth Deformation Constraints. Cardiac motions are smooth, which can be modeled by a Laplacian constraint,

$$\left(\mathcal{T}^{(p-1)}(\boldsymbol{\theta}, \delta\boldsymbol{\theta}) - 2 \cdot \mathcal{T}^{(p)}(\boldsymbol{\theta}, \delta\boldsymbol{\theta}) + \mathcal{T}^{(p+1)}(\boldsymbol{\theta}, \delta\boldsymbol{\theta}) \right) \cdot \widetilde{\mathbf{X}}_n^{(0)} = 0. \quad (11)$$

Again, a first order approximation can be derived,

$$\mathbf{s}_{kn}^{(p)T} \cdot \delta\boldsymbol{\theta} \approx s_{kn}^{(p)}, \quad k = 1, 2, 3. \tag{12}$$

The above constraints also has an intuitive interpretation: The deformation update (left) should make up for any non-smooth deformation (right side) due to the currently estimated deformation $\boldsymbol{\theta}$.

The Cost Function. Finally, by combining (8), (10), and (12), a cost function for 4D coronary tree reconstruction can be written as

$$\mathcal{C}\left(\delta\boldsymbol{\theta}\right) = \sum\nolimits_{f,n,k} \left(\left\| \mathbf{d}_{knf}^T \delta\boldsymbol{\theta} - v_{knf} \right\| + \lambda_s \left\| \mathbf{s}_{kn}^{(p)T} \delta\boldsymbol{\theta} - s_{kn}^{(p)} \right\| + \lambda_c \left\| \mathbf{c}_{kn}^T \delta\boldsymbol{\theta} - c_{kn} \right\| \right) \tag{13}$$

where λ_s and λ_c are weights for smoothness and cyclic constraints respectively. We use L_2 norm in this study. (13) can be solved efficiently using least-squares.

3 Results

The X-ray sequences for our experiments were acquired with a Siemens AXIOM-Artis C-arm system featuring a digital flat panel detector. The system has a constant source intensifier distance (SID), constant cranio/caudal angle and varying anterior/oblique angle, covering a range of 220 degrees. It is run in rotational acquisition mode, which is commonly used to reconstruct CT-like volumes. The C-arm is calibrated so that the perspective projection matrix for each image is known accurately and the acquisition is done under patient breath-hold. A contrast dye is injected into the coronary arteries immediately preceding the acquisition. In addition, the ECG signal is recorded in sync with the image sequence, which allows retrospective gating.

We designed the experiments to test the limits of our 4D reconstruction algorithm along two dimensions. Along the first dimension, we tested the influence of structural perturbation, utilizing 3D models of different quality and detail. The experiments were conducted with four 3D models on three distinct sequences of X-ray images. The first 3D model was constructed using a set of manually labeled vessel centerlines, which resulted in the best quality input 3D model (but still not perfect). The other 3D models were reconstructed fully automatically. The last 3D model contained only two branches that were almost coplanar, an ill-conditioned case for complex deformation models, including the affine model. Ground-truth vessel centerline segmentation was provided for quantitative evaluation of the first two experiments. All GVF fields were automatically computed from vesselness images [9]. We tested the algorithms on four variations: *un-regularized ($\lambda_s = \lambda_c = 0$) rigid* and *affine*, *regularized rigid* and *affine*. For all regularized methods, we used fixed regularization parameters $\lambda_s = 0.1$ and $\lambda_c = 1.0$. A cardiac cycle was divided into 15 discrete cardiac phases, *i.e*, $P = 15$.

Along the second dimension, we studied the influence of noise perturbations. We added zero mean Gaussian noise over 10 noise-levels ($\sigma = 0, 25, \ldots, 225$) to the X-ray images, whereas the input images have a dynamic range of 16 bit and

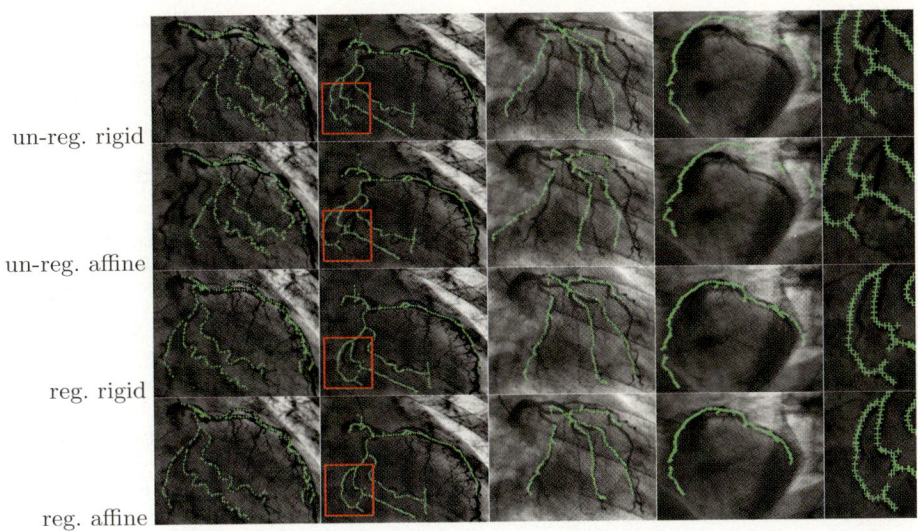

Fig. 1. 4D reconstruction results on the four 3D models. The regularized versions (the last two rows) outperformed the un-regularized versions (the first two rows). The last column shows enlarged views of red box bounded regions of the second column.

the gray value contrast of the major vessels ranged between 50 and 600. For each noise level, we conducted 20 trials of reconstruction using all four methods. For the first two experiments, we conducted 724 reconstructions each.

A qualitative overview of reconstruction results is provided in Figure 1. In general the regularized versions worked better than the non-regularized versions. For the first three cases, we could always find frames that regularized versions succeeded while the non-regularized versions failed, but not the other way around. For the last (ill-conditioned) case, however, we observed that 4D reconstruction using regularized affine was not stable. We could observe rapid shrinkage and expansion of a branch along the true vessel. This was a signature of an over-complex deformation model and noise overfitting.

For the first two experiments, where ground-truth vessel centerlines were available, we measured the 2D projection errors: the distances from projections of points on the 4D model to the nearest centerline point. Overall, 2D projection error has standard deviations about $3.2mm$ for the un-regularized versions and $1.9mm$ for the regularized versions. For the first case, the majority (72%) of the points have a projection error of less than $3mm$. Figure 2 shows errors averaged over all points, all frames and all 20 trials. The black line at the bottom shows the baseline error: average 2D projection error of the *base phase*. We can draw similar conclusions for both experiments. 1) The regularized versions resulted in lower 2D projection errors. 2) With good quality input, a more complex deformation model (affine) resulted in better reconstruction accuracy. 3) Over a large range of noise levels, the reconstruction accuracy did not suffer for the regularized versions. In addition to the effect of the regularization terms, the superior

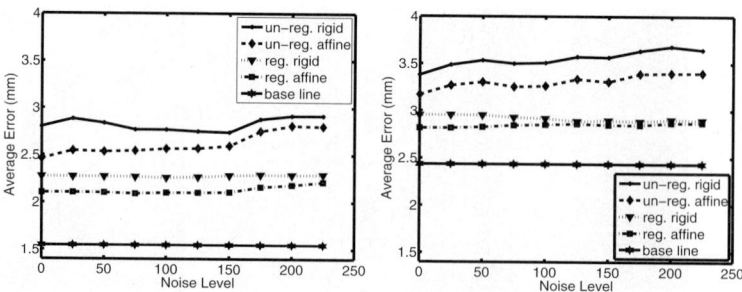

Fig. 2. Average 2D error. Left, using the best 3D model constructed from manually labeled vessel centerlines. Right, starting from a fully automatic 3D reconstruction.

noise-resistance capability of GVF helped. Our experiments show that even a moderate noise perturbation can change centerline extraction dramatically, rendering centerline-based methods [1] unstable.

To further understand how robust the algorithms were with respect to noise perturbation, we studied the variance $\hat{\sigma}^2$ of a reconstructed point $\mathbf{X}_{n,t}^{(p)}$ over all trials t. The variance is then averaged over all points and all three dimensions to give an average measurement. The first observation was that in all cases the simpler rigid model was more stable than the affine model (standard deviation $\hat{\sigma}$ on average 37% smaller). Also, as expected, the regularized versions were much more stable than the un-regularized counterparts ($\hat{\sigma}$ on average 66% smaller). Second and more interestingly, in the ill-conditioned case, regularized affine model resulted in a comparable standard deviation to un-regularized rigid, indicating instability of the former. It can be assumed that models more complex than affine would have suffered even more.

Finally, note that all 3D models contained less than 300 points, providing less than 600 constraints per frame. The B-solid model of Blondel et al. [1] required 1000 variables per frame, far larger than the number of constraints. Very strong regularization terms would be required for their method to succeed on our data. In the first experiment, deformation updates (13) converged in less than 10 seconds for the un-regularized methods, 30 and 90 seconds for regularized rigid and affine respectively, compared to 15 ∼ 30 minutes reported in [1].

4 Conclusions

We proposed a 4D coronary tree reconstruction by deformation tracking method in this paper. Its effectiveness is shown by our extensive experiments. Key elements of our method are 1) GVF as external force; 2) the regularization terms. Fast computation time makes this approach usable in an intra-operative scenario.

We also find that for well-conditioned problems, complex models matching true deformations provide better reconstruction accuracy. However, for ill-posed problems, simpler models or a hierarchical approach are preferred. The right balance between model complexity, data degeneracy and noise-level can be formally addressed by statistical model selection theories, *e.g.*, Geometric-AIC [15], which we leave as a future research topic.

References

1. Blondel, C., Malandain, G., Vaillant, R., Ayache, N.: Reconstruction of coronary arteries from a single rotational X-ray projection sequence. IEEE TMI 25(5), 653–663 (2006)
2. Chen, S., Carroll, J.: 3-D reconstruction of coronary arterial tree to optimize angiographic visualization. IEEE TMI 19(4), 318–336 (2000)
3. Chen, S.Y., Carroll, J.: Kinematic and deformation analysis of 4-D coronary arterial trees reconstructed from cine angiograms. IEEE TMI 22(6), 710–721 (2003)
4. Andriotis, A., Zifan, A., Gavaises, M., et al.: A new method of three-dimensional coronary artery reconstruction from X-ray angiography: validation against a virtual phantom and multislice computed tomography. Catheter Cardio Inte. 71(1), 28–43 (2008)
5. Husmann, L., Leschka, S., Desbiolles, L., et al.: Coronary artery motion and cardiac phases: dependency on heart rate – implications for CT image reconstruction. Radiology 245(2), 567–576 (2007)
6. Hansis, E., Schaefer, D., Doessel, O., Grass, M.: Automatic optimum phase point selection based on centerline consistency for 3D rotational coronary angiography. IJCARS 3(3), 355–361 (2008)
7. Liao, R., Sun, Y., Duong, L.: 3-D symbolic reconstruction of coronary artery tree from multiple views of rotational X-ray angiography. In: Proc. MICCAI-CVII, pp. 80–87 (2008)
8. Xu, C., Prince, J.: Snakes, shapes, and gradient vector flow. IEEE TIP 7(3), 359–369 (1998)
9. Frangi, A.F., Niessen, W.J., Vincken, K.L., Viergever, M.A.: Multiscale vessel enhancement filtering. In: Wells, W.M., Colchester, A.C.F., Delp, S.L. (eds.) MICCAI 1998. LNCS, vol. 1496, pp. 130–137. Springer, Heidelberg (1998)
10. Shechter, G., Devernay, F., Coste-Maniere, E., et al.: Three-dimensional motion tracking of coronary arteries in biplane cineangiograms. IEEE TMI 22(4), 493–503 (2003)
11. Jandt, U., Schäfer, D., Grass, M., Rasche, V.: Automatic generation of time resolved motion vector fields of coronary arteries and 4D surface extraction using rotational x-ray angiography. Phys. Med. Biol. 54(1), 45–64 (2009)
12. Bergen, J.R., Anandan, P., Hanna, K.J., Hingorani, R.: Hierarchical model-based motion estimation. In: Sandini, G. (ed.) ECCV 1992. LNCS, vol. 588, pp. 237–252. Springer, Heidelberg (1992)
13. Hager, G.D., Belhumeur, P.N.: Efficient region tracking with parametric models of geometry and illumination. IEEE TPAMI 20(10), 1025–1039 (1998)
14. Hartley, R.I., Zisserman, A.: Multiple View Geometry in Computer Vision, 1st edn. Cambridge University Press, Cambridge (2000)
15. Kanatani, K.: Statistical Optimization for Geometric Computation: Theory and Practice, 1st edn. North-Holland, Amsterdam (1996)

Automatic Extraction of Mandibular Nerve and Bone from Cone-Beam CT Data

Dagmar Kainmueller[1], Hans Lamecker[2], Heiko Seim[1],
Max Zinser[3], and Stefan Zachow[1]

[1] Zuse Institute Berlin, Germany
kainmueller@zib.de
[2] INRIA Sophia Antipolis, France
[3] Universitätsklinikum Köln, Germany

Abstract. The exact localization of the mandibular nerve with respect to the bone is important for applications in dental implantology and maxillofacial surgery. Cone beam computed tomography (CBCT), often also called digital volume tomography (DVT), is increasingly utilized in maxillofacial or dental imaging. Compared to conventional CT, however, soft tissue discrimination is worse due to a reduced dose. Thus, small structures like the alveolar nerves are even harder recognizable within the image data. We show that it is nonetheless possible to accurately reconstruct the 3D bone surface and the course of the nerve in a fully automatic fashion, with a method that is based on a combined statistical shape model of the nerve and the bone and a Dijkstra-based optimization procedure. Our method has been validated on 106 clinical datasets: the average reconstruction error for the bone is 0.5 ± 0.1 mm, and the nerve can be detected with an average error of 1.0 ± 0.6 mm.

1 Motivation and Contributions

Three-dimensional (3D) imaging has become an important technology for diagnosis and planning in dentistry and maxillofacial surgery [1]. Cone beam computed tomography (CBCT) yields an alternative to conventional CT because of its affordable costs as well as its reduced dose per examination. Thus, CBCT is likely to become a preferred imaging technique for dental practices. One major application for CBCT is dental implantology. Here, a primary concern is an optimal and stable placement of implants within the jaw bone without any impairment of the facial nerves. As a side effect of the low dose, however, the signal to noise ratio is not that high as with CT and soft tissue structures cannot be discriminated clearly. In addition the field of view (FoV) is small compared to conventional CT. This renders the exact localization of the mandibular nerve canal within the alveolar bone highly challenging.

Stein et al. [2] present a Dijkstra and balloon inflation based method for interactively segmenting the nerve canal in CT data, yet report only qualitatively good accordance on five datasets. Hanssen et al. [3] suggest a level-set approach for interactive 3D segmentation of the nerve canals in CBCT data, but do not present any quantitative validation. Rueda et al. [4] propose a semi-automatic system to perform 2D segmentation of the lower cortical and trabecular bone as well as to detect the nerve canal and center in specific 2D slices of conventional CT data. Their method is based on an active appearance model, and requires manual initialization. It yields an accuracy of 1.6 mm for the cortical bone, and 3.4 mm for the dental nerve on 215 single 2D slices in the CT data. More recently, Yau et al. [5] proposed a semi-automatic method to segment the nerve canal from conventional CT data. It requires the user to manually specify a seed point for a subsequent automatic adaptive region-growing approach in consecutive slices of the CT data. However, no quantitative validation was performed.

In contrast to existing work, our method is based on (1) 3D segmentation of the complete mandibular bone surface and (2) localization of the 3D course of the mandibular nerve, both in a fully automatic manner. Instead of relying on conventional CT data, our method operates on CBCT data, an imaging modality increasingly used in clinical routine. Our approach yields an accuracy that significantly surpasses the 2D results of Rueda et al. [4]. It is based on a combined statistical shape model (SSM) of the bone surface and the course of the nerve, which extends the work of Zachow et al. [6]. In order to match the SSM to CBCT data we extend the work of Lamecker et al. [7] in two major ways: (1) We use a modified version of the algorithm presented in Seim et al. [8] to segment the mandibular bone surface. Here, we adapt image feature extraction to the characteristics of mandibular CBCT data. (2) We improve an initial reconstruction of the nerves' position derived from the SSM using a Dijkstra-based tracing algorithm tailored to the specific characteristics of CBCT data.

2 Image Data

CBCT scanners aim for a compromise between image quality and dose, and hence produce images of lesser quality than conventional CT. For our study 106 datasets of complete mandibles were availible from a PACS at the University Hospital of Cologne, Germany, all of which acquired with a Sirona Galileos CBCT at the maxillofacial surgery department (patients of age 16 to 71, 56 female, 50 male). CBCT imaging is performed routinely in cases of suspected orbital floor fractures, mandibular condyle evaluation, wisdom teeth removal, abscesses, etc. Images are taken in seated position with a scan duration of about 15 seconds. All images consist of 512^3 voxels with an isotropic voxel size of 0.3 mm. The FoV is approx. 15 cm^3. The X-ray source is operated at 85 kV with a tube current of 5-7 mA. Fig. 1, right, depicts typical slices through such data. In each dataset the bone as well as the nerve canal were interactively labelled by an experienced dentist using the Amira software.

3 Statistical Shape Model

The SSM is generated on the basis of the CBCT datasets described in Sec. 2. For each mandibular bone a surface model is generated from the labellings, while for

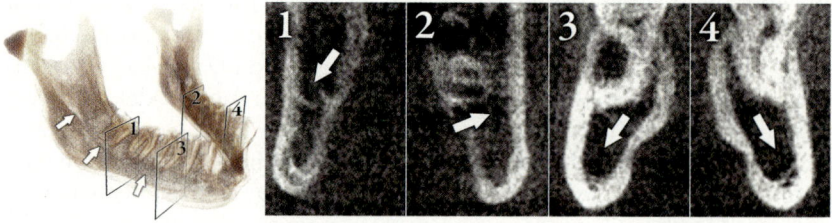

Fig. 1. Volume rendering (left) and coronal slices (right) of CBCT data. Arrows indicate the location of the nerve canal.

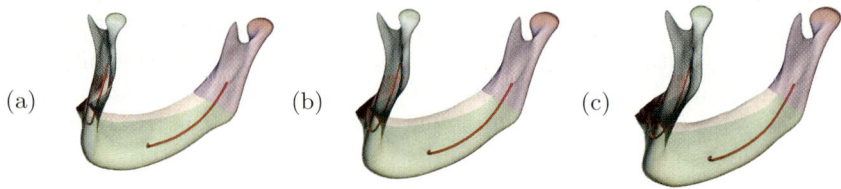

Fig. 2. SSM of mandible bone and nerves: mean shape (b), 1st mode of variation (a/c)

each pair of nerve canals piecewise linear center lines are computed using a skeletonization algorithm [9]. To create the point distribution model underlying the SSM, correspondence must be established between both the bone surfaces and the nerve lines. We use the method of consistent patch decomposition and parameterization to create surface correspondences, see [7] for details. The mandibular surface model is divided into eight patches (Fig. 2) that are bounded by characteristic feature lines, detectable on every mandible. The teeth are not considered in the SSM due to an individually varying dentition state. For the nerves, we consistently resampled the center lines of the segmented nerve canals with a fixed number of points equally spaced starting at the mental foramen. After resampling all 106 mandibular shapes with a common reference mesh (triangulation for bone surface, piecewise linear segments for nerve) and aligning them in a common frame of reference, Principal Component Analysis (PCA) is performed. The SSM is then represented as a bi-linear function $S(b,T) = T(\overline{v} + \sum_k b_k \cdot p_k)$ of the weights b_k of the PCA-eigenmodes p_k, and a global affine transformation T of the coordinates. $\overline{v}$ is the average shape vector, whose dimension is three times the number of bone (8561) and nerve (200) points.

4 SSM-Based Reconstruction of Bone and Nerve

The SSM based method for reconstruction of the mandibular bone and nerves in CBCT data is composed of a preprocessing of the image data with a 3D median filter, a position initialization and a subsequent image driven adaptation of the SSM described in Sec. 3. We adapted an approach for pelvis segmentation [8] to the task of mandible segmentation. Note that only the mandible bone is adapted to image features, while the mandibular nerves are derived from the SSM.

Initialization. The pose initialization of the mandible SSM in CBCT data, that is based on the Generalized Hough Transform (GHT), closely follows a global approach for 3D object detection introduced by Khoshelham [10].

Image Driven SSM Adaptation. Segmentation using the SSM is the task of iteratively finding transformation and shape parameters (b, T) such that the shape $S(b, T)$ approximates the unknown target shape R^* as good as possible. Let $R^i = S(b^i, T^i)$ denote the segmentation in iteration i: A *displacement* vector field ΔR^i is computed that assigns a vector Δr_j to each vertex j of R^i. ΔR^i describes the desired deformation of the model towards R^* in the underlying image data I. Then, both transformation parameters T and shape parameters b are adapted to the target shape $(R^i + \Delta R^i)$, as originally proposed by Cootes et al. [11]. The following paragraph explains how ΔR^i is generated.

Image Features. The displacement vector field ΔR for surface R is computed by analyzing 1D *intensity profiles* in the image data $I : \mathbb{R}^3 \to \mathbb{R}$: For each vertex j of R, I is sampled over a length L along the surface normal u_j at vertex position v_j. A cost function $c_j : P_j \to \mathbb{R}_0^+$ is computed on the set of sampling points $P_j = \{v_j^n := v_j + (\frac{n-1}{N_j-1} - 0.5) \cdot L \cdot u_j \ : \ 1 \leq n \leq N_j\}$. The displacement vector at vertex j is then defined as $\Delta r_j = v_j^* - v_j$, with $v_j^* = \mathrm{argmin}_{v_j^n} c_j(v_j^n)$. Dropping the indices for clarity, we define the cost at a sampling point $c(v) =$

$$\begin{cases} (2i+1)\left(\frac{-g}{dI(v)} + 2\frac{|N-n|}{N}\right) & \text{if } I(v) \in [t+iw, t+(i+1)w] \wedge dI(v) < -g, i = 0, 1, 2 \\ 7\left(\frac{-g}{dI(v)} + 2\frac{|N-n|}{N}\right) & \text{if } I(v) \in [t, t+3w] \text{ and } -g < dI(v) < -0.5 \cdot g \\ 30 + 2\frac{|N-n|}{N} & \text{else.} \end{cases}$$

Here, t and w define an intensity threshold and window width, and g a threshold for gradient magnitude. $dI(v)$ denotes the directional derivative of I along u.

5 Dijkstra-Based Optimization of Nerve Reconstruction

SSM-adaptation as described in Sec. 4 yields an accurate reconstruction of the mandible bone, as well as approximate nerve reconstructions. The SSM-based nerve reconstructions are not based on any image features, but are merely derived by the SSM. We use them as initialization for a Dijkstra-based optimization method. The SSM-based bone reconstruction is also utilized by excluding the area outside the reconstructed bone from the search space for the nerve. The key idea of our method is to build a graph through which the path with minimal cost from source to target is basically the "darkest tunnel" through the image data, while regions where a dark tunnel is surrounded by a brighter border are of particular interest. To achieve this, a graph with weighted edges is built based on the approximate nerve reconstruction as described in the following. Note that all indices used for graph description start at 1, unless stated otherwise.

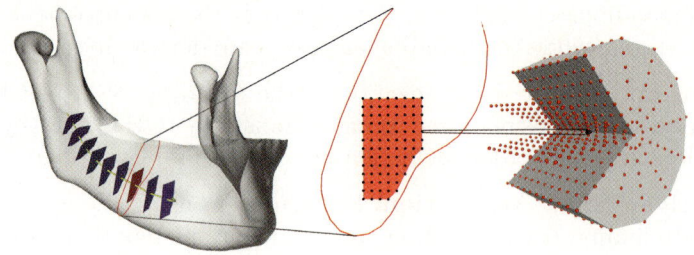

Fig. 3. Dijkstra Optimization. (left) Normal planes along initial nerve reconstruction. (middle) Graph nodes on a normal plane. (right) Sampling cylinder at a graph node.

Graph Nodes. For each point $\boldsymbol{p}_k$ at index k of the piecewise linear initial nerve representation, equidistantly distributed points in the normal plane at $\boldsymbol{p}_k$ serve as graph nodes. Fig. 3 shows some exemplary normal planes (left) and a normal plane with graph nodes (middle). The normal plane at $\boldsymbol{p}_k$ is spanned by two directions perpendicular to the line tangent $\boldsymbol{t}_k$, namely $\boldsymbol{y}_k = \boldsymbol{t}_k \times \boldsymbol{x}_{data}$, where $\boldsymbol{x}_{data}$ is the x-axis of the image data coordinate system, and $\boldsymbol{x}_k = \boldsymbol{y}_k \times \boldsymbol{t}_k$. A graph node is described by k and its indices i, j on the normal plane. Let N_i, N_j be the number of nodes and X, Y the lengths for which the normal plane is considered in x_k- and y_k- direction, respectively. The position of node (k, i, j) is then $\boldsymbol{p}_{k,i,j} = \boldsymbol{p}_k + (\frac{i-1}{N_i-1} - 0.5) \cdot X \cdot \boldsymbol{x}_k + (\frac{j-1}{N_j-1} - 0.5) \cdot Y \cdot \boldsymbol{y}_k$. In addition to these nodes, two "artificial" nodes serve as source and target of the graph.

Graph Edges. The graph contains directional edges from each node (k, i, j) to all nodes $(k+1, i+di, j+dj)$ with $di, dj \in \{-1, 0, 1\}$, as well as directional edges from the source to all nodes with $k = 1$, and from all nodes with $k = N$ to the target, where N is the number of points on the nerve representation.

Edge Weights. For any edge starting at node (k, i, j), a scalar cost function c, evaluated at position $\boldsymbol{p}_{k,i,j}$, serves as edge weight. For edges starting at the source node, the edge weights are 0. The cost $c(\boldsymbol{p}_{k,i,j})$ is computed from intensities sampled inside a cylinder with center $\boldsymbol{p}_{k,i,j}$, orientation $\boldsymbol{t}_k$, some length H and radius R. Fig. 3 (right) shows an exemplary cylinder with its sampling points. A sampling point is described by a length index h, a radius index r, and an angle index a. Let N_h be the number of sampling points in length direction, N_r the number of sampling points along a radius, and N_a the number of angles for which radii are sampled. Then the position of sampling point (h, r, a) is $\boldsymbol{p}_0 + \frac{h-1}{N_h-1} \cdot H \cdot \boldsymbol{t}_k + \frac{r-1}{N_r-1} \cdot R \cdot \boldsymbol{r}_a$ with $\boldsymbol{r}_a$ being a normalized radius vector, rotated by an angle $\frac{a-1}{N_a-1} * 2\pi$ around $\boldsymbol{t}_k$, and $\boldsymbol{p}_0 = \boldsymbol{p}_{k,i,j} - 0.5 \cdot H \cdot \boldsymbol{t}_k$. Note that for $r = 1$, no angle index is necessary to describe the sample point.

To determine the cost $c(\boldsymbol{p}_{k,i,j})$, the unfiltered image intensities at the cylinder sampling points are evaluated as follows: The mean "inner" intensity mi and standard deviation si is computed from all sampling points with r no bigger than an "inner radius index" r_i. For each angle index a, the mean "border" intensity mb_a and standard deviation sb_a is computed from all sampling points

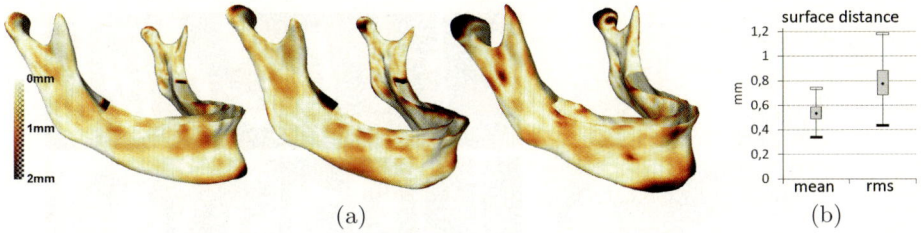

Fig. 4. Surface reconstruction with statistical shape model. (a) Color encodes distance to gold standard surface. from left to right: good, average and bad case. (b) Average surface distance error metrics.

with $r > r_i$ and r no bigger than a "border radius index" r_b. Furthermore, the mean "outside" intensity mo_a is computed for each angle index a from all sampling points with $r > r_b$. The number cf of angle indices is counted for which $mb_a - 0.1 \cdot sb_a > mi + si$ and $mb_a - 0.1 \cdot sb_a > mo_a$. Then the cost is $c(\boldsymbol{p}_{k,i,j}) = mi - 50 \cdot cf$. If a graph node position $\boldsymbol{p}_{k,i,j}$ lies outside the mandibular bone as reconstructed by the SSM, the cost is set to infinity.

6 Results

We evaluated the SSM based reconstruction as well as the Dijkstra based optimization (OPT) described in Sec. 4 and 5 on the 106 CBCT datasets described in Sec. 2. For each dataset, before performing SSM based reconstruction, the respective training shape was removed from the mandible SSM described in Sec. 3, i.e. the evaluation was conducted in a leave-one-out manner. The respective training shape that has been left out serves as gold standard reconstruction for both bone and nerves.

From experiment, we set our method's parameters as follows: SSM adaptation: consider 80 shape modes. Image features: $L = 6$ mm, $t = 350$, $w = 180$, $g = 150/\mathrm{mm}$. Optimization, graph nodes: $X = 12$ mm, $Y = 7$ mm, $N_i = 121$, $N_j = 71$, cylinder: $L = 3$ mm, $R = 2.1$ mm, $N_l = 11$, $N_r = 8$, $N_a = 12$, $r_i = 4$, $r_b = 6$.

The average errors for the mandible surface reconstructions as compared to the respective gold standard surfaces are: mean, root mean square (rms) and maximum surface distance: 0.5 ± 0.1 mm, 0.8 ± 0.2 mm, and 6.2 ± 2.3 mm, see also Fig. 4(b). Fig. 4(a) shows exemplary reconstructions and their distances to the respective gold standard surface. Apart from errors around the teeth, the largest errors occur at the mental protuberance and the condyles, due to the increasing noise towards the fringe of the field of view. The average mean curve distances for the SSM based nerve reconstructions are 1.7 ± 0.7 mm (right nerve), and 2.0 ± 0.8 mm (left nerve).

For the optimized nerve reconstructions, the average mean curve distances to the respective gold standard nerve are 1.0 ± 0.6 mm (right nerve), and 1.2 ± 0.9 mm (left nerve). The average fraction of the optimized reconstruction that lies within the gold standard nerve canal is $80 \pm 24\%$ (right nerve), and $74 \pm$

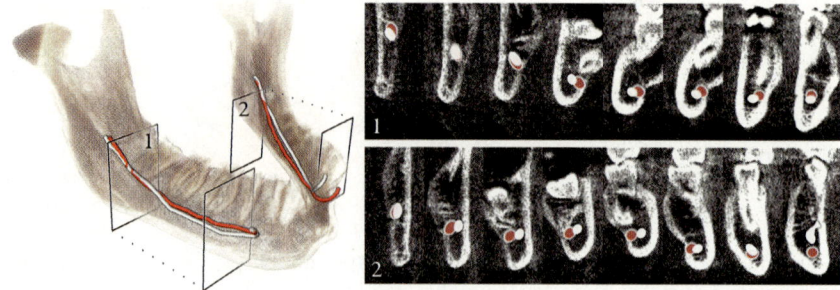

Fig. 5. Reconstruction by optimization, exemplary case for a bad reconstruction. White line: gold standard nerve. Red line: reconstructed nerve. Error measures for this case: Mean distance to gold standard nerve: right 1.5 mm, left 2.1 mm. Fraction that lies within the gold standard nerve canal: right 45%, left 30%.

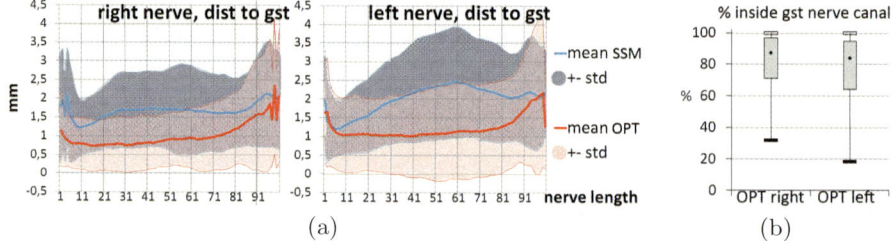

Fig. 6. (a) Average reconstruction error (SSM and OPT) along the nerve from posterior to anterior end (1..100). (b) Nerve fraction within gold standard nerve canal.

27% (left nerve), see also Fig. 6(b). Fig. 5 shows an exemplary optimized nerve reconstruction with high reconstruction error. Fig. 6(a) shows the average curve distance of SSM based and optimized nerve reconstructions per point along the curve. This illustrates that the optimization method is able to reduce the reconstruction error significantly in a region in the middle of each nerve, while the reduction is not that obvious towards the ends of each nerve.

7 Conclusions and Future Work

We presented an accurate and robust method to automatically reconstruct a geometric 3D model of the mandible including the course of the alveolar nerve from CBCT data. There is still room for improvement of the nerve reconstruction, especially concerning the ends of the nerve canal. In this work we chose a conceptually simple approach for nerve detection, yet other methods for tracing tubular structures may be considered, e.g. as described for vessel detection, see for instance [12,13] and references therein.

In future work, the statistical shape model shall be extended to distinguish cortical and trabecular bone as well. Furthermore, a mid-term goal is to find a way to incorporate the teeth, too. This is more challenging since the number of teeth may vary between patients, especially in clinical cases, and it is not quite clear how to incorporate topological changes into the model.

Acknowledgments. D. Kainmueller is funded by the DFG collaborative research center SFB 760.

References

1. Schramm, A., Rücker, M., Sakka, N., Schoen, R., Dueker, J., Gellrich, N.C.: The use of cone beam CT in cranio-maxillofacial surgery. In: Lemke, H., Inamura, K., Doi, K., Vannier, M., Farman, A. (eds.) CARS. Int. Congress Series, vol. 1281, pp. 1200–1204. Elsevier, Amsterdam (2005)
2. Stein, W., Hassfeld, S., Muhling, J.: Tracing of thin tubular structures in computer tomographic data. Computer Aided Surgery 3, 83–88 (1998)
3. Hanssen, N., Burgielski, Z., Jansen, T., Lievin, M., Ritter, L., von Rymon-Lipinski, B., Keeve, E.: Nerves - level sets for interactive 3d segmentation of nerve channels. In: ISBI, pp. 201–204 (2004)
4. Rueda, S., Gil, J.A., Pichery, R., Raya, M.A.: Automatic segmentation of jaw tissues in CT using active appearance models and semi-automatic landmarking. In: Larsen, R., Nielsen, M., Sporring, J. (eds.) MICCAI 2006. LNCS, vol. 4190, pp. 167–174. Springer, Heidelberg (2006)
5. Yau, H.T., Lin, Y.K., Tsou, L.S., Lee, C.Y.: An adaptive region growing method to segment inferior alveolar nerve canal from 3d medical images for dental implant surgery. Computer-Aided Design and Applications 5(5), 743–752 (2008)
6. Zachow, S., Lamecker, H., Elsholtz, B., Stiller, M.: Is the course of the mandibular nerve deducible from the shape of the mandible? Int. J. Computer Assisted Radiology and Surgery 1(1), 415–417 (2006)
7. Lamecker, H., Zachow, S., Wittmers, A., Weber, B., Hege, H.C., Elsholtz, B., Stiller, M.: Automatic segmentation of mandibles in low-dose CT-data. Int. J. Computer Assisted Radiology and Surgery 1(1), 393–395 (2006)
8. Seim, H., Kainmueller, D., Heller, M., Lamecker, H., Zachow, S., Hege, H.C.: Automatic segmentation of the pelvic bones from CT data based on a statistical shape model. In: EG Workshop on VCBM, Delft, Netherlands, pp. 93–100 (2008)
9. Sato, M., Bitter, I., Bende, M., Kaufman, A., Nakajima, M.: TEASAR: Tree-structure extraction algorithm for accurate and robust skeletons. In: Barsky, B.A., Shinagawa, Y., Wang, W. (eds.) Proc. Pacific Graph. Conf. on Comp. Graph. and Application, pp. 281–289. IEEE, Los Alamitos (2000)
10. Khoshelham, K.: Extending generalized hough transform to detect 3d objects in laser range data. In: Rönnholm, P., Hyyppä, H., Hyyppä, J. (eds.) Proc. ISPRS Workshop Laser Scanning and SilviLaser. IAPRS, vol. 36, pp. 206–211 (2007)
11. Cootes, T.F., Taylor, C.J., Cooper, D.H., Graham, J.: Active Shape Models - Their Training and Application. Comput. Vis. Image Underst. 61(1), 38–59 (1995)
12. Wong, W.C., Chung, A.C.: Probabilistic vessel axis tracing and its application to vessel segmentation with stream surfaces and minimum cost paths. Medical Image Analysis 11(6), 567–587 (2007)
13. Poon, K., Hamarneh, G., Abugharbieh, R.: Live-vessel: Extending livewire for simultaneous extraction of optimal medial and boundary paths in vascular images. In: Ayache, N., Ourselin, S., Maeder, A. (eds.) MICCAI 2007, Part II. LNCS, vol. 4792, pp. 444–451. Springer, Heidelberg (2007)

Conditional Variability of Statistical Shape Models Based on Surrogate Variables

Rémi Blanc[1], Mauricio Reyes[2], Christof Seiler[1], and Gábor Székely[1]

[1] Computer Vision Laboratory, ETHZ,
Sternwartstrasse 7, 8092 Zürich, Switzerland
{blanc,szekely}@vision.ee.ethz.ch
[2] ARTORG Center for Biomedical Engineering Research, University of Bern,
Stauffacherstrasse 78, 3014 Bern, Switzerland
{christof.seiler,mauricio.reyes}@artorg.unibe.ch

Abstract. We propose to increment a statistical shape model with surrogate variables such as anatomical measurements and patient-related information, allowing conditioning the shape distribution to follow prescribed anatomical constraints. The method is applied to a shape model of the human femur, modeling the joint density of shape and anatomical parameters as a kernel density. Results show that it allows for a fast, intuitive and anatomically meaningful control on the shape deformations and an effective conditioning of the shape distribution, allowing the analysis of the remaining shape variability and relations between shape and anatomy. The approach can be further employed for initializing elastic registration methods such as Active Shape Models, improving their regularization term and reducing the search space for the optimization.

1 Introduction

Statistical Shape Models [1] (SSM) are increasingly used for medical image analysis. For segmentation purposes, they allow making use of prior anatomical knowledge for compensating low contrast and high noise level in the images. SSM are also used for regularizing elastic registration algorithms [2], so that the estimated shape is both anatomically plausible and matches the image information. Recent extensions use them for predicting unobserved parts of a shape [3,4], or even predicting the shape of one organ from the observation of another [5].

The general idea behind SSM is to perform a linear decomposition of the shape variability by defining modes of deformations through various mathematical criteria. The most commonly used, Principal Component Analysis (PCA), estimates orthogonal directions which iteratively maximize the variance. Other linear decompositions have been proposed, based on Principal Factor Analysis (PFA) methods [6], or Independent Component Analysis (ICA) [7,8] which define modes of deformations which are, among other characteristics, more localized and easier to interpret. However, these modes, resulting from purely mathematical criteria, seldom correspond to deformations which have a direct, anatomically meaningful interpretation [6]. [9]

proposed to estimate the remaining variability of a shape model after fixing a part of it, by calculating the conditional distribution under a multivariate normal assumption. However, due to rank deficiency problems, they had to allow for limited random deviations from the observations, too, in order to allow for any remaining variability. Consequently, the conditional distribution they estimated is strongly dependent on the level of tolerated variability. In the context of surgical simulators, [10] employed a non-linear optimization approach for estimating the most probable shape within a SSM, satisfying exact constraints on characteristic dimensions of the uterus. Nevertheless, the remaining shape variability is not explicitly assessed. The approach neither allows to consider generic patient information such as height, weight or age for restricting the shape model, while these certainly impose morphological constraints, e.g. for bony structures.

We propose in this paper to extend linear SSM description in order to provide with intuitive anatomical control over shape deformations, by explicitly integrating such anatomical information within the model. Section 2 recalls basics about SSM and introduces notations employed throughout the paper. In section 3, we present a method for conditioning the shape distribution based on a set of surrogate variables, in particular for non-parametric kernel densities. In section 4, we apply the method to a shape model of the human femur, and evaluate the effectiveness of the conditioning. Conclusions and perspectives are summarized in Section 5.

2 Statistical Shape Models

Statistical shape models aim at describing the natural variability of a shape, e.g. the morphological manifestations of an organ over different individuals or through time. Such models usually rely on a specific parameterization of a set of training shapes $\mathbf{z}_i, i \in \{1,...,n\}$, e.g. by a set of d landmarks in correspondence across the various shapes [11], usually lying on the shape's outline. Through this parameterization, the k-dimensional shape, $k \in \{2;3\}$, is stored as a column vector with $p = kd$ elements, and can be viewed as a single point in a p-dimensional space. A collection of different instances of a shape, e.g. the same organ observed for different individuals, then corresponds to a point cloud in the parameterized space. This point cloud contains the information about the shape's variability observed from the available samples and can be analyzed using multivariate statistical techniques [12].

The most classical approaches for shape modeling are linear, in the sense that any shape $\mathbf{z}$ is described as a linear combination of a set of r modes of deformations:

$$\mathbf{z} \approx \mathbf{Ub} + \mathbf{m}, \text{ with } \mathbf{m} = \frac{1}{n}\sum_{i=1}^{n}\mathbf{z}_i \text{ and } \mathbf{b} = \mathbf{U}^T(\mathbf{z}-\mathbf{m}) \tag{1}$$

The different existing approach differ in the definition of the modes of deformation $\mathbf{U}$. PCA searches orthogonal modes which iteratively maximize the variance, and can make use of the Singular Value Decomposition to efficiently estimate them. The more general PFA can use other criteria, which usually define orthogonal rotations of the PCA modes. In particular, the varimax rotation [13] intends to cluster the modes of deformations so that each mode has a large influence over only a limited number of variables, and nearly no impact on the others [6]. ICA includes higher order moments, such as skewness or negentropy [8], in order to find directions in which the shape deformations are as independent as possible. It was shown to perform better than PCA when the shape distribution is significantly non-gaussian [7].

Whichever method is chosen, the subspace of admissible shapes is spanned by the r modes of deformation retained by $\mathbf{U}$, and the $r-$ variate distribution of the model parameters $\mathbf{b}_i$, $i \in \{1,...,n\}$ observed on the training samples allow to define compact models for the shape distribution. In the following, we will restrict to PCA, for which the domain of plausible shapes is usually defined by constraining every parameter to be within a $[-3\sigma;3\sigma]$ interval, σ^2 being the corresponding eigenvalue.

3 Conditioning the Shape Distribution with Surrogate Variables

Though a shape is explicitly represented by its parameterization, using either $\mathbf{z}$ or more conveniently the r parameters $\mathbf{b}$, it is more intuitive to describe a shape through a set of anatomically meaningful measures, such as lengths, angles, curvatures, etc. Those measures can be obtained either through an automatic procedure or defined manually as functions of landmarks of a reference shape, taking advantage of established correspondences allowing a consistent definition across the different samples available. It is also possible to include surrogates which are not directly related to the organ's shape, but provide generic information about the patient, such as its age, height or weight, which is likely to correlate with morphology. This set of surrogate variables $\mathbf{x}_i$, $i \in \{1,...,n\}$ offer an easily interpretable description, and can be used for controlling the predicted shape.

By concatenating the surrogates $\mathbf{x}_i$ to the shape parameters $\mathbf{b}_i$, the set of n training examples form samples from the joint multivariate distribution $p(\mathbf{b},\mathbf{x})$, which can be exploited to condition the shape to follow prescribed anatomical constraints. Indeed, the conditional distribution $p(\mathbf{b}|\mathbf{x}=\mathbf{x}_0)$ of the shape parameters given specific values $\mathbf{x}=\mathbf{x}_0$ for the surrogates, is directly given by Bayes theorem:

$$p(\mathbf{b}|\mathbf{x}=\mathbf{x}_0) = \frac{p(\mathbf{b},\mathbf{x}_0)}{p(\mathbf{x}_0)} \quad (2)$$

where $p(\mathbf{x}_0)$ stands for the marginal probability density of $\mathbf{x}$ evaluated at $\mathbf{x}_0$.

Assuming that $p(\mathbf{b},\mathbf{x})$ follows a multivariate Gaussian distribution, with mean $\boldsymbol{\mu}$ and covariance $\boldsymbol{\Sigma}$, the conditional distribution $p(\mathbf{b}|\mathbf{x}=\mathbf{x}_0)$ is known [12 p.87] to be also Gaussian, with mean and covariance given by:

$$\begin{aligned}\boldsymbol{\mu}_{\mathbf{b}|\mathbf{x}_0} &= E\left[\mathbf{b}|\mathbf{x}=\mathbf{x}_0\right] = \boldsymbol{\mu}_\mathbf{b} + \boldsymbol{\Sigma}_{\mathbf{bx}}\boldsymbol{\Sigma}_{\mathbf{xx}}^{-1}(\mathbf{x}_0-\boldsymbol{\mu}_\mathbf{x}) \\ \boldsymbol{\Sigma}_{\mathbf{bb}|\mathbf{x}_0} &= Cov\left[\mathbf{b}|\mathbf{x}=\mathbf{x}_0\right] = \boldsymbol{\Sigma}_{\mathbf{bb}} - \boldsymbol{\Sigma}_{\mathbf{bx}}\boldsymbol{\Sigma}_{\mathbf{xx}}^{-1}\boldsymbol{\Sigma}_{\mathbf{bx}}^T\end{aligned} \quad (3)$$

where the different variables are taken from $\boldsymbol{\mu}$ and $\boldsymbol{\Sigma}$:

$$\boldsymbol{\mu} = \begin{bmatrix}\boldsymbol{\mu}_\mathbf{b} \\ \boldsymbol{\mu}_\mathbf{x}\end{bmatrix} = \begin{bmatrix}E[\mathbf{b}] \\ E[\mathbf{x}]\end{bmatrix} \text{ and } \boldsymbol{\Sigma} = \begin{bmatrix}\boldsymbol{\Sigma}_{\mathbf{bb}} & \boldsymbol{\Sigma}_{\mathbf{bx}} \\ \boldsymbol{\Sigma}_{\mathbf{bx}}^T & \boldsymbol{\Sigma}_{\mathbf{xx}}\end{bmatrix} = \begin{bmatrix}Cov(\mathbf{b},\mathbf{b}) & Cov(\mathbf{b},\mathbf{x}) \\ Cov(\mathbf{x},\mathbf{b}) & Cov(\mathbf{x},\mathbf{x})\end{bmatrix} \quad (4)$$

Unless there are more surrogate variables than available samples in the training set, the only reason for Σ_{xx} not to be invertible is that some surrogates are linear combinations of the others, which means that they could be safely ignored.

Nevertheless, the Gaussian assumption may not always be realistic, especially when considering surrogates related to distances or angles. A non-parametric alternative is to rely on kernel density estimation [14], and to model the joint density $p(\mathbf{x},\mathbf{b})$ as follows, by averaging the contribution of each training sample:

$$p(\mathbf{b},\mathbf{x}) = \frac{1}{n}\sum_{i=1}^{n} K_{\mathbf{H}}(\mathbf{b}_i - \mathbf{b}, \mathbf{x}_i - \mathbf{x}) \tag{5}$$

where $K_{\mathbf{H}}$ is a normalized multivariate kernel function with bandwidth matrix $\mathbf{H}$. Choosing a Gaussian kernel, $K_{\mathbf{H}}$ is the classical Gaussian density, with zero mean and covariance $\mathbf{W} = \mathbf{H}^2$. For this case it can be shown that the conditional mean and conditional covariance are given by:

$$\boldsymbol{\mu}_{\mathbf{b}|\mathbf{x}_0} = \sum_{i=1}^{n} w_i \boldsymbol{\mu}_{\mathbf{b}|\mathbf{x}_0}^{(i)} \;;\; \Sigma_{\mathbf{bb}|\mathbf{x}_0} = \sum_{i=1}^{n} w_i \left(\mathbf{W}_{\mathbf{bb}|\mathbf{x}_0} + \left(\boldsymbol{\mu}_{\mathbf{b}|\mathbf{x}_0}^{(i)} - \boldsymbol{\mu}_{\mathbf{b}|\mathbf{x}_0}\right)\left(\boldsymbol{\mu}_{\mathbf{b}|\mathbf{x}_0}^{(i)} - \boldsymbol{\mu}_{\mathbf{b}|\mathbf{x}_0}\right)^T \right) \tag{6}$$

with,

$$w_i = \frac{K_{\mathbf{H}_x}(\mathbf{x}_0 - \mathbf{x}_i)}{\sum_{j=1}^{n} K_{\mathbf{H}_x}(\mathbf{x}_0 - \mathbf{x}_j)} \;;\; \boldsymbol{\mu}_{\mathbf{b}|\mathbf{x}_0}^{(i)} = \mathbf{b}_i + \mathbf{W}_{\mathbf{bx}} \mathbf{W}_{\mathbf{xx}}^{-1}(\mathbf{x}_0 - \mathbf{x}_i) \;;\; \mathbf{W}_{\mathbf{bb}|\mathbf{x}_0} = \mathbf{W}_{\mathbf{bb}} - \mathbf{W}_{\mathbf{bx}} \mathbf{W}_{\mathbf{xx}}^{-1} \mathbf{W}_{\mathbf{bx}}^T \tag{7}$$

There is a general agreement that the "shape" of the kernel $K_{\mathbf{H}}$ is much less important than the choice of the bandwidth [14 chap.2]. However, full multivariate bandwidth selection is still a difficult issue. A data-driven method has been proposed in [16], where the optimal bandwidth is estimated through a Markov Chain Monte Carlo approach (MCMC). Unfortunately, this approach is still very expensive for high-dimensional distributions. A general rule of thumb for the bandwidth matrix is to choose $\mathbf{H}$ proportional to $\Sigma^{1/2}$ [15 p. 152].

Once the conditional distribution has been calculated, random shapes following the prescribed constraints can be drawn by sampling from $p(\mathbf{b}|\mathbf{x} = \mathbf{x}_0)$. A sample from the conditional distribution can be generated by first selecting i with probability w_i and then drawing a sample from the Gaussian distribution with mean $\boldsymbol{\mu}_{\mathbf{b}|\mathbf{x}_0}^{(i)}$ and covariance $\mathbf{W}_{\mathbf{bb}|\mathbf{x}_0}$.

Such samples are classical shape parameters, and the plausibility of the corresponding shapes can be evaluated by observing their likelihood in the original, unconditional SSM. In the following, we rely on such random samples to evaluate the effectiveness of the conditioning, by comparing the prescribed values of the anatomical parameters with values measured on those shapes.

4 Application to the Human Femur

In this section, we illustrate the concepts developed above on a 3D statistical model of the human femur. The model consists of $n = 170$ femurs obtained from CT scans. The images have been registered using the non-rigid diffeomorphic registration technique proposed by [17]. A mesh, consisting of $d = 23536$ vertices ($p = 70608$), was extracted from the segmentation of the reference bone, and propagated to the other samples using the correspondences obtained during the volumetric registration step. The SSM is defined by this set of meshes. The parameters $\mathbf{b}_i$, $i \in \{1,...,n\}$ were computed using a PCA, keeping 99,9% of the variance ($r = 144$) in order to preserve the shape distribution as much as possible while reducing the dimensionality of the problem and avoiding numerical instabilities in the computations of the densities.

A set of anatomical surrogate variables has been defined as functions of manually selected vertices of our model, based on [18] and as illustrated on Fig. 1. Thanks to the established correspondences, these measurements $\mathbf{x}_i$, $i \in \{1,...,n\}$ are defined in a reproducible way over shapes from the SSM. Additionally, the age (>21 years), height (between 150 and 181 cm) and weight (between 42 and 140 kg) of each subject was recorded. The gender was also recorded (55% males) but not used in the following.

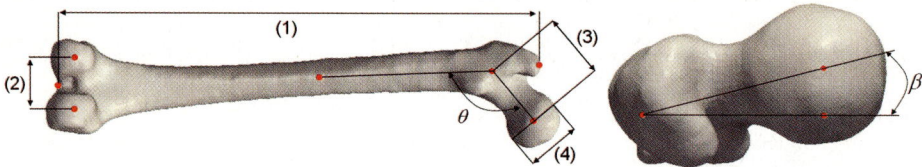

Fig. 1. Reference bone and definition of surrogate variables: femur length **(1)**, inter-condyle distance **(2)**, neck length **(3)**, vertical head diameter **(4)**, collo-diaphysal (neck/shaft) angle θ and anteversion angle β. The distances are stored in *mm*, and the angles in *degrees*.

The joint distribution $p(\mathbf{x}, \mathbf{b})$ was modeled through a gaussian kernel density. Using the rule of thumb presented above, the optimal bandwidth matrix was estimated as $\mathbf{W} = 0.59\,\Sigma$. The retained proportionality factor has been obtained through the optimization of the Kullback-Leibler information criterion, as proposed by [16]. For different combinations of the variables used for conditioning, we estimated the corresponding conditional distribution $p(\mathbf{b}|\mathbf{x} = \mathbf{x}_0)$. Three such combinations used in the following are presented in Table 1. Due to imperfect shape representation through the SSM, a limited number of training shapes, and the fact that the estimation of the conditional distribution does no rely on any known relation between the surrogate variables and the position of the shape vertices, synthetic shapes generated from the conditional distribution may not follow perfectly the prescribed constraints. Consequently, we evaluated the effectiveness of the conditioning by drawing 5000 random shapes from the estimated conditional distribution, and computed the anatomical measurements described on Fig. 1. As can be seen on Table 2, the conditional distributions do not exhibit significant biases and present a low variance, indicating that the conditioning is quite effecitve.

By comparing the traces of the covariance matrices of the joint and conditional distributions for various choices of the conditioning surrogates, their relative influence on the variability of the full shape or of individual morphological parameters can be investigated. This also can provide information about correlations among the surrogates. For example, looking at "Conditions 3", conditioning on the age, weight and height already reduced the shape variability by nearly 50%, especially constraining the femur length while letting the angle β mostly unaffected.

Table 1. Three different choices of the conditioning variables and their values

Surrogates	(1)	(2)	(3)	(4)	θ	β	age	height	weight
Conditions 1	441.75	66.22	72.03	(free)	(free)	9.36	(free)	(free)	(free)
Conditions 2	(free)	63.28	64.52	46.03	115.16	11.07	(free)	(free)	(free)
Conditions 3	(free)	(free)	(free)	(free)	(free)	(free)	40	180	65

Table 2. Effectiveness of the anatomical conditioning. The "% bias" column indicates the observed bias on the prescribed values of the surrogates for the shapes of the conditional distribution. For the variables which were left unconstrained, the observed mean is given instead. The "% var" column indicates the remaining variance of the anatomical measures.

Surrogate variables	Initial distribution		Conditions 1		Conditions 2		Conditions 3	
	mean	std	% bias	% var	% bias	% var	% bias	% var
(1)	426.62	26.63	0.01 %	0.01%	(424.39)	(28.76%)	(458.60)	(32.75%)
(2)	56.68	6.50	-0.07 %	0.61%	0.06 %	0.59%	(58.85)	(54.27%)
(3)	66.34	5.73	0.09 %	0.51 %	0.04 %	0.24 %	(71.22)	(50.45%)
(4)	46.55	4.88	(50.02)	(30.05%)	0.07 %	0.48 %	(48.79)	(46.98%)
θ	115.08	5.48	(112.33)	(34.35%)	-0.08 %	0.63 %	(115.33)	(58.21%)
β	10.87	2.15	1.33 %	1.34 %	0.14 %	1.32 %	(10.71)	(87.10%)
Remaining shape variability			15.03 %		34.06 %		47.74 %	

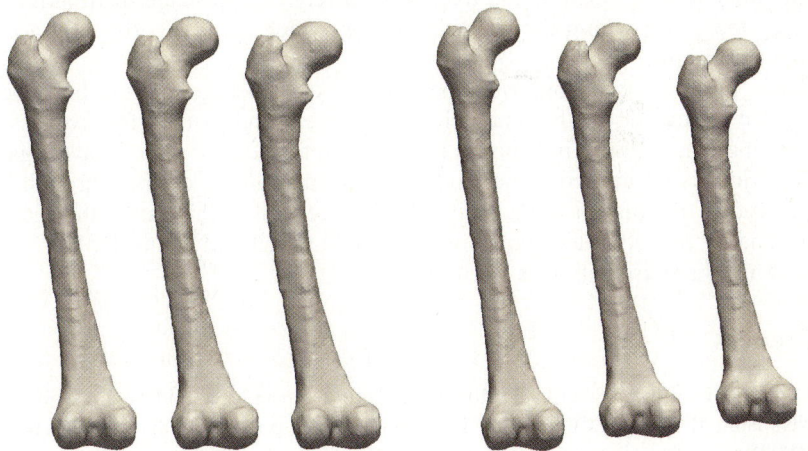

Fig. 2. The three femurs on the left (resp. right) correspond to samples for the Conditional Distribution 1 (resp. 2) defined in Table 1. For both groups, the central bone correspond to the conditional mean, while the bone on the left (resp. right) correspond to variations related to the main mode of the conditional shape covariance, with coefficient -2 (resp. +2).

The conditional covariance matrix $\Sigma_{bb|x_0}$ has been further diagonalized, so as to define orthogonal modes of deformations for the remaining shape variability. For the first two conditional distributions of Table 1, the shape corresponding to the conditional mean and deformations of +/-2 times the standard deviation of the main mode of remaining covariance are represented on Fig. 2. For conditional distribution 1, the femur length remains approximately constant while the remaining variability seems to be mostly related to the unconstrained neck/shaft angle θ. On the other hand, the femur length is clearly dominating the remaining variability of the 2nd distribution, while other parameters do not significantly vary. The obtained shapes were found to be generally plausible – from the initial SSM viewpoint –, as long as the constraints were themselves realistic.

5 Conclusion

In this paper we show how to incorporate explicit anatomical constraints in statistical shape models, in the form of surrogate variables. The conditional shape distribution allows analyzing the remaining shape variability, as well as drawing plausible random shapes following specific anatomical constraints. The method was demonstrated and validated on a statistical shape model of the human femur.

Besides the potential interest for anatomy and morphometry studies, the approach can be further used in conjunction with classical SSM-based registration methods, by providing an initialization of the shape following easily measurable surrogate variables, optimizing the likelihood term used for regularization and reducing the size of the search space. In particular, we plan to adapt the method for SSM of organs subject to respiratory motion, such as the liver, and to rely on the shape distribution conditioned by the phase within the breathing cycle, which could significantly accelerate tracking algorithms.

Finally, in our experiments, we experienced a clear deterioration in both the accuracy of the estimation of the anatomical parameters and in the effectiveness of the conditioning when fewer eigenmodes have been retained. We plan to investigate how this behaviour is influenced if the modes of deformation are defined through PFA or ICA instead of relying on PCA analysis. More generally, this raises the interest for dimensionality reduction techniques which would specifically consider the fidelity of the anatomical representation as a criterion.

References

1. Cootes, T.F., Edwards, G.J., Taylor, C.J.: Active appearance models. In: Burkhardt, H., Neumann, B. (eds.) ECCV 1998. LNCS, vol. 1407, pp. 484–498. Springer, Heidelberg (1998)
2. Kelemen, A., Székely, G., Gerig, G.: Elastic model-based segmentation of 3-D neuroradiological data sets. IEEE Trans. on Medical Imaging 18(10), 828–839 (1999)
3. Rajamani, K.T., Hug, J., Nolte, L.-P., Styner, M.: Bone Morphing with statistical shape models for enhanced visualization. In: Proc. SPIE, vol. 5367, pp. 122–130 (2004)
4. Rao, A., Aljabar, P., Rueckert, D.: Hierarchical statistical shape analysis and prediction of sub-cortical brain structures. Medical Image Analysis 12, 55–68 (2008)

5. Yang, Y.M., Rueckert, D., Bull, A.M.J.: Predicting the shapes of bones at a joint: application to the shoulder. Computer Methods in Biomech. and Biomed. Eng. 11(1), 19–30 (2008)
6. Reyes Aguirre, M., Linguraru, M.G., Marias, K., Ayache, N., Nolte, L.P., Gonzalez Ballester, M.A.: Statistical Shape Analysis via Principal Factor Analysis. In: IEEE International Symposium on Biomedical Imaging (ISBI), pp. 1216–1219 (2007)
7. Üzümcü, M., Frangi, A.F., Sonka, M., Reiber, J.H.C., Lelieveldt, B.: ICA vs. PCA active appearance models: Application to cardiac MR segmentation. In: Ellis, R.E., Peters, T.M. (eds.) MICCAI 2003. LNCS, vol. 2878, pp. 451–458. Springer, Heidelberg (2003)
8. Üzümcü, M., Frangi, A.F., Reiber, J.H.C., Lelieveldt, B.P.F.: Independent Component Analysis in Statistical Shape Models. In: Medical Imaging 2003: Image Processing, Proceedings of SPIE, vol. 5032, pp. 375–383 (2003)
9. Albrecht, T., Knothe, R., Vetter, T.: Modeling the Remaining Flexibility of Partially Fixed Statistical Shape Models. In: Workshop on the Mathematical Foundations of Computational Anatomy, MFCA 2008, New York, USA, September 6 (2008)
10. Sierra, R., Zsemlye, G., Székely, G., Bajka, M.: Generation of variable anatomical models for surgical training simulators. Medical Image Analysis 10, 275–285 (2006)
11. Styner, M.A., Rajamani, K.T., Nolte, L.-P., Zsemlye, G., Székely, G., Taylor, C.J., Davies, R.H.: Evaluation of 3D correspondence methods for model building. In: Taylor, C.J., Noble, J.A. (eds.) IPMI 2003. LNCS, vol. 2732, pp. 63–75. Springer, Heidelberg (2003)
12. Timm, N.H.: Applied Multivariate Statistics. Springer, Heidelberg (2002)
13. Abdi, H.: Factor rotations. In: Lewis-Beck, M., Bryman, A., Futing, T. (eds.) Encyclopedia for research methods for the social sciences, pp. 978–982. Sage, Thousand Oaks (2003)
14. Wand, M.P., Jones, M.C.: Kernel Smoothing. Monographs on Statistics and Applied Probability, vol. 60. Chapman & Hall, Boca Raton (1995)
15. Scott, D.W.: Multivariate Density Estimation: Theory, Practice, and Visualization. J. Wiley & Sons, Chichester (1992)
16. Zhang, X., King, M.L., Hyndman, R.J.: Bandwidth Selection for Multivariate Kernel Density using MCMC. In: Australasian Meetings, p. 120. Econometric Society (2004)
17. Vercauteren, T., Pennec, X., Perchant, A., Ayache, N.: Diffeomorphic Demons: Efficient Non-parametric Image Registration. NeuroImage 45(Suppl. 1), 61–72 (2009)
18. Samaha, A.A., Ivanov, A.V., Haddad, J.J., Kolesnik, A.I., Baydoun, S., Yashina, I.N., Samaha, R.A., Ivanov, D.A.: Biomechanical and system analysis of the human femoral bone: correlation and anatomical approach. Journal of Orthopaedic Surgery and Research 2, 8 (2007)

Surface/Volume-Based Articulated 3D Spine Inference through Markov Random Fields*

Samuel Kadoury and Nikos Paragios

Laboratoire MAS, Ecole Centrale de Paris, France
{samuel.kadoury,nikos.paragios}@ecp.fr
GALEN Group, INRIA Saclay, Ile-de-France, France

Abstract. This paper presents a method towards inferring personalized 3D spine models to intraoperative CT data acquired for corrective spinal surgery. An accurate 3D reconstruction from standard X-rays is obtained before surgery to provide the geometry of vertebrae. The outcome of this procedure is used as basis to derive an articulated spine model that is represented by consecutive sets of intervertebral articulations relative to rotation and translation parameters (6 degrees of freedom). Inference with respect to the model parameters is then performed using an integrated and interconnected Markov Random Field graph that involves singleton and pairwise costs. Singleton potentials measure the support from the data (surface or image-based) with respect to the model parameters, while pairwise constraints encode geometrical dependencies between vertebrae. Optimization of model parameters in a multi-modal context is achieved using efficient linear programming and duality. We show successful image registration results from simulated and real data experiments aimed for image-guidance fusion.

1 Introduction

Spinal deformity pathologies such as idiopathic scoliosis are complex three-dimensional (3D) deformations of the trunk, described as a lateral deviation of the spine combined with asymmetric deformation of the vertebrae. Surgical treatment usually involves correction of the scoliotic curves with preshaped metal rods anchored in the vertebrae with screws and arthrodesis (bone fusion) of the intervertebral articulations. This long procedure can be complex since it requires high level of precision for inserting pedicle screws through the spinal canal [1,2].

With recent advances in medical imaging enabling CT acquisitions during the surgical procedure, real-time fusion of anatomical structures obtained from various modalities becomes feasible. It offers the unique advantage to visualize anatomy during intervention and localize anatomical regions without segmenting operative images. By fusing the 3D volume images such as CT, C-arm CT [2] or

---

* This work was partially supported by an FQRNT grant. The authors would like to thank Philippe Labelle from Sainte-Justine Hospital for data processing.

MR with an accurate preoperative model, the surgeon can see the position and orientation of the instrumentation tools on precise anatomical models in real time. In this work, we take advantage of a personalized preoperative 3D model which reflects the detailed geometry of the patient's spine from standard biplanar X-rays. While the morphology of each vertebra remains identical between initial exam and surgery, intervertebral orientation and translation vary substantially.

Registration of intraoperative fluoroscopic images and preoperative CT/MR images has been proposed to aid interventional and surgical orthopedic procedures [3]. For example in [4,5], 3D models obtained from CT or MR were registered to 2D X-ray and fluoroscopic images using gradient amplitudes for optimizing the correspondence of single bone structures. Similar objective functions using surface normals from statistical PDMs [6] were applied for the femur. In spine registration however, one important drawback is that each vertebra is treated individually instead of as a global shape. An articulated model may allow to account for the global geometrical representation [7] by incorporating knowledge-based intervertebral constraints. These 3D intervertebral transformations were transposed in [8] to accomplish the segmentation of the spinal cord from CT images, but multi-modal registration has yet to be solved. Optimization is also based on gradient-descent, prone to non-linearity and local minimums. These methods require segmentation of 3D data or fluoroscopic image, which itself is a challenging problem and has a direct impact on registration accuracy.

In this paper, we propose a framework for registering preoperative 3D articulated spine models in a standing position to lying intraoperative 3D CT images. The general approach is described as follows. We first use a personalized 3D spine reconstructed from biplanar X-rays to derive an articulated model represented with intervertebral transformations. We then formulate inference through a Markov Random Field (MRF) model, proposing an image-based registration which avoids CT image segmentation, is computational efficient (few seconds) and with known optimality bounds. The optimization integrates prior knowledge to constrain the adjustment of intervertebral links between neighboring objects of the articulated model with pairwise potentials, as well as modular image data-terms. One of the applications is to help surgeons treat complicated deformity cases by fusing high-resolution preoperative models for increased accuracy of pedicle screw insertion, reducing surgery time. Sections 2 and 3 presents the method in terms of geometric modeling and MRF inference. Experiments are showed in Section 4, with a discussion in Section 5.

2 Personalized 3D Reconstruction of Articulated Spines

2.1 Preoperative Spine 3D Reconstruction

From calibrated coronal and sagittal X-ray images of the patient's spine, the personalized 3D model is achieved by means of a reconstruction method merging statistical and image-based models based on the work of [9]. The patient's spine centerline is first embedded onto a 3D database containing scoliotic spines to predict an initial model with 17 vertebrae (12 thoracic, 5 lumbar), 6 points

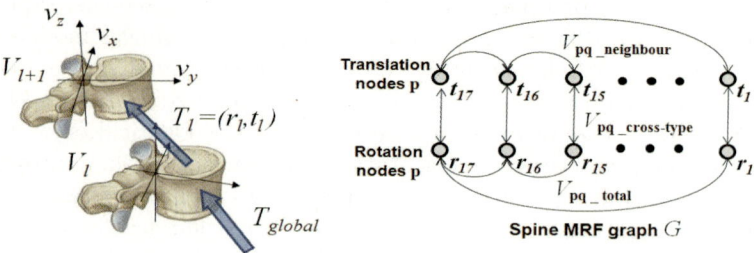

Fig. 1. Articulated spine in an MRF graph, integrating three types of constrained pairwise potentials

per vertebra (4 pedicle tips and 2 endplate midpoints). This crude statistical 3D model is then refined with an individual scoliotic vertebra segmentation approach by extending 2D geodesic active regions in 3D, in order to evolve prior deformable 3D surfaces. An atlas of vertebral meshes $S_i = \{x_{i1}, ..., x_{iN}\}$ with triangles x_j are initially positioned and oriented from their respective 6 precise landmarks s_i composing X_{preop}, and the surface is evolved so that the projected silhouettes of the morphed 3D models would therefore match the 2D information on the biplanar X-rays. At the end of process, the 3D landmark coordinates s_i and corresponding polygonal vertebral meshes S_i are optimal with regards to statistical distribution and image correspondences.

2.2 Articulated Spine Model

The 3D landmarks s_i obtained in the previous section are used to rigidly register each vertebra to its upper neighbor, and the resulting rigid transforms are optimized in the registration problem. Hence, the spine is represented by a vector of local intervertebral rigid transformations $A = [T_1, T_2, \ldots, T_N]$ as illustrated in Fig. 1. To perform global anatomical modeling of the spine, we convert A into an absolute representation $A_{\text{absolute}} = [T_1, T_1 \circ T_2, \ldots, T_1 \circ T_2 \circ \ldots \circ T_N]$ using recursive compositions. The transformations are expressed in the local coordinate system of the lower vertebra, defined by vectors v_x, v_z and $v_y = v_x \times v_z$, where v_x and v_z are the vectors linking pedicle and endplate midpoints respectively. Center of transformation is located at the midpoint of all 4 pedicle tips. The rigid transformations described in this paper are the combination of a rotation matrix R and a translation vector t. We formulate the rigid transformation $T = \{R, t\}$ of a vertebral mesh triangle as $y = Rx + t$ where $x, y, t \in \Re^3$. Composition is given by $T_1 \circ T_2 = \{R_1 R_2, R_1 t_2 + t_1\}$, while inversion as $T^{-1} = \{R^T, -R^T t\}$.

3 Intraoperative Spine Inference from Images with MRFs

Our method reformulates inference as an MRF optimization where a set of labels $L = \{l^1, \ldots, l^i\}$ defined in the quantized space $\Theta = \{\mathbf{d}^1, ..., \mathbf{d}^i\}$ is associated with the set of vertebral transformations T represented by nodes $\mathbf{p}$. One seeks to attribute a label to each node of graph G such that once the corresponding deformation has been applied, the MRF energy measure between the source and target models is optimal for all vertebrae:

$$E_{\text{total}} = \sum_{\mathbf{p} \in G} V_\mathbf{p}(l_\mathbf{p}) + \sum_{\mathbf{p} \in G} \sum_{\mathbf{q} \in \mathcal{N}(\mathbf{p})} V_{\mathbf{pq}}(l_\mathbf{p}, l_\mathbf{q}) \qquad (1)$$

where $V_\mathbf{p}(\cdot)$ are the unary potentials representing the image data term, which can be defined independently from the target imaging modality $g(x)$ such that:

$$V_\mathbf{p}(l_\mathbf{p}) = \int_\Omega \eta_{\text{data}}(g(x), S_i(T_i + \mathbf{d}^\alpha)) dT. \qquad (2)$$

The data term η_{data} seeks to minimize the distance between the multi-modal images. We will discuss the choice of these costs in the next section where two different applications are considered. The right hand side of Eq.(1) are the pairwise potentials representing the smoothness term between vertebrae connected in the MRF (Fig. 1) and help to constrain the vertebrae main directions in the optimization process. Three classes of pairwise neighborhoods $\mathcal{N}$ are defined in this problem: neighboring nodes between levels l and $l+1$ measuring the deviation from the initial pose; deformation magnitudes between interconnected translation and rotation nodes; and consistency in length of the segment. These smoothness terms are described below, with $\lambda_{\mathbf{pq}}$ used as a weighting factor:

$$V_{\mathbf{pq}}(l_\mathbf{p}, l_\mathbf{q}) = \begin{cases} \lambda_{\mathbf{pq}} \|(T_\mathbf{p}^{\text{pre}} \times \mathbf{d}^{l_\mathbf{p}}) - (T_\mathbf{q}^{\text{pre}} \times \mathbf{d}^{l_\mathbf{q}})\|^2, & \text{if } \mathbf{p} \in l \text{ and } \mathbf{q} \in l+1 \\ \lambda_{\mathbf{pq}} (\|\mathbf{d}_{r_z}^{l_\mathbf{p}} + \mathbf{d}_{r_y}^{l_\mathbf{p}}\| - \|\mathbf{d}_{t_x}^{l_\mathbf{p}} + \mathbf{d}_{t_z}^{l_\mathbf{p}}\|), & \text{if } \mathbf{p} \in \Re^t \text{ and } \mathbf{q} \in \Re^R \\ \lambda_{\mathbf{pq}} |(T_\mathbf{p}^{\text{pre}} - T_\mathbf{q}^{\text{pre}}) - (\mathbf{d}^{l_\mathbf{p}} - \mathbf{d}^{l_\mathbf{q}})|, & \text{if } \mathbf{p} \equiv T_{17} \text{ and } \mathbf{q} \equiv T_1. \end{cases} \qquad (3)$$

The optimization strategy for the resulting MRF is based on a primal-dual principle where we seek to assign the optimal labels L to each translation and rotation node $\mathbf{p}$ of the linked vertebrae, so that the total energy of the graph is minimum. We apply a recently proposed method called FastPD [10][1] which can efficiently solve the registration problem in a discrete domain by formulating the duality theory in linear programming. The advantage of such an approach lies in its generality, efficient computational speed, and guarantees the global optimum without the condition of linearity. Two types of inter-modality inferences are explored: 3D surface reconstructed X-ray, and intra-op CT volume images.

4 Experimental Validation

While validating image registration is not a straightforward problem and ground truth data in medical applications is often not available, we assessed the methods performance using both synthetic and real deformations from datasets obtained in scoliosis clinics. To explore the solution space, sparse sampling considering

---
[1] Details of authors implementation: http://www.csd.uoc.gr/~komod/FastPD/

only displacements along the 6 main axis was selected, resulting in $6N+1$ labels in 3D (N is the sampling rate). The smoothness term was set at $\lambda_{\mathbf{pq}} = 0.4$. Tests were performed in C++ on a 2.8 GHz Intel P4 processor and 2 GB DDR memory.

An atlas of 17 generic prior vertebra models obtained from serial CT-scan reconstruction of a cadaver specimen was used to construct the 3D preoperative model. Models were segmented using a connecting cube algorithm [11]. The same six precise anatomical landmarks were added on each model by an expert. The atlas is divided into 3 levels of polygonal mesh catalogues of increasing complexity, to adopt the widely used multi-resolution registration approach where coarse-to-fine geometrical models are applied for optimal convergence.

The method was evaluated with three experiments: (a) simulate synthetic deformations on preoperative spines for ground truth data comparison; (b) evaluate intra-modal registration accuracy on 20 cases with pre- and intra-op 3D X-ray models; and (c) test multi-modal image registration using 12 CT datasets. The data term in (a) and (b) was based on the geometric distance between the reconstructed spine and the inferred one, while in (c) it measures the strength of the edges over the triangles corresponding to the inferred spine.

- **Geometric Inference Support:** the singleton data term potential is defined as $\eta_{\mathrm{RX}} = |S_i \bigcap X_{\mathrm{intra}}|/|S_i \bigcup X_{\mathrm{intra}}|$, which represents the volume intersection between the source S_i and target model X_{intra}.
- **Volume/CT Inference Support:** the singleton data term potential defined as $\eta_{\mathrm{CT}} = \sum_{\mathrm{x}_{ij} \in S_i} (\gamma^2 + \gamma \|\nabla CT(\mathrm{x}_{ij})\|)/(\gamma^2 + \|\nabla CT(\mathrm{x}_{ij})\|^2)$ attracts mesh triangles to target high-intensity voxels in the gradient CT volume without segmentation. The term γ is defined as a dampening factor.

4.1 Ground Truth Validation Using Synthetic Deformations

The first experiment consisted of taking six baseline scoliotic patients exhibiting different types of mild curvatures (15 - 50 deg), and simulating target models by applying synthetic deformations to the spine replicating variations observed intraoperatively. Uniformly distributed random noise (mean 0, SD 2 mm) was added to the target models. In Table 1, we present average translation and rotation errors to ground truth data for all six patients. Direct correspondences of mesh vertices between source and target spines were used to compute the Euclidean distance error, compared to an image gradient-descent method which is equivalent to an optimization without any pairwise constraints. The average 3D error was improved by 7.6 mm compared to gradient-descent. This confirms the advantage of integrating global anatomical coherence of the articulated object during registration instead of straightforward optimization techniques which are sensitive to large deformations and poor initialization. Fig. 2 illustrates good model alignment of the MRF approach with constrained articulations, while gradient-descend may cause vertebra collisions and overlapping.

Table 1. Ground truth errors from 6 synthetic deformation models, with a 3D mean Euclidean distance (MED) comparison of spine models to a gradient-descent approach

Measures / Subject	P1	P2	P3	P4	P5	P6	Average
Translation (T_t) error (mm)	0.41	0.48	0.44	0.76	1.10	0.38	**0.59**
Angular (T_R) error (deg)	0.37	0.34	0.39	0.61	0.92	0.44	**0.51**
3D MED error - MRF method (mm)	0.37	0.57	0.12	0.45	0.89	0.52	**0.48**
3D MED error - Grad. desc. (mm)	7.33	7.94	6.34	8.79	9.15	9.10	**8.11**

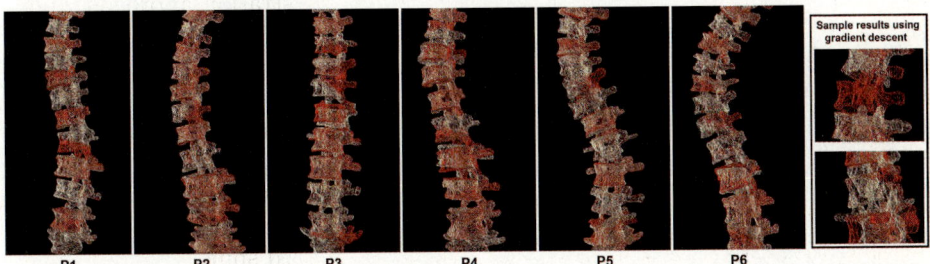

Fig. 2. Ground truth evaluation of multi-level MRF method using synthetic deformations on 6 typical scoliotic cases (target in red). Results show the importance of pairwise intervertebral links in the registration process compared to gradient descent.

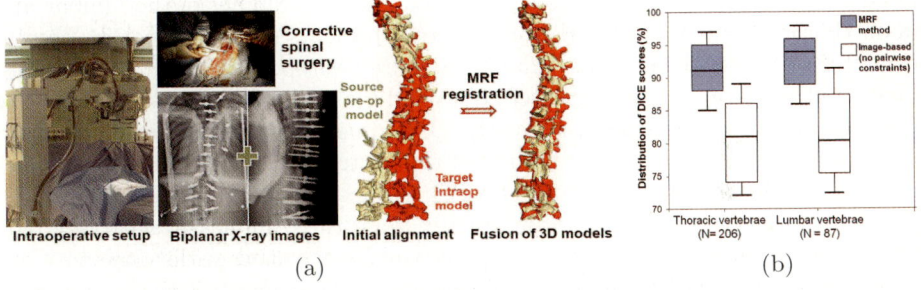

Fig. 3. (a) Operating room configuration for acquiring biplanar reconstructive X-rays. (b) Box-whisker diagrams of DICE scores for the 20 operative patients.

4.2 Validation by Comparison of Intra-op Reconstructed X-Rays

In the next experiment, registration accuracy was determined *in-vivo* in a surgical context using intraoperative 3D models generated from X-ray images. In addition to the patient's preoperative model, the 3D reconstruction was also obtained from X-rays taken during surgery in a setup illustrated in Fig. 3a. A set of 20 operative patients with corresponding pre- and intraoperative biplanar X-rays were selected for this experiment. We compared the average point-to-surface distances and DICE scores between source and target mesh models for all 20 patients and all vertebral levels. For thoracic and lumbar regions respectively, DICE scores were

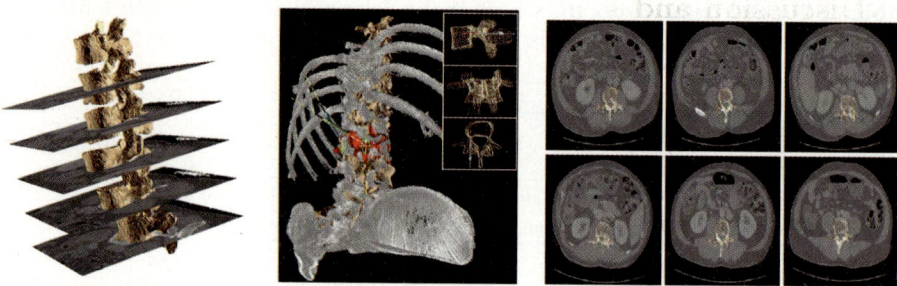

Fig. 4. Visual inspection of registration results. From left to right. Global alignment of preop model with CT images. Fused 3D model for guidance of pedicle screw insertion. Series of CT slices with corresponding geometrical vertebral models.

0.91 and 0.94 (Fig. 3b shows box plots), while the mean distances were of 2.25±0.46 and 2.42±0.87 mm. While these results seem promising and confirm the ability to compensate the shape-pose changes, discrepancies can be explained from the intensity and slight shape variations between both acquisitions, which may influence the statistical shape instantiation.

4.3 Validation through Multi-modal Model Registration

We finally performed multi-modal medical image registration using the articulated MRF method. Data consists of 12 separate CT volumes of the lumbar and main thoracic regions obtained from different patients ($512 \times 512 \times 251$, resolution: 0.8×0.8 mm, thickness: $1-2$ mm), acquired for operative planing purposes. Preoperative X-rays of patients were obtained for initial 3D reconstruction. The CT data was manually annotated with 3D landmarks, corresponding to left and right pedicle tips as well as midpoints of the vertebral body. A coarse initialization is performed using a customized user interface to roughly align both models. Registration is performed to automatically align the CT dataset with $\gamma = 0.05$ and segmentation error is estimated by measuring the average distance with the manually segmented landmarks. Table 2 presents the quantitative evaluation of this experiment with 3D landmark differences, final energy term and registration time. Results for vertebral pedicle landmark errors are 1.62 ± 0.57 mm, which is promising for the required accuracy of surgical screw insertion. Visual registration results of the 3D model with CT is shown in Fig. 4, demonstrating the multi-modal alignment where one could observe accurate superposition of geometrical models on selected CT slices.

Table 2. Quantitative results from multi-modal registration using 12 CT datasets

Subject	1	2	3	4	5	6	7	8	9	10	11	12	Mean
3D landmark diff. (mm)	1.9	2.2	1.6	1.8	2.0	2.7	2.2	3.1	1.8	2.1	2.5	1.7	2.1
Registration time (sec)	3.8	4.5	4.8	3.3	3.7	4.1	3.5	3.5	3.2	4.2	3.8	2.9	4.4

5 Discussion and Future Work

We presented a method for registering preoperative images to intraoperative 3D data for spinal surgery applications. Compared to previous works, our method represents a personalized 3D spine model obtained from baseline X-rays with articulated intervertebral transformations for fast and accurate multi-modal inference through MRFs. We showed results obtained on data acquired in both X-ray and CT experiments, demonstrating good alignment for simulated and natural configurations. Simple modular data terms were able to achieve satisfactory results, although the use of alternative image data costs better capturing the spine properties with bone density could enhance the performance. Introducing prior knowledge with respect to the allowable geometric dependencies between the relative position of vertebrae is also a promising direction. Such a concept could be enhanced through a hierarchical decomposition of the spine using higher order cliques improving the accuracy and the precision of the results. By extending the framework to online cases using tracked dynamic CT, this can help surgeons improve screw insertion accuracy and reduce surgery time.

References

1. Kim, Y., Lenke, L., Cheh, G., Riew, D.: Evaluation of pedicle screw placement in the deformed spine using intraoperative plain radiographs with computerized tomography. Spine 30, 2084–2088 (2005)
2. Lee, C., Kim, M., Ahn, Y., Kim, Y., Jeong, K., Lee, D.: Thoracic pedicle screw insertion in scoliosis using posteroanterior C-arm rotation method. J. Spinal Disord. Tech. 20, 66–71 (2007)
3. Foley, K., Simon, D., Rampersaud, Y.: Virtual fluoroscopy: computer-assisted fluoroscopic navigation. Spine 26, 347–351 (2001)
4. Livyatan, H., Yaniv, Z., Joskowicz, J.: Gradient-based 2-D/3-D rigid registration of fluoroscopic X-ray to CT. IEEE Trans. Med. Imag. 22, 1395–1406 (2003)
5. Markelj, P., Tomazevic, D., Pernus, F., Likar, B.: Robust gradient-based 3-D/2-D registration of CT and MR to X-ray images. IEEE Trans. Med. Imag. 27, 1704–1714 (2008)
6. Zheng, G., Dong, X.: Unsupervised reconstruction of a patient-specific surface model of a proximal femur from calibrated fluoroscopic images. In: Ayache, N., Ourselin, S., Maeder, A. (eds.) MICCAI 2007, Part I. LNCS, vol. 4791, pp. 834–841. Springer, Heidelberg (2007)
7. Boisvert, J., Cheriet, F., Pennec, X., Labelle, H., Ayache, N.: Geometric variability of the scoliotic spine using statistics on articulated shape models. IEEE Trans. Med. Imag. 27, 557–568 (2008)
8. Klinder, T., Wolz, R., Lorenz, C., Franz, A., Ostermann, J.: Spine segmentation using articulated shape models. In: Metaxas, D., Axel, L., Fichtinger, G., Székely, G. (eds.) MICCAI 2008, Part I. LNCS, vol. 5241, pp. 227–234. Springer, Heidelberg (2008)
9. Kadoury, S., Cheriet, F., Labelle, H.: Personalized X-ray 3D reconstruction of the scoliotic spine from statistical and image models. IEEE Trans. Med. Imag. (2009)
10. Komodakis, N., Tziritas, G., Paragios, N.: Performance vs computational efficiency for optimizing single and dynamic MRFs: Setting the state of the art with primal-dual strategies. CVIU 112, 14–29 (2008)
11. Lorensen, W., Cline, H.: Marching cubes: a high resolution 3-D surface construction algorithm. Comput. Graph. 4, 163–169 (1988)

A Shape Relationship Descriptor for Radiation Therapy Planning*

Michael Kazhdan[1], Patricio Simari[1], Todd McNutt[2], Binbin Wu[2], Robert Jacques[3], Ming Chuang[1], and Russell Taylor[1]

[1] Department of Computer Science, Johns Hopkins University, USA
[2] Department of Radiation Oncology and Molecular Radiation Science, Johns Hopkins University, USA
[3] Department of Biomedical Engineering, Johns Hopkins University, USA

Abstract. In this paper we address the challenge of matching patient geometry to facilitate the design of patient treatment plans in radiotherapy. To this end we propose a novel shape descriptor, the Overlap Volume Histogram, which provides a rotation and translation invariant representation of a patient's organs at risk relative to the tumor volume. Using our descriptor, it is possible to accurately identify database patients with similar constellations of organ and tumor geometries, enabling the transfer of treatment plans between patients with similar geometries. We demonstrate the utility of our method for such tasks by outperforming state of the art shape descriptors in the retrieval of patients with similar treatment plans. We also preliminarily show its potential as a quality control tool by demonstrating how it is used to identify an organ at risk whose dose can be significantly reduced.

1 Introduction

In the treatment of patients with malignant tumors, the goal of intensity-modulated radiation therapy (IMRT) is to deliver a high dose of radiation to the tumor volume while sparing nearby organs at risk (OAR). In practice, a pre-treatment computed tomography (CT) scan of the patient is segmented to identify the tumor volume and OAR. The segmented scan is then used by a dosimetrist to guide the settings for each multi-leaf collimator (MLC) on a radiotherapy machine targeting the tumor. This step is referred to as IMRT planning.

The design of a high-quality IMRT plan is one of the most time-consuming and least automated steps of the treatment cycle. The dosimetrist must optimize the MLC settings to achieve a dose distribution that most closely meets a set of physician-driven constraints. For example, in a commonly used treatment protocol for head-and-neck cancer [1] at least 95% of the tumor volume should receive

---

* This research was supported in part by the generosity of Paul Maritz, Philips Radiation Oncology Systems (Madison, WI), and by Johns Hopkins University internal funds.

a dose of at least 70 Gy, while no more than 50% of each parotid should receive more than 30 Gy, and no part of the spinal cord should receive more than 45 Gy. The objective function is non-convex and requires that the dosimetrist perform multiple refinement optimization steps in order to best meet the constraints. Furthermore, computing the dose distribution from a set of MLC settings requires a complex simulation involving the inhomogeneous attenuation and scattering properties within the patient volume, making each individual refinement step computationally expensive. As a result, the process of planning an individual patient usually takes many hours to complete, often resulting in a time-lag of several days between the time that a patient comes in for scanning and when the patient can return for treatment.

We will argue that through shape matching using an appropriate shape relationship descriptor, both the speed and quality of the treatment planning process can be increased. Using a database of previously treated patients, the segmented geometry of the new patient serves as a query into the database, returning the treated patients whose configurations of tumor volume to OAR most closely resemble those of the new patient. Using the treatment plans of these most similar patients, we can facilitate the treatment of new patients, either by directly suggesting a treatment plan for the new patient or by using the retrieved plans as seeds in the optimization. The key challenge in designing such a system is the definition of a shape descriptor that captures not only the geometries of the tumor volume and OAR, but also their configurations relative to each other. Intuitively, the closer an OAR is to the tumor, the harder it is to irradiate the tumor while sparing the OAR.

To this end, we introduce the *Overlap Volume Histogram* (OVH). For each OAR, this 1D histogram describes the distribution of distances of the organ's volume relative to the tumor volume. Since the "spareability" of an organ strongly depends on its proximity to the irradiated tumor, this descriptor provides a simple shape signature that is well-suited to the challenge of treatment plan retrieval. In our results we compare the OVH to several existing state-of-the-art shape descriptors and show significantly improved performance in retrieving patients with similar treatment plans.

2 Related Work

Due to the large size of the databases and guided by the need for real-time performance, many recent techniques for shape retrieval have taken the *shape descriptor* approach. The goal has been to obtain a concise, robust, and discriminating abstraction of the shape geometry that is well-suited for efficient querying. Most typically, the shape descriptor is represented as a vector in a high-dimensional space, dissimilarity of two shapes is measured as the distance between the corresponding descriptors, and database retrieval reduces to finding nearest neighbors in a high-dimensional space.

In whole-object retrieval the challenge is to find the shapes in the database which, up to transformation, are most similar to the query. Since the entire shape

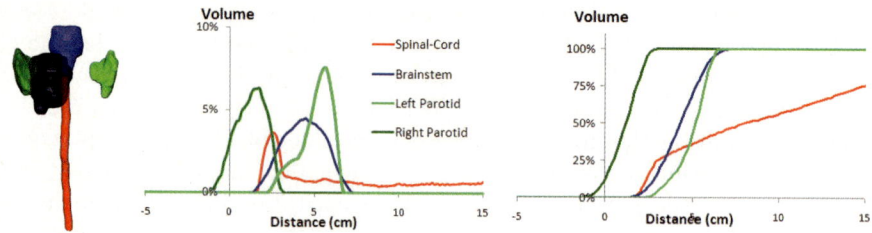

Fig. 1. Visualization of the tumor volume (black) and several OAR (left) and the corresponding OVHs in differential (center) and cumulative (right) forms

is used for retrieval, normalization techniques can be used to remove much of the transformational ambiguity in matching, allowing for the use of the center of mass for removing translational ambiguity, radial-variance or mean-/bounding-radius for removing scaling ambiguity, and principal axes for rotational ambiguity. These methods have included: 1D histograms capturing the distribution of points [2,3,4], crease angles [5], and curvature [6] over the surface; spherical functions characterizing the distribution of surface normals [7], axes of reflective symmetry [8], conformality [9], and angular extent [10]; 3D functions characterizing the rasterization of the boundary boundary points [11] and the distance transform [12]; and even 4D plenoptic functions characterizing the 2D views of a surface [13].

Partial object retrieval is more difficult. The goal is to retrieve shapes containing sub-regions that are a good match to a subset of the query. Because it is not known in advance which subsets of the shapes will be used for matching, global normalization techniques cannot be applied. Instead, partial matching methods represent a shape by a multitude of shape descriptors, each centered at a different point on the shape's boundary and characterizing only the subset of the shape in its vicinity. Using these descriptors, retrieval can be performed by rating target models in terms of the number and quality of matches between the descriptors of the query and the descriptors of the target. Commonly used shape descriptors for partial shape matching have included spin images [14,15], shape contexts [16], and curvature maps [17].

What makes patient retrieval difficult is that the notion of shape similarity required for retrieving treatment plans is not one characterized by either of these two methodologies. The geometric relationship between the tumor and the surrounding anatomy is more important than the detailed shapes of individual structures. The volume of overlap has been suggested for characterizing the relationship between OAR and target [18]. However, this only provides a single value and becomes uninformative when the OAR and target do not overlap.

3 The Overlap Volume Histogram

In designing a shape descriptor, our goal is to capture the proximity of the different OARs to the tumor volume. To this end, we define the *Overlap Volume Histogram*

Algorithm 1. GetOVH($BinaryVoxel\ O$, $BinaryVoxel\ T$)

Require: Binary voxel grids for organ O and tumor T
   $Histogram$ dOVH $\leftarrow 0$
   $Voxel$ DT $\leftarrow$ GetSignedDistanceTransform(T)
   for all $o \in O$ **do** dOVH$[DT(o)] \mathrel{+}= 1/|O|$
   $Histogram$ OVH $\leftarrow$ cumulative(dOVH)
   return OVH

(OVH). This is a one-dimensional distribution associated to each organ at risk, measuring its distance from the tumor.

For a tumor T and organ O, the value of the OVH of O with respect to T at distance t is defined as the volume of the subset of the organ a distance of t or less from the tumor:

$$\text{OVH}_{O,T}(t) = \frac{\left|\{p \in O | d(p,T) \leq t\}\right|}{|O|},$$

where $d(p, T)$ is the signed distance of p from the tumor's boundary and $|O|$ is the volume of the OAR.

In practice, the OVH of an organ with respect to the tumor is efficiently computed from the segmented CT scans. Using the segmented tumor volume, we compute its signed Distance Transform. We iterate over the voxels interior to the organ and for each voxel, we evaluate the distance transform of the tumor, splatting a unit-volume vote into the associated bin. This gives us the differential of the volume which can then be used to compute the final cumulative form in a single pass. Since the signed distance transform can be computed in linear time (e.g. using [19]) the total running time of the algorithm is linear in the size of the CT scan. The algorithm is given in Algorithm 1.

An example of a patient's OVH descriptors is shown in Fig. 1. The image on the left shows the geometry of the tumor volume (black), spinal cord (red), brainstem (blue), and right and left parotid glands (dark and light green respectively). Examining the OVHs, we can quickly identify properties of the geometric configuration of the organs relative to the tumor. For example, the fact that the OVH of the left parotid has non-zero values at negative distances indicates that part of the parotid is overlapped by the tumor volume and therefore it will not be possible to spare the parotid in its entirety when fully irradiating the tumor. Similarly, since the the OVH values for both the spinal cord and brainstem are zero for distance values smaller than one centimeter, we know that no point on the tumor can be within a centimeter of these organs. Therefore, a treatment plan keeping most of the radiation within a centimeter of the tumor is likely to spare them.

To use the OVH for retrieval we need to define a metric on the space of descriptors. Since the differentials of the OVH correspond to distributions, a natural metric is the Earth Mover's Distance (EMD) which measures the amount of work needed to transform one distribution into the other. Although computing this distance in general is computationally difficult, requiring the solution of a

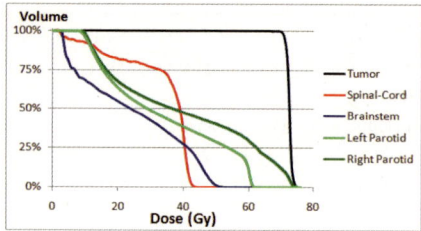

Fig. 2. DVHs for the treatment plan of the patient in Fig. 1

bipartite graph matching problem, it is straightforward to compute in our case. As shown by Rubner et al. [20], in the case that the distributions are normalized and one-dimensional, the EMD between two distributions is the L_1-distance between their cumulative histograms. As a result, run-time retrieval only requires finding the target descriptor(s) in the database minimizing the L_1-distance to the query.

4 Experimental Results

To evaluate the effectiveness of a shape descriptor in patient retrieval, we measure the accuracy with which similarity of descriptors predicts similarity of treatment plans. The challenge in implementing such an experiment is that there does not exist a canonical metric for measuring plan similarity.

After a treatment plan is designed by a dosimetrist, a simulation of the IMRT is performed to determine the resulting dose distribution. In practice, the plan quality is evaluated by considering the *dose-volume histograms* (DVHs) [21] of the different organs and target volumes. These are 1D distributions, whose value at a specific dose is the volume of the organ or tumor that would receive at most that much dose under the proposed plan.

Fig. 2 shows the DVHs derived from the treatment plan for the patient shown in Fig. 1. Since the goal of the treatment is to kill the tumor, the plan results in a DVH for the tumor that has large values for all doses. For serial organs like the spinal cord and brainstem, the goal of the treatment is to ensure that no part of the organ receives a high dose, and the DVHs for both have zero value beyond 50 Gy. Since the parotids are parallel organs that remain functional even after a noticeable fraction of their volume has received high dose, the DVHs for both the left and right parotids show small volumes of the organ receiving doses larger than 60 Gy. Additionally, since the proximity of the left parotid to the tumor makes it hard to spare, the treatment results in more irradiation of this gland, with 10% of the organ receiving as much as 70 Gy.

We evaluate the quality of a descriptor by measuring the effectiveness with which it retrieves patients having similar DVHs. We do this by calculating the variation in DVH distances between a patient and the patient's k nearest neighbors (sorted by descriptor similarity).

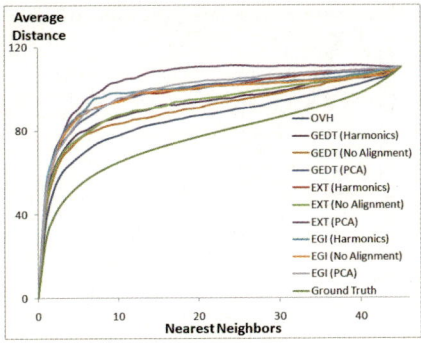

Fig. 3. Plots of the avg. distances from a patient's DVH to the DVHs of its k-nearest neighbors as defined using several different shape descriptors

Given a patient, we compute the sum of squared L_1-distances from the DVH of patient to the DVHs of the patient's k-nearest neighbors, summing over both the nearest neighbors and the different OARs. We repeat the experiment for all patients in the database and average the (root of the) sums. This gives a 1D distribution of the expected distance of a patient's DVH from the DVH of its k nearest-neighbors. In general, we expect descriptors that better predict DVH similarity to give rise to distributions with smaller expected distances. Clearly, the best results are obtained when patients are sorted based on DVH similarity.

Fig. 3 compares the distance distribution obtained with our OVH descriptor with the distributions obtained using several other common shape descriptors, including Extended Gaussian Images (EGI) [7], angular extent functions (EXT) [10], and Gaussian Euclidean Distance Transforms (GEDT) [12]. As a baseline, the figure also shows the results when DVH similarity is used to sort the patients, ("Ground Truth" plot).

For each competing method, we obtained a representation of the organ-tumor relationship by computing the descriptor of the union of the organ and tumor geometries. We also addressed the problem of rotational alignment in three ways. **Harmonic:** We made the descriptors rotation invariant by storing only the magnitudes of the spherical frequencies. **PCA:** We used PCA to align each patient into a canonical pose prior to the computation of the descriptor. And, **No Alignment:** We used the given poses to allow for the possibility of consistent alignment across patients.

As the plots indicate, despite the quality of the traditional descriptors in general shape matching tasks, they are not well-suited patient retrieval, where it is the inter-organ relations that determine similarity. In contrast, our OVH descriptor is specifically designed to capture the proximity of different geometries. Thus it outperforms these methods, more often successfully using organ geometry to identify patients with similar treatment plans. The distance to the ground truth curve implies that, in practice, similarity of patient geometry does not always result in similar treatment. In fact, we have found that in some instances, two patients with nearly identical anatomies receive plans of markedly differing

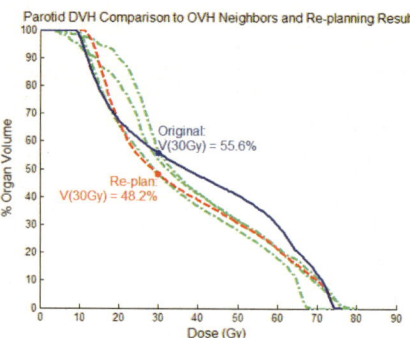

Fig. 4. Parotid DVH (blue) along with the DVHs of its 3 nearest OVH neighbors (dotted green) and the DVH obtained after re-planning (dashed red.) Note the reduction of $V(30Gy)$ from 55.6% to 48.2%.

quality. This is because, given the difficulty of the planning process, physicians can unwittingly approve suboptimal plans.

The OVH can be used as a tool in plan quality assessment by searching the database for similar patients with better plans. As an example, Fig. 4 illustrates a preliminary result in which a parotid's IMRT plan (blue) was automatically flagged as a candidate for replanning because the three database parotids with most similar OVHs (green) received much lower doses. The DVH obtained after replanning is illustrated in dashed red. With the new plan, the $V(30Gy)$ value to the patient's parotid was reduced from 55.6% to 48.2%, crossing the 50% spareability mark in the RTOG protocol. This replanning result is preliminary, since the focus of this paper is the introduction of the OVH and its shape-retrival performance evaluation (Fig. 3). In a related work [22], we focus specifically on the application of our OVH descriptor to IMRT planning. In this study based on sorting the mid-points of OVHs and comparing to the order of DVHs to find outliers, we were able to improve 13 out of 32 patient treatment plans.

5 Conclusion and Future Work

We have introduced the OVH, a novel shape relationship descriptor focused on the characterization of the inter-spacial relationship of different geometries. We have shown it can be computed efficiently and have demonstrated its practical efficacy by showing that it outperforms traditional shape descriptors in retrieving patients with radiotherapy treatment plans similar to the query using geometry alone. We also showed its potential as a quality control tool by demonstrating how it was used to identify an OAR whose dose could be significantly reduced. Based on these encouraging preliminary results, we have begun to explore the use of more complex OVH features and search methods for their application in patient retrieval for radiation therapy.

References

1. Eisbruch, A., Chao, K.C., Garden, A.: Phase I/II study of conformal and intensity modulated irradiation for oropharyngeal cancer (RTOG 0022). Radiation Therapy Oncology Group of the American College of Radiology (2004)
2. Ankerst, M., Kastenmüller, G., Kriegel, H.-P., Seidl, T.: 3D shape histograms for similarity search and classification in spatial databases. In: Güting, R.H., Papadias, D., Lochovsky, F.H. (eds.) SSD 1999. LNCS, vol. 1651, pp. 207–228. Springer, Heidelberg (1999)
3. Osada, R., Funkhouser, T., Chazelle, B., Dobkin, D.: Matching 3D models with shape distributions. In: IEEE International Conference on Shape Modeling and Applications, pp. 154–166 (2001)
4. Osada, R., Funkhouser, T., Chazelle, B., Dobkin, D.: Shape distributions. Transactions on Graphics 21(4), 807–832 (2002)
5. Besl, P.: Triangles as a primary representation. In: Hebert, M., Boult, T., Gross, A., Ponce, J. (eds.) NSF-WS 1994 and ARPA-WS 1994. LNCS, vol. 994, pp. 191–206. Springer, Heidelberg (1995)
6. Zhang, J., Siddiqi, K., Macrini, D., Shokouf, A., Dickinson, S.: Retrieving articulated 3-D models using medial surfaces and their graph spectra. In: Energy Minimization Methods in Computer Vision and Pattern Recognition, pp. 285–300 (2005)
7. Horn, B.: Extended Gaussian images. In: Proceedings of the IEEE, vol. 72, pp. 1656–1678 (1984)
8. Kazhdan, M., Chazelle, B., Dobkin, D., Finkelstein, A., Funkhouser, T.: A reflective symmetry descriptor. In: European Conference on Computer Vision, pp. 642–656 (2002)
9. Wang, S., Wang, Y., Jin, M., Gu, X.D., Samaras, D.: Conformal geometry and its applications on 3d shape matching, recognition, and stitching. IEEE PAMI 29(7) (2007)
10. Vranic, D., Saupe, D.: 3D model retrieval with spherical harmonics and moments. In: DAGM Symposium on Pattern Recognition, pp. 392–397 (2001)
11. Gain, J., Scott, J.: Fast polygon mesh querying by example. SIGGRAPH Technical Sketches, 241 (1999)
12. Funkhouser, T., Min, P., Kazhdan, M., Chen, J., Halderman, A., Dobkin, D., Jacobs, D.: A search engine for 3D models. ACM Transactions on Graphics 22(1), 83–105 (2003)
13. Chen, D., Tian, X., Shen, Y., Ouhyoung, M.: On visual similarity based 3D model retrieval. Computer Graphics Forum 22(3), 223–232 (2003)
14. Johnson, A., Hebert, M.: Efficient multiple model recognition in cluttered 3-D scenes. In: IEEE Conference on Computer Vision and Pattern Recognition, pp. 671–677 (1998)
15. Johnson, A.E., Hebert, M.: Using spin-images for efficient multiple model recognition in cluttered 3-D scenes. IEEE PAMI 21(5), 433–449 (1999)
16. Frome, A., Huber, D., Kolluri, R., Bulow, T., Malik, J.: Recognizing objects in range data using regional point descriptors. In: European Conference on Computer Vision, pp. 224–237 (2004)
17. Gatzke, T., Grimm, C.: Curvature maps for local shape comparison. In: IEEE International Conference on Shape Modeling and Applications, pp. 244–253 (2005)
18. Hunt, M.A., Jackson, A., Narayana, A., Lee, N.: Geometric factors influencing dosimetric sparing of the parotid glands using IMRT. International journal of radiation oncology, biology, physics 66, 296–304 (2006)

19. Saito, T., Toriwaki, J.: New algorithms for euclidean distance transformation of an n-dimensional digitized picture with applications. Pattern Recognition 27(11), 1551–1565 (1994)
20. Rubner, Y., Tomasi, C., Guibas, L.: The earth mover's distance as a metric for image retrieval. International Journal of Computer Vision 40, 99–121 (2000)
21. Drzymala, R., Brewster, L., Chu, J., Goitein, M., Harms, W., Urie, M.: Dose-volume histograms. International Journal of Radiation Oncology, Biology and Physics 21, 71–78 (1991)
22. Wu, B., Ricchetti, F., Sanguineti, G., Kazhdan, M., Simari, P., Chuang, M., Taylor, R., Jacques, R., McNutt, T.: Patient geometry-driven information retrieval for IMRT treatment plan quality control. Medical Physic. (in submission)

Feature-Based Morphometry

Matthew Toews[1], William M. Wells III[1], D. Louis Collins[2], and Tal Arbel[3]

[1] Brigham and Women's Hospital, Harvard Medical School
{mt,sw}@bwh.harvard.edu
[2] Montreal Neurological Institute, McGill University
louis.collins@mcgill.ca
[3] Centre for Intelligent Machines, McGill University
arbel@cim.mcgill.ca

Abstract. This paper presents *feature-based morphometry* (FBM), a new, fully data-driven technique for identifying group-related differences in volumetric imagery. In contrast to most morphometry methods which assume one-to-one correspondence between all subjects, FBM models images as a collage of distinct, localized image features which may not be present in all subjects. FBM thus explicitly accounts for the case where the same anatomical tissue cannot be reliably identified in all subjects due to disease or anatomical variability. A probabilistic model describes features in terms of their appearance, geometry, and relationship to subgroups of a population, and is automatically learned from a set of subject images and group labels. Features identified indicate group-related anatomical structure that can potentially be used as disease biomarkers or as a basis for computer-aided diagnosis. Scale-invariant image features are used, which reflect generic, salient patterns in the image. Experiments validate FBM clinically in the analysis of normal (NC) and Alzheimer's (AD) brain images using the freely available OASIS database. FBM automatically identifies known structural differences between NC and AD subjects in a fully data-driven fashion, and obtains an equal error classification rate of 0.78 on new subjects.

1 Introduction

Morphometry aims to automatically identify anatomical differences between groups of subjects, e.g. diseased or healthy brains. The typical computational approach taken to morphometry is a two step process. Subject images are first geometrically aligned or registered within a common frame of reference or atlas, after which statistics are computed based on group labels and measurements of interest. Morphometric approaches can be contrasted according to the measurements upon which statistics are computed. Voxel-based morphometry (VBM) involves analyzing intensities or tissue class labels [1,2]. Deformation or tensor-based morphometry (TBM) analyzes the deformation fields which align subjects [3,4,5]. Object-based morphometry analyzes the variation of pre-defined structures such as cortical sulci [6].

A fundamental assumption underlying most morphometry techniques is that inter-subject registration is capable of achieving one-to-one correspondence between all subjects, and that statistics can therefore be computed from measurements of the same anatomical tissues across all subjects. Inter-subject registration remains a major challenge, however, due to the fact that no two subjects are identical; the same anatomical structure may vary significantly or exhibit distinct, multiple morphologies across a population, or may not be present in all subjects. Coarse linear registration can be used to normalize images with respect to global orientation and scale differences, however it cannot achieve precise alignment of fine anatomical structures. Deformable registration has the potential to refine the alignment of fine anatomical structures, however it is difficult to guarantee that images are not being over-aligned. While deformable registration may improve tissue overlap, in does not necessarily improve the accuracy in aligning landmarks, such as cortical sulci [7]. Consequently, it may be unrealistic and potentially detrimental to assume global one-to-one correspondence, as morphometric analysis may be confounding image measurements arising from different underlying anatomical tissues [8].

Feature-based morphometry (FBM) is proposed specifically to avoid the assumption of one-to-one inter-subject correspondence. FBM admits that correspondence may not exist between all subjects and throughout the image, and instead attempts to identify local patterns of anatomical structure for which correspondence between subsets of subjects is statistically probable. Such local patterns are identified and represented as distinctive scale-invariant features [9,10,11,12], i.e. generic image patterns that can be automatically extracted in the image by a front-end salient feature detector. A probabilistic model quantifies feature variability in terms of appearance, geometry, and occurrence statistics relative to subject groups. Model parameters are estimated using a fully automatic, data-driven learning algorithm to identify local patterns of anatomical structure and quantify their relationships to subject groups. The local feature thus replaces the global atlas as the basis for morphometric analysis. Scale-invariant features are widely used in the computer vision literature for image matching, and have been extended to matching 3D volumetric medical imagery [11,12]. FBM follows from a line of recent research modeling object appearance in photographic imagery [13] and in 2D slices of the brain [14], and extends this research to address group analysis, and to operate in full 3D volumetric imagery.

2 Feature-Based Morphometry (FBM)

2.1 Local Invariant Image Features

Images contain a large amount of information, and it is useful to focus computational resources on interesting or salient features, which can be automatically identified as maxima of a saliency criterion evaluated throughout the image. Features associated with anatomical structures have a characteristic scale or size which is independent of image resolution, and a prudent approach is thus to identify features in a manner invariant to image scale [9,10]. This can be done by evaluating saliency in an image scale-space $I(x, \sigma)$ that represents the image I at location x and scale σ. The Gaussian scale-space, defined by convolution of the image with the Gaussian kernel, is arguably the most common in the literature [15,16]:

$$I(x,\sigma) = I(x,\sigma_0) * G(x, \sigma - \sigma_0), \quad (1)$$

where $G(x,\sigma)$ is a Gaussian kernel of mean x and variance σ, and σ_0 represents the scale of the original image. The Gaussian scale-space has attractive properties including non-creation and non-enhancement of local extrema, scale-invariance, and causality and arises as the solution to the heat equation [16]. Derivative operators are commonly used to evaluate saliency in scale-space [9,10], and are motivated by models of image processing in biological vision systems [17]. In this paper, geometrical regions $g_i = \{x_i, \sigma_i\}$ corresponding to local extrema of the difference-of-Gaussian (DOG) operator are used [9]:

$$(x_i, \sigma_i) = \underset{x,\sigma}{\text{local argmax}} \left\{ \left| \frac{dI(x,\sigma)}{d\sigma} \right| \right\}. \quad (2)$$

Each identified feature is a spherical region defined geometrically by a location x_i and a scale σ_i, and the image measurements within the region, denoted as a_i.

2.2 Probabilistic Model

Let $F = \{f_1, \ldots, f_N\}$ represent a set of N local features extracted from a set of images, where N is unknown. Let T represent a geometrical transform bringing features into coarse, approximate alignment with an atlas, e.g. a similarity or affine transform to the Talairach space [18]. Let C represent a discrete random variable of the group from which subjects are sampled, e.g. diseased, healthy. The posterior probability of (T, C) given F can be expressed as:

$$p(C,T|F) = \frac{p(C,T)}{p(F)} p(F|C,T) = \frac{p(C,T)}{p(F)} \prod_i^N p(f_i|C,T), \quad (3)$$

where the first equality results from Bayes rule, and the second from the assumption of conditional feature independence given (C,T). Note that while inter-feature dependencies in geometry and appearance are generally present, they can largely be accounted for by conditioning on variables (C,T). $p(f_i|C,T)$ represents the probability of a feature f_i given (C,T). $p(C,T)$ represents a joint prior distribution over (C,T). $p(F)$ represents the evidence of feature set F.

An individual feature is denoted as $f_i = \{a_i, \alpha_i, g_i, \gamma_i\}$. a_i represents feature appearance (i.e. image measurements), α_i is a binary random variable representing valid or invalid a_i, $g_i = \{x_i, \sigma_i\}$ represents feature geometry in terms of image location x_i and scale σ_i, and γ_i is a binary random variable indicating the presence or absence of geometry g_i in a subject image. The focus of modeling is on the conditional feature probability $p(f_i|C,T)$:

$$p(f_i|C,T) = p(a_i, \alpha_i, \gamma_i, g_i|T,C) = p(a_i|\alpha_i)p(\alpha_i|\gamma_i)p(g_i|\gamma_i,T)p(\gamma_i|C), \quad (4)$$

where the 2nd equality follows from several reasonable conditional independence assumptions between variables. $p(a_i|\alpha_i)$ is a density over feature appearance a_i given feature occurrence α_i, $p(\alpha_i|\gamma_i)$ is a Bernoulli distribution of feature occurrence α_i given the occurrence of a consistent geometry γ_i, $p(g_i|\gamma_i, T)$ is a density over feature geometry given geometrical occurrence γ_i and global transform T, and $p(\gamma_i|C)$ is a Bernoulli distribution over geometry occurrence given group C.

2.3 Learning Algorithm

Learning focuses on identifying clusters of features which are similar in terms of their group membership, geometry and appearance. Features in a cluster represent different observations of the same underlying anatomical structure, and can be used to estimate the parameters of distributions in Equation (4).

Data Preprocessing: Subjects are first aligned into a global reference frame, and T is thus constant in Equation (3). At this point, subjects have been normalized according to location, scale and orientation, and the remaining appearance and geometrical variability can be quantified [19]. Image features are then detected independently in all subject images as in Equation (2).

Clustering: For each feature f_i, two different clusters or feature sets G_i and A_i are identified, where $f_j \in G_i$ are similar to f_i in terms of geometry, and $f_j \in A_i$ are similar to f_i in appearance. First, set G_i is identified based on a robust binary measure of geometry similarity. Features f_i and f_j are said to be geometrically similar if their locations and scales differ by less than error thresholds ε_x and ε_σ. In order to compute geometrical similarity in a manner independent of feature scale, location difference is normalized by feature scale σ_i, and scale difference is computed in the log domain. G_i is thus defined as:

$$G_i = \{f_j : ||x_i - x_j||/\sigma_i \leq \varepsilon_x \wedge |\log(\sigma_j/\sigma_i)| \leq \varepsilon_\sigma \}. \tag{5}$$

Next, set A_i is identified using a robust measure of appearance similarity, where f_i is said to be similar to f_j in appearance if the difference between their appearances is below a threshold ε_{a_i}. A_i is thus defined as a function of ε_{a_i}:

$$A_i(\varepsilon_{a_i}) = \{f_j : ||a_i - a_j|| \leq \varepsilon_{a_i}\}, \tag{6}$$

where here $||\ ||$ is the Euclidean norm. While a single pair of geometrical thresholds $(\varepsilon_x, \varepsilon_\sigma)$ is applicable to all features, ε_{a_i} is feature-specific and set to:

$$\varepsilon_{a_i} = \sup\left\{\varepsilon_a \in [0, \infty) : 1 \leq \frac{|A_i(\varepsilon_a) \cap G_i \cap C_i|}{|A_i(\varepsilon_a) \cap \overline{G_i \cap C_i}|}\right\}, \tag{7}$$

where C_i is the set of features having the same group label as f_i, and ε_{a_i} is thus set to the maximum threshold such that A_i is still more likely than not to contain geometrically similar features from the same group C_i. At this point, $G_i \cap A_i$ is a set of samples of model feature f_i, and the informativeness of f_i regarding a subject group C_j is quantified by the likelihood ratio:

$$\frac{p(f_i|C_j, T)}{p(f_i|\overline{C_j}, T)} = \frac{|A_i \cap G_i \cap C_j|}{|A_i \cap G_i \cap \overline{C_j}|}. \tag{8}$$

The likelihood ratio explicitly measures the degree of association between a feature and a specific subject group and lies at the heart of FBM analysis. Features can be sorted according to likelihood ratios to identify the anatomical structures most indicative of a particular subject group, e.g. healthy or diseased. The likelihood ratio is also operative in FBM classification:

$$C^* = \underset{C}{\operatorname{argmax}} \left\{ \frac{p(C,T|F)}{p(\overline{C},T|F)} \right\} = \underset{C}{\operatorname{argmax}} \left\{ \frac{p(C,T)}{p(\overline{C},T)} \prod_i \frac{p(f_i|C,T)}{p(f_i|\overline{C},T)} \right\}, \qquad (9)$$

where C^* is the optimal Bayes classification of a new subject based on a set of features F in the image, and can be used for computer-aided diagnosis.

3 Experiments

FBM is a general analysis technique, which is demonstrated and validated here in the analysis of Alzheimer's disease (AD), an important, incurable neurodegenerative disease affecting millions worldwide, and the focus of intense computational research [20,21,22,23]. Experiments use OASIS [22], a large, freely available data set including 98 normal (NC) subjects and 100 probable AD subjects ranging clinically from very mild to moderate dementia. All subjects are right-handed, with approximately equal age distributions for NC/AD subjects ranging from 60+ years with means of 76/77 years. For each subject, 3 to 4 T1-weighted scans are acquired, gain-field corrected and averaged in order to improve the signal/noise ratio. Images are aligned within the Talairach reference frame via affine transform T and the skull is masked out [23]. In our analysis, the DOG scale-space [9] is used to identify feature geometries (x_i, σ_i), appearances a_i are obtained by cropping cubical image regions of side length $4\sqrt{\sigma_i}$ centered on x_i and then scale-normalizing to $(11 \times 11 \times 11)$-voxel resolution. Features could be normalized according to a canonical orientation to achieve rotation invariance [12], this is omitted here as subjects are already rotation-normalized via T and further invariance reduces appearance distinctiveness. Approximately 800 features are extracted in each $(176 \times 208 \times 176)$-voxel brain volume.

Model learning is applied on a randomly-selected subset of 150 subjects (75 NC, 75 AD). Approximately 12K model features are identified, these are sorted according to likelihood ratio in Figure 1. While many occur infrequently (red curve, low $p(f_i|T)$) and/or are uninformative regarding group (center of graph), a significant number are strongly indicative of either NC or AD subjects (extreme left or right of graph). Several strongly AD-related features correspond to well-established indicators of AD in the brain. Others may provide new information. For examples of AD-related features shown in Figure 1, feature (a) corresponds to enlargement of the extracerebral space in the anterior Sylvian sulcus; feature (b) corresponds to enlargement of the temporal horn of the lateral ventricle (and one would assume a concomitant atrophy of the hippocampus and amygdala); feature (c) corresponds to enlargement of the lateral ventricles. For NC-related features, features (1) (parietal lobe white matter) and (2) (posterior cingulate gyrus)

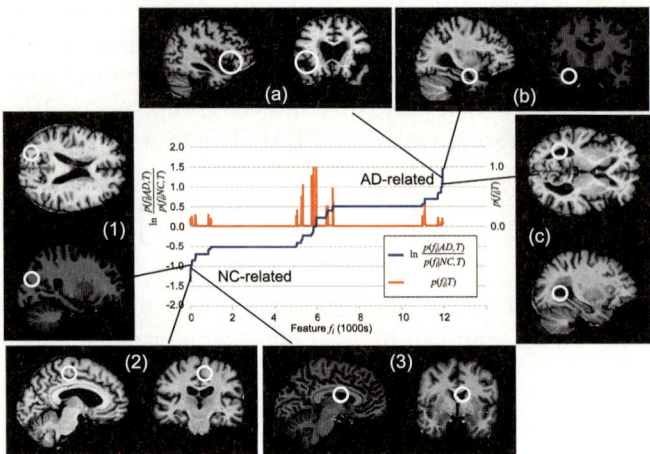

Fig. 1. The blue curve plots the likelihood ratio $\ln \frac{p(f_i|AD,T)}{p(f_i|NC,T)}$ of feature occurrence in AD vs. NC subjects sorted in ascending order. Low values indicate features associated with NC subjects (lower left) and high values indicate features associated with AD subjects (upper right). The red curve plots feature occurrence probability $p(f_i|T)$. Note a large number of frequently-occurring features bear little information regarding AD or NC (center). Examples of NC (1-3) and AD (a-c) related features are shown.

correspond to non-atrophied parenchyma and feature (3) (lateral ventricle) to non-enlarged cerebrospinal fluid spaces.

FBM also serves as a basis for computer-aided diagnosis of new subjects. Classification of the 48 subjects left out of learning results in an equal error classification rate (EER) of 0.78[1]. Classification based on models learned from randomly-permuted group labels is equivalent to random chance (EER $= 0.50$, stdev $= 0.02$), suggesting that the model trained on genuine group labels is indeed identifying meaningful anatomical structure. A direct comparison with classification rates in the literature is difficult due to the availability, variation and preprocessing of data sets used. Rates as high as 0.93 are achievable using support vector machines (SVMs) focused on regions of interest [21]. While representations such as SVMs are useful for classification, they require additional interpretation to explain the link between anatomical tissue and groups [5].

4 Discussion

This paper presents and validates feature-based morphometry (FBM), a new, fully data-driven technique for identifying group differences in volumetric images. FBM utilizes a probabilistic model to learn local anatomical patterns in the form of scale-invariant features which reflect group differences. The primary

---

[1] The EER is a threshold-independent measure of classifier performance defined as the classification rate where misclassification error rates are equal.

difference between FBM and most morphological analysis techniques in the literature is that FBM represents the image as a collage of local features that need not occur in all subjects, and thereby offers a mechanism to avoid confounding analysis of tissues which may not be present or easily localizable in all subjects, due to disease or anatomical variability. FBM is validated clinically on a large set images of NC and probable AD subjects, where anatomical features consistent with well-known differences between NC and AD brains are automatically identified in a set of 150 training subjects. Due to space constraints only a few examples are shown here. FBM is potentially useful for computer-aided diagnosis, and classification of 48 test subjects achieves a classification ERR of 0.78. As validation makes use of a large, freely available data set, reproducability and comparison with other techniques in the literature will be greatly facilitated.

FBM does not replace current morphometry techniques, but rather provides a new complementary tool which is particularly useful when one-to-one correspondence is difficult to achieve between all subjects of a population. The work here considers group differences in terms of feature/group co-occurrence statistics, however most features do occur (albeit at different frequencies) in multiple groups, and traditional morphometric analysis on an individual feature basis is a logical next step in further characterizing group differences. In terms of FBM theory, the model could be adapted to account for disease progression in longitudinal studies by considering temporal groups, to help in understanding the neuroanatomical basis for progression from mild cognitive impairment to AD, for instance. A variety of different scale-invariant features types exist, based on image characteristics such as spatial derivatives, image entropy and phase. These could be incorporated into FBM to model complementary anatomical structures, thereby improving analysis and classification. The combination of classification and permutation testing performed here speaks to the statistical significance of the feature ensemble identified by FBM, and we are investigating significance testing for individual features. FBM is general and can be used as a tool to study a variety of neurological diseases, and we are currently investigating Parkinson's disease. Future experiments will involve a comparison of morphological methods on the OASIS data set.

Acknowledgements. This work was funded in part by NIH grant P41 RR13218 and an NSERC postdoctoral fellowship.

References

1. Ashburner, J., Friston, K.J.: Voxel-based morphometry-the methods. NeuroImage 11(23), 805–821 (2000)
2. Toga, A.W., Thompson, P.M., Mega, M.S., Narr, K.L., Blanton, R.E.: Probabilistic approaches for atlasing normal and disease-specific brain variability. Anat. Embryol. 204, 267–282 (2001)
3. Studholme, C., Drapaca, C., Iordanova, B., Cardenas, V.: Deformation-based mapping of volume change from serial brain MRI in the presence of local tissue contrast change. IEEE TMI 25(5), 626–639 (2006)
4. Chung, M.K., Worsley, K.J., Paus, T., Cherif, C., Collins, D.L., Giedd, J.N., Rapoport, J.L., Evans, A.C.: A unified statistical approach to deformation-based morphometry. Neuroimage 14, 595–606 (2001)

5. Lao, Z., Shen, D., Xue, Z., Karacali, B., Resnick, S.M., Davatzikos, C.: Morphological classification of brains via high-dimensional shape transformations and machine learning methods. Neuroimage 21, 46–57 (2004)
6. Mangin, J., Riviere, D., Cachia, A., Duchesnay, E., Cointepas, Y., Papadopoulos-Orfanos, D., Collins, D.L., Evans, A.C., Regis, J.: Object-based morphometry of the cerebral cortex. IEEE TMI 23(8), 968–983 (2004)
7. Hellier, P., Barillot, C., Corouge, I., Gibaud, B., Le Goualher, G., Collins, D., Evans, A., Malandain, G., Ayache, N., Christensen, G., Johnson, H.: Retrospective evaluation of intersubject brain registration. IEEE TMI 22(9), 1120–1130 (2003)
8. Davatzikos, C.: Comments and controversies: Why voxel-based morphometric analysis should be used with great caution when characterizing group differences. Neuroimage 23, 17–20 (2004)
9. Lowe, D.G.: Distinctive image features from scale-invariant keypoints. IJCV 60(2), 91–110 (2004)
10. Mikolajczyk, K., Schmid, C.: Scale and affine invariant interest point detectors. IJCV 60(1), 63–86 (2004)
11. Cheung, W., Hamarneh, G.: N-sift: N-dimensional scale invariant feature transform for matching medical images. In: ISBI (2007)
12. Allaire, S., Kim, J., Breen, S., Jaffray, D., Pekar, V.: Full orientation invariance and improved feature selectivity of 3d sift with application to medical image analysis. In: MMBIA (2008)
13. Fergus, R., Perona, P., Zisserman, A.: Weakly supervised scale-invariant learning of models for visual recognition. IJCV 71(3), 273–303 (2006)
14. Toews, M., Arbel, T.: A statistical parts-based appearance model of anatomical variability. IEEE TMI 26(4), 497–508 (2007)
15. Witkin, A.P.: Scale-space filtering. In: JCAI, pp. 1019–1021 (1983)
16. Koenderink, J.: The structure of images. Biological Cybernetics 50, 363–370 (1984)
17. Young, R.A.: The gaussian derivative model for spatial vision: I. retinal mechanisms. Spatial Vision 2, 273–293 (1987)
18. Talairach, J., Tournoux, P.: Co-planar Stereotactic Atlas of the Human Brain: 3-Dimensional Proportional System: an Approach to Cerebral Imaging. Georg Thieme Verlag, Stuttgart (1988)
19. Dryden, I.L., Mardia, K.V.: Statistical Shape Analysis. John Wiley & Sons, Chichester (1998)
20. Qiu, A., Fennema-Notestine, C., Dale, A.M., Miller, M.I., Initiative, A.D.N.: Regional shape abnormalities in mild cognitive impairment and alzheimer's disease. Neuroimage 45, 656–661 (2009)
21. Duchesne, S., Caroli, A., Geroldi, C., Barillot, C., Frisoni, G.B., Collins, D.L.: Mri-based automated computer classification of probable ad versus normal controls. IEEE TMI 27, 509–520 (2008)
22. Marcus, D., Wang, T., Parker, J., Csernansky, J., Morris, J., Buckner, R.: Open access series of imaging studies (oasis): Cross-sectional MRI data in young, middle aged, nondemented and demented older adults. Journal of Cognitive Neuroscience 19, 1498–1507 (2007)
23. Buckner, R., Head, D., Parker, J., Fotenos, A., Marcus, D., Morris, J., Snyder, A.: A unified approach for morphometric and functional data analysis in young, old, and demented adults using automated atlas-based head size normalization: reliability and validation against manual measurement of total intracranial volume. Neuroimage 23, 724–738 (2004)

Constructing a Dictionary of Human Brain Folding Patterns

Zhong Yi Sun[1,3], Matthieu Perrot[1,3], Alan Tucholka[1,2,3], Denis Rivière[1,3], and Jean-François Mangin[1,3]

[1] LNAO, Neurospin, I2BM, CEA, Saclay, France
zysun@cea.fr
http://lnao.fr
[2] Parietal, INRIA Saclay, France
[3] IFR 49, France
http://www.ifr49.org/

Abstract. Brain imaging provides a wealth of information that computers can explore at a massive scale. Categorizing the patterns of the human cortex has been a challenging issue for neuroscience. In this paper, we propose a data mining approach leading to the construction of the first computerized dictionary of cortical folding patterns, from a database of 62 brains. The cortical folds are extracted using BrainVisa open software. The standard sulci are manually identified among the folds. 32 sets of sulci covering the cortex are selected. Clustering techniques are further applied to identify in each set the different patterns observed in the population. After affine global normalization, the geometric distance between sulci of two subjects is calculated using the Iterative Closest Point (ICP) algorithm. The dimension of the resulting distance matrix is reduced using Isomap algorithm. Finally, a dedicated hierarchical clustering algorithm is used to extract out the main patterns. This algorithm provides a score which evaluates the strengths of the patterns found. The score is used to rank the patterns for setting up a dictionary to characterize the variability of cortical anatomy.

1 Introduction

With the advances in brain imaging techniques such as MR imaging, human brain can be studied non-invasively. We are in an exciting era, when part of the tedious work of mapping the brain conducted by neuroscientists and neurosurgeons can be handled by computers, integrating anatomical, functional and genetic information. However, this work of mapping the brain cannot be accomplished without better understanding of the brain cortical folding anatomy and its variations.

The cortical folding process is relatively consistent, yet a huge variability exists from one individual to another. The primary sulci that appear early on in development, before the 30th week of gestation, are deeper and more stable [1,2]. The secondary and tertiary folds that form later are more variable from one individual to another [3,4]. The relationship between the sulcation pattern of the cerebral hemispheres and genetics is still controversial despite the efforts of many authors [5,6]. There are evidences that link folding patterns to brain functionality and pathology [3,7]. However, our knowledge of the functionality around the smaller and less stable folds is far from being certain. It is extremely difficult to study the functional implication of these folding patterns, because of the huge variability that exists across individuals.

The standard approach to overcome this variability is to map the individual brains to an average brain, so that group studies can be carried out using a simple voxel-based strategy [8]. The drawback of this approach is that some spatial information concerning the individual brains is averaged out and lost, which is particularly dramatic when studying the folding patterns. A careful alignment of the main gyral patterns is improving the spatial normalization [10,11,12] but is still hiding the existence of incompatible folding patterns, namely patterns that can not be aligned by a smooth warping. The final average brain is made up of the concatenation of the most frequent local patterns. In places where incompatible patterns occur with similar frequencies, the average brain has unpredictable shapes.

In this paper, we set up a different framework that aims at studying these incompatible patterns. The key point is to split the population into subgroups of brains with similar patterns. This leads to clustering analysis, where we try to find representation clusters that summarize the behaviour of the population. Each of these clusters represents a subgroup of the population. In this paper, the patterns defining these clusters are local but the same framework could be applied to infer global patterns. This framework was already proposed in a previous publication [13], but the shape descriptors used were not sufficient to cover all the complexity of the sulcal patterns. The innovation in this paper over the previous work is a new way to describe the sulcal shapes combining the Iterative Closest Point (ICP) and the Isomap algorithms [9,14]. This innovation leads to a much richer dictionary. The same clustering algorithm as in [13,15] is used but we provide a new set of validations dedicated to the new descriptors.

The rest of the paper focuses on our efforts for discovering and mapping the hidden patterns of cortical folding. The goal is to compute the first computerized dictionary of these folding patterns, which is performed from a database of 62 brains. The cortical folds have been extracted using BrainVisa open software. The standard sulci have been manually identified among the folds by human experts. Then these sulci are grouped into 32 different sets with some overlaps. In this paper, we limit the search to these sets. The sulcal sets cover all the regions in the frontal, temporal, parietal and occipital lobes. Some of these regions are defined to address the ambiguities that arise during the labelling process. For example, it is sometimes reported that some brains have two parallel cingulate sulci. Therefore one sulcal set grouping cingulate, intracingulate and paracingulate sulci has been created. The other regions correspond to the gyri which are more intrinsic to the functional organisation than the sulci. For example inferior frontal sulcus and some branches of the Sylvian valley are grouped together to represent Broca's area. Clustering is applied independently to each of these sulcal sets. The method is discussed below and validated using simulated and real datasets. Some results on the real datasets are presented.

2   Clustering Algorithm

The clustering process requires some descriptors of the shape of the sulcal sets. Sophisticated shape descriptors based on 3D moment invariants have been proposed before for this purpose [13]. This approach was based on only 12 general descriptors which is not enough to represent all the complexity of the folding patterns: very different shapes can sometimes lead to similar descriptors which is disturbing the clustering. In order to overcome this weakness, we propose in this paper to describe a shape by a vector of distance to a large number of similar shapes. This approach has been proven to be very efficient to compare shapes in large dimension spaces [14]. Hence the representation of the sulcal set of one subject is consisting of the distances to the same sulcal set in all the other subjects. Each pairwise distance is computed using the simple ICP algorithm after affine global spatial normalization of the brains [8]. Note that performing a global normalisation removes non-interesting patterns induced by global differences in brain size. Our ICP implementation is providing the minimal distance obtained whatever the rotation between the two shapes [9].

The input to the clustering analysis are the feature vectors of dimension 62. The curse of dimensionality is a well-known problem occurring in such situations. Therefore, dimension reduction is applied before clustering using Isomap algorithm. This algorithm has the computational efficiency and global optimality of PCA and MDS, it has also the flexibility to learn a broad class of non-linear manifolds [14]. The input is the distance matrix among the subjects. Linking each point to its K nearest neighbours, a graph is created that is supposed to describe a low dimensional manifold. Isomap first estimates the geodesic distance between points (here the set of sulci of each subject). The geodesic distance is the length of the shortest path in this graph. It is important to choose an appropriate neighbourhood size. When the neighbourhood is too large, too many "short-circuit" edges would be created; when the neighbourhood is too small, the graph becomes too sparse to approximate the geodesic paths. To our knowledge, there is no consensual general way to choose K whatever the problem. In this paper, K has been set to 6 (one tenth of the dataset size). Once the matrix of pairwise geodesic distances has been computed, dimension reduction is achieved using classical MultiDimensional Scaling. This algorithm chooses a N-dimensional configuration minimizing the stress defined by $\Sigma(g_{ij} - d_{ij})^2 / \Sigma d_{ij}^2$ where g_{ij} denotes geodesic distances and d_{ij} denotes pairwise distance in the low dimensional space. In the rest of the paper, N is set to 4. Further work will be carried out to study the dependence of the final patterns on K and N.

The clustering algorithm PCBB is applied to the Isomap result. This algorithm has been recently proposed to perform robust detection of tight clusters in a very noisy environment [15]. In this specific situation PCBB was shown to perform better than GMM (Gaussian Mixture Models [16]). It provides a score evaluating the significance of the set of detected clusters. The clustering algorithm consists of two steps. In the first step, the number of clusters and their size are estimated automatically. This is performed using a modified hierarchical clustering algorithm, where the p-value of the result is estimated by a parametric sampling process. This process is performed many times on bootstrap samples of the original data. The centers of all the clusters detected during the bootstrap are gathered into a new dataset to be clustered in the second step. This two step strategy provides robustness to the clustering. PAM algorithm (Partitioning Around Medoids [17]) is applied to this new dataset to define the final clusters. PAM is an algorithm similar to K-means including estimation of the optimal number of clusters. In our experiments, R cluster toolbox is used [17]. The estimation of the number of clusters performed by PAM in this context has been shown to be reliable [15]. The score of the final result is the average of the p-values provided during the first step of PCBB. This score is inversely proportional to the strength of the underlying patterns.

3 Validation and Results

The motivation for performing dimension reduction with Isomap method is illustrated by Fig 1. A dataset of $3*62$ shapes is generated combining the datasets of three different sulci from our manually labelled database. Dimension reduction of the ICP-based distance matrix is performed with three alternative classical approaches: Isomap, classical MDS and PCA. The result shows that Isomap outperforms the other methods for the separation of sulci.

Next, the performance of the clustering algorithm is evaluated with simulations. Our database of 62 central sulci is used for the generation of simulated datasets. Each of them is composed of 3 simulated tight clusters of 7 sulci plus 41 original central sulci, leading to a total of 62 sulci. For each simulation, three subjects are picked randomly from the original database. Six random variations are generated for each of them. Each variation results from a random transformation applied to the original sulcus. This transformation is an affine transformation endowed with a diagonal of 1 and with 6 random numbers sampled from a Gaussian distribution elsewhere. An example is provided in Fig. 2. 41 additional subjects are picked randomly among the $62-3$ other subjects to

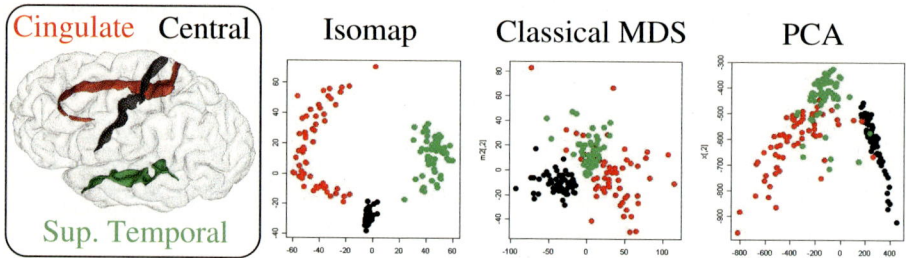

Fig. 1. Comparison of three dimension reduction methods applied on the ICP distance matrix computed for a dataset of 3 x 62 = 186 sulci. The dataset contains 62 different instances of Central (black), Cingulate (red) and Superior Temporal Sulci (green). The dimension is reduced from 186 to 2.

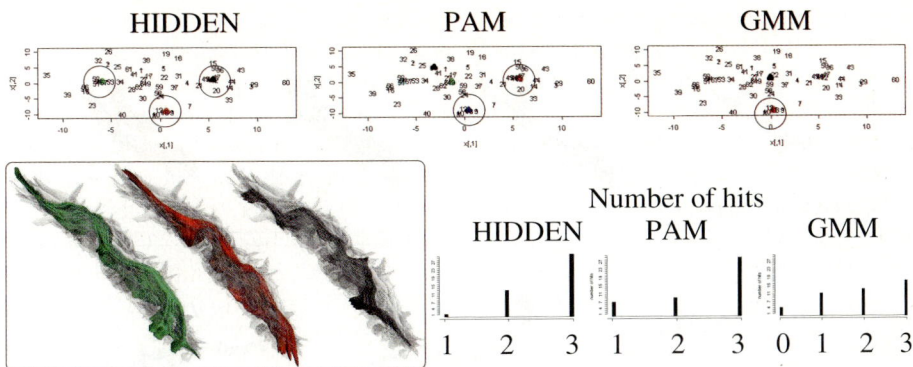

Fig. 2. Validation of the clustering of tight sulcal clusters using 50 simulated datasets. The 62 central sulci of the database are used. Each simulation includes 3 simulated tight clusters of 7 sulci each and 41 original sulci. Each cluster is generated through random deformations of one original sulcus. An example of simulation is provided on the left after ICP-based alignment (0.11 standard deviation, see text). Each color corresponds to one cluster embedded in the 41 transparent original sulci in grey. An example of clustering is provided on top where PCBB detected the three targets, while PAM and GMM missed some. Histograms of the number of hits resulting from 50 simulations are shown on the right.

complete the dataset. Ten different sets of three subjects are picked, and five different standard deviations ranging from 0.11 to 0.15 are used for generating the deformation. A total of 50 simulated datasets are obtained.

For each simulation, the ICP-based distance matrix is computed, Isomap is used for dimension reduction (K=6). Three different clustering methods are applied: PCBB [15], GMM and PAM. GMM involves first fitting a mixture model by expectation-maximization and computation of posterior probabilities [18]. The Bayesian Information Criterion (BIC) provides the number of components. The state-of-the-art Mclust toolbox from R is used to run GMM [16].

The results are evaluated in terms of the number of simulated clusters found. A detected cluster is considered a hit if the distance from its center to the center of the closest simulated cluster is within the radius of this last cluster. The radius is defined as the median of the distances to the center. Extra clusters found are not penalized since it is possible that the real data contains some clusters. Fig 2 shows a typical result and the performance statistics. PCBB outperforms the two other methods. This is not so surprising since PAM and GMM aim at providing a complete partitioning of the dataset. This goal is not always compatible with the detection of tight clusters.

Clustering was applied to the 32 sulcal sets using PCBB. Group of clusters with scores below 0.05 were collected for the dictionary. 13 sets of the left hemisphere and 12 sets of the right hemisphere passed the threshold. Fig. 3 describes three of the items of our first dictionary. Some of the discovered patterns clearly fit our initial idea of incompatibility. For instance the three patterns of left superior temporal sulcus correspond to a simple long sulcus, a Y-shaped

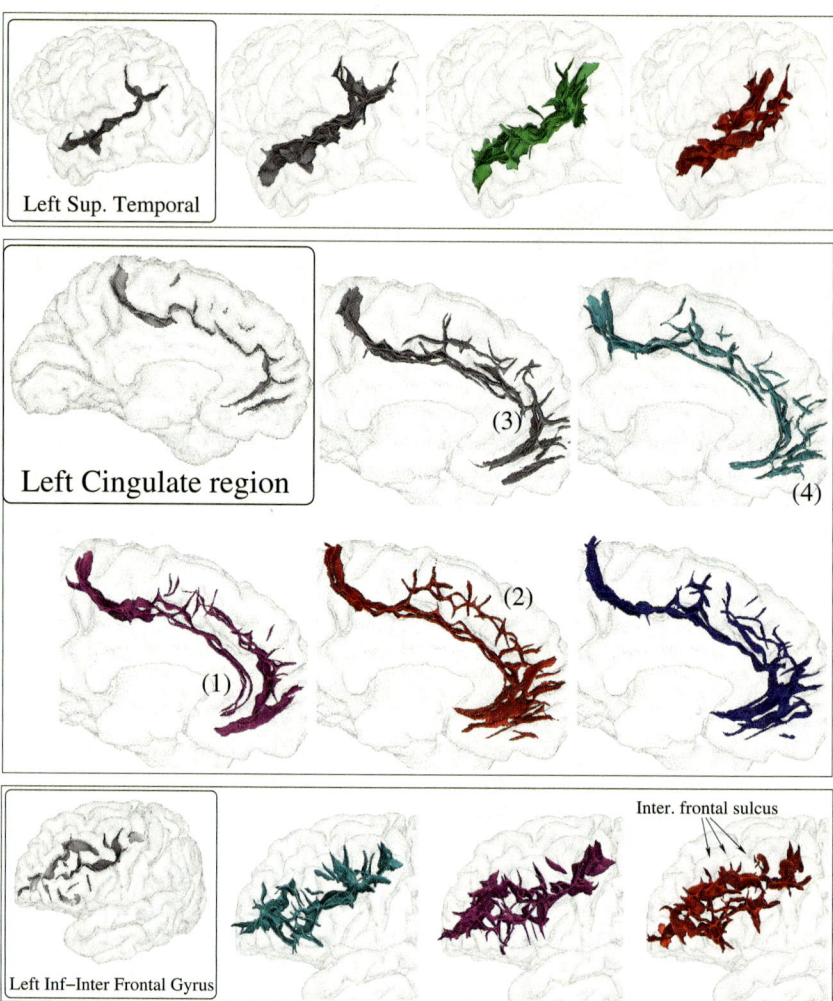

Fig. 3. Three sulcal sets with strong patterns. One example of the sulcal set is shown first. Then for each pattern, three aligned subjects are superimposed in order to highlight the areas of stability making up the patterns. The **left superior temporal sulcus** exhibits three incompatible configurations of its terminal branches. The **left cingulate region** is highly variable. The key features are (1) the development of the intracingulate sulcus (long shallow fold at the bottom of violet pattern), (2) the development of the paracingulate sulcus (series of small folds at the top of red pattern), (3) the interruptions of the cingulate sulcus and (4) the shape of the anterior part of the region. The posterior part is relatively stable. The **left Inf-Inter frontal gyrus** is made up of intermediate precentral and intermediate, marginal, orbitary and inferior frontal sulci. The main difference among the three patterns shown here lies in the different configurations of the intermediate frontal sulcus (small and split: violet, large: red, large and transverse: cyan).

sulcus, and a split sulcus with two parallel folds in the posterior part. These patterns cannot be aligned easily using spatial normalisation. This implies that if a set of brains can be split into 3 groups based on STS patterns, intra and inter group analysis of functional data could reveal new results. A sophisticated analysis including functional data, diffusion-based tractography and post-mortem histology could help us to define the correct match between the three patterns. Hence, the future of spatial normalisation might lie in a multi-template strategy based on the kind of pattern mapping proposed in this paper.

4 Conclusion

The first atlas of the variability of the cerebral sulci was proposed by Ono et al. in 1990 [4]. Tedious and patient manual work was required to collect information about a small database of 20 brains. The patterns highlighted in this seminal book were mainly related to sulcus interruptions and sulcus connexions. Taking into account the geometry of the sulci was not possible because this work was performed from flexible moulds of the brains and not from neuroimaging data using computers. Note that the ICP-based distance used for our pattern definition is not based on nonlinear warping but on the smallest distance provided by the rotation group. Therefore our clustering detects not only what was defined in the introduction as incompatible patterns but also compatible patterns that could be aligned by a nonlinear warping. This second kind of patterns could have some interest for morphometric studies.

The first results presented in this paper show that a computerized approach to the mapping of the sulcal patterns could be much more fruitful than any similar manual work. Comparing brains visually is a very difficult task even if computer graphics replaces moulds. Analysing the variability of the folding patterns is often beyond the capacity of the human visual system. On the other hand, we now have access to thousands of MR brain images that could be mined. Some computer vision softwares like BrainVISA can perform the sulcus recognition automatically. These softwares are not perfect. They do not overcome yet the ambiguities resulting from noncompatible patterns. However, applying the method described in this paper to a very large database, we do think that the quality of the automatic sulcus recognition is enough to perform a large scale mapping of the patterns. Much more sulcal sets could be considered.

Pattern analysis adds a wealth of information to our understanding of the variability that exists. For a long time, morphological variability was considered as a difficulty for functional imaging. This led to the design of the spatial normalisation paradigm. The recent understanding that brain morphology could be used to develop early diagnosis in various diseases has raised some new interests in the study of variability [19]. The research on linking the folding patterns with diseases is ongoing. Environmental and genetic factors can both play a role in early brain development, thus affecting the cortical folding process. Hence it is likely that some patterns could be used to define the signature of some developmental diseases.

References

1. Régis, J., Mangin, J.F., Ochiai, T., Frouin, V., Rivière, D., Cachia, A., Tamura, M., Samson, Y.: "sulcal root" generic model: a hypothesis to overcome the variability of the human cortex folding patterns. Neurol. Med. Chir. (Tokyo) 45, 1–17 (2005)
2. Lohmann, G., von Cramon, D.Y., Colchester, A.C.: Deep sulcal landmarks provide an organizing framework for human cortical folding. Cerebral Cortex 18(6), 1415–1420 (2008)
3. Welker, W.: Why does cerebral cortex fissure and fold? In: Cerebral Cortex, vol. 8B, pp. 3–136. Plenum Press, New York (1988)
4. Ono, M., Kubik, S., Abernathey, C.D.: Atlas of the cerebral sulci. Thieme (1990)
5. Lohmann, G., von Cramon, D.Y., Steinmetz, H.: Sulcal variability of twins. Cerebral Cortex 9, 754–763 (1999)
6. Le Goualher, G., Argenti, A.M., Duyme, M., et al.: Statistical sulcal shape comparisons: application to the detection of genetic encoding of the central sulcus shape. Neuroimage 11(5), 564–574 (2000)
7. Fischl, B., Rajendran, N., Busa, E., et al.: Cortical folding patterns and predicting cytoarchitecture. Cerebral Cortex 18(8), 1973–1980 (2008)
8. Friston, K., Ashburner, J., Poline, J.B., Frith, C.D., Heather, J.D., Frackowiak, R.S.J.: Spatial realignment and normalisation of images. Human Brain Mapping 2, 165–189 (1995)
9. Besl, P.J., McKay, H.D.: A method for registration of 3D shapes. IEEE Trans. PAMI 14(2), 239–256 (1992)
10. Fischl, B., Sereno, M.I., Tootle, R.B., Dale, A.M.: High-resolution intersubject averaging and a coordinate system for the cortical surface. Human Brain Mapping 8(4), 272–284 (1999)
11. Thompson, P.M., Woods, R.P., Mega, M.S., Toga, A.W.: Mathematical / computational challenges in creating deformable and probabilistic atlases of the human brain. Human Brain Mapping 9(2), 81–92 (2000)
12. Lyttelton, O., Boucher, M., Robbins, S., et al.: An unbiased iterative group registration template for cortical surface analysis. Neuroimage 34(4), 1535–1544 (2007)
13. Sun, Z.Y., Rivière, D., Poupon, F., Régis, J., Mangin, J.-F.: Automatic inference of sulcus patterns using 3D moment invariants. In: Ayache, N., Ourselin, S., Maeder, A. (eds.) MICCAI 2007, Part I. LNCS, vol. 4791, pp. 515–522. Springer, Heidelberg (2007)
14. Tenenbaum, J.B., De Silva, V., Langford, J.C.: A global geometric framework for nonlinear dimensionality reduction. Science 290, 2319–2323 (2000)
15. Sun, Z.Y., Rivière, D., Duchesnay, E., Thirion, B., Poupon, F., Mangin, J.F.: Defining cortical sulcus patterns using partial clustering based on bootstrap and bagging. In: 5th Proc. IEEE ISBI, Paris, France, May 2008, pp. 1629–1632 (2008)
16. Fraley, C., Raftery, A.E.: Normal mixture modelling and model-based clustering, Technical Report 504. Department of Statistics, University of Washington (2006)
17. Kaufman, L., Rousseuw, P.J.: In: Finding groups in data. Wiley series in probability and statistics (1990)
18. Duda, R.O., Hart, P.E., Stork, D.G.: In: Pattern Classification. Wiley, Chichester (2000)
19. Ashburner, J., Csernansky, J.G., Davatzikos, C., Fox, N.C., Frisoni, G.B., Thompson, P.M.: Computer-assisted imaging to assess brain structure in healthy and diseased brains. The Lancet Neurology 2, 79–88 (2003)

Topological Correction of Brain Surface Meshes Using Spherical Harmonics

Rachel Aine Yotter, Robert Dahnke, and Christian Gaser

Friedrich-Schiller University, Department of Psychiatry, Jahnstr. 3,
07745 Jena, Germany
{Rachel.Yotter,Robert.Dahnke,Christian.Gaser}@uni-jena.de

Abstract. A brain surface reconstruction allows advanced analysis of structural and functional brain data that is not possible using volumetric data alone. However, the generation of a brain surface mesh from MRI data often introduces topological defects and artifacts that must be corrected. We show that it is possible to accurately correct these errors using spherical harmonics. Our results clearly demonstrate that brain surface meshes reconstructed using spherical harmonics are free from topological defects and large artifacts that were present in the uncorrected brain surface. Visual inspection reveals that the corrected surfaces are of very high quality. The spherical harmonic surfaces are also quantitatively validated by comparing the surfaces to an "ideal" brain based on a manually corrected average of twelve scans of the same subject. In conclusion, the spherical harmonics approach is a direct, computationally fast method to correct topological errors.

1 Introduction

In brain analyses, it is sometimes desirable to deform the grey matter (GM) sheet into a sphere. A brain surface is not required to be homeomorphic with a sphere (e.g., contain no topological errors) before being mapped to a sphere. However, correcting topological defects is a necessary prerequisite for inter-subject analysis. When analyzing inter-subject data, a common coordinate system must be used to extract meaningful comparisons between the subjects. Since a brain surface mesh is roughly spherical, a logical choice is a spherical coordinate system.

There are three common representations of the cortical surface: the interface between GM and white matter (WM); the interface between GM and cerebrospinal fluid (CSF); and the central surface (CS), which is approximately midway between the GM/WM and GM/CSF interfaces. Compared to the other representations, the CS provides an inherently less distorted representation of the cortical surface [1].

Due to noise, partial volume effects, and other problems during the MRI data acquisition process, a brain surface mesh reconstructed from volumetric data often contains topological defects and artifacts. *Topological defects* can include handles and holes that prevent the surface from being homeomorphic with a sphere. *Artifacts* are topologically correct sharp peaks (usually due to noise) that have no relation to brain anatomy. Both types of errors should be repaired before the surface is inflated to a sphere. Artifacts can be minimized via smoothing. However, accurately correcting topology defects is a more complicated endeavor.

Here, we propose to use spherical harmonics for the first time to accurately correct topological defects. Spherical harmonic analysis has recently been applied to brain surface meshes, usually in the realm of shape analysis [2]. It has been applied to quantifying structural differences in subcortical structures [3-6] and full surfaces [7, 8]. Spherical harmonic analysis can be described as a Fourier transform on a sphere that decomposes the brain surface data into frequency components. The surface can also be reconstructed from the harmonic information. Generally, the RMS error of the reconstructed surface decreases as the number of coefficients increases. Furthermore, the coefficients can be weighted to achieve a smoothing effect [9].

A drawback to spherical harmonics is the computation time required to calculate the coefficients. However, a modification of the fast Fourier transform compatible with spherical coordinates significantly decreases the computation time, since it is no longer necessary to directly calculate the coefficients [10, 11].

Previously, there were two general approaches used to correct topology defects. The first approach is to start with a surface with the desired topology and deform it to match the brain surface. This includes active contours or deformable models, and there is a wealth of literature on variations of this method applied to brain data; for a review, see [12, 13]. The second approach is to retrospectively correct the topology after the brain data has been segmented into WM and GM [14-19].

In this paper, we show for the first time that spherical harmonics processing can accurately and quickly repair topological defects. The spherical harmonics approach retrospectively corrects topological errors directly on the brain surface mesh, and results in an accurately reconstructed cortical surface free from topological defects and large artifacts.

2 Methods

Topological correction using spherical harmonics can be subdivided into four processing steps. First, we resample a spherical mapping of the surface mesh and calculate coordinates of location for each sampled point based on its approximate location in the surface mesh. For this step, a spherical mapping of the cortical surface is required. This spherical mapping is not homeomorphic with a sphere, since it still contains the topological defects from the original surface. However, low distortion in the spherical mapping improves the re-parameterization process.

Second, the coordinates of location mapped on the regularly sampled sphere are forward transformed using a Fourier transform to extract the harmonic content. The harmonic content is either left intact or bandwidth-limited using a low-pass Butterworth filter. This creates two sets of data that are passed through a third step, namely an inverse Fourier transform that reconstructs the harmonic data into two distinct surfaces: a high-bandwidth surface and a bandwidth-limited smoothed surface. In the high-bandwidth reconstruction, the topological defects are replaced with a spiked topology. Finally, the spiked topology is corrected by replacing local patches with points from a lower-bandwidth reconstructed surface. The result is a defect-free brain surface that retains a high level of detail and replaces the topological defects with a smoothed, more anatomically accurate representation.

2.1 Spherical Parameterization and Generation of Tensor Fields

To analyze the harmonic content of a spherical surface, the spherical surface needs to have regularly sampled points with respect to θ and ϕ, where θ is the co-latitude and ϕ is the azimuthal coordinate. However, spherical maps of cortical surfaces usually do not have regularly sampled points, so an initial step is a re-parameterization of the spherical surface. In order to accomplish this, points are generated from equally sampled values of θ and ϕ for all members in the sets, such that there are $2B$ points per set, where B is the bandwidth. For each regularly sampled spherical point, the intersecting polygon on the cortical spherical mapping is found. Within that intersecting polygon, a coordinate of location is approximated using barycentric coordinates, e.g., the location of the regularly sampled point within the intersecting polygon on the spherical mapping determines a certain set of barycentric coordinates, and these barycentric coordinates are then used within the corresponding polygon in the original cortical surface to find the cortical location. The result is a regularly sampled spherical map in which every point is associated with a coordinate related to the location on the original cortical surface.

2.2 Harmonic Analysis

The harmonic content of a spherical mesh can be obtained using normalized spherical harmonics $Y_l^m(\theta,\phi)$:

$$Y_l^m(\theta,\phi) = P_l^m(\cos\theta)e^{im\phi}, \qquad (1)$$

where l and m are integers with $|m| \leq l$, and P_l^m is the associated Legendre function defined by:

$$P_l^m(x) = \frac{1}{2^l l!}(1-x^2)^{\frac{m}{2}}\frac{d^{l+m}}{dx^{l+m}}(x^2-1)^l. \qquad (2)$$

A square-integrable function $f(\theta,\phi)$ on the sphere can be expanded in the spherical harmonic basis such that:

$$f(\theta,\phi) = \sum_{l=0}^{B}\sum_{m=-l}^{l}\|Y_l^m\|_2^{-2}\hat{f}(l,m)\cdot Y_l^m, \qquad (3)$$

where the coefficients $\hat{f}(l,m)$ are defined by the inner product $\hat{f}(l,m) = \langle f, Y_l^m \rangle$ and the L2-norm of Y_l^m is given by:

$$\|Y_l^m\|_2^{-2} = \frac{4\pi}{2l+1}\cdot\frac{(l+m)!}{(l-m)!}. \qquad (4)$$

It is possible to solve this system directly by finding the bases first, but a more efficient approach is to use a divide-and-conquer scheme as described in [10].

The calculated coefficients are either left as is or are bandwidth-limited using a 128-order Butterworth low-pass filter in order to exclude the contributions from higher-frequency coefficients. A Butterworth filter reduces ringing artifacts and results in a smoother reconstructed surface. Finally, the harmonic content is processed through an inverse Fourier transform to produce bandwidth-limited coordinates associated with each spherical point. These filtered coordinates are used to reconstruct a cortical mesh without topological defects.

2.3 Refinement of Reconstructed Cortical Meshes

After reconstruction via spherical harmonics, the resulting cortical mesh is homeomorphic with a sphere. However, adjacent to regions formerly containing topological defects, the spherical harmonics reconstructed surface generally replaces the defect with a spiked topology that does not correspond to actual brain anatomy (Figure 1). The spiked appearance is only present if the bandwidth is high enough to admit higher frequencies; if a lower bandwidth is used, the surface near former topological defects is smooth and well-reconstructed, yet some detail is also lost.

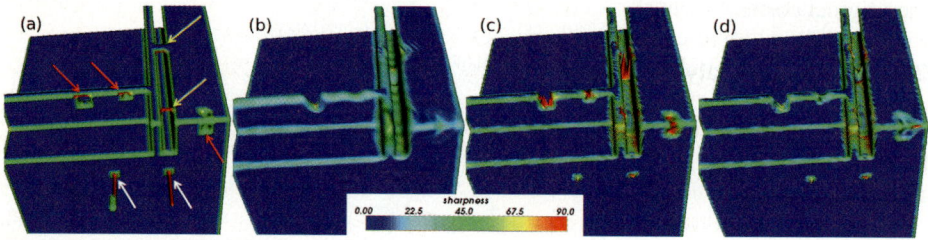

Fig. 1. Topological correction using spherical harmonics relies on a union between a high-bandwidth ($B = 1024$) and bandwidth-limited ($B_l = 64$) surface. A cubic surface (a) contains three holes (red arrows), two bridges (yellow arrows), and two artifacts (white arrows). The bandwidth-limited surface (b) corrects the topological errors but loses detail. The high-bandwidth reconstruction (c) replaces topological defects with sharp spikes. The union of the two surfaces (d) optimizes detail retention and topological error correction. Generally, smaller topological defects are repaired more accurately than larger topological defects.

As a final step, these surfaces are combined such that the regions that exhibit spiked topology in the higher-bandwidth ($B = 1024$) surface are replaced with patches from a bandwidth-limited ($B_l = 64$) cortical reconstruction. The lower bandwidth was chosen such that the spiked regions were smooth but the surface retained the approximate shape of the original cortical surface, such that the union of the two surfaces does not result in large discontinuities.

Topologically spiked regions are found by calculating a sharpness value for each point. The sharpness is the maximum angle between normals of nearest-neighbor polygons. If sharpness is above a threshold, then this point and a set of neighbors are replaced with corresponding points in the bandwidth-limited cortical surface.

Theoretically, optimal defect correction in both the WM and CS should result in the same sharpness threshold, since the bandwidths of the two proposed surfaces are the same. Basing the sharpness threshold on a certain standard deviation within the sharpness histogram is not adequate, since the brain surfaces vary widely in the number and size of their topology defects. Instead, the sharpness threshold should be set to maximize the overlap between the proposed patch area and the defect regions, while minimizing patches outside of the defect regions. It was found that a threshold of $t_s = 110°$ fulfilled these criteria, and separate threshold optimization of the WM and CS surfaces resulted in the same threshold value.

By default, the patch includes the high-sharpness point and the two nearest neighbors. However, it is possible that there may be a discontinuity between the patch and the high-bandwidth surface at the edge. Our approach was to measure the distance between the points surrounding the patch and their corresponding points in the high-bandwidth surface, and to include in the patch any points that were more than 2 mm distant. The union of these two surfaces results in a continuous cortical surface that retains high-frequency information for gyri and sulci, and an anatomically accurate reconstruction of regions that previously contained topological defects.

2.4 Sample Data Set and Verification of Results

Alongside visual validation, we wished to quantitatively assess the validity of the corrected surface. Our approach was to create an "ideal" brain by averaging twelve scans of the same brain. The averaging reduces noise and almost all of the topological defects. The remaining defects were extremely small and corrected manually using publicly available manual editing tools.

The sample data set included 12 brain scans of the same brain. These scans were acquired with a 1mm isotropic resolution on two 1.5T scanners. Each scan was processed to produce WM and CS surface representations for each hemisphere using publicly available software [20, 21]. The CS spherical mappings were additionally postprocessed using in-house tools to improve re-parameterization accuracy.

All topology corrected brain surfaces were then compared to the "ideal" averaged brain surface using mean distance error and outlier reduction percent. The mean distance error d_e is the average minimum distance between a set of points X and a surface S. The minimum distance function $d(p,S)$ between a point $p \in X$ and the surface S can be defined as:

$$d(p,X) = \min_{p' \in S} \|p - p'\|, \quad (5)$$

where p' is a point on surface S. The mean distance error is then defined as follows:

$$d_e = \frac{1}{N_p} \sum_{p \in X} d(p,S), \quad (6)$$

where N_p is the number of points in the set of points X.

Because the distance error histograms are not significantly different, a new metric was developed to quantify the reduction in distance error. The outlier reduction percent represents the fraction of points that remain above a distance error threshold set in the uncorrected brain surface, such that:

$$OP = \left(1 - \frac{N_t}{N_t^o} \cdot \frac{N_p^o}{N_p}\right) \times 100, \quad (7)$$

where N_t° and N_t are the number of points whose distance errors are above threshold in the original brain surface and the corrected surface, respectively, and N_p° and N_p are the total number of mesh points in the original brain surface and the corrected surface, respectively. The threshold is set to include the top 5% points with the largest distance error in the uncorrected brain surface. A value of 100% indicates that all outliers have been removed, while a value of 0% indicates no improvement.

3 Results and Discussion

Visual inspection reveals that the surface reconstructed using spherical harmonics is free from topological defects and is similar to the "ideal" averaged brain surface (Figure 2). The approach is valid for both the central surface and the WM surface. High-bandwidth spherical harmonic reconstruction replaces topological defects with a spiked topology (Figure 2b,f). These regions are repaired by replacing local patches with points from a bandwidth-limited reconstruction (Figure 2c,g). The result is a corrected surface that is closer to the "ideal" averaged surface compared to the original uncorrected surface (Figure 2d,h).

Quantitatively, spherical harmonics generates a corrected surface that has a lower mean distance error (0.5371 for WM; 0.6127 for CS) compared to the uncorrected surface (0.7485 for WM; 0.7757 for CS), when both surfaces are compared to the ideal surface. The outlier reduction percent was 85% for WM and 50% for CS, indicating that points with large errors are significantly reduced.

There is almost no difference between the spherical harmonic surface and the original uncorrected surface in areas that do not contain topological defects or artifacts (Figure 3). It is mostly the corrections in the areas of topological defects that are responsible for the improved distance error metrics.

By using a fast Fourier transformation rather than calculating the spherical harmonic coefficients directly, topology correction using spherical harmonics requires

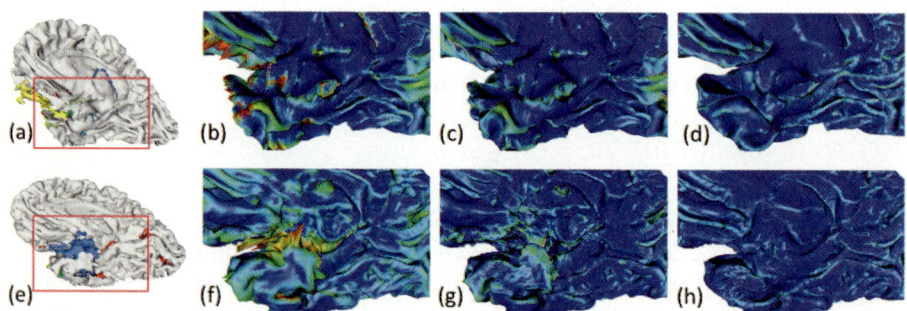

Fig. 2. Spherical harmonic correction of the WM (a-d) and CS (e-h). The original surfaces (a, e) contain holes, handles, and large artifacts (marked for visibility). These are eliminated via spherical harmonics reconstruction. At high bandwidths (b, f), the topological errors are replaced by a spiked topology. By patching these regions, the surface is reconstructed consistent with cortical anatomy (c, g). As a reference, the "ideal" brain surface is shown in (d, h). In (b-d) and (f-h), the colors represent sharpness, with red indicating high sharpness.

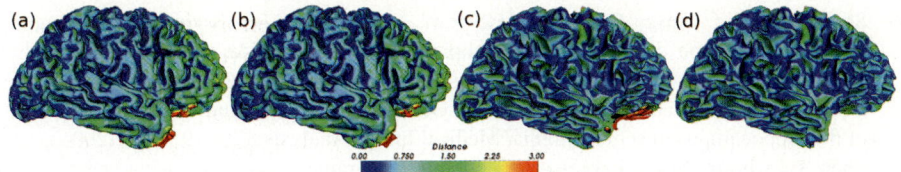

Fig. 3. Away from topological defects, surface information remains unchanged. The uncorrected surfaces for CS (a) and WM (c) are almost identical to the spherical harmonics corrected surfaces for CS (b) and WM (d), except around regions near topological defects (red). The distance in mm is the error between these surfaces and the "ideal" averaged surface.

approximately 5 minutes on a 2.4 GHz iMac for a mesh that contains 150,000 vertices. The resulting mesh contains approximately the same number of vertices.

These results are the raw output from the spherical harmonic reconstruction. There is no post-processing beyond patching the bandwidth-limited reconstruction into the high-bandwidth surface. Reconstruction can be improved by increasing the accuracy of the initial segmentation or via smoothing. Either the full brain or local regions containing high curvature or high sharpness would benefit from smoothing, especially for the CS with its low curvature. The WM surface can be further optimized using a post-refinement process that uses the original T1 data in the correction routines.

4 Conclusion

The spherical harmonics approach is a fast, straightforward method to accurately correct topological defects. We have applied spherical harmonics to cortical surfaces with the goal of correcting topological defects and artifacts, and we have shown that this approach accurately reconstructs the cortical surface. The resulting surfaces have lower mean distance errors to an "ideal" template than the original uncorrected surfaces. The computation time per hemisphere is on the order of a few minutes, suggesting that spherical harmonic reconstruction is a fast, accurate approach for topology error correction. It is highly suitable for inclusion into a processing pipeline for cortical surface analysis.

Acknowledgments. This work was supported by the following grants: BMBF 01EV0709 and BMBF 01GW0740.

References

1. Van Essen, D.C., Maunsell, J.H.R.: Two-dimensional maps of the cerebral cortex. Journal of Comparative Neurology 191(2), 255–281 (1980)
2. Brechbühler, C., Gerig, G., Kübler, O.: Parametrization of closed surfaces for 3-D shape description. Computer Vision and Image Understanding 61(2), 154–170 (1995)
3. Kelemen, A., Szekely, G., Gerig, G.: Elastic model-based segmentation of 3-D neuroradiological data sets. IEEE Transactions on Medical Imaging 18(10), 828–839 (1999)
4. Gerig, G., Styner, M., Jones, D., Weinberger, D., Lieberman, J.: Shape analysis of brain ventricles using SPHARM. In: MMBIA 2001, Kauai, HI, USA, pp. 171–178 (2001)

5. Shenton, M.E., Gerig, G., McCarley, R.W., SzÈkely, G.B., Kikinis, R.: Amygdala-hippocampal shape differences in schizophrenia: the application of 3D shape models to volumetric MR data. Psychiatric Research: Neuroimaging 115(1-2), 15–35 (2002)
6. Styner, M., Lieberman, J.A., Pantazis, D., Gerig, G.: Boundary and medial shape analysis of the hippocampus in schizophrenia. Medical Image Analysis 8(3), 197–203 (2004)
7. Shen, L., Chung, M.K.: Large-scale modeling of parametric surfaces using spherical harmonics. In: 3DPVT 2006, Chapel Hill, NC, pp. 294–301 (2006)
8. Chung, M.K., Shen, L., Dalton, K.M., Davidson, R.J.: Multi-scale voxel-based morphometry via weighted spherical harmonic representation. In: Yang, G.-Z., Jiang, T.-Z., Shen, D., Gu, L., Yang, J. (eds.) MIAR 2006. LNCS, vol. 4091, pp. 36–43. Springer, Heidelberg (2006)
9. Chung, M.K., Dalton, K.M., Li, S., Evans, A.C., Davidson, R.J.: Weighted Fourier series representation and its application to quantifying the amount of gray matter. IEEE Transactions on Medical Imaging 26(4), 566–581 (2007)
10. Healy, D.M., Rockmore, D.N., Moore, S.S.B.: FFTs for the 2-sphere-improvements and variations. Technical Report, Dartmouth College (1996)
11. Kostelec, P.J., Maslen, D.K., Healy, D.M., Rockmore, D.N.: Computational harmonic analysis for tensor fields on the two-sphere. J. Comp. Physics 162(2), 514–535 (2000)
12. McInerney, T., Terzopoulos, D.: Deformable models in medical image analysis: a survey. Med. Image Anal. 1, 91–108 (1996)
13. Montagnat, J., Delingette, H., Ayache, N.: A review of deformable surfaces: topology, geometry and deformation. Image Vis. Comp. 19, 1023–1040 (2001)
14. Fischl, B., Liu, A., Dale, A.M.: Automated manifold surgery: constructing geometrically accurate and topologically correct models of the human cerebral cortex. IEEE Trans. Med. Imaging 20, 70–80 (2001)
15. Shattuck, D.W., Leahy, R.M.: Automated graph-based analysis and correction of cortical volume topology. IEEE Trans. Med. Imaging 20, 1167–1177 (2001)
16. Han, X., Pham, D.L., Tosun, D., Rettmann, M.E., Xu, C., Prince, J.L.: CRUISE: Cortical reconstruction using implicit surface evolution. Neuroimage 23, 997–1012 (2004)
17. Jaume, S., Rondao, P., Macq, B.: Open Topology: A Toolkit for Brain Isosurface Correction. In: MICCAI (2005)
18. Segonne, F., Pacheco, J., Fischl, B.: Geometrically Accurate Topology-Correction of Cortical Surfaces Using Nonseparating Loops. IEEE Trans. Med. Imag. 26, 518–529 (2007)
19. Wood, Z., Hoppe, H., Desbrun, M., Schroder, P.: Removing excess topology from isosurfaces. ACM Trans. Graph. 23, 190–208 (2004)
20. Drury, H.A., Van Essen, D.C., Anderson, C.H., Lee, C.W., Coogan, T.A., Lewis, J.W.: Computerized mappings of the cerebral cortex: A multiresolution flattening method and a surface-based coordinate system. Journal of Cognitive Neuroscience 8(1), 1–28 (1996)
21. Fischl, B., Sereno, M.I., Dale, A.M.: Cortical surface-based analysis: II: Inflation, flattening, and a surface-based coordinate system. Neuroimage 9(2), 195–207 (1999)

Teichmüller Shape Space Theory and Its Application to Brain Morphometry

Yalin Wang[1,2], Wei Dai[3], Xianfeng Gu[4], Tony F. Chan[2], Shing-Tung Yau[5], Arthur W. Toga[1], and Paul M. Thompson[1]

[1] Lab. of Neuro Imaging, UCLA School of Medicine, Los Angeles, CA 90095, USA
[2] Mathematics Department, UCLA, Los Angeles, CA 90095, USA
[3] Mathematics Department, Zhejiang Univ. Hangzhou, China
[4] Comp. Sci. Department, SUNY at Stony Brook, Stony Brook, NY 11794, USA
[5] Department of Mathematics, Harvard University, Cambridge, MA 02138, USA
{ylwang}@loni.ucla.edu

Abstract. Here we propose a novel method to compute Teichmüller shape space based shape index to study brain morphometry. Such a shape index is intrinsic, and invariant under conformal transformations, rigid motions and scaling. We conformally map a genus-zero open boundary surface to the Poincaré disk with the Yamabe flow method. The shape indices that we compute are the lengths of a special set of geodesics under hyperbolic metric. Tests on longitudinal brain imaging data were used to demonstrate the stability of the derived feature vectors. In leave-one-out validation tests, we achieved 100% accurate classification (versus only 68% accuracy for volume measures) in distinguishing 11 HIV/AIDS individuals from 8 healthy control subjects, based on Teichmüller coordinates for lateral ventricular surfaces extracted from their 3D MRI scans.

1 Introduction

In the computational analysis of brain anatomy, volumetric measures of structure identified on 3D MRI have been used to study group differences in brain structure and also to predict diagnosis [1]. Recent work has also used shape-based features [2] to analyze surface changes. In research studies that analyze brain morphometry, many shape analysis methods have been proposed, such as spherical harmonic analysis (SPHARM) [3], medial representations (M-reps) [4], and minimum description length approaches [5], etc.; these methods may be applied to analyze shape changes or abnormalities in subcortical brain structures. Even so, a stable method to compute transformation-invariant shape descriptors would be highly advantageous in this research field. Here we propose a novel and intrinsic method to compute surface Teichmüller space coordinates (shape indices) and we apply it to study brain morphometry in Alzheimers disease (AD) and HIV/AIDS. The computed Teichmüller space coordinates are based on the surface conformal structure and can be accurately computed using the Yamabe flow method.

There are extensive research on brain surface conformal parameterization [6,7,8,9,10,11]. All surfaces may be classified by the conformal equivalence relation. If there exists a conformal map between two surfaces, then they are conformally equivalent. Any two conformally equivalent surfaces have the same conformal invariants and the same Teichmüller space coordinates. By computing and studying Teichmüller space coordinates and their statistical behavior, we can provide a promising approach to describe local changes or abnormalities in anatomical morphometry due to disease or development.

In this work, only genus-zero surfaces with three boundaries are considered. With the discrete surface Ricci flow method [10] (also called the discrete Yamabe flow), we conformally projected the surfaces to the hyperbolic plane and isometrically embedded them in the Poincaré disk. The proposed Teichmüller space coordinates are the lengths of a special set of geodesics under this special hyperbolic metric and can index and compare general surfaces. To the best of our knowledge, it is the first work to apply the Teichmüller space theory to brain morphometry research. For the cerebral cortex surface, first, we converted a closed 3D surface model of the cerebral cortex into a multiple-boundary surface by cutting it along selected anatomical landmark curves. Secondly, we conformally parameterized each cortical surface using the Yamabe flow method. Next, we computed the Teichmüller space coordinates - the lengths of three boundaries (geodesics) on the hyperbolic space - as a 3×1 feature vector. This measure is invariant in the hyperbolic plane under conformal transformations of the original surface, and is the same for surfaces that differ at most by a rigid motion.

We tested our algorithm on cortical and lateral ventricular surfaces extracted from 3D anatomical brain MRI scans. We tested our algorithms on brain longitudinal data to demonstrate the stability of our proposed Teichmüller space coordinate features. Finally, we used a nearest-neighbor classifier together with our feature vector on the lateral ventricular surface data from a group of 11 HIV/AIDS individuals and a group of 8 matched healthy control subjects. Our classifier achieved a 100% accuracy rate and outperformed a nearest neighbor classifier based on lateral ventricle volumes, which achieved an overall 68.42% accuracy rate on the same dataset.

2 Computational Algorithms

This section briefly introduces the computational algorithms in the current work. The theoretic background and definitions were abbreviated due to the page limit. For details, we refer readers to [12] for algebraic topology and [13] for differential geometry.

In this work, only genus-zero surfaces with three boundaries are considered, which are also called as *topological pants*. Let $(S, \mathbf{g})$ be a pair of topological pants with a Riemannian metric $\mathbf{g}$, with three boundaries $\partial S = \gamma_1 + \gamma_2 + \gamma_3$. Let $\tilde{\mathbf{g}}$ be the uniformization metric of S, such that the Gaussian curvature is equal to -1 at every interior point, and the boundaries are geodesics. If the length of the boundary γ_i is l_i under the uniformization metric, then (l_1, l_2, l_3) are the

Teichmüller coordinates of S in the Teichmüller space of all conformal classes of a pair of pants. Namely, if two surface share the same Teichmüller coordinates, they can be conformally mapped to each other.

Figure 1(a) illustrates a pair of pants with the hyperbolic metric and its embedding in Poincaré disk, such that the three boundaries, γ_i, are geodesics. The τ_i are the shortest geodesics connecting γ_j, γ_k, so τ_i is orthogonal to both γ_j and γ_k. The γ_i are divided to two segments with equal lengths by τ_j, τ_k. τ_1, τ_2 and τ_3 split the surface to two identical hyperbolic hexagons, with edge lengths $\frac{\gamma_1}{2}, \tau_3, \frac{\gamma_2}{2}, \tau_1, \frac{\gamma_3}{2}, \tau_2$. Furthermore, all the internal angles are right angles. The lengths of τ_1, τ_2, τ_3 are determined by $\gamma_1, \gamma_2, \gamma_3$. For the mapping in Figure 1(a) to be made, the pair of pants can have any geometry, as long as it has the topology shown. It helps us to study general brain anatomical structures.

In practice, most surfaces are approximated by discrete triangular meshes. Let M be a two-dimensional simplicial complex. We denote the set of vertices, edges and faces by V, E, F respectively. We call the *ith* vertex v_i; edge $[v_i, v_j]$ runs from v_i to v_j; and the face $[v_i, v_j, v_k]$ has its vertices sorted counter-clockwise. Figure 1(b) shows the hyperbolic triangle, and its associated edge lengths l_i, y_i, corner angles θ_i and conformal factors u_i.

A *discrete metric* is a function $l : E \to \mathbb{R}^+$, such that triangle inequality holds on every face, which represents the edge lengths. In this work, we assume all faces are hyperbolic triangles. The *discrete curvature* $K : V \to \mathbb{R}$ is defined as the angle deficit, i.e., 2π minus the surrounding corner angles for an interior vertex, and π minus the surrounding corner angles for a boundary vertex.

Discrete conformal deformation. Suppose the mesh is embedded in $\mathbb{R}^3$, so it has the induced Euclidean metric. We use l_{ij}^0 to denote the initial induced Euclidean metric on edge $[v_i, v_j]$.

Let $u : V \to \mathbb{R}$ be the *discrete conformal factor*. The discrete conformal metric deformation, shown in Figure 1(b), is defined as $\sinh(\frac{y_k}{2}) = e^{u_i} \sinh(\frac{l_k}{2}) e^{u_j}$. The *discrete Yamabe flow* is defined as $\frac{du_i}{dt} = -K_i$, where K_i is the curvature at the vertex v_i.

Let $\mathbf{u} = (u_1, u_2, \cdots, u_n)$ be the conformal factor vector, where n is the number of vertices, and $\mathbf{u_0} = (0, 0, \cdots, 0)$. Then the *discrete hyperbolic Yamabe energy* is defined as $E(\mathbf{u}) = \int_{\mathbf{u_0}}^{\mathbf{u}} \sum_{i=1}^{n} K_i du_i$.

The differential 1-form $\omega = \sum_{i=1}^{n} K_i du_i$ is closed. We use c_k to denote $\cosh(y_k)$. By direct computation, it can be shown that on each triangle, $\frac{\partial \theta_i}{\partial u_j} = A \frac{c_i + c_j - c_k - 1}{c_k + 1}$, where $A = \frac{1}{\sin(\theta_k) \sinh(y_i) \sinh(y_j)}$, which is symmetric in i, j, so $\frac{\partial \theta_i}{\partial u_j} = \frac{\partial \theta_j}{\partial u_i}$.

It is easy to see that $\frac{\partial K_i}{\partial u_j} = \frac{\partial K_j}{\partial u_i}$, which implies $d\omega = 0$. The discrete hyperbolic Yamabe energy is convex. The unique global minimum corresponds to the hyperbolic metric with zero vertex curvatures. This requires us to compute the Hessian matrix of the energy. The explicit form is given as follows: $\frac{\partial \theta_i}{\partial u_i} = -A \frac{2 c_i c_j c_k - c_j^2 - c_k^2 + c_i c_j + c_i c_k - c_j - c_k}{(c_j + 1)(c_k + 1)}$.

The Hessian matrix (h_{ij}) of the hyperbolic Yamabe energy can be computed explicitly. Let $[v_i, v_j]$ be an edge, connecting two faces $[v_i, v_j, v_k]$ and $[v_j, v_i, v_l]$.

Then the edge weight is defined as $h_{ij} = \frac{\partial \theta_i^{jk}}{\partial u_j} + \frac{\partial \theta_i^{lj}}{\partial u_j}$; also for $h_{ii} = \sum_{j,k} \frac{\partial \theta_i^{jk}}{\partial u_i}$, where the summation goes through all faces surrounding v_i, $[v_i, v_j, v_k]$. The discrete hyperbolic energy can be directly optimized using Newton's method. Because the energy is convex, the optimization process is stable.

Given the mesh M, a conformal factor vector **u** is *admissible* if the deformed metric satisfies the triangle inequality on each face. The space of all admissible conformal factors is not convex. In practice, the step length in Newton's method needs to be adjusted. Once the triangle inequality no longer holds on a face, then an edge swap needs to be performed.

3 Experimental Results

We applied our shape analysis to various anatomical surfaces extracted from 3D MRI scans of the brain. In this paper, the segmentations are regarded as given, and result from automated and manual segmentations detailed in other prior works, e.g. Thompson et al. [14,15].

3.1 Feature Stability Study with Longitudinal Brain Imaging Data

To validate the feasibility and efficiency of our proposed shape index, we compute and compare our shape index on a longitudinal brain imaging dataset [14]. The data set consists of a total of 15 pairs of cortex hemisphere surfaces of individuals with Alzheimer's disease (AD). They were scanned at 2 time points about 2 years apart [14]. AD is characterized by gradual tissue loss throughout the brain; the overall hemisphere volume decreases by around 1 percent per year but it is not known how much change there is in the overall cortical surface shape.

We selected a group of 3 landmark curves per hemisphere: the Central Sulcus, Superior Temporal Sulcus, and Primary Intermediate Sulcus. After we cut a cortical surface open along the selected landmark curves, a cortical surface becomes topologically equivalent to an open boundary genus-2 surface, which is topologically equivalent to the topological pant surface (Figure 1(a)). Figure 1 (c)-(e) illustrate a right hemisphere cortical surface and its embedding in the Poincaré disk. The three boundaries are labeled as γ_i and two shortest geodesics that connect boundaries are labeled as τ_i.

We computed the obtained feature vector for two surfaces, for both the left and right sides of the brain, extracted from the same subject scanned at two different times. For each of 15 subjects, we treated left and right hemisphere brain surfaces equivalently at both time-points, computing shape feature vectors $(T1_i, T2_i), i = 1, ..., 30$, where $T1_i$ and $T2_i$ each is a 3×1 vector. We calculated the L^2 norm of the shape difference for a given cortex hemisphere over time, $d_i = \sqrt{\sum_{j=1}^{3}(T1_{i,j} - T2_{i,j})^2}, i = 1, ..., 30$. For comparison, we also computed the L^2 norm of each feature vector, $l_m, m = 1, ..., 60$. The ratio of the median (d_i) and the median of (l_m) was 0.76%. Although this was a relatively small data set, considerable shape differences were found between different cortical hemispheres.

The relatively small difference over time demonstrated the relative stability and efficiency of our proposed feature vector for brain morphometry research.

3.2 Studying Lateral Ventricular Surface Morphometry

The lateral ventricles - fluid-filled structures deep in the brain - are often enlarged in disease and can provide sensitive measures of disease progression [15,16,17,18]. Ventricular changes reflect atrophy in surrounding structures; however, the concave shape, complex branching topology and narrowness of the inferior and posterior horns have made automatic analysis more difficult. To model the lateral ventricular surface, we introduced three cuts on each ventricle (*topology optimization*), in which several horns are joined together at the ventricular "atrium" or "trigone". After modeling the topology in this way, a lateral ventricular surface, in each hemisphere, becomes an open boundary surface with 3 boundaries, a topological pant surface (Figure 1(a)).

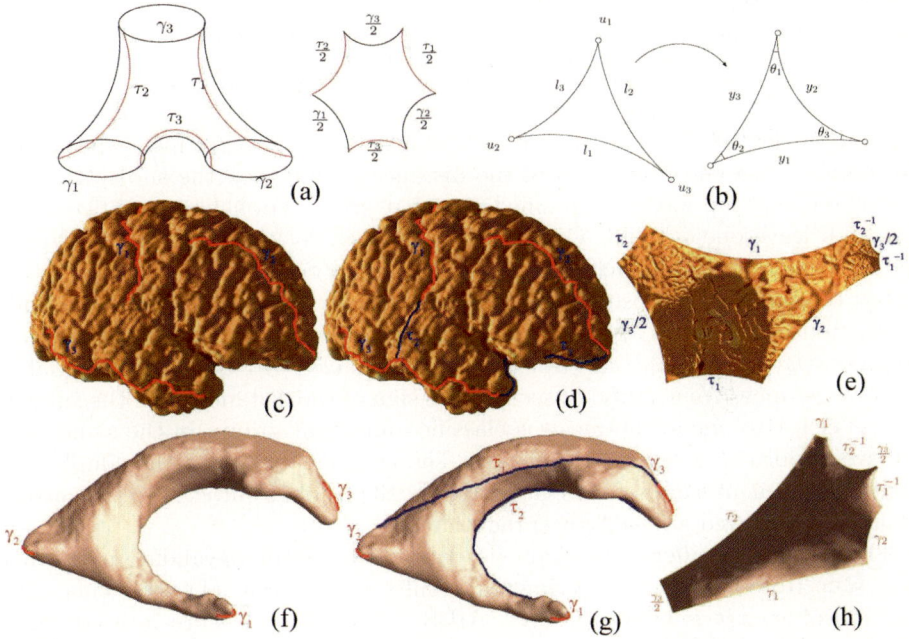

Fig. 1. (a) shows a pair of hyperbolic pants. (b) shows conformal deformation of a hyperbolic triangle. (c)-(e) illustrate how to compute the shape index on a right hemisphere cortical surface with 3 selected landmarks. (f)-(h) illustrate how to compute the shape index on a left ventricular surface. When using it as a feature vector for shape classification, a nearest neighbor classifier achieved a 100% accuracy classification in distinguishing 11 HIV/AIDS individuals from 8 healthy control subjects (versus 68% accuracy for volume measures). The shape index also detected genetic influences more powerfully than volumetric measures in a set of lateral ventricle surfaces from 76 identical twins and 56 same-sex fraternal twins than volume measures.

Figure 1 (f)-(h) illustrates how to compute Teichmüller space coordinates for a lateral ventricle. In Panel (f) and (g), γ_1, γ_2, and γ_3 are labeled boundaries and τ_1 and τ_2 are the shortest geodesics between boundaries. Panel (h) illustrates the surface with the hyperbolic metric that is isometrically flattened onto the Poincaré disk. When we make the topological change, we make sure each new boundary has the same Euclidean length across different surface. As a result, the lengths of each boundary under the Poincaré disk metric are valid metrics for studying lateral ventricular surface morphometry.

In our experiments, we compared ventricular surface models extracted from 3D brain MRI scans of 11 individuals with HIV/AIDS and 8 control subjects. The data was from a prior work [15]. The data collection, MRI image processing and surface construction were done then. We assume the surface data are given in our current work. We automatically perform topology optimization on each ventricular surface and compute their lengths in the Poincaré disk by the Yamabe flow method. For each pair of ventricular surfaces, we obtained a 6×1 vector, $t = (t_1, t_2, ...t_6)$, which consists of 3 boundary lengths for the left ventricular surface and 3 boundary lengths for right ventricular surface. Given this Teichmüller space coordinate based feature vector, we apply a nearest neighbor classifier based on the Mahalanobis distance, $d(t) = \sqrt{(t-\mu_{T_c})^T \Sigma_{T_c}^{-1}(t-\mu_{T_c})} - \sqrt{(t-\mu_{T_a})^T \Sigma_{T_a}^{-1}(t-\mu_{T_a})}$, where μ_{T_c}, μ_{T_a}, Σ_{T_c} and Σ_{T_a} are the feature vector mean and covariance for the two groups, respectively. We classify t based on the sign of the distance of $d(t)$, i.e., the subject that is closer to one group mean is classified into that group. For this data set, we performed a leave-one-out test. Our classifier successfully classified all 19 subjects to the correct group and achieved a 100% accuracy rate.

For comparison, we also tested a nearest neighbor classifier associated with a volume feature vector. For each pair of ventricular surface, we measure their volumes, (v_l, v_r). We also use a nearest neighbor classifier based on the Mahalanobis distance. We classify v based on the sign of the distance, i. e., the subject that is closer to one group mean is classified into that group. In the same data set, we performed a leave-one-out test. The classifier based on the simple volume measurement successfully classified only 13 out of 19 subjects to the correct group and achieved a 68.42% accuracy rate.

The new Teichmüller space shape descriptor requires more validation on other data sets. However, these experimental results suggest that (1) ventricular surface morphometry is altered in HIV/AIDS; (2) volume measures are not sufficient to distinguish HIV patients from controls; and (3) our Teichmüller space feature vector can be used to classify control and patient subjects. Our ongoing work is studying the correlation between the proposed feature vector and clinical measures (e.g., future decline) in an Alzheimer's Disease data set [18].

4 Discussion

An important step in our algorithm is the topology change, i.e. we cut open surfaces along certain curves. It turns a closed surface into a genus-zero open boundary surface that is topologically equivalent to the topological pant surface in Figure 1(a). In our work, they have strong clinical motivations. In modeling the brain's lateral ventricles (which split in a Y-shape), the anatomical motivation is that we introduce cuts at the ends of the anterior, posterior, and inferior horns, which join at the ventricular "atrium" or "trigone" (the center of the Y-shape). The cuts - where the 3 horns join - are automatically located. For the cortical surface, we select landmark curves that consistently appear in all subjects. An automatic algorithm can locate the landmarks as inputs for the cortex work. There are at least two benefits for us to make topology change. First, the cutting boundaries serve as landmark curves for a consistent comparison across surfaces. Secondly, with the introduced artificial cuts, it is possible for us to compute a global conformal parameterization from the entire surface to the hyperbolic space. In the hyperbolic space, we can conveniently compute shape index that continuously depends on the original surface conformal structure. In some sense, it is similar to Fast Fourier Transform (FFT) for signal processing. Our work can discriminate surface structures by computing a valid shape index from the hyperbolic conformal parameterization.

Our algorithm is based on solving elliptic partial differential equations, so the computation is stable. The computation is also insensitive to the surface triangular mesh quality so it is robust to the digitization errors in the 3D surface reconstruction. Overall, it provides an intrinsic and stable way to compute surface conformal structure based shape index for further morphometry study. For a genus zero surface, if we cut along three individual curves on a surface, we achieve a genus-zero surface with three boundaries. The shape index consists of the geodesic lengths $(\gamma_i, i = 1 - 3)$ under the hyperbolic metric in the Poincaré disk. The boundaries are clinically motivated and easy to find automatically; the shape feature is purely determined by the major anatomical features, which are easily identified and consistent across surfaces. For both applications, the shape index is determined by the overall shape so it is not very sensitive to changes in a small neighborhood. Any closed anatomical structure surfaces can be modeled in this way and becomes a topologically equivalent to a topological pant surface. Even we only consider the topological pant surface here, our method is general and can handle all arbitrary topology surfaces with negative Euler numbers. In future, we will explore more general surface applications and compare it with other shape-based surface measures.

Acknowledgments. This work was funded by National Institute of Health through the NIH Roadmap for Medical Research, Grant U54 RR021813 entitled Center for Computational Biology (CCB).

References

1. Botino, C.M., Castro, C.C., Gomes, R.L., Buchpiguel, C.A., Marchetti, R.L., Neto, M.R.: Volumetric MRI measurements can differentiate Alzheimer's disease, mild cognitive impairment and nomral aging. International Psychogeriatrics 14, 59–72 (2002)
2. Li, S., Shi, F., Pu, F., Li, X., Jiang, T., Xie, S., Wang, Y.: Hippocampal shape analysis of Alzheimer's disease based on machine learning methods. American J. of Neuroradiology 28, 1339–1345 (2007)

3. Chung, M., Dalton, K., Davidson, R.: Tensor-based cortical surface morphometry via weighted spherical harmonic representation. IEEE Trans. Med. Imag. 27(8), 1143–1151 (2008)
4. Pizer, S., Fritsch, D., Yushkevich, P., Johnson, V., Chaney, E.: Segmentation, registration, and measurement of shape variation via image object shape. IEEE Trans. Med. Imag. 18(10), 851–865 (1999)
5. Davies, R.H., Twining, C.J., Allen, P.D., Cootes, T.F., Taylor, C.J.: Shape discrimination in the hippocampus using an MDL model. In: Proc. Infor. Proc. Med. Imag, IPMI (2003)
6. Hurdal, M.K., Stephenson, K.: Cortical cartography using the discrete conformal approach of circle packings. Neuroimage 23, 119–128 (2004)
7. Angenent, S., Haker, S., Tannenbaum, A., Kikinis, R.: Conformal geometry and brain flattening. Med. Image Comput. Comput.-Assist. Intervention, 271–278 (September 1999)
8. Gu, X., Wang, Y., Chan, T.F., Thompson, P.M., Yau, S.T.: Genus zero surface conformal mapping and its application to brain surface mapping. IEEE Trans. Med. Imag. 23(8), 949–958 (2004)
9. Wang, Y., Lui, L.M., Gu, X., Hayashi, K.M., Chan, T.F., Toga, A.W., Thompson, P.M., Yau, S.T.: Brain surface conformal parameterization using Riemann surface structure. IEEE Trans. Med. Imag. 26(6), 853–865 (2007)
10. Wang, Y., Gu, X., Chan, T.F., Thompson, P.M., Yau, S.-T.: Brain surface conformal parameterization with algebraic functions. In: Larsen, R., Nielsen, M., Sporring, J. (eds.) MICCAI 2006, Part II. LNCS, vol. 4191, pp. 946–954. Springer, Heidelberg (2006)
11. Wang, Y., Gu, X., Chan, T.F., Thompson, P.M., Yau, S.-T.: Conformal slit mapping and its applications to brain surface parameterization. In: Metaxas, D., Axel, L., Fichtinger, G., Székely, G. (eds.) MICCAI 2008, Part I. LNCS, vol. 5241, pp. 585–593. Springer, Heidelberg (2008)
12. Hatcher, A.: Algebraic Topology. Cambridge University Press, Cambridge (2006)
13. Guggenheimer, H.W.: Differential Geometry. Dover Publications (1977)
14. Thompson, P.M., Hayashi, K.M., Zubicaray, G.D., Janke, A.L., Rose, S.E., Semple, J., Herman, D., Hong, M.S., Dittmer, S.S., Doddrell, D.M., Toga, A.W.: Dynamics of gray matter loss in Alzheimer's disease. J. Neuroscience 23, 994–1005 (2003)
15. Thompson, P.M., Dutton, R.A., Hayashi, K.M., Lu, A., Lee, S.E., Lee, J.Y., Lopez, O.L., Aizenstein, H.J., Toga, A.W., Becker, J.T.: 3D mapping of ventricular and corpus callosum abnormalities in HIV/AIDS. Neuroimage (in Press) (2006)
16. Carmichael, O., Thompson, P., Dutton, R., Lu, A., Lee, S., Lee, J., Kuller, L., Lopez, O., Aizenstein, H., Meltzer, C., Liu, Y., Toga, A., Becker, J.: Mapping ventricular changes related to dementia and mild cognitive impairment in a large community-based cohort. In: 3rd IEEE International Symposium on Biomedical Imaging: Nano. to Macro., April 2006, pp. 315–318 (2006)
17. Ferrarini, L., Palm, W.M., Olofsen, H., van Buchem, M.A., Reiber, J.H., Admiraal-Behloul, F.: Shape differences of the brain ventricles in Alzheimer's disease. NeuroImage 32(3), 1060–1069 (2006)
18. Chou, Y.Y., Leporé, N., Chiang, M.C., Avedissian, C., Barysheva, M., McMahon, K.L., de Zubicaray, G.I., Meredith, M., Wright, M.J., Toga, A.W., Thompson, P.M.: Mapping genetic influences on ventricular structure in twins. Neuroimage 44(4), 1312–1323 (2009)

A Tract-Specific Framework for White Matter Morphometry Combining Macroscopic and Microscopic Tract Features

Hui Zhang, Suyash P. Awate, Sandhitsu R. Das, John H. Woo, Elias R. Melhem, James C. Gee, and Paul A. Yushkevich

Penn Image Computing and Science Laboratory (PICSL), Department of Radiology, University of Pennsylvania, Philadelphia, USA

Abstract. Diffusion tensor imaging plays a key role in our understanding of white matter (WM) both in normal populations and in populations with brain disorders. Existing techniques focus primarily on using diffusivity-based quantities derived from diffusion tensor as surrogate measures of microstructural tissue properties of WM. In this paper, we describe a novel tract-specific framework that enables the examination of WM morphometry at both the macroscopic and microscopic scales. The framework leverages the skeleton-based modeling of sheet-like WM fasciculi using the continuous medial representation, which gives a natural definition of thickness and supports its comparison across subjects. The thickness measure provides a macroscopic characterization of WM fasciculi that complements existing analysis of microstructural features. The utility of the framework is demonstrated in quantifying WM atrophy in Amyotrophic Lateral Sclerosis, a severe neurodegenerative disease of motor neurons. We show that, compared to using microscopic features alone, combining the macroscopic and microscopic features gives a more holistic characterization of the disease.

1 Introduction

Diffusion tensor imaging (DTI) has become an indispensable tool for studying white matter (WM) both in normal populations and in populations with brain disorders because of its unparalleled ability to depict *in vivo* the intricate architecture of WM [1]. Many techniques have been developed recently for localizing WM differences across populations using DTI. The tract-based spatial statistics (TBSS) developed by Smith et al. [2] signficantly advanced the traditional whole-brain voxel-based WM analysis by harnessing the power of statistics on the skeleton structure of WM. However, the whole-brain approach of the TBSS fundamentally limits its anatomical specificity. Recognizing the importance of tract-specific analysis, many groups have recently developed innovative techniques for analyzing individual WM tracts with either tubular geometry [3,4,5] or sheet-like appearance [6].

This recent explosion of advances in tract-specific analysis is in large part made possible by our success in robustly segmenting individual WM tracts using diffusion data. The availability of tract segmentations presents a new opportunity for assessing macroscopic properties of a tract in addition to the standard quantification of microscopic features derived from diffusion data, such as, fractional anisotropy (FA). In this paper, we propose a tract-specific framework that, to the best of our knowledge, enables for the first time the joint analysis of tract morphometry in both macroscopic and microscopic scales. In particular, we leverage the skeleton-based modeling of sheet-like tracts proposed by Yushekvich et al. [6] to derive tract thickness maps. We show how the thickness information can be combined with microstructural features, such as FA, to enhance our understanding changes in WM morphometry. The potential of the proposed framework was illustrated in an application to quantify WM atrophy in Amyotrophic Lateral Sclerosis (ALS), a severe neurodegenerative disease.

The rest of the paper is organized as follows: Sec. 2 describes the proposed framework in detail and discusses its application in ALS. Sec. 3 reports the results from the ALS study that demonstrates the strength of combining information from different scales. Future works are discussed in Sec. 4.

2 Methods

The proposed framework has three components: (1) WM parcellation that segments the tracts of interest in all the study subjects; (2) skeleton surface-based tract modeling and matching that establishes spatial correspondence of the tracts across the study cohort and enables thickness measurement on the tracts; (3) statistical analysis that combines both thickness and standard diffusion measurement. The following discusses each component in detail.

2.1 White Matter Parcellation

We adopt the atlas-based segmentation strategy that has been successfully applied in the literature [7, 6, 3]. It involves WM parcellation in a population-averaged DTI template using fiber tractography. The parcellation in the template is then mapped to individual subjects via spatial correspondence between the template and the subjects established with image registration. If appropriate, an existing template, such as the ICBM-DTI-81 template [8], can be used. Here we choose the more general approach of deriving a population-specific template from the subject data, which simultaneously establishes spatial correspondence between the template and the subjects as part of the construction.

Construction of the Population-Averaged DTI Template. We choose the template construction method described in [9]. The method has been tailored for DT-MR data by employing a high-dimensional tensor-based image registration algorithm shown to improve upon scalar-based alternatives. Briefly, the initial average image is computed as a log-Euclidean mean [10] of the input DT-MR images. The average is then iteratively refined by repeating the following procedure: register the subject images to the current average, then compute a refined average for the next iteration as the mean of the normalized images. This procedure is repeated until the average image converges.

Tract Parcellation in the Template. We follow the approach described in [6] and parcellate the template into individual WM tracts using an established fiber tracking protocol [11]. The validity of such an approach, WM segmentation by tracking in a DTI template like ours, has recently been demonstrated by Lawes et al. [7] in a comparison to classic postmortem dissection. Our framework focuses on the tracts that have a major portion that is sheet-like. As identified in [6], six major tracts fit into this category: corpus callosum (CC), corticospinal tracts (CST), inferior fronto-occipital tracts (IFO), inferior longitudinal tracts (ILF), superior longitudinal tracts (SLF), and uncinates (UNC). White matter tracts that are more appropriately represented by tubular models have been extensively studied in the literature [3, 4, 5] and are not considered here. After fiber tractography, binary 3D segmentations of individual tracts are generated by labeling voxels in the template through which at least one fiber passes.

Tract Parcellation in the Subjects. The tracts of interest in each subject are parcellated by mapping the binary segmentations delineated in the template to the subject space using the spatial correspondence between the template and the subject determined above. In practice, this involves, for each subject, first inverting the transformation that aligns the subject to the template and then using the resulting inverse transformation to warp the template space segmenation into the subject space. The transformations derived from [9] have well-defined inverse since they are constrained to be diffeomorphic with strictly positive Jacobian determinant everywhere in the image domain.

2.2 Skeleton Surface-Based Tract Modeling and Matching

Skeleton surfaces have been shown to be a natural way of modeling sheet-like WM tracts using either direct skeletonization [2] or deformable modeling with the continous medial representation (cm-rep) [6]. In our framework, we choose to adopt the cm-rep approach because its ability to enforce a consistent skeleton topology – a 2D surface patch in our case – across subjects, which the direct skeletonization approach can not. The consistency in skeleton topology is essential for establishing spatial correspondence across subjects.

The cm-reps are models that describe the skeleton and the boundary of a geometrical object as parametric digital surfaces with predefined topology. The models describe the geometrical relationship between the skeleton and the boundary by defining a synthetic skeleton consisting of a parametric medial surface represented as a dense triangular surface mesh and a radial field defined over the surface. The radial field specifies, for each vertex on the mesh, the radius of a sphere centered at the vertex. The boundary of the object represented by the cm-rep is uniquely determined and can be computed from the synthetic skeleton via inverse skeletonization [12].

In our framework, we use the standard deformable fitting algorithm described in [12] to fit the cm-reps to the tract segmentations in the individual subjects and leverage two key feature of the cm-reps. First, the model enables a natural definition of thickness. The sphere associated with a point on the skeleton is tangent to the boundary surface at a pair of points (which may coincide at edges of the skeleton). The thickness at the point can then be estimated as the diameter of the sphere, which is two times the radial field [12]. Second, it establishes spatial correspondence across the subjects via the shape-based coordinate system that parametrizes the entire interior of the model. Because the line segments connecting a point on the skeleton to the points of tangency of the associated sphere, known as the "spokes", are orthogonal to the boundary and no two spokes intersect inside the model, it allows the definition of a coordinate system for interior of the object based entirely on the shape of the object, where two of the coordinate values parametrize the skeleton surface and the third gives the position of a point on the spokes.

2.3 Statistical Analysis of Thickness and Diffusion Features

The deformable modeling of subject-space tract segmentations using the cm-rep approach produces a parametric skeleton surface with an associated thickness map for each tract of each subject. Using the dimensionality reduction approach described in [2,6], diffusion features of interest can be similarly projected onto the same skeleton surface of each subject. We adopt the strategy originally proposed in [2] to minimize the adverse effect of errors in image alignment. Specifically, for each point on the surface, we search along its two spokes, find the location with the highest FA, then assign its diffusion features to the point.

These maps of thickness and diffusion properties computed for each subject in the same shape-based coordinate frame enable a combined analysis of both macroscopic and microscopic features. In our framework, we apply univariate statistical mapping on thickness and diffusion features separately to gain complementary tract information at different scales. A nonparametric statistical mapping of group differences is implemented as described in [6]. Briefly, we compute a two-sample t-test at each point on the skeleton surface of a tract and correct for multiple comparison with the standard permutation-based non-parametric cluster analysis introduced by Nichols et al. [13].

In addition, we utilize a novel multivariate analysis [14] to directly exploit the relationship between thickness and diffusion properties. Specifically, for each subject, we build a joint probability density function (pdf) of thickness and diffusion properties which captures the interdependencies of thickness and diffusion features as provided solely by the data. The pdf of a subject is estimated by determining the fraction of points on its skeleton surface with a particular value of thickness and diffusion properties (See Fig. 2 for an example). We use this pdf as the multivariate high-dimensional descriptor of the associated WM tract to summarize its macroscopic and microscopic properties jointly. Statistical testing for group differeces with these high-dimensional descriptors is then done via the same nonparametric test as the univariate statistical mappings above, except here the test is done in the functional domain of the pdf rather than the spatial domain of the skeleton surface.

2.4 Application: WM Atrophy in ALS

We demonstrate the proposed analysis in an application to identify WM changes in ALS. The present study consisted of 8 ALS patients and 8 healthy controls. Diffusion tensor imaging was performed on a 3T Siemens scanner with a 12-direction diffusion sequence (b = 1000 s/mm^2). For each subject, 40 axial slices with in-plane resolution of 1.72×1.72 mm and thickness of 3.0 mm were acquired. Because of the existing hypothesis that ALS strongly affects the motor pathway, only the left and right CSTs were included in the analysis. Two univariate statistical mappings on thickness and FA were first performed, followed by the multivariate analysis using the joint pdfs of thickness and FA. The clusters with FWE-corrected p-value < 0.05 were deemed significant in all analyses.

3 Results

The results of the two univariate statistical mappings are shown in Fig. 1. Two significant clusters of reduced thickness in ALS compared to healthy controls were found with one on each CST. The cluster on the left CST corresponds to the internal capsule and the one on the right CST maps to Broadmann area (BA) 6, the premotor cortex and supplementary motor cortex. One significant cluster of reduced FA in ALS was found on the left CST, which maps to BA 1, 2 & 3, the primary somatosensory cortex, BA 4, the primary motor cortex. Evidently, the macroscopic changes highlighted by the thickness analysis provides a more complete picture of WM atrophy caused by ALS than the microscopic changes identified by the FA analysis alone.

The results of the multivariate analysis using the joint pdfs of thickness and FA are shown in Fig. 2. The appearance of the joint pdfs is illustrated in Panels (a) and (b) using the joint pdfs of the left CSTs averaged for the healthy controls and the ALS patients, respectively. The two visibly different pdfs indicate that

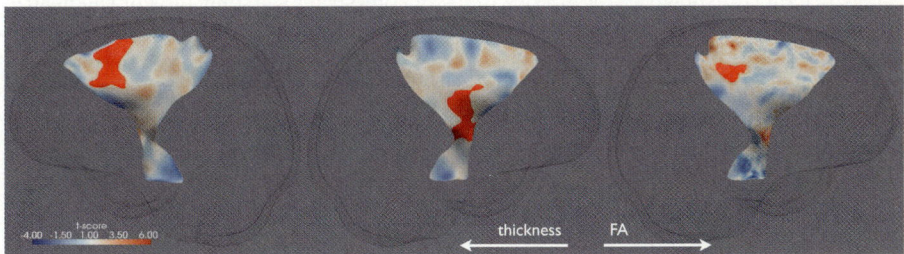

Fig. 1. The significant clusters of reduced thickness and FA in ALS compared to healthy controls (in red) overlaid on the corresponding t-statistics maps on the skeleton surfaces of the CSTs. From left to right: the thickness cluster and t-statistics map for the right CST, the thickness cluster and t-statistics map for the left CST, the FA cluster and t-statistics map for the left CST. Note that image left corresponds to physical right.

the healthy controls have more regions of large FA and thickness while the ALS have more areas of low FA and thickness. A similar pattern is observed for the right CST (not shown). These observations are supported by subsequent non-parametric statistical testing. Panels (c) and (e) show the t-statistics maps of comparing the joint pdfs of the healthy controls to those of the ALS patients. The significant clusters, determined by permutation-based multiple comparison correction, were shown in Panel (d) for the left CST and (f) for the right CST. The red clusters represent the areas of higher density in the healthy controls – high FA, while the blue clusters pinpoint the regions of higher density in the ALS patients – low FA and low thickness.

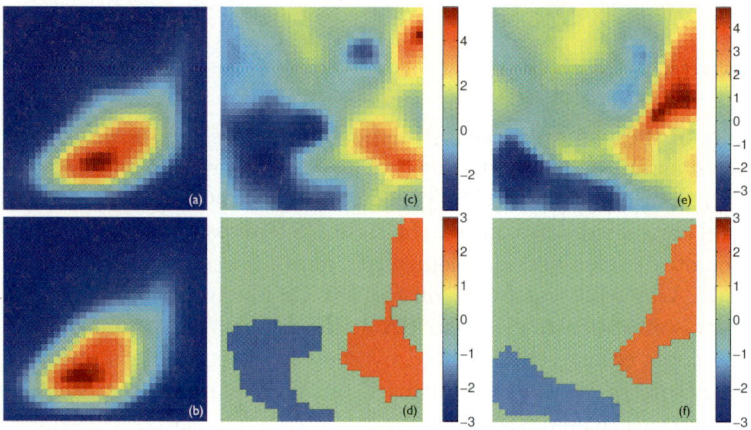

Fig. 2. The joint analysis of thickness and FA. In all panels, FA is plotted along the horizontal axis and varies from 0.1 to 0.7, while thickness is plotted along the vertical axis and varies from 0 to 8 mm. Both values are plotted in linear scale. Panels (a) and (b) show the joint pdfs of the left CST averaged for all the healthy controls and all the ALS patients, respectively, with the hot color corresponding to higher density. Panels (c) and (e) show the t-statistics maps of comparing the joint pdfs of the healthy controls to those of the ALS patients for the left and right CSTs, respectively. Panels (d) and (f) show the significant clusters with z-scores determined via permutation-based non-parametric testing for the left and right CSTs, respectively. The red clusters corresponds to larger density in the healthy controls and the blue clusters higher density in the ALS patients.

The significant clusters from the joint analysis can be better understood by mapping them back into the spatial domain, i.e., onto the skeleton surfaces of the CSTs of the individual subjects. Specifically, for each of the four clusters and for each subject group, we determined a cluster-membership probability map of the corresponding CST skeleton surface. Each of these maps were computed by finding, at each point on the corresponding skeleton surface, the probability of the location with their FA and thickness values falling within the corresponding cluster for the corresponding subject group. For instance, for some point V on

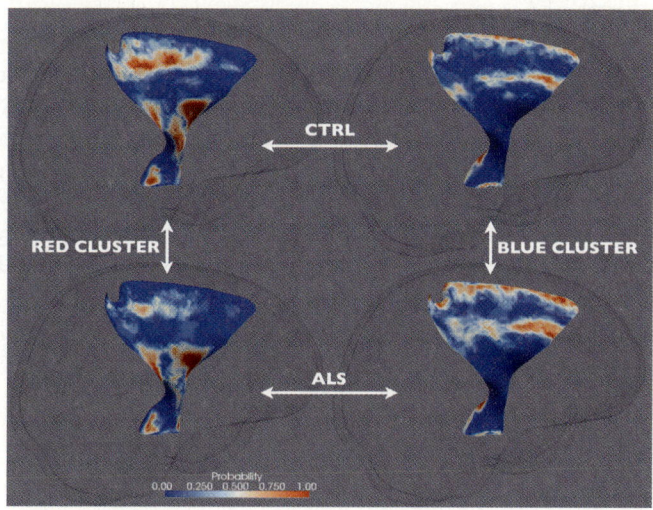

Fig. 3. The cluster-membership probability maps on the left CST for the red cluster and the healthy controls (top left), the red cluster and the ALS patients (bottom left), the blue cluster and the healthy controls (top right), and the blue cluster and the ALS patients (bottom right). See Sec. 3 for details.

the left CST, if 4 out of 8 healthy controls have their FA and thickness values at V fall within the red cluster on the left CST, then the probability map of the healthy controls for the red cluster on the left CST will have a value of 0.5 at V.

The four probability maps corresponding to the two clusters on the left CST are shown in Fig. 3. One striking observation is that, for both the healthy controls and the ALS patients, the red cluster is mapped to almost identical anatomical areas, including, from interior to superior, the cerebral peduncle, the internal capsule, and the primary motor and somatosensory areas (BA 1-4). For these areas, the cluster-membership probability is significantly less in ALS compared to the healthy controls. Because the red cluster corresponds to high FA, this finding indicates that some of the high FA normally found in these areas in the healthy controls are compromised and replaced by lower FA in ALS. Similarly, the blue cluster is mapped to near identical anatomical areas, including the premotor area (BA 6) and the peripheral of the structures. For these areas, the cluster-membership probability is significantly higher in ALS compared to the healthy controls. Since the blue cluster corresponds to low FA and thickness, this finding suggests that some of the normal FA and thickness found in these areas in the healthy controls are compromised and replaced by lower FA and thickness. Similar observations can be made with the probability maps on the right CST (not shown). Compared to the results of the univariate results, these results appear to give a more complete depiction of the extent of WM atrophy in this severe neurodegenerative disease.

4 Discussion

In this paper, we described a new tract-specific framework that supports the evaluation of WM morphometry at both the macroscopic and microscopic scales. The potential of the framework was illustrated with an application to assess WM atrophy in ALS. In the future, we plan to explore extending the novel multivariate analysis framework for tubular WM tracts proposed recently by Goodlett et al. [3] to sheet-like tracts. This should enhance our ability to capture additional patterns of morphological differences in the spatial domain.

Acknowledgments. The authors gratefully acknowledge support of this work by the NIH via grants EB006266, NS045839, DA022897, NS061111, and AG027785.

References

1. Pierpaoli, C., Jezzard, P., Basser, P.J., Barnett, A., Chiro, G.D.: Diffusion tensor MR imaging of the human brain. Radiology 201 (1996)
2. Smith, S.M., Jenkinson, M., Johansen-Berg, H., Rueckert, D., Nichols, T.E., Mackay, C.E., Watkins, K.E., Ciccarelli, O., Cader, M.Z., Matthews, P.M., Behrens, T.E.J.: Tract-based spatial statistics: Voxelwise analysis of multi-subject diffusion data. NeuroImage 31(4) (2006)
3. Goodlett, C.B., Fletcher, P.T., Gilmore, J.H., Gerig, G.: Group analysis of DTI fiber tract statistics with application to neurodevelopment. NeuroImage 45(1), S133–S142 (2009)
4. Niethammer, M., Zach, C., Melonakos, J., Tannenbaum, A.: Near-tubular fiber bundle segmentation for diffusion weighted imaging: segmentation through frame reorientation. NeuroImage 45(1), S123–S132 (2009)
5. O'Donnell, L.J., Westin, C.F., Golby, A.J.: Tract-based morphometry for white matter group analysis. NeuroImage 45(3), 832–844 (2009)
6. Yushkevich, P.A., Zhang, H., Simon, T.J., Gee, J.C.: Structure-specific statistical mapping of white matter tracts. NeuroImage 41(2), 448–461 (2008)
7. Lawes, I.N., Barrick, T.R., Murugam, V., Spierings, N., Evans, D.R., Song, M., Clark, C.A.: Atlas-based segmentation of white matter tracts of the human brain using diffusion tensor tractography and comparison with classical dissection. NeuroImage 39(1), 62–79 (2008)
8. Mori, S., Oishi, K., Jiang, H., Jiang, L., Li, X., Akhter, K., Hua, K., Faria, A.V., Mahmood, A., Woods, R., Toga, A.W., Pike, G.B., Neto, P.R., Evans, A., Zhang, J., Huang, H., Miller, M.I., van Zijl, P., Mazziotta, J.: Stereotaxic white matter atlas based on diffusion tensor imaging in an icbm template. NeuroImage 40, 570–582 (2008)
9. Zhang, H., Avants, B.B., Yushkevich, P.A., Woo, J.H., Wang, S., McCluskey, L.F., Elman, L.B., Melhem, E.R., Gee, J.C.: High-dimensional spatial normalization of diffusion tensor images improves the detection of white matter differences in amyotrophic lateral sclerosis. IEEE TMI 26(11), 1585–1597 (2007)

10. Arsigny, V., Fillard, P., Pennec, X., Ayache, N.: Log-Euclidean metrics for fast and simple calculus on diffusion tensors. MRM 56(2), 411–421 (2006)
11. Wakana, S., Jiang, H., Nagae-Poetscher, L.M., van Zijl, P.C., Mori, S.: Fiber tract-based atlas of human white matter anatomy. Radiology 230(1) (2004)
12. Yushkevich, P.A., Zhang, H., Gee, J.C.: Continuous medial representation for anatomical objects. TMI 25(12), 1547–1564 (2006)
13. Nichols, T., Holmes, A.P.: Nonparametric analysis of PET functional neuroimaging experiments: a primer. HBM 15, 1–25 (2001)
14. Awate, S.P., Yushkevich, P.A., Song, Z., Licht, D., Gee, J.C.: Multivariate high-dimensional cortical folding analysis, combining complexity and shape, in neonates with congenital heart disease. In: Proc. IPMI (2009)

Shape Modelling for Tract Selection

Jonathan D. Clayden, Martin D. King, and Chris A. Clark

Institute of Child Health, University College London, UK
j.clayden@ucl.ac.uk

Abstract. Probabilistic tractography provides estimates of the probability of a structural connection between points or regions in a brain volume, based on information from diffusion MRI. The ability to estimate the uncertainty associated with reconstructed pathways is valuable, but noise in the image data leads to premature termination or erroneous trajectories in sampled streamlines. In this work we describe automated methods, based on a probabilistic model of tract shape variability between individuals, which can be applied to select seed points in order to maximise consistency in tract segmentation; and to discard streamlines which are unlikely to belong to the tract of interest. Our method is shown to ameliorate false positives and remove the widely observed falloff in connection probability with distance from the seed region due to noise, two important problems in the tractography literature. Moreover, the need to apply an arbitrary threshold to connection probability maps is entirely obviated by our approach, thus removing a significant user-specified parameter from the tractography pipeline.

1 Introduction

Probabilistic tractography uses diffusion MRI (dMRI) data to provide estimates of the probability of a connection existing between a seed point, or seed region, and all other points within a brain volume. When the seed region is placed within a white matter tract, areas of high probability are typically found within other sections of the same tract. The first step towards estimating these probabilities of connection is to derive an orientation distribution function (ODF) for each voxel in the brain, which characterises the orientations of local structure. Several alternative methods for calculating such an ODF have been described [1], some of which are based on a specific model of diffusion, while others take a model-free approach. Probabilistic streamlines are then generated by alternating between sampling from these ODFs and stepping along the sampled direction. The probability of connection between the seed region and any other voxel is then estimated as the proportion of these streamlines that visit the target voxel.

Unfortunately, the probabilities of connection estimated by this Monte Carlo method are strongly affected by nuisance characteristics of the basic data, particularly noise, as well as limitations of the applied diffusion model. Streamlines may be deflected away from the tract of interest or prematurely truncated due to the nearby presence of a disparate tract, or due to ambiguity in the estimated

ODFs, or because of noise—and the estimated probability of connection at a given voxel may be affected in turn by any or all of these. The most common method of compensation for these effects is to threshold the visitation map to avoid including pathways which are unlikely to belong to the tract of interest. But this approach is very sensitive to an arbitrary user-specified parameter, the threshold level; and relies on the flawed assumption that false positive pathways are nonrepeatable and spatially dispersed. Moreover, it cannot correct for effects which lead to *underestimation* of the probability of connection, such as the premature termination of streamlines. A method to compensate for the latter has been proposed by Morris *et al.* [2], which uses a "null connection map" to differentiate true connections from chance events, but a threshold is still required, and the technique cannot compensate for the effects of neighbouring pathways.

Seed points or regions may be placed by an observer, or transferred from a reference tract or atlas by registering dMRI data to a standard brain template. In either case, seed regions typically have no special anatomical significance, but are instead located to maximise the chance of reconstructing the tract of interest as fully as possible. Unfortunately, direct transfer of a seed region from an atlas space to diffusion space is generally not a reliable basis for consistent tract reconstruction, although recent work by Clayden *et al.* [3] described how a probabilistic model of tract shape variability can be used to select one or more suitable seed points from within such a region. A related approach was applied to the clustering of deterministic streamlines by Maddah *et al.* [4], whereby a tract trajectory model was used to infer cluster membership.

In this work we describe how the shape modelling approach can be applied not just to the choice of seed points, but also to the selection of streamlines which accurately represent a tract of interest. Using a reference tract for prior information, but also allowing for the topological variability of a given tract between individuals, we demonstrate dramatic improvements in patterns of estimated connectivity, without the need for a user-defined threshold to be applied.

2 Methods

The tract shape model used for this work is based on that described in [3]. Streamlines are represented by uniform cubic B-splines. The knot separation distance is fixed for each tract of interest, but is invariably larger than the typical width of an image voxel, so that small scale directional perturbations are of less importance than the large scale topology of the tract.

Given a set of seed points for a dMRI data set, indexed by i, each of which generates a set of streamlines, indexed by j, a single B-spline is initially fitted to the spatial median of the streamline set. The data, $\mathbf{m}^i$, which are relevant to the model then consist of the lengths of this B-spline either side of the seed point—L_1^i and L_2^i—and the angles, ϕ_u^i, between the straight lines connecting successive knot points, and the corresponding lines in the reference tract. The B-spline is transformed into MNI standard space for the purpose of calculating these lengths and angles only. The location index u is, by convention, negative on one side of the seed point and positive on the other side.

Given the observed data, $\mathbf{m}^i$, for tract i, the model likelihood is given by

$$P(\mathbf{m}^i \mid \Theta) = P(L_1^i \mid L_1^*, \mathbf{L}_1) \, P(L_2^i \mid L_2^*, \mathbf{L}_2) \prod_{u=1}^{\check{L}_1^i} P(\phi_{-u}^i \mid \alpha_u) \prod_{u=1}^{\check{L}_2^i} P(\phi_u^i \mid \alpha_u) \quad (1)$$

where L_1^* and L_2^* are the lengths of the reference tract corresponding to L_1^i and L_2^i respectively; $\check{L}_1^i = \min\{L_1^i, L_1^*\}$ and equivalently for $\check{L}_2^i$; and $\Theta = \{\mathbf{L}_1, \mathbf{L}_2, (\alpha_u)\}$ is a set of model parameters. The distributions over each variable are given by

$$L_1^i \mid L_1^* \sim \text{Multinomial}(\mathbf{L}_1)$$
$$L_2^i \mid L_2^* \sim \text{Multinomial}(\mathbf{L}_2) \quad (2)$$
$$\frac{\cos \phi_u^i + 1}{2} \sim \text{Beta}(\alpha_u, 1) \, .$$

The model parameters are fitted using an Expectation–Maximisation (EM) algorithm, the E-step of which calculates a posterior probability of each tract representing the best match to the reference tract [5]. All tracts are assumed to be *a priori* equiprobable matches. We use the implementation of this algorithm provided by the TractoR software package (http://code.google.com/p/tractor). For the M-step we apply the hyperprior $\alpha_u - 1 \sim \text{Exponential}(\lambda)$, thereby constraining each α_u to ensure that smaller deviations from the reference tract are always more likely (i.e. $\alpha_u \geq 1$), and simultaneously avoiding model overfitting for small data sets. We take $\lambda = 1$ throughout this work.

The fitted model and posterior matching probabilities enable us to select one or more seed points which produce sets of probabilistic streamlines whose medians are accurate representations of the tract of interest for that subject. However, some individual streamlines may not resemble the median, and therefore may not accurately represent the tract of interest. To establish this, we additionally apply the modelling framework described above to streamline selection.

In this streamline-level selection phase, we begin by fitting a B-spline to each streamline, j, individually, and recovering a data vector, $\mathbf{d}^{ij}$, which describes it. This data vector is analogous to $\mathbf{m}^i$ for the median. Treating (1) as a function of the data, with the model parameters fixed to those estimated by the EM algorithm, denoted $\hat{\Theta}$, we calculate the probability of each streamline under the model, which in turn allows us to derive the value

$$\pi^{ij} = \frac{P(\mathbf{d}^{ij} \mid \hat{\Theta})}{P(\mathbf{m}^i \mid \hat{\Theta})} \, . \quad (3)$$

We then retain streamlines probabilistically, such that

$$\Pr(\text{keep streamline } j) = \min\{\pi^{ij}, 1\} \, . \quad (4)$$

Hence, streamline j will be retained with certainty if it has higher probability under the model than the median line itself; otherwise it may be kept if it has not much lower probability. Since heavily truncated streamlines—and those following

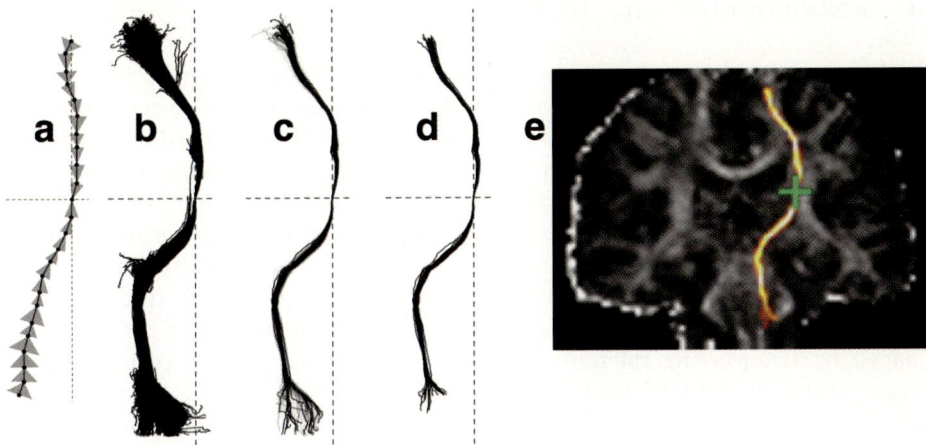

Fig. 1. Stages of the pruning process, shown in coronal projection. The knots of the reference tract are shown with 95% confidence intervals on the orientations of each tract segment (a). We also show a full set of 5000 probabilistic streamlines at full opacity (b), and with the alpha level for streamline j given by π^{ij} (c). The rejection algorithm is applied to the set, and remaining streamlines are then truncated to the length of the reference tract (d). A visitation map is finally calculated from this subset (e).

paths that differ substantially from the reference tract—will be associated with much lower values of π^{ij}, the contributions of such paths to estimates of the probability of connection will be annulled. The final step of our algorithm is to truncate all remaining streamlines to the length of the reference tract in the portions distal to the seed point. This is necessary for consistent results because the reference tract provides no orientational information in these regions, and so inappropriate trajectories have no effect on the value of (3).

This process of streamline pruning is illustrated by Fig. 1 for the left pyramidal tract. The model fitted from the median streamlines embodies the variability in tract topology across the whole data set. The amount of deviation "allowed" by the model over each segment of the reference tract is shown in Fig. 1a, in terms of the 95% confidence intervals on the angular deviation from the reference tract, which is controlled by the α_u parameters in the model. It can be seen that these confidence intervals tend to be wider towards the ends of the tract, particularly at the inferior extreme, due to greater uncertainty or variability in this region of the structure. Mapping the level of transparency to the value of π^{ij} for each streamline in the visualisation makes the effect of the method clear (Fig. 1c): some spread in the trajectories can be observed at the inferior extreme, in line with the greater local uncertainty in the model, but other branching structures are no longer visible. The probabilistic streamline retention algorithm is applied, the streamlines are truncated to the length of the reference, and a visitation map is produced (Fig. 1e).

3 Experiments and Results

Eight young, healthy right-handed volunteers (four male; mean age 31.9±5.3 yr) underwent a dMRI protocol on three separate occasions. Scans were performed on a GE Signa LX 1.5 T clinical scanner using 64 noncollinear diffusion directions at a b value of 1000 s mm^{-2}, and 7 $b = 0$ images. Reconstructed voxel dimensions were $2 \times 2 \times 2$ mm. ODFs were calculated using the Markov chain Monte Carlo method of Behrens et al., and all tractography was performed using the "ProbTrack" algorithm described by the same authors [6]. Reference tracts were created using a published white matter atlas [7], as described in [8].

For each dMRI data set, initial seed points for each tract of interest were placed by transferring reference seeds from MNI standard space to diffusion space, using the FLIRT linear registration algorithm [9]. A neighbourhood of $7 \times 7 \times 7$ voxels (volume 2744 mm^3) centred at this point was then used as a source of seed points for the modelling process. However, seed voxels with a fractional anisotropy (FA) of less than 0.2 were excluded to save time, since such voxels are very likely to be outside white matter. Throughout our experiments, a single seed point from this neighbourhood was retained by the seed-level selection phase for simplicity—although our approach generalises to multiple seed points without modification.

In order to investigate the effects of the streamline-level selection which is the main novelty in this work, we begin by examining the lengths of streamlines retained. Histograms of the streamline lengths in Fig. 1, before and after pruning, are shown in Fig. 2. It is immediately evident from this figure that there is far greater homogeneity in streamline length after the pruning algorithm has been applied. Inferior to the seed point, in particular, the bimodal distribution seen before pruning—due to a short and erroneous pathway followed by a plurality of probabilistic streamlines—is completely absent after pruning.

A significant effect of discarding prematurely truncated streamlines is the removal of the usual dependence of visitation count on distance from the seed point. Fig. 3 shows that while applying a 1% threshold to visitation maps can remove most—though, in this case, not all—false positive pathways, visitation counts are conspicuously reduced at the superior and inferior extremes of the tract. After applying the pruning algorithm this issue disappears (Fig. 3c).

The effect on diffusion tensor parameters of applying each of the three treatments is shown graphically in Fig. 4. It is apparent that the three different treatments produce substantially different patterns of FA and MD across the data set, with greatest dispersion for the untreated case corresponding to Fig. 3a. To further quantify the effects on these widely used parameters, we used a simple random effects model to estimate their group means and variance components under each treatment. Treating equivalent tracts in the two hemispheres as repeated measurements, indexed by n, we model the measurement of FA or mean diffusivity (MD) in the mth scan of the lth subject with $f_{lmn} = \mu + \Delta_l + \delta_{lm} + \varepsilon_{lmn}$, where

$$\Delta_l \sim N(0, \sigma_b^2) \qquad \delta_{lm} \sim N(0, \sigma_w^2) \qquad \varepsilon_{lmn} \sim N(0, \sigma_e^2) \, . \tag{5}$$

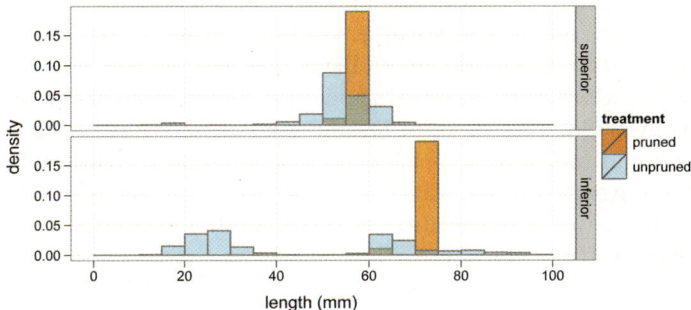

Fig. 2. Histograms showing the lengths of the pruned and unpruned streamline sets from Fig. 1, on the superior (top) and inferior (bottom) sides of the seed point

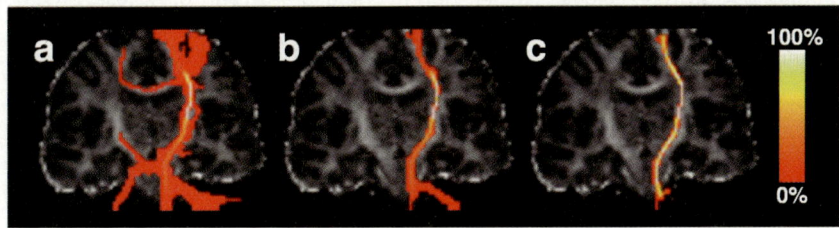

Fig. 3. An untreated visitation map for a left pyramidal tract in the data set (a). Equivalent visitation maps after thresholding at 1% of initiated streamlines (b), and after pruning (c) are also shown. No threshold is applied in the latter case. The colour scale indicates the proportion of streamlines passing through each voxel, with red indicating fewest and yellow most. The underlying images are FA maps.

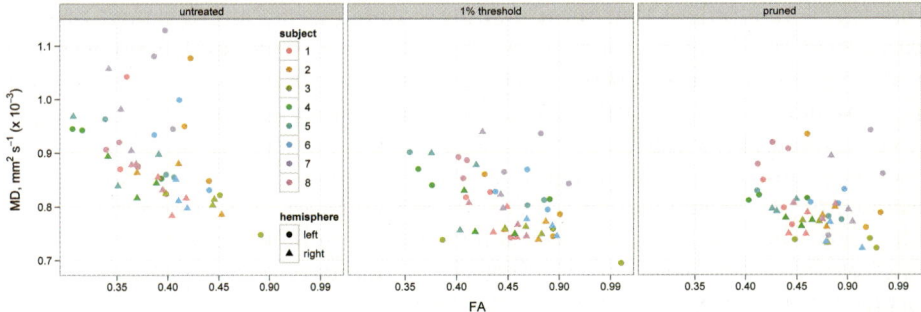

Fig. 4. Scatter plot of FA against MD based on binarised visitation maps for bilateral pyramidal tracts, using different thresholding and pruning strategies on the data

Between-subject (σ_b^2), within-subject (σ_w^2) and error (σ_e^2) variances over the data set are thereby distinguished from one another. This model was fitted using the "nlme" package for the R statistical environment (http://stat.bell-labs.com/NLME/), using the restricted maximum likelihood method [10]. The group mean and error variances for pyramidal tracts and cingulum bundles are summarised in Table 1, using visitation thresholds of 1% and 5% as well as untreated and pruned data. Mean FA and MD vary substantially depending on the threshold level applied, with the untreated results differing noticeably from the rest. The pruning algorithm produces values between those corresponding to thresholds of 1% and 5%, and on average the smallest error variance.

Table 1. Estimated group mean and error standard deviations for two major tracts

	1% threshold		5% threshold		pruned		untreated	
	μ	σ_e	μ	σ_e	μ	σ_e	μ	σ_e
pyramidal tracts, FA	0.448	0.038	0.481	0.038	0.469	0.024	0.389	0.030
pyramidal tracts, MD[†]	0.804	0.044	0.772	0.038	0.798	0.042	0.891	0.067
cingulum bundles, FA	0.374	0.033	0.438	0.045	0.386	0.044	0.285	0.021
cingulum bundles, MD[†]	0.782	0.033	0.740	0.035	0.763	0.030	0.907	0.035

[†] $mm^2 \, s^{-1} \, (\times 10^{-3})$

4 Discussion

We have demonstrated in this work a process by which a model of tract topology, combined with a predefined reference tract, can be used to select seed points for optimal tract segmentation, and also to retain or reject individual streamlines based on their probabilities under the model. The latter "pruning" method is a substantial improvement over standard thresholding approaches.

The absence of any user-specified parameters is a major advantage of the technique. It is rarely advisable to calculate parameters of interest over a region segmented using untreated tractography output (e.g. Fig. 3a), but we observe from Fig. 4 and Table 1 that the absolute recovered values and variances of such parameters are strongly dependent on the chosen threshold level. Moreover, the tacit assumption that erroneous pathways are nonrepeatable is false—as shown by the remaining false positive in Fig. 3b—and so finding a single threshold level which works well for different tracts, or even different parts of a single tract, is essentially impossible. Unlike a simple threshold, our model is sensitive to the meaning of the streamline data, and flexible enough to allow appropriate deviation from the reference tract whilst rejecting streamlines which do not follow its whole length, or branch off it. Since the streamline rejection criterion, (4), is specific to each subject, variation in tract shape from individual to individual is implicitly accounted for. Compared to region-of-interest approaches to streamline selection, our approach is very much less labour-intensive. Although the technique described in [2] also attempts to remove irrelevant tractography output, it is not tract specific and continues to rely upon a user-specified threshold.

In the present study we have limited application of our technique to probabilistic tractography using single seed points. Whilst the method could be directly applied to probabilistic or deterministic fibre tracking output derived from a neighbourhood of seed voxels, it could not, in its present form, be applied to whole-brain deterministic tractography. In addition, our focus has been on segmenting very specific pathways in groups of subjects with very high consistency, rather than covering the entire extent of the complex tracts of interest. These decisions impose some limitations on the immediate scope of this work, but the general approach has broad applicability. All tractography techniques raise the question of validation, but an increasing number of studies are vindicating fibre tracking, and our approach does not make validation any more difficult.

Finally, we have shown that the method ameliorates the usual falloff in connection probability with distance from the seed region. By retaining only sampled streamlines which accurately represent the tract of interest, estimates of connection probability are more robust, and reflect only genuine uncertainty in the tract location, rather than the effects of noise.

Acknowledgments. This work was supported by EPSRC grant EP/C536851/1.

References

1. Jones, D.: Studying connections in the living human brain with diffusion MRI. Cortex 44, 936–952 (2008)
2. Morris, D., Embleton, K., Parker, G.: Probabilistic fibre tracking: differentiation of connections from chance events. NeuroImage 42, 1329–1339 (2008)
3. Clayden, J., Storkey, A., Bastin, M.: A probabilistic model-based approach to consistent white matter tract segmentation. IEEE Trans. Med. Imag. 26, 1555–1561 (2007)
4. Maddah, M., Zöllei, L., Grimson, W., Westin, C.F., Wells, W.: A mathematical framework for incorporating anatomical knowledge in DT-MRI analysis. In: Proc. ISBI, pp. 105–108 (2008)
5. Clayden, J., Storkey, A., Muñoz Maniega, S., Bastin, M.: Reproducibility of tract segmentation between sessions using an unsupervised modelling-based approach. NeuroImage 45, 377–385 (2009)
6. Behrens, T., Woolrich, M., Jenkinson, M., Johansen-Berg, H., Nunes, R., Clare, S., Matthews, P., Brady, J., Smith, S.: Characterization and propagation of uncertainty in diffusion-weighted MR imaging. Magn. Reson. Med. 50, 1077–1088 (2003)
7. Hua, K., Zhang, J., Wakana, S., Jiang, H., Li, X., Reich, D., Calabresi, P., Pekar, J., van Zijl, P., Mori, S.: Tract probability maps in stereotaxic spaces: Analyses of white matter anatomy and tract-specific quantification. NeuroImage 39, 336–347 (2008)
8. Muñoz Maniega, S., Bastin, M., McIntosh, A., Lawrie, S., Clayden, J.: Atlas-based reference tracts improve automatic white matter segmentation with neighbourhood tractography. In: Proc. ISMRM, p. 3318 (2008)
9. Jenkinson, M., Smith, S.: A global optimisation method for robust affine registration of brain images. Med. Image Anal. 5, 143–156 (2001)
10. Bates, D., Pinheiro, J.: Computational methods for multilevel modelling. Technical report, Bell Laboratories (1998)

Topological Characterization of Signal in Brain Images Using Min-Max Diagrams

Moo K. Chung[1,2], Vikas Singh[1], Peter T. Kim[4], Kim M. Dalton[2], and Richard J. Davidson[2,3]

[1] Department of Biostatistics and Medical Informatics
[2] Waisman Laboratory for Brain Imaging and Behavior
[3] Department of Psychology and Psychiatry
University of Wisconsin, Madison, WI 53706, USA
[4] Department of Mathematics and Statistics
University of Guelph, Guelph, Ontario N1G 2W1, Canada
mkchung@wisc.edu

Abstract. We present a novel computational framework for characterizing signal in brain images *via* nonlinear pairing of critical values of the signal. Among the astronomically large number of different pairings possible, we show that representations derived from specific pairing schemes provide concise representations of the image. This procedure yields a "min-max diagram" of the image data. The representation turns out to be especially powerful in discriminating image scans obtained from different clinical populations, and directly opens the door to applications in a variety of learning and inference problems in biomedical imaging. It is noticed that this strategy significantly departs from the standard image analysis paradigm – where the 'mean' signal is used to characterize an ensemble of images. This offers robustness to noise in subsequent statistical analyses, for example; however, the attenuation of the signal content due to averaging makes it rather difficult to identify subtle variations. The proposed topologically oriented method seeks to address these limitations by characterizing and encoding *topological* features or attributes of the image. As an application, we have used this method to characterize cortical thickness measures along brain surfaces in classifying autistic subjects. Our promising experimental results provide evidence of the power of this representation.

1 Introduction

The use of critical values of measurements within classical image analysis and computer vision has been relatively limited so far, and typically appear as part of simple *preprocessing* tasks such as feature extraction and identification of "edge pixels" in an image. For example, first or second order image derivatives may be used to identify the edges of objects (e.g., LoG mask) to serve as the contour of an anatomical shape, possibly using priors to provide additional shape context. Specific properties of critical values as a topic on its own, however, has received less attention. Part of the reason is that it is difficult to construct a streamlined linear analysis framework using critical points, or values of images. Also, the computation of critical values is a nonlinear process and almost always requires the numerical estimation of derivatives. In some applications where this is necessary the discretization scheme must be chosen carefully, and remains an active area of research. It is noticed that in most of these applications, the interest is only in the stable estimation of these points rather than (1) their *properties*, and (2) how these properties vary as a function of images. We note that in brain imaging, on the other hand, the *use* of extreme values has been quite popular in other types of problems. For example, these ideas are employed in the context of multiple comparison correction using random field theory [9]. Recall that in random field theory, the extreme of a statistic is obtained from an ensemble of images, and is used to compute the *p*-value for correcting for correlated noise across neighboring voxels. Our interest in this paper is to take a topologically oriented view of the image data. We seek to interpret the critical values in this context and assess their response as a function of brain image data. In particular, we explore specific representation schemes and evaluate the benefits they afford with respect to different applications.

The calculation of the critical values of a certain function of images (e.g., image intensities, cortical thickness, curvature maps etc.) is the first step of our procedure. This is performed after heat kernel smoothing [3]. It is the second step which is more interesting, and a central focus of the paper. The obtained critical values are paired in a nonlinear fashion following a specific pairing rule to produce so-called min-max diagrams. These are similar to the theoretical construct of persistence diagrams [6] in algebraic topology and computational geometry, but have notable differences (discussed in §2.2). Min-max diagrams resemble scatter plots, and lead to a powerful representation of the key characteristics of their corresponding images. We discuss these issues in detail, and provide a number of examples and experiments to highlight their key advantages, limitations, and possible applications to a wide variety of medical imaging problems.

This paper makes the following contributions: (1) We propose a new topologically oriented data representation framework using the min-max diagrams; (2) We present a new $\mathcal{O}(n \log n)$ algorithm for generating such diagrams without having to modify or adapt the complicated machinery used for constructing persistence diagrams [2] [6]; (3) Using brain MRI, we demonstrate that using the min-max diagram representation, upon choice of a suitable kernel function, the subsequent classification task (e.g., using support vector machines) becomes very simple. In other words, because this representation captures the relevant features of the image nicely, it induces separability in the distribution of clinically different populations (e.g., autism vs. controls). We show that significant improvements can be obtained over existing techniques.

2 Main Ideas

Consider measurements f from images given as

$$f(t) = \mu(t) + \epsilon(t),\ t \in \mathbb{M} \subset \mathbb{R}^d, \tag{1}$$

where μ is the unknown mean signal (to be estimated) and ϵ is noise. The unknown mean signal is estimated *via* image smoothing over $\mathbb{M}$, and denoted as $\widehat{\mu}$. Traditionally, the estimate for the residual $f - \widehat{\mu}$ is used to construct a test statistic corresponding to a hypothesis about the signal. The mean signal may not be able to fully characterize complex imaging data, and as a result, may have limitations in the context of inference. Hence, we propose to use a new topologically motivated framework called the *min-max diagram*, which is the scatter plot of specific pairing of critical values. Intuitively, the collection of critical values of μ can approximately characterize the shape of the continuous signal μ. By pairing critical values in a nonlinear fashion and plotting them, we construct the min-max diagram. We will provide additional details shortly.

2.1 Heat Kernel Smoothing

In order to generate the min-max diagram, we need to find the critical values of μ. It requires estimating the unknown signal smoothly so that derivatives can be computed. We avoid the diffusion equation based implicit smoothing techniques [1] since the approach tend to result in unstable derivative estimation. Instead, we present a more flexible spectral approach called *heat kernel smoothing* that explicitly represents the solution to the diffusion equation analytically [3]. Heat kernel smoothing analytically solves the following equation

$$\frac{\partial F}{\partial \sigma} = \Delta F, \ F(t, \sigma = 0) = f(t).$$

The solution is given in terms of eigenfunctions ψ_k (and the corresponding eigenvalues λ_k) of the Laplace-Beltrami operator, i.e., $\Delta f + \lambda f = 0$. Define the heat kernel K_σ as

$$K_\sigma(t,s) = \sum_{k=0}^{\infty} e^{-\lambda_k \sigma} \psi_k(t) \psi_k(s).$$

The heat kernel smoothing estimate of μ is then given by

$$\widehat{\mu} = \int_\mathbb{M} K_\sigma(t,s) f(s) \, d\eta(s) = \sum_{i=0}^{\infty} e^{-\lambda_k \sigma} f_k \psi_k(t). \tag{2}$$

Examples. For $\mathbb{M} = [0,1]$, with the additional constraints $f(t+2) = f(t)$ and $f(t) = f(-t)$, the eigenfunctions are $\psi_0(t) = 1, \psi_k(t) = \sqrt{2}\cos(k\pi t)$ with the corresponding eigenvalues $\lambda_k = k^2\pi^2$. For simulation in Fig. 1, we used $\sigma = 0.0001$ and truncated the series at the 100-th degree.

For $\mathbb{M} = S^2$, the eigenfunctions are the spherical harmonics $Y_{lm}(\theta, \varphi)$ and the corresponding eigenvalues are $\lambda_l = l(l+1)$. The bandwidth $\sigma = 0.001$ and degree $k = 42$ was used for cortical thickness example in Fig. 2. We found that bandwidths larger than 0.001 smooth out relevant anatomical detail.

The explicit analytic derivative of the expansion (2) is simply given by

$$\mathcal{D}\widehat{\mu} = \sum_{i=0}^{\infty} e^{-\lambda_i \sigma} f_i \mathcal{D}\psi_i(t).$$

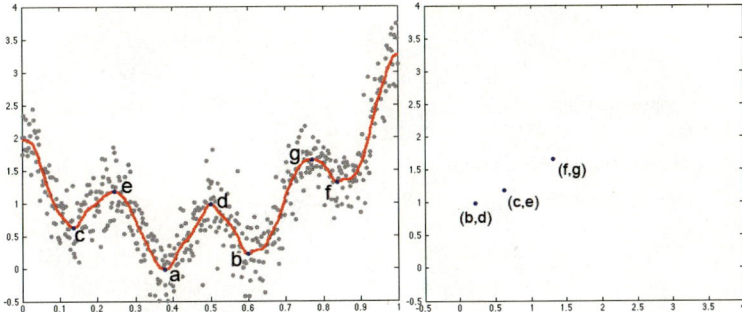

Fig. 1. The birth and death process of sublevel sets. Here $a < b < c < f$ are minimums and $d < e < g$ are maximums. At $y = b$, we add a new component to the sublevel set. When we increase the level to $y = d$, we have the death of the component so we pair them. In this simulation, we pair (f, g), (c, e) and (b, d) in the order of parings generated in Algorithm 1.

where $\mathcal{D}$ is $\frac{\partial}{\partial t}$ for $[0, 1]$ and $(\frac{\partial}{\partial \theta}, \frac{\partial}{\partial \varphi})$ for S^2. For the unit interval, the derivatives are $\mathcal{D}\psi_l(t) = -\sqrt{2}l\pi \sin(l\pi t)$. For S^2, the partial derivatives with respect to θ can be given in slow iterative formulas. To speed up the computation through the paper, the convexity of the first order neighbor of a vertex in a cortical mesh is used in determining a critical point. Fig. 2 shows the result of minimum and maximum detection after heat kernel smoothing.

2.2 Min-Max Diagram

A function is called a Morse function if all critical values are distinct and non-degenerate, i.e., the Hessian does not vanish. For images (where intensities are given as integers), critical values of intensity may not all be distinct; however, the underlying continuous signal μ in (1) can be assumed to be a Morse function. For a Morse function $\widehat{\mu}$, define a sublevel set as $R(y) = \widehat{\mu}^{-1}(-\infty, y]$. The sublevel set is the subset of $\mathbb{M}$ satisfying $\widehat{\mu}(t) \leq y$. As we increase y from $-\infty$, the number of connected components of $R(y)$ changes as we pass through critical values.

Let us denote the local minimums as $g_1, \cdots, g_m$ and the local maximums as $h_1, \cdots, h_n$. Since the critical values of a Morse function are all distinct, we can strictly order the local minimums from the smallest to the largest as $g_{(1)} < g_{(2)} < \cdots < g_{(m)}$ and similarly for the local maximums as $h_{(1)} < h_{(2)} < \cdots < h_{(n)}$ by sorting them. At each minimum, the sublevel set adds a new component while at a local maximum, two components merge into one. By keeping track of the birth and death of components, it is possible to compute topological invariants of sublevel sets such as Euler characteristics and Betti numbers (see [6]).

Simulation. The birth and death processes are illustrated in Fig. 1, where the gray dots are simulated with Gaussian noise with mean 0 and variance 0.2^2 as

$$f(t) = t + 7(t - 1/2)^2 + \cos(8\pi t)/2 + N(0, 0.2^2).$$

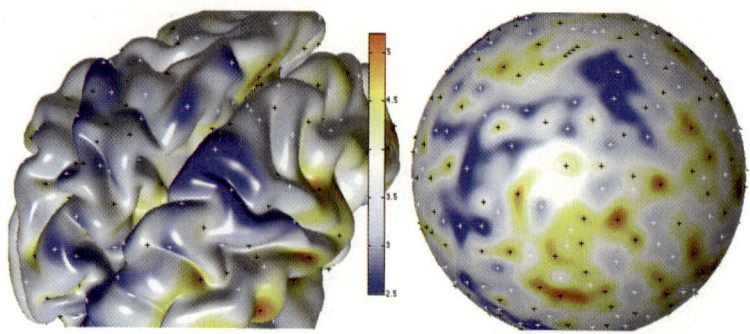

Fig. 2. Heat kernel smoothing of cortical thickness and surface coordinates with $\sigma = 0.001$ and degree $k = 42$. For better visualization, it has been flattened onto the unit sphere. The white (black) crosses are local minimums (maximums). They will be paired in a specific manner to obtain the min-max diagram. The min-max diagram is invariant to whether it is constructed from the cortical surface or from the unit sphere.

The signal is estimated and plotted as the red line using the 1D heat kernel smoothing in §2.1. Let us increase y from $-\infty$ to ∞. At $y = b$, we add a new component to the sublevel set $R(y)$. When we increase the level to $y = d$, we have the death of the component so we pair b and d. In this simulation, we need to pair (b, d), (c, e) and (f, g).

Pairing Rule. *When we pass a maximum and merge two components, we pair the maximum with the higher of the minimums of the two components* [6]. Doing so we are pairing the birth of a component to its death. Note that the paired critical values may not be adjacent to each other. The min-max diagram is then defined as the scatter plot of these pairings.

For higher dimensional Morse functions, saddle points can also create or merge sublevel sets so we also have to be concerned with them. If we include saddle points in the pairing rule, we obtain *persistence diagrams* [2] [6] instead of min-max diagrams. In one dimension, the two diagrams are identical since there are no saddle points in 1D Morse functions. For higher dimensions, persistence diagrams will have more pairs than min-max diagrams. The addition of the saddle points makes the construction of the persistence diagrams much more complex. We note that [10] presents an algorithm for generating persistence diagrams based on filteration of Morse complexes.

Algorithm. We have developed a new simpler algorithm for pairing critical values. Our algorithm generates min-max diagrams as well as persistence diagrams for 1D Morse functions. At first glance, the nonlinear nature of pairing does not seem to yield a straightforward algorithm. The trick is to start with the maximum of minimums and go down to the next largest minimum in an iterative fashion. The algorithm starts with $g_{(m)}$ (step 3). We only need to consider maximums above $g_{(m)}$ for pairing. We check if maximums h_j are in a neighborhood of $g_{(m)}$, i.e. $h_j \sim g_{(m)}$. The only possible scenario of not having any larger

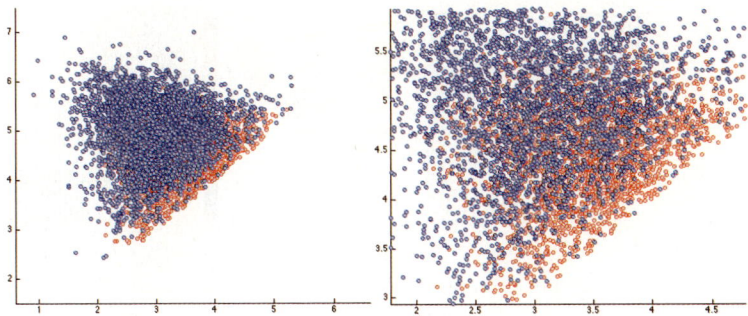

Fig. 3. Min-max diagram for 11 control (blue) and 16 autistic (red) subjects. The pairings for autism often occurs closer to $y = x$ line indicating there is greater high frequency noise in autism. This observation is consistent with the autism literature where it has been found that there is greater anatomical variability in autism subjects than the controls subjects. This figure suggests that the min-max diagram may indeed be useful for discriminating populations.

maximum is when the function is unimodal and obtains the global minimum $g_{(m)}$. In this situation we have to pair $(g_{(m)}, \infty)$. Since ∞ falls outside our 'plot', we leave out $g_{(m)}$ without pairing. Other than this special case, there exists at least one smallest maximum h_m^* in a neighborhood of $g_{(m)}$ (intuitively, if there is a valley, there must be mountains nearby). Once we paired them (step 4), we delete the pair from the set of extreme values (step 5) and go to the next maximum of minimums $g_{(m-1)}$ and proceed until we exhaust the set of all critical values (step 6). Due to the sorting of minimums and maximums, the running time is $\mathcal{O}(n \log n)$. This may also be implemented using a plane-sweep approach [4] which also gives a running time of $\mathcal{O}(n \log n)$. In this case, pairing will be based on how points enter or leave the queue of "events" as the plane (or line) sweeps in the vertical direction.

Algorithm 1. Iterative Pairing and Deletion
1. $H \leftarrow \{h_1, \cdots, h_n\}$.
2. $i \leftarrow m$.
3. $h_i^* = \arg\min_{h_j \in H} \{h_j | h_j > g_{(i)}, h_j \sim g_{(i)}\}$.
4. If $h_i^* \neq \emptyset$, pair $(g_{(i)}, h_i^*)$
5. $H \leftarrow H - h_i^*$.
6. If $i > 1$, $i \leftarrow i - 1$ and go to Step 3.

Higher dimensional implementation is identical to the 1D version except how we define neighbors of a critical point. The neighborhood relationship $\sim$ is established by constructing the Delaunay triangulation on all critical points.

3 Experimental Results

We used an MRI dataset of 16 highly functional autistic subjects and 11 normal control subjects (aged-matched right-handed males). These images were

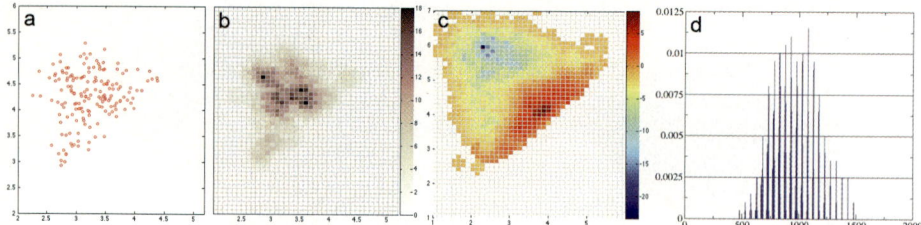

Fig. 4. (a) Min-max diagram of an autistic subject from Fig. 2. (b) The concentration map of the min-max diagram is constructed by discretizing the square $[1, 7]^2$ into 50^2 uniform pixels and evaluating the number of pairs within a circle ($r = 0.2$) centered on the pixel. (c) The t-test statistic (autism - control) shows significant group differences in red regions ($t \geq 3.61$) vs blue ($t \leq -4.05$) regions at level 0.05 (corrected). (d) PDF of the concentration map.

obtained from a 3-Tesla GE SIGNA scanner, and went through intensity nonuniformity correction, spatially normalized into the MNI stereotaxic space, and tissue segmentation. A deformable surface algorithm [7] was used to obtain the inner cortical surface by deforming from a spherical mesh (see Fig. 2). The outer surface $\mathbb{M}$ was obtained by deforming the inner surface further. The cortical thickness f is then defined as the distance between the two surfaces, this measure is known to be relevant for autism. Since the critical values do not change even if we geometrically change the underlying manifold from $\mathbb{M}$ to S^2, the min-max diagram must be topologically invariant as well. Therefore, the min-max diagram is constructed on the unit sphere by projecting the cortical data on to the sphere. Fig. 3 shows the superimposed min-max diagram for 11 control (blue) and 16 autistic (red) subjects. A single subject example is shown in Fig. 4. Pairings for autistic subjects are more clustered near $y = x$ indicating higher frequency noise in autism. More pairing occurs at high and low thickness values in the controls showing additional topological structures not present in autism.

Statistical Inference. We have formally tested our hypothesis of different topological structures between the groups. Given a min-max diagram in the square $[1, 7]^2$, we have discretized the square with the uniform grid such that there are a total of 50^2 pixels (see Fig. 4-b). A concentration map of the pairings was obtained by counting the number of pairs in a circle of radius 0.2 centered at each pixel. The inference at 0.05 level (corrected for multiple comparison) was done by performing 5000 random permutations on the maximum of t-statistic of concentration maps (Fig. 4-c).

If data is white noise, pairings occur close to $y = x$ line. The deviation from $y = x$ indicates signal. In the t-test result, we detected two main clusters of pairing difference. High number of pairings occurs around (2,6) for controls and (4,4) for autism. This is only possible if surfaces have more geometric features/signal in the controls. On the other hand, the autism shows noisier characteristic.

SVM Based Classification. Our final set of experiments were performed to evaluate the usefulness of min-max diagrams for classification at the level of individual subjects. We view the concentration map of each min-max diagram as a PDF (Fig. 4), which allows easy construction of appropriate kernels and making use of Support Vector Machines (SVM). We evaluated linear and Gaussian weighted kernels (using Bhattacharya distance between the two PDFs [5]) and found that the accuracy results were quite similar. To perform our evaluations relative to existing techniques, we used data shared with us by the authors in [8]. We summarize our results next.

For k-fold cross-validation, by varying $k \in \{9, \cdots, 2\}$, and performing 30 random runs for each k value (calculating the mean accuracy), we consistently achieved near perfect accuracy. The algorithm performs exceedingly well for 2-fold cross-validation as well – when only one half of the data is used as the training set. We incrementally decreased the size of the training set (up to 35%) and found that the algorithm still gives more than 96% accuracy. A simple comparison with 90% accuracy reported in [8] that uses the same data suggests that the improvements in accuracy comes primarily from our min-max representation.

4 Conclusions

We have presented a unified framework of the min-max diagram based signal characterization in images. While unconventional, we believe that this representation is very powerful and holds considerable promise for a variety of learning and inference problems in neuroimaging. To demonstrate these ideas, we applied the methods to characterize cortical thickness data in a dataset of autistic and control subjects, *via* the use of a new Iterative Pairing and Deletion algorithm (to generate the min-max diagram). Our results indicate that significant improvements in classification accuracy are possible (relative to existing methods) merely by representing the input data as a set of min-max diagrams. Finally, we note that this paper only scratches the surface, and future research will clearly bring up other applications where these ideas might be useful.

References

1. Cachia, A., Mangin, J.-F., Riviere, D., et al.: A primal sketch of the cortex mean curvature: a morphogenesis based approach to study the variability of the folding patterns. IEEE Transactions on Medical Imaging 22, 754–765 (2003)
2. Chung, M.K., Bubenik, P., Kim, P.T.: Persistence diagrams of cortical surface data. In: Proc. of Information Processing in Medical Imaging, IPMI (2009)
3. Chung, M.K., Dalton, K.M., Shen, L., Evans, A.C., Davidson, R.J.: Weighted fourier representation and its application to quantifying the amount of gray matter. IEEE Transactions on Medical Imaging 26, 566–581 (2007)
4. De Berg, M., Cheong, O., van Kreveld, M.: Computational Geometry: Algorithms and Applications. Springer, Heidelberg (2008)
5. Deza, E., Deza, M.M.: Dictionary of Distances. Elsevier Science, Amsterdam (2006)

6. Edelsbrunner, H., Harer, J.: Persistent homology - a survey. A survey on Discrete and Computational Geometry: Twenty Years Later, 257–282 (2006)
7. MacDonald, J.D., Kabani, N., Avis, D., Evans, A.C.: Automated 3-D extraction of inner and outer surfaces of cerebral cortex from MRI. NeuroImage 12, 340–356 (2000)
8. Singh, V., Mukherjee, L., Chung, M.K.: Cortical surface thickness as a classifier: Boosting for autism classification. In: Proc. of Medical Image Computing and Computer Assisted Intervention (2008)
9. Worsley, K.J., Marrett, S., Neelin, P., Vandal, A.C., Friston, K.J., Evans, A.C.: A unified statistical approach for determining significant signals in images of cerebral activation. Human Brain Mapping 4, 58–73 (1996)
10. Zomorodian, A.J., Carlsson, G.: Computing persistent homology. Discrete and Computational Geometry 33, 249–274 (2005)

Particle Based Shape Regression of Open Surfaces with Applications to Developmental Neuroimaging

Manasi Datar, Joshua Cates, P. Thomas Fletcher, Sylvain Gouttard, Guido Gerig, and Ross Whitaker

Scientific Computing and Imaging Institute
University of Utah
Salt Lake City, Utah

Abstract. Shape regression promises to be an important tool to study the relationship between anatomy and underlying clinical or biological parameters, such as age. In this paper we propose a new method to building shape models that incorporates regression analysis in the process of optimizing correspondences on a set of open surfaces. The statistical significance of the dependence is evaluated using permutation tests designed to estimate the likelihood of achieving the observed statistics under numerous rearrangements of the shape parameters with respect to the explanatory variable. We demonstrate the method on synthetic data and provide a new results on clinical MRI data related to early development of the human head.

1 Introduction

Technologies for shape representation and statistical shape analysis are important for several problems in medical imaging including image segmentation, quantitative analysis of anatomy, and group comparisons. A widely used approach is to evaluating shapes is assign correspondences or landmarks to shapes (curves, or surfaces) and to compare the positions or configurations of these landmarks. This approach has benefitted in recent years from methods for the automatic placement of landmarks in a way that captures the statistical properties of an ensemble of images [1,2,3]. Finding correspondences that minimize description length [2] or entropy [1] has been shown to generate shape models that systematically capture the underlying variability of the population and conform, qualitatively, to the underlying anatomy. This paper extends the method of Cates et al. [1], which uses an variational formulation of ensemble entropy to position dense collections of landmarks, or *particles*.

On the clinical front, quantitative magnetic resonance imaging has significantly advanced our understanding of brain development during childhood and adolescence. Courchesne et al. [4] describe differences in growth patterns in autism compared to controls. However, these studies do not include children below the age of 4 years. Data measured in infants from birth to 4 years are mostly *volumetric measurements*, such as intracranial volume and volumes of brain lobes and subcortical structures [5]. Whereas this selection of previous work demonstrates very active research towards determining brain growth at early stage of development, there is little data on modelling head and brain growth across a continuum of time and almost no work on the study of how development influences shape.

In developmental analyses, such as paediatric neurodevelopment, *shape regression* gives aggregate models of growth, with variability. Thus shape analysis promises to give not only basic insights into the process of development, but also allow comparisons of individuals against normative models. Of course, precise characterizations of these relationships will require shape models that can tease apart those aspects of shape variability that are explained by the underlying variables and those that are not. Likewise, in order to understand the statistical significance of such relationships we will need a systematic, unbiased method for testing these correlations. These are the topics addressed in this paper.

2 Methodology

This section gives a brief overview of the particle-system correspondence optimization method, which is first described in [1]. The general strategy of this method is to represent correspondences as point sets that are distributed across an ensemble of similar shapes by a gradient descent optimization of an objective function that quantifies the entropy of the system. Our proposed extension to this method incorporates a linear regression model into the correspondence optimization. We also present a new methodology for correspondence optimization on open surfaces where surface boundaries are defined by arbitrary geometric constraints—which is important for studying paediatric head shape.

Correspondence Optimization

We define a surface as a smooth, closed manifold of codimension one, which is a subset of $\Re^d$ (e.g., $d = 3$ for volumes). We sample a surface $\mathcal{S} \subset \Re^d$ using a discrete set of N points that are considered random variables $\mathbf{Z} = (\mathbf{X}_1, \mathbf{X}_2, \ldots, \mathbf{X}_N)^T, \mathbf{X} \in \Re^d$ drawn from a probability density function (PDF), $p(\mathbf{X})$. We denote a realization of this PDF with lower case, and thus we have $\mathbf{z} = (\mathbf{x}_1, \mathbf{x}_2, \ldots, \mathbf{x}_N)^T$, where $\mathbf{z} \in \mathcal{S}^N$. The probability of a realization $\mathbf{x}$ is $p(\mathbf{X} = \mathbf{x})$, which we denote simply as $p(\mathbf{x})$.

The amount of information contained in such a random sampling is, in the limit, the differential entropy of the PDF, which is

$$H[\mathbf{X}] = -\int_S p(\mathbf{x}) \log p(\mathbf{x}) dx = -E\{\log p(\mathbf{X})\}, \tag{1}$$

where $E\{\cdot\}$ is the expectation. Approximating the expectation by the sample mean, we have $H[\mathbf{X}] \approx -\frac{1}{Nd}\sum_i \log p(\mathbf{x}_i)$. To estimate $p(\mathbf{x}_i)$, we use a non-parametric Parzen windowing estimation, modified to scale density estimation in proportion to local curvature magnitude. The kernel width σ is chosen adaptively at each $\mathbf{x}_i$ to maximize the likelihood of that position. We refer to the positions $\mathbf{x}$ as *particles*, and a set of particles as a *particle system*.

Now consider an ensemble $\mathcal{E}$, which is a collection of M surfaces, each with their own set of particles, i.e., $\mathcal{E} = \mathbf{z}^1, \ldots, \mathbf{z}^M$. The ordering of the particles on each shape implies a correspondence among shapes, and thus we have a matrix of particle positions $P = \mathbf{x}_j^k$, with particle positions along the rows and shapes across the columns. We model $\mathbf{z}^k \in \Re^{Nd}$ as an instance of a random variable $\mathbf{Z}$, and minimize a combined ensemble and shape cost function

$$Q = H(\mathbf{Z}) - \sum_k H(P^k), \qquad (2)$$

which favors a compact ensemble representation balanced against a uniform distribution of particles on each surface. Given the low number of samples relative to the dimensionality of the space, we use a parametric approach described in [1] for density estimation in the space of shapes. The entropy cost function Q is minimized using a gradient descent strategy to manipulate particle positions (and, thus, also correspondence positions). The surface constraint is specified by the zero set of a scalar function $F(x)$. This optimization strategy balances entropy of individual surface samplings with the entropy of the shape model, maximizing the former for geometric accuracy (a good sampling) and minimizing the latter to produce a compact model.

Any set of implicitly defined surfaces is appropriate as input to this framework. For this paper, we use binary segmentations, which contain an implicit shape surface at the interface of the labeled pixels and the background. To remove aliasing artifacts in these segmentations, we use the r-tightening algorithm given by Williams et al. [6]. Correspondence optimizations are initialized with the splitting strategy described in [1], starting with a single particle on each object. We use a Procrustes algorithm, applied at regular intervals during the optimization, to align shapes with respect to rotation and translation, and to normalize with respect to scale.

Correspondence with Regression Against Explanatory Variables. With the assumption of a Gaussian distribution in the space of shapes, we can introduce a generative statistical model

$$\mathbf{z} = \mu + \epsilon, \epsilon \sim \mathcal{N}(\mathbf{0}, \Sigma) \qquad (3)$$

for particle correspondence positions, where μ is the vector of mean correspondences, and ϵ is normally-distributed error. Replacing μ in this model with a function of an explanatory variable t gives the more general, *regression* model

$$\mathbf{z} = f(t) + \hat{\epsilon}, \hat{\epsilon} \sim \mathcal{N}(\mathbf{0}, \hat{\Sigma}). \qquad (4)$$

The optimization described in the previous section minimizes the entropy associated with ϵ, which is the difference from the mean. In this paper, we propose to optimize correspondences under the regression model in Eqn. 4 by instead minimizing entropy associated with $\hat{\epsilon}$, the residual from the model. Considering particle correspondence to be a linear function of t, given as $f(t) = \mathbf{a} + \mathbf{b}t$, we need an estimate of parameters **a** and **b** to compute $\hat{\epsilon}$. We estimate these with a least-squares fit to the correspondence data,

$$\arg\min_{\mathbf{a},\mathbf{b}} E(\mathbf{a},\mathbf{b}) = \frac{1}{2}\sum_k [(\mathbf{a}+\mathbf{b}t_k)-\mathbf{z}_k]^T \Sigma^{-1} [(\mathbf{a}+\mathbf{b}t_k)-\mathbf{z}_k]. \quad (5)$$

Setting $\frac{\delta E}{\delta \mathbf{a}} = \frac{\delta E}{\delta \mathbf{b}} = 0$ and solving for **a** and **b**, we have $\mathbf{a} = \frac{1}{n}(\sum_k \mathbf{z}_k - \sum_k \mathbf{b}t_k)$, and $\mathbf{b} = (\sum_k t_k \mathbf{z}_k - \sum_k \mathbf{z}_k \sum_k t_k) / (\sum_k t_k^2 - (\sum t_k)^2)$.

The proposed regression model optimization algorithm then proceeds as follows. Correspondences are first optimized under the nonregression model (Eqn 3) to minimize the entropy associated with the total error ϵ, and to establish an initial estimate for **a** and **b**. We then follow the same optimization procedure as described in Section. 2, but replace the covariance of the model with the covariance of the underlying residual relative to the generative model. We interleave the two estimation problems, and thus the parameters **a** and **b** are re-estimated after each iteration of the gradient descent on the particle positions.

Correspondences on Open Surfaces. To compute correspondence positions on a set of *open* surfaces, we propose an extension to the sampling method reviewed in Section. 2. The proposed method is to define the boundary as the intersection of the surface $\mathcal{S}$ with a set of geometric primitives, such as cutting planes and spheres. Our goal is to formulate the interactions with these boundaries so that the positions of these constraints has as little influence as possible on the statistical shape model.

For each geometric primitive, we construct a *virtual* particle distribution that consists of all of the closest points on its surface to the particles $\mathbf{x}_i$ on $\mathcal{S}$. During the gradient descent optimization, particles $\mathbf{x}_i$ interact with the virtual particles, and are therefore effectively repelled from the geometric primitives, and thus from the open surface boundary. The virtual distributions are updated after each iteration as the particles on $\mathcal{S}$ redistribute under the optimization. Because the virtual particles are allowed to factor into the Parzen windowing kernel size estimation, particles $\mathbf{x}_i$ maintain a distance from the

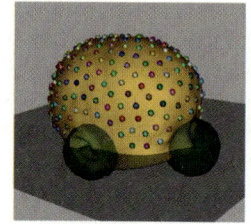

Fig. 1. Particle system with geometric primitives defining the boundary

boundary proportional to their density on the surface $\mathcal{S}$. In this way, features near the boundary may be sampled, but particles are never allowed to lie on the actual boundary itself. One such configuration is shown in Figure. 1

Permutation Test of Significance. Analysis of variance (ANOVA) is the standard parametric test for testing if the explanatory variables have a significant effect in a linear regression. The test statistic used is

$$T = \frac{R^2/(m-1)}{(1-R^2)/(n-m)}, \quad (6)$$

where R^2 is Pearson's coefficient of regression, generally defined as $R^2 = 1 - \frac{SS_{\text{err}}}{SS_{\text{tot}}}$, where SS_{err} is the sum-squared residual error, and SS_{tot} represents total variance in the data. In general, R^2 can be related to the unexplained variance of the generated model, and is used to measure the *goodness-of-fit* for the regression model. When the residuals of the linear model are iid Gaussian, the statistic T follows an F distribution with $m-1$ and $n-m$ degrees of freedom under the null hypothesis.

In this case where the outcome variables are correspondence-optimized shape parameters, the underlying assumptions of the parametric F-test may not hold. Furthermore, optimization with knowledge of the underlying parameter could lead to optimistic estimates of significance, because we are explicitly minimizing the residual. To overcome this, we propose a nonparametric permutation test for significance. Permutation tests for regression work by permuting the values of the explanatory variables. This allows us to compute a distribution of our test statistic under the null hypothesis that the explanatory variable has no relationship to the dependent variable. Given data (z_i, t_i), we generate the kth permuted data set as $(z_i, t_{\pi_k(i)})$, where π_k is a permutation of $1, \ldots, n$. For each permutation we compute a test statistic T_k using (6). Then comparing our unpermuted test statistic T to the distribution of T_k, we can compute the p-value as the percentage of T_k that are greater than T. Notice, that for the case of regression-optimized correspondences, described in Section 2, we perform a the correspondence optimization on *each* permutation separately, and thus *the results of our permutation test are not biased by the correspondence method*.

3 Results and Discussion

This section details experiments designed to illustrate and validate the proposed method. First, we present an experiment with synthetically generated tori to illustrate the applicability of the method and validation based on permutation tests. Next, we present an application to the study of early growth of head shapes extracted from structural MRI data.

To illustrate and validate the proposed methods, we performed two experiments on sets of 40 synthetically generated tori, parameterized by the small radius r and the large radius R. The values for the shape parameters were chosen as independent functions of a uniformly distributed explanatory variable t. The definition of R^2, used to compute the test statistic as explained in Section. 2, is extended to include the two independent variables for this experiment:

$$R^2 = 1 - \frac{(SS_{err})_r + (SS_{err})_R}{(SS_{tot})_r + (SS_{tot})_R}. \tag{7}$$

We examine sets of time-dependent shapes with p-values $\{0.01, 0.1\}$ in order to examine the performance of the system with and without significance. To construct these example data sets, we use the value for the statistic T (look up from the F-distribution) to generate a target R^2. The values of r and R are chosen such that the R^2 of the generated set is approximately equal to the target R^2 for that experiment. Along with explicit correspondences generated from the standard torus parametrization, we use the correspondence methods from Section. 2, optimization with and without an underlying regression model, to optimize correspondences using 256 particles on each shape. An analysis of the resulting models showed that all three sets of correspondences exhibited two pure modes of variation.

Synthetic Data (Tori). Here we present the results of the statistical analysis of the tori test data using permutation tests consisting of 1000 permutations of the explanatory variable t. For the correspondences we compute the test statistics using the two dominant modes from a PCA on the set of correspondences. The procedure described in Section. 2 is then applied to get the corresponding p-values. Table. 1 shows the results of the two permutation tests for the explicit correspondences, and correspondences generated using the proposed methods. A comparison of the parametric p-value with the p-values obtained by the permutation tests confirms that the proposed methods preserve the relationship between the explanatory variable and the dependent variables. The correspondence-based approaches, particularly with the regression model, show greater significance than the parametric case. This might be an inherent property of the statistic or it could be an artifact due to the limited number of example datasets and the limited number of permutations. Future work will include more datasets, more permutations, and a bootstrapping procedure to analyze variability of the p-values computed by the various methods.

Table 1. Results of permutation tests (1000 permutations)

p-value (theory)	p-value (parametric)	Correspondence Type		
		Explicit	Min. Entropy	Regression-based
0.01	0.011	0.011	0.007	0.004
0.1	0.095	0.095	0.067	0.066

Head Shape Regression. The proposed regression-based correspondence method is also used to study the growth of head shape from structural MRI data obtained from clinical studies spanning the age range from neonate to 5 year old. The 40 cases include 1.5T, T1-weighted MRI scans with resolutions of $1mm \times 1mm \times 1mm$ and $0.4mm \times 0.4mm \times 3.6mm$. The scans are preprocessed and segmented to obtain the head surfaces, which are input to the optimization process. Manually placed landmarks on the bridge of the nose and the openings of the left and right ear canals define a cutting plane and a pair of spheres that we use as constraints, as in Section. 2, to repel the correspondences from the neck, face, and ears, in order to restrict the analysis to the cranium, which is most interesting from a neurological point of view. Figure. 1 shows the particle system distributed across one of the head shapes after optimizing 500 particles.

Head size, measured in volume or circumference is well known to correlate with age. This is confirmed by the linear regression plot (size versus log of age) with $p < 2 \times 10^{-16}$, shown in Figure. 2. Next, the shapes were preprocessed using methods mentioned in Section. 2 to remove the effects of size. Changes in head shape along the linear regression line (shape versus *log* of age) are shown in Figure. 3. Note the relative lengthening of the head, and the narrowing at the temples with increasing age. These shape changes are consistent with clinical observations that neonatal brain growth proceeds more rapidly in the forebrain. These results tie head shape to age in the paediatric setting.

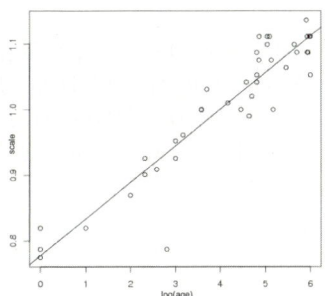

Fig. 2. Changes in head size with age

The permutation tests for both the proposed methods for this example showed that none of 1000 permutations gave a better correlation than the input data. While this $p = 0$ result is not conclusive, it does give strong evidence for significance. Future work will include more permutations to more accurately evaluate the significance.

The experiments were run on a 2GHz processor with run times of approximately 15 minutes for the tori (256 particles) and 40 minutes for the head shapes (500 particles). The permutation tests (1000 permutations) were run as parallel processes on a 16-processor machine.

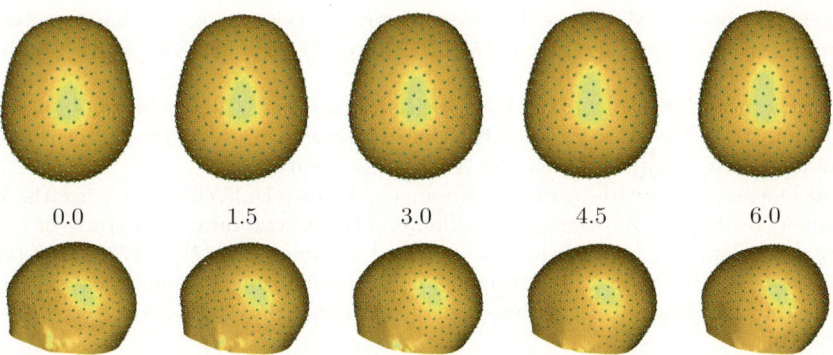

Fig. 3. Overview of head shape regression: Changes in head shape with age

4 Conclusion

This paper describes a method for *shape regression* that accounts for explanatory variables in the placement of correspondences and allows for open surfaces with arbitrary geometric constraints, and presents a mechanism for hypothesis testing of the role of underlying variables in shape. Results from a study of head shape growth indicate that the proposed method can be applied to quantitative characterization of the relationship between age and head shape in young children. Such analysis will generate data beyond the currently established standard of head circumference measurements as an index of growth. Moreover, it will generate normative data as a continuous growth model of shape, which can be useful in building optimal MRI head coils for young infants. The continuous shape model could also find use in population studies where two groups are compared with respect to growth trajectory rather than differences at individual time points.

Acknowledgments. This work was supported by the NIH/NCRR Center for Integrative Biomedical Computing, P41-RR12553-10 and the NIH/NCBC National Alliance for Medical Image Computing, U54-EB005149. We also acknowledge support from the NIMH Silvio Conte Center for Neuroscience of Mental Disorders MH064065 and the BRP grant R01 NS055754-01-02.

References

1. Cates, J.E., Fletcher, P.T., Styner, M.A., Shenton, M.E., Whitaker, R.T.: Shape modeling and analysis with entropy-based particle systems. In: Karssemeijer, N., Lelieveldt, B. (eds.) IPMI 2007. LNCS, vol. 4584, pp. 333–345. Springer, Heidelberg (2007)
2. Davies, R., Twining, C., Allen, P., Cootes, T., Taylor, C.: Shape discrimination in the hippocampus using an MDL model. In: Information Processing in Medical Imaging, pp. 38–50 (2003)
3. Gerig, G., Styner, M., Jones, D., Weinberger, D., Leiberman, J.: Shape analysis of brain ventricles using spharm. In: MMBIA, pp. 171–178. IEEE Press, Los Alamitos (2001)
4. Courchesne, E., Karns, C.M., Davis, H.R., Ziccardi, R., Carper, R.A., Tigue, Z.D., Chisum, H.J., Moses, P., Pierce, K.: Unusual brain growth patterns in early life in patients with autistic disorder: An MRI study. Neurology 57
5. Knickmeyer, R.C., Gouttard, S., Kang, C., Evans, D., Wilber, K., Smith, K.J., Hamer, R.M., Lin, W., Gerig, G., Gilmore, J.H.: A structural MRI study of human brain development from birth to two years. J. Neurosci. 28(47), 12176–12182 (2008)
6. Williams, J., Rossignac, J.: Tightening: curvature-limiting morphological simplification. In: Proc. Ninth ACM Symposium on Solid and Physical Modeling, pp. 107–112 (2005)

Setting Priors and Enforcing Constraints on Matches for Nonlinear Registration of Meshes

Benoît Combès and Sylvain Prima

INSERM, U746, F-35042 Rennes, France
INRIA, VisAGeS Project-Team, F-35042 Rennes, France
University of Rennes I, CNRS, UMR 6074, IRISA, F-35042 Rennes, France
{bcombes,sprima}@irisa.fr
http://www.irisa.fr/visages

Abstract. We show that a simple probabilistic modelling of the registration problem for surfaces allows to solve it by using standard clustering techniques. In this framework, point-to-point correspondences are hypothesized between the two free-form surfaces, and we show how to specify priors and to enforce global constraints on these matches with only minor changes to the optimisation algorithm. The purpose of these two modifications is to increase its capture range and to obtain more realistic geometrical transformations between the surfaces. We conclude with some validation experiments and results on synthetic and real data.

1 Introduction

In medical image analysis, nonlinear registration is a key tool to study the normal and abnormal anatomy of body structures. It allows to spatially normalise different subjects in a common template, to build the average anatomy in a population and to assess the variance about this average, and ultimately to perform group studies via statistical analyses. Many methods have been dedicated to deal with grey level volumes directly, while others have been devised to tackle surfaces representing anatomical structures (*e.g.* after segmentation from MRI or CT) [1]. The last approach allows a more focused analysis of structures of interest, and is the topic of our paper. In Section 2 we show that a simple probabilistic modelling of the registration problem allows to solve it by using standard clustering techniques. In this framework, point-to-point correspondences are hypothesized between the two free-form surfaces, and we show how to specify priors (Section 3) and to enforce global constraints (Section 4) on these matches with only minor changes to the optimisation algorithm. This extends our previous work on the same problem [2]. The purpose of these two modifications is to increase its capture range and to obtain more realistic geometrical transformations between the surfaces. We conclude with some validation experiments and results on synthetic and real data (Section 5).

2   Surface Registration as a Clustering Problem

The problem of interest in this paper is to find the transformation T best superposing two free-form surfaces X and Y (represented by point clouds or meshes). A convenient probabilistic viewpoint on this classical problem is to consider the surface Y as a noised version of $T(X)$. If we note $Y = (y_j)_{j=1...\text{card}(Y)}$ and $X = (x_k)_{k=1...\text{card}(X)}$, and if we hypothesize an isotropic Gaussian noise, a simple way to formulate this viewpoint is to assume that each sample y_j has been drawn independently from any one of card(X) possible 3-variate normal distributions with means $T(x_k)$ and covariance matrices $\sigma^2 I$ (with σ unknown).

This way, the registration problem becomes a *clustering* problem, whose challenge is i) to find the *label* of each point y_j, *i.e.* the one out of card(X) possible distributions from which y_j has been drawn, and ii) to estimate the parameters of these card(X) distributions. The connection between registration and clustering becomes clear when one realises that i) actually amounts to match each point y_j in Y with a point x_k in X, while ii) simply consists in computing T given these matches. This viewpoint is extremely fruitful, as it allows one to refer to classical clustering techniques and especially the maximum likelihood principle to solve the registration problem. Two different paradigms have been especially followed in this context [3]. Let us introduce some notations first:

$\forall k \in 1...\text{card}(X), p_k(.;T) = \mathcal{N}(T(x_k), \sigma^2 I)$
$\forall j \in 1...\text{card}(Y), \forall k \in 1...\text{card}(X), z_{jk} = 1$ if y_j comes from $p_k(.;T)$, 0 else

In the Classification ML (CML) approach, one tries to find the indicator variables z_{jk} and the parameter T so as to maximise the criterion CL [4]:

$$CL = \prod_{y_j \in Y} \prod_{x_k \in X} [p_k(y_j;T)]^{z_{jk}} \quad (1)$$

The problem is typically solved by the Classification EM (CEM) algorithm [5], which can be shown to find an at least local maximum of the criterion CL and proceeds as follows, in an iterative way, starting from an initial value $\tilde{T}$:

EC-step: $\forall j, \tilde{z}_{jk} = 1$ if k maximises $p_k(y_j; \tilde{T})$, 0 else
M-step: $\tilde{T} = \arg\min_T \sum_{jk} \tilde{z}_{jk} ||y_j - T(x_k)||^2$

In other words, the Expectation-Classification (EC) step consists in matching each point y_j of Y with the closest point in $\tilde{T}(X)$, while the Maximisation (M) step consists in computing the transformation best superposing these pairs of matched points. In case T is a rigid-body transformation, this is nothing else than the popular ICP algorithm [6].

In the ML approach, the indicator values z_{jk} are no longer considered as unknown quantities to estimate, but rather as hidden/unobservable variables of the problem. This is actually a drastic and fundamental change of viewpoint, as the focus is no longer on assigning each y_j to one of the distributions p_k

but rather on estimating the parameters of the Gaussian mixture made of these distributions. If we involve priors π_{jk} on the indicator variables ($\forall j, k, 0 < \pi_{jk} < 1$, and $\forall j, \sum_k \pi_{jk} = 1$), the likelihood then simply writes [7]:

$$L = \prod_{y_j \in Y} \sum_{x_k \in X} \pi_{jk} p_k(y_j; T) \qquad (2)$$

In essence, the prior π_{jk} conveys the probability that the point y_j comes from the distribution p_k without knowing anything else. The criterion L can be maximised by using the popular EM algorithm, which converges to an at least local maximum of the likelihood [8]. If we consider the priors π_{jk} as known beforehand and if we introduce the notation γ_{jk} as the posterior probability of the hidden indicator variable z_{jk} to be equal to 1, the EM algorithm writes:

E-step: $\tilde{\gamma}_{jk} = \frac{\pi_{jk} \exp\left[-\|y_j - \tilde{T}(x_k)\|^2 / (2\sigma^2)\right]}{\sum_i \pi_{ji} \exp\left[-\|y_j - \tilde{T}(x_i)\|^2 / (2\sigma^2)\right]}$
M-step: $\tilde{T} = \arg\min_T \sum_{jk} \tilde{\gamma}_{jk} \|y_j - T(x_k)\|^2$

To our knowledge, Granger & Pennec [9] were the first to formulate the problem this way, and they proposed the so-called EM-ICP as a simplified version of the previous algorithm for rigid-body registration, where the priors π_{jk} were considered as uniform. They noted that the parameter σ, which is not estimated in this framework, acts as a scale parameter, and that it can be given an initial value and decreased throughout the iterations for improved performances.

Interpretation & Extensions. Intuitively, the EM approach is a *fuzzy* version of the CEM. It appears clearly from the iterative formulas of both algorithms that the classification likelihood is an "all-or-nothing" version of the likelihood, leading to a "bumpier" and harder-to-maximise criterion, something that is well known by those who are familiar with the ICP algorithm. Note that the ML formulation and the EM algorithm lead to the same iterative formulas that would have resulted from the addition of a barrier function on the indicator variables in the ICP criterion [10]. This formalism is not limited to rigid-body transformations, and can be easily used for any T, the challenge being to choose T such that the M-step remains tractable. In particular, the ML estimation can be easily turned into a MAP problem with only slight modifications to the optimisation scheme, as shown by Green [11]. This allows to view T as a random variable, on which priors (acting as regularisers on T) can be easily specified. Different choices have been proposed for T and associated priors in this context, such as the thin plate splines [10] or locally affine transformations [12]. If $p(T)$ is a prior of the form $p(T) \propto \exp(-\alpha R(T))$ then the optimal transformation can be found using the MAP principle (also termed penalised ML) and the EM algorithm with only a slight modification to the M-step (addition of $\alpha R(T)$).

3 Setting Priors on Matches

3.1 Why Using Priors on Matches?

Most works in this context have been focused on designing transformations and related priors allowing to i) compute realistic deformations between the two surfaces and ii) keep the M-step tractable. Much little has been done to enforce similar constraints on the matches (E-step). Dropping the priors π_{jk}, as done in the ICP of Besl & McKay or the EM-ICP of Granger & Pennec amounts to say that the posteriors γ_{jk} are only estimated using the spatial distance between the points y_j and $T(x_k)$ (E-step). This is unsatisfactory, for two reasons. First, this distance is highly conditioned by the previous estimation of T, which in turn depends on the previous estimation of γ_{jk} and so on. This chicken-and-egg problem limits the capture range of the algorithm, which is likely to converge to a bad solution if no good initial T is given. Second, in medical imaging it is difficult to design a physical model T capturing the expected deformation between two structures. Thus the global maximiser of the ML criterion is likely not to be realistic. By specifying relevant priors π_{jk}, we provide a way to partially alleviate these two limitations. First, it allows to introduce additional information on matches independent of the transformation and thus to compute reliable posteriors even for a bad initial estimate of T. Second, it allows to modify the criterion in a way that its global maximiser is a more realistic transformation.

3.2 Building Priors on Matches

In this section we show how to design the priors π_{jk} to encode very heterogeneous types of a priori knowledge on the matches, such as "two points with similar curvatures are more likely to be matched than others" as well as knowledge of the labels of structures in the objects to be matched (*e.g.* gyri/sulci in cortical registration). In practice, we choose to design $\pi = (\pi_{jk})$ such that $\pi_{jk} \propto \exp(-\beta c(y_j, x_k))$ where $c : X \times Y \to \mathbb{R}^+$ conveys the cost of matching points y_j and x_k, independently of T. The parameter $\beta > 0$ weighs the influence of π_{jk} over $||y_j - T(x_k)||$ during the E-step. Depending on the information to encode (continuous value or label), we propose two approaches to build c.

Using descriptors. c can be computed via the comparison between continuous values (or vectors) $d(x)$ describing the surface around the considered points. To account for potential inaccuracies on $d(.)$, we define the measure as: $c^d(y_j, x_k) = 0$ if $||d(y_j) - d(x_k)|| < \tau$; $= penalty > 0$ else. To the best of our knowledge, there exists no descriptor invariant to any nonlinear transformation. However, one can use some descriptors invariant to more constrained transformations (Fig. 1, left):

- the shape index $sh(x)$ [13] that describes the local shape irrespective of the scale and that is invariant to similarities
- the curvedness $cu(x)$ [13] that specifies the amount of curvature and that is invariant to rigid-body transformations
- the (normalised) total geodesic distance $tgd(x)$ [14] that is invariant to isometries in the shape space (including non-elastic deformations).

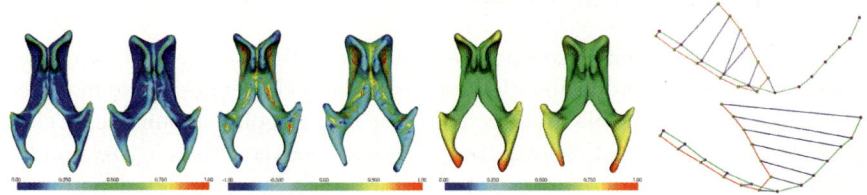

Fig. 1. Left: Mapping of descriptor values: From left to right: curvedness, shape index and total geodesic distance on two lateral ventricles. Homologous anatomical landmarks yield qualitatively the same descriptor values. **Right:** point-based matching (top) vs line-based matching performed by our algorithm (bottom).

Using labels. c can be computed via the comparison between labels on points (cortical sulci/gyri). We define: $c(y_j, x_k) = 0$ if points j and k have compatible labels; $= penalty > 0$ else. In practice, we extract the crest lines from both meshes as they constitute salient features. Each point is given a label depending on whether it belongs to a crest line or not. Then, we define $c_{crest}(y_j, x_k) = 0$ if y_j and x_k have the same label and $c(y_j, x_k) = penalty$ else.

Mixing the two approaches. In practice, we choose to mix the previous four sources of information to build the function c: $c(y_j, x_k) = a_1 c^{sh}(y_j, x_k) + a_2 c^{cu}(y_j, x_k) + a_3 c^{tgd}(y_j, x_k) + a_4 c_{crest}(y_j, x_k)$ with $a_1 + a_2 + a_3 + a_4 = 1$. Parameters a_i allow to weigh the different terms. Their values is application-dependent and will not be studied in this paper, in which we set them to 0.25.

3.3 Efficient Implementation

In practice, we do not consider all points during the computation of γ_{jk} (E-step). For that, we consider $p_k(.; T)$ as a truncated Gaussian pdf with cut-off distance δ. This allows to reduce the computational burden (by the use of a kd-tree) and increase robustness. It can be shown that our algorithm still converges to an at least local maximum of the new (truncated) criterion. The E-Step becomes:

initialise $\gamma = (\gamma_{jk})$ to the null matrix
$\forall x_k \in X$
$\quad S = \{y_j \in Y$ such that $||y_j - \tilde{T}(x_k)||^2 < \delta\}$ (using a kd-tree)
$\quad \forall y_j \in S$
$\quad\quad \gamma_{jk} = \exp(-(||y_j - \tilde{T}(x_k)||^2/(2\sigma^2) + \beta c(y_j, x_k)))$
$\forall j, \forall k, \tilde{\gamma}_{jk} = \gamma_{jk} / \sum_l \gamma_{jl}$ (normalisation)

Moreover, we choose to initialise α (regularisation weight), σ (scale parameter) and β (prior weight) with high values and reduce them throughout iterations.

4 Enforcing Global Constraints on Matches

In the formalism presented so far, the matches in the E-step are performed on an individual basis without any global constraint such as one-to-one matches for instance. Another desirable global constraint is that some geometrical relationships between points in Y should be preserved between their correspondences in X. Thus if we consider each crest line in Y as a set of ordered points, then their correspondences must i) lie on the same crest line in X and ii) be ordered in the same way (up to the orientation of the line) (Fig. 1 right). To enforce these two constraints, let us introduce some notations first. Let L and M be the sets of crest lines of Y and X, each crest line being defined as a set of ordered points. Let $u = (u^{lm})$ be a block matrix whose lines (resp. columns) correspond to the concatenated crest lines of Y (resp. X). Then u_{jk}^{lm} is the indicator variable $u_{jk}^{lm} = 1$ iff y_j in crest line l corresponds to the point x_k in crest line m. The two constraints i) and ii) are specified as follows: the submatrix u^{lm} is either null (the line l does not match with the line m) or contains one 1 per line, with the 1s drawing a "staircase" going to the left or to the right, all "steps" of the staircase having potentially different widths and different heights. Then we propose to maximise the following criterion over T and u having this staircase structure:

$$L-CL = \left[\prod_{y_j \in Y \setminus L} \sum_{x_k \in X \setminus M} \pi_{jk} p_k(y_j|T) \times \prod_{l \in L} \prod_{y_j \in l} \sum_{x_k \in m} [p_k(y_j|T)]^{u_{jk}^{lm}} \right] \times p(T) \quad (3)$$

This criterion is an hybrid between the classification likelihood and the likelihood approaches. Introducing u only modifies the E-step of the algorithm, in which u and γ can be estimated independently. The algorithm becomes:

E-Step: compute $\tilde{\gamma}$ as before
$\forall l$, compute $\tilde{u}^{lm}$ respecting the staircase structure
and maximising $\prod_{y_j \in l} \sum_{x_k \in m} [p_k(y_j|\tilde{T})]^{\tilde{u}_{jk}^{lm}}$
M-Step: $\tilde{T} = \arg\min_T \sum_{y_j \in Y \setminus L, x_k \in X \setminus M} \tilde{\gamma}_{jk} \|y_j - T(x_k)\|^2$
$+ \sum_{l \in L} \sum_{y_j \in l, x_k \in m} \tilde{u}_{jk}^{lm} \|y_j - T(x_k)\|^2 + \alpha R(T)$

To our knowledge, an exhaustive search is the only way to maximise the proposed criterion over u. Instead, we propose to design an heuristic algorithm to do so, that extends the one proposed by Subsol [15] and consists of two steps: i) finding the crest line $m \in M$ that corresponds to each $l \in L$ and ii) starting from different initial potential matches and assigning iteratively each point $y_j \in l$ to a point $x_k \in m$ by keeping the staircase structure of the submatrix u^{lm}.

5 Experiments and Results

In the following we choose to adopt a locally affine regularisation [12] (with only the translational part) because of its ability to perform efficiently ($\sim$ 7min) on large datasets ($\sim$ 50K points).

5.1 Experiments on Synthetic Data

Generation of ground truth data. We first segment a structure X (typically, a pair of lateral ventricles or caudate nuclei, giving surfaces of about 10K points, itksnap.org) from a 3T T1-weighted brain MRI of a healthy subject. Then Y is generated from X by applying a random thin plate spline transformation [2]. Then, we add a uniform Gaussian noise of std 0.5 mm on each point of the deformed surface and remove groups of adjacent vertices to generate holes. This way we generate ground truth pairs of 100 ventricles and 100 caudate nuclei.

Evaluation. We evaluate the error by computing the mean distance between homologous points after registration using different strategies. The results are reported in Tab. 1 and an example is displayed in Fig. 2. They show the strong added value of using priors. The error is further reduced when using constraints, which ensure that the ordering of the points on the lines is kept unchanged, and thus help the algorithm to obtain anatomically coherent matches elsewhere.

Table 1. Experiments on synthetic data (stats). Mean and std (mm) of the registration error for the 100 ventricles and 100 caudate nuclei by varying the parameters.

	no prior/no constraint	prior/no constraint	prior/constraint
ventricle	2.19 ± 0.82	1.43 ± 0.91	1.39 ± 0.93
caudate nuclei	1.54 ± 0.43	1.04 ± 0.57	0.98 ± 0.56

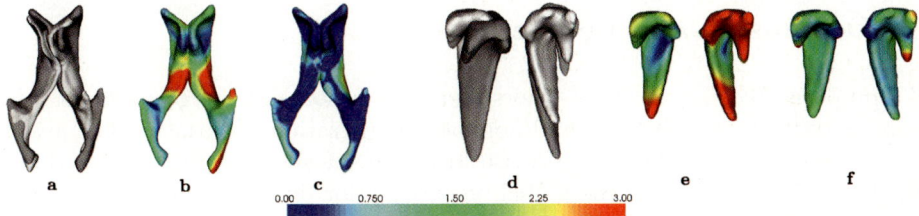

Fig. 2. Experiments on synthetic data. From left to right: Experiments on two different structures: ventricles and caudate nuclei. a) and d) original and deformed; b) and e) mapping of registration error (mm) without using prior/constraint; c) and f) mapping of registration error using prior/constraint.

5.2 Experiments on Real Data

In a first experiment, we choose X and Y as two different lateral ventricles and manually extract a set of 8 anatomical landmarks common to X and Y. We then apply a random affine transformation A to Y, register $A(Y)$ to X with and without using priors/constraints, and evaluate the registration error on landmarks. We perform this experiment 100 times (but we display only 10 on Fig. 3 for better clarity). We observe a mean error of 1.73 ± 1.24mm with the priors/constraints

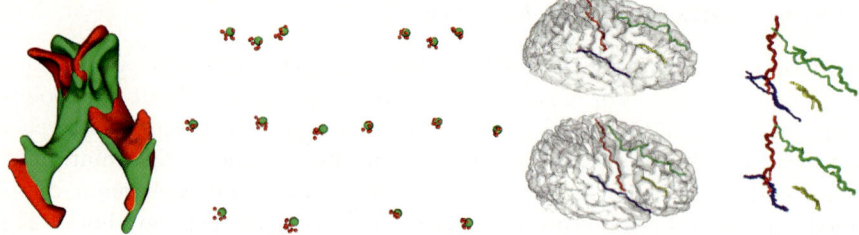

Fig. 3. Experiments on real data. Ventricles: From left to right : X (green) and $A(Y)$ (red) before registration, position of the 8 anatomical landmarks of the 10 random experiments after registration without priors/constraints and with priors/constraints. **Brain:** From left to right and top to bottom: 1) brain 1 (top) and brain 2 (bottom); 2) brain 2 (with sulci shown in transparency) towards brain 1 without (top) and with (bottom) using priors/constraints. The four sulci are the central (red), lateral (blue), superior frontal (green) and inferior frontal (yellow) sulci.

and 2.55 ± 2.46mm without (Fig. 3, left). In a second experiment, we segment the brain from T1-weighted MRI data of two healthy subjects (300,000 points, brainvisa.info), and we extract four sulcal fundus beds (using our algorithm for crest lines) and label them manually for each subject. Then we register the two surfaces with and without using priors/constraints. The distance between the homologous sulci after registration is used as a quality metric. It is evaluated to be 3.3mm in the first case and 6.8mm in the second (Fig. 3, right).

6 Conclusion and Perspectives

We proposed techniques to set priors and enforce some global geometrical constraints on matches for ML-based nonlinear registration of surfaces. The priors on matches give a flexible way to devise structure-specific registration algorithms. They ideally complement the global, generic, prior on the transformation and thus help to obtain a result coherent with the application of interest. In addition, they provide a convenient framework to include additional knowledge (segmentation, landmarks, *etc.*) provided by experts when available. In the future, comparisons with other recent methods, especially landmark-free approaches [16] and others that do not resort to point-to-point correspondences [17] will be led.

References

1. Audette, M.A., Ferrie, F.P., Peters, T.M.: An Algorithmic Overview of Surface Registration Techniques for Medical Imaging. MIA 4, 201–217 (2000)
2. Combès, B., Prima, S.: Prior Affinity Measures on Matches for ICP-Like Nonlinear Registration of Free-Form Surfaces. IEEE ISBI (2009)
3. Marriott, F.H.C.: Separating Mixtures of Normal Distributions. Biometrics 31(3), 767–769 (1975)

4. Scott, A.J., Symons, M.J.: Clustering Methods Based on Likelihood Ratio Criteria. Biometrics 27(2), 387–397 (1971)
5. Celeux, G., Govaert, G.: A Classification EM Algorithm for Clustering and Two Stochastic Versions. Computational Statistics and Data Analysis 14(3), 315–332 (1992)
6. Besl, P., McKay, N.: A Method for Registration of 3-D Shapes. IEEE PAMI 14(2), 239–256 (1992)
7. Day, N.E.: Estimating the Components of a Mixture of Normal Distributions. Biometrika 56(3), 463–474 (1969)
8. Dempster, A.P., Laird, N.M., Rubin, D.B.: Maximum Likelihood from Incomplete Data via the EM Algorithm. Journal of the Royal Statistical Society. Series B (Methodological) 39(1), 1–38 (1977)
9. Granger, S., Pennec, X.: Multi-scale EM-ICP: A fast and robust approach for surface registration. In: Heyden, A., Sparr, G., Nielsen, M., Johansen, P. (eds.) ECCV 2002. LNCS, vol. 2353, pp. 418–432. Springer, Heidelberg (2002)
10. Chui, H., Rangarajan, A.: A Feature Registration Framework Using Mixture Models. In: IEEE MMBIA, pp. 190–197 (2000)
11. Green, P.J.: On Use of the EM for Penalized Likelihood Estimation. Journal of the Royal Statistical Society. Series B (Methodological) 52(3), 443–452 (1990)
12. Combès, B., Prima, S.: New algorithms to map asymmetries of 3D surfaces. In: Metaxas, D., Axel, L., Fichtinger, G., Székely, G. (eds.) MICCAI 2008, Part I. LNCS, vol. 5241, pp. 17–25. Springer, Heidelberg (2008)
13. Koenderink, J.J., van Doorn, A.J.: Surface Shape and Curvature Scales. Image and Vision Computing 10(8), 557–564 (1992)
14. Aouada, D., Feng, S., Krim, H.: Statistical Analysis of the Global Geodesic Function for 3D Object Classification. In: IEEE ICASSP, pp. I-645–I-648 (2007)
15. Subsol, G., Thirion, J.-P., Ayache, N.: A General Scheme for Automatically Building 3D Morphometric Anatomical Atlases: application to a Skull Atlas. MIA 2, 37–60 (1998)
16. Yeo, B.T.T., Sabuncu, M.R., Vercauteren, T., Ayache, N., Fischl, B., Golland, P.: Spherical demons: Fast surface registration. In: Metaxas, D., Axel, L., Fichtinger, G., Székely, G. (eds.) MICCAI 2008, Part I. LNCS, vol. 5241, pp. 745–753. Springer, Heidelberg (2008)
17. Durrleman, S., Pennec, X., Trouvé, A., Ayache, N.: Sparse approximation of currents for statistics on curves and surfaces. In: Metaxas, D., Axel, L., Fichtinger, G., Székely, G. (eds.) MICCAI 2008, Part II. LNCS, vol. 5242, pp. 390–398. Springer, Heidelberg (2008)

Parametric Representation of Cortical Surface Folding Based on Polynomials

Tuo Zhang[1], Lei Guo[1], Gang Li[1], Jingxin Nie[1], and Tianming Liu[2]

[1] School of Automation, Northwestern Polytechnical University, Xi'an, China
[2] Department of Computer Science and Bioimaging Research Center,
The University of Georgia, Athens, GA, USA

Abstract. The development of folding descriptors as an effective approach for describing geometrical complexity and variation of the human cerebral cortex has been of great interests. This paper presents a parametric representation of cortical surface patches using polynomials, that is, the primitive cortical patch is compactly and effectively described by four parametric coefficients. By this parametric representation, the patterns of cortical patches can be classified by either model-driven approach or data-driven clustering approach. In the model-driven approach, any patch of the cortical surface is classified into one of eight primitive shape patterns including peak, pit, ridge, valley, saddle ridge, saddle valley, flat and inflection, corresponding to eight sub-spaces of the four parameters. The major advantage of this polynomial representation of cortical folding pattern is its compactness and effectiveness, while being rich in shape information. We have applied this parametric representation for segmentation of cortical surface and promising results are obtained.

1 Introduction

Quantitative description of the geometrical complexity and variability of the human cerebral cortex has been of great interests. The development of shape descriptors that model the cortical folding pattern is essential to understand brain structure and function. Recent study has shown that cortical folding pattern could be used to predict brain function [1]. Besides, quantitative cortical folding descriptor may help reveal the underlying mechanism of cortical gyrification [2, 3] and provide clues for the understanding of abnormal cortical folding in brain disorders [4, 5].

In order to quantitatively and effectively measure cortical folding, a couple of attempts have been made in literature. In [6], the cortical surface area was compared to its external surface areas to determine the degree of folding. In [7], the gyrification index (GI) was proposed to compute the ratio between the pial contour and the outer contour in successive coronal sections, which has been widely used in many studies [8, 9]. Recently, the GI measurement was extended to 3D [10]. Curvature, which is a 3D parametric measurement, was also widely used as a metric to study cortical folding pattern [11]. These descriptors have their own advantages, but also have their limitations. Novel folding pattern descriptors that incorporate 3D geometric shape pattern information are still to be developed.

In this paper, a compact parametric model with four polynomial coefficients is developed to describe cortical surface patch shape pattern. By this parametric representation, the patterns of cortical patches can be classified by either model-driven or data-driven clustering approaches. In particular, by taking the advantage of symmetry of cortical patch, the model-driven approach is able to classify the patches into one of the eight primitive shape patterns: peak, pit, ridge, valley, saddle ridge, saddle valley, flat and inflection, which altogether cover the 4-dimensional parametric space. In order to show the effectiveness of this method, we have applied this parametric representation for segmentation of cortical surfaces of 80 subjects, and promising results are obtained.

2 Methods

2.1 Parametric Polynomial Model

Our work is inspired by the 2D power function based representation of tectonic folding presented in [12]. Our parametric polynomial surface model is represented as:

$$z = \sum_{i=1}^{m} a_i x^i + \sum_{j=1}^{n} b_j y^j \quad (1)$$

where x, y and z are vertex coordinates, a_i and b_j are coefficients. In order to decide the maximal values of m and n, we fitted the 2D power function to 1000 randomly selected patches along two directions corresponding to two principal curvatures of the central vertex of each patch. The sizes of surface patch are ranging from 1-ring to 7-ring neighborhood. The statistical results of the exponent n are shown in Fig. 1. It is evident that the exponent n is rarely over 3. We have similar results for the exponent m.

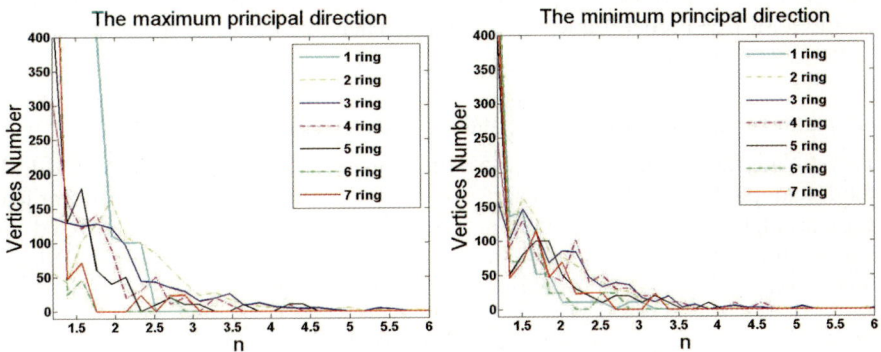

Fig. 1. The statistical distribution of exponent n in power function fitting

Therefore, we present the cortical surface patches by polynomials in the following format:

$$Z = aX^2 + bY^2 + cX^3 + dY^3 \quad (2)$$

where a and b describe the mirror symmetric components of the patch, while c and d represent the rotational symmetric components.

2.2 Model Fitting

We use the Frenet frame as the coordinate system to estimate parameters in Eq. (2). The origin of Frenet frame coincides with the central vertex of the patch, and the central vertex's normal is regarded as the Z-axis of the frame that always points towards outside of the brain. The X-axis and Y-axis are set free in the beginning, and will be determined later by the estimated parameters. So the Frenet frame is called semi-free Frenet frame here (Fig. 2). Eq. (2) is rewritten as $f(\vec{\theta}, \vec{x}) = 0$, and we have:

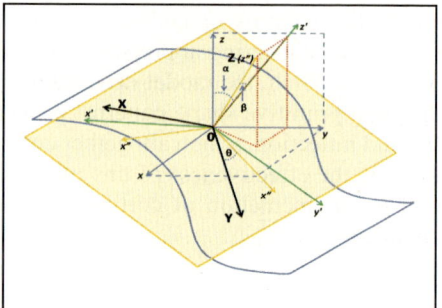

Fig. 2. The semi-free Frenet frame

$$f(\vec{\theta}, \vec{x}) = aX^2 + bY^2 + cX^3 + dY^3 - Z \qquad (3)$$

where $\vec{\theta} = (a, b, c, d)^T$, and $\vec{x} = (X, Y, Z)^T$. It is worth noting that $(X, Y, Z)^T$ is the coordinates in the semi-free Frenet frame. Therefore, all the coordinates of surrounding patch vertices should be rotated as follow:

$$\begin{bmatrix} X \\ Y \\ Z \end{bmatrix} = \begin{bmatrix} 1 & 0 & 0 \\ 0 & \cos\alpha & -\sin\alpha \\ 0 & \sin\alpha & \cos\alpha \end{bmatrix} \begin{bmatrix} \cos\beta & 0 & -\sin\beta \\ 0 & 1 & 0 \\ \sin\beta & 0 & \cos\beta \end{bmatrix} \begin{bmatrix} \cos\theta & -\sin\theta & 0 \\ \sin\theta & \cos\theta & 0 \\ 0 & 0 & 1 \end{bmatrix} \left(\begin{bmatrix} x_i \\ y_i \\ z_i \end{bmatrix} - \begin{bmatrix} x_0 \\ y_0 \\ z_0 \end{bmatrix} \right) \qquad (4)$$

where $[x_0, y_0, z_0]^T$ the coordinate of the central vertex; α and β are two angles between the axes of different coordinates frames; θ is a new parameter introduced to rotate the semi-free Frenet frame on X-Y plane. Then, the Eq. (3) is rewritten as:

$$f(\vec{u}, \vec{x}) = 0 \qquad (5)$$

where parameter $\vec{u} = (a, b, c, d, \theta)^T$, and $\vec{x} = (x_i, y_i, z_i)^T$.

To estimate the parameters in Eq. (5), the non-linear least square fitting (NLLSF) method is adopted to fit the patch. There is no closed-form solution to a non-linear least squares problem. However, the nonlinear problem can be iteratively linearized and becomes a linear least squares problem in each iteration. In order to apply the NLLSF method to our model, Eq. (5) is rewritten in the following way:

$$z = \tilde{f}(\vec{u}, \vec{x}) \qquad (6)$$

Supposing there are n vertices on the patch, the model fitting algorithm is as follows:

Step.1. Initialize parameter $\vec{u}^0$, maximum iteration times N and ε, k = 0;

Step.2. Compute the shift vector $\Delta \vec{u}^k$ by equations written in matrix notation as

$$\Delta \vec{u}^k = (J^T J)^{-1} J^T \Delta \vec{z} \qquad (7)$$

where $\Delta \vec{z} = (z_1 - \tilde{f}(\vec{u}^k, \vec{x}_1), \cdots z_n - \tilde{f}(\vec{u}^k, \vec{x}_n))^T$, and J is the Jacobian matrix.

Step.3. If $\|\Delta \vec{u}^k\| \leq \varepsilon$, or $k > N$, stop iteration and output $\vec{u}^k$; else go to Step.4;

Step.4. $\vec{u}^{k+1} = \vec{u}^k + \Delta \vec{u}^k$, $k = k+1$, go to Step.2.

A critical issue in the polynomial model fitting is the patch size. Generally, the larger the patch is, the more shape information it will enclose. However, if the patch is too large, its folding shape will be too asymmetric to be described by polynomials. By considering the combination of complexity and symmetry degrees of one patch, both qualitative and quantitative experiments show that 3-ring neighborhood is good to maintain the symmetry property of surface patches.

2.3 Model Pattern Classification

As mentioned above, the estimated parameter sets $(a,b,c,d)^T$ will be used to determine the X- and Y- axis as follows. Intuitively, the largest value in a, b, c and d will dominate the shape of a surface patch, as shown in Fig. 3. For example, in the valley shape, the parameter a will be the largest and dominate the patch shape. So for the sake of convenience, we use the X-axis to represent the dominating direction, i.e., the largest absolute value is either a or c, and Y-axis is orthogonal to X-axis. If b or d is of the largest absolute value, we switch a and c with b and d.

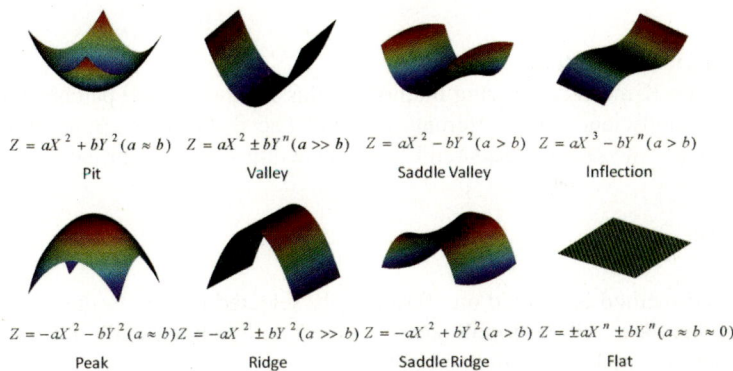

Fig. 3. Eight primitive folding patterns of surface patches

2.3.1 Model-Driven Method

The surface patch patterns represented by above polynomial model are classified into eight primitive fold patterns including peak, pit, ridge, valley, saddle ridge, saddle valley, flat, and inflection as shown in Fig. 3. This classification approach is similar to that in [14]. The decision tree for this model-based classification method is shown in Fig. 4, where the absolute component ratio is defined as:

$$Ratio(\lambda) = \frac{|\lambda|}{|a|+|b|+|c|+|d|}, \lambda \in (a,b,c,d) \qquad (8)$$

This classification method (Fig. 4a) covers the entire four dimensional space of parameter a, b, c and d. The parameter c or d will determines the inflection pattern if any of them is larger than 0.25. Otherwise, the parameter a and b will decide the other shape patterns as shown in Fig. 4b. Currently, all of these thresholds are determined by expert visual inspections.

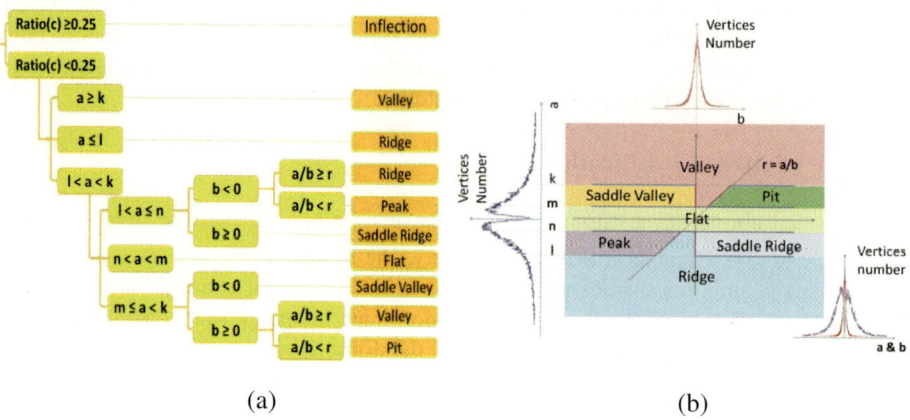

Fig. 4. (a) The clustering decision tree. (b) The parametric subspaces of a and b for different patterns.

2.3.2 Data-Driven Method

We applied the K-means clustering method to classify the surface patches represented by the four coefficients into different patterns. The distance measurement between patches is simply the summed squared Euclidean distance of the four model parameters.

3 Results

The proposed method is applied on 80 randomly selected normal brains in the OASIS MR image database. All the topologically correct and geometrically accurate cortical surfaces are generated via the method in [15].

3.1 Results of Model-Driven Method

The model-driven folding pattern classification method introduced in Section 2.3.1 was applied to 80 cortical surfaces. As an example, Fig. 5 shows the primitive patch shape classification result on a cortical surface. Currently, the thresholds k, l, n, m in Fig. 4a used in this classification are manually determined. Fig. 5 clearly illustrates the distributions of the eight primitive folding patterns over the cortex. Ridges and valleys are commonly distributed on the crests of gyri and at the bottoms of sulci. Pits mostly sit in bowl-shaped sulcal regions. Peaks are more likely to be the joints of connected gyri. Inflections tend to be slender lines separating straight and long slopes where gyral regions meet the sulcal regions. The flats are located on smooth walls beneath the crests of gyri or the plain-shaped gyri crests. Saddle ridges and saddle valleys are distributed relatively evenly. The result in Fig. 5 shows that the proposed cortical patch representation and classification method can properly discriminate the shape differences across the whole cortical surface. Our preliminary results show that the percentage of flats is significantly higher in normal brains than Autism patients.

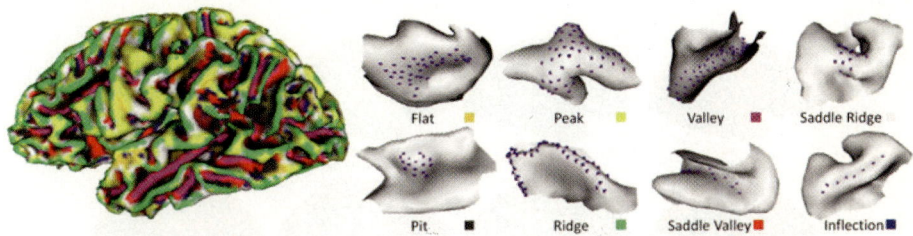

Fig. 5. The model-driven classification result on a cortical surface. Eight primitive folding patterns are represented by different colors. The blue dots on the right patches represent the central vertices of the corresponding patches.

In order to evaluate the accuracy of the folding pattern classification methods, 600 patches randomly selected from 80 cortical surfaces are manually classified into the 8 patterns in Fig. 5 respectively. The automatic classification results are compared with the manual labeling results, and Table 1 summarizes the sensitivity and specificity of the automatic classification method. It is apparent that the automatic folding pattern classification method is quite accurate, given the high sensitivity and specificity over 0.9.

Table 1. The comparison result for model-driven method

Cluster name	Saddle Valley	Inflection	Saddle Ridge	Ridge	Flat	Peak	Pit	Valley
sensitivity	0.8333	0.9091	0.8636	0.9792	0.8438	0.9483	0.8710	0.9792
specificity	0.9929	0.9827	1	0.9762	0.9873	0.9752	0.9926	0.9921

3.2 Results of Data-Driven Method

Fig. 6 shows the data-driven classification results with the number of clusters ranging from 2 to 8. With the increase of cluster numbers, more detailed shape patterns are generated. Especially, the 2-classes clustering results, parcelling cortex into gyral and sulcal regions, is similar to the curvature based parcellation of cortex [13] as shown in the right bottom of Fig. 6. Also, to evaluate the accuracy of the methods, the same 600 surface patches are manually classified into 5 clusters respectively. The data-driven automatic clustering results are compared with the manual labeling, and the results are provided in Table 2. Evidently, the sensitivity and specificity of the data-driven clustering method are quite high.

To investigate the parameter distribution in the data-driven clustering, we take an arbitrary case with 47600 vertices as an example. Distributions of a and b, the two dominant parameter (see Table 3), in each clustering result using different cluster numbers from 2 to 8 are shown in Fig. 7.

Table 2. The comparison result for data-driven method

Cluster index	Cluster 1	Cluster 2	Cluster 3	Cluster 4	Cluster 5
sensitivity	0.9833	0.9661	0.9672	0.9333	0.9000
specificity	0.9958	0.9917	0.9916	0.9833	0.9750

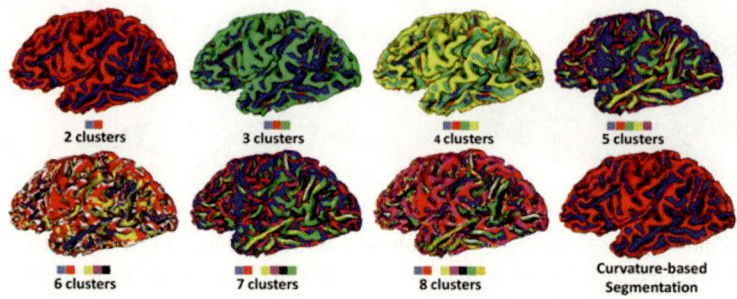

Fig. 6. K-means clustering results with the number of clusters ranging from 2 and 8

Table 3. The numbers of dominant parameters

Dominant parameter	a	b	c	d
Number of vertices	47258	11244	1802	472

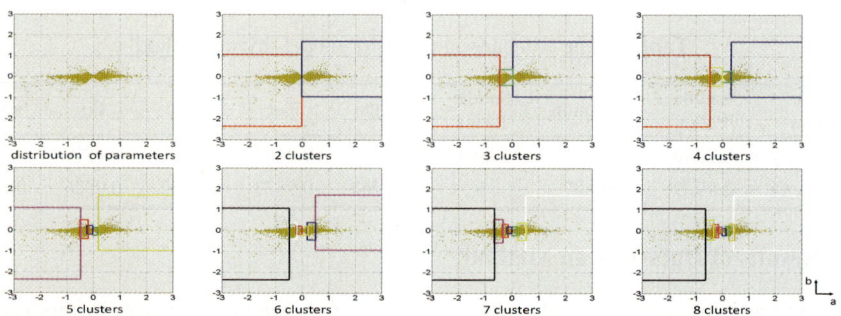

Fig. 7. Distribution of parameter a and b for each cluster across different cluster numbers. The boxes are color coded according to the corresponding clusters in Fig. 6.

4 Discussion and Conclusion

Compared to previous cortical folding descriptors such as curvature and gyrification index, the proposed polynomial parametric representation is able to differentiate cortical surface patches into primitive shape patterns. The major advantage of the polynomial representation of cortical folding pattern is its compactness and effectiveness, while being rich in shape information. However, the polynomial representation in Eq. (2) is not perfect. It requires that the shape of the patch in consideration to be symmetric. As the size of surface patch grows, e.g., larger than 4-ring or 5-ring neighborhood, the symmetry requirement might be violated. Also, the shape complexity of the cortical patch might be beyond the description ability of the polynomial model in Eq. (2). In the future, more factors such as twisting effect should be added into the shape model in Eq. (2) for better description capability of cortical shape patterns. The work presented in this paper demonstrates that parametric shape descriptor is a powerful tool to model cortical folding patterns. Potential applications include automatic parcellation of cortical surface as shown in Fig. 5 and Fig. 6, automatic recognition of cortical structures using folding patterns as features, as well as studies of abnormal folding patterns in brain diseases.

References

1. Fischl, B., Rajendran, N., Busa, E., Augustinack, J., Hinds, O., Yeo, B.T., Mohlberg, H., Amunts, K., Zilles, K.: Cortical Folding Patterns and Predicting Cytoarchitecture. Cereb Cortex 18(8), 1973–1980 (2008)
2. Van Essen, D.C.: A tension-based theory of morphogenesis and compact wiring in the central nervous system. Nature 385, 313–318 (1997)
3. Toro, R., Burnod, Y.: A Morphogenetic Model of the Development of Cortical Convolutions. Cerebral Cortex 15, 1900–1913 (2005)
4. Van Essen, D.C., Dierker, D., Snyder, A.Z., Raichle, M.E., Reiss, A.L., Korenberg, J.: Symmetry of Cortical Folding Abnormalities in Williams Syndrome Revealed by Surface-Based Analyses. J. Neurosci. 26(20), 5470–5483 (2006)
5. Sallet, P.C., Elkis, H., Alves, T.M., Oliveira, J.R., Sassi, E., Campi de Castro, C., Busatto, G.F., Gattaz, W.F.: Reduced Cortical Folding in Schizophrenia: An MRI Morphometric Study. Am. J. Psychiatry 160, 1606–1613 (2003)
6. Elias, H., Schwartz, D.: Surface areas of the cerebral cortex of mammals determined by stereological methods. Science 166, 111–113 (1969)
7. Zilles, K., Armstrong, E., Schleicher, A., Kretschmann, H.J.: The human pattern of gyrification in the cerebral cortex. Anat. Embryol. (Berl) 179, 173–179 (1988)
8. Hardan, A.Y., Jou, R.J., Keshavan, M.S., Varma, R., Minshew, N.J.: Increased frontal cortical folding in autism: a preliminary MRI study. Psychiatry Research 131(3), 263–268 (2004)
9. Neal, J., Takahashi, M., Silva, M., Tiao, G., Walsh, C.A., Sheen, V.L.: Insights into the gyrification of developing ferret brain by magnetic resonance imaging. J. Anat. 210(1), 66–77 (2007)
10. Schaer, M., Cuadra, M.B., Tamarit, L., Lazeyras, F., Eliez, S., Thiran, J.P.: A Surface-based approach to Quantify Local Cortical Gyrification. IEEE Trans. TMI 27(2), 161–170 (2008)
11. Cachia, A., Mangin, J.F., Rivière, D., Kherif, F., Boddaert, N., Andrade, A., Papadopoulos-Orfanos, D., Poline, J.B., Bloch, I., Zilbovicius, M., Sonigo, P., Brunelle, F., Régis, J.: A Primal Sketch of the Cortex Mean Curvature: a Morphogenesis Based Approach to Study the Variability of the Folding Patterns. IEEE Trans. TMI 22(6), 754–765 (2003)
12. Lisle, R.J., Fernández Martínez, J.L., Bobillo-Ares, N., Menéndez, O., Aller, J., Bastida, F.: FOLD PROFILER: A MATLAB—based program for fold shape classification. Computers & Geosciences 32, 102–108 (2006)
13. Li, G., Guo, L., Nie, J., Liu, T.: Automatic cortical sulcal parcellation based on surface principal direction flow field tracking. NeuroImage 46(4), 923–937 (2009)
14. Besl, P.J., Jain, R.C.: Segmentation Through Variable-Order Surface Fitting. IEEE Trans. PAMI 10(2), 167–192 (1988)
15. Liu, T., Nie, J., Tarokh, A., Guo, L., Wong, S.T.: Reconstruction of central cortical surface from brain MRI images: method and application. Neuroimage 40(3), 991–1002 (2007)

Intrinsic Regression Models for Manifold-Valued Data*

Xiaoyan Shi, Martin Styner, Jeffrey Lieberman, Joseph G. Ibrahim, Weili Lin, and Hongtu Zhu

Department of Biostatistics, Radiology, Psychiatry and Computer Science, and Biomedical Research Imaging Center, University of North Carolina at Chapel Hill
Department of Psychiatry, Columbia University

Abstract. In medical imaging analysis and computer vision, there is a growing interest in analyzing various manifold-valued data including 3D rotations, planar shapes, oriented or directed directions, the Grassmann manifold, deformation field, symmetric positive definite (SPD) matrices and medial shape representations (m-rep) of subcortical structures. Particularly, the scientific interests of most population studies focus on establishing the associations between a set of covariates (e.g., diagnostic status, age, and gender) and manifold-valued data for characterizing brain structure and shape differences, thus requiring a regression modeling framework for manifold-valued data. The aim of this paper is to develop an intrinsic regression model for the analysis of manifold-valued data as responses in a Riemannian manifold and their association with a set of covariates, such as age and gender, in Euclidean space. Because manifold-valued data do not form a vector space, directly applying classical multivariate regression may be inadequate in establishing the relationship between manifold-valued data and covariates of interest, such as age and gender, in real applications. Our intrinsic regression model, which is a semiparametric model, uses a link function to map from the Euclidean space of covariates to the Riemannian manifold of manifold data. We develop an estimation procedure to calculate an intrinsic least square estimator and establish its limiting distribution. We develop score statistics to test linear hypotheses on unknown parameters. We apply our methods to the detection of the difference in the morphological changes of the left and right hippocampi between schizophrenia patients and healthy controls using medial shape description.

1 Introduction

Statistical analysis of manifold-valued data has gained a great deal of attention in neuroimaging applications [1], [2], [3], [4], [5], [6], [7], [8], [9]. Examples of

---

* This work was supported in part by NSF grants SES-06-43663 and BCS-08-26844 and NIH grants UL1-RR025747- 01, R01MH08663 and R21AG033387 to Dr. Zhu, NIH grants R01NS055754 and R01EB5-34816 to Dr. Lin, Lilly Research Laboratories, the UNC NDRC HD 03110, Eli Lilly grant F1D-MC-X252, and NIH Roadmap Grant U54 EB005149-01, NAMIC to Dr. Styner.

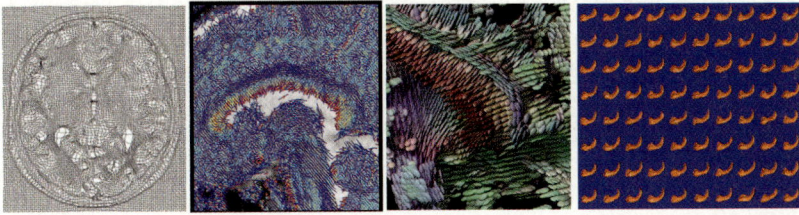

Fig. 1. Four different manifold-valued data (from the left to the right): deformation field reflecting brain deformation obtained from the registration of either diffusion tensor images (DTIs) or T1 magnetic resonance images (T1 MRIs); principal direction (PD) field reflecting fiber orientations obtained from DTIs; diffusion tensor field reflecting water diffusion along fiber tracts from DTIs; medial shape representations of hippocampi from multiple subjects obtained from the segmented T1 MRIs

manifold-valued data that we encounter in medical imaging analysis include the Grassmann manifold, planar shapes, deformation field, symmetric positive definite (SPD) matrices and the medial shape representations (m-rep) of subcortical structures (Fig. 1). Some review papers on the applications of manifold-valued data in medical imaging can be found in a recent special issue of **NeuroImage** [10]. However, the existing statistical methods for manifold-valued data are primarily developed to estimate intrinsic and extrinsic means, to estimate the structure of population variability, to carry out principal geodesic analysis, and to compare intrinsic (or extrinsic) means across two or more groups [11], [9], [12], [13], [14], [15], [16], [17].

Little literature exists for regression analyses of manifold-valued data. The existing parametric and nonparametric regression models for manifold-valued data were primarily developed for 2 (or 3) dimensional directional data [6], [18]. In parametric regression of directional data, parametric distributions, such as the Von Mises distribution, are commonly assumed for directional data, whereas it can be very challenging to assume useful parametric distributions for other manifold-valued data, such as SPD matrices and the m-rep, which can characterize the feature (e.g., shape) of real imaging data [15]. In the nonparametric analysis of manifold-valued data, although smoothing splines have been developed for directional data and planar landmark data, it is computationally difficult to generalize such smoothing splines to other manifold-valued data [6]. Recently, local constant regressions have been developed for manifold-valued data, but these regression models are defined with respect to either the Frechet mean or the geometric median [2], [4].

According to the best of our knowledge, this is the first paper that develops a semiparametric regression model with manifold-valued data as responses on a Riemannian manifold and a set of covariates, such as time, gender, and diagnostic status, in Euclidean space. Our regression model are solely based on the first-order moment, thus avoiding specifying any parametric distributions. We propose an inference procedure to estimate the regression coefficients in this semi-parametric model. We establish asymptotic properties, including consistency and asymptotic normality, of the estimates of the regression coefficients. We develop score statistics to test linear hypotheses on unknown parameters. Finally, we illustrate the application of our statistical methods to the detection of the difference in morphological changes of the hippocampi between schizophrenia patients and healthy controls in a neuroimaging study of schizophrenia.

2 Method

2.1 Review of Regression Models

We consider a dataset that is composed of a response y_i and a $p \times 1$ covariate vector $\mathbf{x}_i$ for $i = 1, \cdots, n$. Responses may be continuous observations in classical linear models, such as age, weight, income, and they may be discrete or ordinal observations, such as differing severity of diseases and disease status (patients v.s. healthy subjects). Covariates may be quantitative, such as age, or qualitative, such as handiness, gender, and presence of risk factors (yes/no).

Regression models often include two key elements: a **link function** $\mu_i(\boldsymbol{\beta}) = g(\mathbf{x}_i, \boldsymbol{\beta})$ and a **residual** $\epsilon_i = y_i - \mu_i(\boldsymbol{\beta})$, where $\boldsymbol{\beta}$ is a $q \times 1$ vector of regression coefficients and $g(\cdot, \cdot)$ is an known mapping from $R^p \times R^q$ to R. Regression models assume that

$$E[\epsilon_i | \mathbf{x}_i] = 0 \quad \text{for all} \quad i = 1, \cdots, n, \tag{1}$$

where the expectation denotes the conditional expectation of ϵ given $\mathbf{x}$. Moreover, nonparametric regressions include a **link function** $\mu_i = g(\mathbf{x}_i)$, in which $g(\cdot)$ is an unknown function, and a **residual** $\epsilon_i = y_i - g(\mathbf{x}_i)$, for which equation (1) holds.

To carry out statistical inference on $\boldsymbol{\beta}$ (or $g(\cdot)$), we need at least three statistical methods. The first one is an estimation method for calculating parameter estimate of $\boldsymbol{\beta}$, denoted by $\hat{\boldsymbol{\beta}}$. Various estimation methods include maximum likelihood estimation, robust estimation, estimating equations, among many others. The second is to prove that $\hat{\boldsymbol{\beta}}$ is a consistent estimator of $\boldsymbol{\beta}$ and has certain asymptotic distribution (e.g., normal). The third is to develop test statistics for testing the hypotheses:

$$H_0 : \mathbf{h}_0(\boldsymbol{\beta}) = \mathbf{b}_0 \quad \text{vs.} \quad H_1 : \mathbf{h}_0(\boldsymbol{\beta}) \neq \mathbf{b}_0, \tag{2}$$

where $\mathbf{h}_0(\cdot)$ is an $r \times 1$ vector function and $\mathbf{b}_0$ is an $r \times 1$ specified vector. In most applications, we are interested in testing $\mathbf{h}_0(\boldsymbol{\beta}) = \mathbf{H}\boldsymbol{\beta} = \mathbf{b}_0$ for a given $r \times q$ matrix $\mathbf{H}$ [18], [7], [8].

2.2 Intrinsic Regression for Manifold-Valued Data

We formally develop an intrinsic regression model for manifold-valued responses and covariates of interest from n observations. Suppose we observe a dataset $\{(S_i, \mathbf{x}_i) : i = 1, \cdots, n\}$, where S_i are points on a Riemannian manifold $\mathcal{S}$ and $\mathbf{x}_i$ are covariates of interest in Euclidean space.

The intrinsic regression model first involves modeling a 'conditional mean' of an manifold-valued response S_i given $\mathbf{x}_i$, denoted by $\mu_i(\boldsymbol{\beta}) = g(\mathbf{x}_i, \boldsymbol{\beta})$, where $g(\cdot,\cdot)$, called **link function**, is a map from $R^p \times R^q$ to the manifold $\mathcal{S}$. Note that we just borrow the term 'conditional mean' from Euclidean space. Given two points $\mathbf{S}_i$ and $\mu_i(\boldsymbol{\beta})$ on the manifold $\mathcal{M}$, the intrinsic regression model also define the **residual** or 'difference' between $\mathbf{S}_i$ and $\mu_i(\boldsymbol{\beta})$ to ensure that $\mu_i(\boldsymbol{\beta})$ is the proper 'conditional mean' of $\mathbf{S}_i$ given $\mathbf{x}_i$. At $\mu_i(\boldsymbol{\beta})$, we have a tangent space of the manifold $\mathcal{S}$, denoted by $T_{\mu_i(\boldsymbol{\beta})}\mathcal{S}$, which is a Euclidean space representing a first order approximation of the manifold $\mathcal{S}$ near $\mu_i(\boldsymbol{\beta})$. Then, we calculate the projection of $\mathbf{S}_i$ onto $T_{\mu_i(\boldsymbol{\beta})}\mathcal{S}$, denoted by $\mathrm{Log}_{\mu_i(\boldsymbol{\beta})}(\mathbf{S}_i)$, which can be regarded as the difference between $\mathbf{S}_i$ and $\mu_i(\boldsymbol{\beta})$ for $i = 1,\cdots,n$. If $\mathcal{S}$ is a Euclidean space, then $\mathrm{Log}_{\mu_i(\boldsymbol{\beta})}(\mathbf{S}_i) = \mathbf{S}_i - \mu_i(\boldsymbol{\beta})$.

The intrinsic regression model for manifold-valued data is then defined by

$$E[\mathrm{Log}_{\mu_i(\boldsymbol{\beta})}(\mathbf{S}_i)|\mathbf{x}_i] = \mathbf{0}, \tag{3}$$

for $i = 1,\cdots,n$, where the expectation is taken with respect to the conditional distribution of $\mathbf{S}_i$ given $\mathbf{x}_i$. Model (3) does not assume any parametric distribution for $\mathbf{S}_i$ given $\mathbf{x}_i$, and thus it allows for a large class of distributions [15]. In addition, our model (3) does not assume homogeneous variance across all i. This is also desirable for the analysis of imaging measures, such as diffusion tensors, because between-subject and between-voxel variability in the imaging measures can be substantial.

2.3 Estimation

We calculate an intrinsic least squares estimator (ILSE) of the parameter vector $\boldsymbol{\beta}$, denoted by $\hat{\boldsymbol{\beta}}$, by minimizing the total residual sum of squares given by

$$G_n(\boldsymbol{\beta}) = \sum_{i=1}^n d(\mathbf{S}_i, \mu_i(\boldsymbol{\beta}))^2 = \sum_{i=1}^n << \mathrm{Log}_{\mu_i(\boldsymbol{\beta})}(\mathbf{S}_i), \mathrm{Log}_{\mu_i(\boldsymbol{\beta})}(\mathbf{S}_i) >>, \tag{4}$$

where $<<\cdot,\cdot>>$ is an inner product of two tangent vectors in $T_{\mu_i(\boldsymbol{\beta})}\mathcal{S}$ and $d(\cdot,\cdot)$ is the Riemannian distance function on $\mathcal{S}$. Thus, let $G_n(\boldsymbol{\beta}) = \sum_{i=1}^n d(\mathbf{S}_i, \mu_i(\boldsymbol{\beta}))^2$, $\hat{\boldsymbol{\beta}}$ solves the estimating equations given by

$$\partial_{\boldsymbol{\beta}} G_n(\boldsymbol{\beta}) = \sum_{i=1}^n \partial_{\boldsymbol{\beta}} d(\mathbf{S}_i, \mu_i(\boldsymbol{\beta}))^2 = \mathbf{0}, \tag{5}$$

where ∂ denotes partial differentiation with respect to a parameter vector, such as $\boldsymbol{\beta}$. The ILSE is closely related to the intrinsic mean $\hat{\mu}_{IM}$ of $\mathbf{S}_1,\cdots,\mathbf{S}_n \in \mathcal{S}$, which is defined as

$$\hat{\mu}_{IM} = \mathrm{argmin}_\mu \sum_{i=1}^n d(\mu, \mathbf{S}_i)^2. \tag{6}$$

In this case, μ_i is independent of i and covariates of interest. Moreover, under some conditions, we can establish consistency and asymptotically normality of $\hat{\boldsymbol{\beta}}$. A Newton-Raphson algorithm is developed to obtain $\hat{\boldsymbol{\beta}}$. Let $\partial_{\boldsymbol{\beta}} G_n(\boldsymbol{\beta})$ and $\partial^2_{\boldsymbol{\beta}} G_n(\boldsymbol{\beta})$, respectively, be the first- and second-order partial derivatives of $G_n(\boldsymbol{\beta})$. We iterates $\boldsymbol{\beta}^{(t+1)} = \boldsymbol{\beta}^{(t)} + \rho\{-\partial^2_{\boldsymbol{\beta}} G_n(\boldsymbol{\beta}^{(t)})\}^{-1}\partial_{\boldsymbol{\beta}} G_n(\boldsymbol{\beta}^{(t)})$, where $0 < \rho = 1/2^{k_0} \leq 1$ for some $k_0 \geq 0$ is chosen such that $G_n(\boldsymbol{\beta}^{(t+1)}) \leq G_n(\boldsymbol{\beta}^{(t)})$. We stop the Newton-Raphson algorithm when the absolute difference between consecutive $\boldsymbol{\beta}^{(t)}$'s is smaller than a predefined small number, say 10^{-4}. Finally, we set $\hat{\boldsymbol{\beta}} = \boldsymbol{\beta}^{(t)}$. In addition, because $-\partial^2_{\boldsymbol{\beta}} G_n(\boldsymbol{\beta}^{(t)})$ may not be positive definite, we use $E[-\partial^2_{\boldsymbol{\beta}} G_n(\boldsymbol{\beta}^{(t)})]$ instead of $-\partial^2_{\boldsymbol{\beta}} G_n(\boldsymbol{\beta}^{(t)})$ in order to stabilize the Newton-Raphson algorithm.

2.4 Hypotheses and Test Statistics

In medical analysis, most scientific questions of interest involve a comparison of manifold-valued data across diagnostic groups or detecting change in manifold-valued data across time [8], [19]. These scientific questions usually can be formulated as follows:

$$H_0 : \mathbf{H}\boldsymbol{\beta} = \boldsymbol{b}_0 \quad \text{vs.} \quad H_1 : \mathbf{H}\boldsymbol{\beta} \neq \boldsymbol{b}_0. \tag{7}$$

We test the null hypothesis $H_0 : \mathbf{H}\boldsymbol{\beta} = \boldsymbol{b}_0$ using a score test statistic W_n defined by

$$W_n = \mathbf{L}_n^T \hat{\mathbf{I}}^{-1} \mathbf{L}_n, \tag{8}$$

where $\mathbf{L}_n = n^{-1/2} \sum_{i=1}^n \hat{\mathbf{U}}_i(\tilde{\boldsymbol{\beta}})$ and $\hat{\mathbf{I}} = n^{-1} \sum_{i=1}^n \hat{\mathbf{U}}_i(\tilde{\boldsymbol{\beta}}) \hat{\mathbf{U}}_i(\tilde{\boldsymbol{\beta}})^T$, in which $\tilde{\boldsymbol{\beta}}$ denotes the estimate of $\boldsymbol{\beta}$ under H_0 and $\hat{\mathbf{U}}_i(\tilde{\boldsymbol{\beta}})$ is associated with $\partial_{\boldsymbol{\beta}} G_n(\boldsymbol{\beta})$. It can be shown that W_n is asymptotically χ^2 distributed.

2.5 Positive Definitive Matrices

We develop an intrinsic regression for SPDs. We introduce the tangent vector and tangent space at any $\mu \in \text{Sym}^+(m)$, the space of SPDs [8]. The tangent space of $\text{Sym}^+(m)$ at μ, denoted by $T_\mu \text{Sym}^+(m)$, is identified with a copy of $\text{Sym}(m)$, the space of symmetric matrices. Then we consider the scaled Frobenius inner product of any two tangent vectors Y_μ and Z_μ in $T_\mu \text{Sym}^+(m)$, which is defined by $<< Y_\mu, Z_\mu >>= \text{tr}(Y_\mu \mu^{-1} Z_\mu \mu^{-1})$. Given the inner product, we can formally construct the Riemannian geometry of $\text{Sym}^+(m)$ [8].

We consider the **link function** $\mu(\mathbf{x}, \boldsymbol{\beta})$ using the Cholesky decomposition of $\mu(\mathbf{x}, \boldsymbol{\beta})$. For the i-th observation, through a lower triangular matrix $\mathbf{C}_i(\boldsymbol{\beta}) = \mathbf{C}(\mathbf{x}_i, \boldsymbol{\beta}) = (C_{jk}(\mathbf{x}_i, \boldsymbol{\beta}))$, the Cholesky decomposition of $\mu(\mathbf{x}_i, \boldsymbol{\beta})$ equals $\mu(\mathbf{x}_i, \boldsymbol{\beta}) = \mu_i(\boldsymbol{\beta}) = \mathbf{C}_i(\boldsymbol{\beta})\mathbf{C}_i(\boldsymbol{\beta})^T$. We must specify the explicit forms of $C_{jk}(\mathbf{x}_i, \boldsymbol{\beta})$ for all $j \geq k$ in order to determine all entries in $\mu_i(\boldsymbol{\beta})$. As an illustration, for $m = 2$, we may choose the 2×2 matrix $\mathbf{C}_i(\boldsymbol{\beta})$ with $C_{11}(\mathbf{x}_i, \boldsymbol{\beta}) = \exp(\mathbf{z}_i^T \boldsymbol{\beta}_{(1)})$, $C_{12}(\mathbf{x}_i, \boldsymbol{\beta}) = 0$, $C_{21}(\mathbf{x}_i, \boldsymbol{\beta}) = \mathbf{z}_i^T \boldsymbol{\beta}_{(2)}$, and $C_{22}(\mathbf{x}_i, \boldsymbol{\beta}) = \exp(\mathbf{z}_i^T \boldsymbol{\beta}_{(3)})$, where $\mathbf{z}_i = (1, \mathbf{x}_i^T)^T$ and $\boldsymbol{\beta}_{(k)}$ for $k = 1, 2, 3$ are subvectors of $\boldsymbol{\beta}$. We introduce a definition of **'residuals'** to ensure that $\mu_i(\boldsymbol{\beta})$ is the proper 'conditional mean' of S_i given $\mathbf{x}_i$. Then, we calculate the **residual** $\text{Log}_{\mu_i(\boldsymbol{\beta})}(S_i)$ given by $\mathbf{C}_i(\boldsymbol{\beta})\log(\mathbf{C}_i(\boldsymbol{\beta})^{-1}S_i\mathbf{C}_i(\boldsymbol{\beta})^{-T})\mathbf{C}_i(\boldsymbol{\beta})^T$. The intrinsic regression is defined in (3).

The first- and second-order derivatives of $G_n(\boldsymbol{\beta})$ are given as follows. The a-th element of $\partial_{\boldsymbol{\beta}}G_n(\boldsymbol{\beta})$ is given by $-2\sum_{i=1}^n \text{tr}\{\mathcal{E}_i(\boldsymbol{\beta})\mathbf{C}_i(\boldsymbol{\beta})^{-1}\partial_{\beta_a}\mu_i(\boldsymbol{\beta})\mathbf{C}_i(\boldsymbol{\beta})^{-T}\}$, where $\mathcal{E}_i(\boldsymbol{\beta}) = \log(\mathbf{C}_i(\boldsymbol{\beta})^{-1}S_i\mathbf{C}_i(\boldsymbol{\beta})^{-T})$ and $\partial_{\beta_a} = \partial/\partial\beta_a$. The (a,b)-th element of $\partial^2_{\boldsymbol{\beta}}G_n(\boldsymbol{\beta})$ is given by $-2\sum_{i=1}^n \text{tr}\{\partial_{\beta_b}\mathcal{E}_i(\boldsymbol{\beta})[\mathbf{C}_i(\boldsymbol{\beta})^{-1}\partial_{\beta_a}\mathbf{C}_i(\boldsymbol{\beta}) + \partial_{\beta_a}\mathbf{C}_i(\boldsymbol{\beta})^T\mathbf{C}_i(\boldsymbol{\beta})^{-T}]\} - 2\sum_{i=1}^n \text{tr}\{\mathcal{E}_i(\boldsymbol{\beta})\partial_{\beta_b}[\mathbf{C}_i(\boldsymbol{\beta})^{-1}\partial_{\beta_a}\mathbf{C}_i(\boldsymbol{\beta}) + \partial_{\beta_a}\mathbf{C}_i(\boldsymbol{\beta})^T\mathbf{C}_i(\boldsymbol{\beta})^{-T}]\}$, where $\partial^2_{\beta_a\beta_b} = \partial^2/\partial\beta_a\partial\beta_b$ and $\partial_{\beta_b}\mathcal{E}_i(\boldsymbol{\beta}) = \int_0^1 \mathbf{h}(s,\boldsymbol{\beta})ds$, in which

$$\mathbf{h}(s,\boldsymbol{\beta}) = \{[\tilde{\mathbf{S}}_i(\boldsymbol{\beta}) - \mathbf{I}_3]s + \mathbf{I}_3\}^{-1}\partial_{\beta_b}\tilde{\mathbf{S}}_i(\boldsymbol{\beta})\{[\tilde{\mathbf{S}}_i(\boldsymbol{\beta}) - \mathbf{I}_3]s + \mathbf{I}_3\}^{-1} \quad (9)$$

and $\tilde{\mathbf{S}}_i(\boldsymbol{\beta}) = \mathbf{C}_i(\boldsymbol{\beta})^{-1}\mathbf{S}_i\mathbf{C}_i(\boldsymbol{\beta})^{-T}$.

2.6 Median Representation

We develop an intrinsic regression for m-reps. An m-rep model consisting of k medial atoms can be considered as the direct product of k copies of $M(1) = R^3 \times R^+ \times S(2) \times S(2)$, that is $M(k) = \prod_{i=1}^k M(1)$, where $S(2)$ is the sphere in R^3 with radius one [5]. We introduce a tangent space $T_PM(1)$ at the point $P = (O, r, \mathbf{n}_0, \mathbf{n}_1)$, where $O \in R^3$, $r \in R^+$, and $\mathbf{n}_0$ and $\mathbf{n}_1 \in S(2)$. The tangent vector $U \in T_PM(1)$ takes the form $U = (U_0, U_r, U_{\mathbf{n}_0}, U_{\mathbf{n}_1})$, where $U_0 \in R^3$, $U_r \in R$, $U_{\mathbf{n}_i} \in R^3$ and $U_{\mathbf{n}_i}^T\mathbf{n}_i = 0$ for $i = 0, 1$. The inner product of any two tangent vectors $U^{(0)}$ and $U^{(1)}$ in $T_PM(1)$ is defined by $<< U^{(0)}, U^{(1)} >>= U^{(0)T}U^{(1)}$. The geodesic distance between P and $P_1 = (O_1, r_1, \mathbf{n}_{0,1}, \mathbf{n}_{1,1})$ in $M(1)$ is uniquely given by

$$\sqrt{(O-O_1)^T(O-O_1) + (\log(r)-\log(r_1))^2 + [\arccos(\mathbf{n}_0^T\mathbf{n}_{0,1})]^2 + [\arccos(\mathbf{n}_1^T\mathbf{n}_{1,1})]^2}.$$

To introduce an intrinsic regression for m-rep, we need to define a **link function** $\mu(\mathbf{x}, \boldsymbol{\beta}) = (\mu_O(\mathbf{x}, \boldsymbol{\beta}), \mu_r(\mathbf{x}, \boldsymbol{\beta}), \mu_0(\mathbf{x}, \boldsymbol{\beta}), \mu_1(\mathbf{x}, \boldsymbol{\beta}))^T \in M(1)$, which is a 10×1 vector. For instance, we may set $\mu_O(\mathbf{x}, \boldsymbol{\beta}) = (\mathbf{x}^T\boldsymbol{\beta}_1, \mathbf{x}^T\boldsymbol{\beta}_2, \mathbf{x}^T\boldsymbol{\beta}_3)^T$ and $\mu_r(\mathbf{x}, \boldsymbol{\beta}) = \exp(\mathbf{x}^T\boldsymbol{\beta}_4)$. A link function for $\mu_k(\mathbf{x}, \boldsymbol{\beta}) = (\mu_{0k}^x(\boldsymbol{\beta}), \mu_{0k}^y(\boldsymbol{\beta}), \mu_{0k}^z(\boldsymbol{\beta}))$ ($k = 0, 1$) is based on the stereographic projection given by

$$\frac{\mu_{0k}^x}{1-\mu_{0k}^z} = g_5(\mathbf{x}^T\boldsymbol{\beta}_{5,k}) \quad \text{and} \quad \frac{\mu_{0k}^y}{1-\mu_{0k}^z} = g_6(\mathbf{x}^T\boldsymbol{\beta}_{6,k}), \quad (10)$$

where $g_5(\cdot)$ and $g_6(\cdot)$ are known link functions and $\boldsymbol{\beta}_{5,k}$ and $\boldsymbol{\beta}_{6,k}$ are subvectors of $\boldsymbol{\beta}$. The **residual** $\text{Log}_{\mu(\mathbf{x},\boldsymbol{\beta})}(P)$ is given by

$$(O - \mu_O(\mathbf{x},\boldsymbol{\beta}), \log(r/\mu_r(\mathbf{x},\boldsymbol{\beta})), \text{Log}_{\mu_0(\mathbf{x},\boldsymbol{\beta})}(U_{\mathbf{n}_0}), \text{Log}_{\mu_1(\mathbf{x},\boldsymbol{\beta})}(U_{\mathbf{n}_1})),$$

where $\text{Log}_{\mu_0(\mathbf{x},\boldsymbol{\beta})}(U_{\mathbf{n}_0}) = \arccos(\mu_0(\mathbf{x},\boldsymbol{\beta})^TU_{\mathbf{n}_0})\mathbf{v}/||\mathbf{v}||_2$, in which $\mathbf{v} = U_{\mathbf{n}_0} - (\mu_0(\mathbf{x},\boldsymbol{\beta})^TU_{\mathbf{n}_0})\mu_0(\mathbf{x},\boldsymbol{\beta})$.

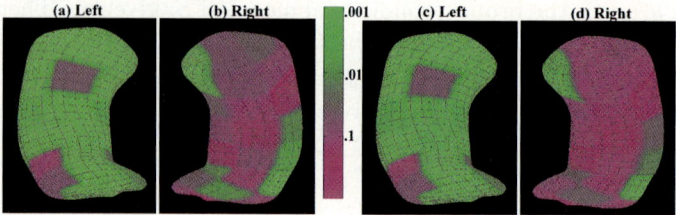

Fig. 2. Results for the m-rep shape analysis result mapped to the surface of the hippocampal schizophrenia study: the color-coded uncorrected p-value maps of the diagnostic status effects for (a) the left hippocampus and (b) the right hippocampus; the corrected p-value maps for (c) the left hippocampus and (d) the right hippocampus after correcting for multiple comparisons

3 Results

To demonstrate our regression method, we applied our methods to the m-rep shape of the hippocampus structure in the left and right brain hemisphere in schizophrenia patients and healthy controls, collected at 14 academic medical centers in North America and western Europe [19]. There were 56 healthy controls and 238 schizophrenia patients who met the following criteria: age 16 to 40 years; onset of psychiatric symptoms before age 35; diagnosis of schizophrenia, schizophreniform, or schizoaffective disorder according to DSM-IV criteria; and various treatment and substance dependence conditions.

We investigated the difference of m-rep shape between schizophrenia patients and healthy controls while controlling for other factors, such as gender and age. The hippocampi m-rep shape at the 24 medial atoms of the left and right brain were used as the response in our intrinsic regression model. Covariates of interest include Whole Brain Volume (WBV), race (Caucasian, African American and others), age (in years), gender, and diagnostic status (patient or control).

We tested the diagnostic status effect on the whole m-rep structure. We presented the color-coded p-values of the diagnostic status effects across the atoms of both the left and right reference hippocampi in Fig 2 (a) and (b) and the corresponding adjusted p-values using false discovery rate were shown in Fig 2 (c) and (d). We observed large significance area in the left hippocampus, and some in the right hippocampus even after correcting for multiple comparisons.

4 Discussion

We have developed an intrinsic regression model for the analysis of manifold-valued data as responses in a Riemannian manifold and their association with a set of covariates. We have developed an estimation procedure to calculate the intrinsic least square estimates. We have developed score statistics for testing linear hypotheses on unknown parameters. We plan to apply our method to other manifold-valued data including the Grassmann manifold, planar shapes, and deformation field.

References

1. Pennec, X.: Intrinsic statistics on riemannian manifolds: Basic tools for geometric measurements. Journal of Mathematical Imaging and Vision 25, 127–154 (2006)
2. Davis, B.C., Bullitt, E., Fletcher, P.T., Joshi, S.: Population shape regression from random design data. In: IEEE 11th International Conference on Computer Vision (2007)
3. Pennec, X., Fillard, P., Ayache, N.: A riemannian framework for tensor computing. International Journal of Computer Vision 66, 41–66 (2006)
4. Fletcher, P.T., Venkatasubramanian, S., Joshi, S.: The geometric median on riemannian manifolds with application to robust atlas estimation. NeuroImage 45, S143–S152 (2009)
5. Yushkevich, P., Fletcher, P., Joshi, S., Thall, A., Pizer, S.M.: Continuous medial representations for geometric object modeling in 2d and 3d. Image and Vision Computing 21, 17–28 (2003)
6. Jupp, P.E., Kent, J.T.: Fitting smooth paths to spherical data. Applied Statistics 36, 34–46 (1987)
7. Schwartzman, A., Robert, F.D., Taylor, J.E.: Cross-subject comparison of principal diffusion direction maps. Magnetic Resonance in Medicine 53, 1423–1431 (2005)
8. Schwartzman, A.: Random ellipsoids and false discovery rates: Statistics for diffusion tensor imaging data. Ph.D. thesis, Stanford University (2006)
9. Huckemann, S., Hotz, T., Munk, A.: Intrinsic shape analysis: Geodesic pca for riemannian manifolds modulo isometric lie group actions (with discussions). Statistica Sinica (2009)
10. Miller, M.I., Qiu, A.: The emerging discipline of computational functional anatomy. NeuroImage 45, S16–S39 (2009)
11. Fletcher, P., Joshi, S., Lu, C., Pizer, S.: Principal geodesic analysis for the study of nonlinear statistics of shape. IEEE Transactions on Medical Imaging 23, 995–1005 (2004)
12. Dryden, I., Mardia, K.: Statistical shape analysis. John Wiley and Sons, New York
13. Dryden, I., Mardia, K.: Multivariate shape analysis. Sankhya 55, 460–480 (1993)
14. Kendall, D.G.: Shape manifolds, procrustean metrics and complex projective spaces. Bull. Lond. Math. Soc. 16, 81–121 (1984)
15. Kent, J.: The complex bingham distribution and shape analysis. Journal of the Royal Statistical Society B 56, 285–299 (1994)
16. Kim, P.T., Koo, J.Y.: Statistical inverse problems on manifolds. Journal of Fourier Analysis and Applications 11, 639–653 (2005)
17. Fréchet, M.: Les éléments aléatoires de nature quelconque dans un espace distancé. Ann. Inst. H. Poincaré 10, 215–230 (1948)
18. Mardia, K., Jupp, P.E.: Directional statistics. Academic Press, John Wiley (1983)
19. Styner, M., Lieberman, J.A., Pantazis, D., Gerig, G.: Boundary and medial shape analysis of the hippocampus in schizophrenia. Medical Image Analysis 4, 197–203 (2004)

Gender Differences in Cerebral Cortical Folding: Multivariate Complexity-Shape Analysis with Insights into Handling Brain-Volume Differences

Suyash P. Awate[1], Paul Yushkevich[1], Daniel Licht[2,*], and James C. Gee[1]

[1] Penn Image Computing and Science Lab (PICSL), University of Pennsylvania
awate@mail.med.upenn.edu
[2] Children's Hospital of Philadelphia, USA

Abstract. This paper presents a study of gender differences in adult human cerebral cortical folding patterns. The study employs a new multivariate statistical descriptor for analyzing folding patterns in a region of interest (ROI) and a rigorous nonparametric permutation-based scheme for hypothesis testing. Unlike typical ROI-based methods that summarize folding complexity or shape by single/few numbers, the proposed descriptor systematically constructs a unified description of *complexity and shape* in a *high-dimensional* space (thousands of numbers/dimensions). Furthermore, this paper presents new mathematical insights into the relationship of intra-cranial volume (ICV) with cortical complexity and shows that conventional complexity descriptors implicitly handle ICV differences in different ways, thereby lending *different meanings* to "complexity". This paper describes two systematic methods for handling ICV changes in folding studies using the proposed descriptor. The clinical study in this paper exploits these theoretical insights to demonstrate that (i) the answer to which gender has higher/lower "complexity" depends on how a folding measure handles ICV differences and (ii) cortical folds in males and females differ significantly in shape as well.

1 Introduction

Cerebral cortical folding forms an underpinning for the cognitive skills and behavioral traits in humans. For the last few decades, magnetic resonance (MR) imaging has enabled in vivo studies of human cortical folding patterns. One class of approaches to folding analysis rely on spatial normalization [1,2] and subsequently perform statistical hypothesis testing at every voxel or surface element in the normalized space. However, the difficulty in finding sufficiently-many homologous features [3,4] may directly affect the normalization and, thereby, the

---

* The authors gratefully acknowledge the support of this work via NIH grants HD042974, HD046159, NS045839, EB06266, DA14129, DA22807, UL1RR024234, K23 NS052380, NS061111, K25 AG027785, the Dana Foundation, the June and Steve Wolfson Family Foundation, and the Institute for Translational Medicine and Therapeutics' (ITMAT) Transdisciplinary Awards Program in Translational Medicine and Therapeutics at the University of Pennsylvania.

reliability of findings in the clinical study. Furthermore, the phenomenon of cortical folding has an inherent large-scale or non-local character. A second class of approaches propose region-based folding descriptors [5,6,7], which avoid the challenges associated with normalization by reducing spatial sensitivity from a voxel to a region of interest (ROI) that can be reliably defined in each individual based on observed homologous features.

Most studies in the literature measure only the complexity of folding, *ignoring* information related to shape, orientation, etc. Although some recent ROI-based approaches propose descriptors incorporating shape information [8], they fail to integrate all the information on shape and complexity in a single descriptor. Furthermore, typical ROI-based approaches produce scalar or low-dimensional summary statistics for the entire ROI, risking serious information loss. This paper builds on a new ROI-based statistical framework for folding analysis [9] relying on a *rich multivariate non-local descriptor that captures the spectrum of complexity and shape*. The proposed descriptor is a joint probability density function (PDF) of two variables, one capturing surface complexity and the other capturing surface shape. The paper proposes a new application of a non-parametric permutation-based approach for statistical hypothesis testing with multivariate cortical descriptors. In these ways, the proposed framework couples the reliability of ROI-based analysis with the richness of the proposed descriptor.

While several folding studies concern neurodevelopmental disorders, studies on *gender* differences, in the normal population, have received very little attention. Moreover, while one study [10] using the fractal-dimension (FD) measure reported higher complexity in adult females, two very recent studies [11,12] using the isoperimetric ratio (IPR) measure report higher complexity in larger adult brains (i.e. males). The study in this paper elucidates these seemingly-conflicting findings. This paper provides new theoretical insights into relationships between folding measures with intra-cranial volume (ICV), pinning them down to the fundamental issues of scale and replication. It shows that standard folding measures in the literature imbibe different meanings of "complexity". It shows that handling ICV differences in folding studies may *not* be as simple as including ICV as a covariate in the underlying statistical test. This paper proposes *two systematic methods for handling ICV changes* in folding studies using the proposed descriptor and shows that while the findings using one method are consistent with [10], those using the other method are consistent with [11,12].

While it is well known [5] that the *shape* of cortical folds is asymmetric, i.e. surface area buried in sulci (predominantly concave areas) being more than that for gyri, the literature on gender differences in folding ignores studies of shape. This paper is, perhaps, the first to demonstrate that the fraction of the cortical surface that is convex (predominantly gyri) is significantly higher in males.

2 Background

This section describes a variety of existing ROI-based folding descriptors summarizing a small part of the complexity-shape spectrum via one or a few numbers.

One class of descriptors quantify surface complexity alone. FD [10] captures the rate of increase in surface area over multiscale representations of the surface. Gyrification index (GI) [13] is the ratio of the lengths of a planar curve to its envelope. Convexity ratio (CR) [6] is the ratio of the area of the surface to the area of the convex hull/envelope of the surface. IPR [6,11,12] is the ratio of the surface area to the two-third power of the volume enclosed by the surface. Average curvedness (AC) [8] measures the deviation of the surface from a plane. Another measure is the 2D centroid of the histogram (HC) of curvature [7].

Some folding descriptors capture a part of the complexity-shape spectrum by summing up specific measures for all surface patches, e.g. intrinsic curvature index (ICI) [5] sums up degrees of hemisphericity, mean curvature norm (MCN) [6] sums up degrees of hemisphericity and cylindricity, Gaussian curvature norm (GCN) [6] sums up degrees of hemisphericity and saddle-likeness, average shape index (AS) [8] sums up shape measures, etc.

3 Methods and Materials

3.1 A Multivariate High-Dimensional Folding Descriptor

This section describes a novel high-dimensional multivariate surface descriptor that captures the spectrum of complexity and shape [9].

At every point m on surface $\mathcal{M}$, the principal curvatures $K_{\min}(m)$ and $K_{\max}(m)$ *completely* describe the local patch geometry. The space $< K_{\min}, K_{\max} >$ can be reparameterized into the orthogonal basis of curvedness C and shape index S [14], meaningfully separating notions of bending and shape (Figure 1).

We propose the following generative model of cortical surfaces. Let us consider $C : \mathcal{M} \to [0, \infty]$ and $S : \mathcal{M} \to [-1, 1]$ as random fields. Let us also consider the joint PDF that captures the dependencies between $C(m)$ and $S(m)$ for a specific class of surfaces. Consider a finite collection $\mathcal{O} = \{d\mathcal{M}^1, \ldots, d\mathcal{M}^T\}$ of T surface

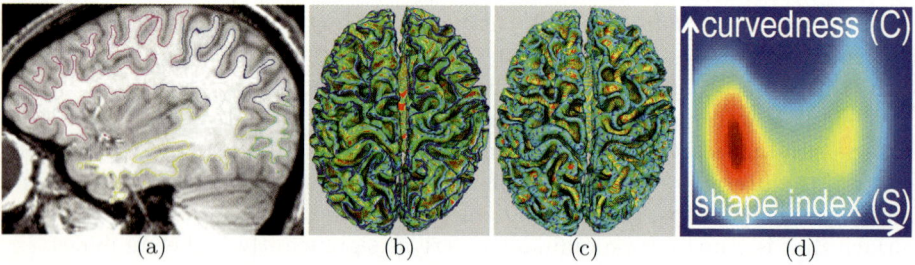

Fig. 1. (a) A sagittal slice of an MR image overlapped with the zero crossing of the level set that represents the cortical surface. (b) Curvedness $C(m)$ values painted on $\mathcal{M}$ (red→blue ≡ low→high). (c) Shape-index $S(m) \in [-1,1]$ values painted on $\mathcal{M}$ (red→blue ≡ $-1 \to 1$). (d) Proposed descriptor $P_{\mathcal{M}}(C,S)$ (blue→red ≡ low→high; for all plots in this paper, horizontal axis ≡ S and vertical axis ≡ C).

patches, located at points $\{m^1, \ldots, m^T\} \in \mathcal{M}$ *uniformly* distributed over the surface $\mathcal{M}$, covering $\mathcal{M}$. Then, $\{(C(m^1), S(m^1)), \ldots, (C(m^T), S(m^T))\}$ is an instantiation of the field of random vectors at locations $\{m^1, \ldots, m^T\}$. We assume that the random field is *stationary*, i.e. each observation $(C(m^t), S(m^t))$, is randomly drawn from a single PDF $P_\mathcal{M}(C, S)$. The complexity and variability in cortical folding suggests that dependencies between random vectors $(C(m^t), S(m^t))$ and $(C(m^s), S(m^s))$ decrease at a fast rate with increasing geodesic distance between locations m^t and m^s. Thus, we assume that the random field is *mixing*.

We propose the joint PDF $P_\mathcal{M}(C, S)$ as the multivariate high-dimensional descriptor of cerebral cortical folding patterns for surface $\mathcal{M}$ (Figure 1(d)). $P_\mathcal{M}(C, S)$ subsumes scalar descriptors like ICI, MCN, GCN, AC, AS, HC. Discretizing $P_\mathcal{M}(C, S)$ on an MxN grid leads to an MN-dimensional descriptor. In this paper $M = N = 64$.

For a given surface $\mathcal{M}$, we propose to estimate the folding pattern descriptor $P_\mathcal{M}(C, S)$ from the sample $\{(C(m^t), S(m^t)) : t = 1, \ldots, T\}$ drawn from a stationary mixing random field. A consistent nonparametric estimate [15] for the folding descriptor is the Gaussian mixture: $P_\mathcal{M}(C, S) \approx \frac{1}{T} \sum_{t=1}^T G_t((C(m^t), S(m^t)), \Sigma_t)$, where $G((\mu_1, \mu_2), \Sigma)$ is a 2D Gaussian kernel with mean (μ_1, μ_2) and covariance Σ. Consistency requires an optimal choice of Σ_t, dependent on the T, and we employ a penalized maximum likelihood scheme [16] to estimate Σ_t; the literature provides many schemes. Figure 1(d) shows a typical $P_\mathcal{M}(C, S)$ that is multimodal and unlike standard parametric PDFs, thus justifying nonparametric PDF estimation for reliability. In practice, typical ROIs yield sample sizes T in the range of thousands or tens of thousands, producing robust estimations.

3.2 A Testing Scheme for Multivariate Histogram Analysis

This section proposes a new application of a known nonparametric permutation-based approach, i.e. statistical nonparametric mapping (SnPM) [17], for statistical hypothesis testing with N multivariate cortical descriptors in a clinical study, i.e. $\{P_{\mathcal{M}^n}(C, S) : n = 1, \ldots, N\}$, Unlike typical usage of SnPM for functions on the image or surface domain, which necessitates spatial normalization, we propose to apply SnPM to discretized versions of the cortical descriptors $P_{\mathcal{M}^n}(C, S)$. Unlike conventional multivariate histogram analysis (e.g. Hotelling T^2), SnPM provides the *locations* (pixels and clusters), in the histogram domain $<C, S>$, for significant differences/effects.

3.3 Complexity and Volume Relationships: New Insights

This section presents new theoretical insights into (i) relationships between folding and ICV and (ii) different meanings of "complexity" underlying descriptors.

In Figure 2, S1 and S2 occupy equal volumes but S2 has finer-scale features than S1. Desirably so, all measures inform that S2 is more complex than S1.

Now consider surfaces occupying different volumes. ICV increase can be associated with two kinds of effects on cortical surfaces: (i) folds are *scaled up/*

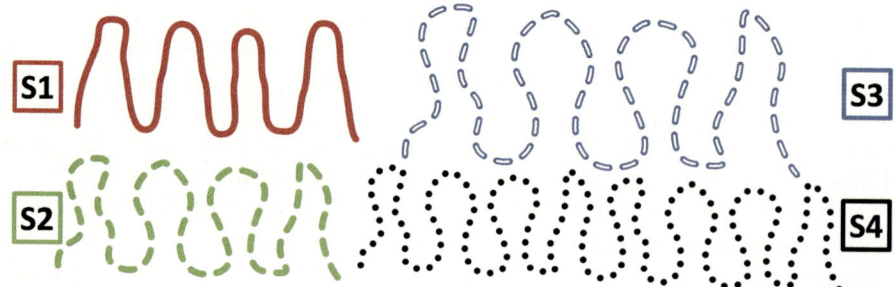

Fig. 2. What does "complexity" mean when volumes differ: issues of scale and replication. S1 and S2 occupy the same volume; S2 is more complex than S1. S3 and S4 occupy larger volumes than S2. S3 enlarges/*scales* the folds in S2. S4 *replicates* the folds in S2. How do we compare the complexities of (i) S3 and S2 and (ii) S4 and S2 ?

enlarged, e.g. comparing S2 and S3, or (ii) folds are *replicated*, e.g. comparing S2 and S4. This section shows that the meaning of "complexity" imbibed in folding descriptors reflects how the descriptors handle scaling and replication.

One class of measures, including GI and CR (both normalized by their convex-hull surface area), are invariant to the aforementioned issues of scale and replication. Thus, GI and CR inform that S2, S3, and S4 have equal complexity.

A second class of measures, including IPR, ICI, MCN, GCN, and AC [6,11,12,8] (all normalized by surface-patch area or, equivalently, ICV$^{2/3}$), is *designed to be invariant to scale*. However, this sacrifices invariance to replication. Thus, these measures inform that S3 and S2 have equal complexity, but S4 is more complex than S2.

A third class of measures, including FD [10], HC [7], and the proposed $P_\mathcal{M}(C, S)$ in Section 3.1, are *invariant to replication*, but *not scale*. Unlike the first two classes, these measures are *not* normalized via area or ICV$^{2/3}$. Thus, they inform that S4 and S2 are equally complex, but S3 is less complex than S2.

We now propose a new scale-invariant descriptor. Enlarging volume by a factor β^3 reduces curvedness by a factor of β. Indeed, unit-area patches in enlarged surfaces appear more planar (Taylor's theorem). Thus, a scale-invariant version of $P_\mathcal{M}(C, S)$ is $P_\mathcal{M}(C\beta, S)$, where β^3 is the ratio of the mean group ICV to the ICV for cortical surface $\mathcal{M}$. Similar to the second class of measures, $P_\mathcal{M}(C\beta, S)$ informs that S3 and S2 have equal complexity, but S4 is more complex than S2.

Subsequent sections denote $P^{\text{replication}} = P_\mathcal{M}(C, S)$ and $P^{\text{scale}} = P_\mathcal{M}(C\beta, S)$.

3.4 Clinical Cohort, Imaging, and Image Analysis

The cohort comprised T1 MR images (1 mm^3 isotropic voxels) of 30 females (age 34.8 ± 9.6 years) and 27 males (age 36 ± 11 years), obtained after enforcing quality-assurance checks on every image in the dataset in [18].

Image analysis: (i) parcellate lobes, (ii) segment tissues [19], (iii) resample segmentations to 0.4^3 mm^3 isotropic voxels, (iv) fit a level set to the cortical gray-white interface $\mathcal{M}$, (v) compute $(C(m), S(m)) \forall m \in \mathcal{M}$, (vi) estimate $P^{\text{replication}}$

(Section 3.1) and P^{scale} (Section 3.3) for all lobes, (vii) cross-sectional test for gender differences via SnPM (Section 3.2). $P^{\text{replication}}$ has been validated in [9].

4 Results and Discussion

4.1 Gender Differences in Cortical Complexity and Shape in Adults

The **proposed replication-invariant folding descriptor** $P^{\text{replication}}$, described in Section 3.1, produces t maps (Figure 3(a)-(d)) indicating larger histogram mass for males (red) in low-curvedness regions (bottom half) and larger histogram mass for males (red) in convex regions (right half). SnPM produces significant clusters for the occipital lobes (Figure 3(e)), but *not* for other lobes. Nevertheless, when the ROI size is increased to a hemisphere, these effects get significantly strengthened; evident in t maps (Figure 3(f),(h)) and significant clusters (Figure 3(g),(i)). These results show that *female cortical surfaces are more complex* based on $P^{\text{replication}}$ (consistent with [10]) and significantly *less convex* than those of males. Figures 3(j)-(k) visualize the complexity differences.

The **proposed scale-invariant folding descriptor** P^{scale}, described in Section 3.3, produces t maps (Figure 4(c)) indicating larger histogram mass for males (red) in high-curvedness regions (top half) for all lobes. Complexity differences are very strong, producing significant locations (Figure 4(d)) and clusters for all lobes, and overwhelm shape differences. These results show that,

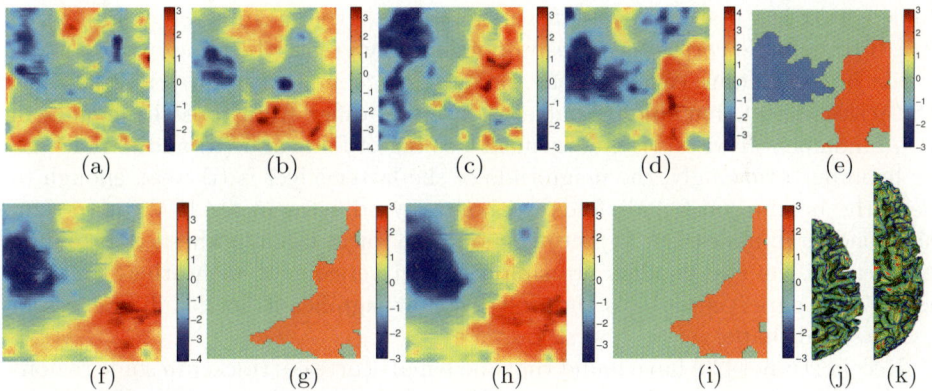

Fig. 3. (a)-(d) Student's t statistics for a cross-sectional study with $P^{\text{replication}}$ (positive t ≡ larger value in males) for frontal, parietal, temporal, and occipital lobes, respectively, in the left hemisphere. Similar patterns exist for lobes in right hemisphere. (e) Significant clusters via SnPM for left occipital lobe. For all plots in this paper, **corrected p values** for significant locations/clusters are indicated by coloring them by the associated z score: e.g. $z(p = 0.05) = 1.65$, $z(p = 0.005) = 2.58$. **(f)-(h)** t statistics and **(g)-(i)** significant clusters for $P^{\text{replication}}$ for left hemisphere (4 lobes) and whole brain (8 lobes), respectively. A similar pattern exists for the right hemisphere. **(j)-(k)** female and male brains, respectively, painted by C values (red→blue ≡ low→high). The female brain appears more blue/cyan (more "complex").

206   S.P. Awate et al.

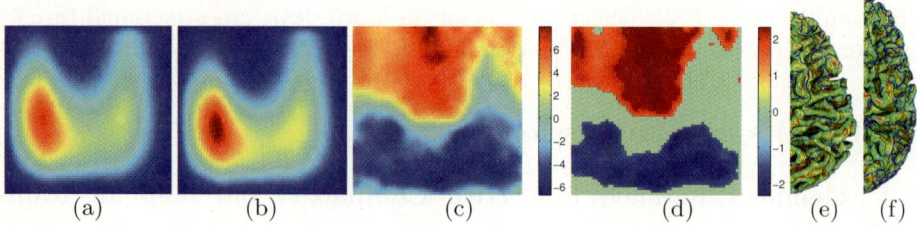

Fig. 4. **(a)-(b)** Average of P^{scale} for males and females, respectively, for the left frontal lobe. **(c)-(d)** t statistics (positive t ≡ larger value in males) and significant *locations*, respectively, for the left frontal lobe. Similar patterns exist for all other lobes. **(e)-(f)** female and male brains, respectively, adjusted for ICV and painted by C values (red→blue ≡ low→high). The female brain appears more red/yellow (less "complex").

when ICV differences have been accounted for (via P^{scale}), *male cortical surfaces are more complex* than those of females. This interpretation is consistent with [11,12]. Figures 4(e)-(f) help visualize the complexity differences.

This paper exploited two new multivariate high-dimensional (65536 dimensional) folding descriptors, unifying complexity and shape information, to provide new mathematical insights into the different meanings of complexity in the context of ICV differences. The paper exploits these insights to resolve two seemingly-contradictory findings in the state of the art on gender-based cortical folding, i.e. [10] and [11,12] differ in which gender has higher "complexity". The cross-sectional clinical study in this paper demonstrates that while the female cortex has more fine-scale features (which is the meaning of "complexity" in [10]), the male cortex has a disproportionately greater bending in proportion to its larger volume (which is the meaning of "complexity" in [11,12]). Thus, the results show that folding patterns in males differ from those in females in two fundamental ways: (i) enlargement/scaling of folds and (ii) additional folds or bending. Amazingly, the magnitude of the latter effect is (i) weak enough to keep the bending in female folds, without any adjustment for ICV, more than the bending in males, but (ii) strong enough to reject the hypothesis that folding patterns in the two genders are simply scaled versions of each other. Furthermore, this paper is perhaps the first to show significant gender differences in gyral/sulcal shape.

Recent studies [20] have found that the female cortex is thicker in some regions even without compensating for lower ICV. After accounting for ICV differences, the entire cortex is significantly thicker in females. The complementary findings concerning cortical complexity, shape, and thickness might help explain the similarities and differences in cognitive skills possessed by both genders.

References

1. Yu, P., Grant, P.E., Qi, Y., Han, X., Segonne, F., Pienaar, R., Busa, E., Pacheco, J., Makris, N., Buckner, R.L., Golland, P., Fischl, B.: Cortical surface shape analysis based on spherical wavelets. IEEE Trans. Med. Imaging 26(4), 582–597 (2007)

2. Nordahl, C., Dierker, D., Mostafavi, I., Schumann, C., Rivera, S., Amaral, D., Van-Essen, D.: Cortical folding abnormalities in autism revealed by surface-based morphometry. Journal of Neuroscience 27(43), 11725–11735 (2007)
3. Mangin, J., Riviere, D., Cachia, A., Duchesnay, E., Cointepas, Y., Papadopoulos-Orfanos, D., Scifo, P., Ochiai, T., Brunelle, F., Regis, J.: A framework to study the cortical folding patterns. NeuroImage 23(1), S129–S138 (2004)
4. Van-Essen, D., Dierker, D.: Surface-based and probabilistic atlases of primate cerebral cortex. Neuron. 56, 209–225 (2007)
5. Van-Essen, D., Drury, H.: Structural and functional analyses of human cerebral cortex using a surface-based atlas. J. Neuroscience 17(18), 7079–7102 (1997)
6. Batchelor, P., Castellano-Smith, A., Hill, D., Hawkes, D., Cox, T., Dean, A.: Measures of folding applied to the development of the human fetal brain. IEEE Trans. Med. Imaging 21(8), 953–965 (2002)
7. Pienaar, R., Fischl, B., Caviness, V., Makris, N., Grant, P.E.: A methodology for analyzing curvature in the developing brain from preterm to adult. Int. J. Imaging Systems Technology 18(1), 42–68 (2008)
8. Awate, S.P., Win, L., Yushkevich, P., Schultz, R.T., Gee, J.C.: 3D cerebral cortical morphometry in autism: Increased folding in children and adolescents in frontal, parietal, and temporal lobes. In: Proc. Int. Conf. Medical Image Computing and Computer Assisted Intervention, vol. 1, pp. 559–567 (2008)
9. Awate, S.P., Yushkevich, P., Song, Z., Licht, D., Gee, J.C.: Multivariate high-dimensional cortical folding analysis, combining complexity and shape, in neonates with congenital heart disease. In: Proc. Information Processing in Medical Imaging (to appear, 2009)
10. Luders, E., Narr, K., Thompson, P., Rex, D., Jancke, L., Steinmetz, H., Toga, A.: Gender differences in cortical complexity. Nat. Neuro. 7(8), 799–800 (2004)
11. Im, K., Lee, J., Lyttelton, O., Kim, S., Evans, A., Kim, S.: Brain size and cortical structure in the adult human brain. Cer. Cor. 18, 2181–2191 (2008)
12. Toro, R., Perron, M., Pike, B., Richer, L., Veillette, S., Pausova, Z., Paus, T.: Brain size and folding of the human cerebral cortex. Cer. Cor. 18, 2352–2357 (2008)
13. Zilles, K., Armstrong, E., Schleicher, A., Kretschmann, H.: The human pattern of gyrification in the cerebral cortex. Anat. Embryol. 179, 173–179 (1988)
14. Koenderink, J., van Doorn, A.: Surface shape and curvature scales. Image and Vision Computing 10(8), 557–565 (1992)
15. Lu, Z., Chen, X.: Spatial kernel regression estimation: weak consistency. Stat. and Prob. Letters 68(2), 125–136 (2004)
16. Chow, Y., Geman, S., Wu, L.: Consistant cross-validated density estimation. Annals of Statistics 11(1), 25–38 (1983)
17. Nichols, T., Holmes, A.: Nonparametric permutation tests for functional neuroimaging: a primer with examples. Human Brain Mapping 15(1), 1–25 (2002)
18. Mortamet, B., Zeng, D., Gerig, G., Prastawa, M., Bullitt, E.: Effects of healthy aging measured by intracranial compartment volumes using a designed MR brain database. In: Med. Imag. Comput. Comp. Assist. Interv, pp. 383–391 (2005)
19. Awate, S.P., Tasdizen, T., Foster, N.L., Whitaker, R.T.: Adaptive Markov modeling for mutual-information-based unsupervised MRI brain-tissue classification. Medical Image Analysis 10(5), 726–739 (2006)
20. Sowell, E., Peterson, B., Kan, E., Woods, R., Yoshii, J., Bansal, R., Xu, D., Zhu, H., Thompson, P., Toga, A.: Sex differences in cortical thickness mapped in 176 healthy individuals between 7 and 87 years of age. Cer. Cor. 17, 1550–1560 (2007)

Cortical Shape Analysis in the Laplace-Beltrami Feature Space

Yonggang Shi, Ivo Dinov, and Arthur W. Toga*

Lab of Neuro Imaging, UCLA School of Medicine, Los Angeles, CA, USA
yshi@loni.ucla.edu

Abstract. For the automated analysis of cortical morphometry, it is critical to develop robust descriptions of the position of anatomical structures on the convoluted cortex. Using the eigenfunction of the Laplace-Beltrami operator, we propose in this paper a novel feature space to characterize the cortical geometry. Derived from intrinsic geometry, this feature space is invariant to scale and pose variations, anatomically meaningful, and robust across population. A learning-based sulci detection algorithm is developed in this feature space to demonstrate its application in cortical shape analysis. Automated sulci detection results with 10 training and 15 testing surfaces are presented.

1 Introduction

The analysis and registration of cortex morphometry is an important area in human brain mapping and has produced valuable findings for the modeling of both normal and pathological brains[1]. With the increasing availability of brain scans from large scale studies[2], manual labeling becomes infeasible and it is thus critical to automate the cortical shape analysis process and robustly resolve its complicated and highly variable convolution pattern. In this paper, we propose a novel feature space derived from the eigenfunction of the Laplace-Beltrami operator to study the cortical surface. This feature space provides an intrinsic and anatomically interesting characterization of locations on the cortical surface and leads to compact modeling of anatomical landmarks invariant to scale and natural pose differences.

One main goal of cortical shape analysis is the automatic labeling of the major sulci that can serve as the landmarks for cortical normalization[1,3]. Various learning-based approaches have been developed to incorporate priors from manual labeling[4,5,6,7,8]. The features used in previous work, however, rely on coordinates in canonical spaces such as the Euclidean space of a brain atlas or the unit sphere to model the position of anatomical landmarks on the cortex, which is not intrinsic and can be sensitive to the image registration results.

---

* This work was funded by the National Institutes of Health through the NIH Roadmap for Medical Research, Grant U54 RR021813 entitled Center for Computational Biology (CCB). Information on the National Centers for Biomedical Computing can be obtained from http://nihroadmap.nih.gov/bioinformatics.

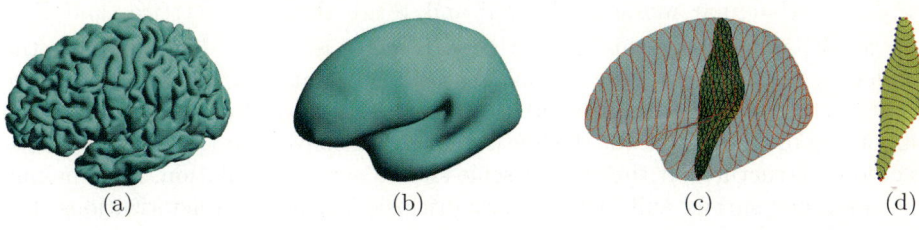

Fig. 1. (a) $\mathcal{M}$. (b) $\widetilde{\mathcal{M}}$. (c) Level contours of f_1 and the surface patches used to define $\mathcal{F}_2$ and $\mathcal{F}_3$. (d) Medial(blue) and lateral(red) points of D_j.

This is especially problematic for pathological brains as they can exhibit large deviations from standard atlases. To overcome this limitation, we propose to characterize the relative locations of cortical landmarks with an intrinsic feature space that has the nice property of being invariant to pose and scale variations. This feature space is computed using the eigenfunction of the Laplace-Beltrami operator[9,10,11,12] of the cortex and a series of surface patches to describe intrinsically the anterior/posterior, superior/inferior, and medial/lateral profile of the cortex. A sulci detection algorithm in the feature space is also developed to demonstrate the application of this feature space in cortical shape analysis.

The rest of the paper is organized as follows. In section 2, we propose the Laplace-Beltrami feature space and develop the algorithm for its numerical computation. In section 3, we develop a learning-based sulci detection algorithm in the feature space to demonstrate its value in analyzing cortical anatomy. Preliminary experimental results are presented in section 4. Finally conclusions are made in section 5.

2 Laplace-Beltrami Feature Space of Cortical Surfaces

For general data analysis, a subset of the Laplacian eigenfunctions were used to form a feature space [13]. To study medical shapes, however, this is not sufficient because it does not take into account the anatomical knowledge of the underlying structure. For elongated structures such as hippocampus, the second eigenfunction of the Laplace-Beltrami operator was used to detect stable anatomical landmarks [14]. In this section, we generalize this approach to cortical surfaces and define a Laplace-Beltrami(LB) feature space $\mathcal{F} = (\mathcal{F}_1, \mathcal{F}_2, \mathcal{F}_3)$, where $\mathcal{F}_i : \mathcal{M} \to \mathbb{R} (i = 1, 2, 3)$ and $\mathcal{M}$ is a cortical surface, to capture the anatomical characteristics of cortex morphometry. We assume all brains are in the neurological orientation to remove ambiguity in the sign of eigenfunctions.

Compared with simple shapes such as hippocampus, the cortical surface is a much more complicated structure. In particular, the highly variable convolution pattern makes the extraction of stable features a challenging problem. To tackle this difficulty, we follow the multi-scale strategy. Given a cortical surface $\mathcal{M}$, we construct its feature space using a surface $\widetilde{\mathcal{M}}$ that represents $\mathcal{M}$ at a coarser scale. For numerical computation, we represent both $\mathcal{M} = (\mathcal{V}, \mathcal{T})$ and $\widetilde{\mathcal{M}} =$

$(\widetilde{\mathcal{V}}, \mathcal{T})$ as triangular meshes, where $\mathcal{V}$ and $\widetilde{\mathcal{V}}$ are the set of vertices and $\mathcal{T}$ is the set of triangles. In this work, the surface $\widetilde{\mathcal{M}}$ is obtained by applying the Laplacian smoothing to the original surface $\mathcal{M}$, thus the vertices in $\widetilde{\mathcal{V}}$ have one-to-one correspondences to vertices in $\mathcal{V}$. As shown in Fig. 1(a) and (b), the smoothing process filters out the fine details in the convolution pattern and keeps geometric structures at the coarser scale shared across population, thus making the smoothed surface suitable to derive intrinsic location characterizations that are stable across population. Using the correspondences between $\widetilde{\mathcal{V}}$ and $\mathcal{V}$, we can then compare detailed cortical features defined on the vertices of $\mathcal{M}$ in the common feature space $\mathcal{F}$ and perform analysis tasks such as sulci and gyri labeling.

For the surface $\widetilde{\mathcal{M}}$, the eigenfunctions of its Laplace-Beltrami operator $\Delta_{\widetilde{\mathcal{M}}}$ are defined as:

$$\Delta_{\widetilde{\mathcal{M}}} f = -\lambda f \tag{1}$$

The eigenvalues of $\Delta_{\widetilde{\mathcal{M}}}$ can be ordered according to their magnitude as $0 = \lambda_0 \leq \lambda_1 \leq \lambda_2 \leq \cdots$. The corresponding eigenfunction of λ_i is denoted as $f_i : \widetilde{\mathcal{M}} \to \mathbb{R}$. By using the weak form of (1) and the finite element method, we can compute the eigenfunctions by solving a generalized matrix eigenvalue problem:

$$Qf = \lambda U f \tag{2}$$

where Q and U are matrices derived with the finite element method.

The first feature function $\mathcal{F}_1$ is defined using the Reeb graph [15] of the second eigenfunction f_1, which minimizes the smoothness measure $\int_{\widetilde{\mathcal{M}}} ||\nabla f|| d\widetilde{\mathcal{M}}$ and can be viewed as the smoothest non-constant projection from $\widetilde{\mathcal{M}}$ to the real line $\mathbb{R}$. As shown in Fig. 1(c), the nodes of the Reeb graph are the level contours of the eigenfunction. Because the eigenfunction is generally a Moss function [16], the Reeb graph of f_1 has a tree structure. Small branches in the Reeb graph are pruned according to the length of the associated level contour such that the final graph has a chain structure. The level contours of the Reeb graph are denoted as $C_i (i = 0, \cdots, N)$ with their order determined by the corresponding value of the eigenfunction f_1. Numerically we represent each contour as a polyline of K points $C_i = [C_{i,1}, C_{i,2}, \cdots, C_{i,K}]$. The linear interpolation relation between these points and the vertices of $\widetilde{\mathcal{M}}$ can be expressed as the following equation:

$$C = A\widetilde{\mathcal{V}} \tag{3}$$

where $C = [C_0, C_1, \cdots, C_N]^T$ and A is the matrix representing the linear interpolation operation. To quantitatively describe the *anterior/posterior* distribution of the cortical surface, we define $\mathcal{F}_1$ on the level contours as $\mathcal{F}_1(C_{i,k}) = -1 + 2 * i/N$. To extend $\mathcal{F}_1$ from the level contours to the vertices of the entire mesh, we solve the following regularized linear inverse problem:

$$||\mathcal{F}_1(C) - A\mathcal{F}_1(\widetilde{\mathcal{V}})||^2 + \beta \mathcal{F}_1(\widetilde{\mathcal{V}})^T Q \mathcal{F}_1(\widetilde{\mathcal{V}}) \tag{4}$$

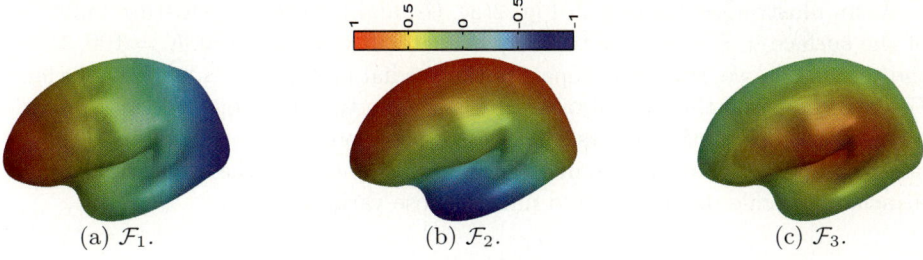

Fig. 2. Feature functions plotted on $\widetilde{\mathcal{M}}$

where $\mathcal{F}_1(C)$ and $\mathcal{F}_1(\widetilde{\mathcal{V}})$ are vectors of the values of $\mathcal{F}_1$ on the level contours and the vertices of the mesh $\widetilde{\mathcal{M}}$, respectively, and the matrix Q is the same as in (2). The regularization term $\mathcal{F}_1(\widetilde{\mathcal{V}})^T Q \mathcal{F}_1(\widetilde{\mathcal{V}})$ encourages smoothness of the feature function. By solving this least square problem, we obtain $\mathcal{F}_1(\widetilde{\mathcal{V}})$ as

$$\mathcal{F}_1(\widetilde{\mathcal{V}}) = (A^T A + \beta Q)^{-1} A^T \mathcal{F}_1(C). \tag{5}$$

To define the second feature function $\mathcal{F}_2$, we first compute a surface patch approximating the minimal surface of each level contour C_i as proposed in [14]. As shown in Fig. 1(c), this surface patch smoothly interpolates the interior of the contour. We use the eigenfunction of each surface patch to define $\mathcal{F}_2$ and characterize the *superior/inferior* profile of cortical surfaces. Let g_1^i denote the second eigenfunction of the Laplace-Beltrami operator of the i-th surface patch. We then compute the Reeb graph of g_1^i by sampling it at $N+1$ level contours $D_j (j = 0, \cdots, N)$ and assign a value $1 - \frac{2L_i(N-j)}{NL_{max}}$ to D_j to describe its superior-to-inferior position on the surface, where L_i is the length of C_i and L_{max} is the maximal length of all level contours. The value of $\mathcal{F}_2$ on the points $C_{i,k}$ is defined using linear interpolation from the values of neighboring level contours of g_1^i. Following the same approach of computing $\mathcal{F}_1$, we can extend the second feature function to the vertices of the entire mesh:

$$\mathcal{F}_2(\widetilde{\mathcal{V}}) = (A^T A + \beta Q)^{-1} A^T \mathcal{F}_2(C) \tag{6}$$

where $\mathcal{F}_2(C)$ and $\mathcal{F}_2(\widetilde{\mathcal{V}})$ are the vectors of values of $\mathcal{F}_2$ on the level contours and the vertices, respectively.

We use the same eigenfunction g_1^i of the surface patches to define the third feature function $\mathcal{F}_3$ to characterize the *medial/lateral* distribution of the cortical surface. Using the assumption that the cortical surface is in the neurological orientation, we denote the two end points of the level contour D_j as the medial and lateral point of D_j by comparing the magnitude of their x-coordinates, which are plotted as the blue and red dots in Fig. 1(d). For the medial point of D_j, we assign a value $\frac{(|2j-N|-N)L_i}{NL_{max}}$. For the lateral point of D_j, we assign a value $\frac{(N-|2j-N|)L_i}{NL_{max}}$. The same interpolation procedure of computing $\mathcal{F}_2$ is then applied to extend these values to the entire mesh and obtain the feature function $\mathcal{F}_3$.

As an illustration, we plot in Fig. 2(a), (b) and (c) the three feature functions of the surface in Fig. 1(b) with the parameter $\beta = 1, N = 100, K = 100$. Using the sign of $\mathcal{F}_3$, we can easily separate the medial and lateral side of the surface. For each point on the medial or lateral side, the two functions $(\mathcal{F}_1, \mathcal{F}_2)$ provide an intrinsic description of its relative location on the cortex. With the only assumption that the brain is in neurological orientation, these descriptions are invariant to scale differences and natural pose variations.

3 Sulci Detection in the Feature Space

In this section, we demonstrate the application of the LB feature space in cortical shape analysis by applying it to the automated detection of major sulci. To illustrate the advantage of the LB feature space in describing the location on cortical surfaces, we show in Fig. 3(a) two cortical surfaces in the Euclidean space and their central and pre-central sulcus in Fig. 3(b). After we compute the LB feature functions, we project the sulci of both surfaces into the common space $(\mathcal{F}_1, \mathcal{F}_2)$. From the result in Fig. 3(c), we can see the sulci are much better aligned in the feature space than in the original space. This shows the invariance of LB features and suggests their ability of building more compact sulcal models.

For automated sulci detection, we follow the learning-based approach in [8] by first generating a sample space of candidate curves in the feature space and then finding the most likely curve as the projection of the detected sulci in $\mathcal{F}$. Due to space limitation, we describe our method briefly in the following. To learn the prior model of a sulcus in the feature space, we assume a training set of cortical surfaces with manually labeled sulcal curves and compute the feature functions for each surface to project the sulcus into the feature space. Using these projected training curves, we estimate a density function $p(\overrightarrow{x}, \overrightarrow{v})$ with the Parzen window method, where $\overrightarrow{x}$ represents a point of a curve in the feature space and $\overrightarrow{v}$ is the tangent vector of the curve at the point $\overrightarrow{x}$. For a curve in the feature space, we can then compute its likelihood of being part of the major sulcus as the integral of the density function on this curve divided by its length. Besides this local model, we also apply the principal component analysis (PCA) [17] to the set of projected training curves to capture their global characteristics.

There are four main steps in our sulci detection algorithm. Using the central sulcus as an example, we illustrate the result generated from each step in Fig. 4. Given a cortical surface $\mathcal{M}$, we first construct the skeletal representation of the

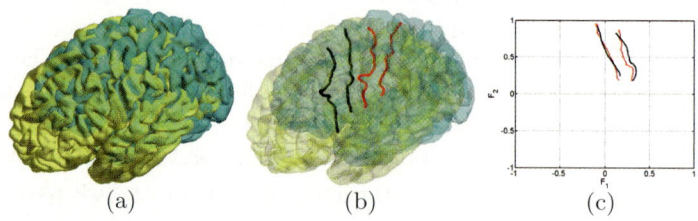

(a)   (b)   (c)

Fig. 3. Sulci in the Euclidean and LB feature space

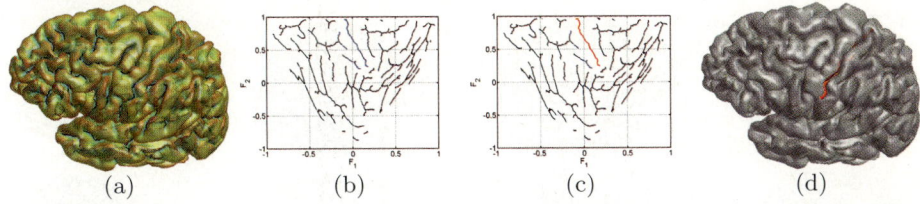

Fig. 4. (a) Hamilton-Jacobi skeletons of sulcal regions. (b) Skeletons in the LB feature space. (c) The most likely path (red) in the LB feature space. (d) The detected central sulcus on the original cortical surface.

folding pattern by computing the Hamilton-Jacobi skeleton of the sulcal regions [18] as shown in Fig. 4(a). After that, we compute the feature space $(\mathcal{F}_1, \mathcal{F}_2, \mathcal{F}_3)$. For major sulci on the lateral surface, we then project all skeletal branches with $\mathcal{F}_3 > 0$ onto the feature space $(\mathcal{F}_1, \mathcal{F}_2)$. Similarly, skeletal branches with $\mathcal{F}_3 < 0$ will be processed for major sulci on the medial surface. We divide each skeletal branch into curve segments of fixed length and compute their probability of being on the major sulcus of interest using the density function $p(\vec{x}, \vec{v})$. Curve segments with the probability greater than a threshold, which we set as 0.01 in all our experiments, are then chosen as candidate segments on the major sulcus, which we plot in blue in Fig. 4(b). In the third step, we follow the sample space generation algorithm in [8] to construct a graph model from these curve segments and generate a set of candidate curves via random walking on the graph model. For each candidate curve, we compute its likelihood of being the major sulcus as the product of the probability obtained from the density function and the PCA model to account for both local and global information. The most likely path, as shown in red in Fig. 4(c), is chosen as the projection of the detected sulcal curve in the feature space. Finally we connect the skeletal segments of the most likely path with curvature-weighted geodesics on the original surface $\mathcal{M}$ as the automatically generated major sulcus shown in Fig. 4(d).

4 Experimental Results

In this section, we present preliminary experimental results on the detection of two major sulci: the central and precentral sulcus using the LB feature space. The data set is composed of 25 right hemispherical cortical surfaces of spherical topology[19]. We manually labeled the two sulci on 10 of the 25 surfaces and use them as the training data. The projection of these training curves in the feature space is shown in the upper left of Fig. 5. From these training curves, we learn the density function and PCA model. Using these prior models, we tested our sulci detection algorithm on the other 15 cortical surfaces. The automatically detected sulcal curves on these surfaces are plotted in Fig. 5.

From the results we can see that our method is able to successfully detect the two major sulci on all testing surfaces. Even though the brains vary quite significantly in terms of shape and orientation, our method is robust to such pose

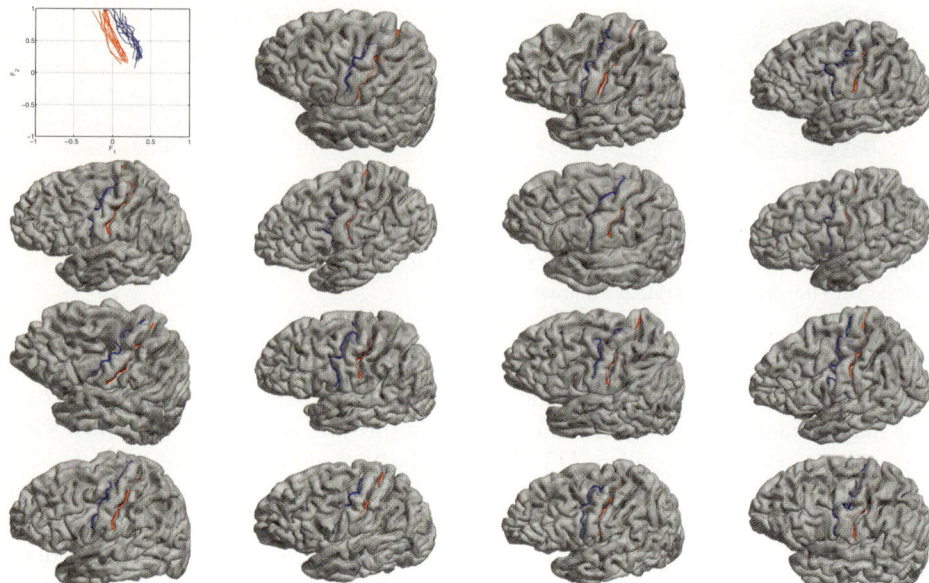

Fig. 5. Training data (upper left) and sulci detection results on the 15 testing surfaces (red: central sulcus; blue: pre-central sulcus)

and geometric variations because it is designed in the space of intrinsic eigenfeatures. In our future work, we will incorporate Markovian priors of neighboring sulci in the feature space for the detection of multiple sulci and validate on larger data sets of different populations.

5 Conclusion

In this paper, we proposed a novel approach of constructing feature spaces for cortical shape analysis using the eigenfunction of the Laplace-Beltrami operator. The LB feature space provides an intrinsic and anatomically meaningful way of characterize locations on the cortical surfaces. We demonstrated its application in automated sulci detection and preliminary experimental results have been presented.

References

1. Thompson, P.M., Hayashi, K.M., Sowell, E.R., Gogtay, N., Giedd, J.N., Rapoport, J.L., de Zubicaray, G.I., Janke, A.L., Rose, S.E., Semple, J., Doddrell, D.M., Wang, Y., van Erp, T.G.M., Cannon, T.D., Toga, A.W.: Mapping cortical change in alzheimer's disease, brain development, and schizophrenia. NeuroImage 23, S2–S18 (2004)
2. Mueller, S., Weiner, M., Thal, L., Petersen, R., Jack, C., Jagust, W., Trojanowski, J., Toga, A., Beckett, L.: The Alzheimer's disease neuroimaging initiative. Clin. North Am. 15, 869–877 (2005)

3. Van Essen, D.C.: A population-average, landmark- and surface-based (PALS) atlas of human cerebral cortex. NeuroImage 28(3), 635–662 (2005)
4. Lohmann, G., Cramon, D.: Automatic labelling of the human cortical surface using sulcal basins. Med. Image. Anal. 4, 179–188 (2000)
5. Tao, X., Prince, J., Davatzikos, C.: Using a statistical shape model to extract sulcal curves on the outer cortex of the human brain. IEEE Trans. Med. Imag. 21(5), 513–524 (2002)
6. Rivière, D., Mangin, J.F., Papadopoulos-Orfanos, D., Martinez, J., Frouin, V., Régis, J.: Automatic recognition of cortical sulci of the human brain using a congregation of neural networks. Med. Image. Anal. 6, 77–92 (2002)
7. Tu, Z., Zheng, S., Yuille, A., Reiss, A., Dutton, R.A., Lee, A., Galaburda, A., Dinov, I., Thompson, P., Toga, A.: Automated extraction of the cortical sulci based on a supervised learning approach. IEEE Trans. Med. Imag. 26, 541–552 (2007)
8. Shi, Y., Tu, Z., Reiss, A., Dutton, R., Lee, A.D., Galaburda, A., Dinov, I., Thompson, P.M., Toga, A.W.: Joint sulcal detection on cortical surfaces with graphical models and boosted priors. IEEE Trans. Med. Imag. 28(3), 361–373 (2009)
9. Qiu, A., Bitouk, D., Miller, M.I.: Smooth functional and structural maps on the neocortex via orthonormal bases of the Laplace-Beltrami operator. IEEE Trans. Med. Imag. 25(10), 1296–1306 (2006)
10. Reuter, M., Wolter, F., Peinecke, N.: Laplace-Beltrami spectra as Shape-DNA of surfaces and solids. Computer-Aided Design 38, 342–366 (2006)
11. Niethammer, M., Reuter, M., Wolter, F.E., Bouix, S., Koo, N.P.M.S., Shenton, M.: Global medical shape analysis using the laplace-beltrami spectrum. In: Ayache, N., Ourselin, S., Maeder, A. (eds.) MICCAI 2007, Part I. LNCS, vol. 4791, pp. 850–857. Springer, Heidelberg (2007)
12. Shi, Y., Lai, R., Krishna, S., Sicotte, N., Dinov, I., Toga, A.W.: Anisotropic Laplace-Beltrami eigenmaps: Bridging Reeb graphs and skeletons. In: Proc. MMBIA (2008)
13. Belkin, M., Niyogi, P.: Laplacian eigenmaps for dimensionality reduction and data representation. Neural Computation 15(6), 1373–1396 (2003)
14. Shi, Y., Lai, R., Kern, K., Sicotte, N.L., Dinov, I.D., Toga, A.W.: Harmonic surface mapping with laplace-beltrami eigenmaps. In: Metaxas, D., Axel, L., Fichtinger, G., Székely, G. (eds.) MICCAI 2008, Part II. LNCS, vol. 5242, pp. 147–154. Springer, Heidelberg (2008)
15. Reeb, G.: Sur les points singuliers d'une forme de Pfaff completement integrable ou d'une fonction nemérique. Comptes Rendus Acad. Sciences 222, 847–849 (1946)
16. Uhlenbeck, K.: Generic properties of eigenfunctions. Amer. J. of Math. 98(4), 1059–1078 (1976)
17. Cootes, T., Taylor, C., Cooper, D., Graham, J.: Active shape models-their training and application. Computer Vision and Image Understanding 61(1), 38–59 (1995)
18. Shi, Y., Thompson, P., Dinov, I., Toga, A.: Hamilton-Jacobi skeleton on cortical surfaces. IEEE Trans. Med. Imag. 27(5), 664–673 (2008)
19. Dale, A.M., Fischl, B., Sereno, M.I.: Cortical surface-based analysis i: segmentation and surface reconstruction. NeuroImage 9, 179–194 (1999)

Shape Analysis of Human Brain Interhemispheric Fissure Bending in MRI

Lu Zhao[1], Jarmo Hietala[2], and Jussi Tohka[1]

[1] Department of Signal Processing, Tampere University of Technology,
FIN-33101, Tampere, Finland
lu.zhao@tut.fi
[2] Department of Psychiatry, University of Turku, FIN-20014, Turku, Finland

Abstract. This paper introduces a novel approach to analyze Yakovlevian torque by quantifying the bending of human brain interhemispheric fissure in three-dimensional magnetic resonance imaging. It extracts the longitudinal medial surface between the cerebral hemispheres, which are segmented with an accurate and completely automatic technique, as the shape representation of the interhemispheric fissure. The extracted medial surface is modeled with a polynomial surface through least-square fitting. Finally, curvature features, e.g. principal, Gaussian and mean curvatures, are computed at each point of the fitted medial surface to describe the local bending of the interhemispheric fissure. This method was applied to clinical images of healthy controls (12 males, 7 females) and never-medicated schizophrenic subjects (11 males, 7 females). The hypothesis of the normal interhemispheric fissure bending (rightward in the occipital region) was quantitatively demonstrated. Moreover, we found significant differences ($p < 0.05$) between the male schizophrenics and healthy controls with respect to the interhemispheric fissure bending in the frontal and occipital regions. These results show that our method is applicable for studying abnormal Yakovlevian torque related to mental diseases.

1 Introduction

The left and right hemispheres of human brain are roughly equal in volume, weight and density, however, the tissue distribution differs notably between the two hemispheres. Among the most prominent observations of structural asymmetry of human brain are the right frontal and left occipital petalias [1]. Petalias are the greater protrusion of one hemisphere relative to the other at the frontal and occipital regions.

The right frontal and left occipital petalias were revealed from computed tomography (CT) and magnetic resonance imaging (MRI) scans with width measurements [2,3]. Bilder et al. [4] conducted the first volumetric study for petalias in MRI using manual outlining of lobar volumes. Recently, automatic image analysis methods have been applied to investigate the petalias of human brain in MRI with respect to local volumetric asymmetry. The voxel-wise interhemispheric differences in tissue volume [5] and tissue density [6] was studied using the reflection-based registration. In [7] and [8], the reflection method was extended to produce low dimensional maps showing interhemispheric differences in tissue volume in an array of column orthogonal to the mid-plane (two-dimensional) and profiles of coronal slice volumes (one-dimensional). Thirion et al. [9] quantified the regional volume differences between homologous structures in opposite brain hemispheres by nonrigidly co-registering the two hemispheres with each other.

Another prominent geometric distortion of the brain hemispheres, known as Yakovlevian torque, is that the right frontal lobe is torqued forward the left, and the left occipital lobe extends across the midline (over the right occipital lobe) and skews the interhemispheric fissure towards the right [1]. In this work, we developed an automatic shape analysis method to analyze the interhemispheric fissure bending of human brain in three-dimensional (3D) MRI using curvature features. This method can provide morphological interpretations of brain asymmetry that are easy to understand. To our knowledge, no previous studies of Yakovlevian torque by quantifying the interhemispheric fissure bending exist.

2 Methods

2.1 Image Preprocessing

The cerebral hemispheres (CH) are extracted and segmented in MR brain images in the acquisition space by using an automatic CH segmentation technique [10,11]. For inter-subject comparisons, the segmented CH volumes are normalized into the ICBM152 space (dimension: $91 \times 109 \times 91$ voxels, voxel size: $2 \times 2 \times 2$ mm^3) [12] with a 12-parameter affine transformation in SPM5 [13].

2.2 Representation of the Interhemispheric Fissure Shape

The interhemispheric fissure of human brain refers to the narrow groove separating the left and right CH. We use a medial interhemispheric surface to represent the shape of the interhemispheric fissure. Denote the lateral, longitudinal and vertical axes of the image space as X, Y and Z, respectively, the normalized segmented left and right CH as lCH and rCH, the Euclidean distances from a image voxel (x, y, z) to lCH and rCH as $D_l(x, y, z)$ and $D_r(x, y, z)$. We define the medial interhemispheric surface as a longitudinal surface S where each surface point is located with its projection (y, z) on the YZ plane. The lateral magnitude x_S of S at (y, z) is found as

$$x_S(y, z) = \arg\min_x \{|\ D_l(x, y, z) - D_r(x, y, z)\ |\}. \tag{1}$$

To build a mathematical model of S, a two-variable polynomial of degree k

$$\hat{x}_S(y, z) = \sum_{i=0}^{k} \sum_{j=0}^{i} a_{ij} y^{i-j} z^j \tag{2}$$

is used to fit it, where $\hat{x}_S$ is the approximation of the lateral magnitude x_S at (y, z). Because the curvature features will be computed based on the second fundamental form of the fitted surface, the polynomial must be two-times differentiable, i.e. $k \geq 2$. In addition, k should not be very large, since the fitted surface needs to be smooth enough to present the global bending tendency of the interhemispheric fissure. The coefficients a_{ij} are estimated with the least-square fitting approach. In the image space, let $\mathbf{x}_S$ be the column vector containing the x_S values of all surface points, B be the matrix whose each row consists of the values of item $y^{i-j}z^j$ in Eq.2 for all (y, z). The least-square solutions of a_{ij}, written in a column vector $\mathbf{a}$, are

$$\mathbf{a} = (B^T B)^{-1} B^T \mathbf{x}_S. \tag{3}$$

2.3 Curvature Feature Computation

We compute the 2×2 Hessian matrix

$$\mathcal{H} = \begin{pmatrix} \frac{\partial^2 \hat{x}_S}{\partial y^2} & \frac{\partial^2 \hat{x}_S}{\partial y \partial z} \\ \frac{\partial^2 \hat{x}_S}{\partial y \partial z} & \frac{\partial^2 \hat{x}_S}{\partial z^2} \end{pmatrix}, \tag{4}$$

based on the approximation (Eq.2) of S. Through $\mathcal{H}$, a number of curvature features can be computed at each point of S. The two eigenvalues of $\mathcal{H}$, κ_1 and κ_2, are the principal curvatures, which describe the maximum and minimum curvatures. The tangent directions of the principal curvatures, called principal directions, are given by the orthogonal eigenvectors of $\mathcal{H}$. The Gaussian curvature $K = \kappa_1 \kappa_2$ and mean curvature $H = (\kappa_1 + \kappa_2)/2$. The diagonal elements of $\mathcal{H}$, $C_{XY} = \frac{\partial^2 \hat{x}_S}{\partial y^2}$ and $C_{XZ} = \frac{\partial^2 \hat{x}_S}{\partial z^2}$, are the curvatures in XY and XZ planes, respectively. The above curvature features, except Gaussian curvature and principal directions, are taken to be positive if the relative curve turns in the same direction as the surface's chosen normal, and otherwise negative.

We also define the integrated average of the curvature features in regions of interest (ROIs). ROIs were extracted by masking S with the projection of the LONI Probabilistic Atlas (LPBA40) [14] on its mid-sagittal plane. The employed version of LPBA40 is LPBA40/SPM5, which was constructed by transforming the manual delineations into the ICBM152 template where the longitudinal median plane is the mid-sagittal plane. Because the image containing the normalized CH volumes is digital and has voxel size of $2 \times 2 \times 2~mm^3$, the projection of each ROI on the mid-sagittal plane consists of a number of square cells with size of $2 \times 2~mm^2$. Thus, the integrated average ξ_f of a curvature feature f in a ROI is

$$\xi_f = \frac{\sum_{c_i} \int_{y_i^0}^{y_i^0+2} \int_{z_i^0}^{z_i^0+2} f(y,z) \sqrt{(\frac{\partial \hat{x}_S}{\partial y})^2 + (\frac{\partial \hat{x}_S}{\partial z})^2 + 1}\, dydz}{\sum_{c_i} \int_{y_i^0}^{y_i^0+2} \int_{z_i^0}^{z_i^0+2} \sqrt{(\frac{\partial \hat{x}_S}{\partial y})^2 + (\frac{\partial \hat{x}_S}{\partial z})^2 + 1}\, dydz}, \tag{5}$$

where $c_i = [y_i^0, y_i^0 + 2) \times [z_i^0, z_i^0 + 2)$ is a single cell in the projection of the ROI on the mid-sagittal plane; y_i^0 and z_i^0 are the Y and Z coordinates of the origin of c_i; the numerator is the total value of f in the ROI; and the denominator is the total area of the ROI. In this work, the numerical integrations in Eq.5 were solved with the two-dimensional Simpson's rule [15].

2.4 Statistical Shape Analysis

We introduce two alternative ways to conduct the statistical shape analysis of the curvature features of the interhemispheric surface between two subject populations. The first is *point-to-point* analysis. The average of the normalized segmented CH volumes of all studied subjects is computed. The projection of this averaged volume on the ICBM152 template's mid-sagittal plane are used to locate the points of interest (POIs) on the fitted medial interhemispheric surface. Because the probability distribution types of the curvature features are unknown, the nonparametric Wilcoxon Rank Sum test is used to assess the differences in the curvature features between two populations at each POI. The second way is *ROI-to-ROI* analysis. The computation of the integrated average curvatures in ROIs includes a large amount of integration (see Eq.5). Therefore, due to the central limit theorem, we can assume that the integrated average curvatures are approximately Gaussian distributed. For each ROI, the integrated average curvatures are analyzed between groups with t-test. For both the *point-to-point* and *ROI-to-ROI* analyses, the significance level is set to 0.05.

3 Experiments and Results

3.1 Materials

The proposed method was applied to clinical T1-weighted MR images (voxel size: $1.5 \times 1.5 \times 1.0\ mm^3$; dimension: $256 \times 256 \times 150$ or $256 \times 256 \times 170$ voxels) of 18 schizophrenic subjects (11 males, 7 females) and 19 healthy controls (12 males, 7 females) [16]. All the subjects were right-handed. The schizophrenic patients were never-medicated, i.e. the brain asymmetry patterns in these subjects were not affected by antipsychotic drugs.

3.2 Quantification for Interhemispheric Fissure Bending

The degree of the polynomial used for surface fitting (Eq.2) was 4, because it is the lowest degree for the curvature features, computed based on the second fundamental form of the fitted surface, to remain nonlinear w.r.t to (y, z). Employing polynomial surfaces with a higher degree would produce more accurate surface fitting, but it would also produce non-essential shape information (noise) for analyzing the interhemispheric fissure bending. In MRI, the laterally-oriented interhemispheric fissure bending caused by Yakovlevian torque is mainly observed in the transverse view (XY planes), and the geometric interpretations of the Gaussian and principal curvatures are complicated. Therefore, we only considered the mean curvature H and the curvature in the XY plane C_{XY} in the presented experiments. Because the projections of chosen normals on X axis at each point of the fitted medial interhemispheric surface were always rightward, positive values of H and C_{XY} indicated laterally rightward bending, and negative values indicated leftward bending. Figs.1 and 2 illustrate medial interhemispheric surface extraction, fitting and the corresponding H and C_{XY} values at POIs.

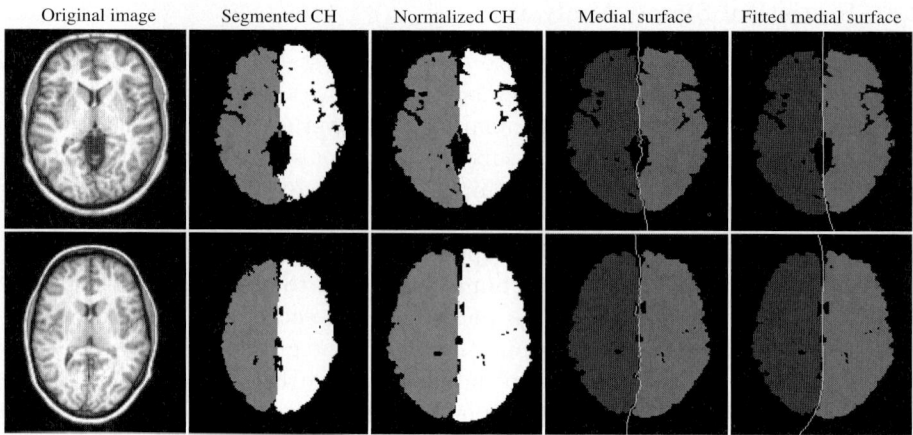

Fig. 1. Medial interhemispheric surface extraction and fitting. The first and second rows respectively show examples for subjects with normal (rightward) and abnormal (leftward) interhemispheric fissure bending. Original images were in neurological convention, namely the left (or right) hemisphere was in the left (or right). The extracted medial interhemispheric surfaces and fitted surfaces are visualized as longitudinal lines in the transverse view.

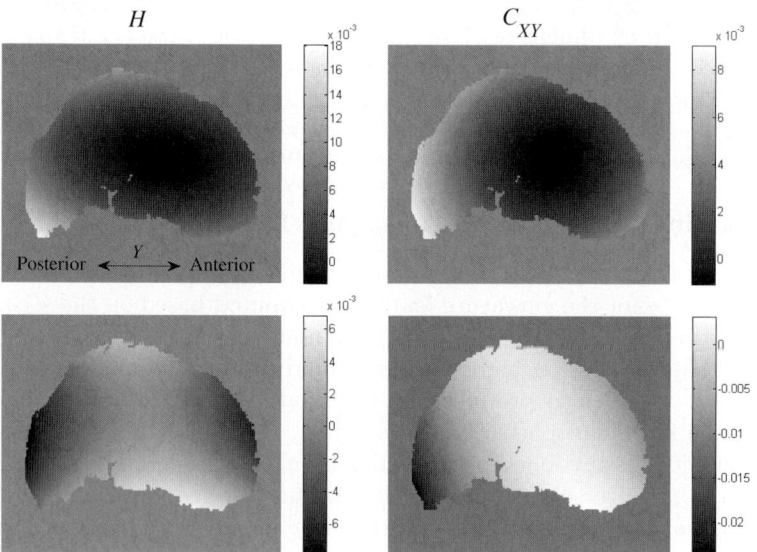

Fig. 2. Visualization in the sagittal view (YZ plane) for the values of H and C_{XY} at POIs. The first and second rows respectively correspond to the subjects shown in the first and second rows in Fig.1.

Table 1. Means of ξ_H and $\xi_{C_{XY}}$ in the frontal and occipital regions for male controls (MC), female controls (FC), male schizophrenics (MS), and female schizophrenics (FS)

	MC	FC	MS	FS
	Frontal region			
mean of ξ_H	7.8 e-4	-2.8 e-4	-8.2 e-4	7.5 e-5
mean of $\xi_{C_{XY}}$	7.5 e-4	-3.4 e-4	-5.3 e-4	3.9 e-4
	Occipital region			
mean of ξ_H	1.8 e-3	2.4 e-4	8.9 e-4	8.3 e-4
mean of $\xi_{C_{XY}}$	2.6 e-3	9.6 e-4	1.1 e-3	1.6 e-3

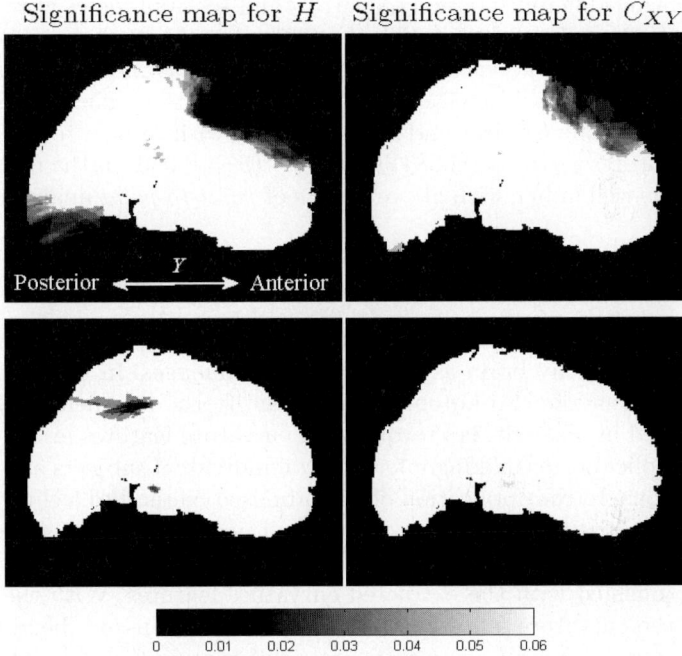

Fig. 3. Statistically significant results of *point-to-point* analysis (uncorrected $p < 0.05$) for comparison between controls and schizophrenics with respect to H and C_{XY}. The first and second rows respectively present the results for males and females.

We calculated the integrated average values of H and C_{XY}, denoted as ξ_H and $\xi_{C_{XY}}$, in ROIs corresponding to the frontal and occipital regions. For every subject, the accuracy of the proposed method to automatically detect the lateral direction of interhemispheric fissure bending with curvature features was evaluated by comparing the bending direction indicated by the sign of ξ_H or $\xi_{C_{XY}}$ in the occipital region against the bending direction manually identified in the transverse slices of the original image. For all the 37 studied subjects, the proposed method obtained correct detection for 34 subjects with ξ_H and for 36 subjects with $\xi_{C_{XY}}$. The means of ξ_H and $\xi_{C_{XY}}$ for different populations are tabulated in Table 1. In all populations, the means of ξ_H and $\xi_{C_{XY}}$ in the occipital region were positive, and their absolute values were always notably greater than their counterparts in the frontal region. This indicates that, in average, the interhemispheric fissure bending of right-handed subject mainly occurs in the occipital region and is laterally rightward. This re-confirms the hypothesis of interhemispheric fissure bending caused by normal Yakovlevian torque [1].

3.3 Statistical Shape Analysis between Controls and Schizophrenics

The results of statistical comparison between controls and schizophrenics with *point-to-point* analysis are shown in Fig.3. It can be seen that, for males, POIs of the significant difference between controls and schizophrenics were mainly located in the superior frontal region for H and C_{XY}, and in the inferior occipital region for II. Pointwise differences between female controls and schizophrenics were not as great as in males. From the *ROI-to-ROI* analysis, we found significant difference between male controls and schizophrenics with respect to the integrated average curvatures ξ_H ($p = 0.0084$) and $\xi_{C_{XY}}$ ($p = 0.036$) in the frontal region. This finding is well in line with above results of *point-to-point* analysis.

4 Conclusion

The traditional methods based on width and volume measurements have limited capabilities to quantify brain asymmetry in neuroimages. In this paper, we developed a novel method to automatically quantify the interhemispheric fissure bending caused by Yakovlevian torque with curvature features in 3D MRI. This method is applicable for making inferences on individual subjects as well as subject populations. In the application of the proposed method to a clinical data set containing MR images of healthy controls and never-medicated schizophrenics, the hypothesis of normal rightward interhemispheric fissure bending was quantitatively confirmed with the extracted curvature features. With the statistical analysis of the curvature features, the interhemispheric fissure bending of male schizophrenics was found to be significantly different from male controls' in the frontal and occipital regions.

Acknowledgements. This work was supported by the Academy of Finland, (application number 129657, Finnish Programme for Centres of Excellence in Research 2006- 2011), and the STATCORE cluster of the University Alliance Finland. Thanks to Dr. Saku Suuriniemi for help with numerical analysis.

References

1. Toga, W., Thompson, P.: Mapping brain asymmetry. Nature Reviews Neuroscience 4(1), 37–48 (2003)
2. LeMay, M., Kido, D.: Asymmetries of the cerebral hemispheres on computed tomograms. J. Comput. Assist. Tomogr. 2, 471–476 (1978)

3. Kertesz, A., Polk, M., Black, S., Howell, J.: Sex, handedness, and the morphometry of cerebral asymmetries on magnetic resonance imaging. Brain Res. 530, 40–48 (1990)
4. Bilder, R., Wu, H., Bogerts, B., Degreef, G., Ashtari, M., Alvir, J., Snyder, P., Lieberman, J.: Absence of regional hemispheric volume asymmetries in first-episode schizophrenia. Am. J. Psychiatry 151(10), 1437–1447 (1994)
5. Good, C., Johnsrude, I., Ashburner, J., Henson, R., Friston, K., Frackowiak, R.: Cerebral asymmetry and the effects of sex and handedness on brain structure: a voxel-based morphometric analysis of 465 normal adult human brains. NeuroImage 14, 685–700 (2001)
6. Watkins, K., Paus, T., Lerch, J., Zidjenbos, A., Collins, D., Neelin, P., Taylor, J., Worsley, K., Evans, A.: Structural asymmetries in the human brain: a voxel-based statistical analysis of 142 MRI scans. Cereb. Cortex 11, 868–877 (2001)
7. Mackay, C., Barrick, T., Roberts, N., DeLisi, L., Maes, F., Vandermeulen, D., Crow, T.: Application of a new image analysis technique to the study of brain asymmetry in schizophrenia. Psychiatry Res. NeuroImaging 124(1), 25–35 (2003)
8. Barrick, T., Mackay, C., Prima, S., Maes, F., Vandermeulen, D., Crow, T., Roberts, N.: Automatic analysis of cerebral asymmetry: an exploratory study of the relationship between brain torque and planum temporale asymmetry. NeuroImage 24(3), 678–691 (2005)
9. Thirion, J.P., Prima, S., Subsol, G., Roberts, N.: Automatic analysis of cerebral asymmetry. Med. Image Anal. 4, 111–121 (2001)
10. Zhao, L., Tohka, J., Ruotsalainen, U.: Accurate 3D left-right brain hemisphere segmentation in MR images based on shape bottlenecks and partial volume estimation. In: Ersbøll, B.K., Pedersen, K.S. (eds.) SCIA 2007. LNCS, vol. 4522, pp. 581–590. Springer, Heidelberg (2007)
11. Zhao, L., Tohka, J.: Automatic compartmental decomposition for 3D MR images of human brain. In: 30th Annual International Conference of the IEEE Engineering in Medicine and Biology Society, Vancouver, Canada, pp. 3888–3891 (2008)
12. Evans, A., Collins, D., Neelin, P., MacDonald, D., Kamber, M., Marrett, T.: Three-dimensional correlative imaging: applications in human brain mapping. In: Huerta, M. (ed.) Functional Neuroimaging: Technical Foundations, pp. 145–162. Academic Press, San Diego (1994)
13. Ashburner, J., Friston, K.: Nonlinear spatial normalization using basis functions. Human Brain Mapping 7(4), 254–266 (1999)
14. Shattuck, D., Mirza, M., Adisetiyo, V., Hojatkashani, C., Salamon, G., Narr, K., Poldrack, R., Bilder, R., Toga, A.: Construction of a 3D probabilistic atlas of human cortical structures. NeuroImage 39, 1064–1080 (2008)
15. Süli, E., Mayers, D.: An Introduction to Numerical Analysis. Cambridge University Press, Cambridge (2003)
16. Laakso, M., Tiihonen, J., Syvälahti, E., Vilkman, H., Laakso, A., Alakare, B., Räkköläinen, V., Salokangas, R., Koivisto, E., Hietala, J.: A morphometric MRI study of the hippocampus in first-episode, neuroleptic-naive schizophrenia. Schizophr Res. 50(1-2), 3–7 (2001)

Subject-Matched Templates for Spatial Normalization

Torsten Rohlfing[1], Edith V. Sullivan[2], and Adolf Pfefferbaum[1,2]

[1] Neuroscience Program, SRI International, Menlo Park, CA, USA
torsten@synapse.sri.com, dolf@synapse.sri.com
[2] Department of Psychiatry and Behavioral Sciences, Stanford University, Stanford CA, USA
edie@stanford.edu

Abstract. Spatial normalization of images from multiple subjects is a common problem in group comparison studies, such as voxel-based and deformation-based morphometric analyses. Use of a study-specific template for normalization may improve normalization accuracy over a study-independent standard template (Good et al., NeuroImage, 14(1):21-36, 2001). Here, we develop this approach further by introducing the concept of subject-matched templates. Rather than using a single template for the entire population, a different template is used for every subject, with the template matched to the subject in terms of age, sex, and potentially other parameters (e.g., disease). All subject-matched templates are created from a single generative regression model of atlas appearance, thus providing a priori template-to-template correspondence without registration. We demonstrate that such an approach is technically feasible and significantly improves spatial normalization accuracy over using a single template.

1 Introduction

A essential task in group comparison studies is the normalization of all individual anatomies in a subject population to a joint template, which provides the reference coordinate system for statistical analysis. Hundreds such studies haven been published in the fields of voxel-based morphometry [1] and deformation-based morphometry [2] alone, and others come from functional and diffusion tensor magnetic resonance (MR) imaging studies.

As noted by Good *et al.* [3], it is typically advantageous to use a template generated from the population specific to a study itself, rather than a generic template shared by many different studies. Despite many years of research, the image registration algorithms used for normalization are still imperfect. In particular, these algorithms tend to produce less accurate coordinate correspondences when the images to register are very different, be it in terms of morphology or image intensities. Thus, it is not surprising that a study comparing the brains of younger adults would achieve better normalization using a template representing a younger brain than one representing an older brain.

This example can be considered an application of a minimum deformation template (MDT) [4]. The fundamental principle of MDT is to construct a template that minimizes, on average, the deformation applied to all individual images when they are deformed to that template, thus increasing the average registration accuracy as deformation is minimized.

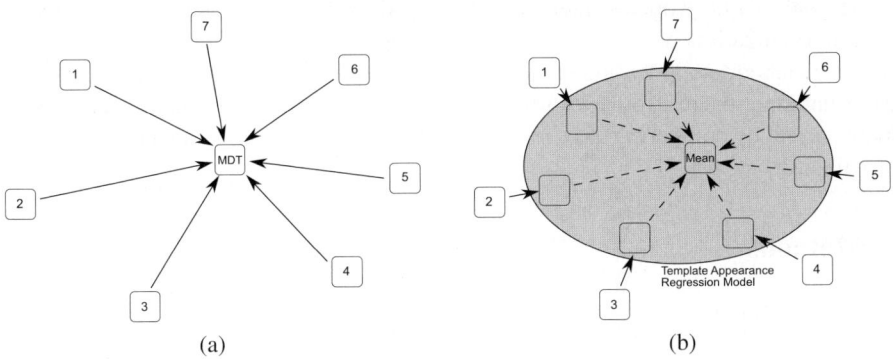

Fig. 1. Illustration of the difference between a minimum-deformation template and subject-matched templates from a single regression appearance model. *(a)* Each subject image (numbered 1 through 7) is registered to the Minimum Deformation Template. *(b)* Each subject image is registered to its own subject-matched template. All subject-matched templates relate to the model mean template via known transformations (dashed arrows), which do not need to be computed by registration.

One problem with study-specific templates is that their unique quality poses a serious challenge for comparison of results across studies. We have recently suggested, albeit not experimentally demonstrated, a technique [5], to address this problem by generating study-appropriate templates, rather than study-specific ones, from a single study-independent appearance model of brain anatomy, so that all different templates remain compatible via *a priori* dense correspondences between them. The appearance model itself is created by a regression-based modeling framework, which is similar to the shape-regression framework by Davis *et al.* [6].

Our contribution in this paper is to take the idea of study-specific or study-appropriate templates further by using subject-matched individual templates. In other words, we propose to use a different template for normalization of each subject's images, such that the subject demographic parameters (e.g., age, sex) match the corresponding template parameters. As all templates are generated from the same regression appearance model, they all relate to a common "mean model" via *a priori* coordinate transformations. The mean model provides a natural reference system for all studies that use instances of the same model as their templates.

The concept of using subject-matched instances of an appearance model as templates is similar to registration using an active appearance model [7], wherein registration is performed by varying model parameters until the generated model instance optimally matches the target image. Our approach is substantially different, however, in that it decouples the model parameter determination, which we achieve directly by using a regression-based rather than PCA-based model, from the residual nonrigid registration. The ultimate normalization transformation for each subject is thus a concatenation of a transformation from mean template to subject-matched template, which is defined by the appearance model, with a second transformation from subject-matched template to subject image, which is determined via registration. This is illustrated in Fig. 1.

The goal of our proposed method is to improve registration accuracy and achieve better normalization of all subjects by reducing the residual deformations between subject-matched templates and subject images. We demonstrate the effect in this paper by normalizing images from 64 normal subjects to subject-matched as well as per-study templates and by comparing the overlaps of tissue segmentations as a measure of spatial normalization accuracy.

2 Methods

2.1 Test Subjects

To test spatial normalization, MR images from 64 normal controls, 30 men and 34 women, age range 22.4 to 79.2 years (mean±std.dev. = 50.5±15.2 years) were acquired as part of an ongoing study in our laboratory. For each subject, a T_1-weighted three-dimensional image with 256×256×124 pixels (pixel size 0.9375×0.9375×1.25) was acquired on a 3T GE clinical scanner using a SPoiled Gradient Recalled echo (SPGR) sequence. All images were bias-field corrected [8] using in-house software, skull stripped using FSL BET [9], and segmented into three tissue classes (gray matter: GM, white matter: WM, cerebrospinal fluid: CSF) using FSL FAST [10].

2.2 Template Model Generation

The template model was created from MR images of 36 normal subjects (none of them part of the above test set) scanned at 3T. Skull-stripped SPGR images from all subjects were aligned using a simultaneous groupwise nonrigid registration algorithm [11]. A regression appearance model was then created that relates the two independent variables age and sex to anatomical shape and image intensities. Details of the regression appearance modeling procedure and the input data used here can be found in Rohlfing et al. [5].

In short, all input images were first aligned using template-free, unbiased groupwise nonrigid image registration. Template shape was then modeled analogous to the active deformation model [12], but using generalized multi-linear regression instead of principal components analysis. The resulting model relates each subject's image space to a common template space, where the latter depends on the independent variables of the model. To create actual atlas images in template space, image intensity at each pixel was also modeled via the same regression model, rather than simple averaging [13]. The result of the modeling procedure is an appearance model than can be instantiated for arbitrary values of the independent variables. For the model used here, each such instance represents a brain of given age and sex, but all instances are related to each other via known coordinate transformations defined by the regression model.

2.3 Experimental Procedure

The SPGR image of each of the 64 test subjects was registered independently to: a) each of seven mixed-sex template, instantiated for ages 20, 30, 40, 50, 60, 70, and 80 years, b) a template that matched subject age and sex, c) a mixed-sex template that matched subject

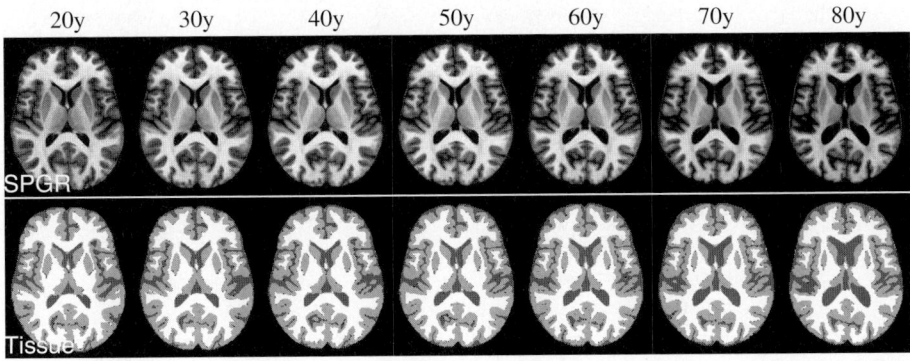

Fig. 2. Templates created from the continuous atlas regression model for ages 20 through 80 years in 10 year increments. *Top row:* SPGR channel; *bottom row:* three-class tissue segmentation.

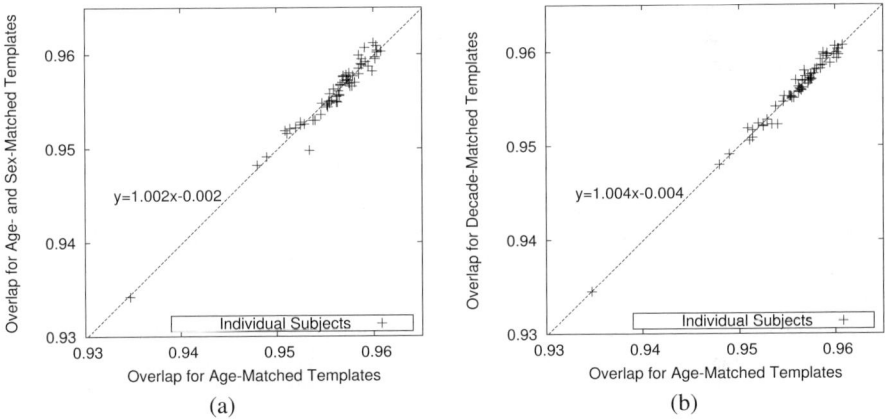

Fig. 3. Scatter plots and linear regression fits of tissue overlaps for (a) age-matched vs. age- and sex-matched templates, and (b) age-matched vs. decade-matched templates.

age, and d) a mixed-sex template that matched the age of the subject by closest decade[1]. All registrations were computed via a variant of the algorithm by Rueckert *et al.* [14] with a multi-resolution deformation strategy and 2.5 mm final control point spacing.

For each template that was needed for registration, SPGR and tissue segmentation images were created at 1 mm isotropic resolution (shown in Fig. 2 for the decade atlases). The SPGR channel was used for registration to the subject SPGR images, the tissue segmentation channel was used for computing the overlaps (in terms of fraction of matching pixels) between the template tissue image and the subject tissue.images,

---

[1] Registration to the template with the closest age by decade was already covered by the registrations mentioned in a), but for the decade-matched template evaluation we grouped the results differently.

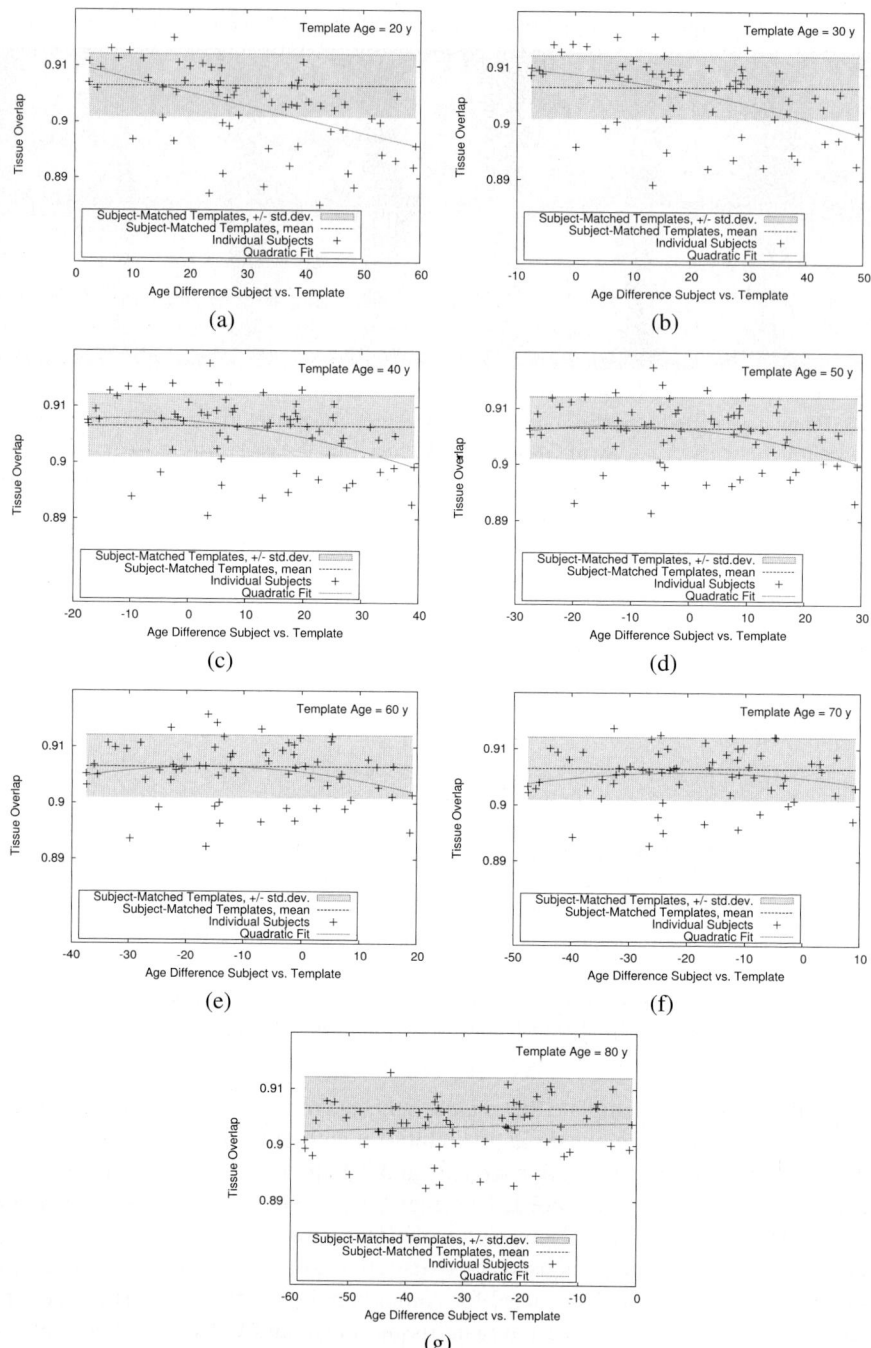

Fig. 4. Tissue overlaps plotted vs. subject-template age difference. (a)–(g), results for mixed-sex templates instantiated for ages 20, 30, 40, 50 60, 70, and 80 years. See text for details.

after reformatting the latter into template space. To make the results comparable across templates, tissue images of all subjects were actually reformatted, via concatenation of transformations, into the space of the model mean template (mixed-sex, age=52.2 years) and overlaps computed in that space.

3 Results

The different subject matching techniques (age matched, age and sex matched, decade matched) are compared via scatter plots in Fig. 3. These results suggest that all three matching strategies work comparably well. Because including sex and matching the exact subject age each increase the number of templates that need to be generated from the atlas appearance model, we limit further consideration to the decade-matched templates as the more computationally efficient option.

The influence of age difference between subject and template on tissue overlap is illustrated in Fig. 4. In each plot, the mean of overlaps for the decade-matched templates is shown for comparison as a dashed horizontal line, and the range of ±1 standard deviation as a gray box. Each plot also shows a second-order polynomial regression line fitted to the individual overlaps via nonlinear least squares. These plots, in particular the incremental tilt of the regression lines, suggest that indeed normalization accuracy decreases with increasing age difference, although it appears that younger subjects are more easily registered to an older template than the other way around.

As Fig. 5 shows, the average performance of middle-aged templates comes close to the performance of the decade-matched templates. Going back to Fig. 4, however, it is clear that the situation would be more favorable for the decade-matched templates if we excluded the middle-aged subjects from the test set and compared only the very young and the very old.

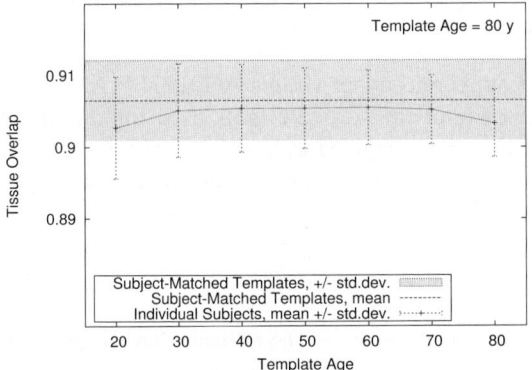

Template	Overlap mean±std.dev.	t-test vs. Decade
Decade	0.9065±0.0056	—/—
20 y	0.9027±0.0071	1.8×10^{-9}
30 y	0.9051±0.0065	3.8×10^{-4}
40 y	0.9054±0.0061	1.3×10^{-4}
50 y	0.9054±0.0056	5.3×10^{-6}
60 y	0.9055±0.0052	6.6×10^{-5}
70 y	0.9052±0.0048	5.0×10^{-5}
80 y	0.9033±0.0047	3.6×10^{-10}

Fig. 5. Comparison of tissue overlaps over all subjects vs. template age. *Left:* mean±standard deviation of overlap vs. template age. For comparison, the dashed line and gray box show mean ± standard deviation for decade-matched templates. *Right:* Actual numerical values represented by the plot on the left, including results of two-sided, paired t-tests of overlap values by subject for each of the single atlases vs. decade-matched subject-specific atlases.

4 Discussion

This paper has introduced the concept of using individually age-matched templates for spatial normalization of neuroimage data. Because all matched templates were generated from a single, regression-based appearance model, they were all related to each other through known spatial correspondences without the need for template-to-template registration.

Using test data from 64 subjects and a model from a separate set of 36 subjects we have demonstrated that matched templates can slightly, but significantly, increase the accuracy of spatial normalization. By excluding middle-aged subjects from the test set, we could have made the results appear even more favorable, but chose not to do so because it is important to investigate the performance of our method even in less-than-ideal circumstances.

Likewise, using a weaker nonrigid (or even an affine) registration algorithm for testing would have amplified the superiority of our method, because clearly a perfect registration algorithm would deliver perfect label overlaps regardless of the template used. Instead, we still observed an improvement in label overlap using a registration algorithm [14] that has been found to be at least on par with all other currently available algorithms ("IRTK", see [15]).

Using matched templates for normalization incurs only moderate additional computational complexity once the appearance model for template generation has been created. It is particularly encouraging to note that we achieved essentially the same results using templates matched to subjects only by age rounded to the nearest decade, which greatly reduces the number of templates needed to cover a subject population.

Fundamental problems with our approach could arise in situations where, for example, the actual ages of subjects do not match their "brain ages," e.g., due to neurodegenerative disorders. The obvious solution to this problem would be to create subject-matched templates using a more appropriate regression model. Using a model that includes disease factors as additional independent variables would then allow subjects to be matched to templates in terms of these variables as well, in addition to age and sex.

Acknowledgments. This work was supported under Grants AG019717, AA017923, AA005965, and AA017347. Source code of the software tools used for registration and modeling is available in the Computational Morphometry Toolkit (CMTK), http://nitrc.org/projects/cmtk/, supported by the NIBIB under Grant EB008381.

References

1. Ashburner, J., Friston, K.J.: Voxel-based morphometry — the methods. NeuroImage 11(6), 805–821 (2000)
2. Ashburner, J., Hutton, C., Frackowiak, R., Johnsrude, I., Price, C., Friston, K.: Identifying global anatomical differences: Deformation-based morphometry. Hum. Brain Map. 6(5-6), 348–357 (1998)
3. Good, C.D., Johnsrude, I.S., Ashburner, J., Henson, R.N.A., Friston, K.J., Frackowiak, R.S.J.: A voxel-based morphometric study of ageing in 465 normal adult human brains. NeuroImage 14(1), 21–36 (2001)

4. Kochunov, P., Lancaster, J.L., Thompson, P., Woods, R., Mazziotta, J., Hardies, J., Fox, P.: Regional spatial normalization: toward an optimal target. J. Comput. Assist. Tomogr. 25(5), 805–816 (2001)
5. Rohlfing, T., Sullivan, E.V., Pfefferbaum, A.: Regression models of atlas appearance. In: Prince, J.L., Pham, D.L., Myers, K.J. (eds.) IPMI 2009. LNCS, vol. 5636, pp. 151–162. Springer, Heidelberg (2009)
6. Davis, B.C., Fletcher, P.T., Bullitt, E., Joshi, S.: Population shape regression from random design data. In: IEEE 11th International Conference on Computer Vision, ICCV, October 2007, pp. 1–7 (2007)
7. Cootes, T.F., Beeston, C.J., Edwards, G.J., Taylor, C.J.: A unified framework for atlas matching using active appearance models. In: Kuba, A., Sámal, M., Todd-Pokropek, A. (eds.) IPMI 1999. LNCS, vol. 1613, pp. 322–333 Springer, Heidelberg (1999)
8. Likar, B., Viergever, M.A., Pernus, F.: Retrospective correction of MR intensity inhomogeneity by information minimization. IEEE Trans. Med. Imag. 20(12), 1398–1410 (2001)
9. Battaglini, M., Smith, S.M., Brogi, S., De Stefano, N.: Enhanced brain extraction improves the accuracy of brain atrophy estimation. NeuroImage 40(2), 583–589 (2008)
10. Zhang, Y., Brady, M., Smith, S.: Segmentation of brain MR images through a hidden Markov random field model and the expectation-maximization algorithm. IEEE Trans. Med. Imag. 20(1), 45–57 (2001)
11. Balci, S.K., Golland, P., Shenton, M., Wells, W.M.: Free-form B-spline deformation model for groupwise registration. In: MICCAI 2007 Workshop Statistical Registration: Pair-wise and Group-wise Alignment and Atlas Formation, pp. 23–30 (2007)
12. Rueckert, D., Frangi, A.F., Schnabel, J.A.: Automatic construction of 3-D statistical deformation models of the brain using nonrigid registration. IEEE Trans. Med. Imag. 22(8), 1014–1025 (2003)
13. Guimond, A., Meunier, J., Thirion, J.P.: Average brain models: A convergence study. Comput. Vision Image Understanding 77(2), 192–210 (2000)
14. Rueckert, D., Sonoda, L.I., Hayes, C., Hill, D.L.G., Leach, M.O., Hawkes, D.J.: Nonrigid registration using free-form deformations: Application to breast MR images. IEEE Trans. Med. Imag. 18(8), 712–721 (1999)
15. Klein, A., Andersson, J., Ardekani, B.A., Ashburner, J., Avants, B., Chiang, M.C., Christensen, G.E., Collins, L.D., Gee, J., Hellier, P., Song, J.H., Jenkinson, M., Lepage, C., Rueckert, D., Thompson, P., Vercauteren, T., Woods, R.P., Mann, J.J., Parsey, R.V.: Evaluation of 14 nonlinear deformation algorithms applied to human brain MRI registration. NeuroImage 46(3), 786–802 (2009)

Mapping Growth Patterns and Genetic Influences on Early Brain Development in Twins

Yasheng Chen[1], Hongtu Zhu[2], Dinggang Shen[1], Hongyu An[1], John Gilmore[3], and Weili Lin[1]

[1] Dept. of Radiology, [2] Biostatistics and [3] Psychiatry
Univ. of North Carolina at Chapel Hill, Chapel Hill, NC 27599, USA
yasheng_chen@med.unc.edu, hzhu@bios.unc.edu,
dgshen@med.unc.edu, hongyuan@med.unc.edu,
john_gilmore@med.unc.edu, weili_lin@med.unc.edu

Abstract. Despite substantial progress in understanding the anatomical and functional development of the human brain, little is known on the spatial-temporal patterns and genetic influences on white matter maturation in twins. Neuroimaging data acquired from longitudinal twin studies provide a unique platform for scientists to investigate such issues. However, the interpretation of neuroimaging data from longitudinal twin studies is hindered by the lacking of appropriate image processing and statistical tools. In this study, we developed a statistical framework for analyzing longitudinal twin neuroimaging data, which is consisted of generalized estimating equation (GEE2) and a test procedure. The GEE2 method can jointly model imaging measures with genetic effect, environmental effect, and behavioral and clinical variables. The score test statistic is used to test linear hypothesis such as the association between brain structure and function with the covariates of interest. A resampling method is used to control the family-wise error rate to adjust for multiple comparisons. With diffusion tensor imaging (DTI), we demonstrate the application of our statistical methods in quantifying the spatiotemporal white matter maturation patterns and in detecting the genetic effects in a longitudinal neonatal twin study. The proposed approach can be easily applied to longitudinal twin data with multiple outcomes and accommodate incomplete and unbalanced data, i.e., subjects with different number of measurements.

1 Introduction

Longitudinal neuroimaging studies have grown rapidly for better understanding the progress of neuropsychiatric and neurodegenerative disorders or the normal brain development, and typical large-scale longitudinal studies include ADNI (Alzheimer's Disease Neuroimaging Initiative) and the NIH MRI study of normal brain as in [1]. Compared with cross-sectional neuroimaging studies, longitudinal neuroimaging follow-up may allow characterization of correlation between individual change in neuroimaging measurements (e.g., volumetric and morphometric) and the covariates of interest (such as age, diagnostic status, gene, and gender). Longitudinal design may also allow one to examine a causal role of time-dependent covariate (e.g., exposure) in disease process. A distinctive feature of longitudinal neuroimaging data is the temporal order of the imaging measures (see more discussions in [2, 3]). Particularly, imaging measurements of the same individual usually exhibit positive correlation and the strength of the correlation may decrease with prolonged time separation.

Twin neuroimaging studies are invaluable for disentangling the effects of genes and environments on brain functions and structures. The twin design typically compares the similarity of monozygotic twins (MZ, who are developed from a single fertilized egg and therefore share 100% of their genes) to that of dizygotic twins (DZ, who are developed from two fertilized eggs and therefore share on average 50% of their alleles). These known differences in genetic similarity, together with the assumption of equal environments for MZ and DZ twins allows us to explore the effects of genetic and environmental variance on a phenotype, such as brain structure. The current neuroimaging twin studies have focused upon locating the brain regions subject to either environmental factors or genetic factors. For instance, high heritability was found in intracranial volume, global gray and white matter volume [4], cerebral hemisphere volume [5]. Cortical thickness in sensorimotor cortex, middle frontal cortex and anterior temporal cortex were found to be under the influence of genetic factors [6]. High heritabilities were also located in paralimbic structures and temporal/parietal neocortical regions [7].

The longitudinal twin neuroimaging studies, which combine both the longitudinal design and the twin design, provide a unique platform for examining the effects of gene and environment on the development of brain functions and structures. To properly analyze the longitudinal twin imaging measures, any image processing and statistical tools must account for three key features: the temporal correlation among the repeated measures, the different genetic and environmental effects among MZ and DZ twins, and the spatial correlation between each twin pair. Failure to account for these three features can result in misleading scientific inferences [2]. However, advanced image processing and statistical tools designated to complex and correlated image data along with behavioral and clinical information remains lacking. The cross-sectional image processing and statistical tools may be useful for longitudinal twin imaging data, but they are not statistically optimal in power. To the best of our knowledge, most existing neuroimaging software platforms including SPM, AFNI, and FSL do not have any valid methods to process and analyze neuroimaging data from longitudinal twin studies.

We propose two statistical methods for the analysis of neuroimaging data from longitudinal twin studies. We develop second-order generalized estimating equations (GEE2) for jointly modeling univariate (or multivariate) imaging measures with covariates of interest in longitudinal twin studies (including genetic and environmental factors, behavioral and clinical variables). Compared with the structural equation modeling (SEM) for twin neuroimaging data, GEE2 avoids the assumption that latent genetic and environmental variables follow a Gaussian distribution. We develop a score test statistic to test linear hypotheses such as the associations between brain structure and function and covariates of interest. In order to adjust for multiple comparisons, a resampling method is used to control the family-wise error rate. We demonstrate the utility of the proposed approach in analyzing diffusion tensor imaging (DTI) data to quantify spatiotemporal patterns and detect genetic influences on early postnatal white matter development.

2 Methods

2.1 Image Acquisition and Preprocessing

Our study is approved by the institutional review board. A total of 30 pairs of same sex twins were recruited with the consents of parents. These subjects were followed longitudinally at the time close to birth, at 1 year and 2 years after birth. With missing data, a total of 142 datasets were obtained. All subjects were fed and calmed to sleep on a warm blanket inside the scanner wearing proper ear protection. All images were acquired using a 3T Allegra head only MR system with 6 encoding gradient directions with an istropic voxel size of 2 mm^3. Two DTI parametric maps including fractional anisotropy (FA) and mean diffusivity (MD) were computed with the diffusion tensor tool box in FSL (http://www.fmrib.ox.ac.uk/fsl/). In order to construct voxel based atlas, the FA images from all subjects were co-registered towards a template of a two-year old FA image (not a subject in this study) with a widely used elastic registration method HAMMER [8], which relies on neighborhood intensity distribution and edge information for image alignment instead of image intensity alone.

2.2 Generalized Estimating Equations

We observe imaging, behavioral and clinical data from n twins at m_i time points t_{ij} for $i=1,...,n, j=1,...,m_i$ in a longitudinal study. Let $x_{ij} = (x_{ij,1},...x_{ij,q})^T$ be a $q \times 1$ covariate vector, which may contain age, gender, height, gene, and others. Note that the number of time points for the i-th twin m_i may differ across twins. There are a total $\sum_{i=1}^{n} m_i = N$ sets of images in this study. Based on observed image data, we compute neuroimaging measures, denoted by $Y_i = \{y_{ij}(d) : d \in D, j=1,...,m_i\}$ across all m_i time points from the i-th twin, where d represents a voxel (or a region of interest) on D, a specific brain area. For simplicity, we assume that imaging measure $y_{ij}(d) = (y_{ij,1}(d), y_{ij,2}(d))^T$ at voxel d is a 2×1 vector consisting of the same measure from two subjects within each twin.

We apply the second-order GEE method for jointly modeling univariate (or multivariate) imaging measures with covariates of interest in longitudinal twin studies (such as behavioral, clinical variables or genetic and environmental effects). The GEE2 explicitly introduces two sets of estimating equations for regression estimates on original data and covariance parameters, respectively. For notational simplicity, d is dropped from our notation temporarily.

To study the growth trajectories for imaging measures in healthy neonatal/pediatric subjects, we assume that the model for $y_{ij,k}$ at the j-th time point for the i-th twin is

$$E(y_{ij}) = u_{ij} = x_{ij,1}\beta_{1,k} + ... + x_{ij,q}\beta_{q,k} = x_{ij}^T \beta_{\Box k} \qquad (1)$$

for $i=1,...,n, j=1,...,m_i$ where $x_{ij,1}$ is usually set to 1, $x_{ij,k}$ ($k \geq 2$) can be chosen as time, gender, gene, and others, and β is a $q \times 1$ vector.

For all measurements from the i-th twin, we can form a $2m_i \times 1$ vector $Y_i = (y_{i1,1}, y_{i1,2}, ..., y_{im_i,1}, y_{im_i,2})^T$ and $U_i(\beta) = (u_{i1,1}, u_{i1,2}, ..., u_{im_i,1}, u_{im_i,2})^T$. To solve the regression coefficients in $\beta = (\beta_{\Box 1}, \beta_{\Box 2})^T$, we construct a set of estimating equations given by

$$\sum_{i=1}^{n} D_i' V_i^{-1}(Y_i - u_i(\beta)) = 0 \qquad (2)$$

where $D_i = \partial u_i(\beta)/\partial \beta$ and V_i is a working covariance matrix such as autoregressive structure. To study the genetic and environmental effects on imaging measures, we assume that

$$y_{ij} - u_{ij} = a_{0:i} + d_{0:i} + c_{0:i} + t_{ij} a_{s:i} + t_{ij} d_{s:i} + t_{ij} c_{s:i} + \varepsilon_{ij} \qquad (3)$$

where $\varepsilon_{ij,k}$ is random error, $a_{0:i,k}$, $d_{0:i,k}$ and $c_{0:i,k}$ are, respectively, the additive genetic, dominance genetic, and environmental residual random effects (so called ADE model in twin study) associated with intercept. $a_{s:i,k}$, $d_{s:i,k}$ and $c_{s:i,k}$ are the additive genetic, dominance genetic, and environmental residual random effects associated with time, respectively. We assume that $\varepsilon_{ij,k}$, $a_{0:i,k}$, $d_{0:i,k}$, $c_{0:i,k}$, $a_{s:i,k}$, $d_{s:i,k}$ and $c_{s:i,k}$ are independently distributed with zero mean and variances σ_e^2, $\sigma_{0,a}^2, \sigma_{0,d}^2, \sigma_{0,c}^2, \sigma_{s,a}^2, \sigma_{s,d}^2$, and $\sigma_{s,c}^2$, respectively. According to ADE models, we assume that $\text{cov}(a_{0:i,1}, a_{0:i,2}) = \sigma_{0,a}^2/2$, $\text{cov}(d_{0:i,1}, d_{0:i,2}) = \sigma_{0,a}^2/4$, $\text{cov}(a_{s:i,1}, a_{s:i,2}) = \sigma_{s,a}^2/2$ and $\text{cov}(d_{s:i,1}, d_{s:i,2}) = \sigma_{s,a}^2/4$ for DZ, and $\text{cov}(a_{0:i,1}, a_{0:i,2}) = \sigma_{0,a}^2$, $\text{cov}(d_{0:i,1}, d_{0:i,2}) = \sigma_{0,a}^2$, $\text{cov}(a_{s:i,1}, a_{s:i,2}) = \sigma_{s,a}^2$ and $\text{cov}(d_{s:i,1}, d_{s:i,2}) = \sigma_{s,a}^2$ for MZ. For model identifiability, we may drop either dominance genetic effect or environmental effect from the model.

Based on these assumptions, we calculate the covariance between $\tilde{y}_{ij,k} = y_{ij,k} - u_{ij,k}$ and $\tilde{y}_{ij',k'} = y_{ij',k'} - u_{ij',k'}$ for any j, j' and k, k'. Specifically, $E(\tilde{y}_{ij,k}\tilde{y}_{ij',k'})$ can be expressed as

$$\sigma_{i,(j,j'),(k,k')} = z_{i,1}\sigma_{0,a}^2 + z_{i,2}\sigma_{0,d}^2 + \sigma_{0,c}^2 + t_{ij}t_{ij'}(z_{i,1}\sigma_{s,a}^2 + z_{i,2}\sigma_{s,d}^2 + \sigma_{s,c}^2) \qquad (4)$$

in which $(z_{i,1}, z_{i,2})$ takes $(1,1)$ for either $k = k'$ or MZ and $(0.5, 0.25)$ for DZ. For all products between $\tilde{y}_{ij,k}$ and $\tilde{y}_{ij,k}$, we can form a $m_i(2m_i+1) \times 1$ vector $S_i = (\tilde{y}_{i1,1}^2, \tilde{y}_{i1,1}\tilde{y}_{i1,1}, ..., \tilde{y}_{im_i,2}^2)^T$ and $S_i(\sigma) = (\sigma_{i,(1,1),(1,1)}, ..., \sigma_{i,(m_i,m_i),(2,2)})^T$.

To solve the regression coefficients in σ, we construct a set of estimating equations given by

$$\sum_{i=1}^{n} \tilde{D}_i' V_{S,i}^{-1}(S_i - S_i(\sigma)) = 0, \qquad (5)$$

Where, $\tilde{D}_i = \partial S_i(\sigma)/\partial \sigma$ and $V_{S,i}$ is a working covariance matrix.

Applying GEE2 methods has many attractive advantages. *First*, this model proposed above is very flexible and free of distribution assumption. *Second*, the GEE2 estimator is consistent even we mis-specify the covariance structure V_i and $V_{S,i}$. *Third*, our inferences using the empirical standard errors are robust even if our knowledge of the covariance structure is imperfect. *Fourth*, our GEE2 method avoids modeling the high order moments of imaging measures. *Finally*, it is computationally straightforward to compute GEE2 estimators $\hat{\beta}$ and $\hat{\sigma}$ by iterating between Eq. (2) and Eq. (5).

2.3 Hypothesis and Test Statistics

In longitudinal twin studies, one is interested in answering various scientific questions involving the asessment of brain development across time and the testing of genetic influences on brain structure and function. These questions concerning brain development can often be reformulated as either testing linear hypothesis of β as follows:

$$H_0 : R\beta = b_0 \text{ vs. } H_1 : R\beta \neq b_0 \tag{6}$$

where R is an $r \times 2q$ matrix of full row rank and b_0 is an $r \times 1$ specified vector. The question concerning genetic effect on brain are usually formulated as testing

$$H_{0,S} : R_s\sigma = 0 \text{ vs. } H_{1,S} : R_s\sigma > 0 \tag{7}$$

where R_s is an $kx7$ of full row rank. For instance, if we are interested in testing the genetic effect $a_{0:i,k}$, then we choose $R_s\sigma = a_{0,a}^2$. To test these hypotheses in Eq. (6) and [7], we use the score test statistics with appropriate asymptotic null distributions [9]. A wild boostrap method was used to control for multiple comparisons. The proposed test procedure is computationally much more efficient than the permutation method.

3 Results

3.1 Growth Patterns

In the longitudinal analysis of the DTI images using GEE2 (Eq. (2) for growth pattern quantification), covariates of interest including intercept, age, age*age, zygote (0 for MZ and 1 for DZ) and zygote * times were tested for significance (Eq. (8)).

$$E(y_{ij}) = u_{ij} = \beta_1 + \beta_2 * age + \beta_3 * age^2 + \beta_4 * zygote + \beta_5 * zygote * age \tag{8}$$

Significant contributions were only found for β_1, β_2 and β_3. Thus, nonlinear changing patterns were observed in early postnatal stages for FA and MD. But no zygote related significance was detected. Squared ROIs with a fixed size (2x2 pixels) were drawn in axial view at posterior limb of internal capsules, external capsules bilaterally and at the centers of genu and splenium. The growth patterns of FA and MD from these regions are given in Fig. 1 for both MZ and DZ twins. There is a slight difference existed between the growth curves between MZ and DZ twins. Among these brain regions, external capsule and internal capsule respectively have the lowest FA and MD values in this period of time (Fig. 1).

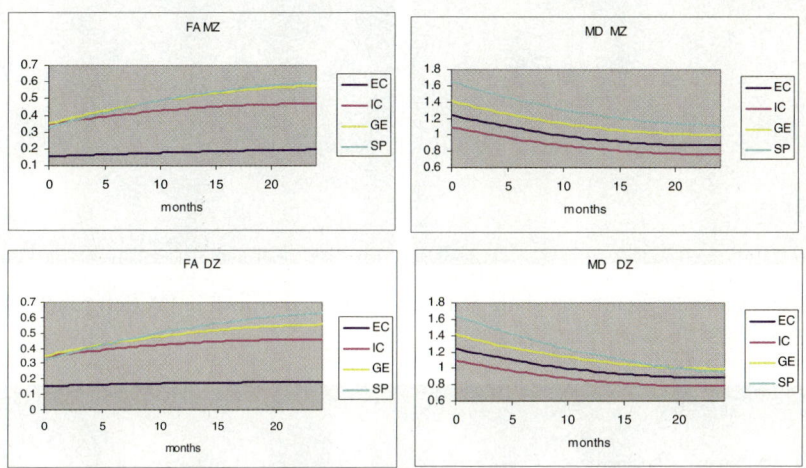

Fig. 1. Temporal growth patterns for FA (nonlinear increase, left panel) and MD (nonlinear decrease, right panel) in both MZ (top panel) and DZ (bottom panel) twins in external capsule (EC), posterior limb of internal capsule (IC), genu (GE) and splenium (SP)

3.2 Genetic Influence

For model identifiability, we use AE model to estimate genetic influences on brain development. Since each twin pair share similar nurturing environment, the squared difference (sqd=$[(y_{ij',1} - u_{ij',1}) - (y_{ij',2} - u_{ij',2})]^2$) between the DTI images from the same twin pair should exclude the environmental effect from analysis. In such a situation, Eq. (4) can be shortened as in Eq. (9). In our current implementation, statistical testing was performed with Eq. (10).

$$E(sqd) = \beta_1 \sigma_{0,a}^2 + \beta_2 \sigma_{1,a}^2 * age^2 \qquad (9)$$

$$E([y_{ij,1} - y_{ij,2}]^2) = \beta_1 + \beta_2 * zygote + \beta_3 * zygote * age^2 \qquad (10)$$

In Eq. (10), the two zygote related terms can be tested for the significance of static and dynamic genetic influences upon early brain development separately. Significant regions were found in left parietal white matter with FA, and significant regions in basal gangalia and right frontal white matter were identified with MD for term *zygote* in Eq. (10). Thus, these regions demonstrate static genetic influence (Fig. 2). Furthermore, brain regions with significant genetic influence on growth were identified with MD in frontal, occipital and parietal white matter for term $zygote * age^2$, which demonstrates dynamic genetic influence (Fig. 3).

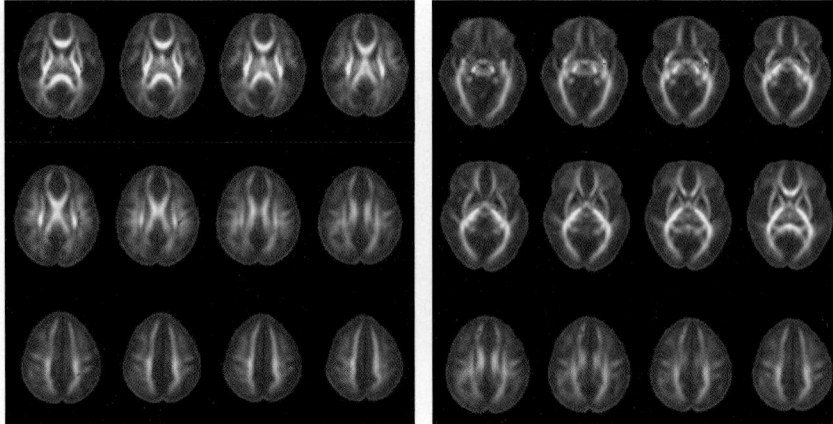

Fig. 2. Regions under significant static genetic influence on growth in FA (left panel) and MD (right panel)

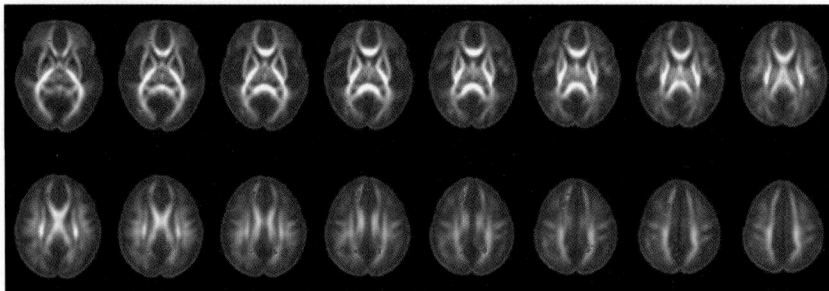

Fig. 3. Regions under significant dynamic genetic influence on growth in MD

4 Discussion

In this study, we have demonstrated the potentials of using GEE2 based statistical methods in analyzing twin images in a longitudinal study. This work may be the first study to identify the growth patterns of DTI parameters in longitudinal twin study. Our preliminary results demonstrated that genetic influences upon brain development can be identified with the squared difference images under the assumption of equal environmental exposure. Furthermore, our approach may suggest the existence of dynamic component of genetic influences on brain development in this early postnatal stage.

There are several potential improvements can be made to the current approach. One is to use the two GEE equations (Eq. (2) and (5)) iteratively for joint estimation of growth patterns and genetic influences. Another extension is to use multivariate analysis to improve the sensitivity in detecting genetic related influences. At last, from imaging registration end, the statistical analysis will benefit from an improved registration of the DTI images across different ages.

References

1. Almli, C.R., Rivkin, M.J., McKinstry, R.C.: The NIH MRI Study of Normal Brain Development (Objective-2): Newborns, Infants, Toddlers and Preschoolers. IEEE-TMI 35, 308–325 (2007)
2. Diggle, P., Heagerty, P., Liang, K.Y., Zeger, S.: Analysis of Longitudinal Data, 2nd edn. Oxford University, Oxford (2002)
3. Liang, K.Y., Zeger, S.L.: Longitudinal Data Analysis Using Generalized Linear Models. Biometrika 73, 13–22 (1986)
4. Baare, W.F., Hulschoff, H.E., Boomsma, D.I., Posthuma, D., Schnack, H.G., van Haren, N.E., van Oel, C.J., Kahn, R.S.: Quatitative Genetic Modeling of Variation in Human Brain Morphology. Cereb. Cortex. 11, 816–824 (2001)
5. Geschwind, D.H., Miller, B.L., DeCarli, C., Carmelli, D.: Heritability of Lobar Brain Volumes in Twins Supports Genetic Models of Cerebral Laterality and Handedness. PNAS 99, 3176–3181 (2002)
6. Thompson, P.M., Cannon, M.D., Narr, K.L., van Erp, T., Poutanen, V.P., Huttunen, M., Lonnqvist, J., Standerskjoid-Nordestam, C.G., Kaprio, J., Khaledy, M., Dail, R., Zoumalan, C.L., Toga, A.W.: Genetic influences on Brain Structure. Nat. Neurosci. 4, 1253–1258 (2001)
7. Wright, I.C., Sham, P., Murray, R.M., Weinberger, D.R., Bullmore, E.T.: Genetic Contributions to Regional Variability in Human Brain Structure: Methods and Preliminary Results. Neuroimage 17, 256–271 (2002)
8. Shen, D.: Image Registration by Local Histogram Matching. IEEE Trans. Med. Imaging 40, 1161–1172 (2007)
9. Zhu, H., Li, Y.M., Tang, N.S., Bansal, R., Hao, X.J., Weissman, M.M., Peterson, B.S.: Statistical Modelling of Brain Morphometric Measures in General Pedigree. Statistica Sinica 18, 1554–1569 (2008)

Tensor-Based Morphometry with Mappings Parameterized by Stationary Velocity Fields in Alzheimer's Disease Neuroimaging Initiative

Matías Nicolás Bossa, Ernesto Zacur, and Salvador Olmos

GTC, Aragon Institute of Engineering Research (I3A), University of Zaragoza, Spain
{bossa,zacur,olmos}@unizar.es

Abstract. Tensor-based morphometry (TBM) is an analysis technique where anatomical information is characterized by means of the spatial transformations between a customized template and observed images. Therefore, accurate inter-subject non-rigid registration is an essential prerequisite. Further statistical analysis of the spatial transformations is used to highlight some useful information, such as local statistical differences among populations. With the new advent of recent and powerful non-rigid registration algorithms based on the large deformation paradigm, TBM is being increasingly used. In this work we evaluate the statistical power of TBM using stationary velocity field diffeomorphic registration in a large population of subjects from Alzheimer's Disease Neuroimaging Initiative project. The proposed methodology provided atrophy maps with very detailed anatomical resolution and with a high significance compared with results published recently on the same data set.

1 Introduction

Alzheimer's disease (AD) is the most common form of dementia and one of the most serious health problems in the industrialised world. Dementia affects approximately 1–5% of the population over 65 years of age, and 20–40% of the population over 80 years of age. Mild cognitive impairments (MCI) may affect 10 times as many individuals.

The Alzheimer's Disease Neuroimaging Initiative (ADNI) [1] is a large multi-site longitudinal magnetic resonance imaging (MRI) and fluorodeoxyglucose positron emission tomography (FDG-PET) study of 800 adults, ages 55 to 90, including 200 elderly controls, 400 subjects with mild cognitive impairment, and 200 patients with AD. The primary goal of ADNI has been to test whether serial MRI, PET, other biological markers, and clinical and neuropsychological assessment can be combined to measure the progression of MCI and early AD. Determination of sensitive and specific markers of very early AD progression is intended to aid researchers and clinicians to develop new treatments and monitor their effectiveness, as well as lessen the time and cost of clinical trials.

Tensor-based morphometry (TBM) is a relatively new image analysis technique that identifies regional structural differences in the brain, across groups or over time, from the gradients of the deformation fields that warp images to a common anatomical template. The anatomical information is encoded in the spatial transformation. Therefore, accurate inter-subject non-rigid registration is an essential tool. With the new advent of recent and powerful non-rigid registration algorithms based on the large deformation paradigm, TBM is being increasingly used [2,3,4]. Further statistical analysis of the spatial transformations is used to highlight some useful information, such as local statistical differences among populations. The simplest and most common feature is given by the Jacobian determinant $|J|$ which can be interpreted as a local atrophy/expansion factor. More complete descriptors are the Jacobian matrix, or other invariant features, such as $\sqrt{J^T J}$ [2].

By diffeomorphic registration we mean algorithms where the transformation can be arbitrarily large, and still keeping smoothness and invertibility. Most of these methods use time-varying velocity fields either to update or to characterize the warpings. The first approach was based on viscous-fluid methods [5]. Later, regularization was obtained by minimizing the length of a path on the group of diffeomorphisms [6]. Among the benefits of the latter approach is that its parametrization lives in a metric linear space allowing statistical analysis. The main limitation of these methods is their large computational complexity. In order to alleviate this computational requirement some algorithms were proposed [7,8,9] using a stationary velocity field parameterization.

The aim of this study was to evaluate the performance of stationary velocity field (SVF) diffeomorphic registration on a TBM study.

2 Materials and Methods

2.1 Subjects

In this study we selected the same subset of subjects as in [10] in order to allow an easier comparison. To summarize, MRI screening scans of 120 subjects, divided into 3 groups: 40 healthy elderly individuals, 40 individuals with amnestic MCI, and 40 individuals with probable AD. Each group of 40 subjects was well matched in terms of gender and age. Likewise [10], an independent second group of normal subjects, age- and gender-matched to the first group of controls, was selected to test whether analysis techniques correctly detects no differences when no true differences are present. More details about criteria for patient selection and exclusion can be found in [10] and in the ADNI protocol [1,11].

In addition, a larger set of subjects was analyzed including 231 control subjects, 200 AD patients and 405 MCI patients from the ADNI study at screening stage. During the clinical follow up 127 MCI subjects converted to AD group. The MCI group was divided into converters (MCIc) and non-converters (MCInc).

2.2 MRI Acquisition, Image Correction and Preprocessing

High-resolution structural brain MRI scans were acquired at multiple ADNI sites using 1.5 Tesla MRI scanners using the standard ADNI MRI protocol.

For each subject, two T1-weighted MRI scans were collected using a sagittal 3DMP-RAGE sequence with voxel size of $0.94 \times 0.94 \times 1.2 mm^3$. The images were calibrated with phantom-based geometric corrections to ensure consistency among scans acquired at different sites Additional image corrections included geometric distortion correction, bias field correction and geometrical scaling. The pre-processed images are available to the scientific community and were downloaded from the ADNI website.

2.3 Stationary Velocity Fields (SVF) Diffeomorphic Registration

A diffeomorphism $\varphi(x)$ (smooth and invertible mapping) characterized by a stationary velocity field v is obtained as the solution at time $t = 1$ of

$$\frac{d}{dt}\phi_t(x) = v(\phi_t(x)), \qquad \phi_0(x) = Id(x), \tag{1}$$

i.e. $\varphi(x) \equiv \phi_1(x)$ and $v(x)$ is a smooth vector field. Several efficient numerical scheemes can be used to compute the exponential mapping $\exp(tv) \equiv \phi_t$ [12]. Note that the inverse mapping is $\varphi^{-1} = \phi_{-1} = \exp(-v)$.

Many registration methods can be formulated as a variational problem, where the cost function to be minimized contains an image term measuring matching between a template T and a target image I and a regularization term

$$E(I, T, v) = \frac{1}{\sigma^2} \|T(\varphi^{-1}) - I\|^2 + \langle v, v \rangle_V. \tag{2}$$

In this work the regularization term is of the form: $\langle v, v \rangle_V = \langle Hv, v \rangle_{L^2}$, with H the linear differential operator $H = (Id - \alpha\triangle)^2$, where $\triangle$ is the Laplacian operator. The gradient of this functional is (see [6])

$$\nabla_v E(I, T, v) = 2v - \frac{2}{\sigma^2} H^{-1} \int_0^1 |D\phi_{1-t}| \big(T(\phi_{-t}) - I(\phi_{1-t})\big) \nabla_x T(\phi_{-t}) dt \tag{3}$$

Different strategies have been proposed to minimize the energy functional defined by (2) [13,8,7,9]. In [7] the derivative of $\exp(v)$ was approximated by $\partial_h \exp(v) \approx h$ for $v \approx 0$, resulting in a simplified gradient $\nabla_v E(I, T, v) = 2v - \frac{2}{\sigma^2} H^{-1}\big((T(\phi_{-1}) - I)\nabla_x T(\phi_{-1})\big)$ which reduces significatively the computational complexity when using gradient descent.

2.4 Unbiased Average Template

An average template is one of the key components of TBM studies. It provides a coordinate system where all image samples will be registered. In order to make automatic registration easier and more robust, the template must represent common intensity and geometric features from the group of subjects. Population templates should not be biased toward any particular image or sub-group of images.

In this work the unbiased template T was estimated from images of the normal group, likewise in [10]. An initial affine average atlas was estimated by means of global affine registration of all intensity-normalized normal group images I^i to the ICBM53 template and voxel-wise averaging. Next, an iterative process was used to estimate the template, including three stages for each iteration: nonlinear registration of the affine-alligned images ($N = 40$) to the current estimated template; computing the bi-invariant mean $\overline{\varphi} = \exp(\overline{v})$ [14] of all warpings $\varphi^i = \exp(v^i)$, and finally image intensities are averaged after subtracting the mean warping $T = 1/N \sum_i I^i(\varphi^i \circ \exp(-\overline{v}))$.

2.5 Voxel-Wise Statistical Analysis of Brain Atrophy

To quantify spatial distribution of brain atrophy in MCI and AD compared to the normal group, all individual brains were non-linearly registered to the normal group template. Hypothesis testing is usually performed on logarithm of Jacobian determinants to assess effect size and statistical significance of local brain atrophy between patient groups. Statistical maps that visualize the patterns of significant expansion factors between groups were computed by means of t-test.

2.6 Regions of Interest Statistical Analysis

In order to summarize the information of hypothesis testing from the voxel level to the region of interest (ROI) level, a scalar descriptor of the ROI, such as a weighted average, the maximum value or many others, can be used. Similarly to [10], we used the average Jacobian determinant, which is equivalent to the

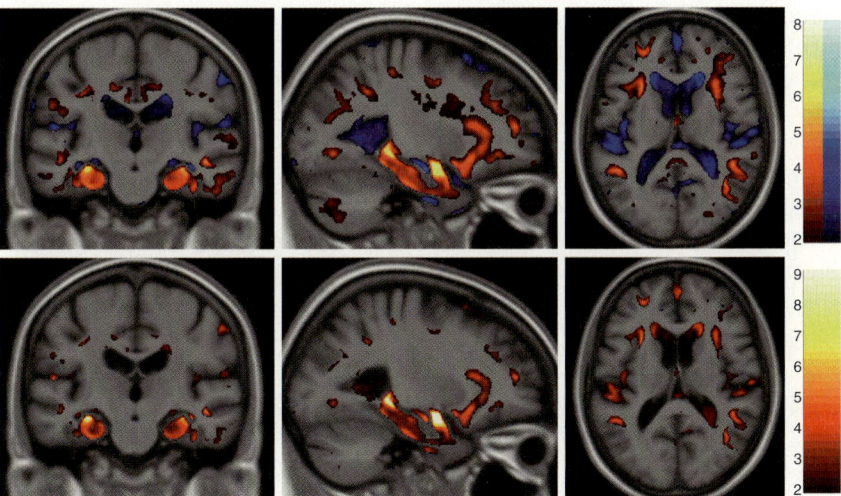

Fig. 1. Statistical maps of brain atrophy in the selected population (*N=120*) of AD versus Normal group. Top: Student's t-test map (blue/red denotes expansion/contraction respectively. Bottom: corresponding significance map ($-log_{10} p$).

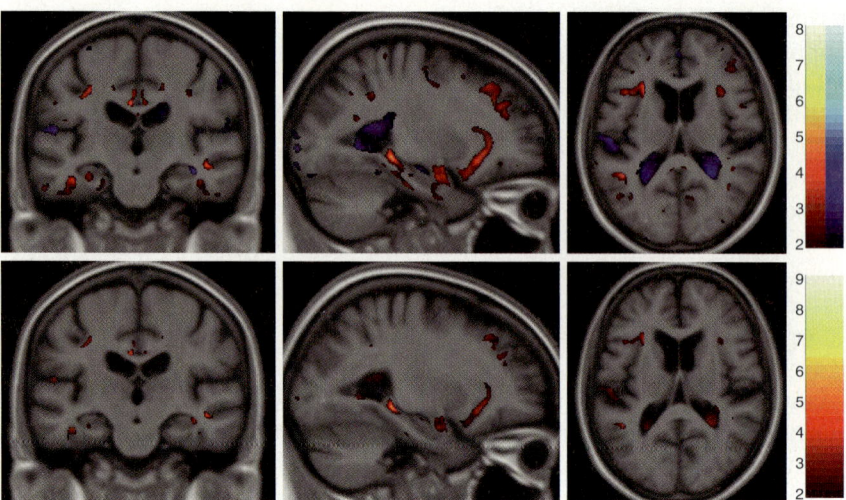

Fig. 2. Statistical maps of brain atrophy in the selected population ($N=120$) of MCI versus Normal group. See legend of Fig. 1.

overall volume change of the ROI. In this work the following ROIs were considered: hippocampus, amygdala, caudate nucleus, thalamus, nucleus accumbens and lateral ventricles. These subcortical nuclei were automatically segmented at the normal template using the tool FIRST [15] from FSL package.

3 Results

The statistical significance (p-value) and Student's t-test maps in Fig. 1(2) illustrate the atrophy pattern observed in the AD(MCI) groups compared to the normal group. AD patients showed larger areas affected by more severe brain atrophy specially at the hippocampus and amygdala. In contrast, brain atrophy in MCI patients affects smaller regions with a less pronounced effect size. Note that detected areas have a well defined anatomical boundary compared to previous results using the same data set [10]. The statistical map under the null hypothesis (between the two independent normal groups) did not show any significant region.

Table 1. ROI analysis: Student's t-test on large population ($N=836$)

Groups\ROI	LAccu	LAmyg	LHipp	LLate	LThal	RAccu	RAmyg	RHipp	RLate	RThal
Nor vs AD	4.07	13.84	6.47	-6.48	4.68	4.17	13.57	9.66	-7.07	5.21
Nor vs MCIc	2.69	10.16	5.40	-5.12	3.68	2.54	8.98	6.96	-5.13	3.77
Nor vs MCInc	2.86	6.59	4.88	-3.49	3.69	2.45	5.78	6.07	-2.86	3.91
AD vs MCIc	-0.81	-2.29	-0.42	0.86	-0.45	-1.00	-2.58	-1.27	1.40	-0.55
AD vs MCInc	-1.44	-7.65	-2.18	3.15	-1.41	-1.98	-8.13	-4.26	4.38	-1.71
MCI c vs nc	-0.39	-4.31	-1.44	1.89	-0.76	-0.62	-4.16	-2.21	2.43	-0.83

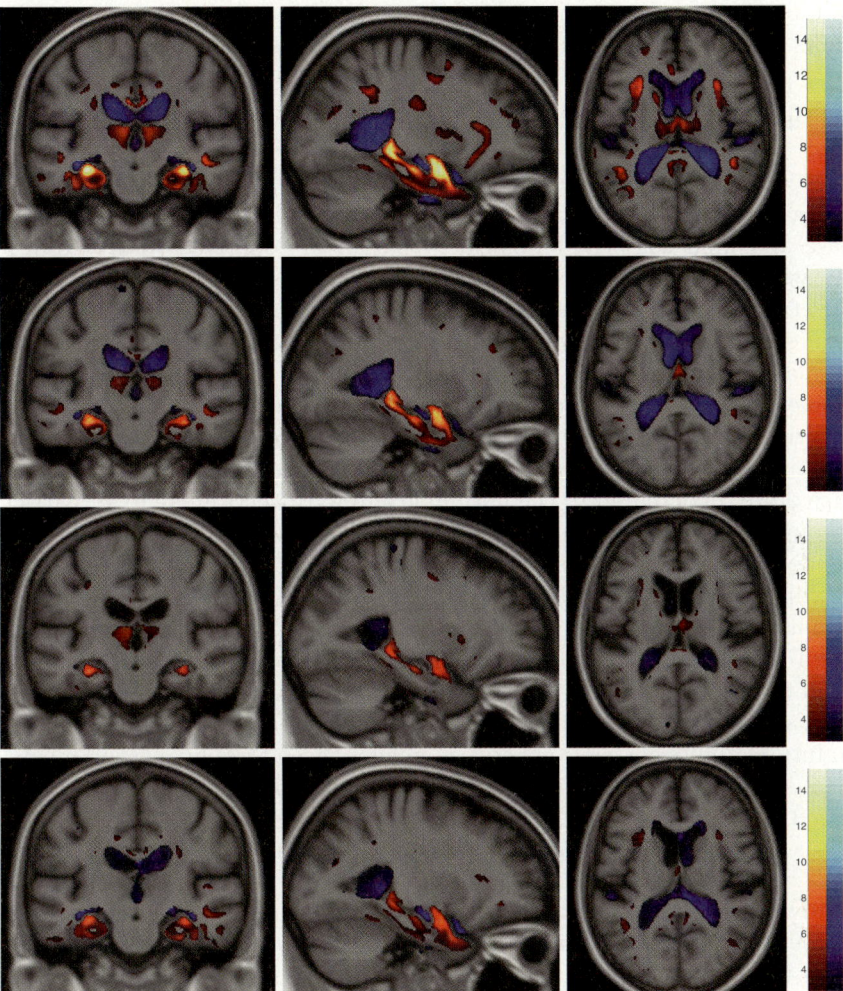

Fig. 3. Student's t-test maps of brain atrophy in the large population ($N=836$). From top to bottom: AD versus Normal group; converter MCI versus Normal group; non-converter MCI versus Normal group; AD vs non-converter MCI group.

If the TBM analysis is performed on the larger population (N=836), very similar anatomical patterns of atrophy are obtained (see Fig. 3) but with a much higher statistical significance due to the larger number of subjects in the analysis. Interestingly, the brain atrophy map in the MCInc group was closer to the normal group, while the MCIc group was closer to the AD group.

The Jacobian determinant was spatially averaged within each ROI and subject. Student's t-test was performed on these scalar descriptors to assess the statistical significance between mean atrophy levels. Table 1 contains the Student's t-test statistic for each ROI on the complete set of subjects ($N=836$).

Again hippocampus and amygdala obtained the most significant volumetric differences between groups, in agreement with previous studies.

4 Discussion and Conclusions

In this study a large deformation registration method was used in a cross-sectional TBM study in order to localize brain atrophy regions in Alzheimer's disease and mild cognitive impairment patients. Compared to a recent TBM study with the same data set of 120 images at baseline from ADNI [10], our brain atrophy patterns presented a higher spatial resolution with a larger statistical significance. In our opinion, the improved performance obtained in this work may be due to the higher spatial resolution of the registration algorithm.

The evaluation was also extended to 836 subjects from ADNI corroborating brain atrophy patterns shown in the subset of subjects with stronger significance. Interestingly, brain atrophy patterns between converters and non-converters subgroups of MCI compared to the normal group were very different. In particular, non-converters were much close to normal group, while converters were much closer to AD group. Our first preliminary results found brain atrophy at amygdala, hippocampus, entorhinal cortex, cingulate gyrus, posterior parts of the thalamus, frontal regions of the insular cortex, and superior temporal sulcus, all of them involved in Alzheimer's Disease. To our knowledge, this is the first time that all these structures are jointly identified in a brain morphometry study with such anatomical detail.

In future studies correlation between image-driven atrophy measurements and clinical variables (including cognitive tests, genotypes and biomarkers) will be assessed as it is proposed in [16], prediction of conversion to AD, single-subject analysis and evaluation of atrophy rates using longitudinal images.

Acknowledgments. This work was partially funded by research grants TEC2006-13966-C03-02 from CICYT and PI100/08 from DGA, Spain. Data used in the preparation of this article were obtained from the Alzheimer's Disease Neuroimaging Initiative (ADNI) database (www.loni.ucla.edu/ADNI). The Principal Investigator of this initiative is Michael W. Weiner, M.D., VA Medical Center and University of California - San Francisco. ADNI is the result of efforts of many co-investigators from a broad range of academic institutions and private corporations.

References

1. Mueller, S.G., Weiner, M.W., Thal, L.J., Petersen, R.C., Jack, C., Jagust, W., Trojanowski, J.Q., Toga, A.W., Beckett, L.: The Alzheimer's Disease Neuroimaging Initiative. Neuroimaging Clinics of North America 15(4), 869–877 (2005)
2. Lepore, N., Brun, C., Chou, Y.Y., Chiang, M.C., Dutton, R., Hayashi, K., Luders, E., Lopez, O., Aizenstein, H., Toga, A., Becker, J., Thompson, P.: Generalized Tensor-Based Morphometry of HIV/AIDS Using Multivariate Statistics on Deformation Tensors. IEEE Transactions on Medical Imaging 27(1), 129–141 (2008)

3. Chiang, M.C., Dutton, R.A., Hayashi, K.M., Lopez, O.L., Aizenstein, H.J., Toga, A.W., Becker, J.T., Thompson, P.M.: 3D pattern of brain atrophy in HIV/AIDS visualized using tensor-based morphometry. NeuroImage 34(1), 44–60 (2007)
4. Lee, A.D., Leow, A.D., Lu, A., Reiss, A.L., Hall, S., Chiang, M.C., Toga, A.W., Thompson, P.M.: 3D pattern of brain abnormalities in Fragile X syndrome visualized using tensor-based morphometry. NeuroImage 34(3), 924–938 (2007)
5. Christensen, G., Rabbitt, R., Miller, M.: Deformable templates using large deformation kinematics. IEEE Transactions on Image Processing 5(10), 1435–1447 (1996)
6. Beg, M.F., Miller, M.I., Trouve, A., Younes, L.: Computing Large Deformation Metric Mappings via Geodesic Flows of Diffeomorphisms. International Journal of Computer Vision 61(2), 139–157 (2005)
7. Hernandez, M., Bossa, M., Olmos, S.: Registration of Anatomical Images Using Paths of Diffeomorphisms Parameterized with Stationary Vector Fields Flows. International Journal of Computer Vision (2009)
8. Ashburner, J.: A fast diffeomorphic image registration algorithm. NeuroImage 38(1), 95–113 (2007)
9. Vercauteren, T., Pennec, X., Perchant, A., Ayache, N.: Symmetric log-domain diffeomorphic registration: A demons-based approach. In: Metaxas, D., Axel, L., Fichtinger, G., Székely, G. (eds.) MICCAI 2008, Part I. LNCS, vol. 5241, pp. 754–761. Springer, Heidelberg (2008)
10. Hua, X., Leow, A.D., Lee, S., Klunder, A.D., Toga, A.W., Lepore, N., Chou, Y.Y., Brun, C., Chiang, M.C., Barysheva, M., Jack Jr., C.R., Bernstein, M.A., Britson, P.J., Ward, C.P., Whitwell, J.L., Borowski, B., Fleisher, A.S., Fox, N.C., Boyes, R.G., Barnes, J., Harvey, D., Kornak, J., Schuff, N., Boreta, L., Alexander, G.E., Weiner, M.W., Thompson, P.M., The Alzheimer's Disease Neuroimaging Initiative: 3D characterization of brain atrophy in Alzheimer's disease and mild cognitive impairment using tensor-based morphometry. NeuroImage 41(1), 19–34 (2008)
11. Mueller, S.G., Weiner, M.W., Thal, L.J., Petersen, R.C., Jack, C.R., Jagust, W., Trojanowski, J.Q., Toga, A.W., Beckett, L.: Ways toward an early diagnosis in Alzheimer's disease: The Alzheimer's Disease Neuroimaging Initiative (ADNI). Alzheimers Dement 1(1), 55–66 (2005)
12. Bossa, M., Zacur, E., Olmos, S.: Algorithms for computing the group exponential of diffeomorphisms: Performance evaluation. In: Proc. IEEE Computer Society Conference on Computer Vision and Pattern Recognition (CVPR), June 23-28, pp. 1–8 (2008)
13. Hernandez, M., Olmos, S.: Gauss-Newton optimization in Diffeomorphic registration. In: Proc. 5th IEEE International Symposium on Biomedical Imaging (ISBI), May 14-17, pp. 1083–1086 (2008)
14. Arsigny, V.: Processing Data in Lie Groups: An Algebraic Approach. Application to Non-Linear Registration and Diffusion Tensor MRI. PhD Thesis, École polytechnique (November 2006)
15. Patenaude, B.: Bayesian Statistical Models of Shape and Appearance for Subcortical Brain Segmentation. PhD thesis, University of Oxford (2007)
16. Hua, X., Leow, A.D., Parikshak, N., Lee, S., Chiang, M.C., Toga, A.W., Jack Jr., C.R., Weiner, M.W., Thompson, P.M.: Tensor-based morphometry as a neuroimaging biomarker for Alzheimer's disease: An MRI study of 676 AD, MCI, and normal subjects. NeuroImage 43(3), 458–469 (2008)

High-Quality Model Generation for Finite Element Simulation of Tissue Deformation

Orcun Goksel and Septimiu E. Salcudean

Department of Electrical and Computer Engineering
University of British Columbia, Vancouver, Canada
{orcung,tims}@ece.ubc.ca

Abstract. In finite element simulation, size, shape, and placement of the elements in a model are significant factors that affect the interpolation and numerical errors of a solution. In medical simulations, such models are desired to have higher accuracy near features such as anatomical boundaries (surfaces) and they are often required to have element faces lying along these surfaces. Conventional modelling schemes consist of a segmentation step delineating the anatomy followed by a meshing step generating elements conforming to this segmentation. In this paper, a one-step energy-based model generation technique is proposed. An objective function is minimized when each element of a mesh covers similar image intensities while, at the same time, having desirable FEM characteristics. Such a mesh becomes essential for accurate models for deformation simulation, especially when the image intensities represent a mechanical feature of the tissue such as the elastic modulus. The use of the proposed mesh optimization is demonstrated on synthetic phantoms, 2D/3D brain MR images, and prostate ultrasound-elastography data.

1 Introduction

The finite element method (FEM) is a common technique for medical simulations. Its speed and accuracy depend on the number of nodes/elements used and their shape and placement in the domain. In this paper, a single-step and fully-automatic variational modelling approach is presented to produce good FEM meshes for given tissue domains in both 2D and 3D. The method, which aligns FEM elements to group similar intensities while still keeping element shapes relatively *good* for FEM, is applicable on most medical imaging modalities. Its use becomes particularly important if the input image represents a mechanical feature distribution of the tissue such as Young's modulus.

In the conventional modelling methods for tissue FEM simulation, a discrete representation of the anatomy of interest is obtained from an intensity image/volume by employing two steps, *segmentation* and *meshing*. Segmentation, which consists of *recognition* and *delineation* of anatomy, has been studied in several medical contexts using numerous different approaches. Although automatic segmentation techniques do exist, recognition is not a computationally well-defined problem and thus is usually achieved with manual intervention leading to semi-automatic implementations. In contrast, delineation, which in many cases can be stated roughly as *grouping similar pixels*, allows for algorithmic approaches. Nonetheless, segmentation overall often requires some *a priori* information about both the anatomy and the medical imaging modality.

The result of segmentation is a representation of the organ boundary, which is often in an explicit form such as a surface mesh, although implicit representations are also viable. This anatomical boundary is then supplied to a meshing scheme, which tiles the space with elements while ensuring some geometrical measures of such elements meet given or well-known criteria. Popular meshing schemes include octree-based methods, Delaunay approaches, and advancing fronts, most of which were developed and tuned for modelling of mechanical structures and systems [1]. The final mesh is then used for simulating tissue deformation for procedures such as laparoscopic surgery, brain surgery, and brachytherapy.

Most segmentation methods require some sort of a manual intervention not only demanding the scarcely available time of health professionals but also preventing an automatic modelling for FEM. The surface mesh generated during the segmentation is often left unchanged by the meshing software since this surface is used as a boundary constraint for meshing. Thus, for a meshing scheme to guarantee good FEM elements using a limited number of nodes/elements, these surfaces should either be inherently FEM-friendly delineations or should be *fixed* using some intermediate steps. Furthermore, boundary conforming meshes, when the inside and outside of an anatomical feature are to be discretized with no element faces cutting the boundary, present a challenge for otherwise successful schemes such as Delaunay tessellation [1]. The technique presented in this paper intrinsically overcomes these issues producing high-quality FEM elements that are also aligned with the features in a given image.

2 Methods

2.1 Element Shape Optimization

Let $u(x)$ be the deformation of a point x within a continuous domain $\mathcal{M} \subset \mathbb{R}^n$, where this deformation is approximated using the FEM by a piece-wise linear discrete function $g_\mathcal{T}(x)$ over a tessellation $\mathcal{T}$. During such modelling of deformation, the two main sources of error are the *interpolation errors* for the approximation to the function and its gradient (which is strain for deformation), and the *numerical errors* during the solution of the approximation [2].

Variational (energy-minimization based) methods were shown to produce successful meshes for various applications including meshes suitable for FEM [1]. Recent studies showed that a primal mesh energy definition is superior to the Voronoi-based approaches [3]. It was also shown that the following error [1]:

$$E_G = \|u(\mathbf{x}) - g_\mathcal{T}(\mathbf{x})\| = \frac{1}{n+1} \sum_i \mathbf{x}_i^2 |\Omega_i| - \int_\mathcal{M} \mathbf{x}^2 d\mathbf{x} \tag{1}$$

is minimized by the following two operations: a Delaunay tessellation of given node locations, and a relocation of a node $\mathbf{x}_i$ to the weighted average of the

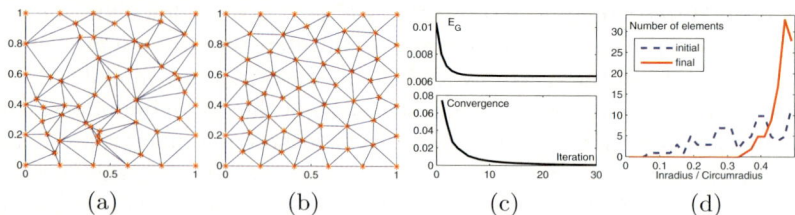

Fig. 1. A random mesh initialization (a), its optimized configuration (b), the energy and convergence during this optimization (c), and the initial/final ρ distributions (d)

element circumcenters in its 1-ring neighbourhood Ω_i, where the weighting is the element volume. Consequently, a (local) minimizer mesh for E_G is found using Lloyd's relaxation by alternately re-tessellating and relocating the nodes [1]. Figure 1(a-b) shows an initial mesh of randomly-distributed 61 nodes and its optimized configuration after having converged. The energy E_G and the nodal position convergence $\|\mathbf{x}_i^{t+1} - \mathbf{x}_i^t\|/\|\mathbf{x}_i^t\|$ at iteration t are presented in Fig. 1(c).

Comparing two meshes using merely a single error measure is an attractive approach, not only simply to choose the *better* mesh, but also to formulate energy definitions that can derive variational schemes. No such single measure has been developed in the literature. For predicting the worst interpolation-error in a single element, various measures were proposed in [2]. The inradius-to-circumradius ratio ρ, which was presented in [1] as the *fairest* comparison in 3D that punishes all types of poor-geometry elements including slivers, is used in this paper. This ratio is maximized at $1/2$ for the equilateral triangle and at $1/3$ for the regular tetrahedron. Similarly to [1], normalized histograms of this ratio are used to compare meshes, where a desired mesh has a histogram more compacted towards higher ratios as displayed in Fig. 1(d) for the initial and optimized meshes presented above. Since a qualitative comparison of curves can be difficult, we propose the following measures in this paper: (i) mean quality error $mean(\frac{1}{n} - \rho)$, (ii) harmonic-mean quality error $1/\sum \frac{1}{\frac{1}{n}-\rho}$, ($iii$) $\mathcal{L}_2$-norm quality error $|\frac{1}{n} - \rho|^2$, and (iv) worst quality error $max(\frac{1}{n} - \rho)$. All these quality errors improve during the sample optimization above as seen in Table 1.

Table 1. The inradius-to-circumradius ratios for each row corresponding to the meshes presented in Figs. 1(a,b), Figs. 2(a,c,d), and Figs. 3(c,d), respectively

Error measures based on ρ	i	ii	iii	iv
Initial mesh with uniform background in Fig. 1(a)	0.1576	0.1029	3.6807	0.4335
Final mesh with uniform background in Fig. 1(b)	0.0405	0.0274	0.2671	0.1558
Initial mesh for synthetic phantom in Fig. 2(a)	0.0858	0.0858	1.4424	0.0858
$k_D = 0.05$ mesh for synthetic phantom in Fig. 2(c)	0.0399	0.0301	0.4789	0.1418
$k_D = 0.30$ mesh for synthetic phantom in Fig. 2(d)	0.0438	0.0251	0.6910	0.2467
Initial mesh for prostate elastography in Fig. 3(c)	0.0859	0.0856	1.4532	0.0922
Final mesh for prostate elastography in Fig. 3(d)	0.0372	0.0232	0.4668	0.1595

2.2 Modelling a Known Background Distribution

The methods above assume isotropic meshing of a uniform domain. Anisotropic meshes [3] and effective adjustment of element sizes throughout the mesh [1] have been studied in the literature by incorporating these in the energy definition in (1). However, it is not clear from these and other work, how the information about a feature distribution through the tissue (e.g. distribution of elastic modulus) can be incorporated into the mesh generation, assuming this distribution is known in the continuum *a priori*. There exist well-established methods, as part of the *post-processing* stage of FEM simulations, that can refine or modify a mesh based on a computed simulation output such as element strains during deformation. However, this requires the cumbersome process of first running the simulation, which in turn requires *a priori* knowledge of the boundary conditions such as the fixed and the excited nodes of a mesh during deformation. These boundary conditions may not be known during meshing. Furthermore, their location and nature may change substantially from simulation to simulation such as encountered when a medical tool interacts with different parts of an organ and/or in different directions. Moreover, post-process refinement approaches aim to minimize interpolation error by adjusting node/element density locally. However, such refinement techniques do not formulate an optimum placement for an element intrinsically and refining elements may worsen stiffness matrix conditioning. Also, unlike mechanical engineering, where higher accuracy around high-strain contact areas is desired, medical simulations often require higher accuracy around organ surfaces or anatomical features such as tumors or an overall accuracy in the entire domain. In addition, for a non-uniform property distribution, refining a high-strain element may not always be the right strategy: Consider a 1D example of two elements, one covering a homogeneous soft region and the other one covering an overall stiffer region which internally consists of two disjoint sections with slightly-different elastic properties. Note that, for mesh refinement, subdividing the former element may not necessarily be the optimal strategy despite its higher strain. As a result, we propose the following method based on an error definition that encourages element placement consistent with a given background distribution.

Due to mesh discretization, the FEM models a feature $h(\mathbf{x}), \mathbf{x} \in \tau_j$ of the entire space within an element τ_j using a single value $\tilde{h}_j$. An error associated with the fitness of this single-value approximation is suggested intuitively to be the $\mathcal{L}_2$-norm of the difference between this approximation value and the known background distribution, i.e. $\int_{\tau_j} \left(h(\mathbf{x}) - \tilde{h}_j \right)^2 d\mathbf{x}$. This is derived below from the elastic strain energy of a linear element, where the known tissue feature is Young's modulus $\mathcal{E}$. For a linear stress-strain relationship, the strain energy of an element can be written in terms of the four corner displacements $\mathbf{u}^j$, the constant partial-derivative matrix B^j (found from the corner positions), and the material stiffness matrix C as $E_{strain}^j(\mathbf{u}^j) = \frac{1}{2} \int_{\tau_j} \mathbf{u}^{j^T} B^{j^T} C B^j \mathbf{u}^j \, d\mathbf{x}$ [4]. In the conventional derivation, C is constant as each element is modeled with a single set of material properties. With C constant, this integration results in the

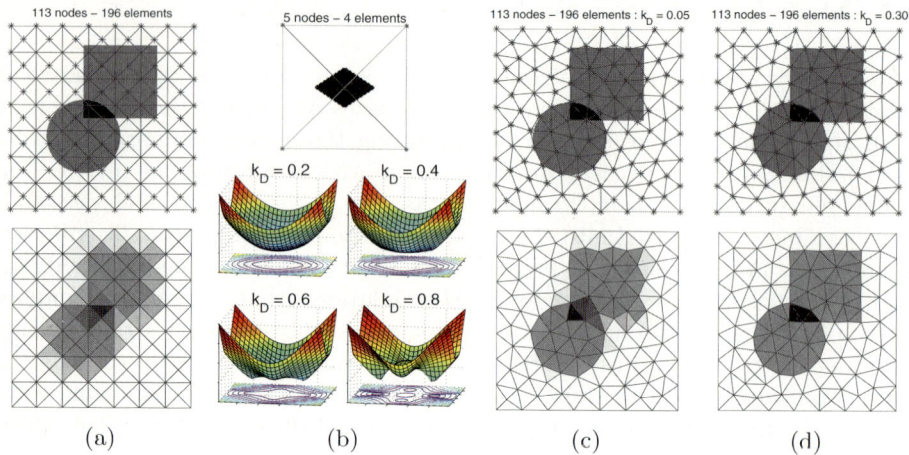

Fig. 2. An initial synthetic phantom with its discretization (a), the combined error E as a function of center node position for a simple 4-element mesh (b), and the two optimized versions of the initial phantom mesh using $k_D = 0.05$ (c) and $k_D = 0.3$ (d)

element volume v^j. However, C is indeed a linear function of Young's modulus $\mathcal{E}$, the distribution of which is assumed to be known in this paper (i.e., $C = \mathcal{E}(\mathbf{x})C'$). Then, the strain energy can be written for a non-uniform element as:

$$E^j_{strain}(\mathbf{u}^j) = \frac{1}{2}\mathbf{u}^{jT} B^{jT} C' B^j \mathbf{u}^j \int_{\tau^j} \mathcal{E}(\mathbf{x})\,dx = \frac{1}{2}\mathbf{u}^{jT} B^{jT} C' B^j \mathbf{u}^j\, \tilde{\mathcal{E}}_j v^j \quad (2)$$

which is satisfied when $\tilde{\mathcal{E}}_j$ is the mean of the distribution within the element.

The above observations show that a single-value equivalent of a known background distribution within an element is its mean value. This is presented in Fig. 2(a) with a uniform mesh overlaid on a synthetic phantom, where the element colors represent the mean value of the underlying image pixels.

In this paper, an $\mathcal{L}_2$-norm discretization error measure E_D for a single-value approximation $\tilde{h}_j$ and the actual known distribution $h(\mathbf{x})$ is defined as:

$$E_D = \sum_j \int_{\tau_j} \left|h(\mathbf{x}) - \tilde{h}_j\right|^2 dx = \sum_j v^j \mathbf{Var}\left(h(\mathbf{x}) : \mathbf{x} \in \tau_j\right) \quad (3)$$

where **Var** is the second-moment of a distribution around its mean. Then, the two error measures E_G and E_D above are combined into a single error definition in order to derive a variational scheme trading off between element geometry and image representation as:

$$E = (1 - k_D)E_G + k_D E_D \quad (4)$$

where $k_D \in [0, 1)$ is a weighting factor. This energy is plotted in Fig. 2(b) as a function of the center node position, which defines a unique four-triangle mesh over the simple image presented. Note the change of priority from better element-geometry to lower element-variance as k_D increases.

A good approximate initial configuration for geometry error E_G can easily be defined as a uniform mesh of regular elements throughout the domain, although it is difficult to define a good initial approximation for E_D. Therefore, an initial uniform mesh is chosen to start the optimization process. Note that the combined error E depends on how the given image is partitioned by the current tessellation and hence it does not have a simple closed-form expression. In order to minimize this error, a gradient descent search with numerical derivatives has been implemented, where a given node $\mathbf{x}_i$ is relocated at each iteration using the error E_{Ω_i} in its 1-ring neighbourhood Ω_i, calculated for perturbations in each coordinate axis by a given *step length*. Sub-step length updates are further achieved using a parabola fit in each individual axis. In our implementation, the step length is defined as a ratio of the distance to the closest element centroid.

3 Results

The initial 2D mesh of the synthetic phantom in Fig. 2(a) was optimized using two different energy weighting factors yielding the meshes and their discretizations shown in Fig. 2(c-d). The ρ-error definitions for this initial mesh and its two different optimized configurations are presented in Table 1. Note that all measures, except for the worst element error (iv), were improved, meaning that even for a higher k_D value the mesh geometry overall is not worsened while modelling a background image.

The feasibility of our method was next studied on MR images of the brain. An MR slice is first discretized using an initial regular mesh with 128 nodes and 224 triangles as seen in Fig. 3(a). This mesh is next optimized for $k_D = 0.2$ resulting in the discretization in Fig. 3(b) in 20 iterations. Although the mesh still remains coarse, a substantial improvement in the representation of the given image is observed once a mesh is optimized using the technique presented. The mesh optimization method was also applied on prostate elastography images. Several methods of tissue parameter identification from displacement estimations have been proposed in the literature [5]. For the purpose of this paper, a simple approximation to the tissue elastic modulus from a tissue strain map $e(x)$ was derived as $1/e(x)$ [6]. An initial 2D mesh with 113 nodes and 196 triangles in Fig. 3(c) takes the form seen in Fig. 3(d) after an optimization taking 15 iterations using $k_D = 0.3$. A preliminary result of this mesh optimization in 3D is presented in Fig. 3(e-f), where 1078 nodes and 3900 tetrahedra were employed.

The geometric quality of elements, which is traded off in this work for a better discretization of an image, is a major contributor to stiffness matrix conditioning. In this paper, the conditioning k of the stiffness matrices compiled using the initial and final meshes presented have also been studied in order to show that it does not increase significantly, which would negatively affect a simulation. The maximum eigenvalue λ of such matrices was proposed in [2] as a good estimate to

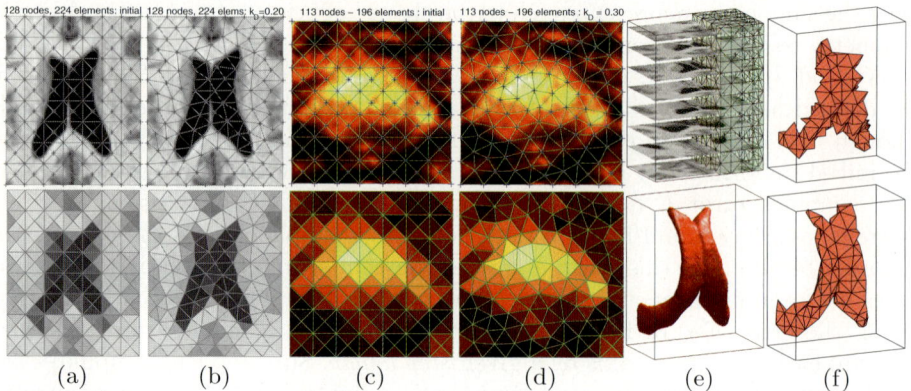

Fig. 3. Initial and optimized meshes of ventricles in brain MR images (a-b) and sagittal approximate-stiffness images from prostate elastography (c-d). Slices from a 3D brain MR dataset are shown embedded in an initial 3D mesh (only, part of the mesh is plotted) and the ventricle surface extracted from this volume is presented for comparison purposes (e). Initial and optimized 3D meshes of this MR volume (f). For better 3D visualization, only the largest connected-set of tetrahedra j with $\tilde{h}_j$ lower than a chosen threshold are displayed.

the conditioning assuming that the volume of the minimum element is not much smaller than the other elements', which is the case for our nearly uniform-size meshes. The increase in λ and k after optimization were 16% and 7%, respectively. These expected increases were observed to be within acceptable range so as not to introduce numerical instabilities to an FEM application. Furthermore, it was desired to see whether the aggregate strain energy $E_{strain}^{\mathcal{T}}$ would decrease for a tessellation $\mathcal{T}$ that is optimized as a better discretization of an image using our method. Note that the discretized energy $E_{strain}^{\mathcal{T}}$ is an overlaid approximant to the exact continuous strain energy and hence bounded below. To compute k and E_{strain}, the top of the meshes were fixed while the bottom was compressed using a plane-stress model. E_{strain} was observed to be reduced by 5% for the given constraints after the mesh optimization for the prostate. This agrees with our expectation of improving the strain energy approximation by better aligning the elements with a given parameter distribution.

4 Discussion

Some active-contours segmentation approaches that move a parametric surface minimizing the variance inside and outside this surface [7] use a variance-based energy definition similar to our method. However, in contrast to such techniques, where a surface can be evolved at any of its points, linear FEM element faces cannot be modified arbitrarily but instead they are expressed through a connectivity of the mesh nodes. Therefore, an explicit relation between given FEM node relocations and the resulting variance change within elements does not exist. Furthermore, there are no longer just two regions, namely *inside* and *outside*, but instead multiple disjoint but neighbouring simplex-shaped regions, the FEM *elements*. Consequently, image feature resolution that a mesh can resolve now depends on the FEM element size. Only uniform meshes were implemented in this paper. Nonetheless, the definition of E_G can easily be modified to incorporate a desired local mesh-size information [1] to produce smaller elements that model small anatomical features or higher strain regions, where needed.

Note that the conditioning and strain energy measures presented do not depend only on the mesh and its parametrization, but also are tightly bound by the boundary conditions applied to the FEM. Meshes are optimized by our method assuming that there is no *a priori* knowledge of the boundary constraints and hence this boundary information is not incorporated into our variational approach. Nevertheless, considering both measures above, an optimized mesh is still expected to rank well for a range of different boundary conditions, one of which was presented in this paper by simply constraining the top and the bottom surface for the prostate mesh. This choice was to model the pubic bone and the ultrasound probe motion during a trans-rectal prostate biopsy.

Although a re-tessellation of nodes ensures a decrease in E_G, it may possibly increase E_D and hence the total energy since it changes the nature of the problem for E_D. Nonetheless, allowing for re-tessellation is essential to yield geometrically good elements, therefore, re-tessellations are enabled in our optimization scheme during the first n_t number of iterations, after which the element connectivity is fixed so the combined energy can be minimized consistently. Alternatively, a tessellation can be accepted only if it decreases the combined energy. In this paper, the initial nodes distributed regularly on the domain boundary are kept fixed during the optimization process and only the position of the internal nodes are optimized. This constraint can be relaxed in various ways to yield better meshes, such as letting these nodes move tangential to the boundary [1]. Note that the errors E_G and E_D may be in different scales given the image, mesh, and domain dimensions. For similar results among different optimizations using a given k_D, these error values were normalized to their values in the initial mesh.

5 Conclusions

In this paper, an error definition based on FEM interpolation error is combined with a proposed image-representation error and the combined error is optimized to produce high-quality FEM elements that also discretize a given image successfully. With the emerging fields of elastography imaging and tissue parameter identification, this method becomes essential for optimal meshes conforming to such parameters. Note that such an optimized discretization can further be used for a fast approximate segmentation since optimized elements represent an image using far fewer degrees-of-freedom than the underlying pixels. In future work, other optimization techniques will be studied in order to improve on the current descent-based approach. The methods presented do not rely on any assumptions of 2D and they extend to 3D easily, as shown by our ventricle-meshing example.

References

1. Alliez, P., Cohen-Steiner, D., Yvinec, M., Desbrun, M.: Variational tetrahedral meshing. ACM Trans. on Graphics (procs. of SIGGRAPH) 24(3), 617–625 (2005)
2. Shewchuk, J.R.: What is a good linear element? interpolation, conditioning, and quality measures. In: Eleventh International Meshing Roundtable (2002)
3. Chen, L., Xu, J.: Optimal Delaunay triangulation. Journal of Computational Mathematics 22(2), 299–308 (2004)
4. Zienkiewicz, O.C., Taylor, R.L.: The Finite Element Method. Butterworth-Heinemann (2000)
5. Greenleaf, J.F., Fatemi, M., Insana, M.: Selected Methods for Imaging Elastic Properties of Biological Tissues. Annual Review of Biomed. Eng. 5, 57–78 (2000)
6. Ophir, J., Céspedes, I., Ponnekanti, H., Yazdi, Y., Li, X.: Elastography: a method for imaging the elasticity of biological tissues. Ultrasonic Img. 13(2), 111–134 (1991)
7. Chan, T.F., Vese, L.A.: Active contours without edges. IEEE Trans. Image Processing 10(2), 266–277 (2001)

Biomechanically-Constrained 4D Estimation of Myocardial Motion

Hari Sundar, Christos Davatzikos, and George Biros

Section for Biomedical Image Analysis, Department of Radiology,
University of Pennsylvania

Abstract. We propose a method for the analysis of cardiac images with the goal of reconstructing the motion of the ventricular walls. The main feature of our method is that the inversion parameter field is the active contraction of the myocardial fibers. This is accomplished with a biophysically-constrained, four-dimensional (space plus time) formulation that aims to complement information that can be gathered from the images by *a priori* knowledge of cardiac mechanics. *Our main hypothesis is that by incorporating biophysical information, we can generate more informative priors and thus, more accurate predictions of the ventricular wall motion.* In this paper, we outline the formulation, discuss the computational methodology for solving the inverse motion estimation, and present preliminary validation using synthetic and tagged MR images. The overall method uses patient-specific imaging and fiber information to reconstruct the motion. In these preliminary tests, we verify the implementation and conduct a parametric study to test the sensitivity of the model to material properties perturbations, model errors, and incomplete and noisy observations.

1 Introduction

Medical Imaging can help in the diagnosis of cardiac masses, cardiomyopathy, myocardial infarction, and valvular disease. Advances in medical imaging methods have enabled us to acquire high-resolution 4D images of the heart that capture the structural and functional characteristics of individual hearts. Our long term goal is the integration of the proposed framework with cine magnetic resonance imaging (cine-MRI), which is emerging as the method of choice for diagnosing a variety of cardiovascular disorders [1,2]. However, our framework can be used with any cardiac modality that gives spatio-temporal information, for example tagged cine-MRI, stimulated echo, CT. Computational challenges limit analysis to 3D (2D × time) motion estimation, where in fact 4D analysis would be preferable [3,4]. Segmentation of the ventricles and the myocardium is the first step toward quantitative functional analysis of cine-MRI data. However, segmentation is time consuming, thereby limiting clinical throughput [5]. Moreover, sometimes accuracy is limited by long-axis motion, and inter and intra-observer variability.

Related Work. To address these problems in motion reconstruction, one of the main thrusts in recent research has been 4D motion estimation using biomechanical models. There is significant work on the integration of imaging with cardiovascular mechanics. In [6], a piecewise linear composite biomechanical model was used to determine active forces and the strains in the heart based on tagged MRI information. In [7] MR images were combined with biomechanical models for cardiac motion estimation. Interactive segmentation was combined with a Bayesian estimation framework that was regularized by an anisotropic, passive, linearly elastic, myocardium model. The authors recognized the importance of neglecting active contraction of the left ventricle. In [8], the need for realistic simulations and the need for inversion and data assimilation was outlined. In [9], Kalman filters were used to recover the initial state of the heart and spatial abnormalities. That method however, is difficult to generalize to nonlinear inversion with time-dependent inversion parameters.

Overview of the Method. Given 4D imaging data of cardiac motion the main steps in our framework are the following: (**1**) segment the end-diastolic frame to myocardium, blood pool, and surrounding tissue; (**2**) register the segmented frame with a cardiac atlas in order to assign material properties and fiber-orientation information [10]; and (**3**) solve an inverse problem for forces along the fibers in the myocardium by minimizing an image-similarity functional, which is constrained by the biomechanical model of the heart. In this way, we explicitly couple raw image information with cardiac mechanics.

Contributions. We propose a biomechanically-constrained motion estimation algorithm that has the potential to address intra-individual motion estimation problems. We discuss formulation, numerical implementation, and we present preliminary verification tests that confirm the potential of the method. *The novelty of our approach is in the formulation and the algorithms (solvers and parallel implementation).* The main features of our scheme are (1) a patient-specific image-based inversion formulation for the active forces; (2) a octree-based, adaptive finite-element forward solver that incorporates anatomically-accurate fiber information; (3) an adjoint/Hessian-based inversion algorithm; and (4) a 4D coupled inversion for all images. This work builds on our previous work on parallel octree-based methods [11].

2   Formulation of the Inverse Problem

The basic premise of our formulation is the following: The heart motion is induced by the active forces in the myocardium. If we knew the exact biomechanical model for the myocardial tissue (constitutive law, geometry, fiber orientations, material properties for the heart and surrounding tissues, endocardial tractions due to blood flow) and the active stretching time-space profile, then we could solve a system of partial differential equations (PDEs) that describe the motion of the myocardial tissue for the displacements given the fiber forces; we refer to this system of PDEs (typically nonlinear elasticity) as the *"forward problem"*. Similarly, if we knew the displacements at certain locations in the myocardium, we could solve the so-called *"inverse problem"* to reconstruct active forces so that the motion due to the reconstructed forces matches the observed one. More generally, we have imaging data, typically cine-MRI, but not the displacements. We can still invert for the displacements; by solving a biomechanically-constrained image registration problem. In this context, an abstract formulation of the myocardium motion estimation problem is given by

$$\min_{u,s} \mathcal{J}(I_t, I_0, u) \quad \text{subject to} \quad \mathcal{C}(u,s) = 0. \qquad (1)$$

Here, $I_t := I_t(x,t)$ is the cine-MR image sequence with x,t denoting the space-time coordinates, $I_0 := I(x,0)$ is the end-diastolic frame, $u := u(x,t)$ is the *displacement* (motion), $s = s(x,t)$ is the active fiber contraction, and $\mathcal{C}$ is the forward problem operator. Also, $\mathcal{J}$ is an image similarity measure functional. This is a classical PDE-constrained inverse problem. Notice that there is no need for elastic, fluid, or any kind of regularization for u. It is constrained through the biomechanical model $\mathcal{C}$.[1]

Objective Function. (Operator $\mathcal{J}$). Different image similarity metrics can be used depending on the modality, like sum of squared differences and mutual information [12]. In this paper for simplicity, we consider point correspondences. We compute point-correspondences for all time frames, i.e., $d_j(t) := u(x_j,t)_{i=1}^M$ at M points. Then, the objective function is given by

$$\mathcal{J} := \int_0^1 (Qu - d)^2 \, dt := \int_0^1 \sum_{i=1}^M (u(x_j,t) - d_j(t))^2 \, dt, \qquad (2)$$

where Q is the so called spatial observation operator.

Forward Problem. (Operator $\mathcal{C}$). We make several approximations in our biophysical model. We assume a linear isotropic inhomogeneous elastic material for the myocardium; we ignore the geometric nonlinearities in both material response and active forces; we model the blood pool as an incompressible material with very small stiffness and large dissipation. We recognize that these are very strong assumptions but the model is meant to be driven by image data and assist in the motion reconstruction. More complex models, in particular nonlinear elasticity, will be incorporated in the future, if necessary. In addition to the constitutive assumptions, we assume a model for the active forces: given the fiber contractility s as a function of space and time, we define the active stretch tensor $U = \mathbf{I} + s\, n \otimes n$, whose divergence results in a distributed active force of the form $\text{div}(s\, n \otimes n)$; here $\mathbf{I}$ is the 3D identity matrix. Taken together, these assumptions result in the following form for $\mathcal{C}$:

$$M\ddot{u}(t) + C\dot{u}(t) + Ku(t) + As(t) = 0 \quad t \in (0,1). \qquad (3)$$

Using a Ritz-Galerkin formulation, with ϕ and ψ basis functions for u and s respectively, the expressions for M, K and $A(n)$ are given by $M_{ij} = \int \mathrm{I}(\phi_i \phi_j)$,

---

[1] However, one can show that the problem is ill-posed on s. Here we regularize by discretization of s.

$K = \int (\lambda + \mu) \nabla \phi_i \otimes \nabla \phi_j + \mu I (\nabla \phi_i \cdot \nabla \phi_j)$, $A_{ij} = \int (n \otimes n) \nabla \phi_i \psi_j$, and $C = \alpha M + \beta K$, with α and β viscous-damping parameters. Here, $\otimes$ is the outer vector product, and λ and μ are the Lamé constants. Equation (3) is derived by the Navier linear elastodynamics equation [13]. The domain of spatial integration (for M, K, and A) is the unit cube, corresponding to the image domain. In our formulation, we solve for the motion of *all the tissue* in the MR images. At the outer boundaries of the cube we impose homogeneous Neumann boundary conditions(zero traction). Also, we assume zero displacements and velocities as initial conditions.

Inverse Problem. The inverse problem is stated by (1) where $\mathcal{J}$ is given by (2) and $\mathcal{C}$ is given by (3). By introducing Lagrange multipliers p, the first-order optimality conditions for (1) can be written as:

$$M\ddot{u}(t) + C\dot{u}(t) + Ku(t) + As(t) = 0, \quad \dot{u}(0) = u(0) = 0,$$
$$M\ddot{p}(t) - C\dot{p}(t) + Kp(t) + Q^T(Qu - d) = 0, \quad \dot{p}(1) = p(1) = 0, \quad (4)$$
$$A^T p(t) = 0.$$

Equation (4) consists of a system of partial-differential equations for u (cardiac motion), p (adjoints), and s (active fiber contraction). It is a 4D boundary value problem since we have conditions prescribed at both $t = 0$ and $t = 1$.

Discretization and Solution Algorithms. We discretize the forward and adjoint problems in space using a Ritz-Galerkin formulation. We have developed a parallel data-structure and meshing scheme, discussed in [11]. The basis functions are trilinear, piecewise continuous polynomials. In time, we discretize using a Newmark scheme. The overall method is second-order accurate in space and time. The implicit steps in the Newmark scheme are performed using the method of Conjugate Gradients (CG) combined with a domain-decomposition preconditioner in which the local preconditioners are incomplete factorizations. The solver and the preconditioner are part of the PETSc package [14].

For these particular choices of objective function and forward problem the inverse problem (4) is linear in p, u, and s. We use a reduced space approach in which we employ a matrix-free CG algorithm for the Schur-complement of s; also called the (reduced) Hessian operator. Each matrix-vector multiplication with the Hessian requires one forward and one adjoint cardiac cycle simulation. One can show that the Hessian is ill-conditioned and the overall cost of the method can be quite high. Although, there are ways to accelerate the calculations, here we report results from a simple CG method. To reduce the computational cost for the calculations in the present paper, we used a reduced-order model for s in which ψ is a product of B-splines in time and radial functions in space (Gaussians). The activation s is parmeterized only when we solve the inverse problem. For the forward problem, we use the underlying finite element basis.

3 Results

We first describe the set of experiments performed to validate the motion estimation framework using synthetic datasets. This is followed by results using MR tagged images.

Tests on Synthetic Datasets for Verification. In order to assess the parametrized model of the forces, we use an ellipsoidal model of the left ventricle. The fiber orientations are generated by varying the elevation angle between the fiber and the short axis plane between $+60°$ and $-60°$ from the endocardium to the epicardium [15]. For this model we selected a Poisson's ratio $\nu = 0.45$ and a Young's modulus of 10 kPa for the myocardial tissue and 1 kPa for the surrounding tissue and ventricular cavity[2]. Raleigh damping ($C = \alpha M + \beta K$) was used with parameters $\alpha = 0$ and $\beta = 7.5 \times 10^{-4}$. In order to drive the forward model, we generated forces by propagating a synthetic activation wave from the apex to the base of the ventricles. The number of time steps were set to be 50. The motion field obtained by solving the forward problem was used to drive the inverse estimation. The relative residual tolerance for the forward solver (CG) was set to 10^{-8} and to 10^{-4} for the inverse solver.

Table 1. Error in recovery of activation for increasing number of radial basis functions. By changing the inversion solver accuracy, we can accelerate the calculation without compromising accuracy (e.g., the 4^3 calculation).

Basis Size	Relative Error (%)	Time
2^3	13.1	36 mins
4^3	5.67	≈ 5 hrs
4^3	11.2	108 mins
8^3	9.66	141 mins

Table 2. Error in the recovery of activation with partial observations of the displacements. Errors are reported on the ellipsoidal model for a grid size of 32 with 4^3 basis functions.

Observations	Relative Error (%)
Full	5.36×10^{-2}
1/8	6.21×10^{-2}
1/64	8.51×10^{-2}

We calculated the error in the estimation of the activations for different degrees of parametrization using the radial basis. In all cases, the time dependence of the force was parametrized by five B-splines. The relative error in the estimation of the activation for a 64^3 grid was computed for spatial parametrizations of 2^3, 4^3 and 8^3 and is tabulated in Table 1. In addition, we investigated the error in the estimation when only partial observations are available. We compared estimations based on full and sparse observations with 12% and 6% samples against the analytical solutions. These results are tabulated in Table 2. In order to assess the sensitivity of the motion estimation framework, we estimated the motion for the synthetic model of the heart at a grid size of 64 with a radial basis parametrization of 4^3 by adding noise to the system. We added a 5% random error on the estimates of the fiber orientation and to the material properties of

---

[2] We treat the blood pool as an incompressible solid with low shear resistance.

the myocardium. In addition, we added a 1% noise to the true displacements. The system converged and the relative error, in the L^2 norm, increased from 5.67×10^{-2} to 9.43×10^{-2}. Overall, the solution is not sensitive to the errors in the material properties (due to the well-posedness of the forward problem) and on the noise (due to the presence of model regularization).

Validation using Tagged MR Images. We acquired tagged MR sequences for 5 healthy volunteers, on a Siemens Sonata 1.5T^{TM} scanner, in order to validate our motion estimation algorithm. Three short axis and a single long axis grid tagged, segmented k-space breath-hold cine TurboFLASH images with image dimensions of 156x192 pixels and with pixel size of 1.14x1.14 mm^2 were acquired. The slice thickness was $8mm$. The displacements (observations) at the tag intersection points within the myocardium were computed manually. An average of 70-tag intersection points were selected over the left and right ventricles on each plane resulting in around 300 observations in space. Three independent observers processed all five datasets to get three sets of observations. To account for observer variability, we treated the mean location of the landmark as the ground truth observations.

The fiber orientations required for the biomechanical model were obtained using using *ex-vivo* DTI data and a tensor mapping method [10]. The end-diastolic MR image was segmented manually to assign material properties to the myocardial tissue, the blood and the surrounding tissue.

In three separate experiments, we used 70%, 50%, and 20% of the ground truth observations (selected per slice) as the data for the inversion. The observations that are not used during the inversion are the control observations and are used for assessing the goodness of the inversion. We used the B-spline and the radial bases to reduce the parameter space. We used a total of 4^3 spatial parameters, each with 5 B-spline temporal parameters, giving us a total of 320 parameters. We used a grid size of 64^3 for all inversions.

After inversion, one additional forward solve was performed using the dense estimates of the fiber contractions to obtain dense estimates of myocardial displacements. These displacements were compared with the ground truth displacements at the tag-intersection points. The relative error (as a percentage) and the absolute error in millimeters for all observations and restricted to only the control observations are shown in Table 3. The RMS errors over time for different levels of partial observations are plotted in Figures 1a-1c.

An alternate way of interpreting the results is to analyze the left-ventricular volume, obtained using manual segmentation and by the using the motion estimates, as seen for one particular subject in Figure 1d. The volume estimates using 70% and 50% observations are in general agreement with those obtained using manual segmentation. The volume estimated using 20% observations does not match very well with the manual segmentation, although the general trend is captured even when using only 20% observations.

Table 3. Results from tagged data using a 64^3 forward mesh size and an inverse parametrization of 4^3 spatial parameters and 5 temporal B-spline parameters. The percentage specifies the percentage of total observations that were used to drive the inverse optimization. The control observations are the remaining observations that were not used during the inverse optimizations and are used for validation purposes.

	Error (%) All obs.	Error (%) Control obs.	Error (mm) All obs.	Error (mm) Control Obs.
Observers	9.21	8.41	1.39	1.26
Algorithm 70%	12.46	14.22	1.88	2.13
Algorithm 50%	16.37	21.02	2.47	3.15
Algorithm 20%	41.61	51.19	6.28	7.67

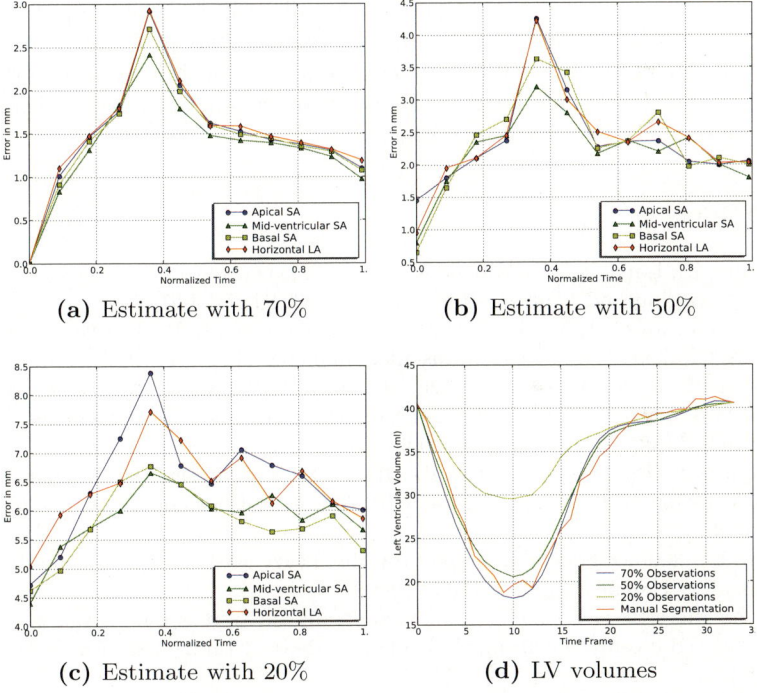

(a) Estimate with 70%   (b) Estimate with 50%

(c) Estimate with 20%   (d) LV volumes

Fig. 1. Comparison of the RMS errors over time for the motion estimation algorithm using partial observations. Motion estimation was performed using (a)70%, (b)50% and (c)20% partial observations, and the errors are plotted as a function of time for each of the partial observation cases. (d) Left ventricular volume of a selected subject, segmented automatically and by manually over all frames in a cardiac cycle.

4 Conclusions

We presented a method for cardiac motion reconstruction. We integrate tagged-MR images and a biomechanical model that accounts for inhomogeneous tissue properties, fiber information, and active forces. We presented an inversion algorithm. Using only a total of 320 parameters we were able to reconstruct the 4D cardiac motion quite accurately.

The limitations of our current implementation (but not the method) is the assumptions of linear geometric and material response and the potential bias due to template-based fibers that does not account for anatomical variability, that is still requires some preprocessing of the initial frame to assign material properties and fiber orientation, that assumes zero residual stresses and initial conditions, and that it does not include an electrophysiology model.

Our on-going work includes transition to an intensity-based image-registration inversion (in which case we need to solve a nonlinear inversion) and its clinical validation by reconstructing motions of normal and abnormal populations and conducting statistical analysis. Among the many open problems are the level of required model complexity for clinically relevant motion reconstructions, the bias of the fibers, the sensitivity to the values of the material properties, and the sensitivity to the image similarity functional.

References

1. Castillo, E., Lima, J.A.C., Bluemke, D.A.: Regional myocardial function: Advances in MR imaging and analysis. Radiographics 23, S127–S140 (2003)
2. Shah, D.J., Judd, R.M., Kim, R.J.: Technology insight: MRI of the myocardium. Nature Clinical Practice Cardiovascular Medicine 2(11), 597–605 (2005)
3. O'Donnell, T., Funka-Lea, G., Tek, H., Jolly, M.P., Rasch, M., Setser, R.: Comprehensive cardiovascular image analysis using MR and CT at Siemens Corporate Research. IJCV 70(2), 165–178 (2006)
4. Sampath, S., Prince, J.L.: Automatic 3D tracking of cardiac material markers using slice-following and harmonic-phase MRI. Magnetic Resonance Imaging 25(2), 197–208 (2007)
5. Axel, L.: Biomechanical dynamics of the heart with MRI. Annual Review of Biomedical Engineering 4, 321–347 (2002)
6. Hu, Z., Metaxas, D., Axel, L.: In vivo strain and stress estimation of the heart left and right ventricles from MRI images. Medical Image Analysis 7(4), 435–444 (2003)
7. Papademetris, X., Sinusas, A.J., Dione, D.P., Constable, R.T., Duncan, J.S.: Estimation of 3-D left ventricular deformation from medical images using biomechanical models. IEEE Trans. on Medical Imaging 21(7), 786 (2002)
8. Sermesant, M., Moireau, P., Camara, O., Sainte-Marie, J., Andriantsimiavona, R., Cimrman, R., Hill, D., Chapelle, D., Razavi, R.: Cardiac function estimation from MRI using a heart model and data assimilation: Advances and difficulties. Medical Image Analysis 10(4), 642–656 (2006)
9. Moireau, P., Chapelle, D., Le Tallec, P.: Joint state and parameter estimation for distributed mechanical systems. Computer Methods in Applied Mechanics and Engineering 197, 659–677 (2008)

10. Sundar, H., Sampath, R.S., Biros, G.: Bottom-up construction and 2:1 balance refinement of linear octrees in parallel. SIAM Journal on Scientific Computing 30(5), 2675–2708 (2008)
11. Sundar, H., Sampath, R.S., Adavani, S.S., Davatzikos, C., Biros, G.: Low-constant parallel algorithms for finite element simulations using linear octrees. In: ACM/IEEE SCXY Conference Series (2007)
12. Zitová, B., Flusser, J.: Image registration methods: a survey. Image Vision Comput. 21(11), 977–1000 (2003)
13. Gurtin, M.E.: An Introduction to Continuum Mechanics. Academic Press, London (1981)
14. Balay, S., Buschelman, K., Gropp, W.D., Kaushik, D., Knepley, M.G., McInnes, L.C., Smith, B.F., Zhang, H.: PETSc home page (2001), http://www.mcs.anl.gov/petsc
15. Sachse, F.B.: Computational Cardiology. LNCS, vol. 2966. Springer, Heidelberg (2004)

Predictive Simulation of Bidirectional Glenn Shunt Using a Hybrid Blood Vessel Model

Hao Li[1,2], Wee Kheng Leow[1,2], and Ing-Sh Chiu[3]

[1] Dept. of Computer Science, National University of Singapore, Singapore
[2] Image & Pervasive Access Lab (IPAL), UMI CNRS Singapore
[3] Dept. of Surgery, National Taiwan University Hospital, Taipei, Taiwan
{lihao,leowwk}@comp.nus.edu.sg, ingsh@ntu.edu.tw

Abstract. This paper proposes a method for performing predictive simulation of cardiac surgery. It applies a hybrid approach to model the deformation of blood vessels. The hybrid blood vessel model consists of a reference Cosserat rod and a surface mesh. The reference Cosserat rod models the blood vessel's global bending, stretching, twisting and shearing in a physically correct manner, and the surface mesh models the surface details of the blood vessel. In this way, the deformation of blood vessels can be computed efficiently and accurately. Our predictive simulation system can produce complex surgical results given a small amount of user inputs. It allows the surgeon to easily explore various surgical options and evaluate them. Tests of the system using bidirectional Glenn shunt (BDG) as an application example show that the results produced by the system are similar to real surgical results.

1 Introduction

Many cardiac surgeries for correcting congenital heart defects, such as arterial switch operations and bidirectional Glenn shunt [1], involve complex operations on the cardiac blood vessels. At present, cardiac surgeons mostly rely on echocardiography, cardiac catheterization and CT images of a patient's heart to examine the specific anatomical anomalies of the patient. Without appropriate surgical planning and visualization tool, they often resort to manual drawings to visualize the surgical procedures and the expected surgical results. This approach is imprecise and is impossible to provide details of the possible outcome of the surgical procedures. To improve the precision and effectiveness of cardiac surgery planning, novel surgical simulation systems are desired.

Among existing surgical simulation systems, *reactive* systems (e.g., [2,3]) attempt to simulate real-time displacement and deformation of body tissues in response to user inputs that emulate surgical operations. They are useful for training and navigational planning of surgical operations. However, to use a reactive system to predict results of complex surgeries, the surgeon would need to go through all the detailed surgical steps, which is tedious and time-consuming.

In contrast, *predictive* simulation systems (e.g., [4]) aim at efficiently producing complex surgical results based on the physical properties of the anatomies and a small amount of user inputs that indicate the surgical options. In this way, the surgeon can easily explore various surgical options and evaluate the predicted surgical results without going through the surgical details.

This paper illustrates a predictive simulation system for bidirectional Glenn shunt (BDG), which is a very important cardiac surgery for the treatment of several congenital heart defects (Sec. 3). In the predictive simulation of BDG, as in the simulation of other surgical procedures that involve soft tissues, the model objects should deform according to their physical properties. In addition, the deformation of the blood vessels should comply with an additional constraint: they should not be overly stretched or twisted to avoid obstruction of blood flow. This constraint translates to the requirement of modeling global strains such as bending, stretching and twisting of the blood vessels.

Blood vessel deformation can be modeled using 3D finite elements [5] or thin shell models [6,7]. These methods are in general computationally expensive. For reactive simulation, mass spring model has been applied to the simulation of cardiac tissue and blood vessel deformation [2,3]. However, its simulation accuracy highly depends on careful placements of springs between mass points, which may not have physical correlates. More importantly, these general surface/volume deformation methods do not explicitly model global bending and twisting, which are important characteristics of blood vessels.

To meet the requirement of modeling global strains in the predictive simulation of BDG, this paper presents a hybrid approach for modeling blood vessel deformation (Sec. 2). The hybrid blood vessel model binds a surface mesh elastically to a reference Cosserat rod [8]. The mesh model represents the surface details of the blood vessel while the reference rod models global bending, stretching, twisting and shearing of the vessel. Deformation of the hybrid model is accomplished by first deforming the reference rod according to Cosserat theory, then deforming the mesh according to its binding to the rod and its surface elastic energy. This approach allows the blood vessel to deform in a physically correct manner in relation to its global strains. It also allows the surface to deform realistically and efficiently. Moreover, the hybrid model provides structural information of the blood vessel, thus reducing the amount of user inputs that indicate surgical options (Sec. 3). Experimental results (Sec. 4) confirm the effectiveness of our model in the predictive simulation of BDG. Note that although the example application in this paper is BDG, our blood vessel model is general enough for the predictive simulation of other complex cardiac surgeries.

In comparison to our work, existing reactive simulation systems of cardiac surgery [2,3] focus on low-level operations such as incision and retraction of the heart [2,3] and suturing of ventricular septal defect [2], rather than complex operations on the cardiac blood vessels. For predictive simulation of cardiac surgery, Li et al. [4] applied differential geometry approach to predict the surgical results of aorta reconstruction. The predictive simulation idea is in spirit similar to that of this paper. However, the deformation approach adopted in [4] is a pure geometrical approach, which is not necessarily accurate. Moreover, it took into consideration only the surface elastic energies and did not model the global strains of blood vessels. Although torsion energy can be approximated as described in [9], it is nontrivial to incorporate the torsion energy term to affect the behavior of the blood vessel model.

2 Hybrid Blood Vessel Model

Our hybrid model of a blood vessel consists of a reference Cosserat rod and a surface mesh of the blood vessel (Fig. 2.1). For a given surface mesh of a blood vessel, we construct the hybrid model by fitting a reference rod to the centerline of the surface using the technique described in [9,10]. A binding relationship between the surface model and the reference rod is then established. The deformation of the blood vessel is achieved by first deforming the reference rod according to Cosserat theory [8] (Sec. 2.1), then deforming the mesh model according to the surface elastic energy in terms of surface bending and stretching, and the established binding relationship to the reference rod (Sec. 2.2).

2.1 Cosserat Rod

A Cosserat rod C [8] is represented by a 3D curve $\mathbf{r}(s)$ and orthonormal directors $\mathbf{d}_k(s)$, with $k \in \{1, 2, 3\}$ and the arc length parameter $s \in [0, L]$. $\mathbf{d}_3(s)$ is normal to the cross-sectional plane $\mathcal{X}_s$ of the rod at s. $\mathbf{d}_1(s)$ and $\mathbf{d}_2(s)$ are in $\mathcal{X}_s$ and point at two material points on the rod's surface (Fig. 2.1).

The strains of a Cosserat rod are expressed as *linear strain vector* $\boldsymbol{v}(s)$ and *angular strain vector* $\boldsymbol{u}(s)$ [8] such that

$$\boldsymbol{v}(s) = \partial_s \mathbf{r}(s), \quad \partial_s \mathbf{d}_k(s) = \boldsymbol{u}(s) \times \mathbf{d}_k(s), \quad k \in \{1, 2, 3\}. \tag{1}$$

The strain vectors $\boldsymbol{u}(s)$ and $\boldsymbol{v}(s)$ can be resolved into three components by the directors $\mathbf{d}_k$ to yield the *strain variables* u_k and v_k:

$$u_k = \boldsymbol{u} \cdot \mathbf{d}_k, \quad v_k = \boldsymbol{v} \cdot \mathbf{d}_k, \quad k \in \{1, 2, 3\}. \tag{2}$$

Together with global translation and rotation of the rod, u_k and v_k define the rod's configuration, i.e., $\mathbf{r}$ and $\mathbf{d}_k$. The components u_1 and u_2 are the curvatures along $\mathbf{d}_1$ and $\mathbf{d}_2$ which measure the bending of the rod, while u_3 measures twisting. The components v_1 and v_2 measure shear, and v_3 measures stretching. Let us denote

$$\mathbf{u} \equiv [u_1, u_2, u_3]^\top, \quad \mathbf{v} \equiv [v_1, v_2, v_3]^\top. \tag{3}$$

Assuming the Kirchhoff constitutive relations, the couple (i.e., inner torque) $\mathbf{m}(s)$ and stress $\mathbf{n}(s)$ experienced by the rod are

$$\mathbf{m}(s) = \mathbf{J}(s)(\mathbf{u}(s) - \mathbf{u}^0(s)), \quad \mathbf{n}(s) = \mathbf{K}(s)(\mathbf{v}(s) - \mathbf{v}^0(s)), \tag{4}$$

where $\mathbf{J}(s)$ and $\mathbf{K}(s)$ are stiffness matrices that depend on the geometric moments of inertia and material properties of the rod, and $\mathbf{u}^0(s)$ and $\mathbf{v}^0(s)$ are the strain values in the initial configuration. The potential energy of the rod is [8]:

$$\mathcal{E} = \frac{1}{2} \int_0^L \left[\left(\mathbf{u}(s) - \mathbf{u}^0(s)\right)^\top \mathbf{m}(s) + \left(\mathbf{v}(s) - \mathbf{v}^0(s)\right)^\top \mathbf{n}(s) \right] ds. \tag{5}$$

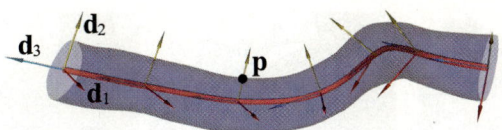

Fig. 1. A hybrid blood vessel model with its reference rod, directors and surface mesh

Given boundary conditions on the positions $\mathbf{r}$ or the directors $\mathbf{d}_k$, the deformed configuration $C^t = \{\mathbf{r}^t, \mathbf{d}_k^t\}$ is the equilibrium state of the rod, with minimum potential energy $\mathcal{E}$ that minimizes the difference between the strains.

2.2 Blood Vessel Surface Deformation

Binding Surface to Cosserat Rod. If the cross-sections do not change, the surface of a blood vessel can be considered as a shape function defined by the reference Cosserat rod. For each mesh vertex $\mathbf{p}$, there exists an s such that $\mathbf{p}$ is on the cross-section $\mathcal{X}_s$ of the blood vessel at s. A one-to-one mapping function $\mathbf{f}$ can then be established between the local coordinates (x, y, z) in the directors $\mathbf{d}_k$ at s and the global coordinates $\mathbf{p}$:

$$\mathbf{p} = \mathbf{f}(s, x, y, z) = \mathbf{r}(s) + x\,\mathbf{d}_1(s) + y\,\mathbf{d}_2(s) + z\,\mathbf{d}_3(s). \qquad (6)$$

In the initial configuration, the local coordinates (x, y, z) for each mesh vertex are computed from the initial reference rod. When the reference Cosserat rod deforms, function $\mathbf{f}$ defines the reference binding position $\mathbf{p}'$ of the mesh vertex $\mathbf{p}$ in the deformed configuration. The elastic binding energy between the surface mesh and the reference Cosserat rod can then be defined as:

$$E_c(\mathbf{p}) = k_c \|\mathbf{p} - \mathbf{p}'\|_2^2, \qquad (7)$$

where k_c is the corresponding binding coefficient.

Surface Bending and Stretching. When a blood vessel deforms, its surface undergoes stretching and bending, which incur stretching and bending energies. For discrete meshes, various techniques have been presented to approximate the energies (e.g., [7]). Since stretching and bending are essentially non-linear characteristics, the resulting deformable model are usually non-linear, which may be computationally costly.

One efficient way to approximate the bending energy is to use Laplacian operators [11,12]. Since Laplacian is a linear operator, it is rotation variant. Traditional ways of achieving rotation-invariant Laplacian is to approximate the rotation of Laplacian from known handle vertices [12] or by using multi-resolution hierarchies [11]. In our model, rotation-invariance is achieved by measuring the Laplacians with respect to the directors of the reference rod, which are intrinsic properties of the rod. This is a more natural approach to achieving rotation invariance of Laplacian for tubular objects like blood vessels. Therefore, the reference Cosserat rod serves the important roles of modeling global strains of

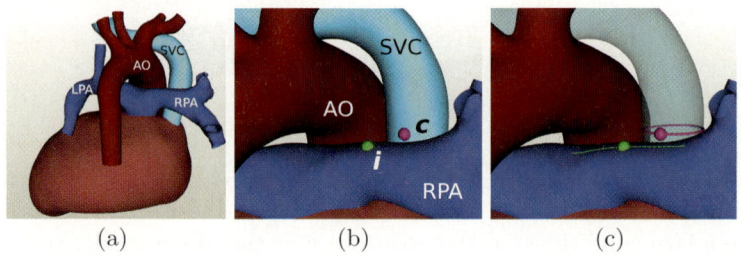

(a) (b) (c)

Fig. 2. Models and inputs. (a) Heart and blood vessel models reconstructed from a patient's CT images. (b) User input points to indicate surgical options. (c) Cross-sectional cut path and incision path generated by the system.

the blood vessel, as well as achieving rotation-invariant Laplacians. The surface bending energy at a vertex $\mathbf{p}$ with its Laplacian $\mathbf{l}(\mathbf{p})$ is:

$$E_b(\mathbf{p}) = k_b \|\mathbf{l}(\mathbf{p}) - \mathbf{R}(\mathbf{p})\,\mathbf{l}^0(\mathbf{p})\|_2^2, \qquad (8)$$

where $\mathbf{l}^0(\mathbf{p})$ is the Laplacian of $\mathbf{p}$ in the initial configuration, $\mathbf{R}(\mathbf{p})$ is the rotation of the corresponding directors, and k_b is the bending stiffness.

Surface stretching energy is measured by the change of edge lengths similar to [7]. For an edge $\mathbf{e}$ that connects vertices $\mathbf{p}_i$ and $\mathbf{p}_j$, the stretching energy is:

$$E_s(\mathbf{e}) = k_s \left(\|\mathbf{p}_i - \mathbf{p}_j\| - \|\mathbf{p}_i^0 - \mathbf{p}_j^0\|\right)^2, \qquad (9)$$

where k_s is the stretching stiffness related to the Young's modulus, and $\|\mathbf{p}_i^0 - \mathbf{p}_j^0\|$ is the edge length in the initial configuration.

The total surface deformation energy to be minimized is thus:

$$E = E_c + E_b + E_s. \qquad (10)$$

Note that the binding and bending terms are both linear. The stretching term, although non-linear, can be solved efficiently in an iterative way described in [13]. Hence, the overall surface deformation can be achieved efficiently.

3 Predictive Simulation of Bidirectional Glenn Shunt

Bidirectional Glenn shunt (BDG) is a very important operation involved in the treatment of several congenital heart detects such as tricuspid atresia, hypoplastic left heart syndrome, and single ventricle anomalies [1]. It is performed by first detaching the superior vena cava (SVC) from the heart through a cross-sectional cut on the SVC, then making an incision on the top side of the right pulmonary artery (RPA), and connecting the distal end of the SVC to the top side of RPA. After BDG, venous blood from the head and upper limbs will pass directly to the lungs, bypassing the right ventricle such that the volume load on the ventricle will be decreased and the oxygen saturation will be improved.

In the surgical planning of BDG, the surgeon needs to decide: a) the position of the cross-sectional cut on the SVC to detach it from the heart; b) the incision path on the top side of the RPA; c) the correspondence between the two joining boundaries to join the SVC and RPA with minimum twisting.

These decisions should be carefully made for every patient to reduce the potential risk (e.g., obstruction of blood flow) and to improve the long-term outcome. In addition, the surrounding cardiac structures (e.g., the aorta and the heart) limit the desirable deformation of the SVC and RPA, making the surgical decisions very crucial.

3.1 Predictive Simulation Algorithm

Our predictive simulation system allows the user to simply pick a point on the SVC and RPA respectively to indicate the surgical decision (Fig. 2(b)). It then automatically predicts the result of BDG with minimum blood vessel deformation. The simulation algorithm consists of the following three steps:

Step 1. Given the cut position **c** on the SVC (Fig. 2(b)), the algorithm computes its projection to the reference rod of SVC to get the parameter s and the cross-sectional plane $\mathcal{X}_s$ of the reference rod (Fig. 2(c)). The surface is cut by this cross-sectional plane and the reference rod is split into two parts.

Step 2. Given the incision point **i** on the RPA (Fig. 2(b)), an incision path is drawn on RPA's surface (Fig. 2(c)) such that it is parallel to RPA's reference rod and the mid-point of the path is the input point **i**. The length of the incision path is determined by the perimeter of the distal end of the cut SVC.

Step 3. The point correspondence between the two joining boundaries is established such that the center of the distal end of SVC is aligned with point **i**, and the director $\mathbf{d}_3$ is normal to the surface of RPA. Next, the deformation algorithm is applied to solve for the final configuration that minimizes the Cosserat rod energy $\mathcal{E}$ (Eq. 5), the surface energy E (Eq. 10), and an additional spring energy introduced to join the corresponding points of the two boundaries.

The final configuration illustrates the expected surgical results based on the given surgical decision, which is the minimally deformed configuration. In addition, the system also illustrates a way of cutting and joining the blood vessels with minimum deformation.

4 Tests and Discussions

For testing our hybrid model, a straight tube (Fig. 3(a)) was constructed to model a real elastic tube that the surgeon uses to emulate blood vessels during surgery planning. Figure 3(b, c) compares the bending and twisting deformation of the model and that of the real tube, which was manipulated by hand at its two ends. The similarity of our tube model to the real tube shows the correctness of our hybrid approach in simulating tubular object deformation. Figure 3(d)

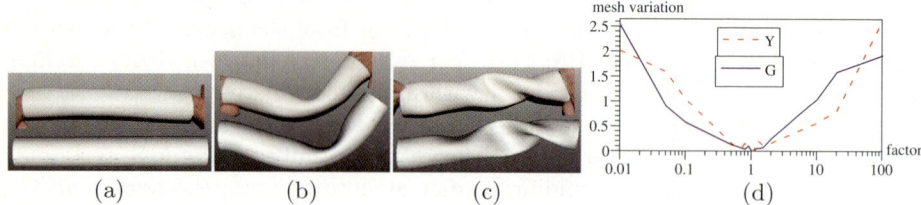

Fig. 3. Deformation of hybrid model (lower) in comparison with real elastic tube manipulated by hand (upper). (a) Initial configuration, (b) bending, (c) twisting. (d) Mesh variation with respect to change of Young's (Y) and shear (G) moduli.

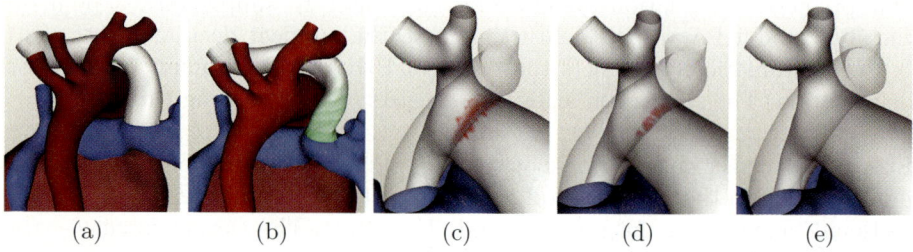

Fig. 4. Predicted surgical results of various surgical options. (a) Desired result, free of congestion and twisting. (b) Result with undesirable twisting indicated in green. (c–e) Different selections of cut points on SVC result in different amount of pressure due to collision with aorta. SVC's are made semi-transparent to illustrate the pressure in red.

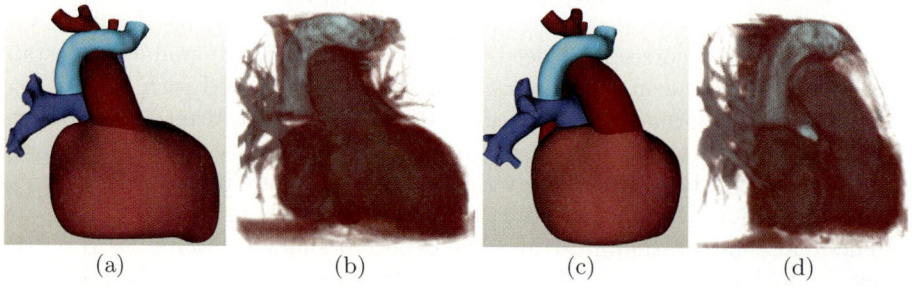

Fig. 5. Comparison of (a, c) simulation results with (b, d) volume rendering of postoperative CT data. (a, b) Frontal view. (c, d) Side view.

illustrates mesh variation with respect to change of material property in simulating the twisting example (Fig. 3(c)). The Young's and shear moduli varied from their default values with a factor ranging from 0.01 to 100. Figure 3(d) shows that the deformation algorithm is robust, i.e., produces small mesh variation with small change of material property. The slight fluctuation of the curves for factors close to 1 may be attributed to the non-linear behavior of the model and numerical error in discrete optimization.

For testing the predictive simulation algorithm, 3D mesh models of the heart, aorta, pulmonary artery and superior vena cava were segmented and reconstructed from a patient's CT images (Fig. 2(a)), and the hybrid models were constructed. For blood vessels with branches such as the aorta and pulmonary trunk, the major branches can also be modeled using the hybrid model with reference rods connected to the reference rod of the main trunk, thus constructing a tree structure of rods. The BDG simulation algorithm was performed on the blood vessel models to join the SVC to the RPA. Various surgical options were tested as inputs for evaluating the predicted surgical results.

Figure 4(a) shows a desired surgical result which is free of congestion and twisting. Explicit modeling of global strains in our model allows strain values to be easily visualized. For example, by intentionally rotating the distal end of SVC, undesirable twisting of SVC was produced and visualized (Fig. 4(b)). The selection of the cut position on the SVC is crucial since it affects the length of the cut SVC. As shown in Figure 4(c–e), when the cut SVC was too short, it collided with the aorta thus resulting in pressure on both vessels (Fig. 4(c)). The pressure decreased with increasing SVC length (Fig. 4(d)), and became zero when the cut SVC was long enough to avoid collision (Fig. 4(e)).

Note that quantitative validation of the predictive simulation system is difficult to achieve because the reconstructed 3D models cannot be exact due to errors in CT scanning and image segmentation. Moreover, the blood vessel shape is affected by other factors such as blood pressure. Therefore, this paper presents only a qualitative validation by comparing the simulation result with the volume data of the patient's postoperative CT rendered by VTK [14]. Frontal and side views of the volume rendering were selected such that the SVC and aorta can be clearly seen. Figure 5 shows that the shapes of the blood vessels in our simulation result are similar to those in the volume data. The heart model differs somewhat from the real heart due to segmentation error and rendering effects.

The above tests were carried out on a 2.33 GHz Core 2 Duo PC. The execution time for BDG simulation is on average 10 seconds, with the blood vessel models containing a total of 24,393 vertices (AO: 8,995, PA: 9,824, VC: 5,574).

5 Conclusion

This paper presented a predictive simulation system for bidirectional Glenn shunt (BDG) in cardiac surgery. The system uses a hybrid approach to model blood vessel deformation. The hybrid model binds a reference Cosserat rod and a surface mesh elastically. The reference rod models the global strains of the blood vessel in a physically correct manner, while the 3D mesh models the surface details of the blood vessel. In this way, blood vessel deformation can be achieved accurately and efficiently. Our blood vessel model also provides structural information that facilitates predictive simulation procedure. Experiments and qualitative validation confirm the feasibility and effectiveness of the hybrid blood vessel model for the predictive simulation of BDG.

References

1. Gardner, T.J., Spray, T.L.: Operative Cardiac Surgery, 5th edn. Arnold (2004)
2. Sørensen, T.S., Greil, G.F., Hansen, O.K., Mosegaard, J.: Surgical simulation - a new tool to evaluate surgical incisions in congenital heart disease? Interact. CardioVasc. Thorac. Surg. 5(5), 536–539 (2006)
3. Mosegaard, J.: LR-spring mass model for cardiac surgical simulation. In: Proc. MMVR, pp. 256–258 (2004)
4. Li, H., Leow, W.K., Chiu, I.S.: Modeling torsion of blood vessels in surgical simulation and planning. In: Proc. MMVR, pp. 153–158 (2009)
5. Nealen, A., Müller, M., Keiser, R., Boxermann, E., Carlson, M.: Physically based deformable models in computer graphics. In: Proc. Eurographics, pp. 71–94 (2005)
6. Terzopoulos, D., Platt, J., Barr, A., Fleischer, K.: Elastically deformable models. In: Proc. ACM SIGGRAPH, pp. 205–214 (1987)
7. Grinspun, E.: A discrete model of thin shells. In: SIGGRAPH Courses (2006)
8. Antman, S.S.: Nonlinear Problems of Elasticity. Springer, Heidelberg (1995)
9. Li, H., Leow, W.K., Qi, Y., Chiu, I.S.: Predictive surgical simulation of aorta reconstruction in cardiac surgery. In: Proc. MMVR, pp. 159–161 (2009)
10. Kirchberg, K.J., Wimmer, A., Lorenz, C.H.: Modeling the human aorta for MR-driven real-time virtual endoscopy. In: Proc. MICCAI, pp. 470–477 (2006)
11. Botsch, M., Sorkine, O.: On linear variational surface deformation methods. IEEE Trans. on Visualization and Computer Graphics 14(1), 213–230 (2008)
12. Masuda, H., Yoshioka, Y., Furukawa, Y.: Interactive mesh deformation using equality-constrained least squares. Computers & Graphics 30(6), 936–946 (2006)
13. Weng, Y., Xu, W., Wu, Y., Zhou, K., Guo, B.: 2D shape deformation using non-linear least squares optimization. The Visual Computer 22(9), 653–660 (2006)
14. Kitware, Inc.: The Visualization Toolkit, http://www.vtk.org

Surgical Planning and Patient-Specific Biomechanical Simulation for Tracheal Endoprostheses Interventions

Miguel A. González Ballester[1], Amaya Pérez del Palomar[2],
José Luís López Villalobos[3], Laura Lara Rodríguez[1], Olfa Trabelsi[2], Frederic Pérez[1],
Ángel Ginel Cañamaque[3], Emilia Barrot Cortés[3], Francisco Rodríguez Panadero[3],
Manuel Doblaré Castellano[2], and Javier Herrero Jover[1,4]

[1] Alma IT Systems, Barcelona, Spain
[2] Group of Structural Mechanics and Material Modelling, University of Zaragoza, Spain
[3] Medico-Surgical Dept. of Respiratory Diseases, Virgen del Rocío Hospital, Seville, Spain
[4] Centro Médico Teknon, Barcelona, Spain
Miguel.Gonzalez@alma3d.com

Abstract. We have developed a system for computer-assisted surgical planning of tracheal surgeries. The system allows to plan the intervention based on CT images of the patient, and includes a virtual database of commercially available prostheses. Automatic segmentation of the trachea and apparent pathological structures is obtained using a modified region growing algorithm. A method for automatic adaptation of a finite element mesh allows to build a patient-specific biomechanical model for simulation of the expected performance of the implant under physiological movement (swallowing, sneezing). Laboratory experiments were performed to characterise the tissues present in the trachea, and movement models were obtained from fluoroscopic images of a patient. Results are reported on the planning and biomechanical simulation of two patients that underwent surgery at our hospital.

1 Introduction

A number of pathologies affecting the trachea exist, both benign and malignant, leading to the obstruction of the airways and, ultimately, to asphyxia. Tracheostomy consists in performing an orifice in the trachea, distal to the obstruction, to ensure access to the air. This type of procedures – reported as early as 3.600 b.C. – have evolved towards new therapeutic variants, leading to the design of modern tracheal endoprostheses and stents 1.

Preoperative planning of tracheal surgery is performed nowadays on CT or MR images of the patient. Planning includes the selection of the material, type and placement of the prosthesis, and these choices are largely influenced by the previous experience of the surgeon. Further, planning based on a single static image of the patient does not portray the behaviour of the implant under stress conditions derived from physiological movements (swallowing, sneezing, etc.).

We have developed a system for computer-aided planning and simulation, allowing to explore the anatomy of the patient and automatically segment the trachea and any apparent pathological structures. A database of models of commercially available tracheal implants permits to select and virtually position the implant of choice. Finally, the established plan is used as initial condition for biomechanical simulations of swallowing movement. Prior to such simulations, laboratory experiments were performed to characterise the tissues present in the trachea and thus build realistic constitutive models.

We present our framework for surgical planning (section 2) and biomechanical simulation (section 3). Results are presented on data from 2 patients that underwent tracheal surgery with the implantation of an endoprosthesis (section 4).

2 Surgical Planning

We have developed a software for surgical planning of tracheal implants. The tool supports full connectivity to PACS systems and DICOM conformance, as well as professional 2D, MPR and 3D volume rendering capabilities for the exploration of the data sets. We have implemented an implant database integrated into the GUI of the application, allowing to explore the full range of implant models and sizes commercially available, and including CAD models of each of them for virtual placement. Intuitive manipulation tools allow to fine tune the selection and placement of the implant, and determine potential complications due to factors such as the distance to the vocal chords and the tracheal wall.

2.1 Automatic Segmentation of the Trachea

Several segmentation methods for automatic identification and delineation of the trachea in CT images have been tested, ranging from basic thresholding algorithms

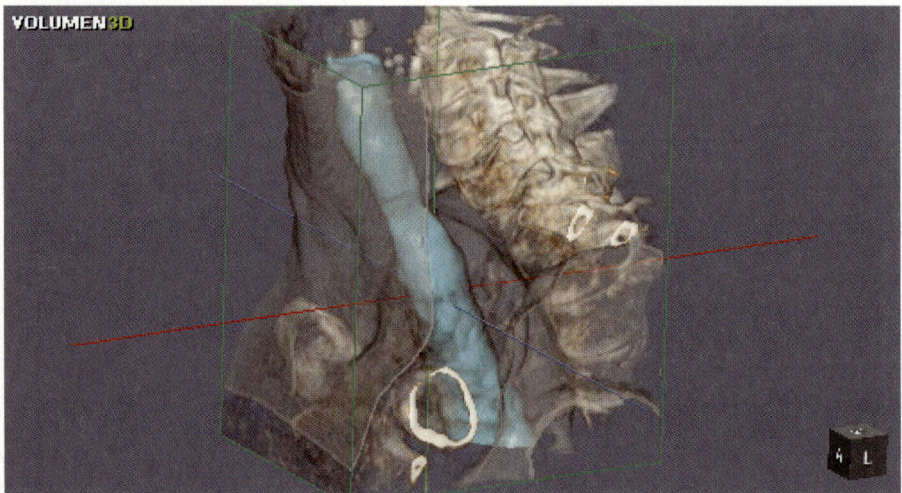

Fig. 1. Automatic segmentation of the trachea (shown in blue) based on anisotropic diffusion, region growing and morphological operations. An alternative approach based on level sets was tested and yielded similar results at higher computational cost.

to sophisticated level-set evolution techniques 2. Based on criteria such as speed, robustness and minimum user interaction, we designed an adapted region growing method consisting of the following steps:

1) anisotropic diffusion 3;
2) adaptive region growing 4;
3) morphological operations for segmentation refinement 5.

Segmentation results were validated by surgeons on 30 cases, via detailed visual inspection. An example of the application of this algorithm to one of our datasets is shown in figure 1.

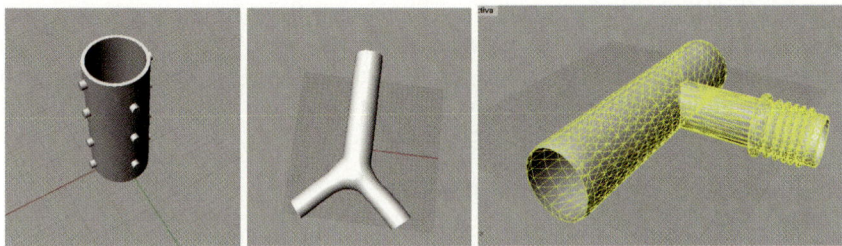

Fig. 2. A database of virtual models of commercially available tracheal endoprostheses was implemented. This allows to make multiple simulations using different implant models and sizes.

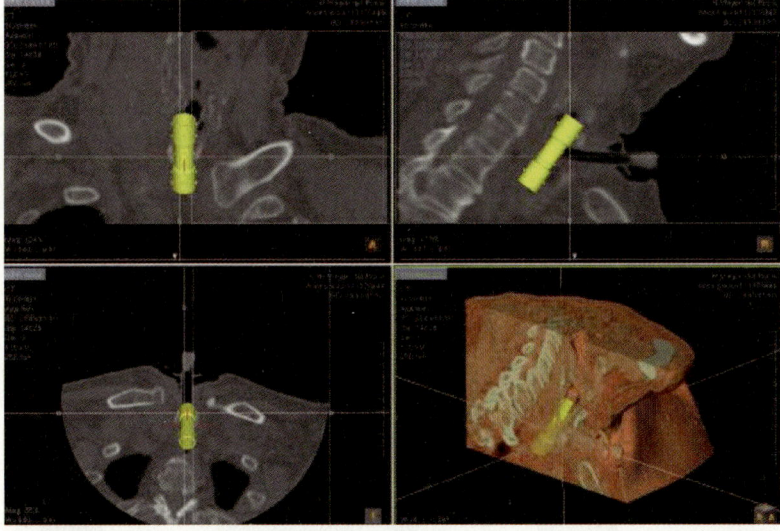

Fig. 3. Planning module for virtual placement of tracheal implants. A preoperative CT scan is used as reference to plan the position and orientation of the chosen implant. The plan is stored and further used for biomechanical simulations.

2.2 Implant Database and Virtual Placement

We have created 3D models of a total of 93 prostheses of different models and sizes (figure 2). These models have been incorporated into our software as a "virtual catalogue". Once a model has been selected, the 3D representation of the implant is shown on the patient's image data. An intuitive 3D interface allows to virtually position and align the prosthesis (figure 3).

3 Biomechanical Simulation

The choice of implant model, size and position has been made based on a single static CT image of the patient. However, as part of its normal function, the trachea undergoes demanding physiological movements that have an important effect on the performance and lifespan of the prosthesis. To take this into account, we create a patient-specific biomechanical model of the trachea and the implant, and perform finite element simulations to predict the dynamic behaviour and thus identify possible risks due to excessive stress on the tracheal walls.

3.1 Patient-Specific Models of the Trachea

We built a detailed finite element mesh including all tissues present in the trachea. This model was constructed from a CT data set of a subject with no tracheal pathology, using the segmentation method described above and the commercial meshing software packages: PATRAN (MSC, Santa Ana, USA) and I-DEAS (Siemens PLM, Plano, USA). The resulting mesh contains 28.350 hexahedral elements, grouped into 3 groups: membrane, tracheal muscle, and cricoid and thyroid cartilage (figure 4, left).

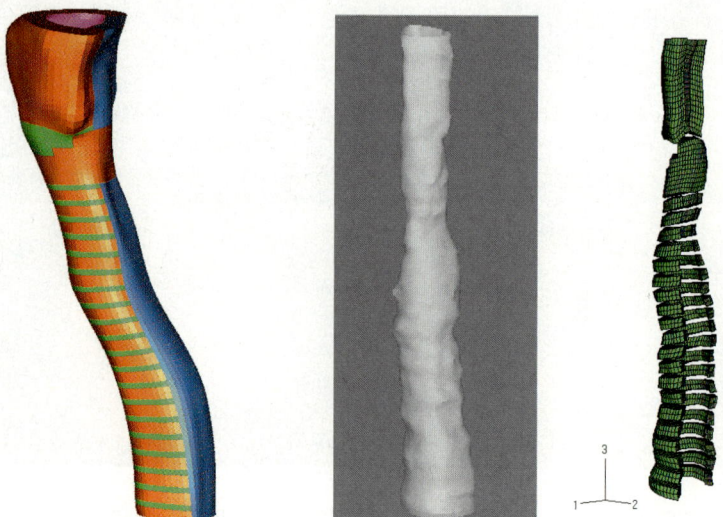

Fig. 4. Complete finite element model of the human trachea, including cartilage (red), muscle (blue), internal membrane (green). On the right, automatic adaptation of the finite element mesh (cartilage is shown) to a new tracheal geometry, in this case with a stenosis, obtained by deforming the mesh to the segmented tracheal surface of a patient (middle).

This mesh can be adapted to the particular patient's anatomy by deforming it to match the segmented internal and external surfaces of the patient's trachea. To this end, first a surface matching process is used to find correspondences between these surfaces and the nodes of the mesh defining the internal and external surfaces in the model. Using these correspondences, a simple elastic transformation is applied to deform the complete mesh (solved as a linear perturbation problem using the commercial software ABAQUS, DSS, Providence, USA). Thus, an automatic procedure can be followed to construct finite element models of each patient in a matter of seconds. An example of this mesh adaptation can be seen in Fig. 4.

3.2 Tissue Characterization

Laboratory experiments were performed to characterise the two main tissues in the trachea: cartilage and muscle. There is no possibility of taking samples of internal membrane out of the trachea, but its structure is similar to the muscular membrane, so, its mechanical behaviour will be assumed to be the same. A blinded controlled trial on 20 patients was performed as follows. An experimental study consisting of an extension test 67 (up to 5% deformation) of the cartilage was used to determine its elastic behaviour. A Neo-Hookean 8 curve regression was fitted to the experimental results, yielding to a value of C=0.56 MPa for the stiffness of the cartilage. In order to determine the anisotropy of the material, histology was performed on several cuts over various tracheal rings. These observations allowed to confirm that tracheal cartilage is a material in which collagen fibres are randomly distributed.

Regarding the tracheal muscle, histology showed that it consists of two families of orthogonal fibres. In order to optimise computational time, we opted for building two different models, based on traction experiments of transversal and longitudinal tissue cuts. A Neo-Hookean material was assumed, and validated by curve fitting on the extension curves. The resulting parameters were C=0.032715 MPa for the longitudinal and C=0.008984 MPa for the transversal directions. For simulations of swallowing movement the longitudinal model was used, as this is the predominant direction of the movement. Conversely, the transversal model was used for simulations of sneezing movements.

Finally, the tracheal prosthesis was assumed to be elastic, since it is usually made of silicone.

3.3 Simulation of Swallowing Movement

Fluoroscopic image sequences were used to build a realistic model of the physiological swallowing movement. Several images were available, portraying both normal and pathological movement patterns, including explorations of patients after the implantation of endoprostheses. We adopted the movement of a healthy subject as the base for our simulations, as this is the movement that ideally would be recovered after the intervention. Further, it has been clinically seen that the movement of the trachea among different patients is not very different, because the glottis has to close to let the food going through the oesophagus.

Key anatomical landmarks (e.g. crycoid) are identified and tracked in the fluoroscopic images, and the resulting displacement fields are taken to the finite element analysis using correspondences on the deformed mesh. The finite element simulation, incorporating the models for the trachea and the implant, and reproducing the established movement pattern, was performed using ABAQUS.

4 Results

The framework was tested on data from 2 patients that underwent tracheal surgery. For each patient, two simulations were run, one on the data prior to the intervention and without incorporating the implant, and another one including the implant as positioned by the clinical expert using our tools. For the first patient (62 y.o., male, 83 kg), we obtained a global displacement of the thyroid cartilage of 27.89 mm, which is within the normal physiological range of 20-35 mm, and a maximum principal tension of 0.487 MPa, when simulating without implant. Running the same simulation including the prosthesis led to a maximum displacement of 5.69 mm and a maximum principal tension of 0.61 MPa, meaning that the movement was reduced to only 20.4% of the original one, but the tension was 1.25 times higher.

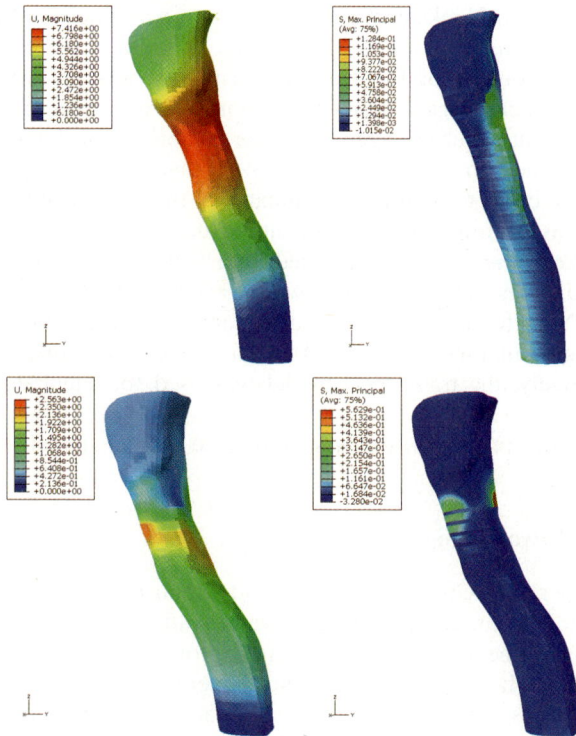

Fig. 5. Simulation of swallowing movement for patient 2, first without the implant (top row) and then simulating the implantation and the interaction with the tracheal wall (bottom row). For each case, we show the norm of the displacement (left) and the maximum tension (right).

For the second patient (28 y.o., male, 75 kg), the simulation without implant yielded a displacement of the reference cartilage of 7.41 mm, with a maximum principal tension of 0.128 MPa. Incorporating the implant we obtained a displacement of 2.56 mm and a maximum principal tension of 0.563 MPa (figure 5).

The results support the clinical hypothesis that tracheal implants lead to a loss of roughly 50% of the ability to swallow, and generate a damage (due to the increase in tension around the edges of the implant) that leads to the creation of granulomas in the tracheal wall 9.

5 Conclusions

We have developed a software for surgical planning of tracheal interventions, combining image segmentation, a database of virtual models of implants, and patient-specific biomechanical simulations of physiological movements to predict implant performance. Laboratory experiments were performed to characterise the tissue elements in the model, and adaptation of a detailed finite element mesh to fit the patient data was implemented. The method was tested on data from 2 patients, and results are clinically sound.

Several issues remain to be further explored. In future work, we plan to continue on the evaluation of the method an quantitatively evaluate its performance. That is, we will define clinical surrogates that can be measured from post-operative data and compared to the simulations. This is work in progress.

On the methodological side, one of the issues to be refined is the establishment of suitable movement models for different physiological processes. In addition to swallowing, sneezing movement simulations are underway. Further, movement models are currently obtained from fluoroscopic data of one patient (or normal subject). One of the approaches we are exploring is the construction of a parametric movement model, or even a statistical 4D model, such as the ones built for breathing movements 10.

We believe that the results presented in this paper are promising and contribute to the development of novel therapies based on patient-specific virtual models including physiological simulations, which are bound to replace current ad-hoc surgical planning procedures and lead to principled evidence-based patient care.

Acknowledgments. This work was in part supported by Grant PI07/90023 of the Instituto de Salud Carlos III, Spain.

References

1. Smuk, P., Tiberiu, E., Evron, S., Roth, Y., Katz, J.: A brief history of tracheostomy and tracheal intubation, from the bronze age to the space age. Intensive Care Med. 34, 222–228 (2008)
2. Manniesing, R., Velthuis, B.K., van Leeuwen, M.S., van der Schaaf, I.C., van Laar, P.J., Niessen, W.J.: Level set based cerebral vasculature segmentation and diameter quantification in CT angiography. Medical image analysis 10(2), 200–214 (2006)
3. Perona, P., Malik, J.: Scale-space and edge detection using anisotropic diffusion. IEEE Transactions on Pattern Analysis and Machine Intelligence 12(7), 629–639 (1990)

4. Chang, Y.L., Li, X.: Adaptive image region-growing. IEEE Transactions on Image Processing 3(6), 868–872 (1994)
5. Gonzalez, R.C., Woods, R.E.: Digital Image Processing, 2nd edn. Pearson, London (2001)
6. Teng, Z., Ochoa, I., Bea, J.A., Doblaré, M.: Theoretical and experimental studies on the nonlinear mechanical property of the tracheal cartilage. In: Procs. of 29th International Conference of the IEEE Engineering in Medicine and Biology, pp. 1058–1061 (2007)
7. Teng, Z., Ochoa, I., Li, Z., Lin, Y., Rodríguez, J., Bea, J., Doblaré, M.: Nonlinear mechanical property of tracheal cartilage: A theoretical and experimental study. Journal of Biomechanics 41(9), 1995–2002 (2008)
8. Holzapfel, G.A., Gasser, T.C., Ogden, R.W.: A new constitutive framework for arterial wall mechanics and a comparative study of material models. Journal of Elasticity 61, 1–48 (2000)
9. Noppen, M., Stratakos, G., D'Haese, J., Meysman, M., Vinken, W.: Removal of covered self-expandable metallic airway stents in benign disorders: indications, technique, and outcomes. Chest 127(2), 482–487 (2005)
10. von Siebenthal, M., Székely, G., Lomax, A., Cattin, P.C.: Inter-subject modelling of liver deformation during radiation therapy. In: Ayache, N., Ourselin, S., Maeder, A. (eds.) MICCAI 2007, Part I. LNCS, vol. 4791, pp. 659–666. Springer, Heidelberg (2007)

Mesh Generation from 3D Multi-material Images*

Dobrina Boltcheva, Mariette Yvinec, and Jean-Daniel Boissonnat

GEOMETRICA – INRIA Sophia Antipolis, France

Abstract. The problem of generating realistic computer models of objects represented by 3D segmented images is important in many biomedical applications. Labelled 3D images impose particular challenges for meshing algorithms because multi-material junctions form features such as surface pacthes, edges and corners which need to be preserved into the output mesh. In this paper, we propose a feature preserving Delaunay refinement algorithm which can be used to generate high-quality tetrahedral meshes from segmented images. The idea is to explicitly sample corners and edges from the input image and to constrain the Delaunay refinement algorithm to preserve these features in addition to the surface patches. Our experimental results on segmented medical images have shown that, within a few seconds, the algorithm outputs a tetrahedral mesh in which each material is represented as a consistent submesh without gaps and overlaps. The optimization property of the Delaunay triangulation makes these meshes suitable for the purpose of realistic visualization or finite element simulations.

1 Introduction

Motivation. Advanced medical techniques frequently require geometric representations of human organs rather than grey-level MRI or CT-scan images. The precondition for extracting geometry from a medical image is usually to *segment* it into multiple regions of interest (materials). This paper focuses on the next step: the automatic generation of meshes from 3D labelled images. These meshes are either surface meshes approximating the boundaries of anatomical structures or volume meshes of these objects.

The generation of geometric models from segmented images presents many challenges. In particular, the algorithm must handle arbitrary topology and multiple junctions. Multi-material junctions form *surface patches* (2-junctions), *edges* (1-junctions) and *corners* (0-junctions) which are expected to be accurately represented in the output mesh. However, it is still very challenging to construct a good mesh where each feature (surface patch, edge or corner) is accurately represented.

---

* This research was supported by the FOCUS K3D Coordination Action, EU Contract ICT-2007.4.2 contract number 214993.

In this paper, we present a Delaunay refinement algorithm which addresses this issue. In a matter of seconds, the algorithm outputs a high-quality tetrahedral mesh where each anatomical structure is represented by a submesh with conforming boundaries.

Related work. There are only a few meshing strategies which directly provide volume meshes from multi-material images. Early grid-based methods deal with tetrahedral elements that are created from the original rectilinear volume subdivision [1,2]. More recently, an octree-based method has been proposed [3] that outputs tetrahedral or hexahedral meshes with consistent multi-material junctions. However, like the other grid-based methods, this algorithm does not offer a mesh quality control and elements of poor quality are always generated along boundaries. Quality improvement techniques are usually used as a post-processing step to deliver acceptable meshes.

Another powerful strategy based on Delaunay refinement, has been proposed for meshing smooth surfaces [4] and volumes bounded by smooth and piecewise smooth surfaces [5,6]. The refinement process is controlled by highly customizable quality and size criteria on triangular facets and on tetrahedra. Pons et al. [7] have adapted this mesh generation strategy to labelled images and have shown that the sizing criteria can be tissue-dependent leading to high-quality volume meshes of the different materials. However, in this work, 1- and 0-junctions are not explicitly handled and they are not accurately represented in the output mesh. It is well recognized that the presence of edges where different surface patches meet forming small angles, jeopardize the termination of Delaunay refinement in 3D [8]. A recent method [9] deals with this problem using the idea of protecting small angle regions with balls so that during the refinement no point is inserted into these protecting balls.

Very recently, Mayer et al. [10] proposed a sampling strategy for labelled images based on a dynamic particle system which explicitly samples corners, edges, and surface patches. The resulting set of well-distributed points is adapted to the underlying geometry of multi-material junctions. From these surface points, Delaunay-based meshing scheme outputs high-quality surface meshes. However, this sampling approach relies on heavy pre-processing computations and takes between 3 and 12 hours for small medical images.

Our contribution. In this paper, we propose a feature (edge and corner) preserving extension of the Delaunay refinement algorithm introduced by Pons et al. [7]. The basic idea is to explicitly sample 1- and 0-junctions before launching the Delaunay refinement and to constrain the latter to preserve these features. The algorithm first extracts, from the input 3D image, all multi-material junctions where 3 or more materials meet. Then it samples and protects these junctions with protecting balls as in [9]. The Delaunay refinement is then run using a weighted Delaunay triangulation, with the protecting balls as initial set of data points. This allows to preserve 0-junctions (corners) and to reconstruct accurately the 1-junctions (edges) with a sequence of mesh edges. In contrast to Mayer et al. [10], we sample only 0- and 1-junctions and not the 2-junctions which are meshed by the Delaunay refinement algorithm according to user-given quality and sizing criteria. Our multi-material junction detection and sampling algorithm is very fast and has little influence on the computation time of the Delaunay refinement algorithm.

The remainder of this paper is organized as follows: Section 2 gives a brief background and recalls the Delaunay refinement algorithm. Our multi-material junction detecting and protecting strategy is presented in Section 3. Section 4 reports some results and numerical experiments which demonstrate the effectiveness of our approach for segmented medical 3D images.

2 Delaunay Refinement Mesh Generation from 3D Images

The method is related to the concept of *restricted Delaunay triangulation*, borrowed from computational geometry.

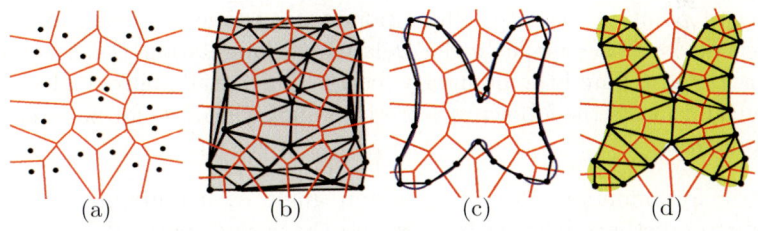

Fig. 1. (a) A set of points in the plane and its Voronoi diagram. (b) The dual Delaunay triangulation. (c) The Delaunay triangulation restricted to the blue curve is plotted with a black line. (d) The Delaunay triangulation restricted to the yellow region is composed of triangles whose circumcentres are inside the region.

Background. Let $E = \{p_0, ..., p_n\}$ be a set of points in $\mathbb{R}^3$ called *sites* hereafter. The *Voronoi cell*, denoted $Vor(p_i)$, associated to the site p_i is the locus of points that are closer to p_i than to any other site in E. The *Voronoi diagram* of E, denoted $Vor(E)$, is the partition of space induced by the Voronoi cells $Vor(p_i)$. The Delaunay complex is the dual of the Voronoi diagram defined as follows: for esch subset of sites $T \subset E$, the convex hull $conv(T)$ is a cell of the Delaunay complex if and only if the intersection $\cap_{p \in T}(Vor(p))$ of the Voronoi cells of sites in T is non empty. When the set E is in general position, i.e. there are no 5 sites lying on the same sphere, the Delaunay complex is a simplical complex called the *Delaunay triangulation* of E, denoted $Del(E)$.

Let us now consider a subset $\Omega \subset \mathbb{R}^3$ and a set of points E. We call Delaunay triangulation of E *restricted* to Ω, and denote $Del(E)|\Omega$, the subcomplex of $Del(E)$ composed of Delaunay simplices whose dual Voronoi faces intersect Ω. Fig.1 gives an example of these notions in 2D.

Let us consider a multi-material 3D image I as a function $F : \mathbb{Z}^3 \to J$, where $J = \{0, ..., n\}$ is a set of labels where 0 represents the background and 1...n the other materials. Each label i defines a characteristic function $f_i : \mathbb{Z}^3 \to \{0,1\}$ such as $f_i(p) = 1$ iff $F(p) = i$ and 0 otherwise. Let $\tilde{f}_i : \mathbb{R}^3 \to \{0,1\}$ be the trilinear interpolation of f_i. Then we define the extension $\tilde{F} : \mathbb{R}^3 \to J$ of the image function F, as follows: $\tilde{F}(p) = i$ iff $\tilde{f}_i(p) = max_{j \in J}\{\tilde{f}_j(p)\}$. $\tilde{F}$ defines a partition of the domain to be meshed $\Omega = \cup_{i \neq 0}\Omega_i$, where $\Omega_i = \tilde{F}^{-1}(i), i \in J$. We call B_i the boundary of Ω_i and $B = \cup B_i$ denotes the locus of multi-material junctions including surface patches, edges and corners.

The Delaunay refinement meshing algorithm presented in the next section samples a set of points $E \in \mathbb{R}^3$ and builds the Delaunay triangulation of E restricted to Ω. The algorithm outputs $Del(E)|\Omega = \cup_{i \in J, i \neq 0} Del(E)|\Omega_i$ where $Del(E)|\Omega_i$ is the set of tetrahedra whose circumcentres are contained in Ω_i. In other words, each tetrahedron is labelled according to the material in which its circumcentre lies. We call *boundary facets* the facets incident to two tetrahedra with different labels. These boundary facets form a watertight non-manifold surface mesh that approximates surface patches where two material meet.

Delaunay refinement algorithm. The algorithm starts by sampling a small initial set of points E on $\cup B_i$. Three points per connected component of $\cup B_i$ are sufficient. Next it calculates the Delaunay triangulation $Del(E)$ and its restrictions $Del(E)|\Omega_i$ and the boundary fecets. This initial approximation is then refined until it meets the following user-given quality criteria for boundary facets and tetrahedra:

- criteria for boundary facets: minimum angle α; maximum edge length l; maximum distance between a facet and the surface patch d;
- criteria for tetrahedra: ratio between tetrahedron cirumradius and shortest edge length β; maximum edge length L.

Thus, the mesh refinement criteria are given by the 5-uplet (α, l, d, β, L). A *bad element* is an element that does not fulfil criteria. *Bad facets* are removed from the mesh by inserting their *surface centres*. The *surface centre* of a boundary facet is the point of intersection between its dual Voronoi edge and a surface patch.

Bad tetrahedra are removed from the mesh by inserting their circumcentres. The algorithm inserts refinement points one by one and maintains the current set E, $Del(E)$, $Del(E)|\Omega$ and boundary facets. The refinement procedure is iterated until there is no bad element left.

After the refinement, degenerated tetrahedra with small dihedral angles (slivers) are removed from the mesh using a *sliver exudation* algorithm [11].

It is proven in [6] that for appropriate choices of refinement criteria, the algorithm terminates. It delivers surface and volume meshes which form a good approximation of the image partition as soon as E is a "sufficiently dense" sample of its boundaries and volumes. However, 0- and 1-junctions are not handled explicitly and they are poorly reconstructed in the output mesh. As shown on Fig.2(1) the 1-junctions are zigzagging and the 0-junctions are not preserved.

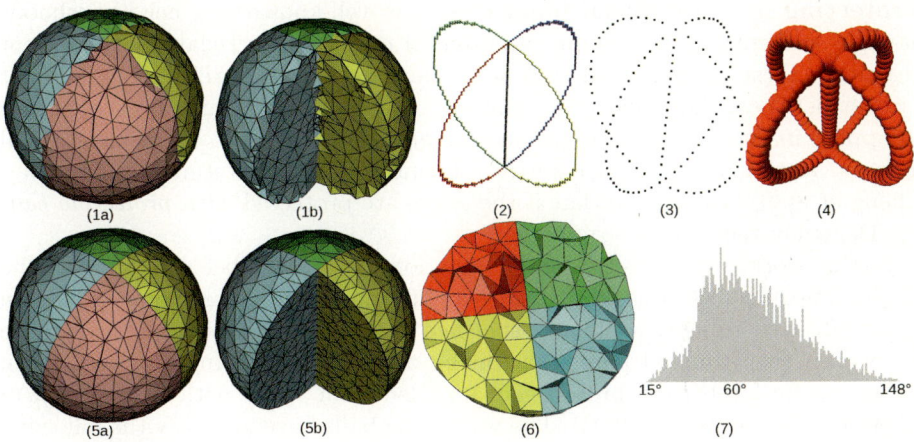

Fig. 2. (1) Delaunay refinement 3D mesh. (2) Multimaterial junctions: five 1-junctions and two 0-junctions. (3) Sampled points on junctions. (4) Protecting balls. (5) Edge preserving Delaunay refinement 3D mesh. (6) A cut of the tetrahedral mesh. (7) Dihedral angles distribution.

3 Feature Preserving Extension

In order to constrain the Delaunay refinement algorithm to mesh properly 0- and 1-junctions, firstly we need to extract these junctions from the input image.

Multi-material junction extraction. Here, we extend the image function $F : \mathbb{Z}^3 \to J$ into a function $\tilde{F} : \mathbb{R}^3 \to J$ using the the concept of *continuous analog*, borrowed from digital geometry and topology [12,13]. Following this concept, for any point $p \in \mathbb{R}^3$, $\tilde{F}(p) = F(p_i)$, where p_i is the point of $\mathbb{Z}^3$ closest to p. As before, this function $\tilde{F}$ defines a partition of the domain to be meshed $\Omega = \cup_{i \neq 0} \Omega_i$ but now $\Omega_i = \tilde{F}^{-1}(i), i \in J$ is a set of cubic voxels with the same label. As before, $B = \cup B_i$ denotes the multi-material junctions which are composed of:

- 2-junctions S (surface patches composed of voxel faces) which correspond to the intersection of exactly 2 materials;
- 1-junctions L (composed of voxel edges) which are defined at the intersection of exactly 3 or 4 materials;
- 0-junctions P (defined by voxel vertices) which correspond to the intersection of 4 or more materials (at maximum 8).

As it has been stressed before, our multi-material junction extraction algorithm delivers only 0- and 1-junctions because the Delaunay refinement algorithm handles surface patches well. The result is a 1D cellular complex composed of edges $\{L_i\}$ and their end points $\{P_i\}$. Fig.2(2) shows the 1D complex obtained for the multi-material sphere which is composed of five edges and two corners.

Protecting multi-material junctions. It is well known that neighbourhoods of edges and corners are regions of potential problems for Delaunay refinement algorithm. First, as we have already seen, the usual Delaunay refinement does not reconstruct these sharp features accurately. Secondly, if we constrain these edges to appear in the mesh and if the surface patches incident to them make small dihedral angles, the usual Delaunay refinement may not terminate. However, Cheng et al.[9] have shown that if the edges are protected with *protecting balls* the Delaunay refinement terminates.

In this work, we protect 0- and 1-junctions with balls before launching the mesh refinement. We first keep all corners in $\{P_i\}$ and then we sample points on edges $\{L_i\}$ according to some user-specified density (see Fig.2(3)). This distance d between two sampled points should be at most the maximum edge length parameter for facets l. We protect each sampled point $p \in L_i$ with a ball $b = (p, r)$ where $r = 2/3 * d$ (see Fig.2(4)). The protecting balls have to satisfy the following properties:

- each edge L_i is completely recovered by the protecting balls of its samples
- any two adjacent balls on a given edge L_i overlap significantly without containing each other's centres
- any two balls on different edges L_i and L_j do not intersect
- no three balls have a common intersection

After the sampling and protection step, we use the previous Delaunay refinement algorithm as follows: Each protecting ball $b = (p, r)$ is turned into a weighted point (p, r) and inserted into the initial set of points E. The Delaunay triangulation is turned into a *weighted* Delaunay triangulation where the Euclidean distance is replaced by the *weighted distance*. The weighted distance from a point $x \in \mathbb{R}^3$ to a weighted point (p, r) is defined as $||x - p||^2 - r^2$. All the other points inserted during the refinement are considered as points of weight zero.

The protecting balls and the weighted Delaunay triangulation guarantee two important properties. First, the segment between two *adjacent* points on any protected edge L_i remains connected with restricted Delaunay edges (see Fig.2(5)). Secondly, since the algorithm will never try to insert a refinement point into the union of protecting ball, its termination is guaranteed (see [9] for more detail).

In practice, when a multi-material 3D image is the input, the algorithm outputs high-quality tetrahedral meshes of different materials which are consistent with each other. In particular, 1-junctions are properly reconstructed with edges whose vertices lie on these junctions (see Fig.2(5)).

4 Results and Conclusion

The Delaunay refinement algorithm and its feature preserving extension have been implemented upon robust primitives to compute the Delaunay triangulation provided by the CGAL library [14].

We have tested our meshing algorithm on synthetic labelled images and on segmented medical images provided by IRCAD [15]. Figure 3 shows the meshes

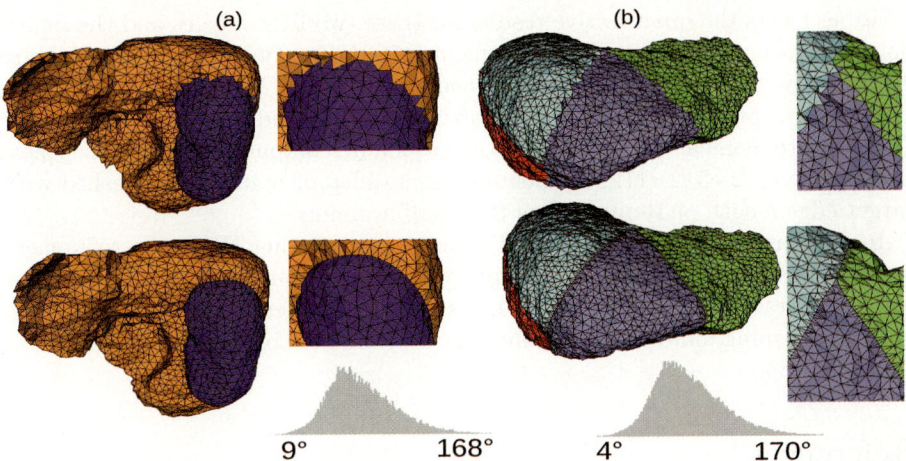

Fig. 3. Meshes generated from labelled liver images: (a) A liver adjacent to a right kidney and a zoom on their edge. (b) A liver segmented into 4 anatomical regions and a zoom on one of the corners. The first raw shows meshes obtained with the usual Delaunay refinement. The second raw shows meshes resulting from our feature preserving extension and histograms of their dihedral angles distributions.

Table 1. Quantitative results and parameters for three different 3D images. The α in the refinement criteria is given in $degree$ and l, d and L are given in mm. The four last raws give the computation times of different algorithm steps in seconds.

Experiment	sphere	liver-kidney	liver segments
Image size	62×62×62	512×512×112	402×356×238
Image resolution (mm)	1×1×1	0.67×0.67×2	2×2×2
Refinement criteria (α, l, d, β, L)	(20,10,3,4,10)	(30,12,2,4,14)	(25,14,4,4,18)
# vertices	964	6142	12381
# boundary facets	1431	5439	9646
# tetrahedra	4434	31043	64485
Junction Extraction (sec)	0.72	4.56	21.35
Surface meshing (sec)	1.74	9.99	11.04
Volume meshing (sec)	1.13	5.82	17.23
Sliver exudation (sec)	3.75	13.82	48.64

generated from two labelled liver datasets by the Delaunay refinement strategy with and without the feature preserving extension. Figure 3(a) displays the mesh of a liver adjacent to a right kidney and the 1-junction produced at the intersection of these two objects and the background. In this case, the 1-junction is a simple closed curve which has been protected with balls of radius $6mm$. Figure 3(b) shows the mesh of a liver which has been cut into 4 anatomical regions. There are 8 1-junctions and 4 0-junctions produced at the intersection of these anatomical regions which have been protected with balls of radius $3mm$.

Table 1 lists the quantitative results for these two liver images and the multi-material sphere on Fig.2. The refinement criteria for Delaunay refinement are given as the 5-uplet (α, l, d, β, L) defined in section 2. Note that our edge extraction and protection algorithm takes few seconds and does not penalize the Delaunay refinement which also has a reasonable computation time. A typical liver image (512×512×112) segmented into 4 different materials is meshed with target edge length of 10mm in less than half a minute.

In conclusion, we have proposed a feature preserving Delaunay refinement meshing strategy to generate conforming 3D meshes from labelled images. These meshes are targeted towards applications in the finite element methods which require conforming multi-material junctions to avoid instabilities and errors during the simulation.

References

1. Nielson, G.M., Franke, R.: Computing the separating surface for segmented data. In: VIS, pp. 229–233 (1997)
2. Hartmann, U., Kruggel, F.: A fast algorithm for generating large tetrahedral 3d finite element meshes from magnetic resonance tomograms. In: WBIA (1998)
3. Zhang, Y., Hughes, T., Bajaj, C.L.: Automatic 3d mesh generation for a domain with multiple materials. In: Meshing Roundtable, pp. 367–386 (2007)
4. Oudot, S., Rineau, L., Yvinec, M.: Meshing volumes bounded by smooth surfaces. In: Meshing Roundtable, pp. 203–219 (2005)
5. Rineau, L., Yvinec, M.: A generic software design for delaunay refinement meshing. Comput. Geom. Theory Appl. 38, 100–110 (2007)
6. Rineau, L., Yvinec, M.: Meshing 3d domains bounded by piecewise smooth surfaces. In: Meshing Roundtable, pp. 443–460 (2007)
7. Pons, J.-P., Ségonne, F., Boissonnat, J.-D., Rineau, L., Yvinec, M., Keriven, R.: High-quality consistent meshing of multi-label datasets. In: Karssemeijer, N., Lelieveldt, B. (eds.) IPMI 2007. LNCS, vol. 4584, pp. 198–210. Springer, Heidelberg (2007)
8. Shewchuk, J.R.: Mesh generation for domains with small angles. In: SCG, pp. 1–10. ACM, New York (2000)
9. Cheng, S.W., Dey, T.K., Ramos, E.A.: Delaunay refinement for piecewise smooth complexes. In: SODA, Philadelphia, PA, USA, pp. 1096–1105 (2007)
10. Meyer, M., Whitaker, R., Kirby, R.M., Ledergerber, C., Pfister, H.: Particle-based sampling and meshing of surfaces in multimaterial volumes. Visualization and Computer Graphics 14(6), 1539–1546 (2008)
11. Cheng, S.W., Dey, T.K., Edelsbrunner, H., Facello, M.A., Teng, S.H.: Sliver exudation. In: SCG, pp. 1–13 (1999)
12. Latecki, L.: 3d well-composed pictures. Graph. Models Image Process 59(3) (1997)
13. Françon, J., Bertrand, Y.: Topological 3d-manifolds: a statistical study of the cells. Theoretical Computer Science, 233–254 (2000)
14. CGAL: Computational Geometry Algorithms Library, http://www.cgal.org
15. IRCAD: Institut de Recherche contre les Cancers de l'Appareil Digestif, http://www.ircad.fr

Interactive Simulation of Flexible Needle Insertions Based on Constraint Models

Christian Duriez[1], Christophe Guébert[1], Maud Marchal[2], Stephane Cotin[1], and Laurent Grisoni[1]

[1] INRIA Nord-Europe (University of Lille), France
[2] INRIA Bretagne Nord-Atlantique (IRISA-INSA), France
christian.duriez@inria.fr

Abstract. This paper presents a new modeling method for the insertion of needles and more generally thin and flexible medical devices into soft tissues. Several medical procedures rely on the insertion of slender medical devices such as biopsy, brachytherapy, deep-brain stimulation. In this paper, the interactions between soft tissues and flexible instruments are reproduced using a set of dedicated complementarity constraints. Each constraint is positionned and applied to the deformable models without requiring any remeshing. Our method allows for the 3D simulation of different physical phenomena such as puncture, cutting, static and dynamic friction at interactive frame rate. To obtain realistic simulation, the model can be parametrized using experimental data. Our method is validated through a series of typical simulation examples and new more complex scenarios.

1 Introduction

Needles, electrode or biopsy tools are some examples of thin and flexible medical tools used in a clinical routine. Several medical applications are concerned by the use of these tools, such as biopsy, brachytherapy or deep brain stimulation. As these objects are often thin and flexible, the accuracy of their insertion into soft tissues can be affected. Moreover, different physical phenomena, such as puncture, friction or cutting through heterogeneous tissues could alter the procedure. The simulation of the insertion of thin and flexible medical tools into various tissues can enable useful clinical feedback, such as training but also planning. We chose the example of a needle to explain our methodology but our method can be generalized to thin and flexible instruments.

Pioneering works concerning needle insertion were presented by Di Maio *et al.* [1] and Alterovitz *et al.* [2]. They proposed modeling methods based on FEM for the interaction between a needle and soft tissues. A recent survey proposed by Abolhassani *et al.* [3] summarizes the different characteristics of the existing methods in the literature. Remeshing process of tissue models remains an obstacle to obtain interactive simulations. In [4], the authors simulate the insertion of several rigid needles in a single soft tissue (such as during brachytherapy procedures). The interaction model between needle and tissue is the most challenging part as it combines different physical phenomena. Different studies based on experimental data are proposed in the literature to identify the forces occuring during the needle insertion [5]. Three different types of force are often underlined: puncture force, cutting force and friction force. Recent studies use experimental data to perform an identification of the model parameters [6,7,8].

In this paper, a new generic method based on the formulation of several constraints is proposed in order to simulate the insertion of thin and flexible medical devices into soft tissues. Any classical deformation model of both tissue and needle can be used with our approach. For this study, we obtain interactive frame rate while modeling the geometrical non-linearities of the tissue and needle deformations. Contrary to existing methods, no remeshing process is needed, even if Finite Element Method (FEM) is used for the tissue simulation. Our method can handle complex scenarios where needle steering, non-homogeneous tissues and interactions between different needles can be combined.

The paper is divided into five sections. In Section 2, the formulation of our modeling method is presented. Section 3 details the simulation process. Section 4 shows the results obtained with the new modeling method. Section 5 draws conclusions and discusses future works.

2 Constraint-Based Modeling of Needle Insertion

In this work, we propose a new model for the interactions that take place at the surface of a needle during its insertion in soft tissues. The formulation relies on a constraint formulation which is independent of both needle and tissue models that are used to simulate deformations. We highlight two different aspects: Firstly, for the *constraint positioning*, no remeshing is necessary. Secondly, we present several new *constraint laws*, based on complementarity theory [9]. These laws capture in a unified formalism all the non-smooth mechanical phenomena that occur during insertion.

2.1 How to Avoid Remeshing?

The *constraint positioning* is defined by two points: one on the tissue volume P and one on the needle curve Q. For each constraint, δ measures the distance between these two points along a defined constraint direction $\mathbf{n}$. The points can be placed anywhere in the volume of the soft tissue and anywhere on the needle curve. The displacements of these points are mapped with the same interpolation than the deformable models (see Fig. 1). The variation of δ can be mapped on the displacements of deformable model nodes $\Delta \mathbf{q}_n$ (needle) and $\Delta \mathbf{q}_t$ (tissue):

$$\Delta \delta = \mathbf{n}^T(\mathbf{u}_n - \mathbf{u}_t) = \mathbf{n}^T(\mathbf{J}_n \Delta \mathbf{q}_n - \mathbf{J}_t \Delta \mathbf{q}_t) = \mathbf{H}_n \Delta \mathbf{q}_n + \mathbf{H}_t \Delta \mathbf{q}_t \qquad (1)$$

In the following, λ represents the force used to solve the constraint (applied by the tissue on the needle). To map this force on the deformable model nodes, we use the virtual work principle ($\lambda^T \Delta \delta = \mathbf{f}_t^T \Delta \mathbf{q}_t + \mathbf{f}_n^T \Delta \mathbf{q}_n$). We obtain:

$$\mathbf{f}_t = \mathbf{H}_t^T \lambda \qquad \text{and} \qquad \mathbf{f}_n = \mathbf{H}_n^T \lambda \qquad (2)$$

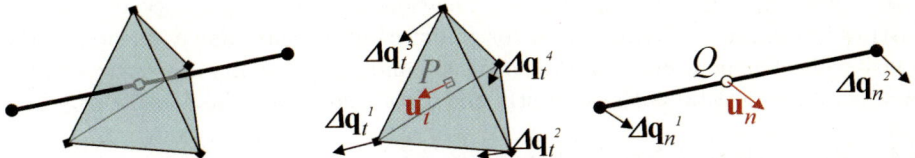

Fig. 1. Example of mapping for a constraint point. A linear interpolation is used on tetrahedra for the soft tissue model, the displacement $\mathbf{u}_t$ of a tissue constraint point placed inside a tetrahedron is given by the barycentric coordinates and the displacement $\Delta \mathbf{q}_t$ of the 4 nodes $\mathbf{u}_t = \mathbf{J}_t \Delta \mathbf{q}_t$. The displacement of the needle point $\mathbf{u}_n$ is mapped using the interpolation of the needle deformation model $\mathbf{u}_n = \mathbf{J}_n \Delta \mathbf{q}_n$.

2.2 Puncturing Soft Tissue

Puncturing illustrates the interest of using complementarity theory to model the constraint: three successive steps of the interaction can be defined with a set of inequalities, as illustrated in Fig. 2. Here, Q is the tip of the needle and P is the contacting point (or the penetration point) on the tissue surface. $\mathbf{n}$ is the surface normal vector at point P.

The puncture constraint can be applied several times during the simulation if the needle passes through different tissue layers: different values for the threshold f_p can be defined in order to simulate different tissue behaviors. If the tip of the needle hits a bone for example, f_p is very high and never reached by λ_p: the needle slips along the surface of the bone. The constraint is associated with an other constraint on each lateral direction: friction constraint when contact is established (step 2), and tip path constraint (see section 2.4) when puncture states are activated (step3).

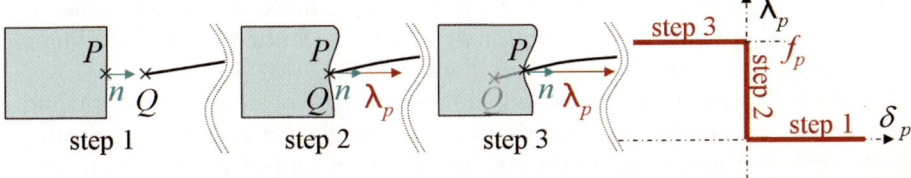

Fig. 2. Puncturing steps. During **step 1**, Q is only approaching the tissue surface. The gap δ is positive ($\delta_p \geq 0$) and the interaction force must be null ($\lambda_p = 0$). During **step 2**, Q is touching without puncturing the tissue surface. The gap between P and Q is null ($\delta_p = 0$) and the interaction force is necessarily positive in the direction of the surface normal ($\lambda_p \geq 0$). The value of this force is strictly less than a puncturing force threshold $\lambda_p \leq f_p$. During **step 3**, the needle tip enters in the tissue, the gap along the constraint direction is negative ($\delta_p \leq 0$) and the constraint force is equal to the threshold ($\lambda_p = f_p$).

2.3 Cutting through Different Layers

The cutting force f_c is the force needed to traverse a tissue structure. As for f_p, it can be tuned to different values from a layer to another. This force disappears if the needle is re-inserted at the same location. The constraint used to simulate cutting is similar to the one used for puncturing, except that δ_c measures the relative displacement between the needle tip and the extremity of a curve created by a previous cutting path. λ_c is still the force that solves the constraint.

2.4 Tip Path and Needle Steering

A direction is associated to the needle tip in order to constrain its lateral motion. To obtain needle steering due to bevel-tip needle, a specific orientation of the cutting direction in the tip frame is defined (Fig. 3(a)) and the displacement of the tip is tangential to this direction ($\delta_t = 0$). In that case, whether the needle is being pushed or pulled, the constraint is not aligned in the same direction (Fig. 3(b)). During needle insertion, the path of the tip inside the soft tissues is followed by the rest of the needle. This behavior is modeled using additional constraints: we impose a null relative displacement δ_t between the needle and the organ along the tangential directions of the needle curve (Fig. 3(c)). Here λ_t will provide the force necessary to solve this equality constraint.

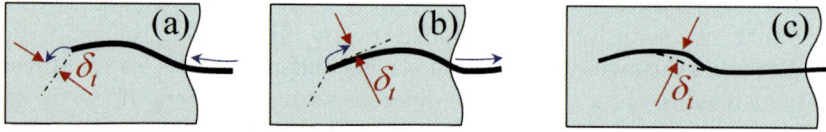

Fig. 3. Needle model is constrained on the path defined by the needle tip

2.5 Friction

Dry friction resists to the motion when the needle is inserted but also retracted. The complementarity constraint for the friction defines two states: adherence (stick) when there is no relative motion $\delta_f = 0$ due to static friction and dynamic friction (slip) when the relative motion is not null $\delta_f \neq 0$ (Fig. 4).

A threshold $\mu.p$ is used to limit adherence: μ is the coefficient of friction and p is the pressure exerted by the soft tissue on the needle. Currently, this pressure is estimated from the stiffness of the soft tissue and remains constant. To model it more accurately, we plan to use stress measures based on the soft tissue deformable model. The value of the friction resistance r, given by the graph (Fig. 4) is integrated along the inserted surface of the needle. Each constraint point owns a part of the needle curve and computes the friction force by using the length l of this curve part ($\lambda_f = l\pi d.r$ where d is the diameter of the cross-section).

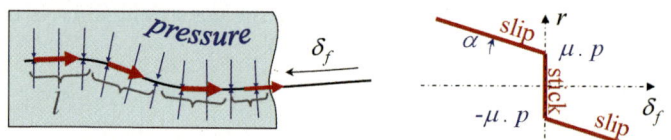

Fig. 4. Friction model: static and dynamic friction are included

3 Simulation of Tissue and Needle Interaction

In this section, we describe how we combine, using Lagrangian mechanics, the previously defined insertion constraints with the deformation models of the needle and the soft tissues. Let's consider the dynamic deformation models of the needle n and the soft tissue t. We use the synthetic formulation:

$$\mathbf{M}_n \dot{\mathbf{v}}_n = \mathbf{p}_n - \mathbb{F}_n(\mathbf{q}_n, \mathbf{v}_n) + \mathbf{H}_n^T \lambda \qquad (3)$$

$$\mathbf{M}_t \dot{\mathbf{v}}_t = \mathbf{p}_t - \mathbb{F}_t(\mathbf{q}_t, \mathbf{v}_t) + \mathbf{H}_t^T \lambda \qquad (4)$$

where $\mathbf{q} \in \mathbb{R}^n$ is the vector of generalized degrees of freedom, $\mathbf{M}$ is the mass matrix, $\mathbf{v} \in \mathbb{R}^n$ is the vector of velocity. $\mathbb{F}$ represents internal visco-elastic forces, and $\mathbf{p}$ gathers external forces. λ is the vector of the constraint forces that is multiplied by matrices $\mathbf{H}_n^T$ and $\mathbf{H}_t^T$ presented on section 2.1.

To allow a stable interaction between models, implicit integration is used with backward Euler scheme. The simulation is realized in three steps: during the first step, constraint forces are ignored to obtain what we call a *free motion* of each model. During the second step, constraint forces λ are computed as described in the following. Then when λ is known, a correction of the motion of each model is performed in order to respect equations (3) and (4).

The computation of the contact forces, during step 2, relies on solving the *constraint laws* presented on section 2 with the following equation:

$$\boldsymbol{\delta} = \left[\underbrace{\mathbf{H}_n \left(\frac{\mathbf{M}_n}{h^2} + \frac{d\mathbb{F}_n}{h d\mathbf{v}_n} + \frac{d\mathbb{F}_n}{d\mathbf{q}_n} \right)^{-1} \mathbf{H}_n^T}_{\mathbf{W}_n} + \underbrace{\mathbf{H}_t \left(\frac{\mathbf{M}_t}{h^2} + \frac{d\mathbb{F}_t}{h d\mathbf{v}_t} + \frac{d\mathbb{F}_t}{d\mathbf{q}_t} \right)^{-1} \mathbf{H}_t^T}_{\mathbf{W}_t} \right] \lambda + \boldsymbol{\delta}^{\text{free}} \qquad (5)$$

where h is a time step and $\left(\frac{\mathbf{M}}{h^2} + \frac{d\mathbb{F}}{h d\mathbf{v}} + \frac{d\mathbb{F}}{d\mathbf{q}} \right)$ is the dynamic tangent matrix. We note that depending on the deformation model, the computation of matrices $\mathbf{W}$ could be time consuming (see discussion on section 4). To find the constraint force value, we propose to use a Gauss-Seidel like algorithm. Considering a constraint α, among m instantaneous constraints, one can rewrite equation (5):

$$\delta_\alpha - [\mathbf{W}_{\alpha,\alpha}]\lambda_\alpha = \underbrace{\sum_{\beta=1}^{\alpha-1} [\mathbf{W}_{\alpha,\beta}]\lambda_\beta + \sum_{\beta=\alpha+1}^{m} [\mathbf{W}_{\alpha,\beta}]\lambda_\beta + \delta_\alpha^{\text{free}}}_{\delta_\alpha^-} \qquad (6)$$

where $[\mathbf{W}_{\alpha,\beta}]$ is the value of the matrix $\mathbf{W} = \mathbf{W}_n + \mathbf{W}_t$ at line α and column β. It models the coupling between constraint points α and β. At each iteration of the Gauss-Seidel solver, each constraint α is visited and a new estimate of λ_α is performed while "freezing" the contributions of λ_β with $\alpha \neq \beta$. The new estimate of λ_α is found at the intersection of the characteristic graph of each *constraint law* described in section 2 with the line of equation (6). Note that for all mechanical models, the local compliance of a point is always positive :

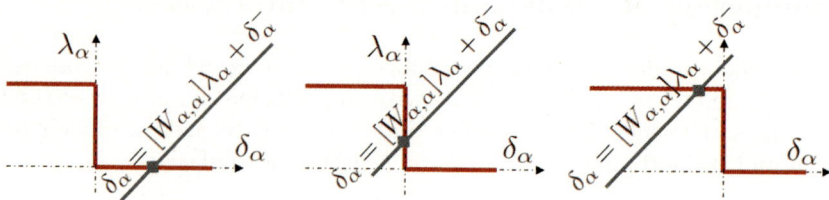

Fig. 5. Example of graph intersection to find λ_α on a given constraint graph

$[W_{\alpha,\alpha}] > 0$, so we obtain a unique solution for λ_α (see Fig 5). We stop the algorithm when the error on the values of vector $\boldsymbol{\delta}$ reach a given threshold.

In our approach, the sampling of the constraints is important for both accuracy and convergence of the constraint solver. Namely, if there are more constraints than degrees of freedom involved, the problem is over-constrained. However, if the space between the constraints points is too large, the accuracy decreases. In practice, we use a regular sampling of the constraint points along the needle curve that corresponds to the discretization of the needle deformation model. During the insertion and the withdrawal of the needle, constraint points are dynamically inserted and removed to obtain a sufficient number of constraints along the needle curve.

4 Results

4.1 Deformable Models

In this work, the needle model that relies on a series of beam elements can handle deformations with large displacements. The parameters of the model are mainly: E, the Young Modulus, ν the poisson ratio, and A the area of the cross section (hollow needles can be simulated). The computation is optimized using a band tri-diagonal solver: $\mathbf{W}_n$ value is obtained at high refresh rate (few milliseconds) with a precise discretization of the needle (50 beams).

The soft tissues of the human anatomy often have a visco-elastic anisotropic behavior which leads to complex FEM models if high precision is needed. However, to assess our constraint-based model of the interaction between the needle and the soft tissues during insertion, we use basic shapes and simple tissue model. The simulated soft tissue can only undergo large displacements with small deformations. We use Hooke's constitutive law: deformations are considered to be isotropic and elastic and the Poisson ratio is tuned to quasi incompressibility ($\nu = 0.49$). A viscous behavior is obtained using Rayleigh model. It provides an attenuation that is proportionally related to both elastic and inertial forces. Using this model, we can obtain a very fast estimation of the compliance matrix $\mathbf{W}_t$ [10] that leads to the ability of obtaining real-time simulation of the needle insertion. Once again, this tissue model is only used in a preliminary approach, to validate the constraints used for needle insertion. More complex model could be used.

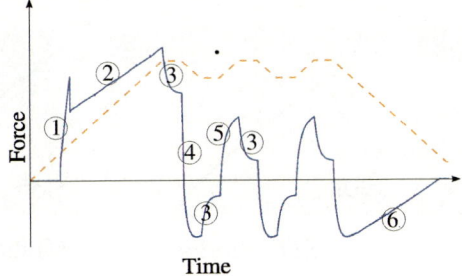

Fig. 6. Insertions and pullbacks. Stippled line represents the motion imposed to the needle. At step (1), the needle punctures the tissue surface. During step (2), friction is increasing with the penetration distance and (3) is the relaxation. After being partially retracted (4), the needle is inserted again along the same path (5); therefore no cutting force is applied. During the last and complete pullback (6), the friction force decreases.

4.2 Experiments

Our first experiment consists in inserting and pulling back multiple times the needle in a 3D soft tissue. This experiment is similar to the measurements proposed in [8], and the results obtained with our simulation (presented in Fig. 6) match the previous work.

Then we propose a second experiment based on the 3D simulation of an obstacle avoidance using needle steering. Indeed, surgeons sometimes use thin and flexible needles with beveled tip to reach the target with a curved path. However, flexible needle insertion and navigation deep into the tissue complicate the procedure [11]. The experiment is close to the one presented in [12], except that their tissue phantom was considered as rigid and here the tissue is deformable. The Fig. 7 shows a real-time simulation of needle steering in a deformable object (we obtain an average of 28 frames per second).

In-vivo tissues are inherently non-homogeneous and thin medical tools can be deflected by harder regions inside overall soft tissues. We simulate this phenomenon using a 3D volume mesh composed of two regions with different stiffnesses. During its insertion, a needle collides with the surface of the stiff region: as the force at the tip is lower than the puncture threshold, the needle slides along the surface of this object. Using the same parameters, but with an

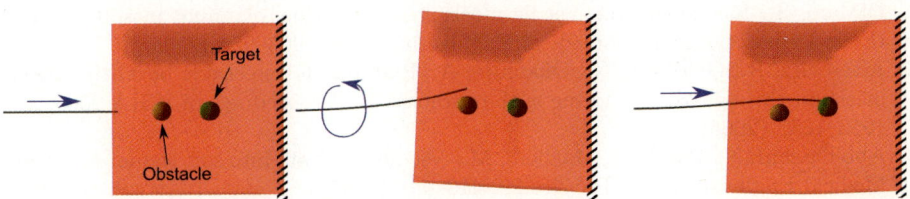

Fig. 7. The needle is first inserted one half of the distance into the phantom, then spun 180 degrees, and finally inserted the remaining distance

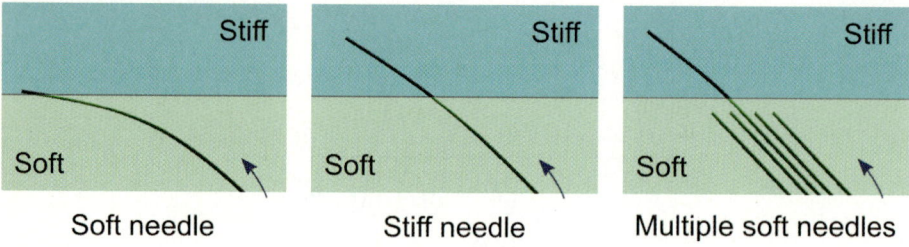

Fig. 8. Needle deviation when puncturing nonhomogeneous layers. (Left) the needle cannot penetrate the harder inclusion. (Center) First solution: by increasing the stiffness of the needle, it can now puncture the second region. (Right) Second solution: additional needles are inserted into the soft tissue, the flexible needle can penetrate.

increase of its stiffness, the needle punctures the stiff region, as shown in Fig. 8. The soft region can also be rigidified by the insertion of other needles. It allows for a precise insertion of the flexible needle without increasing its stiffness. This technique is commonly used for brachytherapy.

5 Conclusion and Future Work

In this paper, we demonstrate the interest of using complementarity constraints for the simulation of the insertion of flexible needles into soft tissue. The presented model can be parameterized using previous work experiments, and also allows for the simulation of more complex scenarios.

We plan to complete our simulations using more realistic constitutive laws for the deformation of the anatomy. In the near future, we will perform some validations on experiments to assess the precision on scenarios that are closer to clinical procedures. We aim at using the simulation as a planning tool for some therapeutic protocols that rely on the insertion of slender medical instruments.

Acknowledgments. This work is supported by ANR project 06-MDCA-015 VORTISS.

References

1. DiMaio, S., Salcudean, S.: Needle steering and motion planning in soft tissues. IEEE Transactions on Biomedical Engineering 19(6), 965–974 (2005)
2. Alterovitz, R., Goldberg, K., Okamura, A.: Planning for steerable bevel-tip needle insertion through 2d soft tissue with obstacles. In: Proceedings of ICRA 2005, pp. 1652–1657 (2005)
3. Abolhassani, N., Patel, R., Moallem, M.: Needle insertion into soft tissue: A survey. Medical Engineering and Physics 29, 413–431 (2007)
4. Marchal, M., Promayon, E., Troccaz, J.: Comparisons of needle insertion in brachytherapy protocols using a soft tissue model. In: Proceedings of the Third International Conference Surgetica 2007, pp. 153–160 (2007)

5. Okamura, A., Simone, C., O'Leary, M.: Force modeling for needle insertion into soft tissue. IEEE Transactions on Biomedical Engineering 51(10), 1707–1716 (2004)
6. Crouch, J.R., Schneider, C.M., Wainer, J., Okamura, A.M.: A velocity-dependent model for needle insertion in soft tissue. In: Duncan, J.S., Gerig, G. (eds.) MICCAI 2005. LNCS, vol. 3750, pp. 624–632. Springer, Heidelberg (2005)
7. Hing, J., Brooks, A., Desai, J.: A biplanar fluoroscopic approach for the measurement, modeling and simulation of needle and soft-tissue interaction. Medical Image Analysis 11, 62–78 (2007)
8. Dehghan, E., Wen, X., Zahiri-Azar, R., Marchal, M., Salcudean, S.: Needle-tissue interaction modeling using ultrasound-based motion estimation: Phantom study. Computer Aided Surgery 13(5), 265–280 (2008)
9. Murty, K.G.: Linear Complementarity, Linear and Nonlinear Programming, Internet edition. (1988)
10. Saupin, G., Duriez, C., Cotin, S., Grisoni, L.: Efficient contact modeling using compliance warping. In: Proceedings of CGI 2008 (2008)
11. Glozman, D., Shoham, M.: Flexible needle steering and optimal trajectory planning for percutaneous therapies. In: Barillot, C., Haynor, D.R., Hellier, P. (eds.) MICCAI 2004. LNCS, vol. 3217, pp. 137–144. Springer, Heidelberg (2004)
12. Webster, R., Kim, J., Cowan, N., Chirikjian, G., Okamura, A.: Nonholonomic modeling of needle steering. International Journal of Robotics Research 5(6), 509–525 (2006)

Real-Time Prediction of Brain Shift Using Nonlinear Finite Element Algorithms

Grand Roman Joldes[1], Adam Wittek[1], Mathieu Couton[1,3], Simon K. Warfield[2], and Karol Miller[1]

[1] Intelligent Systems for Medicine Laboratory, The University of Western Australia
35 Stirling Highway, 6009 Crawley/Perth, Western Australia, Australia
[2] Computational Radiology Laboratory, Children's Hospital Boston and Harvard Medical School
300 Longwood Avenue, Boston, MA02115, USA
[3] Institut Francais de Mechanique Avancee IFMA
Clermont Ferrand, 63175 Aubiere Cedex, France
grandj@mech.uwa.edu.au

Abstract. Patient-specific biomechanical models implemented using specialized nonlinear (i.e. taking into account material and geometric nonlinearities) finite element procedures were applied to predict the deformation field within the brain for five cases of craniotomy-induced brain shift. The procedures utilize the Total Lagrangian formulation with explicit time stepping. The loading was defined by prescribing deformations on the brain surface under the craniotomy. Application of the computed deformation fields to register the preoperative images with the intraoperative ones indicated that the models very accurately predict the intraoperative positions and deformations of the brain anatomical structures for limited information about the brain surface deformations. For each case, it took less than 40 s to compute the deformation field using a standard personal computer, and less than 4 s using a Graphics Processing Unit (GPU). The results suggest that nonlinear biomechanical models can be regarded as one possible method of complementing medical image processing techniques when conducting non-rigid registration within the real-time constraints of neurosurgery.

1 Introduction

Distortion of the preoperative anatomy due to surgical intervention and misalignment between the actual position of pathology and its position determined from the preoperative images are one of the key challenges facing image-guided neurosurgery. A typical example is the craniotomy-induced brain shift that results in movement of the pathology (tumor) and critical healthy tissues. As the contrast and spatial resolution of the intraoperative images are typically inferior to the preoperative ones [1], the high-quality preoperative data need to be aligned to the intraoperative brain geometry to retain the preoperative image quality during the surgery. Accurate alignment requires taking into account the brain deformation, which implies nonrigid registration. In recent years image-based methods for nonrigid registration have been improved by including the biomechanical models that take into account the mechanical properties of anatomical structures depicted in the image, and, therefore, ensure plausibility of the predicted intraoperative deformation field [2-4]. In most practical cases, such models utilize the finite element method to solve sets of partial differential equations of solid mechanics governing the behavior of continua. In the vast majority of biomechanical models for nonrigid registration linear finite element procedures were used [2, 3, 5]. In these procedures, the brain deformation is assumed to be infinitesimally small, i.e. the equations of solid mechanics are integrated over the initial (undeformed) brain geometry. It has been reported in several studies, that linear finite element procedures can facilitate computations of brain deformation within the real-time constraints of neurosurgery (below 60 s according to [6]). For instance, Warfield et al. [2] reported the computation time of around 15 s and Skrinjar et al. [5] – time of 80 s.

However, the brain surface deformations due to craniotomy can exceed 20 mm [7] which is inconsistent with the infinitesimally small deformation assumption. Therefore, in several studies [4, 8], finite element models utilizing geometrically nonlinear (i.e. finite deformations) formulation of solid mechanics have been used to compute the deformation field within the brain for neuroimage registration. Despite facilitating accurate predictions of the brain deformations, the nonlinear biomechanical models have been, so far, of little practical importance as the algorithms used in such models led to computation times appreciably exceeding the real-time constraints of neurosurgery [9].

Recently, however, specialized nonlinear finite element algorithms and solvers for real-time computation of soft organ deformation for image registration have become available [10-11]. In this study, we use them to compute brain deformation in five cases of craniotomy-induced brain shift. We demonstrate that biomechanical models using specialized nonlinear finite element algorithms facilitate accurate prediction of deformation field within the brain for computation times below 40 s on a standard personal computer and below 4 s on a Graphics Processing Unit (GPU).

2 Methods

2.1 Analyzed Cases

To account for various types of situations that occur in neurosurgery, we analyzed five cases of craniotomy-induced brain shift with tumor (and craniotomy) located anteriorly (cases 1 and 2), laterally (case 3) and posteriorly (cases 4 and 5) (Fig. 1).

2.2 Construction of Finite Element Meshes for Patient-Specific Brain Models

Three-dimensional patient-specific brain meshes were constructed from the segmented preoperative magnetic resonance images (MRIs). The segmentation was done using seed growing algorithm followed, in some cases, by manual corrections.

Because of the stringent computation time requirements, the meshes had to be constructed using low order elements that are not computationally expensive. The linear under-integrated hexahedron is the preferred choice. Many algorithms are now available for fast and accurate automatic mesh generation using tetrahedral elements, but not for automatic generation of hexahedral meshes [12]. Template based meshing algorithms could not be used here because of the presence of irregularly placed and

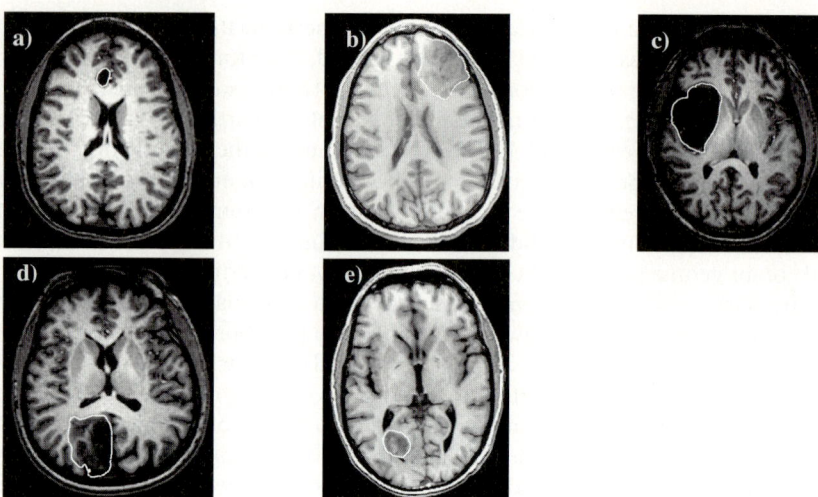

Fig. 1. Preoperative T1 MRIs (inferior view) showing tumor location in the cases analyzed in this study. White lines indicate the tumor segmentations. a) Case 1; b) Case 2; c) Case 3; d) Case 4; and e) Case 5.

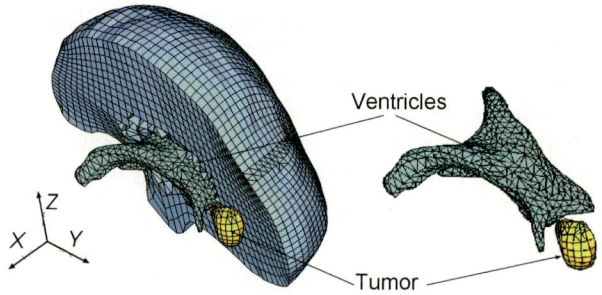

Fig. 2. Typical example (Case 1) of a patient-specific brain mesh built in this study. In this example the ventricles were discretized using tetrahedral elements only.

Table 1. Summary of the patient-specific brain meshes built in this study

	Case1	Case2	Case3	Case4	Case5
Number of Hexahedral Elements	14447	10258	10127	9032	8944
Number of Tetrahedral Elements	13563	20316	23275	23688	21160
Number of Nodes	18806	15433	15804	14732	14069
Number of Degrees of Freedom	55452	45315	46896	43794	42018

shaped tumors. Therefore, to partly automate the meshing, we used mixed meshes consisting of both linear hexahedral and tetrahedral elements (Fig. 2, Table 1). As the brain parenchyma is typically regarded as either incompressible or nearly incompressible [13, 19], the linear tetrahedral elements with average nodal pressure ANP formulation [14] were used to prevent volumetric locking. The meshes were built using IA-FEMesh (a freely available software toolkit aimed at hexahedral mesh generation developed at the University of Iowa [15]) and HyperMesh (a high-performance commercial finite element mesh generator by Altair of Troy, MI, USA).

2.3 Biomechanical Model for Brain Shift Computation

Loading and Boundary Conditions. There are always uncertainties in patient-specific properties of the living tissues. To reduce the effects of such uncertainties, we loaded the models by prescribing displacements on the exposed (due to craniotomy) part of the brain surface. It has been suggested in [9] that for this type of loading, the unknown deformation field within the brain depends very weakly on the mechanical properties. The displacements for loading the models were determined from the segmented preoperative and intraoperative cortical surfaces. The correspondences between the preoperative and intraoperative surfaces were determined by applying the vector-spline regularization algorithm described in [16] to the surface curvature maps.

To define the boundary conditions for the remaining nodes on the brain model surface, a contact interface was defined between the rigid skull model and the part of the brain surface where nodal displacements were not prescribed. Contact formulation described in [17] was used. This formulation prevents the brain surface from penetrating the skull while allowing for frictionless sliding and separation between the brain and skull.

Mechanical Properties for the Models. It has been reported in [9] that, when the geometrical nonlinearity is taken into account, constitutive model of the brain tissue exerts negligible effects on the brain shift prediction. Therefore, we used the simplest hyperelastic model: the neo-Hookean one [18]. Based on the published experimental data [13] a value of 3000 Pa was used for the parenchyma Young's modulus. The Young's modulus of the tumor was designated a value two times larger than that of the parenchyma, which is consistent with the experimental data of Sinkus et al. [20]. Following [8], we used Poisson's ratio of 0.49 for the brain parenchyma and tumor.

Solution Algorithms. We described the details of the applied algorithms (including their verification and validation) in our previous publications [10, 11, 14, 21]. Therefore, only a brief summary is given here. Computational efficiency of the algorithms for integrating the equations of solid mechanics used in this study have been achieved through application of the following two means: 1) Total Lagrangian (TL) formulation [10, 11] for updating the calculated variables; and 2) Explicit Integration in the time domain combined with mass proportional damping. In the Total Lagrangian formulation, all the calculated variables (such as displacements and strains) are referred to the original configuration of the analyzed continuum. The decisive advantage of this formulation is that all derivatives with respect to spatial coordinates can be pre-computed [10]. As indicated in [10], this greatly reduces the computation time in comparison to Updated Lagrangian formulation used in vast majority of commercial finite element solvers (such as e.g. LS-DYNA, ABAQUS).

In explicit time integration, the displacement at time $t+\Delta t$ (where Δt is the time step) is solely based on the equilibrium at time t. Therefore, no matrix inversion and iterations are required when solving nonlinear problems. In consequence, application of explicit integration can reduce the time required to compute the brain deformations by an order of magnitude in comparison to implicit integration typically used in commercial finite element codes for steady state solutions [8].

Accuracy Evaluation. Universally accepted "gold standards" for validation of nonrigid registration techniques have not been developed yet [22]. Objective metrics of the images' alignment can be provided by automated methods using image similarity metrics (such as e.g. Mutual Information and Normalized Cross-Correlation). One of the key deficiencies of such metrics is that they quantify the alignment error in terms that do not have straightforward geometrical (in Euclidean sense) interpretation.

To provide an error measure that enables such interpretation, we compared X, Y and Z bounds of the ventricles determined from the intraoperative segmentations and obtained by registration (i.e. warping using the predicted deformation field) of the preoperative data. The bounds provide six numbers that can be geometrically interpreted as the X, Y and Z coordinates of vertices P_1 and P_2 defining a cuboidal box bounding the ventricles (see Fig. 3). The difference between the coordinates of these vertices determined from the intraoperative MRIs and predicted by our biomechanical models was used as a measure of the alignment error. The coordinates of the vertices P_1 and P_2 can be determined automatically, which makes such difference less prone to subjective errors than the measures based on anatomical landmarks selected by experts. We provide no error measure for the tumor registration as we were not able to reliably quantify the intraoperative bounds of tumors due to limited quality of the intraoperative images.

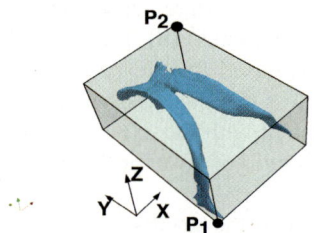

Fig. 3. Definition the ventricles' bounds. Vertices P1 and P2 define a cuboidal box that bounds the ventricles. The box faces are formed by planes perpendicular to X, Y and Z axes.

3 Results

The maximum displacement of the cortical surface was 7.7 mm (Case 2), and the brain maximum (Green) strain predicted by our models was 30%. The computation times on a PC (Intel E6850 dual core 3.00 GHz processor, 4 GB of internal memory, and Windows XP operating system) varied from 30 s (Case 1) to 38 s (Case 5). Following our earlier work [23] on application of Graphics Processing Units (GPUs) for scientific computations, we also implemented our algorithms using the NVIDIA Compute Unified Device Architecture (CUDA). Non-trivial details of this implementation are given in [24]. For the NVIDIA CUDA implementation of our algorithms, the computation times were under 4 s for all the craniotomy cases analyzed in this study. The maximum errors when predicting the intraoperative bounds of the ventricles were 1.6 mm in X (lateral) direction, 1.6 mm in Y (i.e. anterior-posterior) direction and 2.2 mm in Z (inferior-superior) direction (Table 2). These errors compare well with the voxel size (0.86x0.86x2.5 mm^3) of the intraoperative images. Detailed comparison of the contours of ventricles in the intraoperative images and the ones predicted by the finite element brain models developed in this study indicate some local misregistration. However, the overall agreement is remarkably good (Fig. 4).

In Table 2, the computation results are presented to one decimal place as it has been reported in the literature [8] that this is approximately the accuracy of finite element computations using the type of finite element algorithms applied in this study.

Table 2. Error in predicting the X, Y, and Z coordinates (in millimeters) of vertices P1 and P2 defining the bounds of the ventricles in the intraoperative MRIs (see Fig. 3). The directions of the X, Y, and Z axes are as in Fig. 3. The numbers in bold font indicate the maximum errors.

	X Coordinate Error [mm]		Y Coordinate Error [mm]		Z Coordinate Error [mm]	
	P1	P2	P1	P2	P1	P2
Case 1	0.3	0.2	0.7	1.3	0.7	0.2
Case 2	0.0	0.5	1.2	0.5	0.6	0.5
Case 3	**1.6**	0.4	0.6	**1.6**	**2.2**	0.1
Case 4	0.5	0.0	0.5	0.4	0.1	0.7
Case 5	0.1	0.4	0.5	1.5	1.1	0.4

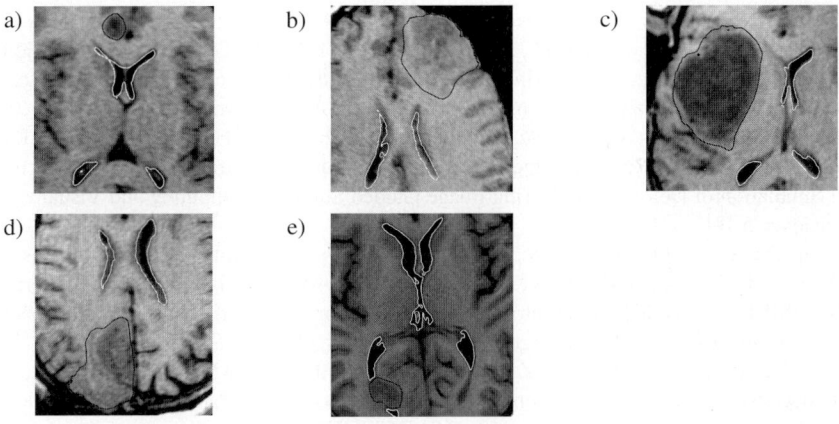

Fig. 4. The registered (i.e. deformed using the calculated deformation field) preoperative contours of ventricles and tumor are imposed on the intraoperative images. The images were cropped and enlarged. a) Case 1; b) Case 2; c) Case 3; d) Case 4; and e) Case 5.

4 Discussion

Instead of relying on unrealistic linearization (i.e. assumption about infinitesimally small brain deformation during craniotomy and linear stress–strain relationship of brain tissue) used so far in biomechanical models to satisfy real-time constraints of neurosurgery, we applied specialized fully nonlinear (i.e. including both geometrical and material nonlinearities) finite element procedures and predicted deformation field within the brain due to craniotomy-induced brain shift in less than 40 s using standard personal computer with a single dual-core processor, and less than 4 s using Graphics Processing Unit.

Thus, our results indicate that accurate computations of deformation field within the brain by means of state-of-the-art finite element procedures utilizing fully nonlinear formulation of solid mechanics can be achieved in real time without advanced computer hardware. This is an important step in enabling application of such formulation in neuroimage registration practice. However, before nonlinear computational biomechanical models can become a part of clinical systems for image-guided neurosurgery, reliability and accuracy of such models must be confirmed against much larger data sample than five cases of craniotomy-induced brain shift analyzed in this study.

Acknowledgments. The financial support of the Australian Research Council (Grants DP0664534, DP1092893, DP0770275 and LX0774754), National Institute of Health (Grants R03 CA126466, R01 RR021885, R01 GM074068 and R01 EB008015), CIMIT, and Australian Academy of Science is gratefully acknowledged. We thank Prof. Ron Kikinis of Brigham and Women's Hospital for very helpful suggestions.

References

1. Warfield, S.K., Haker, S.J., Talos, I.F., Kemper, C.A., Weisenfeld, N., Mewes, A.U.J., Goldberg-Zimring, D., Zou, K.H., Westin, C.F., Wells, W.M., Tempany, C.M.C., Golby, A., Black, P.M., Jolesz, F.A., Kikinis, R.: Capturing Intraoperative Deformations: Research Experience at Brigham and Womens's Hospital. Medical Image Analysis 9, 145–162 (2005)
2. Warfield, S.K., Talos, F., Tei, A., Bharatha, A., Nabavi, A., Ferrant, M., Black, P.M., Jolesz, F.A., Kikinis, R.: Real-Time Registration of Volumetric Brain MRI by Biomechanical Simulation of Deformation During Image Guided Surgery. Computing and Visualization in Science 5, 3–11 (2002)
3. Archip, N., Clatz, O., Whalen, S., Kacher, D., Fedorov, A., Kot, A., Chrisochoides, N., Jolesz, F., Golby, A., Black, P.M., Warfield, S.K.: Non-Rigid Alignment of Pre-Operative MRI, fMRI, and DT-MRI with Intra-Operative MRI for Enhanced Visualization and Navigation in Image-Guided Neurosurgery. NeuroImage 35, 609–624 (2007)
4. Hu, J., Jin, X., Lee, J.B., Zhang, L.Z., Chaudhary, V., Guthikonda, M., Yang, K.H., King, A.I.: Intraoperative Brain Shift Prediction Using a 3D Inhomogeneous Patient-Specific Finite Element Model. Journal of Neurosurgery 106, 164–169 (2007)
5. Skrinjar, O., Nabavi, A., Duncan, J.: Model-Driven Brain Shift Compensation. Medical Image Analysis 6, 361–373 (2002)
6. Gobbi, D.G.: Brain Deformation Correction Using Interactive 3D Ultrasound Imaging. PhD Thesis. Faculty of Medicine, University of Western Ontario, London, Canada (2003)
7. Roberts, D.W., Hartov, A., Kennedy, F.E., Miga, M.I., Paulsen, K.D.: Intraoperative Brain Shift and Deformation: A Quantitative Analysis of Cortical displacement in 28 Cases. Neurosurgery 43, 749–758 (1998)
8. Wittek, A., Miller, K., Kikinis, R., Warfield, S.K.: Patient-Specific Model of Brain Deformation: Application to Medical Image Registration. Journal of Biomechanics 40, 919–929 (2007)

9. Wittek, A., Hawkins, T., Miller, K.: On the Unimportance of Constitutive Models in Computing Brain Deformation for Image-Guided Surgery. Biomechanics and Modeling in Mechanobiology 8, 77–84 (2009)
10. Miller, K., Joldes, G., Lance, D., Wittek, A.: Total Lagrangian Explicit Dynamics Finite Element Algorithm for Computing Soft Tissue Deformation. Communications in Numerical Methods in Engineering 23, 121–134 (2007)
11. Joldes, G.R., Wittek, A., Miller, K.: Suite of Finite Element Algorithms for Accurate Computation of Soft Tissue Deformation for Surgical Simulation. Medical Image Analysis (in press) (2008), doi:10.1016/j.media.2008.12.001
12. Viceconti, M., Taddei, F.: Automatic Generation of Finite Element Meshes from Computed Tomography Data. Critical Reviews in Biomedical Engineering 31, 27–72 (2003)
13. Miller, K., Chinzei, K.: Mechanical Properties of Brain Tissue in Tension. Journal of Biomechanics 35, 483–490 (2002)
14. Joldes, G.R., Wittek, A., Miller, K.: Non-locking Tetrahedral Finite Element for Surgical Simulation. Communications in Numerical Methods in Engineering (in press) (2008), doi: 10.1002/cnm.1185
15. Grosland, N.M., Shivanna, K.H., Magnotta, V.A., Kallemeyn, N.A., DeVries, N.A., Tadepalli, S.C., Lisle, C.: IA-FEMesh: An Open-Source, Interactive, Multiblock Approach to Anatomic Finite Element Model Development. Computer Methods and Programs in Biomedicine (in press, 2009), doi: 10.1016/j.cmpb.2008.12.003
16. Arganda-Carreras, I., Sorzano, C.O.S., Marabini, R., Carazo, J.M., Ortiz-de-Solorzano, C., Kybic, J.: Consistent and elastic registration of histological sections using vector-spline regularization. In: Beichel, R.R., Sonka, M. (eds.) CVAMIA 2006. LNCS, vol. 4241, pp. 85–95. Springer, Heidelberg (2006)
17. Joldes, G., Wittek, A., Miller, K., Morriss, L.: Realistic and Efficient Brain-Skull Interaction Model for Brain Shift Computation. In: Computational Biomechanics for Medicine III (MICCAI 2008 Associated Workshop), pp. 95–105 (2008)
18. Yeoh, O.H.: Some Forms of Strain-Energy Function for Rubber. Rubber Chemistry and Technology 66, 754–771 (1993)
19. Miller, K., Chinzei, K.: Constitutive Modeling of Brain Tissue: Experiment and Theory. Journal of Biomechanics 30, 1115–1121 (1997)
20. Sinkus, R., Tanter, M., Xydeas, T., Catheline, S., Bercoff, J., Fink, M.: Viscoelastic Shear Properties of In Vivo Breast Lesions Measured by MR Elastography. Magnetic Resonance Imaging 23, 159–165 (2005)
21. Joldes, G.R., Wittek, A., Miller, K.: An Efficient Hourglass Control Implementation for the Uniform Strain Hexahedron Using the Total Lagrangian Formulation. Communications in Numerical Methods in Engineering 24, 1315–1323 (2008)
22. Chakravarty, M.M., Sadikot, A.F., Germann, J., Bertrand, G., Collins, D.L.: Towards a Validation of Atlas Warping Techniques. Medical Image Analysis 12, 713–726 (2008)
23. Walsh, T.: Hardware Finite Element Procedures. Internal Report. Intelligent Systems for Medicine Laboratory, The University of Western Australia, Crawley, Australia (2004)
24. Joldes, G.R., Wittek, A., Miller, K.: Real-Time Nonlinear Finite Element Computations on GPU Using CUDA - Application to Neurosurgical Simulation. Computer Methods in Applied Mechanics and Engineering (submitted, 2009)

Model-Based Estimation of Ventricular Deformation in the Cat Brain

Fenghong Liu[1], S. Scott Lollis[2], Songbai Ji[1], Keith D. Paulsen[1,3], Alexander Hartov[1,3], and David W. Roberts[2,3]

[1] Thayer School of Engineering, Dartmouth College, Hanover, NH 03755 USA
[2] Department of Neurosurgery, Dartmouth-Hitchcock Medical Center, Lebanon, NH 03756 USA
[3] Norris Cotton Cancer Center, Lebanon, NH 03756 USA
keith.paulsen@dartmouth.edu

Abstract. The estimation of ventricular deformation has important clinical implications related to neuro-structural disorders such as hydrocephalus. In this paper, a poroelastic model was used to represent deformation effects resulting from the ventricular system and was studied in 5 feline experiments. Chronic or acute hydrocephalus was induced by injection of kaolin into the cisterna magna or saline into the ventricles; a catheter was then inserted in the lateral ventricle to drain the fluid out of the brain. The measured displacement data which was extracted from pre-drainage and post-drainage MR images were incorporated into the model through the Adjoint Equations Method. The results indicate that the computational model of the brain and ventricular system captured 33% of the ventricle deformation on average and the model-predicted intraventricular pressure was accurate to 90% of the recorded value during the chronic hydrocephalus experiments.

1 Introduction

The cerebral ventricles in the brain are cavities filled with cerebrospinal fluid (CSF). The deformation of the ventricular system is related to diseases such as hydrocephalus and edema but may also occur as the result of a space occupying lesion. Together with the compression of the white matter adjacent to the ventricles, these diseases can cause serious neurological problems including cognitive impairment and even death.

Different research groups have been studying the mathematical modeling of the ventricular system in the brain. Drake's approach represents the brain as a lumped-parameter system [1], but given that the brain is a sponge-like material, a more realistic poroelastic model has been investigated to incorporate the fluid distribution in the parenchyma. Nagashima et al. [2] modeled the brain and ventricles based on Biot's consolidation theory [3]. A 2D finite element model of the parenchyma was created using computed tomography (CT) scans. Pena et al. further studied the poroelastic model to represent the stress concentrations and ventricular anatomy more accurately [4, 5]. Several groups have attempted to improve the boundary conditions and material parameters used in the poroelastic model [6, 7, 8]. Miller et al. proposed a nonlinear viscoelastic representation [9]. Kyriacou et al. compared it with the linearly elastic approach and concluded that the viscoelastic model is more suitable to capturing high stain rates [10]. Considering the fact that ventricular deformation is related to CSF flow and is not representative of high stain rate deformation, we modeled the brain as an elastic porous medium to allow the flow of the interstitial fluid into and out of the extracellular space through the ventricular walls. We represented the ventricular system through mixed boundary conditions and used sparse measurement data to estimate the driving fluid pressure required to deform the brain during the induction and release of pressure-induced ventriculomegaly. The importance of the work is that we show for the first time an algorithm that is able to successfully estimate the unknown pressure parameters in the boundary conditions from displacement data that allows the fluid-filled ventricles to be represented by their surface, rather than directly including them within the discretized computational domain in which case a phase change would need to be incorporated into the mechanical equations describing brain deformation that is far more complicated to implement numerically.

2 Materials and Methods

2.1 Experimental System

A group of five felines was studied with MR imaging for *in vivo* observation of the progression of ventricle deformation. Chronic or acute hydrocephalus was first induced by injection of kaolin into the cisterna magna or saline into the ventricle as a control. Following that, a catheter was inserted into the lateral ventricle to drain fluid out of the brain, which caused the enlarged ventricles to shrink. The model simulated the ventricular shrinking process.

Five adult female domestic felines were quarantined for three days prior to the beginning of the experiment. On the day of cisternal injection, general anesthesia was induced and a peripheral intravenous catheter was placed. All animals underwent baseline magnetic resonance imaging (MRI) of the brain. Animals then underwent cisternal injection of kaolin or saline. Each animal was placed prone on a heated operating table with the neck partially flexed. A pediatric spinal needle was inserted in the midline, under fluoroscopic guidance, into the occiput-C1 interspace until clear CSF was returned (Figure 1, left). The needle was secured using a mobile clamp affixed to the table (Figure 1, right). The kaolin dose was 10 -50 mg mixed in sterile saline. Slow injection of kaolin was completed over 10 minutes.

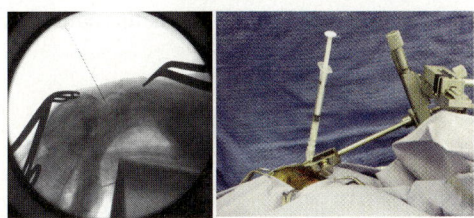

Fig. 1. Lateral fluoroscopic view of injection via occiput-C1 interspace (left) and operative photograph of 1 cc syringe affixed to stabilizing clamp (right) [11]

Once ventriculomegaly was confirmed, a ventricular catheter connected to a subcutaneous reservoir was placed in the right frontal region, to enable subsequent measurement of intracranial pressure (ICP). The catheter-reservoir construct was inserted into the right lateral ventricle using a central stylet. [11]

Another MRI session was scheduled between 7 and 17 days after the initial injection. Cats were anesthetized and the animal's head was fixed on the exam table as shown in Figure 2(a). After the ventricles were enlarged, a series of MR images were taken (Figure 2(b)). These images are referred to as pre-drainage MR. Intraventricular pressures (IVP) were measured after induction of hydrocephalus. One hour later, the fluid was drained out of the ventricle through the catheter. The enlarged ventricle shrunk markedly. Another set of images (Figure 2(c)) were acquired at this point which are called post-drainage MR. IVPs were measured again at this stage.

By comparing the two sets of images, substantial ventricular shrinkage was observed. We attempted to drain the ventricles in stages, for example, by removing fluid in 0.5 cc increments but observed a threshold effect whereby either no observable deformation occurred (if too little fluid was removed) or no additional deformation resulted (if more fluid was removed after an initial amount sufficient to cause an immediate and measurable reduction in ventricular size was taken). The images were acquired with a 3.0 T MRI (Philips) system and had a resolution of 256×256×24 voxels and a voxel size of 0.3125 mm×0.3125 mm×1.2 mm.

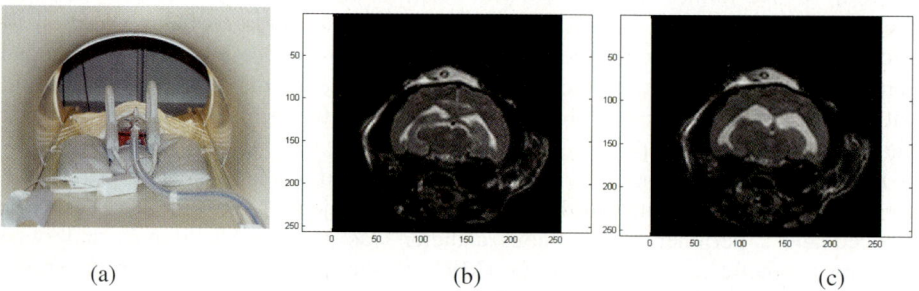

(a)   (b)   (c)

Fig. 2. (a) The cat was anesthetized and the head was fixed on the exam table. (b) Pre-drainage MR. (c) Post-drainage MR of the same cat brain.

2.2 Computational Model

The biomechanical model was based on Biot's consolidation theory, and the brain was modeled as poroelastic material [3, 12]. The mathematical description is [13, 14]:

$$\nabla \cdot G \nabla \mathbf{u} + \nabla \frac{G}{1-2v}(\nabla \cdot \mathbf{u}) - \alpha \nabla p = \mathbf{f}$$
$$\alpha \frac{\partial}{\partial t}(\nabla \cdot \mathbf{u}) + \frac{1}{S}\frac{\partial p}{\partial t} - \nabla \cdot k \nabla p = \Psi$$
(1)

where

    $\mathbf{f}$ body force (e.g., gravity) per unit volume (N/m^3);

    Ψ pressure source strength (Pa/s);

G   shear modulus (Pa);
v   Poisson's ratio;
u   displacement vector (m);
p   pore fluid pressure (Pa);
α   ratio of fluid vol. extracted to vol. change of the tissue under compression;
k   hydraulic conductivity ($m^3 s/kg$);
1/S   amount of fluid which can be forced into the tissue under constant vol. ($1/Pa$).

By using the finite element method (FEM), these equations can be solved with the adjoint equations method (AEM) [15] to incorporate the intraoperative measurements.

2.3 Model Generation

The FEM discretization process begins with segmentation of the region of interest. A semi-automatic method was used to segment the cat brain and ventricles from the pre-drainage MR images. A surface description consisting of triangular patches was generated from the segmented brain and ventricles. Then, a 3-D tetrahedral mesh was created to define the computational domain. The volume mesh contained about 11,000 nodes and 53,000 elements. Given the boundary conditions and material properties, and the input of measured displacement data around the ventricle, the biomechanical model can be solved with FEM. The original mesh was deformed using the displacement results and the pre-drainage MR images were morphed to predict the post-drainage MR status. Figure 3 illustrates the entire procedure.

The ventricles were modeled as a cavity since they only include CSF which is treated as a void in the consolidation equations. Approximate boundary conditions were imposed to simulate the physical conditions. The upper brain surface was specified as stress free and allowed free flow of CSF. The ventricle surface was set to be stress free to allow displacements, and pressure was handled by a mixed (type 3)

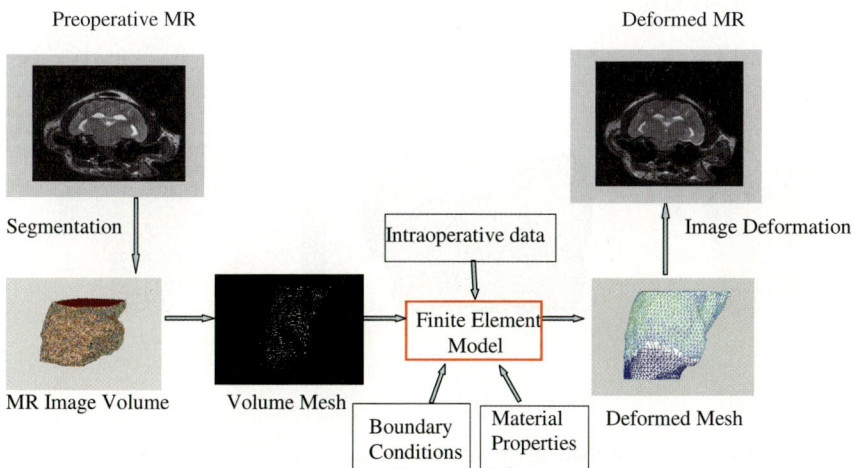

Fig. 3. Illustration of the modeling procedure for the ventricular system in the brain

boundary condition, $\frac{\partial p}{\partial n} = k(p - p_v)$ where p is the brain tissue interstitial pressure, n is the normal to the boundary of the ventricle, p_v is the ventricle fluid pressure and k is the conductivity coefficient. This condition specifies the drainage through the ventricle surface as a function of the interstitial pressure and permeability of the ventricular wall. The flow of fluid is determined by the hydraulic conductivity and the pressure difference between the interstitial and ventricular fluid pressures. The lower part of the brain was modeled as brainstem which was assumed to have no displacements and free flow of CSF.

Reliable tissue properties are important to the biomechanical modeling. There are many studies on the mechanical properties of brain tissue. The material properties deployed here were Young's modulus E = 3240 Pa, Poisson's ratio v = 0.45 and the hydraulic conductivity, $k = 1 \times 10^{-7} m^3 s/kg$ [14, 16].

3 Results

The first cat was a control animal. Saline was infused into the ventricle before the pre-drainage stage of the experiment. Fluid was drained from the ventricle before the post-drainage MR session. In Figure 4(a), the red arrows around the ventricles show the 31 sparse data points which were incorporated into the model. They were evenly distributed around the ventricles, except in areas where unreliable displacements were measured. In the quantitative validation, the number of validation data points was 1105. The brain configuration and ventricle deformation are presented in Figure 4(b), which shows that the maximum displacement is about 3 mm. In Figure 4(c), the gray color is the pre-drainage ventricle, the brown color is the measured post-drainage ventricular shape (after shrinkage), and the green is the model estimate of the post-drainage ventricle. The 3D view shows that the model results match the measured ones very well. In order to better visualize the model results, four 2D slices were generated to produce an overlay of the ventricle boundary in the 3 experimental states.

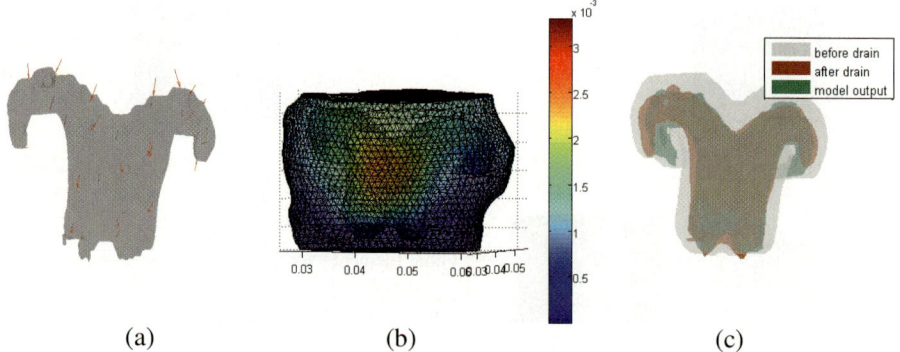

Fig. 4. (a) Sparse data distribution around the ventricle used for data assimilation in cat 1. (b) Displacement results of the cat brain surface. (c) Overlay of the pre-drainage ventricle (gray), post-drainage ventricle (brown) and model estimated post drainage ventricle (green).

In Figure 5 (left), the blue line is the pre-drainage ventricle, background MR shows the post-drainage ventricle, and the red dots represent the model estimate of the post-drainage ventricle. The pre-drainage ventricle (blue) is large as seen from the 2D slices. After the fluid was drained, its size shrunk. The model result (red) matches the measurement (MR) better in the slices compared to the pre-drainage ventricle (blue).

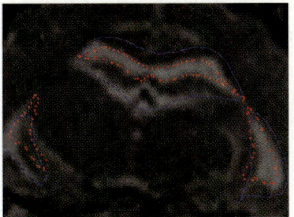 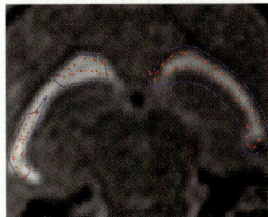

Fig. 5. Overlays of the predrainage ventricle (blue), postdrainage ventricle (background MR) and model deformed ventricle (red) for cat 1(left) and cat 2 (right)

The second cat was also a control animal. There were 48 sparse data around the ventricle used in this case and 710 data were deployed for validation. The results are shown in Figure 5 right. The 2D overlay indicates the model made certain improvements for cat 2. For both of the control animals, the model-estimated intraventricular pressure was less than 1000 Pa, which is lower than the measured 3000 Pa pressure. This may have occurred because of the leakage of fluid around the catheter, an effect which was observed during the injection in the experiments. Another possible explanation is that the fluid can flow out the lateral ventricle through the third ventricle, and therefore, reduce the pressure around the lateral ventricles which are modeled in the study.

The remaining three cats underwent hydrocephalus experiments. Hydrocephalus was induced by injection of kaolin into the cisterna magna. The intraventricular pressure was different in the pre-drainage state, but it was the same post-drainage and equaled 500 Pa. The difference in the measured intraventricular pressure between the two stages was 1000 Pa, 700 Pa and 600 Pa for cat 3, cat 4 and cat 5, respectively.

The displacement results for cat 3, cat 4 and cat 5 are reported in Figure 6 left, middle and right, respectively. The number of sparse data was 35, 31 and 41 and number of validation points was 414, 381 and 719 in each case, respectively. Points

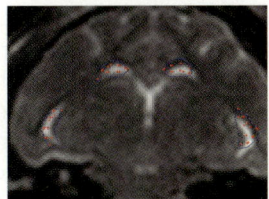 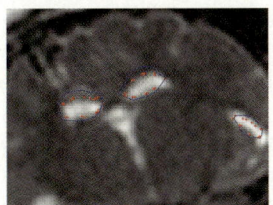 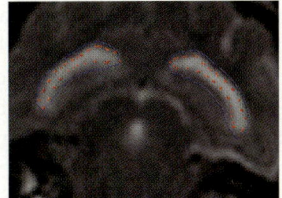

Fig. 6. Overlays of the pre-drainage ventricle (blue), post-drainage ventricle (background MR) and model deformed ventricle (red) for cat 3 (left), cat 4 (middle) and cat 5 (right)

were evenly distributed around the ventricle. The model estimations achieved different levels of success. Both the displacement and pressure results from the model match the measurements. The model estimations of IVP were 900Pa, 730Pa and 570 Pa, respectively. Compared to the measured pressure differences of 1000 Pa, 700 Pa and 600 Pa, the model estimates were accurate to 90% in all three experiments.

A quantitative comparison of the displacement results is shown in Table 1. The data indicates that in all five cases, the model captured 33% of the deformation on average. The misfit reported in Table 1 is the average distance between the measured and model estimated ventricles for each cat.

Table 1. The misfit before and after the model prediction for five cat studies

	Mean Misfit (before) (mm)	Mean Misfit (after) (mm)	Improvements (%)
Cat1	1.27	0.786	38.0
Cat2	0.799	0.555	30.5
Cat3	0.616	0.419	32.0
Cat4	0.515	0.349	32.8
Cat5	0.725	0.364	29.9

4 Discussion

The results showed that the computational method was able to estimate ventricular deformation in the cat brain within 1 mm through type 3 boundary condition representation of the ventricular surface which holds promise for improving modeling accuracy as well as avoiding the need of implementing the more complicated mechanical modeling framework that would be required to represent the fluid phase of the ventricles, if they are discretized directly within the computational domain. The quantitative analysis indicates that the model captured 33% of the ventricular deformation on average in five cat experiments and the model estimated IVP to be accurate within 90% compared to the measured value in the chronic hydrocephalus experiments.

Although the mathematical representation of the ventricles has produced relatively good results, in some respects the average percentage of deformation capture (33%) is disappointing. Here, it is important to recognize that the overall deformation in the cat brain was very small (~ 1mm), placing a premium on the fidelity of the image processing and displacement data extraction procedures that were used in the study. Further investigations are needed to explore the extent to which the modeling errors are, in part, a result of imperfections in the data analysis techniques. For example, in the segmentation and surface and volume meshing processes, error is accumulated and can be reduced. The nonrigid motion of the ventricles was also approximated through Iterative Closest Point to determine displacements. In order to provide better guidance and improve model-data mismatch, more accurate displacement measurements are needed. The brain mechanical properties employed in this study were taken from the literature whereas material properties determined experimentally for each feline brain will likely contribute to improved modeling accuracy.

The methodology can be extended to human clinical studies. Since the CSF pressure in the intraventricular space is measurable during the neurosurgery, data on both displacement and pressure will be available. The measurements can then be used as data for the model computed brain deformation. Incorporating the ventricle structure and the pressure data will help to further develop the model to yield more accurate estimates of the state of the brain during surgery and can help the surgeon to optimize the planned surgical path. Additional clinical studies are needed for future validation at the human scale but the *in vivo* results presented here in the cat brain appear promising and suggest that the approach will be successful in humans as well.

References

1. Drake, J., Kestle, J., Milner, R.: Randomized clinical trials of cerebrospinal fluid shunt design in pediatric hydrocephalus. Neurosurgery 43, 294–305 (1998)
2. Nagashima, T., Tamaki, N., Matsumoto, S., Horwitz, B., Seguchi, Y.: Biomechanics of hydrocephalus: a new theoretical model. Neurosurgery 21, 898–903 (1987)
3. Biot, M.: General theory of three-dimensional consolidation. Journal of Applied Physics 12, 155–164 (1941)
4. Pena, A., Bolton, M.D., Whitehouse, H., Pickard, J.D.: Effects of brain ventricular shape on periventricular biomechanics: a finite element analysis. Neurosurgery 45, 107–118 (1999)
5. Pena, A., Harris, N.G., Bolton, M.D., Czosnyka, M., Pickard, J.D.: Communicating hydrocephalus: the biomechanics of progressive ventricular enlargement revisited. Acta Neurochir. Suppl. 81, 59–63 (2002)
6. Kaczmarek, M., Subramaniam, R., Neff, S.: The hydromechanics of hydrocephalus: steady state solution for cylindrical geometry. Bull. Math. Biol. 59, 295–323 (1997)
7. Tenti, G., Sivaloganathan, S., Drake, J.: Brain biomechanics: steady-state consolidation theory of hydrocephalus. Can. Appl. Maths (1998)
8. Taylor, Z., Miller, K.: Reassessment of brain elasticity for analysis of biomechanisms of hydrocephalus. J. Biomech. 37, 1263–1269 (2004)
9. Miller, K., Chinzei, K.: Constitutive modelling of brain tissue: experiment and theory. J. Biomech. 30, 115–1121 (1997)
10. Kyriacou, S., Mohamed, A., Miller, K., Neff, S.: Brain mechanics for neurosurgery: modeling issues. Biomech. Mod. Mechanobiol. 1, 151–164 (2002)
11. Lollis, S., Hoopes, P., Bergeron, J., Kane, S., Paulsen, K., Weaver, J., Roberts, D.: Low-dose kaolin-induced feline hydrocephalus and feline ventriculostomy: An updated model. Protocol (2007)
12. Nagashima, T., Tamaki, N., Takada, M., Tada, Y.: Formation and resolution of brain edema associated with brain tumors. A comprehensive theoretical model and clinical analysis. Acta Neurochirurgica Suppl. 60, 165–167 (1994)
13. Paulsen, K., Miga, M., Kennedy, F., Hoopes, P., Hartov, A., Roberts, D.: A computational model for tracking subsurface tissue deformation during stereotactic neurosurgery. IEEE Transactions on Biomedical Engineering 46, 213–225 (1999)
14. Miga, M.: Development and Quantification of a 3D Brain Deformation Model for Model-Updataed Image-Guided Stereotactic Neurosurgery, Phd thesis, Thayer School of Engineering, Dartmouth College, Hanover, NH (September 1998)
15. Lynch, D.R.: Numerical Partial Differential Equations for Environmental Scientists and Engineers - A First Practical Course, 2nd edn. Springer, Heidelberg (2004)
16. Chinzei, K., Miller, K.: Compression of swine brain tissue; experiment in vitro. J. Mech. Eng. Lab. 50, 19–28 (1996)

Contact Studies between Total Knee Replacement Components Developed Using Explicit Finite Elements Analysis

Lucian G. Gruionu[1], Gabriel Gruionu[2], Stefan Pastrama[3], Nicolae Iliescu[3], and Taina Avramescu[1]

[1] University of Craiova, A.I.Cuza 13, Craiova, Romania
 lucian.gruionu@imst.ro
[2] Indianapolis University Purdue University, 420 University Blvd. Indianapolis, IN, USA
[3] University Politehnica of Bucharest, Splaiul Independentei 313, Bucharest, Romania

Abstract. A pneumatic simulator of the knee joint with five DOF was developed to determine the correlation between the kinematics of the knee joint, and the wear of the polyethylene componenet of a TKR prosthesis. A physical model of the knee joint with total knee replacement (TKR) was built by rapid-prototyping based on CT images from a patient. A clinically-available prosthesis was mounted on the knee model. Using a video analysis system, and two force and contact pressure plates, the kinematics and kinetics data were recorded during normal walking of the patient. The quadriceps muscle force during movement was computed using the Anybody software. Joint loadings were generated by the simulator based on recorded and computed data. Using the video analysis system, the precise kinematics of the artificial joint from the simulator was recorded and used as input for an explicit dynamics FE analysis of the joint. The distribution of the contact stresses in the implant was computed during the walking cycle to analyze the prosthesis behavior. The results suggest that the combination of axial loading and anterior-posterior stress is responsible for the abrasive wear of the polyethylene component of the prosthesis.

1 Introduction

At present, the short life cycle of TKR represent a great concern for both orthopedic surgeons and prosthesis designers. Loosening of the tibial component is an important cause of TKR failure [1]. During the gait cycle, the forces developed in the knee have a cyclic pattern with values between 10 and 30 MPa, resulting in high stress values and wear of the artificial joint components. The mechanisms responsible for TKR wear are delamination, scratching, pitting and abrasion [1-3].

The present study used clinical investigation, engineering and computational methods: non-invasive imaging methods to collect data directly from the patient, a newly developed knee simulator to reproduce the physical forces acting on the joint during movement, and finite element analysis to integrate the clinical observations and experimental data and to compute the resulting stresses in the joint. The purpose of the study was to determine the correlation between the kinematics of the knee joint, and the stress distribution in the polyethylene componenent of the TKR during the gait cycle.

2 Materials and Methods

The three-dimensional computational joint reconstruction (Fig. 1, a) was achieved from CT serial sections of the patient's leg and radiographic images of the joint with TKR. Images have been acquired in DICOM format and converted to JPEG using the MRIco software. The three-dimensional CAD model of the patient's knee joint was used to develop an artificial human knee by rapid prototyping using an Objet Eden 260 3D printer. The femoral metallic components and the tibial metallic tray with polyethylene plate were mounted on the plastic components (Fig. 1, b) using medical cement. Five HBM LY strain gages were placed on both components of the joint for data recording during the simulation (Fig. 1,c).

A new 5DOF simulator for the knee joint was designed and developed in our labs to study the biomechanical changes in different pathological cases and to establish the efficacy of the type of osteotomy with different fixation systems and prostheses.

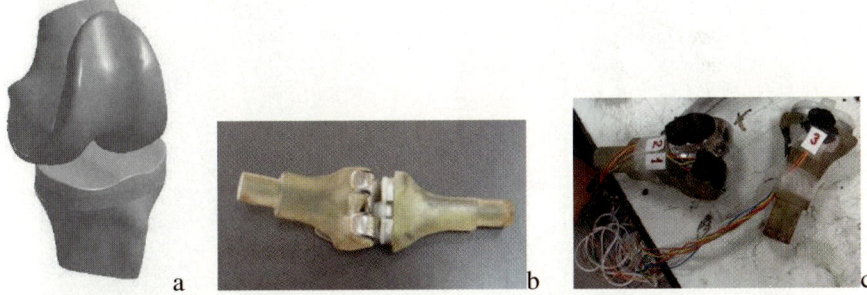

Fig. 1. Three-dimensional CAD models of the TKR joint of the patient (a), the prosthesis components and the artificial joint with implants mounted (b), the artificial femur and tibia with artificial prosthesis and strain markers (c)

The knee simulator is based on the general principles of the Purdue Knee Simulator with several novel patent-pending improvements. The new design allows an unconstrained flexion/extension motion between femur and tibia, with the hip and ankle joints attached to the frame (Fig. 2). The loads on the knee are: the simulated quadriceps muscle action (quadriceps load), and the applied external loads at the simulated hip (body weight) and ankle (vertical rotation torque and medial-lateral translation load) (Fig. 2, b). This particular design can simulate the natural behavior of the joint by varying the applied loads and articular geometry of the knee.

There are two DOF between the femur and simulator frame: vertical translation of the hip and flexion/extension/rotation relative to the translating hip sled. The hip sled is constrained by two vertical precision rails attached to the frame, and the load that simulates the body weight (max. 200 kgf) is provided by a pneumatic cylinder. The flexion-extension rotation (±65°) is imposed through the quadriceps muscle simulated by an actuator fixed to the femur. The action of the quadriceps actuator cause an extension moment about the knee that extended the hip as well. The ankle sled provides four degrees of freedom between the tibia and the ground. A universal joint gives the

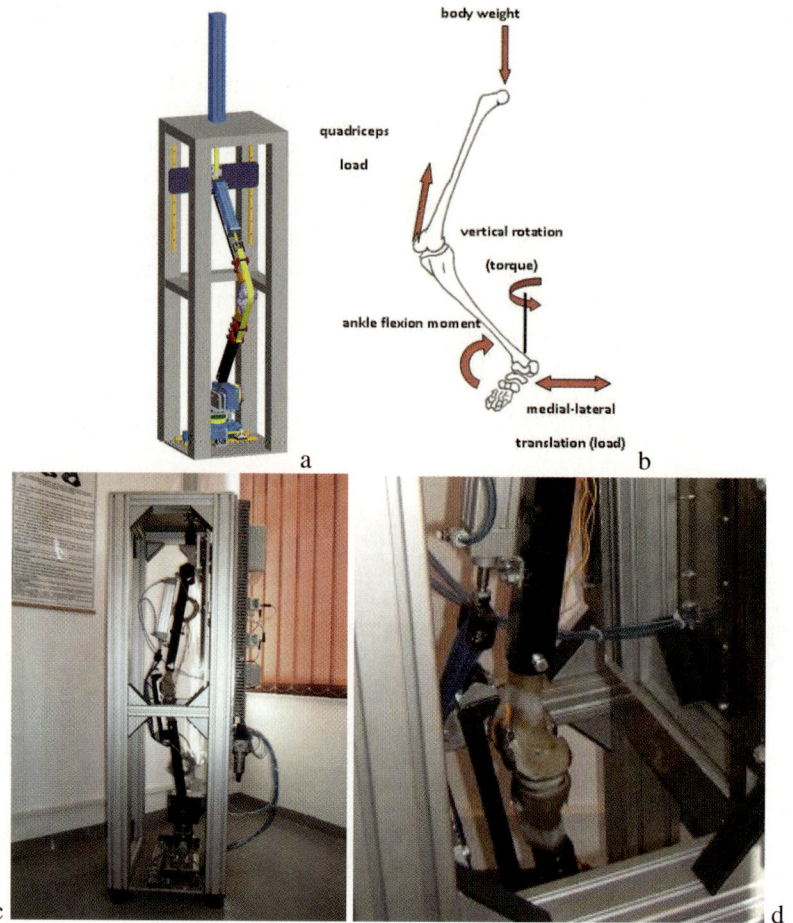

Fig. 2. The CAD design (a), resultant loads diagram on the joint (b), the newly developed knee simulator (c) and close-up of the knee joint region (d)

flexion-extension and adduction-abduction of the tibia at the ankle. The universal joint also rotate about a vertically oriented axis (±20°). The ankle assembly is free to move on a medial/lateral direction (±7.5 mm). The motion of the ankle sled is controlled by the adduction-abduction load actuator (max. 1000N).

The tibia is free to abduct/adduct. Its motion is dependent on the medial-lateral translation of the ankle sled since the femur is fixed to the frontal plane. Internal-external rotation of the tibia is controlled by a rotational actuator (max. 45 Nm) in a vertical axis translating with respect to the ankle sled.

The ankle flexion moment induced by a rotational actuator (max. 55 Nm), applies a torque between the tibia and the ankle sled relative to the flexion-extension axis. The actuator translates in the medial-laterally direction, and rotates relative to the vertical axis of the tibia.

Mechanical Testing of the Knee Joint. The testing was performed on an artificial knee implanted with a clinically-available prosthesis. The plastic femur and tibia were mounted on stainless steel tubes in the aluminum fixture. Both tubes include a three-axis force and a torque sensor allowing a closed-loop feedback control.

The load profile on the ankle joint from the medial-lateral translation, and the torque movement were obtained directly from the patient using coupled AMTI/RSSCAN force/pressure plates. The values of the quadriceps load and ankle flexion moment during walking cycle were computed using the Anybody and Gait Model (Aalborg Univ.) software packages (Fig. 3). The patient lower member segments dimensions, body weight and foot center of pressure constitute the input data for the Anybody model.

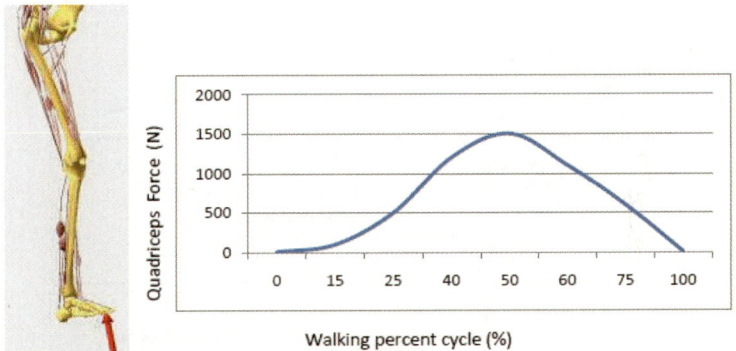

Fig. 3. Anybody model and quadriceps muscle values (N) during the walking cycle

The force generated by all pneumatic actuators were set to half of the measured values during the walking cycle to prevent damage to the artificial plastic model, which has a lower mechanical strength compared to the natural bone. The pressure values were also adjusted to account for differences in congruency between the synthetic and biological component surfaces during movement.

The movement of the joint in the simulator was recorded using two high speed (100f/s) Basler cameras and an image acquisition and analysis system, SIMI Motion (SIMI Reality Motion Systems GmbH). The kinematics data for the artificial joint have been obtained and the kinematics curves have been plotted (Fig. 4, a, b).

The finite element model of surface of the TKR prosthesis has been developed on the three-dimensional model using Ansys/LS-DYNA software (Fig. 4, c).

To decrease the computational burden and facilitate the analysis, the femoral implant and polyethylene tibial element were separated from the model.

The contact/impact conditions were simulated based on the assumption that at the time of contact the two surfaces have the same distortion speed in the direction of the impact. In this way, the impact was separated from the rest of the dynamic analysis.

The values (solutions) of the serial impulse equations were propagated over the impact, and generate initial conditions for the subsequent steps of the analysis. The erosion of the polyethylene component was estimated by calculating the quantity of material removed by friction for a given contact pressure. Experimentally, the degree of erosion can be assessed by weighing the polyethylene component after a large number of movement cycles and observing its microstructure under the microscope.

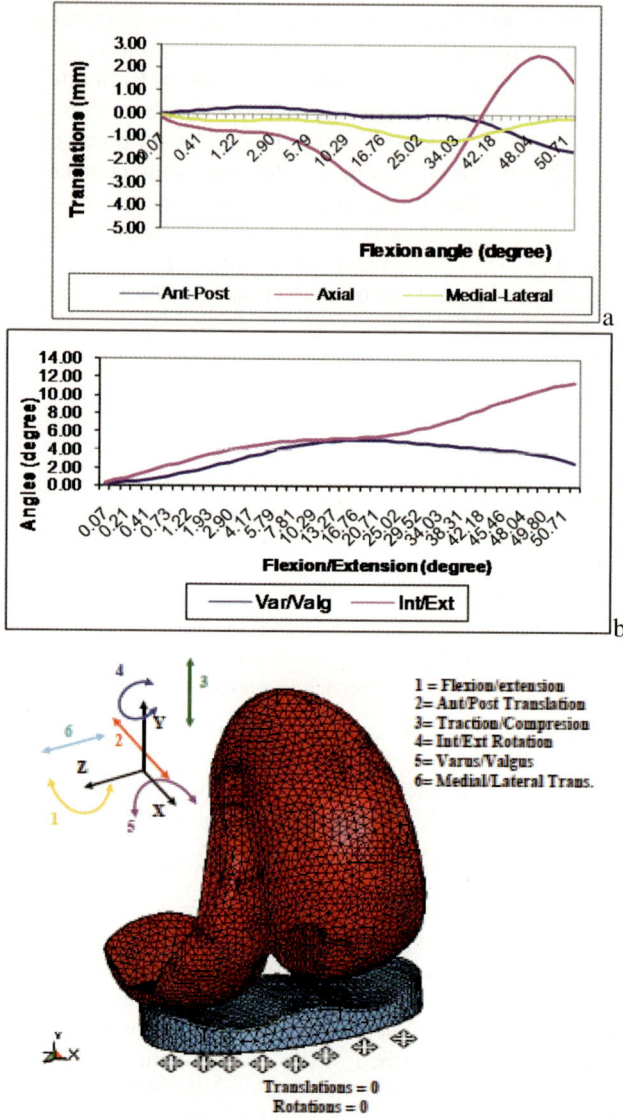

Fig. 4. The knee joint kinematics obtained with the simulator, and analyzed with the SIMI Motion software: translations (a) and rotations (b). The 3D finite elements model of the femoral component, tibial polyethylene and boundary conditions (c).

3 Results

The correlation between the TKR kinematics and tibial polyethylene loading was computed for two different ankle flexion moments, 15° and 20° flexion, corresponding to mid stance during the gait cycle (Fig. 5).

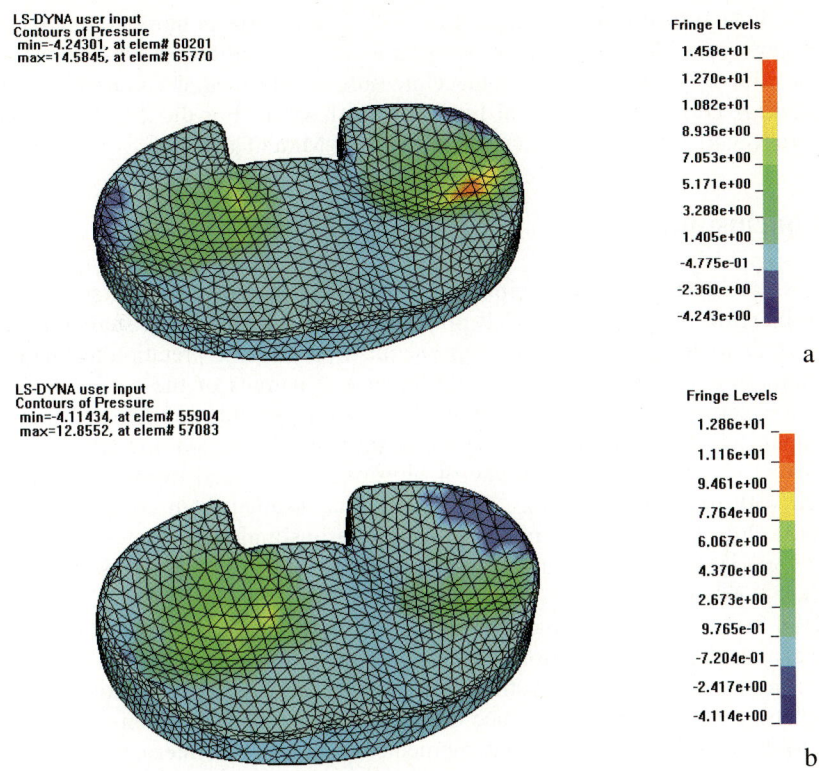

Fig. 5. Contact pressure (in MPa) for 15^0 (a) and 20^0 (b) flexion angles

Table 1. Contact pressure (in MPa), shear stress, anterior-posterior stress, axial stress, medial-lateral stress and peripheral stress

		15° of flexion	20° of flexion
Contact pression	Internal compartment	14, 5	9,46
	External compartment	8,9	7,76
Shear stress	Internal compartment	3,2	2,97
	External compartment	2,49	1,98
A – P stress	Internal compartment	12,8	6,79
	External compartment	8,4	5,21
Axial loading	Internal compartment	14,01	9,29
	External compartment	11,7	7,45
M – L stress	Internal compartment	8,07	7,97
	External compartment	8,07	4,11
Peripheral loading	Internal compartment	7, 05	4,3
	External compartment	4,24	2,4

Polyethylene loadings were highest for 15° flexion corresponding to the mid stance of the gait cycle. For comparison we used a second position of 20° flexion. For the first position (15° flexion), the contact pressure in the medial compartment is 14.5 MPa, and is correlated with axial loading (14.01 MPa). For the 20° flexion, contact pressure is 9.46 MPa and the axial loading is 9.29 MPa (Table 1).

4 Conclusions

The present paper used interdisciplinary engineering methods to understand the clinical problem of the wear of the TKR prostheses. The novelty of the study comes from using a new knee joint simulator, image acquisition and interpretation techniques, but also numerical methods to simulate the inverse dynamics of the patient lower limb and finite elements models to determine the explicit dynamics of the stress and strain. The input data for the computational simulations was collected directly from the patient (joint geometry and magnitude of physical forces), and from experiments performed with the joint simulator. The output data resulted from computation can be verified using strain markers on the artificial joint in simulator.

The relationship between axial loading and anterior-posterior stress is responsible for the initiation of abrasive wear of polyethylene. The stress in this direction is maximal in the internal compartment for a 15° flexion. The delamination of polyethylene can result from association at the same level of shear and axial forces.

The same pattern of stress distribution is observed in the external compartment but the values are lower. The difference between medial and lateral compartments is related to the presence of the various moments at the level of internal compartment in the unipodal weight bearing.

The presented simulator and the overall research methodology were designed for the study of the biomechanical behavior of bone components of the knee joint in different pathological cases and different types of movement. This system can also be used for fatigue and wear studies of some types of the prosthesis and osteotherapy devices.

The simulator can be used for research, prosthetics testing, and orthopedic surgeon training. Future studies using the knee simulator are needed to continue to determine and the regions where the physical forces produce wear and fatigue into the TKRimplant.

References

1. Nordin, M., Frankel, V.H.: Basic Biomechanics of the Musculoskeletal System, p. 400. Lippincott Williams & Wilkins (2001)
2. De Lima, D.D., Chen, P.C., Colwell, C.W.: Polyethylene contact stresses, articular congruity, and knee alignment. Clin. Orthop., 232–238 (2001)
3. Perie, D., Hobatho, M.C.: In vivo determination of contact areas and pressure of the femorotibial joint using non-linear finite element analysis. Clin. Biomech. (Bristol, Avon) 13, 394–402 (1988)
4. Waldman, S.D., Bryant, J.T.: Dynamic contact stress and rolling resistance model for total knee arthroplasties. J. Biomech. Eng. 119, 254–260 (1997)

A Hybrid 1D and 3D Approach to Hemodynamics Modelling for a Patient-Specific Cerebral Vasculature and Aneurysm

Harvey Ho[1], Gregory Sands[1], Holger Schmid[2], Kumar Mithraratne[1], Gordon Mallinson[3], and Peter Hunter[1]

[1] Bioengineering Institute, University of Auckland, New Zealand
{harvey.ho,g.sands,p.mithraratne,p.hunter}@auckland.ac.nz
[2] Department of Continuum Mechanics, RWTH Aachen University, Germany
schmid@km.rwth-aachen.de
[3] Department of Mechanical Engineering, University of Auckland, New Zealand
g.mallinson@auckland.ac.nz

Abstract. In this paper we present a hybrid 1D/3D approach to haemodynamics modelling in a patient-specific cerebral vasculature and aneurysm. The geometric model is constructed from a 3D CTA image. A reduced form of the governing equations for blood flow is coupled with an empirical wall equation and applied to the arterial tree. The equation system is solved using a MacCormack finite difference scheme and the results are used as the boundary conditions for a 3D flow solver. The computed wall shear stress (WSS) agrees with published data.

1 Introduction

Intracranial aneurysms are dilated arterial lesions in the brain. The majority of them are saccular shaped and arise from the Circle of Willis (CoW), the ring of vessels formed at the skull base (Fig. 1a). When a cerebral aneurysm ruptures, blood will flow into the subarachnoid space causing subarachnoid hemorrhage (SAH), which has a high mortality and morbidity rate [1]. Although the mechanisms underlying the formation of aneurysms are still not fully understood, it has been suggested that haemodynamic factors play an important role in their genesis and development [2].

To better understand these factors, many research groups have studied the flow patterns in cerebral aneurysms e.g. in [2,3,4,5]. The techniques used include non-invasive *in vivo* MR imaging [3], *in vitro* phantom experiments [4], and three-dimensional (3D) computational fluid dynamics (CFD) modelling [2], or a combination of these techniques [5]. Among these methods, well validated CFD has the advantage of being able to predict flow at locations where *in-vivo* flow data are difficult to obtain. The problem of 3D CFD models, however, is that a huge number of computational elements are generally required to capture complex flow patterns in tortuous vessels and bifurcations, therefore making 3D modelling for large vasculatures computationally infeasible. On the other hand,

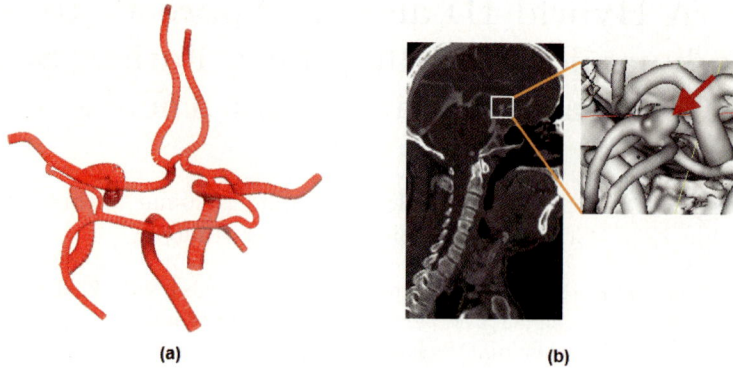

Fig. 1. (a) Circle of Willis (posterior view); (b) A CTA image: the arrow indicates an aneurysm at the anterior communicating artery (ACoA)

blood flow in a vasculature can be modelled with reduced 1D formulations of the governing equations, as used to model flow in cerebral and coronary arterial trees e.g. in [6,7]. However, the 1D models are not capable of capturing complex flow patterns, such as vortices, flow separation and reattachment, or flow reversal as in 3D models.

To absorb the strength from both 1D and 3D modelling strategies, some research groups have investigated *hybrid* or *multidimensional* modelling strategies [8,9]. The philosophy is to employ a 3D CFD model to analyze the flow in the vessel of interest in high detail, and use the 1D CFD model for the remaining part of the arterial tree. The result is a reduced number of parameters and substantially decreased computational cost [9].

This work takes a similar approach i.e. by applying a hybrid 1D/3D modelling technique to haemodynamic analysis in a patient-specific cerebral aneurysm, which grows at the anterior communication artery (ACoA) (Fig. 1b). The difference between our work and that of [8,9] is that both the 1D arterial tree and the 3D aneurysm in our model are digitized from a 3D CTA image, and therefore reflect the actual vascular anatomy.

2 Method

2.1 Vascular Model Construction

Arterial Tree. The 3D CT Angiography (CTA) image of Fig. 1(b) contains 421 slices of 378 × 336 pixels. The spatial resolution of the image is 0.488 × 0.488 × 0.7 mm. Using the open source imaging and visualization tool CMGUI we manually select 175 key points along the centre line of large blood vessels as *nodes*. The radius at each node is defined as a *field* for that particular node. These nodes are then connected by 1D cubic Hermite elements. Cylinders are constructed along these elements to represent the major arteries supplying blood to the brain. Fig. 2 depicts this digitization process.

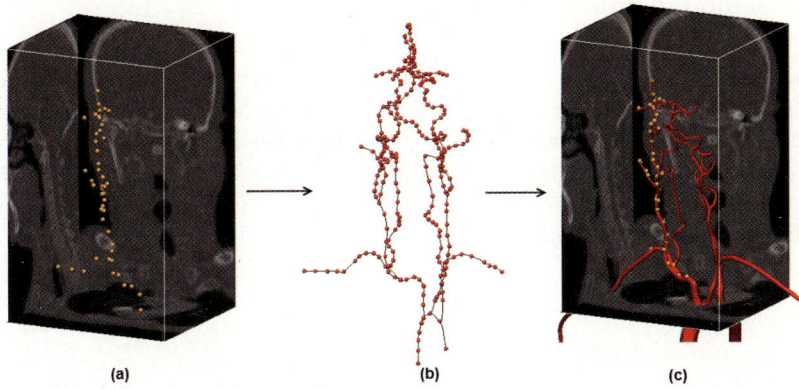

Fig. 2. Vascular tree construction pipeline: (a) Node selection; (b) 1D elements construction; (c) Cylinder simulation incorporating radius information

Aneurysm Models. Using CMGUI, the isosurface of the aneurysm lumen is extracted from the volume image as an isovalue of the image intensity at the lumen boundary. The initial isosurface (triangular mesh) is further repaired by mesh smoothing or decimation algorithms, which are available in CMGUI. Fig. 3(a) and 3(b) show the initial triangular mesh extracted from the volume image, and the surface mesh after repairing.

Computational Grid Generation. As with other Finite Element Analysis software, the geometrical model must be split into a finite set of elements, the so-called *computational grid*, to be used for flow analysis. In this work we employ a commercial grid generator ANSYS ICEM and use the octree method, which results in the grid shown in Fig. 3(c).

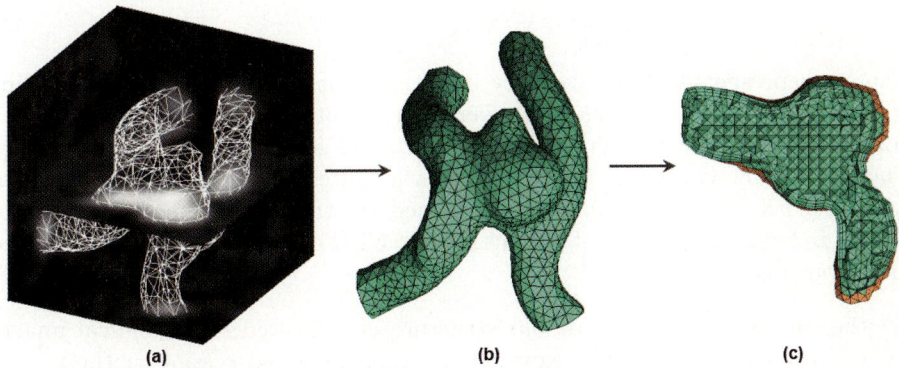

Fig. 3. (a) Isosurface extracted from volume image; (b) Surface triangular mesh after repairing; (c) Computational grid at the cross-section of aneurysm

2.2 Haemodynamics Modelling

1D Model. In large arteries, the relative size of red blood cell to vessel diameter is small and blood can be modeled as an incompressible, homogeneous, Newtonian fluid [6,7,8]. If we further assume that the flow in the circumferential direction is negligible and that the radial velocity is small compared to axial velocity, then the governing equations can be reduced to two equations. By further including a constitutive wall equation [7] we get:

$$\frac{\partial R}{\partial t} + V\frac{\partial R}{\partial x} + \frac{R}{2}\frac{\partial V}{\partial x} = 0 \qquad (1)$$

$$\frac{\partial V}{\partial t} + (2\alpha - 1)V\frac{\partial V}{\partial x} + 2(\alpha - 1)\frac{V^2}{R}\frac{\partial R}{\partial x} + \frac{1}{\rho}\frac{\partial p}{\partial x} = -2\frac{\upsilon\alpha}{\alpha - 1}\frac{V}{R^2} \qquad (2)$$

$$p(R) = G_o\left[\left(\frac{R}{R_o}\right)^\beta - 1\right] \qquad (3)$$

where P, R, V, ρ and υ represent pressure, inner vessel radius, velocity, blood density and viscosity respectively. The parameter α specifies axial velocity profile. G_o is a stiffness reference, R_o is the unstressed radius, and β is the wall elasticity coefficient. The hyperbolic set of nonlinear partial differential equations (1-3) is solved numerically using a second order MacCormack finite difference method. Furthermore, a bifurcation model is incorporated to predict flow distribution, velocity and pressure gradient across branches, and thus the whole arterial tree [7].

3D Model. The full 3D version of the governing Navier-Stokes equation can be expressed in a vector form:

$$\nabla \cdot \mathbf{v} = 0 \qquad (4)$$

$$\rho(\frac{\partial \mathbf{v}}{\partial \mathbf{t}} + \mathbf{v} \cdot \nabla \mathbf{v}) = -\nabla p + \nabla \cdot \tau \qquad (5)$$

where $\mathbf{v}$ represents the flow velocity in 3D. The practice of 3D CFD modelling is to discretize the equations (4-5) over the computational mesh of the physical domain (in this case the cerebral aneurysm), and solve the system numerically. The flow solver employed in this work is a finite volume based CFD solver, ANSYS CFX [10], which has a well defined interface with the grid generator ICEM. In brief, the process of patient specific CFD modelling can be streamlined into a pipeline:

(a) the surface mesh of a vascular structure is extracted from medical images (e.g. by using a threshold isovalue, or other image processing methods);
(b) the initial surface mesh is repaired, improved and translated into a format (e.g. the stereolithography format STL) acceptable to a grid generator;
(c) a computational grid is generated (e.g. by using ICEM) and exported to a 3D flow solver (e.g. CFX-Pre);

(d) the flow and domain configuration, the initial and boundary conditions plus solver parameters are specified (e.g. in CFX-Pre);
(e) the (transient) flow is solved (e.g. by using CFX);
(f) the results are post-processed (e.g. in CFX-Post or CMGUI).

Steps (a)-(c) in the pipeline constitute the pre-processing block, (d)-(e) the solver block and (f) the post-processing block.

Coupling of 1D/3D Solvers. The 1D and 3D solvers are coupled in step (d) of the pipeline. The flow solver CFX allows transient waveforms to be prescribed as boundary conditions and these waveforms must be expressed as functions of time. The waveforms calculated from the 1D model, however, are not analytical functions but discrete numeric values. Hence, we perform Fourier analysis for these waveforms and supply their leading ten harmonics to CFX.

3 Results

1D Model. When solving the governing equations, the density ρ and viscosity ν of the blood are set as $1.05 g/cm^3$ and $3.2 cm^2/s$ respectively. The initial velocity and pressure at all vessel segments are 0mm/s and 10.6kPa (80mmHg) respectively. The spatial and temporal step of the finite difference grid is set as 1mm and 0.1 millisecond, respectively. A physiological pulsatile pressure (80mmHg-120mmHg) is prescribed from the inlet i.e. the ascending aorta. The pressure at outlets is fixed at 80mmHg. The pressure gradient between the inlet and outlets therefore drives blood flow through the arterial tree. It takes about three minutes to compute the flow during a cardiac cycle using a laptop PC (1.73 GHz, Intel Pentium Dual-Core) and the resulting pressure distribution at four distinct phases of a cardiac cycle is shown in Fig. 4a. The velocity profiles at three locations of the aneurysm region are shown in Fig. 4b and the data from sites **B** and **C** will be passed to the 3D model as boundary conditions.

3D Model. The computational grid of Fig. 3c contains about 129,500 elements, which have a combination of tetrahedra and pentahedra. The boundary conditions are set as follows: the velocities computed from the 1D model (at sites **B** and **C** of Fig. 4b) are used as the inflow boundary conditions for the 3D model. The zero pressure boundary condition is prescribed from outlets. The viscoelastic properties of vessel wall are ignored and the no-slip wall boundary condition is applied. The flow type is defined as laminar which is justified by the highest Reynolds number (754) which occurs at the ventricular ejection phase. The computational results include important flow data such as pressure, velocity in the whole fluid domain and wall shear stress (WSS) at the vessel wall. The distribution of WSS at time steps 0.15s, 0.3s, 0.5s and 0.9s are visualized in Fig. 5a. These time steps represent four different phases of cardiac cycle as illustrated in the pressure profile chart of Fig. 5. The streamlines in Fig. 5b which bears the flow velocity information visualize the pathway of blood flow.

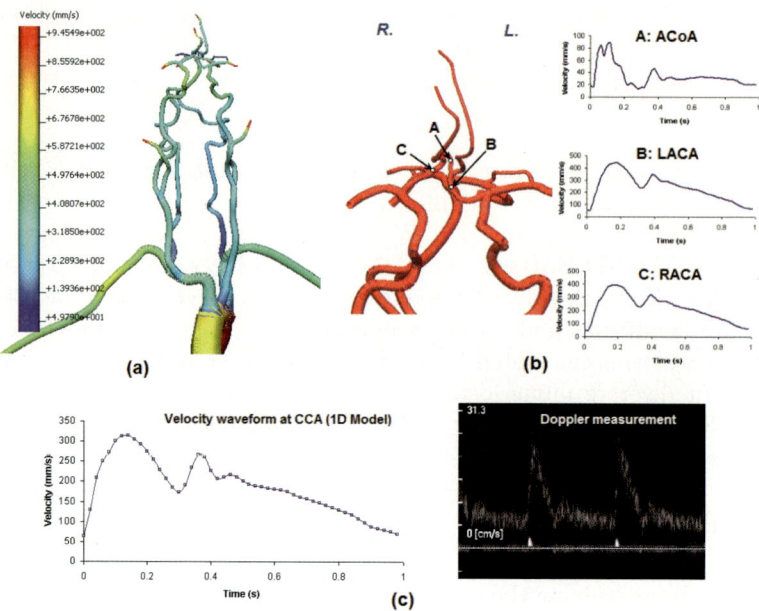

Fig. 4. Haemodynamics modelling in the cerebral vasculature: (a) Velocity distribution in the arterial tree at 0.2s; (b) A closer look at cerebral arteries: A - the communicating artery where the aneurysm grows; B,C - two inlets on ACA; (c) Velocity waveform at CCA: Left-1D model; Right-Doppler measurement

Model Validation. A LogicScan 128 ultrasound scanner (TELEMED Ltd., Lithuania) is used to detect the flow velocity at the inner carotid artery to validate the 1D result. The measured waveform, which varies between 55mm/s to 310mm/s during a cardiac cycle, is shown in Fig. 4c. A comparison with the 1D model indicates that the largest velocity (about 31-32 cm/s, occurs at systole) of the simulation matches that of the ultrasonic data. However, our model overestimates the flow velocity at diastole. Overall, we consider the simulation result is within the acceptable physiological range of *in vivo* measurement.

We also compare the computed WSS data with the results published by other research groups e.g. in [2,5]. The comparison is tabulated in Table 1 and it shows that our result agree favourably with the published data.

4 Discussion

A number of *in vivo*, *in vitro* measurements and CFD modellings (e.g. in [2,3,4,5]) have been performed to study the WSS induced by blood flow and its relationship with aneurysm genesis. The problem with the CFD approach is that a huge computational cost is required for full 3D analysis of a large vasculature. In this work we adopt a hybrid 1D/3D approach to a patient-specific cerebral vasculature and aneurysm. The benefits of such a strategy are obvious: (1) the difficulties arising

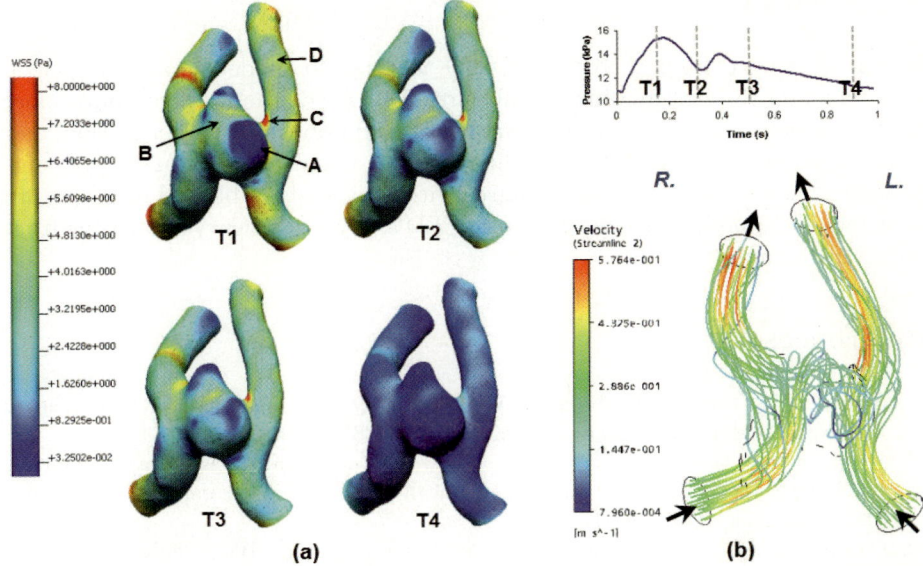

Fig. 5. Postprocessing of data for the aneurysm (posterior view). (a) WSS on vessel wall at 4 time steps, postprocessed in CMGUI; (b) Streamline in the fluid domain, postprocessed in CFX-Post.

Table 1. Comparison of flow data in literatures

Time step	Our model at selected sites				Shojima et al [2]			Steinman et al [5]	
	A(Dome)	B	C(Neck)	D	Dome	Sac	Neck	Dome	Sac
T1	0.35	2.65	9.87	5.73	-	-	-	-	-
T2	0.86	2.77	6.52	4.03	-	-	-	-	-
T3	0.71	2.78	6.98	4.34	-	-	-	-	-
T4	0.24	0.55	1.68	0.84	-	-	-	-	-
Average	0.54	2.18	6.26	7.52	0.3-0.5	1 - 5	8 - 10	0.4-0.8	1.6-2

from the treatment of boundary conditions for 3D models are handled naturally from the 1D model; and (2) the computational cost is substantially reduced [9]. At regions of interest, the 3D model reveals more flow information (e.g. the streamline in Fig. 5b) which cannot be captured by a pure 1D model.

It is worth noting that in this work we assumed that the arterial wall is elastic in the 1D model but rigid in the 3D model. That is to say, we ignored the wall deformation during a cardiac cycle in 3D modelling. This is an acceptable approximation for intracranial arteries because they are stiffer than extracranial arteries [5,6]. However, the same assumption may not hold true for carotid arteries and certainly not for the aorta. In the latter case, a more complex deformable wall model and an Arbitrary Lagrangian Eulerian (ALE) formation of the governing equations need to be solved, and this remains as our future work.

5 Conclusion

In this study we used a hybrid 1D/3D method to model a patient-specific aneurysm and the surrounding vasculature. We have developed a computational pipeline which starts from vascular model construction, to grid generation, and to 1D/3D CFD modelling. The pipeline leads to a substantial reduction of computational cost. The initial results agree with previously published data. Future work include applying such a pipeline to CFD analysis of aneurysms arising from other (intracranial) arteries.

References

1. Suarez, J.I., Tarr, R.W., Selman, W.R.: Aneurysmal subarachnoid hemorrhage. The New England Journal of Medicine 354(4), 387–396 (2006)
2. Shojima, M., Oshima, M., Takagi, K., Torii, R., Hayakawa, M., Katada, K., Morita, A., Kirino, T.: Magnitude and role of wall shear stress on cerebral aneurysm. Stroke 35, 2500–2505 (2004)
3. Cebral, J., Yim, P.J., Lohner, R., Soto, O., Choyke, P.L.: Blood flow modeling in carotid arteries with computational fluid dynamics and MR imaging. Academic Radiology 9(11), 1286–1299 (2002)
4. Liou, T., Li, Y., Juan, W.: Numerical and experimental studies on pulsatile flow in aneurysms arising laterally from a curved parent vessel at various angles. Journal of Biomechanics 40, 1268–1275 (2007)
5. Steinman, D., Milner, J., Norley, C.J., Lownie, S.P., Holdsworth, D.W.: Image-based computational simulation of flow dynamics in a giant intracranial aneurysm. American Journal of Neuroradiology, 559–566 (2003)
6. Alastruey, J., Parker, K., Peiro, J., Byrd, S., Sherwin, S.: Modelling the circle of willis to assess the effects of anatomical variations and occlusions on cerebral flows. Journal of Biomechanics 40, 1794–1805 (2007)
7. Smith, N.P., Pullan, A.J., Hunter, P.J.: An anatomically based model of transient coronary blood flow in the heart. SIAM Journal of Applied Mathematics 62(3), 990–1018 (2000)
8. Formaggia, L., Gerbeau, J.F., Nobile, F., Quarteroni, A.: On the coupling of 3d and 1d navier-stokes equations for flow problems in compliant vessels. Computer Methods in Applied Mechanics and Engineering 191, 561–582 (2001)
9. Urquiza, S.A., Blanco, P.J., Venere, M.J., Feijoo, R.: Multidimensional modelling for the carotid artery blood flow. Computer Methods in Applied Mechanics and Engineering 195, 4002–4017 (2006)
10. ANSYS: ANSYS CFX-Solver, Release 10.0: Theory. ANSYS Europe Ltd (2005)

Incompressible Cardiac Motion Estimation of the Left Ventricle Using Tagged MR Images

Xiaofeng Liu[1], Khaled Z. Abd-Elmoniem[3], and Jerry L. Prince[1,2,*]

Departments of [1]Computer Science, [2]Electrical and Computer Engineering,
[3]Radiology and Radiological Science
Johns Hopkins University, Baltimore, MD USA

Abstract. Interpolation from sparse imaging data is typically required to achieve dense, three-dimensional quantification of left ventricular function. Although the heart muscle is known to be incompressible, this fact is ignored by most previous approaches that address this problem. In this paper, we present a method to reconstruct a dense representation of the three-dimensional, incompressible deformation of the left ventricle from tagged MR images acquired in both short-axis and long axis orientations. The approach applies a smoothing, divergence-free, vector spline to interpolate velocity fields at intermediate discrete times such that the collection of velocity fields integrate over time to match the observed displacement components. Through this process, the method yields a dense estimate of a displacement field that matches our observations and also corresponds to an incompressible motion.

1 Introduction

To measure regional function in the heart, magnetic resonance tagging [1] generates images that can be processed to find two-dimensional in-plane motion at every pixel location, and when short-axis and long-axis images are combined, three-dimensional (3D) motion of each point in the left ventricle (LV) can be inferred through interpolation of the sparse imaging data. Although dense methods for directly imaging 3D myocardial motion have been developed, they require too much time for routine acquisition of dense, three-dimensional myocardial motion in scientific research or clinical medicine. Therefore, interpolation methods are likely to be required in practice and may well be the critical element in promoting routine imaging of dense, 3D myocardial function in the heart. It is widely accepted that the volume change of myocardium during the cardiac cycle is no more than 4% [2]. Since materials that are incompressible undergo deformations that preserve volumes at all scales and have divergence-free velocity fields, it is natural to assume that one can improve interpolation by exploiting this constraint. Song et al. [3] first applied this property in building the 3D velocity of the heart from cine CT images. Denney et al. [4] directly applied the divergence-free constraint to reconstruct the 3D displacement field of the LV

---
* This work was supported by NIH grant R01HL047405.

in an estimation theoretic approach. Recently, Bistoquet et al. [5] constructed nearly incompressible cardiac motion field from non-tagged MR images using a vector spline with a divergence-free matrix-valued function. There is a key problem with these approaches, however. Because the temporal resolution of the image sequences, the deformation between two neighboring time frames may be large. A velocity field that is approximated as the displacement field divided by the time interval is not theoretically predicted to be divergence-free. When this fact is ignored and the underlying field is interpolated in a divergence-free fashion this can lead to considerable errors when reconstructing motion fields in a time sequence since the errors in earlier time frames propagate to later time frames. In [5], this error was reduced by interpolating both forwards and backwards in time and then computing a weighted average of these solutions. However, solutions generated this way do not yield motions that have divergence-free velocity fields or correspond to incompressible motions. In this paper, we present a new approach to reconstruct a 3D, dense, incompressible deformation field in the LV of the heart from tagged MR images based on divergence-free vector spline with incomplete data samples. A key novelty of our approach is that, instead of computing divergence-free displacement field, we seek a sequence of divergence-free velocity fields from which the final displacement field is computed by integration. We also adopt a multi-resolution strategy and adaptive smoothing to reduce the computation and improve the accuracy. Our method was validated using both numerical simulation and *in vivo* cardiac experiments.

2 Background

2.1 Smoothing Divergence-Free Vector Spline

Given N points in space $\mathbf{x}_n = [x_n, y_n, z_n]^T$, $n = 1, \ldots, N$, and vector-valued observations $\mathbf{v}_n$, $n = 1, \ldots, N$, at these points, *vector splines* (VS) [6] interpolates a smooth vector field over the whole space. Specifically, the smoothing VS finds a vector field $\mathbf{v}(\mathbf{x})$ that minimizes

$$C(\mathbf{v}) = \rho J_{\alpha,\beta}(\mathbf{v}(\mathbf{x})) + \frac{1}{N}\sum_{n=1}^{N}||\mathbf{v}(\mathbf{x}_n) - \mathbf{v}_n||^2, \quad \text{with} \tag{1}$$

$$J_{\alpha,\beta}(\mathbf{v}) = \int [\alpha||\nabla^k(\text{div}\mathbf{v}(\mathbf{x}))||^2 + \beta\sum_{i=1}^{3}||\nabla^k(\text{rot}\mathbf{v}(\mathbf{x}))_i||^2]d\mathbf{x} \tag{2}$$

where ρ is the smoothing parameter, α and β are the weighting coefficients, div yields the divergence of a vector field, and rot yields the curl. It has been shown that (1) has the closed form solution [6] $\mathbf{v}(\mathbf{x}) = \sum_{n=1}^{N} \mathbf{K}(\mathbf{x} - \mathbf{x}_n) \cdot \mathbf{c}_n + \mathbf{p}(\mathbf{x})$, where $\mathbf{c}_n$ are the unknown vectorial coefficients and $\mathbf{K}(\mathbf{x})$ is the matrix-valued kernel function given by

$$\mathbf{K}_{\text{VS}}(\mathbf{x}) = [\frac{1}{\beta}\triangle \mathbf{I} + (\frac{1}{\alpha} - \frac{1}{\beta})\nabla\nabla^T]h(\mathbf{x}) \tag{3}$$

where I is the identity matrix, $h(\mathbf{x}) = ||\mathbf{x}||^{2k+1}$ is the solution to $\triangle^{k+1} h(\mathbf{x}) = \delta(\mathbf{x})$ and $\triangle$ is the Laplace operator. $\mathbf{p}(\mathbf{x})$ is a polynomial of order k. The coefficients in the smoothing VS can be solved using known vector values at the sample points.

As a special case, the VS can be used to interpolate the divergence-free vector field by constraining the vector field to be divergence-free, i.e., div$\mathbf{v}(\mathbf{x}) = 0$. The *divergence-free vector spline* (DFVS) solution is similar to that of VS except that the kernel matrix becomes $\mathbf{K}_{\text{DFVS}}(\mathbf{x}) = [\triangle \mathbf{I} - \nabla \nabla^T] h(\mathbf{x})$, and $\mathbf{p}(\mathbf{x})$ is also constrained to be divergence-free.

2.2 Smoothing VS from Incomplete Samples

In some applications—such as the displacement computed from tagged MR images—only selected components of the vector field are observed at the sample points. This incomplete sample data can be written as: $\{\mathbf{x}_n, \mathbf{l}_n, w_n\}$ for $n = 1, 2, \ldots, N$, where $\mathbf{l}_n$ is a normal vector representing a projection direction, and $w_n = \mathbf{l}_n \cdot \mathbf{v}(\mathbf{x}_n)$ is the projection of $\mathbf{v}(\mathbf{x}_n)$ on $\mathbf{l}_n$. The minimization problem of a smoothing VS given incomplete data can be expressed as

$$\arg\min_{\mathbf{v}} C(\mathbf{v}) = \rho J(\mathbf{v}(\mathbf{x})) + \frac{1}{N} \sum_{n=1}^{N} (\mathbf{l}_n^T \mathbf{v}(\mathbf{x}_n) - w_n)^2. \quad (4)$$

Arigovindan [7] showed that the solution to this problem is

$$\mathbf{v}(\mathbf{x}) = \sum_{n=1}^{N} \mathbf{K}(\mathbf{x} - \mathbf{x}_n) \mathbf{l}_n c_n + \mathbf{p}(\mathbf{x}), \quad (5)$$

where the coefficients c_n are scalars, and $\mathbf{K}(\mathbf{x})$ and $\mathbf{p}(\mathbf{x})$ are the same as in VS. By replacing $\mathbf{K}$ with $\mathbf{K}_{\text{DFVS}}$, Eqn. (5) describes the solution to smoothing DFVS with incomplete samples.

3 Method

3.1 Experiments and Data Processing

We acquired CSPAMM cardiac image sequences using a breath-hold scenario on a Phillips 3T Achieva MRI scanner (Philips Medical Systems, Best, NL). An approved IRB protocol was used and informed consent was obtained. Both short axis (SA) and radial long axis (LA) images were acquired on a healthy subject. Two sets of images with orthogonal tag directions were acquired separately on each SA slice. The LA images were tagged in a direction perpendicular to the SA image planes. The imaging parameters were: tag spacing = 12 mm, pixel spacing = 1.25 mm, temporal resolution = 30 msec, time frames=20. We acquired twelve SA image slices with a 4 mm slice separation, and six LA image slices. The SA slices were divided into two interleaved groups (even and odd slice numbers) so that the slice separation within each group is 8 mm. The first group of six SA slices and all six LA slices were used to reconstruct a 3D, dense, incompressible displacement field of LV. The slices in the second group were used for validation. The relative locations of the slices used in the motion reconstruction are illustrated in Fig. 1.

All of the images were first processed using the harmonic phase (HARP) method [8] to yield sequences of HARP images. Let us define the time that the tags are just applied and have not deformed as the reference time t_0. At t_0, the tagging phase ϕ is a linear function of the point's coordinate $\mathbf{x}$, and wrapped to the range $[-\pi, \pi)$, i.e., $\phi(\mathbf{x}, t_0) = W(k\mathbf{x} \cdot \mathbf{l} + \phi_0)$, where k is the known tagging frequency, $\mathbf{l}$ is a unit vector representing the tagging orientation, ϕ_0 is an unknown phase offset, and W is a phase wrapping operator. By assuming the tags do not deform much at the first time frame, ϕ_0 can be estimated from the HARP images at the first time frame [9]. Therefore, the tissue points at each time frame can be tracked back to t_0 using HARP tracking [8]. For tagging direction $\mathbf{l}$ and a 3D spatial point $\mathbf{x_j}$ imaged at t, if it comes from $\mathbf{X}_j = \mathbf{x}_j(t) - \mathbf{u}(\mathbf{x}_j(t), t)$ at t_0, then HARP tracking computes the projection of its displacement $\mathbf{u}(\mathbf{x}, t)$ onto $\mathbf{l}$ as:

$$w_j = \mathbf{l} \cdot \mathbf{u}(\mathbf{x_j}, t) = \mathbf{l} \cdot (\mathbf{x}_j - \mathbf{X}_j). \tag{6}$$

Because the SA images are acquired with two tag orientations, two projections of the displacement of each point are computed. For tissue points in the LA images, only one projection is computed. Therefore except for points at the intersections of LA and SA image planes, only partial knowledge of the displacement is available for any other pixel on the observed images. (Of course, no observations are available at 3D points that do not lie on an observed image plane.)

Intermediate image frames are not used to assist in tracking later frames because the observed tissues are not the same, primarily due to through-plane motion; thus the Lagrangian framework that is used to carry out incompressible interpolation (see next section) cannot take advantage of these observations.

3.2 3D Incompressible Displacement Field Reconstruction

The myocardium can be considered incompressible because it is composed mainly of water. For an incompressible elastic body subjecting to a deformation $\mathbf{x} = \mathbf{X} + \mathbf{u}(\mathbf{X})$, the Jacobian determinant of the deformation satisfies $\det(\mathbf{I} + \nabla_{\mathbf{X}} \mathbf{u}(\mathbf{X})) = 1$ for any material point $\mathbf{X}$, where $\nabla_{\mathbf{X}}$ is the material gradient operator. As well, the spatial velocity field $\mathbf{v}(\mathbf{x})$ giving rise to such a deformation must be divergence free, i.e., $\mathrm{div}\,\mathbf{v}(\mathbf{x}) = 0$. Based on this physical property of the heart, we propose an approach based on DFVS to reconstruct the displacement field of the LV of the heart. HARP tracking provides N incomplete and non-uniform data samples $\{\mathbf{x}_n, \mathbf{l}_n, w_n\}$ at any time frame. Our goal is to reconstruct the 3D, incompressible displacement field $\mathbf{u}(\mathbf{x})$ such that $\mathbf{l}_n \cdot \mathbf{u}(\mathbf{x}_n) = w_n$.

The deformation is calculated through the integration of the velocity. Let us define the integration variable as s, which takes on values in the interval $[0, 1]$, and let the velocity of $\mathbf{x}$ at s be $\mathbf{v}(\mathbf{x}(s), s)$. We define

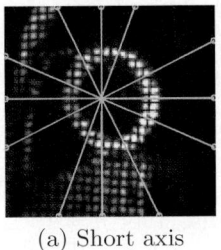 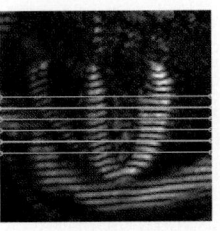

(a) Short axis (b) Long axis

Fig. 1. A tagged (a) SA and (b) LA image. For visualization purposes, the SA image shown is the product of the separately acquired horizontal and vertical tagged images. The overlaying lines depict the geometry of the (a) LA and (b) SA images.

$$\mathbf{w}(\mathbf{x}, s) = \int_0^s \mathbf{v}(\mathbf{x}(\tau), \tau) d\tau, \quad \text{and} \quad \mathbf{v}(\mathbf{x}(\tau), \tau) = \frac{d\mathbf{w}(\mathbf{x}, \tau)}{d\tau}, \qquad (7)$$

with $\mathbf{x}(s) = \mathbf{x} + \mathbf{w}(\mathbf{x}, s)$. Then the displacement field $\mathbf{u}(\mathbf{x}) = \mathbf{w}(\mathbf{x}, 1)$. The problem can be reduced to a finite-dimensional problem by dividing the integration into discrete steps, i.e., $s_m = m\delta$ for $m = 0, 1, \ldots, M$ with $\delta = 1/M$. When M is reasonably large, the velocity is assumed constant within each interval, so $\mathbf{u}(\mathbf{x}) = \mathbf{w}(\mathbf{x}, 1) = \delta \sum_{m=0}^{M-1} \mathbf{v}(\mathbf{x}(s_m), s_m)$. Note $\mathbf{v}$ is not the true myocardial velocity, but rather a computational tool for the estimation of the displacement.

We use DFVS from incomplete data samples to interpolate the divergence-free velocity fields separately over each interval. The velocity fields are computed sequentially starting from $s_0 = 0$ through $s_M = 1$. Let us denote $r_n(s_m) = \mathbf{l}_n \cdot \mathbf{v}(\mathbf{x}_n(s_m), s_m)$ for any step s_m, and the data samples at s_m are written as $\{\mathbf{x}_n(s_m), \mathbf{l}_n, r_n(s_m)\}$ for $n = 1, \ldots, N$. The velocity at any sample point $\mathbf{x}_n(s_m)$ at s_m is approximated by taking the first order expansion

$$\mathbf{u}(\mathbf{x}_n) - \mathbf{w}(\mathbf{x}_n(s_m), s_m) = \mathbf{v}(\mathbf{x}_n(s_m), s_m)(1 - \delta m), \qquad (8)$$

so that

$$r_n(s_m) = \mathbf{l}_n \cdot \mathbf{v}(\mathbf{x}_n(s_m), s_m) = \frac{w_n - \mathbf{l}_n \cdot \mathbf{w}(\mathbf{x}_n(s_m), s_m)}{1 - \delta m}. \qquad (9)$$

With the N data samples, the continuous velocity field $\mathbf{v}(\mathbf{x}, s_m)$ is interpolated with smoothing DFVS using Eqns. (4) and (5).

From Taylor's expansion, the first order approximation of the velocity is accurate up to the order $(1-\delta m)^2$. Therefore, it is less accurate at smaller s and more smoothing is required at earlier steps. So the smoothing parameter ρ should be chosen to be large at small s and grow smaller as s approaches 1. At s_{M-1}, ρ should be set to 0 so that the final displacement $\mathbf{w}(\mathbf{x}_n, 1)$ matches the original data samples exactly—i.e., $\mathbf{l}_n \cdot \mathbf{u}(\mathbf{x}_n) = \mathbf{l}_n \cdot \mathbf{w}(\mathbf{x}_n, 1) = w_n$ for $n = 1, \ldots, N$. In practice, we choose the smoothing parameter as $\rho_m = \frac{M-m-1}{M-1}\rho_0$, where ρ_0 is determined empirically.

To reduce computation time, a multi-resolution scheme is adopted. For smaller m, the sample points are downsampled so that only a subset of the samples is used in the interpolation. Since the computation time is dominated by solving the coefficients from Eqn. (5) with complexity $O(N^3)$, the multi-resolution scheme can greatly reduce the computation while not affecting the accuracy of the displacement field reconstruction.

The algorithm can be summarized as follows.

Algorithm 1: Dense 3D incompressible displacement field reconstruction
Given the data samples $\{\mathbf{x}_n, \mathbf{l}_n, w_n\}$, and $w_n = \mathbf{l}_n \cdot \mathbf{u}(\mathbf{x}_n)$ for $n = 1, \ldots, N$, and a dense 3D grid of data points $\mathbf{y}_k$ for $k = 1, \ldots, K$ of which the 3D displacement vectors are to be computed, carry out the following steps:

1. Initialize ρ_0, M, $\mathbf{y}_k(0) = \mathbf{y}_k$, $\mathbf{w}(\mathbf{y}_k, 0) = 0$, and $\mathbf{w}(\mathbf{x}_n, 0) = 0$ for all k and n.
2. for $m = 0$ to $M - 1$
   (a) set $s_m = m\delta$, $\rho_m = \rho_0(M - m - 1)/(M - 1)$;
   (b) downsample the data points $\mathbf{x}(s_m)$ if needed;
   (c) compute $r_n(s_m)$ using Eqn. (9) for all sample points;
   (d) compute the interpolating coefficients with samples $\{\mathbf{x}_n(s_m), \mathbf{l}_n, r_n(s_m)\}$ and $\rho = \rho_m$;
   (e) compute the velocities $\mathbf{v}(\mathbf{y}_k(s_m), s_m)$ and $\mathbf{v}(\mathbf{x}_n(s_m), s_m)$ using Eqn. (5);
   (f) set $\mathbf{w}(\mathbf{x}_n, s_{m+1}) = \mathbf{w}(\mathbf{x}_n, s_m) + \delta \mathbf{v}(\mathbf{x}_n(s_m), s_m)$, $\mathbf{w}(\mathbf{y}_k, s_{m+1}) = \mathbf{w}(\mathbf{y}_k, s_m) + \delta \mathbf{v}(\mathbf{y}_k(s_m), s_m)$, $\mathbf{x}_n(s_{m+1}) = \mathbf{x}_n(s_m) + \mathbf{w}(\mathbf{x}_n, s_{m+1})$, and $\mathbf{y}_k(s_{m+1}) = \mathbf{y}_k(s_m) + \mathbf{w}(\mathbf{y}_k, s_{m+1})$;
3. Set $\mathbf{u}(\mathbf{x}_n) = \mathbf{w}(\mathbf{x}_n, s_M)$ and $\mathbf{u}(\mathbf{y}_k) = \mathbf{w}(\mathbf{y}_k, s_M)$, and the algorithm ends.

4 Results

4.1 2D Numerical Simulation

A 2D incompressible vector field was simulated using second order polynomials:
$$u_x = \frac{1}{90}(\frac{8}{281}x + y)^2 + \frac{1}{15}(x - 0.5y) - 15$$
$$u_y = \frac{1}{900}(\frac{8}{281}x + y)^2 + \frac{1}{15}(2x - y) - 3$$

on an image with ranges $x \in [-50, 50]$ and $y \in [-50, 50]$. This vector field is incompressible because $\det(\mathbf{I} + \nabla \mathbf{u}) = 1$. The two displacement components are shown in Figs. 2(a) and (b). We picked a grid of sample points, shown in Fig. 2(c), and assumed the vectors on these sample points were known. To mimic the tagged image acquisition, these points were distributed densely in one dimension and sparsely in the other. Our method was then applied to reconstruct the 2D motion field in the whole image with $M = 20$ and $\rho = 0.1$.

The reconstructed motion field was then compared with the closed-form solution. In this simulation the mean interpolation error was 0.064 pixel, and the standard deviation was 0.036 pixel. Fig. 2(d) shows the Jacobian determinant of the deformation. The average error of Jacobian determinant of the reconstructed deformation from 1 was 0.0046. For comparison, we also reconstructed the motion field using the direct divergence-free interpolation approach of Bistoquet et al. [5]. This approach yielded a mean interpolation error of 0.95 pixel and a mean error of Jacobian determinant (Fig. 2(e)) of 0.099.

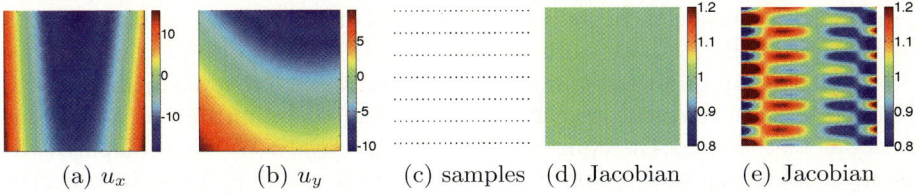

Fig. 2. (a) The x and (b) y components of the simulated motion. The (c) sample points used in the interpolation. The Jacobian determinant from the motion field constructed using (d) our method and (e) one step divergence-free interpolation.

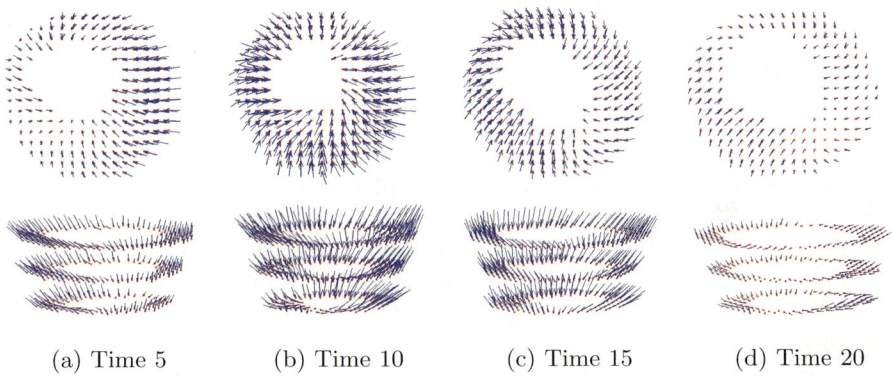

Fig. 3. The 3D displacement field illustrated using three SA slices. From top to bottom: two different views; From left to right: the displacement field at different time frames.

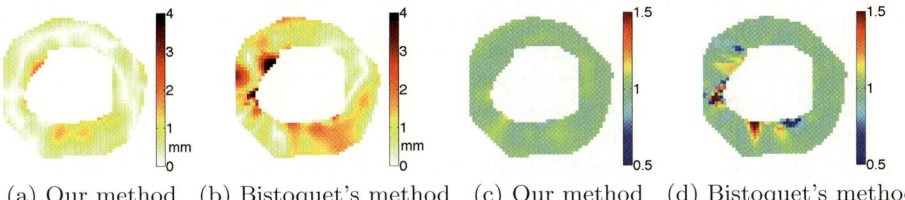

Fig. 4. The displacement error map on one slice using (a) our method and (b) Bistoquet's method. The Jacobian determinant of the deformation field computed on the same slice from (c) our method and (d) Bistoquet's method.

4.2 Cardiac Motion Experiments

We applied Algorithm 1 to the cardiac images shown in Fig. 1 using a smoothing parameter $\rho_0 = 0.1$ and $M = 20$ integration steps. The reconstructed 3D displacement field in the LV regions of three SA slices are shown in two views in Fig. 3 at different times. The reconstructed displacements of points on the LV in the validation slices were compared with the 2D displacement projection computed using HARP. Over all time frames, the mean displacement error was 0.446 mm, and the standard deviation was 0.310 mm. For comparison, we also computed the displacement field using Bistoquet's approach, i.e., direct DFVS interpolation with backward-forward averaging [10]. The mean displacement error was 0.803 mm, and the standard deviation was 0.652 mm. Figs. 4(a) and (b) show the displacement error maps on the 5th validation slice at time frame 10 of our method and Bistoquet's method, respectively. We also compared the incompressibility of the reconstructed motion fields. At time frame 10 when the heart deforms the most, the average absolute difference between the Jacobian determinant and unity of our approach was 0.030. The difference was mainly caused by both spatial and temporal discretization. The average absolute difference of Bistoquet's method was 0.067. Figs. 4(c) and (d) show the Jacobian determinants at the 5th validation slice.

5 Conclusion

We presented an approach to reconstruct a 3D, dense, incompressible displacement field of the left ventricle of the heart using tagged MR images. Our method uses a divergence-free vector spline on incomplete and non-uniform sample data to interpolate the velocity fields at discrete integration steps, and the displacement field is achieved by integrating these velocity fields. Our method was validated with both numerical simulation and *in vivo* cardiac experiment.

References

1. Axel, L., Dougherty, L.: MR imaging of motion with spatial modulation of magnetization. Radiology 171, 841–845 (1989)
2. Yin, F., Chan, C., Judd, R.: Compressibility of perfused passive myocardium. Amer. J. Physiol.-Heart Circ. Physiol. 8, 1864–1870 (1996)
3. Song, S.M., Leahy, R.M.: Computation of 3-D velocity fields from 3-d cine CT images of a human heart. IEEE Trans. Med. Imag. 10(3), 295–306 (1991)
4. Denney, T., Prince, J.L.: Reconstruction of 3D left ventricular motion from planar tagged cardiac MR images: an estimation theoretic approach. IEEE Trans. Med. Imag. 14(4), 625–635 (1995)
5. Bistoquet, A., Oshinski, J., Skrinjar, O.: Myocardial deformation recovery from cine MRI using a nearly incompressible biventricular model. Med. Imag. Anal. 12, 69–85 (2008)
6. Amodei, L., Benbourhim, M.N.: A vector spline approximation. J. Approx. Theo. 67(1), 51–79 (1991)
7. Arigovindan, M.: Variational reconstruction of vector and scalar images from non-uniform samples. PhD thesis, École Polytechnique Federale de Lausanne (2005)
8. Osman, N.F., Kerwin, W.S., McVeigh, E.R., Prince, J.L.: Cardiac motion tracking using CINE harmonic phase (HARP) magnetic resonance imaging. Magn. Reson. Med. 42, 1048–1060 (1999)
9. Tecelao, S.R., Zwanenburg, J.J., Kuijer, J.P., Marcus, J.T.: Extended harmonic phase tracking of myocardial motion: improved coverage of myocardium and its effect on strain results. J. Magn. Reson. Imag. 23(5), 682–690 (2006)
10. Bistoquet, A., Oshinski, J., Skrinjar, O.: Left ventricle deformation recovery from cine MRI using an incompressible model. IEEE Trans. Med. Imag. 26(9), 1136–1153 (2007)

Vibro-Elastography for Visualization of the Prostate Region: Method Evaluation

Seyedeh Sara Mahdavi[1], Mehdi Moradi[1], Xu Wen[1], William J. Morris[2], and Septimiu E. Salcudean[1]

[1] Department of Electrical and Computer Engineering,
University of British Columbia, Vancouver, Canada
tims@ece.ubc.ca
[2] British Columbia Cancer Agency Vancouver, Canada

Abstract. We show that vibro-elastography, an ultrasound-based method that creates images of tissue viscoelasticity contrast, can be used for visualization and segmentation of the prostate. We use MRI as the gold standard and show that VE images yield more accurate 3D volumes of the prostate gland than conventional B-mode imaging. Furthermore, we propose two novel measures characterizing the strength and continuity of edges in noisy images. These measures, as well as contrast to noise ratio, demonstrate the utility of VE as a prostate imaging modality. The results of our study show that in addition to mapping the visco-elastic properties of tissue, VE can play a central role in improving the anatomic visualization of the prostate region and become an integral component of interventional procedures such as brachytherapy.

1 Introduction

Segmentation of the prostate is required in prostate cancer treatment. In low dose rate brachytherapy, permanent radioactive seeds must be accurately placed in the prostate and peri-prostatic tissue. In high dose rate brachytherapy, temporary catheters must be repeatedly and accurately placed for radiation fraction delivery. Thus accurate visualization and segmentation of the prostate is important in treatment planning and delivery, and can reduce the possible treatment side effects such as impotence, rectal bleeding, and urinary incontinence.

Image-based guidance for prostate interventions is an active area of research [1,2]. Ultrasound (B-mode) is the primary imaging modality used for radiation treatment planning and delivery. While safe, accessible and real-time, ultrasound B-mode imaging does not delineate the prostate reliably [3].

In our prior work, we have introduced *ultrasound vibro-elastography* (VE) to generate patient-specific viscoelastic models of the prostate region, and have shown, based on phantom images and a few patient images, that the method has promise in delineating the prostate and anatomical details such as the urethra [4]. In this paper, we show the effectiveness of VE-based segmentation quantitatively by analyzing data from a more extensive patient study in novel ways. First, we use volume-based measures to compare the overall shape of the gland as seen in VE and B-mode images, with MRI images as the gold standard. We then evaluate the performance of VE-based segmentation by computing the contrast to noise ratio (CNR) of the prostate relative to the background in VE and standard B-mode images, and show that VE is vastly superior. Finally, because CNR measures are not appropriate for relatively uniform images that may present strong edges, we propose a third measure based on the strength of the prostate edges. The conventional methods for characterizing edge strength in images include using the maximum of a gradient-based edge detector [5] and measuring the changes in the distribution of image features such as brightness and texture on the two sides of the edge. These approaches have met with little success in the case of ultrasound images due to speckle and image artifacts. Therefore, we propose a new correlation-based index of edge continuity and a model-based statistical approach that relates the edge strength with stationarity of the edge intensity profile.

2 Vibro-Elastography

A brachytherapy stepper (EXII, CIVCO Medical Solutions) was modified to enable the acquisition of 3D vibro-elastography (VE) images during conventional prostate brachytherapy. A shaker was mounted on the transducer cradle in order to vibrate the transducer radially. The cradle rotation was motorized, and a control system and interface were developed to enable the application of compression waves ($0-10\ Hz$ frequency, $0-3$ mm amplitude) to the rectal wall with probe rotation from -45 to 50 degrees from the sagittal plane. Synchronized with the probe motion, ultrasound B-mode and high-frequency RF data images were acquired from a Sonix RP machine with the sagittal array of a dual plane linear/microconvex broadband $5-9$ MHz endorectal transducer (Ultrasonix Medical Corp.). The RF data, collected at the approximate rate of 40 fps, was processed to compute the tissue motion resulting from the applied compression. A measure of strain energy was computed in the frequency domain to show tissue stiffness contrast [6]. Our studies involving 14 patients show that the average normalized correlation (NC) of tissue displacement estimation in the vibro-elastography approach is around 0.95 and the average coherence function is over 0.8. This is a clear sign of the reliability of the estimation.

Since elastography measures the mechanical properties of tissue, it can be used for biopsy guidance [7] and to create tissue elasticity models used for needle insertion planning. However, the goal of this paper is to evaluate the VE performance in prostate visualization and segmentation.

3 Data Acquisition

The images analyzed in this paper were collected from patients going through the standard prostate brachytherapy procedure at British Columbia Cancer Agency in Vancouver, with additional MR and VE image acquisition. After obtaining informed consent, MR images (slice spacing 4 mm, pixel size 0.27×0.27 mm)

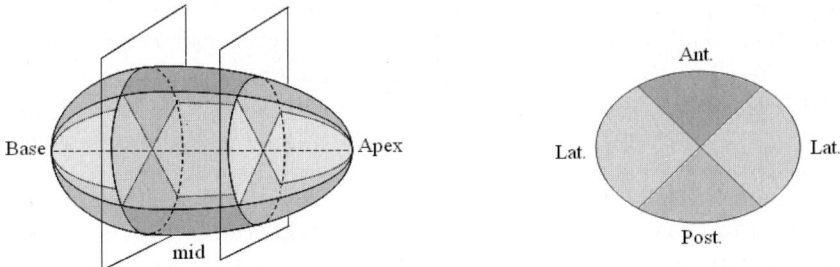

Fig. 1. Transverse planes divide the prostate into base, mid and apex regions. Within each transverse view the prostate is divided to anterior, posterior and lateral sectors.

were collected at the UBC Hospital with a Philips Achieva 3.0 Tesla MRI scanner 1-2 weeks prior to the brachytherapy intervention. A pelvic coil was used for patient comfort and to minimize the deformation of the gland. Transverse B-mode images (slice spacing 5 mm, pixel size 0.156 × 0.156 mm) were obtained as part of the standard treatment planning using an ultrasound machine (B&K Pro-Focus System B-Series machine with the MFI Biplane Transducer). Intra-operatively, 3D VE images showing the tissue stiffness contrast were acquired at the beginning of the brachytherapy intervention. The sagittal VE images were converted to transverse views via interpolation. For each patient, this process results in 128 transverse images (slice spacing 0.43 mm, pixel size 0.5 × 0.5 mm). So far data from seven patients has been acquired and included in the reported results. MRI images are available from five patients.

4 Evaluation Methods

3D reconstructions have been generated through delineating the prostate in B-mode, VE and MRI transverse images by an expert. Two types of measures have been used for the evaluation of VE images; volume-based measures and 2D edge/contrast measures. Volume-based measures include "volume difference" and "volume error." 2D edge/contrast measures are the contrast-to-noise ratio, edge strength and edge continuity. The following subsections describe the details of each method. To best represent the critical regions surrounding the prostate, edge evaluation was carried out on the nine distinct regions of the prostate depicted in Figure 1. Division of the prostate in the transverse plane produces three anterior, posterior and lateral sectors and axial division results in the apex, base and mid sectors.

4.1 Comparison of the Volumes

Since boundaries of the prostate are more visible in MRI, this modality has been selected as the gold standard. The volume of the prostate gland is an important parameter used in planning the dose distribution in prostate brachytherapy. Volume difference measures the difference between this volume computed from the

B-mode and VE imaging with that from the gold standard (MRI). Volume error, on the other hand, measures the volume between two registered reconstructed surfaces from VE/B-mode and MRI. Volume error determines how well the extracted "3D shape" from VE/B-mode matches with that of the gold standard.

The VE and B-mode shapes were registered to the MRI by first matching the centers of the volumes and applying a rotation to align the two superior-inferior axes. Then, the point-based Iterative Closest Point (ICP) method [8] was applied to the two surfaces to fine-tune the registration. Due to the clarity of the boundaries in the mid portion of the gland in all three modalities, this region has been selected for volume error calculation. A comparison between the volume-difference of the total gland and volume-error of the mid portion can provide additional information about the base and apex regions.

4.2 Evaluation of the Contrast - the CNR

The higher the contrast-to-noise ratio of an image object with respect to the image background, the more distinguishable the object is. To compare the contrast of B-mode and VE images, the CNR was calculated using [9]:

$$CNR = \frac{2(m_t - m_b)^2}{\sigma_t^2 + \sigma_b^2} \tag{1}$$

in which m and σ^2 are the mean and variance of the target, t, and background, b, pixel intensities in a region of interest (ROI). The target and background ROI's are selected as regions with the best visible contrast, the target being an area inside the prostate close to the boundary and the background being an area outside the prostate close to the target ROI. Histogram stretching was performed on B-mode and VE images to ensure that the range of intensities in both modalities match.

Because an object may have a low CNR but still be visually distinguishable due to a strong edge, characterization of edges is also required in order to compare the segmentation of the prostate gland in B-mode and VE images.

4.3 Edge Continuity - A Correlation-Based Measure

An important characteristic of a good edge is "continuity". We propose a new measure based on the correlation of neighboring edge profiles.

In transversal images, we extended radii in polar coordinates from the center of the prostate. The intersections r_{θ_i}, $i = 1, ..., N_\theta$ of these radii with the boundary of the prostate were manually identified for each θ_i, and a radial edge intensity profile function $I_{\theta_i}(r)$ was computed for a window $r \in [r_\theta - \Delta, r_\theta + \Delta]$. The normalized cross-correlations $R_{\theta, \theta_i \pm \delta\theta}(r)$ of $I_{\theta_i}(r)$ and $I_{\theta_i \pm \delta\theta}(r)$ and the average $c(\theta_i)(r) = \frac{1}{2}[R_{\theta,\theta_i+\delta\theta} + R_{\theta,\theta_i-\delta\theta}]$ were computed from these edge intensity profiles. The parameters used in implementation were $\Delta = 0.3\ cm$, $N_\theta = 12$ and $\delta\theta = 2°$. For a strong edge at θ_i, the function $c(\theta_i)(r)$ should have a shape similar to a Gaussian distribution with a large peak and small standard deviation indicating high similarity of the two profiles. Thus, we let $P(\theta_i)$ and $\sigma(\theta_i)$ be

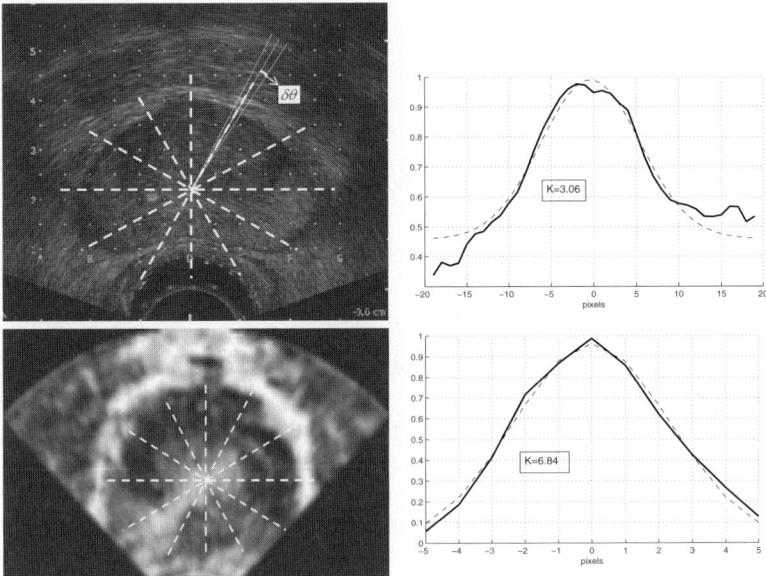

Fig. 2. B-mode (top row) and VE (bottom row) images along with the cross-correlation curve for the specified edge

the peak and standard deviation of a Gaussian function fitted to $c(\theta_i)$ and we define a measure of edge profile consistency, $K(\theta_i)$, as:

$$K(\theta_i) = \frac{P^2(\theta_i)}{\sigma(\theta_i)} \ . \tag{2}$$

The average over the dataset of K value was computed for each of the nine regions defined in Figure 1. Figure 2 shows $c(\theta_i)(r)$, the fitted Gaussian function, and the calculated K for a strong edge in both B-mode and VE images.

4.4 Edge Strength - A Model-Based Statistical Measure

Apart from being continuous, a good edge should also exhibit high contrast normal to it. Gradient-based edge detectors do not work well in B-mode images as they are plagued by local minima. Therefore, we propose a new approach that models the difference of the radial edge intensity profile as an autoregressive process. The edge strength is characterized based on the degree of stationarity of this process.

In each image, each edge profile $I(\theta_k)(r)$ was considered as a time series $I(i) := I(\theta_k)(\delta r\, i)$, where the discretized radius distance i replaces the usual time index. For the edge profile I, the first order difference is calculated as: $D_I(i) = I(i) - I(i-1)$. We model D_I as a first order autoregressive (AR(1)) processes of the form:

$$D_I(i) = \phi D_I(i-1) + e(i) \tag{3}$$

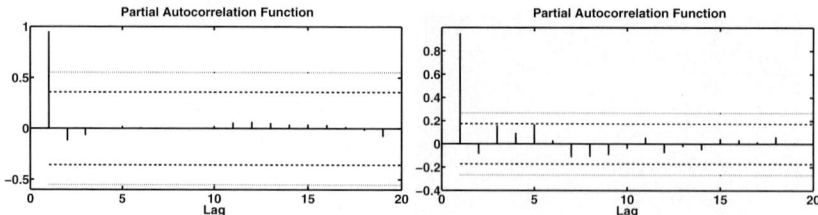

Fig. 3. Typical PACF of the differenced intensity profiles from VE (left) and B-mode (right). The horizontal lines mark the 5% and 10% significance levels.

where $e(i)$ is white noise and ϕ is the model parameter, estimated based on Yule-Walker equations [10]. The length of the edge profiles is 2 cm. In order to show that an AR(1) model is sufficient for modeling D_I, we compute the partial autocorrelation function (PACF) of D_I. The PACF of an AR(1) process only has significant values at lag=1. In 78% of the edge profiles extracted from both B-mode and VE images, at the significance level of 0.05, the PACF function only has significant values at lag=1. Figure 3 shows typical PACF functions for D_I extracted from B-mode and VE images.

If a strong edge exists, D_I is expected to have a strong peak at the edge. This "trend" of existence of a strong peak means that D_I is non-stationary (a signal with a trend can not be stationary, since its statistical moments depend on time, or in our model, on distance). On the other hand, if the radial edge profile does not pass through a strong edge, its derivative is more likely to be trend-free. For an AR(1) model, the condition for stationarity is $|\phi| < 1$. Therefore, in our model, larger $|\phi|$ values indicate strong edges. We also performed the Augmented Dickey Fuller (ADF) test [11] to statistically evaluate the edge profiles for their stationarity. The ADF test examines the null hypothesis of non-stationarity against the hypothesis of stationarity.

5 Results

Volume measures. Table 1 shows the percentage of volume error (VE/MRI vol. error % = $100 \times (non\text{-}overlapping\ vol.\ from\ VE\ and\ MRI)/(V_{MRI}+V_{VE})$) and volume difference (VE/MRI vol. difference % = $100 \times (V_{VE} - V_{MRI})/V_{MRI}$) between 3D reconstructed prostate shapes from B-mode/MRI and VE/MRI of five patients. The average volume error over the five patients, which is calculated for the mid-region, is similar in both cases (5.1% vs. 5.2%). However, the percentage of volume difference between B-mode and MRI, calculated on the whole volume, is higher than that between VE and MRI (5% vs. 9.6%). Since the volume error in the mid sections are fairly similar, the volume differences over the entire gland should be mainly originating from the base and apex.

Contrast evaluation. The CNR of VE and B-mode images, averaged over the three sections of the prostate, is shown in Table 2. In all three regions the CNR of VE is clearly higher than that of B-mode.

Table 1. Percentage of vol. error and vol. difference for VE/B-mode and MRI

%	P1 P2 P3 P4 P5
VE/MRI volume error	4.0 3.0 7.9 5.6 4.4
B-mode/MRI volume error	6.8 2.7 5.8 4.7 6
VE/MRI volume difference	1.8 -5.1 -2.7 8.9 -6.6
B-mode/MRI volume difference	6.0 9.7 9.7 14.6 8.1

Table 2. CNR comparison of VE and B-mode images (data from seven patients)

	Base	Mid	Apex
CNR VE	21.2±10.2	24.5±11.6	25.4±15.2
CNR B-mode	4.8±1.9	1.3±0.6	1.8±1.2

Table 3. Edge continuity measure for nine sectors of the prostate (seven patients)

	Base	Mid	Apex		Base	Mid	Apex
Ant.	1.43±1.56	1.29±1.1	0.67±0.79	Ant.	0.78±0.64	1.03±0.82	0.78±0.54
Lat.	0.86±0.88	1.11±0.94	0.48±0.57	Lat.	0.69±0.58	0.94±0.71	0.75±0.65
Post	0.85±0.73	0.87±0.81	0.38±0.54	Post	0.34±0.38	0.33±0.41	0.52±0.44
(a) B-mode				(b) VE			

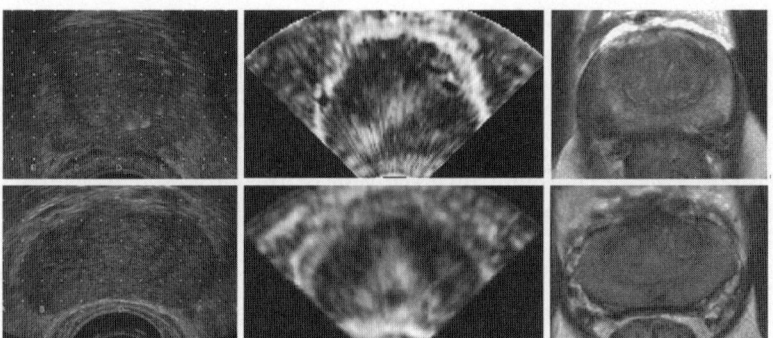

Fig. 4. B-mode, VE and MRI sample images from two patients

Edge continuity: Tables 3a and 3b show the mean and standard deviation of the edge continuity measure, K, for nine sectors of the prostate. The B-mode and VE images of seven patients have been used. The overall mean value of K for VE images is larger than that of B-mode in the apex of the gland. However, K values for VE images degrade in the mid and base sections.

Edge strength based on the AR model and ADF test. The absolute value of AR(1) coefficient $|\phi|$ for the difference edge profiles (D_I) was significantly larger in VE images than in B-mode images in all nine areas ($|\phi| = 0.59 \pm 0.19$ for VE images and $|\phi| = 0.19 \pm 0.11$ for B-mode images). The ADF test shows that in VE images, the stationarity hypothesis is rejected ($p < 0.1$) for 94% of the edge profiles. Whereas, in B-mode images, the stationarity hypothesis is rejected only in 23% of the profiles. In other words, more than 77% of the B-mode edge profiles are stationary, suggesting that there is no strong trend in the profile which goes against having a strong edge.

6 Discussion and Conclusions

In this paper, vibro-elastography (VE) is evaluated as an imaging modality to visualize and segment prostate. A visual comparison of VE and B-mode in more than 20 patients scanned so far clearly shows that VE imaging is a promising modality for prostate interventions (Figure 4). Quantitative results presented in this paper also confirm this observation. We showed that VE is successful in extracting the 3D shape of the prostate specially in the base and apex region, with MRI as the gold standard. The regional CNR of VE images is significantly higher than that of B-mode. In order to compare the edge qualities in B-mode and VE images, novel measures have been proposed that show stronger edges in VE images, characterized by non-stationarity of the edge profiles in VE modality. Our proposed measure of edge continuity indicates more consistent edges, compared to B-mode, in VE images of the apex region. In other areas, specially in the posterior region near the transducer, VE images deteriorate. Potential causes to this problem are transducer slip, which deteriorates the image close to the probe, and the use of only axial strain estimation [6] in determining prostate elasticity. This can generate known "softening" artifacts. Understanding this shortcoming and the visualization of other anatomical details, e.g. urethra and the cavernosal nerve plexi, are the subject of future research. Also, as a future goal, we plan to carry out a more thorough investigation of the proposed measures of edge strength and continuity on simulated ultrasound data.

Acknowledgments. We would like to thank Dr. T. Pickles, Dr. M. McKenzie, the staff at the BC Cancer Agency, Mr. O. Goksel and Mr. R. Zahiri Azar. Financial support from NIH grant R21 CA120232-01 is gratefully acknowledged.

References

1. Jain, A., Deguet, A., Iordachita, I., Chintalapani, G., Blevins, J., Le, Y., Armour, E., Burdette, C., Song, D., Fichtinger, G.: Intra-operative 3D guidance in prostate brachytherapy using a non-isocentric c-arm. Med. Image Comput. Comput. Assist Interv. Int. Conf. Med. Image Comput. Comput. Assist. Interv. 10(Pt 2), 9–17 (2007)
2. Wei, Z., Ding, M., Downey, D., Fenster, A.: 3D TRUS guided robot assisted prostate brachytherapy. Med. Image Comput. Comput Assist. Interv. Int. Conf. Med. Image Comput. Comput. Assist. Interv. 8(Pt 2), 17–24 (2005)
3. Smith, S., Wallner, K., Merrick, G., Butler, W., Sutlief, S., Grimm, P.: Interpretation of pre- versus postimplant TRUS images. Med. Phys. 30(5), 920–924 (2003)

4. Salcudean, S.E., French, D., Bachmann, S., Zahiri-Azar, R., Wen, X., Morris, W.J.: Viscoelasticity modeling of the prostate region using vibro-elastography. Med. Image Comput. Comput. Assist. Interv. Int. Conf. Med. Image Comput. Comput. Assist. Interv. 9(Pt 1), 389–396 (2006)
5. Canny, J.: A computational approach to edge detection. IEEE Transactions on Pattern Analysis and Machine Intelligence 8(6), 679–698 (1986)
6. Zahiri-Azar, R., Salcudean, S.E.: Motion estimation in ultrasound images using time domain cross correlation with prior estimates. IEEE Trans. Biomed. Eng. 53(10), 1990–2000 (2006)
7. Pesavento, A., Lorenz, A.: Real time strain imaging and in-vivo applications in prostate cancer. In: Proc. IEEE Ultrasonics Symposium, vol. 2, pp. 1647–1652 (2001)
8. Besl, P.J., McKay, H.D.: A method for registration of 3D shapes. IEEE Trans. Pattern Analysis and Machine Intelligence 14(2), 239–256 (1992)
9. Bilgen, M., Insana, M.F.: Predicting target detectability on acoustic elastography. In: IEEE Ultrasonics Symposium, pp. 1427–1430 (1997)
10. Shumway, R.H., Stoffer, D.S.: Time Series Analysis and Its Applications: With R Examples. Springer Texts in Statistics. Springer, Heidelberg (2006)
11. Dickey, D.A., Fuller, W.A.: Distribution of the estimators for autoregressive time series with a unit root. Journal of the American Statistical Association 74(366), 427–431 (1979)

Modeling Respiratory Motion for Cancer Radiation Therapy Based on Patient-Specific 4DCT Data

Jaesung Eom[1], Chengyu Shi[2], Xie George Xu[1], and Suvranu De[1]

[1] Department of Mechanical, Aerospace and Nuclear Engineering,
Rensselaer Polytechnic Institute, Troy, NY 12180, USA
{eomj,xug2,des}@rpi.edu
[2] Department of Radiation Oncology,
University of Texas Health Science Center at San Antonio, San Antonio, TX 78229, USA
shic@uthscsa.edu

Abstract. Prediction of respiratory motion has the potential to substantially improve cancer radiation therapy. A nonlinear finite element (FE) model of respiratory motion during full breathing cycle has been developed based on patient specific pressure-volume relationship and 4D Computed Tomography (CT) data. For geometric modeling of lungs and ribcage we have constructed intermediate CAD surface which avoids multiple geometric smoothing procedures. For physiologically relevant respiratory motion modeling we have used pressure-volume (PV) relationship to apply pressure loading on the surface of the model. A hyperelastic soft tissue model, developed from experimental observations, has been used. Additionally, pleural sliding has been considered which results in accurate deformations in the superior-inferior (SI) direction. The finite element model has been validated using 51 landmarks from the CT data. The average differences in position is seen to be 0.07 cm (SD = 0.20 cm), 0.07 cm (0.15 cm), and 0.22 cm (0.18 cm) in the left-right, anterior-posterior, and superior-inferior directions, respectively.

1 Introduction

Respiratory motions have a profound impact on the radiation treatment planning of cancer in the lung and adjacent tissues. In external beam radiation treatment, for example, a lethal radiation dose is delivered through precisely conformed radiation to the target. The current radiation treatment paradigm, however, is largely based on an assumption that both tumor location and shape are well known and remain unchanged during the course of radiation delivery. Such a favorable rigid-body relationship does not exist in anatomical sites such as the thoracic cavity and the abdomen, owing predominantly to respiratory motions. When the tumor-bearing normal organs move during radiation therapy, discrepancies between planned and actually delivered radiation doses can be quite significant. As a result, although higher radiation doses have shown better local tumor control, organ motions have sometimes required less aggressive treatment strategies having relatively large dose margins to tolerate potential targeting errors.

One previous approach to account for respiration caused target movement is to consider a larger planning target volume which covers a composite of 3D volumes of the moving target defined by the entire respiratory cycle. A relatively new approach is based on an image-guided technique which aligns and delivers the radiation according to a gated time and position or follows the tumor's trajectory during the respiratory cycle, to allow for a smaller and more conformal treatment volume. Hence, it is important to be able to predict the pattern of the lung motion as part of radiation therapy and know the tumor location in real time.

Discrepancies between the Deformable Image Registration (DIR) and physics based modeling methods are apparent when comparing motion field estimates. The question arises as to what motion field is more realistic and physiologically correct. There are several attempts to include the physiology in non-linear registration based methods [1, 2]. The basic assumptions of DIR often concern image-related aspects, and hence physiological and anatomical processes are not taken into consideration. As a result, gray values of anatomically corresponding voxels are treated to be constant over time. More accurate physics based techniques have also been reported more recently [3-5]. However, in most of the existing models the physiological data is ignored both in applying the boundary conditions and in using appropriate material models for the lung tissue.

To investigate these issues, a patient-specific non-linear finite element (FE) lung model is developed in this study by considering vigorous physiological conditions in the modeling. During inspiration, the diaphragm and the external intercostals contract with each other, resulting in an increased the thoracic volume. The resulting decrease in alveolar pressure causes the air to enter the lung. Expiration, on the other hand, is passive and the diaphragm relaxes, leading to a reduced thoracic volume and an increased pressure. The chest pressure-volume (PV) curve can be constructed by plotting lung volumes against pleural pressures that are estimated from esophageal pressures and body plethysmography [6]. Such PV curve data is used to drive the lung motion which simulates the breathing. Additionally, we take advantage of the sophisticated Computer Aided Engineering (CAE) concept in the geometric modeling of organs. The CAD surface reconstruction procedure affords more interactive mesh control and preserves the original geometric features of organs obtained from 4D CT image data.

This paper introduces the CAD surface reconstruction procedure using 4D CT data and then briefly discusses the outline of a nonlinear finite element modeling including the application of boundary and contact/sliding conditions. The advantage of the proposed geometric modeling procedure over conventional smoothing for the purposes of improving the accuracy of the respiratory simulation is presented.

2 Methods and Materials

2.1 Geometric Modeling

4D respiration gated CT images were acquired using a 16 Slice Brilliance CT Big Bore Oncology configuration (Philips). Breathing information was obtained using the associated Pneumo Chest bellows (Lafayette Instruments). Each Image slice has a resolution of 0.98 mm x 0.98 mm and a thickness of 2 mm. The categorized 10 phases of images were contoured into different ROIs (regions of interest) as [7]. According to the volume of each phase, the end of expiration (EE) state and the end of inspiration

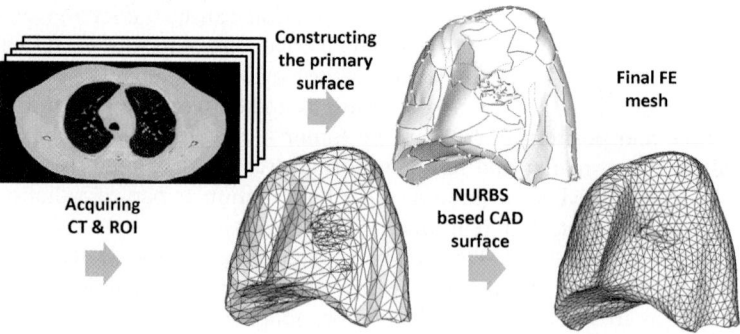

Fig. 1. Geometric modeling procedure using the CAD surface reconstruction (Reverse engineering)

(EI) states were selected. For accurate simulations, a uniform mesh of "good quality" must be used. However, for patient-specific geometric modeling, the characteristic features of the 4D CT image data must be preserved. It is noted that, in most previous studies [4, 5, 8], combination of mesh decimation and Laplacian smoothing were used to reduce the number of elements from the highly dense but non-regular mesh to the more uniform mesh acceptable in FE simulations. The problem of this procedure is that details of the mesh topology are lost. Also, the procedure is not interactive as multiple steps are involved. In this study, we used a CAD surface reconstruction approach to convert the ROIs into FE meshes as depicted in Figure 1. Primary surfaces are generated from ROI contour lines in Rhinoceros 3D (Robert McNeel & Associates, Seattle, WA). From these surfaces, NURBS-based CAD surfaces are reconstructed and converted into suitable FE meshes using HYPERMESH (Altair Engineering, Troy, MI). The surface that closely fits the tessellated surface is generated. This approach greatly simplifies the procedure of FE mesh generation and from CT scanned image data without losing the geometric details.

2.2 Physiologically-Based Respiratory Motion Modeling

The motion of the lungs during inhalation is physiologically caused by the expansion of the thoracic cavity. This expansion is induced by contraction of the diaphragm and outer intercostal muscles. These movements cause the pressure to change in the pleural cavity surrounding the lungs and the alveoli and, as a result, the air flows from the atmosphere into the lungs. This in turn causes a change in the intrapleural pressure which exerts force on the lung surface. Hence, the lung expands and the visceral pleura slides against the internal surface of the thoracic cavity with nearly frictionless contact due to lubrication of pleural liquid [9].

To model the motion of the lungs between EE to EI, a quasi-static nonlinear finite element model has been developed. A distributed time-varying pressure load was applied to the surface of the geometric lung model. The current paper outlines a physiologically-based modeling approach. The pressure amplitudes have been computed by comparing CT image data and FEM results. For now, the pressure history was assumed to follow the sinusoidal curve [10] according to the body plethysmography and the parameterized P-V curve [11]. We limited the expansion to a geometry defined by the lung shape at the end of inspiration phase. Pleural sliding is treated as a contact-friction model. Any contact between the lungs and the ribcage is modeled without friction—an approach that is justified as there is an incompressible and friction-minimizing pleural fluid in and between the visceral and parietal pleural.

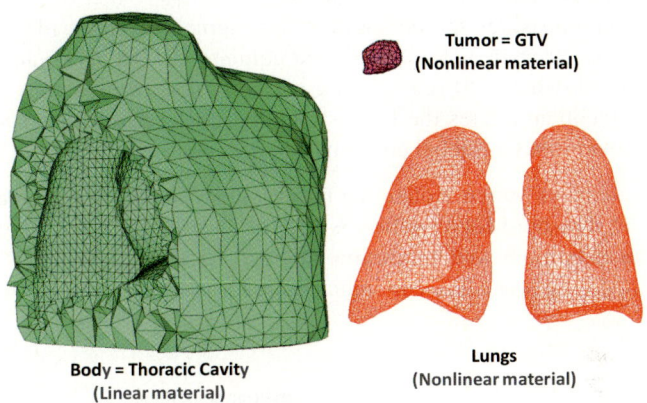

Fig. 2. Finite element models including a thoracic cavity, a tumor (gross target volume for radiation treatment purposes) and lungs

The FE model, which has 66704 tetrahedral elements and 55947 degrees of freedom in total, is composed of the thoracic cavity and the lungs with an embedded tumor in the right lung as seen in Figure 2. The lungs and thoracic cavity are fixed at the root of lungs according to anatomy.

The lung tissue was modeled as a hyperelastic material with the following expression for the strain energy per unit volume [12]

$$\rho_0 W = \frac{1}{2} c \exp\left(a_1 E_{xx}^2 + a_2 E_{yy}^2 + 2a_4 E_{xx} E_{yy}\right) + \frac{1}{2} c \exp\left(a_1 E_{xx}^2 + a_2 E_{zz}^2 + 2a_4 E_{xx} E_{zz}\right) + \frac{1}{2} c \exp\left(a_1 E_{zz}^2 + a_2 E_{yy}^2 + 2a_4 E_{zz} E_{yy}\right) \quad (1)$$

where c, a_1, a_2, a_4 are material constants derived from experiments, and E_{xx}, E_{xy} etc. are the components of the Green strain. For simplicity, lung tissue was assumed to be homogeneous and thoracic cavity was assumed to be linear elastic material (E = 6.0kPa Poisson's ration = 0.4 from [5]). Simulations, using Abaqus (Dassault Systèmes Simulia Corp., Providence, RI), have been carried out on an Intel Core2 Quadcore 2.83 GHz CPU machine with 8 GB RAM for 2.1 hours.

3 Results and Discussion

3.1 Comparison on Laplacian Smoothing vs. CAD Surface Reconstruction

To assess the advantage of the CAD surface reconstruction procedure over conventional mesh preparation using multiple Laplacian smoothing and decimating [6], we compared the geometric quality of the elements. Four mesh quality indices, commonly used in CAE [13] are used:

(a) *Aspect ratio*: This is the ratio of the longest edge of an element to its shortest edge.
(b) *Maximum and minimum interior angles*: These maximum and minimum values are evaluated independently for triangle facet.
(c) *Jacobian*: This measures the deviation of an element from its ideal or "perfect" shape, such as a triangle's deviation from equilateral. The Jacobian value ranges from 0.0 to 1.0, where 1.0 represents a perfectly shaped element. The determinant of the Jacobian relates the local stretching of the parametric space which is required to map it to the global coordinate space.

In Figure 3, elements which violate the mesh quality indices for each approach are color-coded. The threshold for violation is 0.9 for Jacobian, 2.0 for aspect ratio, 80° and 50° for the maximum and minimum interior angle, respectively. The volume change under modeling procedure can indicate the loss of geometric feature. It is clear

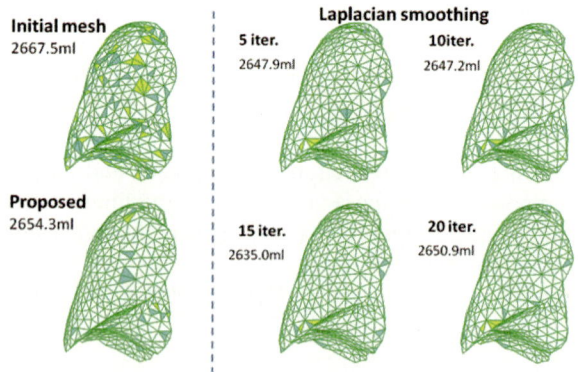

Fig. 3. Comparison of relaxing (Laplacian smoothing) vs. proposed CAD surface reconstruction procedure showing changes in mesh volume and elements that are close to or violating the quality indices using the following color coding : *light blue* = warning that an index is close to threshold and *yellow* = failure.

Table 1. Percentage of elements violating threshold criteria

Mesh	Jacobian (0.9)	Aspect Ratio (2.0)	Max angle (>80°)	Min angle (<50°)
Initial	21.1%	0.2%	49.9%	83.7%
Laplacian Smoothing				
5 Iterations	4.2%	0.2%	28.3%	66.9%
10 Iterations	4.1%	0.2%	27.7%	66.0%
15 Iterations	3.4%	0.2%	24.7%	63.7%
20 Iterations	3.9%	0.2%	27.6%	66.2%
Proposed model	3.0%	0.0%	21.3%	59.3%

that the proposed geometric modeling procedure preserves initial geometry of the CT scan data. Laplacian smoothing is an algorithm to smooth a polygonal mesh. For each vertex in the mesh, a new position is chosen based on local information (such as the position of neighbors) and then the vertex is moved. Laplacian smoothing focuses on moving point locations to improve triangulation without any guarantees on the preservation of the original geometric features.

In previous studies, 10 iterations of Laplacian smoothing and additional 10 smoothing iterations with decimation were used to prepare the computational mesh[5, 8]. Table 1 shows that 10 cycles of smoothing iterations reduce the original volume by 20.3 ml and the relaxing operations fail to enhance the mesh quality indices, while our proposed approach has achieved better meshes with 13.2 ml of volume loss.

3.2 Validation Based on Landmarks

The procedure to evaluate the modeling accuracy was based on the patient specific models and 4D CT image data. As shown in Figure 4, anatomical points that represent the bifurcation of vessels and airways were chosen on the exhale and inhale images. A total of 51 such landmarks were chosen from the CT images. The motion of the corresponding points in the FE model provides a measure of our modeling accuracy.

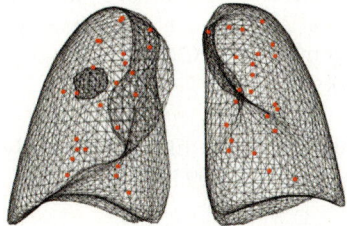

Fig. 4. Landmark bifurcation positions inside the lungs determined by radiologists

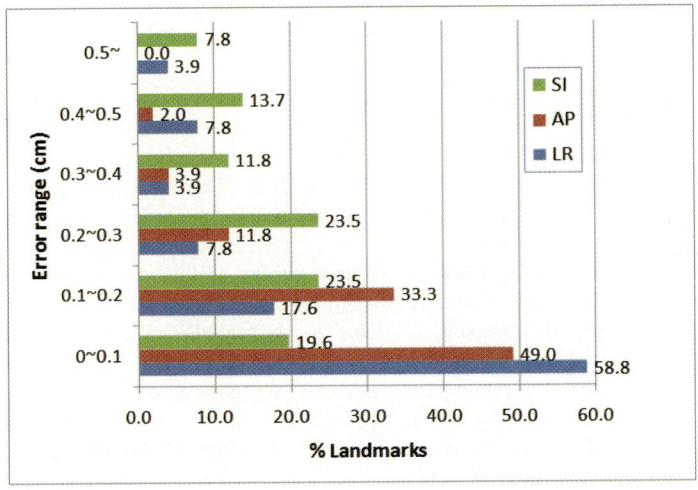

Fig. 5. Histogram of errors at landmarks at end of inhalation

We observe that the mean deviations $\left(P_{FEM} - P_{CT}\right)$ of our FE model predictions from the CT data are 0.07cm (SD = 0.20cm), 0.07cm (SD = 0.15 cm), and 0.22 cm (SD = 0.18 cm) in left-right (LR), anterior-posterior (AP), and superior-inferior (SI) directions, respectively. On the majority of landmarks the displacement errors are less than 2 mm (Figure 5). It should be noted that the landmarks are located in regions where effects of heterogeneity of the lung tissue are not negligible. Considering this, the accuracy of our homogeneous model is remarkable.

4 Conclusions

We present a nonlinear finite element model of respiratory motion during full breathing cycle based on patient-specific pressure-volume relationship and 4D CT data. For geometric modeling of the lungs and ribcage we have constructed an intermediate CAD surface between 4D CT scanned images and meshes for FE computation. This avoids multiple geometric smoothing procedures and increases the quality of the FE mesh while preserving geometric features of the CT scans. For a patient-specific FE lung model we have used pressure-volume (PV) relationship of lungs as physiological conditions and hyperelastic soft tissue model [12]. The PV relationship provides physiologically relevant boundary conditions over the entire breathing cycle. Validation using 51 landmarks from the CT image has been performed and our proposed model shows excellent agreement with CT data with a position error of less than 2 mm for most of the landmarks.

Acknowledgments. The authors would like to gratefully acknowledge the funding support from NIH/NLM grant R01LM009362.

References

1. McClelland, J., Blackall, J., Tarte, S., Chandler, A., Hughes, S., Ahmad, S., Landau, D., Hawkes, D.: A continuous 4D motion model from multiple respiratory cycles for use in lung radiotherapy. Medical Physics 33, 3348 (2006)
2. Sarrut, D., Boldea, V., Miguet, S., Ginestet, C.: Simulation of four-dimensional CT images from deformable registration between inhale and exhale breath-hold CT scans. Medical Physics 33, 605 (2006)
3. Zhang, T., Orton, N.P., Mackie, T.R., Paliwal, B.R.: Technical note: A novel boundary condition using contact elements for finite element deformable image registration. Medical Physics 31, 2412–2415 (2004)
4. Al-Mayah, A., Moseley, J., Brock, K.: Contact surface and material nonlinearity modeling of human lungs. Physics in Medicine and Biology 53, 305 (2008)
5. Brock, K., Sharpe, M., Dawson, L., Kim, S., Jaffray, D.: Accuracy of finite element model-based multi-organ deformable image registration. Medical Physics 32, 1647 (2005)
6. West, J.: Respiratory Physiology: The Essentials. Williams & Wilkins (2007)
7. Lin, L., Shi, C.T., Liu, Y., Swanson, G., Papanikolaou, N.: Development of a novel post-processing treatment planning platform for 4D radiotherapy. Technology in Cancer Research & Treatment 7, 125–132 (2008)

8. Villard, P., Beuve, M., Shariat, B., Baudet, V., Jaillet, F.: Lung mesh generation to simulate breathing motion with a finite element method. In: Proceedings of Eighth International Conference on Information Visualisation. IV 2004, pp. 194–199 (2004)
9. D'Angelo, E., Loring, S., Gioia, M., Pecchiari, M., Moscheni, C.: Friction and lubrication of pleural tissues. Respiratory Physiology & Neurobiology 142, 55–68 (2004)
10. Lujan, A.E., Larsen, E.W., Balter, J.M., Ten Haken, R.K.: A method for incorporating organ motion due to breathing into 3D dose calculations. Medical Physics 26, 715–720 (1999)
11. Santhanam, A.: Modeling, Simulation, And Visualization of 3d Lung Dynamics. University of Central Florida Orlando, Florida (2006)
12. Zeng, Y., Yager, D., Fung, Y.: Measurement of the mechanical properties of the human lung tissue. Journal of Biomechanical Engineering 109, 169–174 (1987)
13. Bathe, K.: Finite element procedures. Englewood Cliffs, New Jersey (1996)

Correlating Chest Surface Motion to Motion of the Liver Using ε-SVR – A Porcine Study

Floris Ernst[1], Volker Martens[1], Stefan Schlichting[2], Armin Beširević[2], Markus Kleemann[2], Christoph Koch[3], Dirk Petersen[3], and Achim Schweikard[1]

[1] Institute for Robotics and Cognitive Systems, University of Lübeck, DE
{ernst,martens,schweikard}@rob.uni-luebeck.de
[2] Clinic for Surgery, University Hospital Schleswig-Holstein, Lübeck, DE
{stefan.schlichting,armin.besirevic,markus.kleemann}@uk-sh.de
[3] Institute for Neuroradiology, University Hospital Schleswig-Holstein, Lübeck, DE
koch@neuroradiologie.uni-luebeck.de, dirk.petersen@uni-luebeck.de

Abstract. In robotic radiosurgery, the compensation of motion of internal organs is vital. This is currently done in two phases: an external surrogate signal (usually active optical markers placed on the patient's chest) is recorded and subsequently correlated to an internal motion signal obtained using stereoscopic X-ray imaging. This internal signal is sampled very infrequently to minimise the patient's exposure to radiation. We have investigated the correlation of the external signal to the motion of the liver in a porcine study using ε-support vector regression. IR LEDs were placed on the swines' chest. Gold fiducials were placed in the swines' livers and were recorded using a two-plane X-ray system. The results show that a very good correlation model can be built using ε-SVR, in this test clearly outperforming traditional polynomial models by at least 45 and as much as 74 %. Using multiple markers simultaneously can increase the new model's accuracy.

1 Introduction

In recent years, it has become possible to irradiate tumours in the whole body without using respiratory coaching, gating or stereotactic fixation. The CyberKnife® [1] system – a robotic device used to detect and compensate for respiratory motion in radiosurgery – records optical markers placed on the patient's chest and correlates them to the position of landmarks, i.e. gold fiducials, obtained during stereoscopic X-ray imaging [2]. This model is subsequently used to guide a γ-radiation source. That this correlation indeed exists has been evaluated before [3,11]. Currently, this model is built using 10-20 measurements of internal fiducials acquired during the first couple of breathing cycles. The model is checked and updated periodically. This is typically done once every 2-5 minutes by taking another X-ray shot. Furthermore, the markers (currently three) are placed on the patient's chest at those points showing the greatest excursion. The currently employed correlation model is either linear, curvilinear, dual-curvilinear or a mixture of those and is based on the principal directional component of motion of each individual chest LED [4].

We propose to improve the CyberKnife by modifying the correlation model employed in clinical practice. We compute the correlation using all three dimensions of movement of the LEDs as well as their first and second derivatives. This is done with a novel correlation model we have developed which is based on ε-support vector regression (ε-SVR) [5]. With this model it is also possible to use multiple LEDs as input surrogates.

2 Materials and Methods

For this work, four gold fiducials were implanted into the liver of a living swine under US guidance. Respiratory motion of the liver was recorded in two sessions while the swine was ventilated manually using a bag valve mask. The swine was killed minutes prior to the experiments. An ethics proposal has been approved.

2.1 Data Acquisition

To acquire the fiducials' 3D position, a two-plane X-ray imaging device (Philips Allura Xper FD20/10, Fig. 1a) at the Institute for Neuroradiology (University Hospital Schleswig-Holstein, Lübeck) was connected to a high resolution/high speed frame grabbing system (Matrox Helios XA) to allow the capturing of live fluoroscopic video streams. The X-ray system takes images at a frame rate of 15 Hz. To record the swine's chest surface motion, a net of 19 IR LEDs (see [6] and Fig. 1b) was placed on the swine's abdomen. The LEDs were tracked using the atracsys accuTrack compact system, effectively delivering a recording frame rate of 216 Hz for each LED. The signals were then downsampled to 15 Hz to match the acquisition speed of the X-ray cameras.

To determine the geometric relation between the two X-ray imaging units and the tracking camera, a custom calibration rig was used: an acrylic box (10x7x5 cm^3) with twelve embedded metallic spheres and eight LEDs was built. The system was calibrated by simultaneously acquiring an image of the calibration

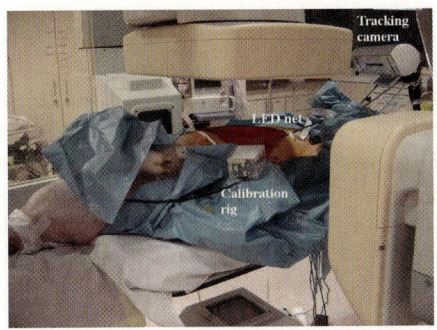   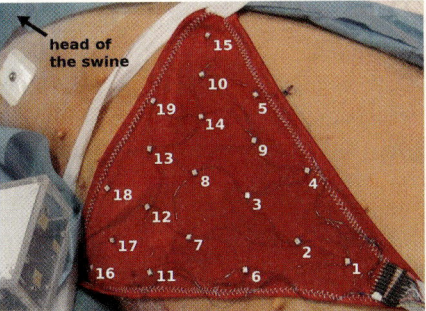

       (a) Experimental setup   **(b)** The LED net

Fig. 1. X-ray device, tracking camera, calibration rig and LED net

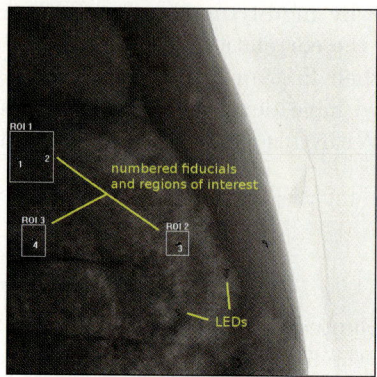 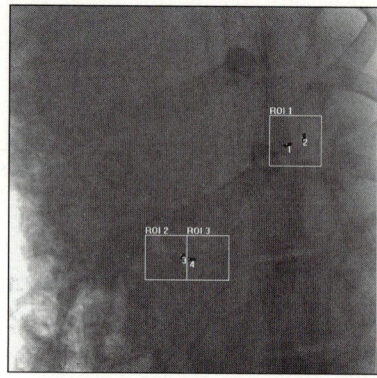

Fig. 2. The tracking GUI. Both the fiducials and the LEDs are clearly visible. The regions used for segmentation are marked with white rectangles.

rig with the X-ray devices and determining the rig's position using the tracking camera. The actual calibration was performed using the POSIT algorithm [7], resulting in a projection error of less than one pixel (RMS). Both the LEDs and the metal spheres could be detected with sub-millimetre accuracy.

The frame grabber and the IR tracking system are connected to one machine (Intel Q9450, 8 GiB RAM, ubuntu 8.04 x64). To track the gold fiducials in the X-ray images, we developed a graphical tool kit written in C++ to perform region-of-interest based segmentation of ellipsoidal objects and triangulate the 3D position of the fiducials (Fig. 2).

2.2 Correlation Methods

To compute the 3D position of the gold fiducials from the surrogate signal, the following methods were investigated:

- The polynomial models traditionally used in the CyberKnife, see [4]
- Our correlation model based on ε-SVR machines

These correlation algorithms were developed and implemented in MATLAB. The SVR machines were built using LibSVM [8].

Let us assume that N is the number of samples we have taken. To build the correlation model, the input signal is divided into two parts: a training part $\mathcal{T} = \{1, \ldots, m\}$ and an evaluation part $\mathcal{E} = \{m+1, \ldots, N\}$. On the training part, we select points $\mathcal{M} \subseteq \mathcal{T}$ representative of the breathing pattern (i.e., points at maximum inspiration and expiration as well as points halfway between). Now let $\mathbf{L}_{i,j,n}$ be the time series of the 19 IR LEDs ($i = 1, \ldots, 19$ is the number of the LED, $j = 1, \ldots, 3$ are the spatial coordinates and n is the temporal index) and let $\mathbf{F}_{k,j,n}$ be the time series of the four gold fiducials ($k = 1, \ldots, 4$ is the fiducial number, j and n as before).

The polynomial models given in [4] are used to find coefficients of a linear or quadratic polynomial relating the principal directional component of motion of one LED to the principal directional component of motion of the fiducial. Additionally, the model supports breathing hysteresis by building two polynomials, one for inspiration and one for expiration. Both the simple quadratic model as well as the so-called bilinear and biquadratic models can also be blended to the simple linear model outside the values seen in the training data set $\mathcal{M}$.

We introduce a new correlation model based on ε-support vector regression. We do not only use the LEDs' principal directional component of motion as the polynomial models but all three dimensions. Second, information about the direction of breathing is directly built into the model by creating vectors $\mathbf{D}_i$ indicating the direction of breathing:

$$\mathbf{D}_{i,n} = \begin{cases} -1 & \text{for } \tilde{\mathbf{L}}_{i,\cdot,n} - \tilde{\mathbf{L}}_{i,\cdot,n-1} < -0.05mm \\ 0 & \text{for } -0.05mm \leq \tilde{\mathbf{L}}_{i,\cdot,n} - \tilde{\mathbf{L}}_{i,\cdot,n-1} \leq 0.05mm \\ 1 & \text{for } \tilde{\mathbf{L}}_{i,\cdot,n} - \tilde{\mathbf{L}}_{i,\cdot,n-1} > 0.05mm \end{cases}, \quad n = 2, \ldots, N.$$

Here, $\tilde{\mathbf{L}}_{i,\cdot,n}$ denotes the n-th sample of the principal directional component of the point cloud $\mathbf{L}_{i,\cdot}$. Third, we incorporate information about the signal's speed and acceleration by also bringing in the first and second derivatives $\mathbf{L}^{(1)}$ and $\mathbf{L}^{(2)}$ of the LEDs' positions. These derivatives are computed using central differences.

Now let $\mathbf{x}_{i,m} = \left(\mathbf{L}_{i,\cdot,m}^{\mathrm{T}}, {\mathbf{L}_{i,\cdot,m}^{(1)}}^{\mathrm{T}}, {\mathbf{L}_{i,\cdot,m}^{(2)}}^{\mathrm{T}}, \mathbf{D}_{i,m} \right)^{\mathrm{T}} \in \mathbb{R}^9 \times \{-1, 0, 1\}$. Then for each $i = 1, \ldots, 19$, $j = 1, \ldots, 4$ and $m \in \mathcal{M}$ we create training samples $s_m^{i,j} = \left\{ \mathbf{x}_{i,m}, \tilde{F}_{j,\cdot,m} \right\}$, i.e., the samples $s_m^{i,j}, m \in \mathcal{M}$, describe the relation between LED i and $\tilde{F}_{j,\cdot}$, the principal directional component of motion of fiducial j. These samples are then used to train ε-SVR machines which in turn serve as correlation models. The SVR machines are built using a linear kernel function.

2.3 Evaluation

The correlation models outlined above were applied to two groups of signals (120 s and 590 s duration) recorded during the ventilation of the swine. During both tests, not all LEDs were visible. In the first test, only LEDs 11, 14 and 16 to 19 were visible; in the second test, LEDs 6 to 14 and 16 to 19 were visible. The models were built using the first 20 s of motion. The ε-SVR's parameters were set to $C = 1$ and $\varepsilon = 0.2$ (signal 1) and $\varepsilon = 0.15$ (signal 2).

We also evaluated the influence of LED selection on correlation accuracy: first, which LED yields the best result and second, if the correlation model can be improved by using more than one LED at the same time.

3 Results

Analysis of LED motion shows that it is not only in one direction and does exhibit strong hysteresis relative to fiducial motion. This is the first indication that the simple polynomial models are not adequate.

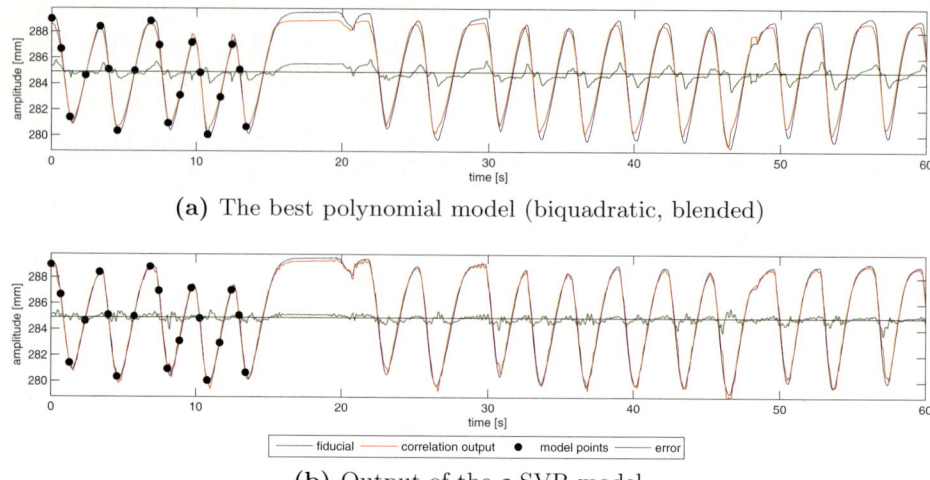

(a) The best polynomial model (biquadratic, blended)

(b) Output of the ε-SVR model

Fig. 3. First test run, results of the correlation process. First 60 s are shown. Fiducial motion is shown in blue, training points used in black and the correlation output in red. The residual error is plotted in green. The respiratory pause around $t = 20$ s is accidental and not connected to the correlation model.

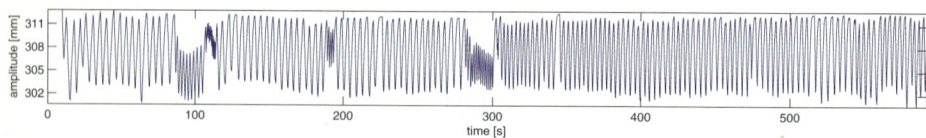

Fig. 4. Second test run. The signal shows variations in breathing frequency and amplitude.

The correlation plots of all the polynomial correlation models are given in Fig. 5. Ideally, the red curves would cover all blue dots. Clearly, the simple polynomial models don't fit the data very well, the bipolynomial models' matching is better. The actual numbers are given in Tab. 1.

Evaluation results for the best polynomial model (biquadratic with blending) and for the ε-SVR model are given in Fig. 3. The polynomial model does not only incur a larger RMS error (see Tab. 1) but also suffers from periodic errors at the inspiration and expiration peaks. The reason for this is that the model does not adequately capture correlation in the regions marked with black dotted rectangles in Fig. 5g.

Evaluation of the ε-SVR correlation model shows a much better matching: Fig. 6 shows the correlation plots of the three axes of LED eleven versus the principal directional component of fiducial one. Clearly, the red dots (output of the correlation model) correspond very well to the blue dots (actual correlation). This is also reflected in the numbers given in Tab. 1: the SVR approach outperforms the best (bi)polynomial model by 45 % (signal 1) or 38 % (signal

Table 1. RMS errors, 75 % and 95 % confidence intervals of the correlation models. Eleventh LED to first fiducial.

model	RMS error [mm]		75 % CI [mm]		95 % CI [mm]		max [mm]	
	sig. 1	sig. 2	sig. 1	sig. 2	sig. 1	sig. 2	sig. 1	sig. 2
linear	1.06	1.05	1.33	1.23	2.01	2.09	2.26	2.84
quadratic	1.03	1.04	1.32	1.22	1.90	2.04	2.14	2.80
quadratic, blended	1.03	1.04	1.32	1.22	1.90	2.04	2.14	2.80
bilinear	0.78	0.96	0.91	1.16	1.61	1.90	4.36	5.88
bilinear, blended	0.79	0.96	0.93	1.15	1.61	1.90	1.86	2.57
biquadratic	0.55	0.95	0.57	1.16	1.13	1.85	4.36	5.88
biquadratic, blended	0.50	0.95	0.52	1.14	1.05	1.85	1.71	2.54
ε-SVR	0.28	0.59	0.28	0.64	0.52	1.12	1.48	4.14

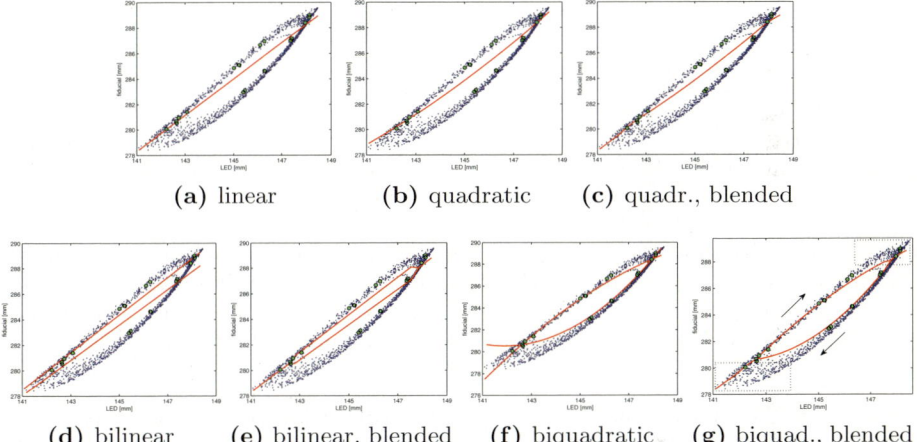

(a) linear (b) quadratic (c) quadr., blended

(d) bilinear (e) bilinear, blended (f) biquadratic (g) biquad., blended

Fig. 5. The polynomial models. The x-axis shows the principal directional component of the motion of LED 11, the y-axis shows the principal directional component of motion of the first fiducial. Model points are marked with green circles, the model output is shown in red. In Subfig. (g), the dotted boxes show the areas corresponding to maximum inspiration and expiration; the arrows indicate the breathing direction.

2). Furthermore, the SVR model does not suffer from systematic errors like the polynomial models.

3.1 Selection of LEDs and Using Multiple LEDs

We also investigated the influence of LED selection on the quality of the correlation model. When selecting different LEDs as input surrogates, we see that on the first signal, the RMS error ranges from 0.27 mm to 0.38 mm whereas on the second signal, it ranges from 0.36 mm to 1.91 mm. Since the ε-SVR correlation model has been designed such that it can use input from more than one LED at a time, we evaluated the model for all possible pairs (triplets, quadruplets, ...). The results are shown in Fig. 7. We can see that on the first signal, using more

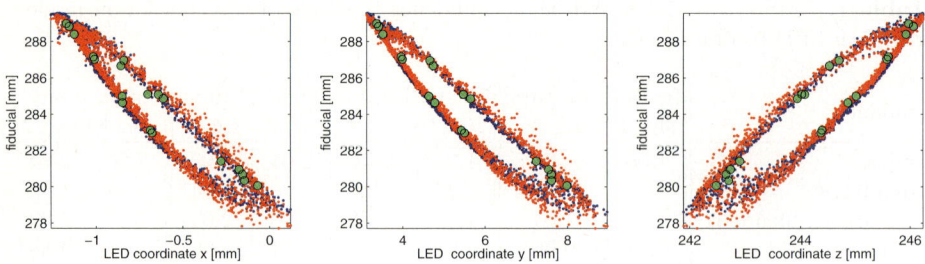

Fig. 6. The ε-SVR model. The x-axes show the motion of LED 11, the y-axes show the principal directional component of motion of the first fiducial. Model points are marked with green circles, the model output is shown in red.

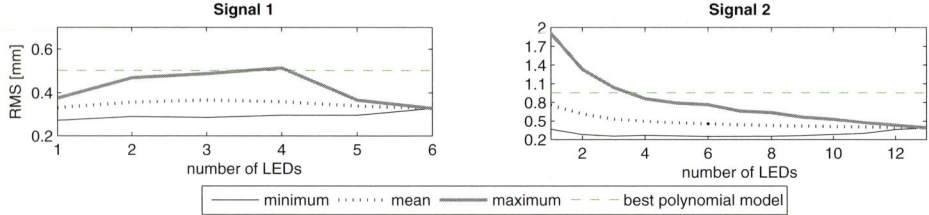

Fig. 7. The plots show the range (minimum and maximum values) and mean of the RMS error when using multiple LEDs. Read: when using six LEDs (1716 possibilites) to build the correlation model on signal two, the resulting RMS error is, depending on the selected sixtet, between 0.25 and 0.77 mm with a mean of 0.45 mm.

than one LED does not noticeably improve correlation results, possibly due to overfitting. On the second signal, however, the best attainable correlation model uses six LEDs and outperforms the best model using one LED by 32 %: the RMS value drops from 0.36 mm to 0.25 mm. In this case, the best polynomial model is outperformed by as much as 74 %. Additionally, the 95 % CI drops to 0.47 mm. We believe that in this case we can clearly see that in this case the model using more LEDs is capable of catching the changing characteristics of the signal. Note that on signal one, only 19 and on signal two, only 17 samples are used to build the model which is evaluated on 1,876 and 8,588 samples, respectively.

4 Discussion

The fact that correlation on the second signal (with a length of 590 s) can be improved significantly by using multiple LEDs is due to the signal's complexity: ventilation speed was varied as was the ventilation volume such as to mimick changing breathing patterns. It seems that especially the changes in breathing mode cannot be adequately covered by using one single LED.

We also went beyond the work presented in [9,10] and [11]. In [9], the internal position of the tumour was measured with NDI's magnetic tracking system using biopsy needles inserted into the swine. This approach suffers from poor temporal and spatial resolution and also from possibly altering the organ's motion patterns due to the insertion of biopsy needles. In [10], the evaluation of the correlation was done retrospectively on lung tumour patients where the tumour was located using stereoscopic fluoroscopy at changing angles and the external motion was recorded using a laser-based measuring device. The disadvantages in this study are the relatively short duration of the recordings (just over one minute in average) and the fact that the laser-based measuring system can only record distances and does not show the 3D displacement of a single point in space. In [11], the authors use very poor temporal resolution (4-5 Hz) and only compute the leave-one-out error of their correlation model. Furthermore, their model is built using all signal points but one and no long-term evaluation of the model is done.

In the near future, we plan to continue this study with more swines either under mechanical lung ventilation or breathing freely. We also hope to see this new correlation model implemented in the CyberKnife to perform tests under real conditions. Also, further investigation needs to be done as to where to place the LEDs on which the model is built, since this placement significantly influences the correlation accuracy.

5 Conclusion

It has been shown that the polynomial models used in determining the tumour position from chest marker positions are not very accurate, delivering RMS errors of up to 0.95 mm, depending on the complexity of the input signal. On the other hand, the correlation model based on ε-SVR can achieve far better results: for both signals tested, RMS errors of 0.3 mm or less are feasible, a reduction of 40 to 75 %.

References

1. Adler, J.R., Schweikard, A., Murphy, M.J., Hancock, S.L.: Image-guided stereotactic radiosurgery: The CyberKnife. In: Image-guided neurosurgery: clinical applications of surgical navigation, pp. 193–204. Quality Medical Publishing (1998)
2. Schweikard, A., Glosser, G., Bodduluri, M., et al.: Robotic motion compensation for respiratory motion during radiosurgery. J. Comput. Aided Surg. 5(4), 263–277 (2000)
3. Gierga, D.P., Brewer, J., Sharp, G.C., et al.: The correlation between internal and external markers for abdominal tumors: Implications for respiratory gating. Int. J. Radiat. Oncol. Biol. Phys. 61(5), 1551–1558 (2005)
4. Sayeh, S., Wang, J., Main, W.T., et al.: Respiratory Motion Tracking for Robotic Radiosurgery. In: Urschel, H.C. (ed.) Robotic Radiosurgery. Treating Tumors that Move with Respiration, 1st edn., pp. 15–30. Springer, Berlin (2007)
5. Drucker, H., Burges, C.J.C., Kaufman, L., et al.: Support vector regression machines. In: Advances in Neural Information Processing Systems. NIPS, vol. 9, pp. 155–161. MIT Press, Cambridge (1997)

6. Knöpke, M., Ernst, F.: Flexible Markergeometrien zur Erfassung von Atmungs und Herzbewegungen an der Körperoberfläche. In: 7. CURAC Jahrestagung, Leipzig, Germany, September 24-26, pp. 15–16 (2008)
7. DeMenthon, D.F., Davis, L.S.: Model-based object pose in 25 lines of code. Int. J. Comput. Vision 15(1-2), 123–141 (1995)
8. Chang, C.C., Lin, C.J.: LibSVM: a library for support vector machines (2001), http://www.csie.ntu.edu.tw/~cjlin/libsvm
9. Tang, J., Dieterich, S., Cleary, K.: Respiratory motion tracking of skin and liver in swine for CyberKnife motion compensation. In: Galloway Jr., R.L. (ed.) Medical Imaging 2004: Visualization, Image-Guided Procedures, and Display. vol. 5367, pp. 729–734. SPIE, San Diego (2004)
10. Seppenwoolde, Y., Berbeco, R.I., Nishioka, S., et al.: Accuracy of tumor motion compensation algorithm from a robotic respiratory tracking system: A simulation study. Med. Phys. 34(7), 2774–2784 (2007)
11. Khamene, A., Warzelhan, J.K., Vogt, S., Elgort, D., Chefd'Hotel, C., Duerk, J.L., Lewin, J.S., Wacker, F.K., Sauer, F.: Characterization of internal organ motion using skin marker positions. In: Barillot, C., Haynor, D.R., Hellier, P. (eds.) MICCAI 2004. Part II. LNCS, vol. 3217, pp. 526–533. Springer, Heidelberg (2004)

Respiratory Motion Estimation from Cone-Beam Projections Using a Prior Model

Jef Vandemeulebroucke[1,2,3], Jan Kybic[3], Patrick Clarysse[1], and David Sarrut[1,2]

[1] University of Lyon, CREATIS-LRMN; CNRS UMR5220; INSA-Lyon, France
[2] University of Lyon, Léon Bérard Cancer Center, F-69373, Lyon, France
[3] Center for Machine Perception, Czech Technical University in Prague, Czech Republic

Abstract. Respiratory motion introduces uncertainties when planning and delivering radiotherapy for lung cancer patients. Cone-beam projections acquired in the treatment room could provide valuable information for building motion models, useful for gated treatment delivery or motion compensated reconstruction. We propose a method for estimating 3D+T respiratory motion from the 2D+T cone-beam projection sequence by including prior knowledge about the patient's breathing motion. Motion estimation is accomplished by maximizing the similarity of the projected view of a patient specific model to observed projections of the cone-beam sequence. This is done semi-globally, considering entire breathing cycles. Using realistic patient data, we show that the method is capable of good prediction of the internal patient motion from cone-beam data, even when confronted with interfractional changes in the breathing motion.

1 Introduction

In radiotherapy, breathing motion causes uncertainties in the dose delivered to the tumor. The existing approaches to take respiratory motion into account include adding safety margins to ensure target coverage, breath-hold, gating, or tracking of the target [1]. An important prerequisite to plan and evaluate treatment when using these techniques is a detailed knowledge of the motion. Four-dimensional (4D) computed tomography imaging [2] or cone-beam (CB) CT [3], consisting of three dimensional (3D) frames each representing a breathing phase, can provide additional motion information. However, no intercycle variability can be measured as they represent a single respiratory cycle.

Breathing motion occurs predominantly in cranio-caudal direction and tends to be larger for the lower lobes [1]. Trajectories of tumors and organs can be subject to hysteresis [4], i.e. a different path is followed during inhalation and exhalation. Cycles can differ from one another in breathing rate and level [5]; the latter influencing the amplitude of the motion. Variations in the mean tumor position (baseline) between and during fractions have also been reported [4,6].

Previously, 4D CT [7] and cine CT volume segments covering multiple cycles [8] have been used to model breathing motion. The small amount of acquired breathing cycles limits their ability to model intercycle variability. 4D MRI [9] covering more cycles could offer a solution to this problem. Regardless of the chosen approach, one should be able to detect and correct for interfractional changes in breathing motion that occur frequently between treatment sessions [4,6].

A CB projection sequence consists of a series of wide angle X-ray projections taken from viewpoints orbiting the patient. CBCT is routinely acquired for patient setup in many institutions, immediately before treatment, with the patient in the treatment position. Zijp et al. [10] have a fast and robust method for extracting a respiratory phase signal from a CB projection sequence. By establishing a relation to a prior 4D CT, Rit et al. [11] obtained a motion model that proved suitable for motion compensated CB reconstruction. Zeng et al. [12] estimated motion from a projection sequence by deforming a reference CT image so that its projection views match the CB sequence. Optimization of the large number of parameters of a B-spline based deformation model required adding aperiodicity penalties to the cost function to regularize the problem.

This article deals with *in situ* motion estimation from CB projection data for radiotherapy of lung cancer. With respect to [12] we incorporate prior knowledge in the form of a patient-specific model, significantly reducing the number of parameters to be identified. No intercycle regularization is required and we obtain improvement in speed and robustness. Within-cycle smoothness is guaranteed automatically, through the use of a B-spline temporal model.

2 Method

First, a parametric patient-specific motion model with a small number of degrees of freedom is built from a 4D CT image routinely acquired preoperatively for the irradiation treatment planning of the considered patient group. The model is able to represent changes in the breathing phase in addition to small variations in breathing pattern. The model is then fitted to the CB projection sequence by optimizing the model parameters to maximize the similarity between the acquired 2D CB projections and simulated projection views of the model. Individual cycles are processed separately and a smooth motion estimate is found by simultaneously considering the whole cycle with suitable boundary conditions.

2.1 Motion Model

Using the demons algorithm [13], we deformably register a manually chosen reference frame f_* to all other frames f_ϑ of the 4D CT, where $\vartheta \in [0;1)$ is the breathing phase. f_* should be chosen as to contain as little artifacts as possible. End-exhale is usually a good choice. Let $g_\vartheta(\mathbf{x})$ be the resulting deformation vector field, mapping f_* to f_ϑ. All deformation fields are averaged and a *mean position image* $\bar{f}$ is created by backward warping of f_* [14] (Figure 1a).

$$\bar{f}(\mathbf{x}) = f_* \left(\bar{g}^{-1}(\mathbf{x}) \right) \quad \text{with} \quad \bar{g}(\mathbf{x}) = \frac{1}{b} \sum_{\theta=1}^{b} g_\theta(\mathbf{x}) \qquad (1)$$

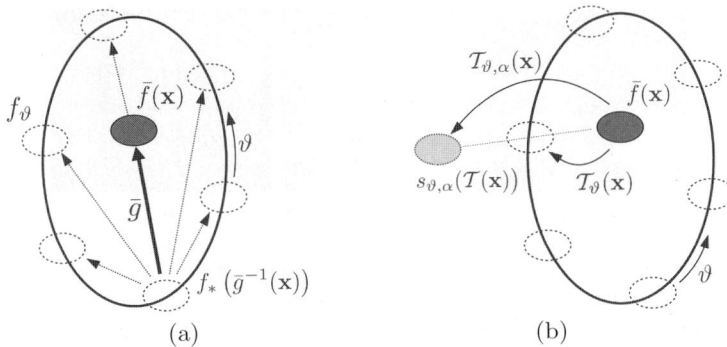

Fig. 1. (a) The procedure for obtaining a mean position image $\bar{f}$. (b) A schematic representation of the representable space for the proposed model. Consider a point with position **x** in in the image $\bar{f}$ (*dark oval*). Its position in all frames of the 4D CT (*white ovals*) is interpolated yielding the estimated breathing trajectory (*bold curve*). The amplitude parameter α allows to reach breathing states $s_{\vartheta,\alpha}$ off the trajectory.

All structures appear at their time-weighted mean position in the image $\bar{f}$ [15]. Next, $\bar{f}$ is registered to the original frames f_ϑ. The resulting deformation fields are approximated using B-splines as

$$\mathcal{T}_{\vartheta,\alpha}(\mathbf{x}) = \mathbf{x} + \alpha \sum_i \sum_j a_{ij}\, \beta^{n_\mathbf{x}}\!\left(\frac{\mathbf{x} - \mathbf{x_i}}{\Delta_\mathbf{x}}\right) \beta^{n_\vartheta}\!\left(\frac{\vartheta - \vartheta_j}{\Delta_\vartheta}\right). \quad (2)$$

where $\beta^n(.)$ are B-splines placed at positions $\mathbf{x_i}$, ϑ_j with uniform spacing $\Delta_\mathbf{x}$, Δ_ϑ; a_{ij} are the B-spline coefficients. As ϑ varies from 0 to 1, the deformation model produces a motion corresponding to an entire breathing cycle starting from end-exhalation. Note that this allows to model hysteresis. The second parameter α is an instantaneous amplitude (it can vary with ϑ) and helps to model variations of the trajectory shape and breathing level. We chose cubic spline interpolation for phase space ($n_\vartheta=3$). For the spatial dimension however, since dense deformation fields are available, a fast nearest neighbor ($n_\mathbf{x} = 0$) is employed. The coefficients a_{ij} are found quickly using digital filtering [16]. Image $s_{\vartheta,\alpha}$ for a particular breathing state described by ϑ,α (Figure 1b) is obtained through forward warping [14] (where the subscript for $\mathcal{T}$ was omitted)

$$s_{\vartheta,\alpha}(\mathcal{T}(\mathbf{x})) = \bar{f}(\mathbf{x}). \quad (3)$$

2.2 Cost Function and Optimization Strategy

We propose to optimize the parameters of the model together for each breathing cycle. This renders the method more robust with respect to simply considering each projection separately (see Section 3), but is computationally more tractable than a truly global optimization (over many breathing cycles). Since breathing cycle extrema can usually be identified well, the accuracy is not compromised.

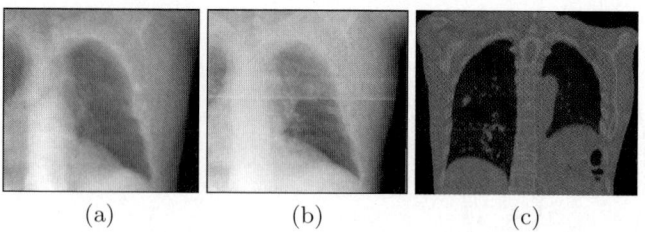

Fig. 2. (a) A simulated CB projection view calculated from the mean position image $\bar{f}$ and (b) a true CB projection of the same patient from the same viewpoint. Note that the images are very similar except for a horizontal reinforcement of the treatment table visible in the true CB projection. (c) Color overlay of preregistered end-inhalation frames from the two 4D CT acquisitions of patient 1.

Given a CT volume f, an ideal cone-beam projection image p can be calculated using a linear projection operator $\mathcal{P}_\phi$ where the parameter ϕ fully describes the (known) camera position and orientation:

$$p = \mathcal{P}_\phi f \qquad (4)$$

Figure 2a and 2b show a CB projection view of a mean position image $\bar{f}$ compared with a CB projection of the same patient. We measure similarity between an observed CB projection $\hat{p}$ and a modeled breathing state $s_{\vartheta,\alpha}$ by calculating the normalized correlation coefficient (NCC) in the 2D projection space:

$$J(\vartheta, \alpha; \phi) = \mathrm{NCC}(\hat{p}, \mathcal{P}_\phi s_{\vartheta,\alpha}) \ . \qquad (5)$$

In a first step, we detect the approximate time positions (projection indexes) t_e corresponding to extreme breathing phases [10]. The method is based on taking image derivatives and analyzing 1D projections of the obtained image. Second, we refine the parameters $\vartheta(t_e)$ and $\alpha(t_e)$ by minimizing

$$J\left(\vartheta(t_e), \alpha(t_e); \phi\right) + w\left(\vartheta(t_e) - \vartheta_e\right) \quad \text{with} \quad w(y) = \begin{cases} 0 & \text{for} |y| \leq h \\ \delta |y|^2 & \text{otherwise} \end{cases}. \qquad (6)$$

Note we are favoring solutions near the expected phase value ϑ_e. Powell-Brent [17] multidimensional search was used with $h = 0.1$ and $\delta = 20$ with initial values $\alpha(t_e) = 1$ and $\vartheta(t_e) = \vartheta_e = \vartheta_{ee}$ or ϑ_{ei} for end-exhalation and end-inhalation, respectively. The values for both ϑ_{ee} and ϑ_{ei} were determined by applying the extrema detection method [10] to simulated projections of the model with slowly varying phase.

Let t_e and $t_{e'}$ be the two end-inhalation positions, the beginning and end of a breathing cycle. We have just shown how to get ϑ and α at $t_e, t_{e'}$, what remains is to obtain the estimates also for frames $t_{e+1}, \ldots, t_{e'-1}$. Assuming temporal smoothness, we propose to represent ϑ as

$$\vartheta(t) = \sum_{i=0}^{k} c_i \, \beta^{n_{\vartheta_t}}\left(\frac{t - t_i}{\Delta_{\vartheta_t}}\right) \quad \text{for} \quad t_e < t < t_{e'} \ . \qquad (7)$$

where k is the number of control points, t_i are the temporal position of the knots, Δ_{ϑ_t} is the knot spacing and c_i are the B-spline coefficients. Fixing the value for $\vartheta(t_e)$ we can express the boundary coefficient c_0 as

$$c_0 = \frac{\vartheta(t_e) - \sum_{i=1}^{k} c_i \beta^{n_{\vartheta_t}}\left(\frac{t_e - t_i}{\Delta_{\vartheta_t}}\right)}{\beta^{n_{\vartheta_t}}\left(\frac{t_e - t_0}{\Delta_{\vartheta_t}}\right)}. \qquad (8)$$

and similarly for c_k. A B-spline expansion with coefficients d_j is used to represent $\alpha(t)$. By summing the contributions for m different time instances within the cycle and using equations (5),(7–8), we obtain the following similarity measure:

$$J^t(\mathbf{c}, \mathbf{d}) = \frac{1}{m} \sum_{t=1}^{m} J\left(\vartheta(t_e + t), \alpha(t_e + t); \phi(t_e + t)\right). \qquad (9)$$

We find the coefficients $\mathbf{c} = [c_1, \ldots, c_k]$, $\mathbf{d} = [d_1, \ldots, d_l]$ by minimizing J^t, using a Nelder-Nead downhill simplex algorithm [17], which performed well in this high dimensional search space, requiring less iterations than Powell-Brent and yielding comparable results. A linear progression is used as a starting point. We use a quadratic B-spline representation ($n_{\vartheta_t} = n_{\alpha_t} = 2$) with $k = l = 4$.

3 Experiments and Results

Accurately evaluating the 2D-3D motion estimation is very difficult, as no ground truth is available. In this work we use pairs of 4D CT sequences acquired for three lung cancer patients using a Philips Brilliance BigBore 16-slice CT scanner (Philips Medical Systems, Cleveland, OH). The time between acquisitions ranged from 20 minutes (patient 1 and 2) to 3 days (patient 3). Patients 1 and 2 were asked to stand up from the acquisition table and walk around for 10

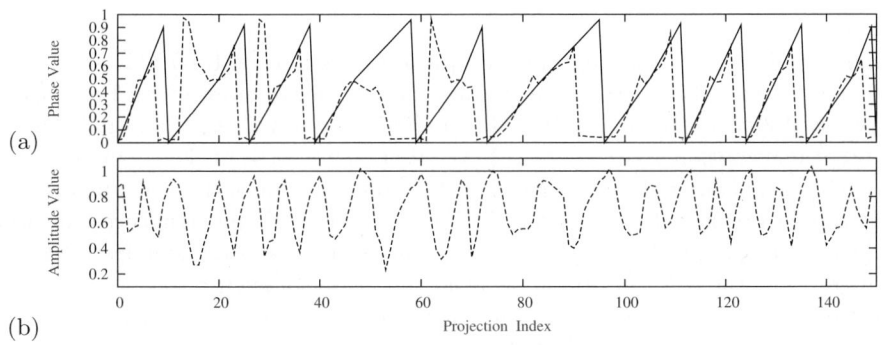

Fig. 3. Results of sequential motion estimation for patient 1: the recovered phase (a) and amplitude (b) (*dashed line*) together with the parameters used to generate the CB sequence (*full line*). The reference amplitude is a constant, $\alpha = 1$.

Table 1. Results of the semi-global motion estimation. The residual misalignment (*residual*) between the found and the true motion: the mean (μ), standard deviation (σ) and maximum (*max*) is compared to the original motion with respect to $\bar{f}$ (*original*).

(mm)	original			residual		
	μ	σ	max	μ	σ	Max
Patient 1	3.8	2.1	17.1	1.1	0.6	8.3
Patient 2	2.8	1.7	16.1	1.6	0.8	11.0
Patient 3	3.7	1.6	13.8	1.3	0.7	5.8

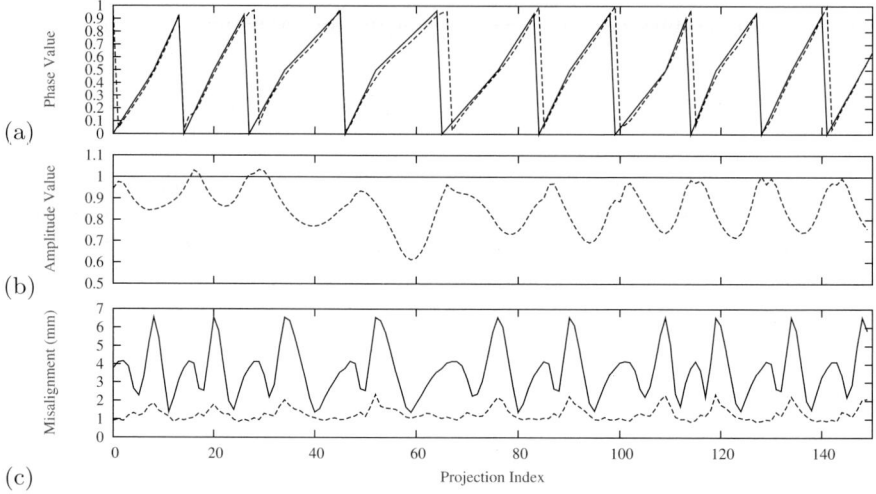

Fig. 4. Results of the semi-global motion estimation for Patient 3: the recovered phase (a) and amplitude (b) (*dashed line*) are shown together with the parameters used to generate the CB sequence (*full line*). The reference amplitude is a constant, $\alpha = 1$. (c) The resulting residual misalignment (*dashed line*) is shown in comparison with the original misalignment with respect to the mean position image (*full line*).

minutes before repositioning and acquisition of the second 4D CT. In spite of the small time between the acquisitions, substantial difference can be observed between the two subsequent 4D CT acquisitions due to interfractional changes in breathing motion (see Figure 2c). We used the first 4D CT sequence to construct a patient model as described in Section 2.1. The second acquisition was first rigidly registered to the first 4D CT to align the bony structures. In order to have a ground truth available, we took the mean position image from the first sequence and the deformation fields from the second sequence to get a simulated reference 4D CT sequence. A respiratory trace was randomly generated [5] and a piece-wise linear phase signal $\vartheta(t)$ with variable breathing rate was derived. We simulated the first 90° of a CB acquisition protocol in our institute by calculating 150 projections for evenly spaced angles from the reference 4D CT with varying phase value over a period of 30 s.

When optimizing separately for each projection the criterion (5) with respect to ϑ and α, we obtained bad results when confronted to interfractional changes in breathing motion (see Figure 3, results for other patients were similar). Note that an optimal result doesn't necessarily mean recovering identical parameter values as they correspond to different deformation fields. In this case however, we can observe how intermediate phases during inhalation ($\vartheta \approx 0.2$) and exhalation ($\vartheta \approx 0.8$) are confused, due to limited hysteresis and unfavorable projection angle and are accompanied with strong variations in amplitude.

The phase and amplitude found for Patient 3 using our semi-global criterion (9) are shown in Figure 4a and 4b, together with the parameters used to generate the CB sequence. To evaluate the accuracy we calculate the residual geometric misalignment (i.e. the norm of the difference between deformation vector fields) between the estimated motion and the true motion. This measure is averaged over the lower lung, where the largest motion tends to occur. For comparison, the original misalignment, i.e. the motion with respect to the mean position image, is also given. Table 1 contains the average over all projections for each patient. Figure 4c shows this mean misalignment as a function of the projection index for Patient 3. Note that while displacement might locally attain 3cm, the average motion as seen from the mean position does not exceed 1cm.

4 Discussion and Conclusion

We achieved a smooth motion estimation from a CB projection sequence using B-splines and by considering the complete movement in a respiratory cycle and obtained a considerable reduction of the original misalignment for all patients.

To our knowledge this is the first time a respiratory motion model is tested against clinical data containing real interfractional changes in breathing motion. Some additional challenges presented by real CB data will include dealing with scatter [12] and detecting and correcting for rigid misalignment (setup errors).

As a consequence of generating the ground truth, baseline shifts were not present in our patient data. Changes in breath rate, breathing level or trajectory shape were however present. It is expected that the method will be able to cope with small shifts ($< 20\%$ of the motion amplitude). For larger shifts, a prior shift estimation can be performed, e.g. from a 4D CBCT [6].

In this work we exploited only acquisitions already acquired for treatment purposes. More preoperative data, such as breath hold CT scans [8,12] or MRI data [9], could further improve the prior model, rendering it's construction more robust to artifacts and providing prior information on the intercycle variation.

Acknowledgments. Jef Vandemeulebroucke was funded by the EC Marie Curie grant WARTHE, Jan Kybic was sponsored by the Czech Ministry of Education, Project MSM6840770012.

References

1. Keall, P.J., Mageras, G.S., Balter, J.M., Emery, R.S., Forster, K.M., Jiang, S.B., Kapatoes, J.M., Low, D.A., Murphy, M.J., Murray, B.R., Ramsey, C.R., Herk, M.B.V., Vedam, S.S., Wong, J.W., Yorke, E.: The management of respiratory motion in radiation oncology report of AAPM task group 76. Med. Phys. 33(10), 3874–3900 (2006)
2. Ford, E.C., Mageras, G.S., Yorke, E., Ling, C.C.: Respiration-correlated spiral CT: a method of measuring respiratory-induced anatomic motion for radiation treatment planning. Med. Phys. 30(1), 88–97 (2003)
3. Sonke, J., Zijp, L., Remeijer, P., van Herk, M.: Respiratory correlated cone beam CT. Med. Phys. 32(4), 1176–1186 (2005)
4. Seppenwoolde, Y., Shirato, H., Kitamura, K., Shimizu, S., van Herk, M., Lebesque, J.V., Miyasaka, K.: Precise and real-time measurement of 3D tumor motion in lung due to breathing and heartbeat, measured during radiotherapy. Int. J. Radiat. Oncol. Biol. Phys. 53(4), 822–834 (2002)
5. George, R., Vedam, S.S., Chung, T.D., Ramakrishnan, V., Keall, P.J.: The application of the sinusoidal model to lung cancer patient respiratory motion. Med. Phys. 32(9), 2850–2861 (2005)
6. Sonke, J.J., Lebesque, J., van Herk, M.: Variability of four-dimensional computed tomography patient models. Int. J. Radiat. Oncol. Biol. Phys. 70(2), 590–598 (2008)
7. Zhang, Q., Pevsner, A., Hertanto, A., Hu, Y.C., Rosenzweig, K.E., Ling, C.C., Mageras, G.S.: A patient-specific respiratory model of anatomical motion for radiation treatment planning. Med. Phys. 34(12), 4772–4781 (2007)
8. McClelland, J.R., Blackall, J.M., Tarte, S., Chandler, A.C., Hughes, S., Ahmad, S., Landau, D.B., Hawkes, D.J.: A continuous 4D motion model from multiple respiratory cycles for use in lung radiotherapy. Med. Phys. 33(9), 3348–3358 (2006)
9. von Siebenthal, M., Székely, G., Gamper, U., Boesiger, P., Lomax, A., Cattin, P.: 4D MR imaging of respiratory organ motion and its variability. Phys. Med. Biol. 52(6), 1547–1564 (2007)
10. Zijp, L., Sonke, J., van Herk, M.: Extraction of the respiratory signal from sequential thorax cone-beam X-ray images. In: 14th International Conference on the Use of Computers in Radiation Therapy, Seoul, Korea (May 2004)
11. Rit, S., Wolthaus, J., van Herk, M., Sonke, J.-J.: On-the-fly motion-compensated cone-beam CT using an a priori motion model. In: Metaxas, D., Axel, L., Fichtinger, G., Székely, G. (eds.) MICCAI 2008, Part I. LNCS, vol. 5241, pp. 729–736. Springer, Heidelberg (2008)
12. Zeng, R., Fessler, J.A., Balter, J.M.: Estimating 3-D respiratory motion from orbiting views by tomographic image registration. IEEE Trans. Med. Imaging 26(2), 153–163 (2007)
13. Thirion, J.P.: Image matching as a diffusion process: an analogy with Maxwell's Demons. Med. Image Anal. 2(3), 243–260 (1998)
14. Wolberg, G.: Digital image warping. IEEE Computer Society Press, Los Alamitos (1990)
15. Wolthaus, J.W.H., Sonke, J.J., van Herk, M., Damen, E.M.F.: Reconstruction of a time-averaged midposition CT scan for radiotherapy planning of lung cancer patients using deformable registration. Med. Phys. 35(9), 3998–4011 (2008)
16. Unser, M.: Splines: A perfect fit for signal and image processing. IEEE Signal Processing Magazine 16(6), 22–38 (1999)
17. Press, W.H., Flannery, B.P., Teukolsky, S.A., Vetterling, W.T.: Numerical Recipes in C, 2nd edn. Cambridge University Press, Cambridge (1992)

Heart Motion Abnormality Detection via an Information Measure and Bayesian Filtering

Kumaradevan Punithakumar[1], Shuo Li[1], Ismail Ben Ayed[1], Ian Ross[2], Ali Islam[3], and Jaron Chong[4]

[1] GE Healthcare, London, ON, Canada
[2] London Health Science Center, London, ON, Canada
[3] St. Joseph's Health Care, London, ON, Canada
[4] University of Western Ontario, London, ON, Canada

Abstract. This study investigates heart wall motion abnormality detection with an information theoretic measure of heart motion based on the Shannon's differential entropy (SDE) and recursive Bayesian filtering. Heart wall motion is generally analyzed using functional images which are subject to noise and segmentation inaccuracies, and incorporation of prior knowledge is crucial in improving the accuracy. The Kalman filter, a well known recursive Bayesian filter, is used in this study to estimate the left ventricular (LV) cavity points given incomplete and noisy data, and given a dynamic model. However, due to similarities between the statistical information of normal and abnormal heart motions, detecting and classifying abnormality is a challenging problem which we proposed to investigate with a global measure based on the SDE. We further derive two other possible information theoretic abnormality detection criteria, one is based on Rényi entropy and the other on Fisher information. The proposed method analyzes wall motion quantitatively by constructing distributions of the normalized radial distance estimates of the LV cavity. Using 269×20 segmented LV cavities of short-axis magnetic resonance images obtained from 30 subjects, the experimental analysis demonstrates that the proposed SDE criterion can lead to significant improvement over other features that are prevalent in the literature related to the LV cavity, namely, mean radial displacement and mean radial velocity.

1 Introduction

Early detection of motion abnormality is the utmost importance in the diagnosis of coronary heart disease – the most common type of cardiovascular disease. Unfortunately, early detection by visual inspection is limited due to vast amount of information and uncertainty associated with heart motion. Computer-aided detection systems, which can analyze extensive amount of information associated with the heart motion, have attracted research attention in recent years [1,2,3]. Computer-aided abnormality detection primarily consists of two components: preprocessing and classification.

The preprocessing, centered around image segmentation, is in itself challenging due to the difficulties inherent to cardiac images [4]. Additionally, the classification is also difficult because of similarities between the statistical information associated with normal and abnormal heart motion. Fig. 1 depicts typical examples of normal and abnormal heart motion, along with the corresponding distributions of motion measurements over time. The significant overlap between these distributions makes the classification problem difficult, and the use of distribution moments, for instance the mean [2], may not be sufficient to separate normal and abnormal motions. To tackle the classification problem, we propose an information theoretic measure of heart motion. In order to take full advantage of the information related to cardiac motion, we propose to use the Shannon's differential entropy (SDE) [5], which provides a *global*, theoretically grounded measure of distributions – rather than relying on elementary measurements or a fixed set of moments, the SDE measures a global distribution information and, as such, has more discriminative power in classifying distributions. The typical examples in Fig. 1 illustrate the potential of the SDE in the classification problem: the means of abnormal and normal motion distributions are very close, whereas, the SDEs are relatively different.

We further derive two other possible information theoretic abnormality detection criteria, one is based on Rényi entropy and the other on Fisher information [5]. Although widely used in physics [6], computer vision [7,8], communications [9], and many other fields, the application of information theoretic concepts is still in its early stage in medical image analysis. Few notable exceptions include

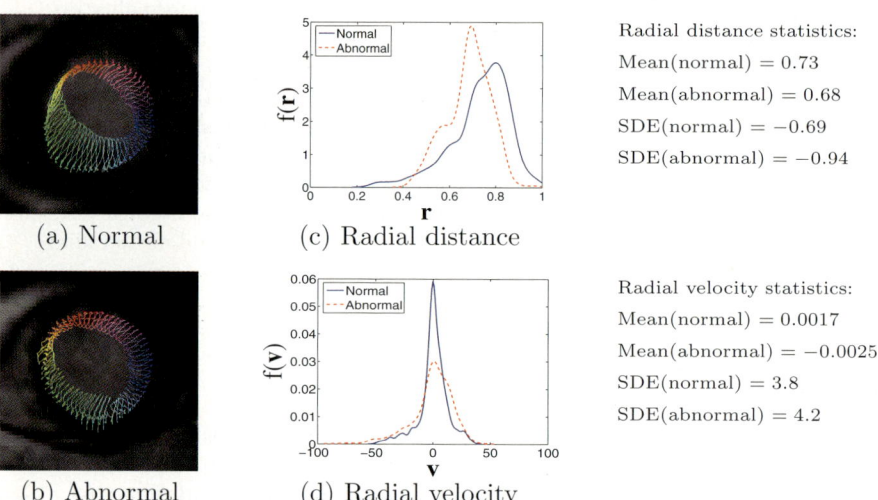

Fig. 1. The potential of the SDE measure in detecting abnormal motion. (a) typical normal motion, (b) typical abnormal heart, (c) and (d) corresponding distributions of radial distances and radial velocities. A significant overlap exists between normal and abnormal motion distributions, and the corresponding first moments are approximately the same, whereas the SDEs are relatively different.

using cross and joint entropy for image registration [10,11], the Rényi entropy for measuring the heart rate Gaussianity [12], and the Shannon entropy for analyzing heart period variability [13].

To tackle image preprocessing, an overlap prior based left ventricle (LV) segmentation [4], which does not require a training, is used, and the segmentation results are subsequently processed with recursive Bayesian filtering. The latter, which provides a temporal smoothing of the dataset given a suitable model, is shown to be very effective when the data is less reliable. Specifically, a cyclic model is used to characterize the dynamics of sample points of the segmented LV cavity and the Kalman filter [14] is used for state estimation. The filter estimates are subsequently analyzed to build an information theoretic classifier of heart motion.

Using 269 image sequences, each consisting of 20 segmented LV cavities of short-axis magnetic resonance functional images, obtained from 30 subjects, the experimental analysis demonstrates that the proposed information theoretic measure of heart motion can lead to significant improvement over other features that are prevalent in the literature related to the LV cavity, namely, the mean radial displacement and mean radial velocity [2]. Furthermore, an analysis based on Bhattacharyya distance (cf. plots in Fig. 3), which measures the separability of classes in classification problems, show that the SDE yields better classification ability amidst the stochastic nature of the cardiac motion and image segmentation inaccuracies.

2 The Recursive Bayesian Filtering

The analysis is performed by sampling a set of points along the segmented LV cavity. We assume a cyclic state-space model for the dynamics of sample points that characterize the temporal evolution of the points for a periodic heart motion. Let $\mathbf{x}_k^i = [\bar{x}_k^i \ x_k^i \ \dot{x}_k^i \ \bar{y}_k^i \ y_k^i \ \dot{y}_k^i]^T$ be the state vector, consisting of mean position $(\bar{x}_k^i, \bar{y}_k^i)$, current position (x_k^i, y_k^i) and velocity $(\dot{x}_k^i, \dot{y}_k^i)$ of sample point i, respectively, in x and y coordinate directions at time step k (for $k = 1, \ldots, K$). The state transition equation for cyclic motion is given by

$$\mathbf{x}_k^i = F_{k-1}\mathbf{x}_{k-1}^i + v_{k-1}^i \qquad \text{for } i = 1, \ldots, N \qquad (1)$$

where $F_k = \begin{bmatrix} A_k & \mathbf{0}_{3\times 3} \\ \mathbf{0}_{3\times 3} & A_k \end{bmatrix}$, $A_k = \begin{bmatrix} 1 & 0 & 0 \\ 1 - \cos(\omega T) & \cos(\omega T) & \frac{1}{\omega}\sin(\omega T) \\ \omega \sin(\omega T) & -\omega \sin(\omega T) & \cos(\omega T) \end{bmatrix}$, $\{v_{k-1}^i\}$

is a zero-mean Gaussian noise sequence with covariance Q_k, ω the reciprocal of period of heart cycle, and T the interval between two subsequent image frames. The additive noise in the dynamic model is an approximation, and is included to accommodate significant differences between the modeling and real motion of the LV cavity points.

The measurement equation is given by

$$\mathbf{z}_k^i = H_k \mathbf{x}_k^i + w_k^i \qquad \text{for } i = 1, \ldots, N \qquad (2)$$

where $H_k = \begin{bmatrix} B_k & \mathbf{0}_{1\times 3} \\ \mathbf{0}_{1\times 3} & B_k \end{bmatrix}$, $B_k = \begin{bmatrix} 0 & 1 & 0 \end{bmatrix}$ and $\{w_k^i\}$ is a zero-mean Gaussian noise sequence with covariance R_k. The measurements are obtained by sampling the segmented LV cavities. The measurement equation indicates the fact that only the current position of a sample point is measured.

The Kalman filter, which yields an optimal estimate for linear/Gaussian systems, is applied for state estimation. In some very rare cases, the segmentation results of the LV deviate significantly, and such inconsistencies are detected by gating the center of the segmented LV. The segmentation results are ignored in such cases, and the sample points were only predicted using the dynamic model, i.e., they were not updated by filter.

In order to find the sequence of corresponding points over time, the *symmetric nearest neighbor correspondences* [15] is applied by sampling a set of equally-spaced points along the LV boundary. The construction of a sequence of points is essential to analyze wall motion regionally. Using spline interpolation, N_s points were sampled along the LV cavity in each frame, and N points were chosen as measurements to the filter. A kernel density estimation based on normal kernel function is applied to obtain the probability density. The radial distance for each dataset is normalized with respect to maximum value, which allows analyzing different long-axis segments, namely, apical, mid and basal, without additional processing.

3 The SDE of Normalized Radial Distance

We define the following normalized radial distance r_k^i by

$$r_k^i = \frac{\sqrt{(\hat{x}_k^i - \frac{1}{N}\sum_i \hat{x}_k^i)^2 + (\hat{y}_k^i - \frac{1}{N}\sum_i \hat{y}_k^i)^2}}{\max_i \sqrt{(\hat{x}_k^i - \frac{1}{N}\sum_i \hat{x}_k^i)^2 + (\hat{y}_k^i - \frac{1}{N}\sum_i \hat{y}_k^i)^2}}, \quad (3)$$

where $\hat{x}_k^i$ and $\hat{y}_k^i$ are the estimates of x_k^i and y_k^i, respectively. Let $\mathbf{r} \in \mathbb{R}$ be a random variable. The kernel density estimate of the normalized radial distance is given by

$$f(\mathbf{r}) = \frac{\sum_{i,k} \mathcal{K}(r_k^i - \mathbf{r})}{NK}, \quad (4)$$

where $\mathcal{K}(y) = \frac{1}{\sqrt{2\pi\sigma^2}} \exp(-\frac{y^2}{2\sigma^2})$ is the Gaussian kernel. In this study, we derive the SDE measure of heart motion as follows

$$S_f = -\int_{\mathbf{r}\in\mathbb{R}} \frac{\sum_{i,k} \mathcal{K}(r_k^i - \mathbf{r})}{NK} \left(\ln \sum_{i,k} \mathcal{K}(r_k^i - \mathbf{r}) - \ln NK \right) d\mathbf{r} \quad (5)$$

We further derive two other information theoretic criteria to measure the *global* information associated with heart motion, one is based on the Rényi entropy

$$R_f^\alpha = \frac{1}{1-\alpha} \ln \int_{\mathbf{r}\in\mathbb{R}} \left(\frac{\sum_{i,k} \mathcal{K}(r_k^i - \mathbf{r})}{NK} \right)^\alpha d\mathbf{r} \quad \text{for } 0 < \alpha < \infty, \, \alpha \neq 1 \quad (6)$$

and the other on Fisher information

$$I_f = 4 \int_{\mathbf{r} \in \mathbb{R}} |\nabla g(\mathbf{r})|^2 d\mathbf{r}, \qquad (7)$$

where

$$g(\mathbf{r}) = \sqrt{\frac{\sum_{i,k} \mathcal{K}(r_k^i - \mathbf{r})}{NK}}. \qquad (8)$$

4 Experiments

The data contain 269 short-axis image sequences, each consisting of 20 functional 2D-images acquired from 20 normal and 10 abnormal hearts. The data were acquired on 1.5T MRI scanners with fast imaging employing steady state acquisition (FIESTA) image sequence mode. The Kalman filter positions and velocities were initialized using *two-point initialization* [14], and mean positions were initialized using all the measurements in the sequence.

The experiments compare the proposed information theoretic measure based on the SDE with other classifier elements, namely, the mean radial displacement and mean systolic radial velocity, as well as other information measures, namely, Rényi entropy ($\alpha = 2$) and Fisher information. Radial velocity computations are based on the systolic phase of cardiac cycle. The results were compared with ground truth classification of the cine MRI sequences by experienced medical professionals. A heart is considered to be abnormal in an image sequence if any of its segments [16] is abnormal.

We used two criteria to measure the performance of each classifier element, namely, classification accuracy via *leave-one-subject-out* method[1] and the receiver operating characteristic (ROC) curves with corresponding area under the curves (AUCs). Furthermore, we used the Bhattacharyya measure to assess the discriminative power of each classifier elements. Table 1 summarizes the results.

The ROC and AUC. The ROC curves for classifier elements is shown in Fig. 2. The more inclined the curve towards the upper left corner, the better the classifier's ability to discriminate between abnormal and normal hearts. The figure shows that the proposed SDE has superior classifying ability than other classifier elements. The AUCs that correspond to the ROC curves in Fig. 2 are reported in Table 1. The AUC represents the average of the classifier sensitivity over false-positive resulting from considering different threshold values, and gives an overall summary of the classification accuracy. The SDE yielded the highest AUC and, therefore, has the best performance.

The Bhattacharyya measure. We used the Bhattacharyya distance metric to evaluate the overlap between the distributions of classifier elements over normal and abnormal motions. The Bhattacharyya metric [17] is given by

$$\mathcal{B} = \sqrt{1 - \sum_{y \in \mathbb{R}} \sqrt{f_N(y) f_A(y)}} \qquad (9)$$

---

[1] Each subject is classified given the information learned from other subjects.

where f_N and f_A are the distributions over, respectively, normal and abnormal hearts. The higher $\mathcal{B}$, the lesser the overlap (Refer to Fig. 3 for an illustration) and, therefore, the better the discriminative ability of the classifier. The SDE yielded the highest $\mathcal{B}$ as reported in Table 1 and, therefore, the best discriminative ability. This is consistent with the previous findings based on ROC/AUC evaluations.

Classification accuracy. Evaluating the percentage of correctly classified hearts using *leaving-one-subject-out* method, the proposed SDE yielded 90.5% true positive (TP) and 78.6% true negative (TN), i.e., 90.5% of abnormal hearts and 78.6% of normal hearts were classified correctly, which is the best overall performance among the reported classifier elements in Table 1.

Table 1. The area under the curve corresponding to Fig. 2, Bhattacharyya distance metric of normal/abnormal distributions given in Fig. 3, and the percentage of classification accuracy using leaving-one-subject-out method for classifier elements

Classifier element	AUC (%)	Bhattacharyya distance metric ($\mathcal{B}$)	Classification accuracy Abnormal (%)	Normal (%)
Mean systolic velocity	70.8	0.32	79.4	54.9
Mean radial displacement	87.3	0.53	76.2	70.9
Fisher information	89.3	0.59	84.1	85.0
Rényi entropy	90.8	0.60	87.3	84.5
Shannon's differential entropy	90.9	0.62	90.5	78.6

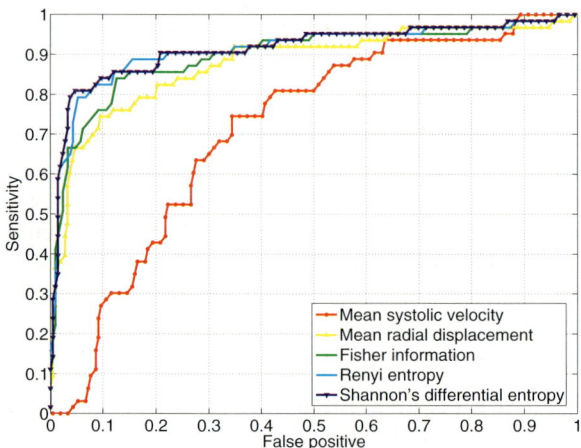

Fig. 2. Receiver operating characteristics of classifier elements. The closer the curve to the left hand top corner, the better the classification performance. *The proposed information theoretic measure based on the SDE outperforms other classifier elements.*

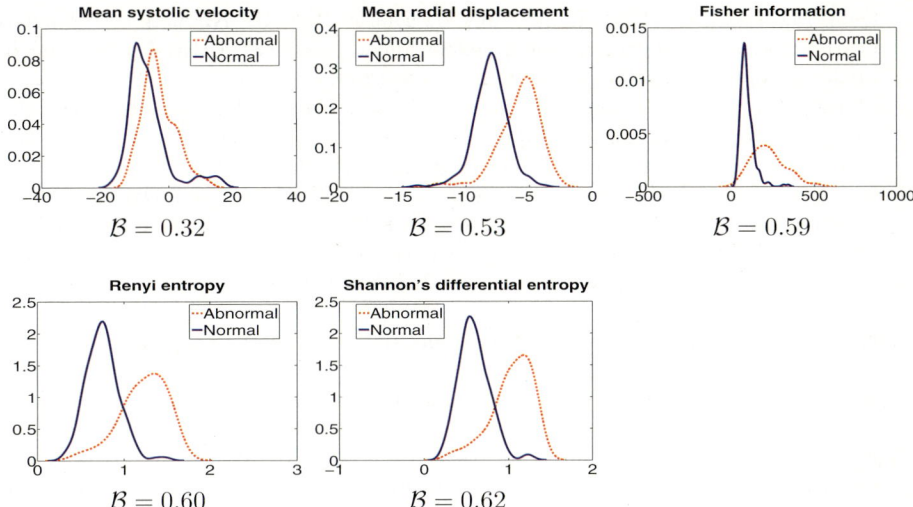

Fig. 3. Distribution of normal and abnormal hearts categorized using classifier elements. The Bhattacharyya distance metric show that information theoretic measure based on the SDE has better discriminative ability over other classifier elements.

5 Conclusions

This study investigates heart wall motion abnormality detection, which primarily consists of two components: preprocessing and classification. In preprocessing, an overlap prior based segmentation is used to generate left ventricular (LV) contours and the results are subsequently processed using Kalman filter, given a cyclic dynamic model. More importantly, we propose an information theoretic measure based on the Shannon's differential entropy (SDE) for classification. The proposed method analyzes wall motion quantitatively by constructing distributions of the radial distance estimates of the LV cavity. We further derive two other possible information theoretic abnormality detection criteria, one is based on Rényi entropy and the other on Fisher information. The experimental analysis is performed using 269×20 short-axis magnetic resonance images obtained from 30 subjects. The results, based on receiver operating characteristics, area under the curves, Bhattacharyya distance metrics and *leave-one-subject-out* cross validation, show that the proposed SDE criterion can lead to significant improvement over other prevalent classifier elements.

References

1. Qian, Z., Liu, Q., Metaxas, D.N., Axel, L.: Identifying Regional Cardiac Abnormalities from Myocardial Strains Using Spatio-temporal Tensor Analysis. In: Metaxas, D., Axel, L., Fichtinger, G., Székely, G. (eds.) MICCAI 2008, Part I. LNCS, vol. 5241, pp. 789–797. Springer, Heidelberg (2008)

2. Qazi, M., Fung, G., Krishnan, S., Bi, J., Bharat Rao, R., Katz, A.: Automated heart abnormality detection using sparse linear classifiers. IEEE Engineering in Medicine and Biology Magazine 26(2), 56–63 (2007)
3. Mansor, S., Noble, J.: Local wall motion classification of stress echocardiography using a Hidden Markov Model approach. In: 5th IEEE International Symposium on Biomedical Imaging: From Nano to Macro., pp. 1295–1298 (2008)
4. Ben Ayed, I., Lu, Y., Li, S., Ross, I.: Left Ventricle Tracking Using Overlap Priors. In: Metaxas, D., Axel, L., Fichtinger, G., Székely, G. (eds.) MICCAI 2008, Part I. LNCS, vol. 5241, pp. 1025–1033. Springer, Heidelberg (2008)
5. Cover, T.M., Thomas, J.A.: Elements of Information Theory. Wiley-Interscience, New York (1991)
6. Frieden, B.R.: Physics from Fisher Information: a Unification. Cambridge University Press, Cambridge (1998)
7. Ben Ayed, I., Li, S., Ross, I.: Tracking distributions with an overlap prior. In: IEEE Conference on Computer Vision and Pattern Recognition, pp. 1–7 (2008)
8. Kim, J., Fisher III, J.W., Cetin, A., Yezzi, A., Cetin, M., Willsky, A.: A nonparametric statistical method for image segmentation using information theory and curve evolution. IEEE Transactions on Image Processing 14(10), 1486–1502 (2005)
9. Biglieri, E., Proakis, J., Shamai, S.: Fading channels: information-theoretic and communications aspects. IEEE Transactions on Information Theory 44(6), 2619–2692 (1998)
10. Studholme, C., Hill, D.L.G., Hawkes, D.J.: An overlap invariant entropy measure of 3D medical image alignment. Pattern Recognition 32(1), 71–86 (1999)
11. Zhu, Y.M.: Volume image registration by cross-entropy optimization. IEEE Transactions of Medical Imaging 21, 174–180 (2002)
12. Lake, D.E.: Renyi entropy measures of heart rate Gaussianity. IEEE Transactions on Biomedical Engineering 53(1), 21–27 (2006)
13. Porta, A., Guzzetti, S., Montano, N., Furlan, R., Pagani, M., Malliani, A., Cerutti, S.: Entropy, entropy rate, and pattern classification as tools to typify complexity in short heart period variability series. IEEE Transactions on Biomedical Engineering 48(11), 1282–1291 (2001)
14. Bar-Shalom, Y., Li, X.R., Kirubarajan, T.: Estimation with Applications to Tracking and Navigation. Wiley-Interscience, New York (2001)
15. Papademetris, X., Sinusas, A., Dione, D., Constable, R., Duncan, J.: Estimation of 3-D left ventricular deformation from medical images using biomechanical models. IEEE Transactions on Medical Imaging 21(7), 786–800 (2002)
16. Cerqueira, M.D., Weissman, N.J., Dilsizian, V., Jacobs, A.K., Kaul, S., Laskey, W.K., Pennell, D.J., Rumberger, J.A., Ryan, T., Verani, M.S.: Standardized Myocardial Segmentation and Nomenclature for Tomographic Imaging of the Heart: A Statement for Healthcare Professionals From the Cardiac Imaging Committee of the Council on Clinical Cardiology of the American Heart Association Circulation. 105, 539–542 (2002)
17. Comaniciu, D., Ramesh, V., Meer, P.: Kernel-based object tracking. IEEE Transactions on Pattern Analysis and Machine Intelligence 25(5), 564–577 (2003)

Automatic Image-Based Cardiac and Respiratory Cycle Synchronization and Gating of Image Sequences

Hari Sundar, Ali Khamene, Liron Yatziv, and Chenyang Xu

Siemens Corporate Research, Princeton NJ, USA

Abstract. We propose a novel method to detect the current state of the quasi-periodic system from image sequences which in turn will enable us to synchronize/gate the image sequences to obtain images of the organ system at similar configurations. The method uses the cumulated phase shift in the spectral domain of successive image frames as a measure of the net motion of objects in the scene. The proposed method is applicable to 2D and 3D time varying sequences and is not specific to the imaging modality. We demonstrate its effectiveness on X-Ray Angiographic and Cardiac and Liver Ultrasound sequences. Knowledge of the current (cardiac or respiratory) phase of the system, opens up the possibility for a purely image based cardiac and respiratory gating scheme for interventional and radiotherapy procedures.

1 Introduction

Image synchronization and gating are problems faced during the imaging and subsequent processing of organs with quasi-periodic motion, like the heart. The two most common sources of organ motion during imaging are respiratory and cardiac motion. The deformations caused by cardiac and respiratory motion make it difficult to image organs in the thorax and the abdomen. This severely limits the efficacy and efficiency of interventional and radiotherapy procedures performed in this region.

Different approaches have been devised to overcome cardiac and respiratory motion. Cardiac motion is usually handled by ECG gating whereas respiratory motion is usually handled by the use of markers placed on the patients body [1]. The problem with these approaches is that the ECG requires additional hardware, long setup times and in most cases there is a delay between the ECG signal and the image acquisition which makes it hard to make them synchronized. As far as the detection of respiratory phase is concerned, the placement of markers is usually impractical in a clinical setting; furthermore it is difficult to set up and prolongs the overall acquisition procedure. In addition most laboratories and existing image databases do not contain either ECG or respiratory information. Additionally, since the end goal is to perform image gating, detecting the phase using the images should be more reliable and robust compared to cases where an external signal is used.

Another strategy for reducing respiratory motion is to acquire images using breath-hold techniques [2]. Although this reduces breathing motion by relatively simple and natural means, it is, nonetheless, restricted by the patient's ability to perform a supervised breath hold during the treatment [3]. A third class of strategies addresses the problem of respiratory motion correction by incorporating suitable motion models. Manke et al. [4] proposed a linear parametric model describing the relation between the variation of the diaphragmatic position and the respiratory-induced motion derived from image-intensity based registration for cardiac-triggered 3D MR imaging. King et al. [5] present an affine model which is based on the tracked motion of the diaphragm to compensate for respiratory motion in real-time X-ray images. The main drawback of these approaches is that they require manual landmark selection for diaphragm tracking.

Related Work. Prior work in this area is fairly limited, with [6] presenting an approach for retrospective gating of Intra coronary ultrasound (ICUS) sequences using feature extraction and classification. The method is computationally expensive and requires processing the whole sequence together as some of the features are temporal. In [7], the authors propose a method to analyze images in the sequence and retrieve the cardiac phase by using average image intensity and absolute image difference between the consecutive frames. The method is not very robust and has not been shown to work with real datasets. In [8], the authors propose to detect the respiration (phase) using mutual information. The mutual information (MI) is calculated between the fluoroscopic image and a reference angiogram. The MI calculation is performed only on selected regions of interest (ROI) and the results are variable depending on the choice of ROIs. A similar approach using Normalized MI is presented in [9]. A review of the effects of respiratory motion is presented in [10] and highlights the importance and need for reliable detection of the respiratory phase, specifically for the target organ. In [11], Berbeco et al. detect the breathing phase information by analyzing the fluoroscopic intensity fluctuations in the lung. However, the approach requires the selection of region of interest(ROI) in a section of the middle of the lung that does not contain the tumor.

Contributions. We propose a novel method to detect the current state of the quasi-periodic system which in turn will enable us to synchronize/gate image sequences to obtain images of the organ system at similar configurations. The proposed method is applicable to 2D and 3D time varying sequences and all imaging modalities. We demonstrate its effectiveness on 2D X-Ray Angiographic and 3D Liver and intra-cardiac Ultrasound sequences.

2 Methods

Let $I_t(x, y)$ represent the image at time t of a scene changing with time. According to the phase correlation technique [12], if we represent the Fourier transform of $I_t(x, y)$ by $\mathcal{F}(\xi, \eta)$, and assume that objects in the scene exhibit only translations, then for $I_{t+1}(x, y) = I_t(x - x_t, y - y_t)$, we have

$$\mathcal{F}_{t+1}(\xi, \eta) = e^{-j2\pi(\xi x_t + \eta y_t)} \mathcal{F}_t(\xi, \eta). \tag{1}$$

By inverse transforming the ratio of the cross-power spectrum of I_{t+1} and I_t to its magnitude,

$$\frac{\mathcal{F}_{t+1}\mathcal{F}_t^*}{\|\mathcal{F}_{t+1}\mathcal{F}_t^*\|} = \exp(-j2\pi(\xi x_t + \eta y_t)),$$

we obtain a peak at (x_t, y_t). If we consider a simple 1D example as shown in Figure 1, we have the original image represented by the blue sinusoidal curve, and applying a translation to the image produces a phase shift in the spectrum.

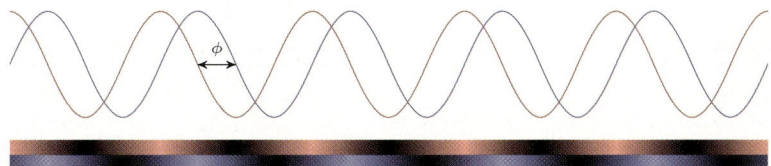

Fig. 1. The Relationship between object motion and the phase shift (ϕ)

This approach was used in [13] to compensate for translational motion in coronary angiogram sequences.

It is important to realize that image features can be thought of as being a combination of signals at different frequencies, and that calculating the phase shift of the different frequencies in an image amounts to measuring the motion of image features corresponding to those frequencies. Measuring the phase shift in the frequency domain allows us to estimate the overall motion within an image without explicitly solving the problem of correspondence detection. The phase shift can be calculated in the Fourier domain [14]. The overall change in the energy within the object being imaged can be estimated by integrating over the phase shift, which is the same as the energy change only due to the motion in the spatial domain because of Parsevals Theorem [14]. It is important to note that this energy is not affected by changes in intensity which might happen as a result of varying levels of contrast agent and differing acquisition parameters. In addition, the proposed method is relatively insensitive to noise, as long as the spectrum of the noise is similar in successive images. As in this usually the case with image sequences acquired on the same scanner during the same acquisition session, the phase detection is robust to the noise levels during acquisition.

We estimate the energy change of the system being imaged by analyzing consecutive frames. The energy change in the system is computed in the spectral domain making the system more robust to outliers that might be introduced in the scene. Common examples are catheters, contrast agents, needles etc. The energy change in the scene is given by,

$$E = \int \frac{\mathcal{F}(I_t)^* \cdot \mathcal{F}(I_{t+1})}{|\mathcal{F}(I_t)^*| |\mathcal{F}(I_{t+1})|} df, \qquad (2)$$

where, $\mathcal{F}(I_t)$ represents the Fourier transform of the image I at time t.

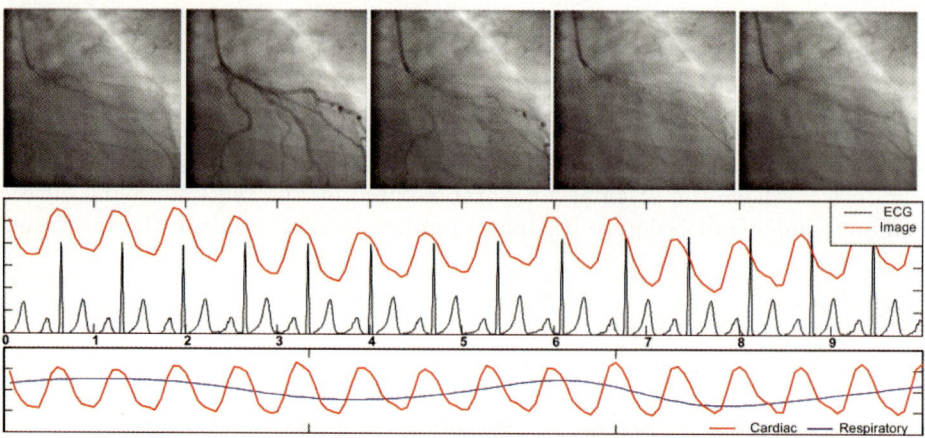

Fig. 2. Results of Phase detection in X-Ray sequences. The estimated phase is overlaid with the actual ECG signal. The low frequency variation in the phase corresponds to the respiratory cycle. The cardiac and respiratory cycles are also shown in this figure are separated using high and low pass filters respectively.

This energy is used as an estimate of the current phase of the organ. The extrema of this signal can be easily detected to detect the cardiac and the respiratory phases. Additionally, if separate cardiac and respiratory signals are required, then a band pass filter centered at 1Hz should recover the cardiac signal, whereas a low pass filter will recover the respiratory signal. The system can be used with N-dimensional by computing the appropriate higher order Fourier transform.

3 Results

In order to test the efficacy and accuracy of the proposed method, we tested it on X-Ray and ultrasound(US) images and compared it against ground truth data. ECG signals were treated as ground truth for the detection of the cardiac cycle, and breathing phase obtained using a magnetic tracking system was treated as ground truth for respiratory motion.

Validation on Cardiac X-Ray Angiography images. We validate our method by comparing it against ECG signals embedded within 20 X-Ray angiographic and fluoroscopic images acquired on a biplane C-arm system (AXIOM Artis, Siemens Medical Solutions, Erlangen, Germany). The minima of the image-based phase correspond to end-diastole and therefore, we compared the alignment of this minima with the P-wave on the ECG signal. Additionally, for the cases where a mismatch existed, a visual comparison of images gated using the 2 methods yielded no obvious winner. An example of the detected phase overlaid on the ECG signal and with sample images is shown in Figure 2. Figure 2 also illustrates the separation of cardiac and respiratory signals from the combined phase signal.

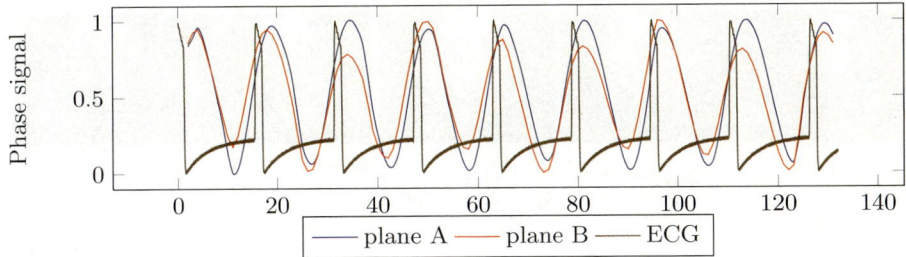

Fig. 3. Simple validation using biplane sequences. Normalize phase signals from a biplane Xray sequence are plotted along with the normalized ECG signal. It can clearly be seen that the phase is correctly calculated from both views independently.

We also compared the image-based phase signals from biplane X-Ray images. Since the two images are basically projections of the same heart, the phase signals should match, in spite of differences due to the projection angles. In Figure 3 we illustrate one such case in which the phase signals from both planes are plotted with the ECG QRS trigger signal. As can be seen, although there are small variations in the signals from the two planes, they are in overall agreement regarding the cardiac phase.

Validation on Liver 3D Freehand Ultrasound Images. In order to test the efficacy of the system on detecting respiratory motion, we used a Siemens ACUSON Sequoia 512 ultrasound machine (Siemens Ultrasound, Mountain View, CA) with abdominal curved-array probe, and a MicroBird magnetic tracking system (Ascencion Technology Corp., Burlington VT). "Tracked ultrasound" recordings were made in free breathing, with the transducer moving arbitrarily to image any longitudinal and transversal planes of the liver. A second MicroBird magnetic position sensor was attached to the chest and was tracked. The dominant translation of the tracked sensor was treated as a measure of the breathing phase [15]. This was tested on four volunteers and in all cases the image based phase was in agreement with the tracked sensor. An example of this is shown in Figure 4.

Table 1. Correlation ratio of the detected phase against ground truth for angiography and liver ultrasound datasets

Modality	Compared with	Correlation
2D Angiography	ECG	0.92
3D Liver US	Respiratory tracker	0.88

Validation on Intracardiac Echocardiography images. In order to test the image-based phase detection method on highly dynamic images, we applied it on Intracardiac Echocardiography (ICE) images acquired using a Siemens ACUSON AcuNav[TM] catheter[16]. The images were acquired within the left atrium. Being inside the heart the image acquired by the ICE catheter changes rapidly and

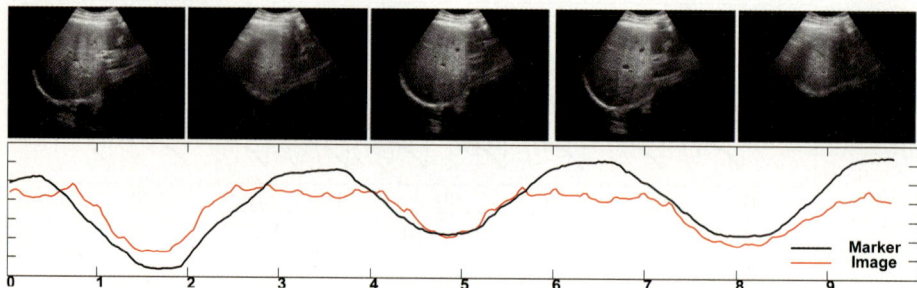

Fig. 4. Results of Phase detection in Liver ultrasound sequences. The estimated phase is overlaid with the dominant translation of a magnetic marker placed on the chest.

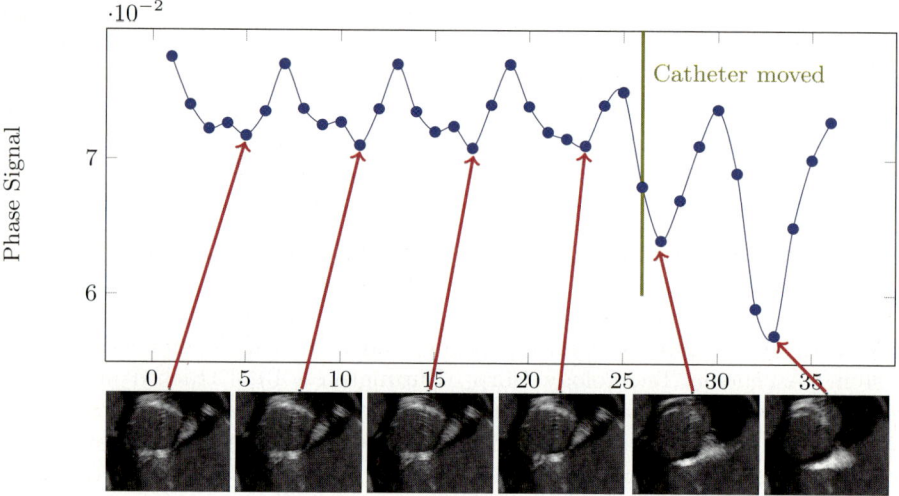

Fig. 5. Results of Phase detection in intra cardiac ultrasound sequences. The end-diastolic image are detected using the image-based phase detection algorithm. The figure also highlights the effect of a quick catheter move on the image-based phase signal.

is especially pronounced when the catheter is moved. The phase detection does however manage to detect the phase correctly, although in some cases there phase is lost when the catheter is moved rapidly. An example of the phase detection on ICE images is shown in Figure 5. The figure also illustrates the effect of a rapid catheter move.

4   Implementation and Performance Considerations

The major use of the proposed algorithm will be in real time interventional applications requiring a motion phase signal. Additionally, one of the main problems in using external triggers like ECG signals or displacement transducers is that the delay between the systems can be substantial and will limit the acquisition frequency. For any image based phase detection method to be practical, performance is as important as the accuracy with which the phase can be detected. The proposed algorithm is very fast, and we tested its performance using optimized code written using the Intel Integrated Performance Primitives for computing the Fourier transforms. We also tested using an implementation using nVidias CUDA library. The performance was evaluated on a Intel Core 2 Duo 2.2GHz notebook with a nVidia Quadro FX 5500 graphics card. We tested using a 1024×1024 angiographic sequence having 132 frames. The optimized software implementation took on an average 2.3 secs, implying a 60 fps capability with 1024×1024 images. The GPU implementation worked slightly faster on the same dataset, taking on an average 1.84 secs to process all 132 frames. Additionally, since the complexity of the proposed algorithm is dependent on Fourier transform of the input images, one easy way to speed up the algorithm further is to define regions of interest.

5 Conclusion

In this paper, we presented a novel algorithm for the automatic detection of the phase of a moving organ system directly from images. The algorithm is able to detect cardiac and respiratory phases from images of different imaging modality. We validated the algorithm on XRay angiographic, liver US and intra cardiac echocardiography images. ECG signals were used to validate the detection of the cardiac phase, and magnetic markers attached to the chest were used to validate the detection of the respiratory phase. The algorithm is very fast and can process images of size 1024×1024 at rates in excess of 60 fps.

The algorithm should be particularly useful in cardiac and abdominal interventional procedures where cardiac and respiratory motion make localization difficult and challenging. Current attempts at image fusion for such procedures are limited for these reasons. The availability of a reliable image-based phase detection algorithm should make it possible to compensate for intra-operative cardiac and/or respiratory motion. It is possible to use the signal for not only gating but also for real-time dynamic compensation. Real-time dynamic compensation is not currently available mainly because of the high computational complexity of most motion compensation algorithms. Since a pre-operative compensation for different phases of cardiac/respiratory motion can be performed, and the results simply recalled based on the current phase of the system, the image-based phase detection should be most useful for dynamic roadmapping applications for cardiac interventions.

References

1. Khamene, A., Warzelhan, J., Vogt, S., Elgort, D., Chefd Hotel, C., Duerk, J., Lewin, J., Wacker, F., Sauer, F.: Characterization of internal organ motion using skin marker positions. LNCS, pp. 526–533. Springer, Heidelberg (2004)
2. Paling, M.R., Brookeman, J.R.: Respiration artifacts in MR imaging: reduction by breath holding. J. Comput. Assist. Tomogr. 10(6), 1080–1082 (1986)

3. Mageras, G.S., Yorke, E.: Deep inspiration breath hold and respiratory gating strategies for reducing organ motion in radiation treatment. Semin. Radiat. Oncol. 14(1), 65–75 (2004)
4. Manke, D., Rosch, P., Nehrke, K., Bornert, P., Dossel, O.: Model evaluation and calibration for prospective respiratory motion correction in coronary MR angiography based on 3-d image registration. IEEE Trans. on Medical Imaging 21(9), 1132–1141 (2002)
5. King, A.P., Boubertakh, R., Rhode, K.S., Ma, Y.L., Chinchapatnam, P., Gao, G., Tangcharoen, T., Ginks, M., Cooklin, M., Gill, J.S., Hawkes, D.J., Razavi, R.S., Schaeffter, T.: A subject-specific technique for respiratory motion correction in image-guided cardiac catheterisation procedures. Med. Image. Anal. 13(3), 419–431 (2009)
6. de Winter, S., Hamers, R., Degertekin, M., Tanabe, K., Lemos, P., Serruys, P., Roelandt, J., Bruining, N.: A novel retrospective gating method for intracoronary ultrasound images based on image properties. Computers in Cardiology, 13–16 (September 2003)
7. Zhu, H., Oakeson, K., Friedman, M.: Retrieval of cardiac phase from IVUS sequences. In: Proceedings of SPIE, vol. 5035, pp. 135–146 (2003)
8. Martin-Leung, B., Eck, K., Stuke, I., Bredno, J., Aach, T.: Mutual information based respiration detection. In: International Congress Series, vol. 1256, pp. 1085–1092. Elsevier, Amsterdam (2003)
9. Moser, T., Biederer, J., Nill, S., Remmert, G., Bendl, R.: Detection of respiratory motion in fluoroscopic images for adaptive radiotherapy. Physics in Medicine and Biology 53(12), 3129–3145 (2008)
10. Webb, S.: Motion effects in (intensity modulated) radiation therapy: a review. Physics in Medicine and Biology 51(13), 403 (2006)
11. Berbeco, R., Mostafavi, H., Sharp, G., Jiang, S.: Towards fluoroscopic respiratory gating for lung tumours without radiopaque markers. Physics in Medicine and Biology 50(19), 4481 (2005)
12. Kuglin, C., Hines, D.: The phase correlation image alignment method. In: Proc. Int. Conf. on Cybernetics and Society, vol. 4, pp. 163–165 (1975)
13. Wu, Q., Bones, P., Bates, R.: Translational motion compensation for coronary angiogram sequences. IEEE Transactions on Medical Imaging 8(3), 276–282 (1989)
14. Kaplan, W.: Advanced Calculus, 4th edn. Addison-Wesley, Reading (1992)
15. Wein, W., Cheng, J.Z., Khamene, A.: Ultrasound based respiratory motion compensation in the abdomen. In: MICCAI 2008 Workshop on Image Guidance and Computer Assistance for Soft-Tissue Interventions (September 2008)
16. Wein, W., Camus, E., John, M., Diallo, M., Duong, C., Al-Ahmad, A., Fahrig, R., Khamene, A., Xu, C.: Towards guidance of electrophysiological procedures with real-time 3d intracardiac echocardiography fusion to c-arm ct. In: Yang, G.-Z., et al. (eds.) MICCAI 2009, Part I. LNCS, vol. 5761, pp. 9–16. Springer, Heidelberg (2009)

Dynamic Cone Beam Reconstruction Using a New Level Set Formulation

Andreas Keil[1], Jakob Vogel[1], Günter Lauritsch[2], and Nassir Navab[1,*]

[1] Computer Aided Medical Procedures, TU München, Germany
keila@cs.tum.edu
[2] Siemens AG, Healthcare Sector, Forchheim, Germany

Abstract. This paper addresses an approach toward tomographic reconstruction from rotational angiography data as it is generated by C-arms in cardiac imaging. Since the rotational acquisition scheme forces a trade-off between consistency of the scene and reasonable baselines, most existing reconstruction techniques fail at recovering the $3D + t$ scene.

We propose a new reconstruction framework based on variational level sets including a new data term for symbolic reconstruction as well as a novel incorporation of motion into the level set formalism. The resulting simultaneous estimation of shape and motion proves feasible in the presented experiments. Since the proposed formulation offers a great flexibility in incorporating other data terms as well as hard or soft constraints, it allows an adaption to a wider range of problems and could be of interest to other reconstruction settings as well.

1 Introduction

The clinical motivation for providing a 3D($+t$) reconstruction of the coronary arteries from rotational angiography data is to provide the physician with intra-interventional 3D data. Currently, patients with chest pain and other symptoms for a cardiac infarction either get a conventional CT (for a definite rule-out) or are directly sent to the catheter lab where diagnosis and intervention are performed at once using a C-arm system. In the former case, the physician may obtain a 3D reconstruction which is not intra-interventional whereas in the latter case, there are only series of 2D X-rays available for diagnosis and navigation.

Bringing the two worlds together requires a reconstruction from calibrated angiographic projections which can be obtained during a rotational run (190°) of the C-arm around the patient (see Fig. 1). Such a run takes about 4 s to 5 s which is a hard limit for technical as well as security reasons. Therefore, a human heart beats about 4 to 7 times during imaging. The resulting inconsistent projection data inhibits 3D reconstruction. This is the reason why a simultaneous

---

[*] The authors thank Moritz Blume, Jan Boese, and Martin Brokate for valuable discussions. Credits also go to Tobias Klug and the Chair "LRR" at TUM for providing the high performance hardware and to Christopher Rohkohl for the phantom data. This work was funded by Siemens AG, Healthcare Sector, Forchheim, Germany.

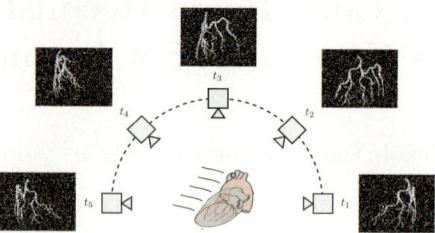

Fig. 1. Rotational angiography of a dynamic scene. (Image is derived from work by Patrick J. Lynch, medical illustrator; C. Carl Jaffe, MD, cardiologist. http://creativecommons.org/licenses/by/2.5/)

reconstruction of shape and motion is needed in order to compensate for the heart motion during the reconstruction of the shape.

The ill-posedness of a direct tomographic 4D reconstruction suggests to seek a symbolic/binary reconstruction first and then use the recovered motion for a later tomographic reconstruction. Such a symbolic reconstruction is performed on the coronaries since they are contrasted and cover the motion in the relevant area around the patient's heart.

2 Related Work

To the authors' knowledge, all previous work on cardiac cone beam CT makes strong use of the assumption that the heart motion can be grouped into several phases (usually defined by a percentage value between two adjacent R-peaks). Within such a phase (e.g. 10% − 20%), the heart is assumed to re-position to the same state in each of the phase's images. This permits a retrospective gating using the simultaneously recorded ECG signals. Based on this, Blondel et al. [1], Hansis et al. [2], and Movassaghi et al. [3] mostly rely on epipolar geometry and triangulation. Temporally distant but spatially consistent projections (yielding a wider baseline) are used to reconstruct 3D points and track them over time. Using traditional computed tomography solutions (like filtered back projection [4] or algebraic reconstruction [5,6]) Prümmer et al. [7] and Schäfer et al. [8] perform phase-wise tomographic reconstructions. These phase-wise reconstructions can then be fused if the motion between cardiac phases is somehow known. [8] focuses on the motion-compensated FDK-reconstruction algorithm assuming a known motion field whereas [7] also proposes to do multiple sweeps for acquiring enough projection data.

For the following reasons we propose a level set framework for symbolic reconstruction instead of using tomographic- or triangulation-based methods: Due to the bad image quality of contrasted angiographic X-ray projections, an algorithm not explicitly using correspondences but just a soft coupling of points in 3D space would be desirable. Although healthy hearts beat in a more or less regular manner, assuming exact re-positioning and perfectly periodic ECG signals is a quite strong requirement. This is in particular problematic for patients with pathologies like congenital cardiac defects or a prior bypass-surgery. To this end, a soft coupling in time domain could also prove to be advantageous. Level sets have the further advantage of being able to handle the unknown tree structure.

Although we will present novel data terms and a new space-time coupling, we still want to point the reader to the following works which we share some ideas with: Yoon et al. [9] perform a CT-like reconstruction from X-ray data using multiphase level sets. This work enables the reconstruction of piece-wise constant tissue from very few projections but does not deal with motion. Rathi et al. [10] and Cremers et al. [11] perform deformable tracking on 2D images using active contours which is related to our time-coupling.

Additionally, there is a lot of related work on 3D reconstruction from optical images using level sets, graph cuts, or voxel occupancy techniques. For the sake of brevity, we do not delve into this field but just want to mention Franco et al. [12] who give a nice derivation and solution to the problem of 3D reconstruction from probabilistic silhouette images in a *synchronized* multi-view environment.

3 Methods

Having laid out our motivation for developing a level set framework (offering the desired soft coupling) for symbolic reconstruction we now proceed to its modeling. The main theoretical contributions of this paper are the development of energy terms, fitting a level set function to the given image data, and its usage with a dynamic[1] level set function.

3.1 Dynamic Level Sets

Since we seek to obtain a symbolic or binary reconstruction of our 3D scene over time, we have chosen to model the "inside" and "outside" of reconstructed objects using a level set function

$$\Phi_0 : \begin{cases} \mathbb{R}^3 \to \mathbb{R} \\ \boldsymbol{x}_0 \mapsto \Phi_0(\boldsymbol{x}_0) \end{cases} \qquad (1)$$

on some reference domain with coordinates $\boldsymbol{x}_0$ and the convention $\Phi(\boldsymbol{x}_0) < 0$ for "inside" or reconstructed points. In order to establish a temporal relationship of the reconstruction frames, this level set function is made dynamic by introducing a warping transformation $\boldsymbol{\varphi}$. Similar to what was presented in [13], this transformation maps points from location $\boldsymbol{x}$ at time t to coordinates $\boldsymbol{x}_0$ in the reference frame where the shape is reconstructed using one single level set function Φ_0. For the experiments presented in this paper, we modeled a rigid motion over time using 6 temporal B-splines (with 10 degrees of freedom each) for the time-dependent rotation matrix $\boldsymbol{R}$ and translation vector $\boldsymbol{T}$ yielding coefficients $\boldsymbol{\alpha} \in \mathbb{R}^{6 \times 10}$:

---

[1] "Dynamic" in this context means the deformation of the level set function over the real time variable t (as opposed to an evolution of the level set function over artificial time during iterations).

$$\varphi : \begin{cases} \mathbb{R}^3 \times \mathbb{R} \times \mathbb{R}^{6 \times 10} \to \mathbb{R}^3 \\ (\boldsymbol{x}, t, \boldsymbol{\alpha}) \mapsto \boldsymbol{R}(t, \boldsymbol{\alpha}) \cdot \boldsymbol{x} + \boldsymbol{T}(t, \boldsymbol{\alpha}) \end{cases} \tag{2}$$

Note that the reference frame is arbitrary and not fixed to any point in time. This way, we avoid any bias toward a specific time.

Putting together equations (1) and (2), we obtain the dynamic level set function $\Phi : \mathbb{R}^3 \times \mathbb{R} \times \mathbb{R}^{6 \times 10} \to \mathbb{R}$

$$\Phi(\boldsymbol{x}, t, \boldsymbol{\alpha}) = \Phi_0\bigl(\varphi(\boldsymbol{x}, t, \boldsymbol{\alpha})\bigr) . \tag{3}$$

Note that one could also choose to directly model a 4D level set function $\Phi(\boldsymbol{x}, t)$. But using a dynamic warping function φ has several advantages:

- The shape reconstruction is implicitly regularized over time, since there is only one shape model.
- The motion can be recovered directly, simplifying its later use in a tomographic reconstruction as well as enabling a direct motion regularization.
- Memory requirements are much lower compared to a 4D grid if φ is parametrized.

3.2 Reconstruction Energies

Having built a model for the shape and motion to be reconstructed, we now proceed to setting up an energy functional that fits the reconstruction parameters Φ_0 and $\boldsymbol{\alpha}$ to the given L projection images I_l acquired at times t_l, $1 \le l \le L$. The projection images' pixels are assumed to contain intensity values in $[0, 1]$ corresponding to the probability that the associated ray hit a vessel. Imposing penalties on false positive and false negative reconstructed points in space works in a manner similar to what was first presented by Chan and Vese [14] but taking into account the projective character of the imaging device:

Let V be the reconstruction volume, $\boldsymbol{P}_l : \mathbb{R}^3 \to \mathbb{R}^2$ the projection operator for frame l, and H the Heaviside step function (or rather a mollified version of it, see [14] for examples). The false positive term then is

$$E_{\text{FP}}(\Phi_0, \boldsymbol{\alpha}) = \sum_{l=1}^{L} \int_V S_{\text{FP}}\bigl(I_l(\boldsymbol{P}_l(\boldsymbol{x}))\bigr) \cdot \bigl[1 - H\bigl(\Phi_0(\varphi(\boldsymbol{x}, t_l, \boldsymbol{\alpha}))\bigr)\bigr] \cdot \bigl[1 - I_l(\boldsymbol{P}_l(\boldsymbol{x}))\bigr] \, \mathrm{d}\boldsymbol{x} , \tag{4}$$

where $S_{\text{FP}}(i) = H\left(\frac{1}{2} - i\right)$ is a switching function, enabling the false positive penalty for low intensities/probabilities $i \in [0, \frac{1}{2}]$ only. In this formula, the first two factors filter out the false (1st factor) positive (2nd factor) reconstructions, whereas the 3rd factor is a weighted penalty. This way, reconstructed points are penalized every time they are hit by a "non-vessel ray".

Penalizing false negatives works in a similar way. However, the big difference is that we cannot accumulate penalties in volume space. Due to the images being probabilistic projections, we may only impose a false negative penalty if, and only if, no object is reconstructed along the whole ray corresponding to a high intensity pixel.[2] Thus, whole rays have to be considered instead of single points:

$$E_{\text{FN}}(\Phi_0, \boldsymbol{\alpha}) = \sum_{l=1}^{L} \int_A S_{\text{FN}}(I_l(\boldsymbol{p})) \cdot H\left(\min_{\boldsymbol{x} \in X_l(\boldsymbol{p})} \Phi_0(\varphi(\boldsymbol{x}, t_l, \boldsymbol{\alpha}))\right) \cdot I_l(\boldsymbol{p}) \, \mathrm{d}\boldsymbol{p} \quad (5)$$

Here, $A \subset \mathbb{R}^2$ is the projection image space, $X_l(\boldsymbol{p})$ is the set of volume points corresponding to pixel $\boldsymbol{p}$ in image l, and $S_{\text{FN}}(i) = H\left(i - \frac{1}{2}\right)$ is the switching function enabling the term for falsely reconstructed points only. The three factors here are responsible for selecting pixels which indicate a vessel to be reconstructed on the ray to pixel $\boldsymbol{p}$ (1st factor), selecting rays where all Φ values are positive, i.e. there is no object reconstructed (2nd factor), and adding a weighted penalty (3rd factor), respectively.

The two data terms seem to be of very different type. This is remedied by either appropriately weighting them or reformulating the false negative term to a volume integral using the coarea formula.

3.3 Regularization

In terms of regularization we only need to care about shape regularization at this point since the motion parameters are inherently regularized due to the usage of B-Splines with an appropriate number of knots. For obtaining a smooth shape reconstruction in the reference frame, we use

$$E_{\text{shape}}(\Phi_0) = \int_{V_0} \delta(\Phi_0(\boldsymbol{x})) \cdot \|\nabla \Phi_0(\boldsymbol{x})\| \, \mathrm{d}\boldsymbol{x} \quad (6)$$

for penalizing the level set surface and thereby favoring reconstructions with low surface curvatures.

3.4 Implementation

Optimizing the system

$$E(\Phi_0, \boldsymbol{\alpha}) = \lambda_{\text{FN}} \cdot E_{\text{FN}}(\Phi_0, \boldsymbol{\alpha}) + \lambda_{\text{FP}} \cdot E_{\text{FP}}(\Phi_0, \boldsymbol{\alpha}) + \lambda_{\text{shape}} \cdot E_{\text{shape}}(\Phi_0), \quad (7)$$

resulting from putting together the terms (4)–(6), is rather complex as two sets of parameters must be computed simultaneously, namely the shape model Φ_0 and the deformation parameters $\boldsymbol{\alpha}$. The former is minimized using the variational derivative of $\frac{\delta E}{\delta \Phi_0}$, the latter by calculating the gradient $\nabla_{\boldsymbol{\alpha}} E$. Computing these terms from their analytic forms involves deriving the minimum functional from equation (5), several numerical approximations, and a step size management during gradient descent for Φ_0 and α.

---

[2] Note that another approach would be to focus on a point in space and impose a false negative penalty iff *all* projected intensities enforce an object. However, this would favor "empty" reconstructions due to the initially inconsistent data.

The most demanding issue to solve is the computation of E_{FN} and its derivative. It involves ray casting (customized to using 3×4 projection matrices and applying the estimated motion for every sample point) for computing the minimum contained in the equation's second factor. Updates to Φ_0 have to be applied at the sample points (which are in general not at grid locations of Φ_0) and thus be "backward-interpolated".

Several approaches to implement such a scheme are possible, including GPU-based methods. After considering aspects related to memory usage and speed of computation, we decided to use a CPU-based procedure, optimized using the OpenMP framework. Even though GPUs appear to be a natural choice for ray casting, their bad support for arbitrary writes disqualifies them for this algorithm.

4 Experiments and Discussion

We tested our method using synthetic and phantom data. The "synthetic" data was created by modeling tubes of considerable diameter clearly visible in the projection images (see Fig. 2(a) and (b)) while the "phantom" data was physically built, scanned, reconstructed (without motion) and segmented. It contains thin vessels of just 1 or 2 voxels diameter as visible in Fig. 2(d). In both cases, we used 3×4 projection matrices, obtained from the calibration of a real stationary C-arm, to generate synthetic views of the data. During the virtual image acquisition process we applied a dynamic but rigid motion with realistic intervals

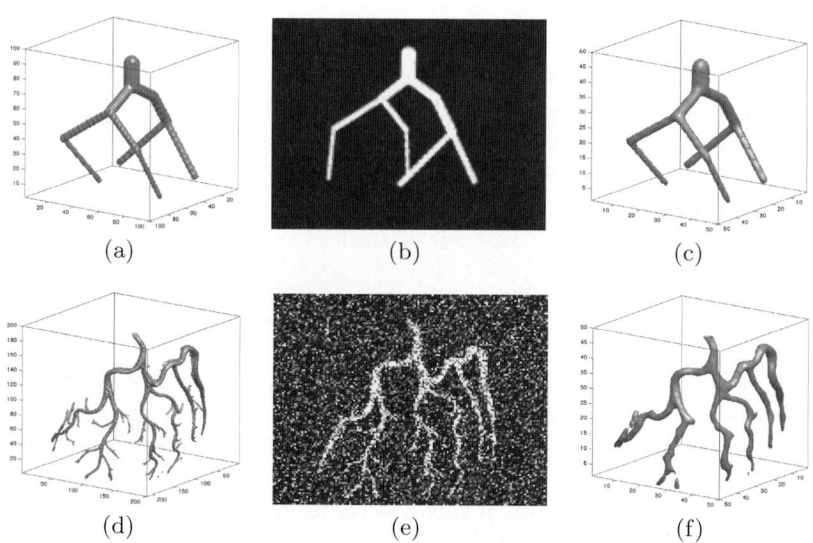

Fig. 2. Two examples of the imaging and reconstruction process. Top row: "Synthetic" data without noise. Bottom row: "Phantom" data with 50 % noise. From left to right: Ground truth models, exemplary projection, and the final reconstruction. Note that the projections do not show a static setting, but a snapshot of a moving artery tree.

Table 1. Comparison of the reconstruction errors. The two data sets "Synthetic" and "Phantom" were reconstructed at three different noise levels. All errors are given in mm and have been evaluated for a series of 5-10 experiments.

Data Set	Noise	Mean	St.D.	Max.	Med.	Data Set	Noise	Mean	St.D.	Max.	Med.
Synthetic	0%	0.54	0.30	2.19	0.47	Synthetic	0 – 50%	1.20	1.70	11.73	0.64
Synthetic	25%	0.68	0.36	3.14	0.60	Phantom	0 – 50%	1.98	2.22	9.79	1.03
Synthetic	50%	2.36	2.53	11.73	1.18	both	0%	0.81	0.47	4.41	0.72
Phantom	0%	0.91	0.48	4.41	0.82	both	25%	0.83	0.45	4.37	0.75
Phantom	25%	0.88	0.46	4.37	0.81	both	50%	3.68	2.77	11.73	3.07
Phantom	50%	4.15	2.70	9.79	3.86						

and amplitudes. An image inhancement step as necessary in the real application could be omitted grace to the use of symbolic ground truth data. Instead, we randomly added Gaussian noise (with zero mean and standard deviations of 25 % and 50 % of the full intensity range) to the projection images in order to test the proposed algorithm's sensitivity to noise. Sample projections with different magnitudes of noise are shown in Fig. 2.

As a result of these steps, we obtained a series of projection images of the moving artery tree, and their corresponding projection matrices. In order to speed up testing, we worked on rather coarse data using 48 projections at 155×120 pixels each (compared to 200-400 images at 620×480 pixels each in a real setting). The reconstruction volume V covered a cube of size $(15\text{cm})^3$, discretized as grid of 50^3 voxels.

All experiments have been run on high-performance hardware, including quad-core and 24-core equipment. The execution time depends on several factors such as noise and complexity of both motion and image content. For the 24-core machine, an average execution time of roughly 5 min for 100 iterations has been attained, after which the result was stable.

In order to compute a meaningful error measure, we collected all spatial points $\boldsymbol{X}_{k=1..K}$ corresponding to vessel voxels in the ground truth data. Afterwards, for each moment t_l, we warped these points using both the ground truth motion $\widehat{\boldsymbol{R}}(t_l)$, $\widehat{\boldsymbol{T}}(t_l)$ and the reconstructed motion $\boldsymbol{R}(t_l, \boldsymbol{\alpha})$, $\boldsymbol{T}(t_l, \boldsymbol{\alpha})$ and computed the reconstruction error

$$\left\| [\widehat{\boldsymbol{R}}(t_l) \cdot \boldsymbol{X}_k + \widehat{\boldsymbol{T}}(t_l)] - [\boldsymbol{R}(t_l, \boldsymbol{\alpha}) \cdot \boldsymbol{X}_k + \boldsymbol{T}(t_l, \boldsymbol{\alpha})] \right\|_2 \tag{8}$$

for every point $\boldsymbol{X}_k$ at every moment t_l.

A comparison of errors for two data sets and three noise levels is given in Table 1. Obviously, the algorithm supports a fair amount of noise. Still, low-noise images (25 %) compare best to the segmented vessel images to be used in the final application. The phantom data set performs worse than the synthetic model. However, this problem can most likely be traced to the coarse resolution we used despite the fine structures of this data set (see Fig. 2, bottom row). Nevertheless, the motion was usually still well estimated, in these cases. The average errors for reasonably posed problems with max. 25 % noise does not exceed 1 mm (and thus is sub-voxel accurate) even though we downsampled all data by factor four in space and time compared to the real setting.

5 Conclusion

The presented method is a promising alternative to other cone beam reconstruction procedures. Its major benefit is that it does not depend on hard constraints such as perfect ECG signals (although they may be included as a soft constraint later) or an exact re-positioning of cardiac anatomy between heart beats.

However, the motion description does not yet cover all possible motions that one encounters in the clinical setting. Future work will thus aim at more universal descriptions providing more degrees of freedom, such as affine transformations and fully deformable models. Especially in the latter case, application-specific soft constraints (e. g. relating ECG and motion) will become necessary.

References

1. Blondel, C., Malandain, G., Vaillant, R., Ayache, N.: Reconstruction of coronary arteries from a single rotational X-ray projection sequence. IEEE TMI 25(5), 653–663 (2006)
2. Hansis, E., Schäfer, D., Dössel, O., Grass, M.: Projection-based motion compensation for gated coronary artery reconstruction from rotational x-ray angiograms. Phys. Med. Biol. 53 (2008)
3. Movassaghi, B., Schaefer, D., Grass, M., Rasche, V., Wink, O., Garcia, J.A., Chen, J.Y., Messenger, J.C., Carroll, J.D.: 3D reconstruction of coronary stents in vivo based on motion compensated X-ray angiograms. In: Larsen, R., Nielsen, M., Sporring, J. (eds.) MICCAI 2006. LNCS, vol. 4191, pp. 177–184. Springer, Heidelberg (2006)
4. Feldkamp, L.A., Davis, L.C., Kress, J.W.: Practical cone-beam algorithm. J. Opt. Soc. Am. A 1(6), 612–619 (1984)
5. Gordon, R., Bender, R., Herman, G.T.: Algebraic reconstruction techniques (ART) for three-dimensional electron microscopy and X-ray photography. J. Theor. Biol. 29(3) (1970)
6. Andersen, A.H., Kak, A.C.: Simultaneous algebraic reconstruction technique (SART): A superior implementation of the ART algorithm. US Imag. 6(1) (1984)
7. Prümmer, M., Wigström, L., Hornegger, J., Boese, J., Lauritsch, G., Strobel, N., Fahrig, R.: Cardiac C-arm CT: Efficient motion correction for 4D-FBP. In: NSS and MIC, pp. 1–20. Springer, Heidelberg (2006)
8. Schäfer, D., Borgert, J., Rasche, V., Grass, M.: Motion-compensated and gated cone beam filtered back-projection for 3-D rotational X-ray angiography. IEEE TMI 25(7), 898–906 (2006)
9. Yoon, S., Pineda, A.R., Fahrig, R.: Level set reconstruction for sparse angularly sampled data. In: NSS and MIC, vol. 6, pp. 3420–3423 (2006)

10. Rathi, Y., Vaswani, N., Tannenbaum, A., Yezzi, A.: Particle filtering for geometric active contours with application to tracking moving and deforming objects. In: CVPR, vol. 2, pp. 2–9. IEEE, Los Alamitos (2005)
11. Cremers, D.: Dynamical statistical shape priors for level set-based tracking. IEEE Trans. PAMI 28(8), 1262–1273 (2006)
12. Franco, J.S., Boyer, E.: Fusion of multi-view silhouette cues using a space occupancy grid. In: ICCV, vol. 2, pp. 1747–1753 (2005)
13. Blume, M., Keil, A., Navab, N., Rafecas, M.: Blind motion compensation for positron-emission-tomography. In: SPIE Med. Imag. Proc. of the SPIE (2009)
14. Chan, T.F., Vese, L.A.: Active contours without edges. In: IEEE TIP, vol. 10(2) (2001)

Spatio-temporal Reconstruction of dPET Data Using Complex Wavelet Regularisation*

Andrew McLennan and Michael Brady

Department of Engineering Science, University of Oxford, UK
andrew.mclennan@new.ox.ac.uk, jmb@robots.ox.ac.uk

Abstract. Traditionally, dynamic PET studies reconstruct temporally contiguous PET images using algorithms which ignore the inherent consistency between frames. We present a method which imposes a regularisation constraint based on wavelet denoising. This is achieved efficiently using the Dual Tree – Complex Wavelet Transform (DT-CWT) of Kingsbury, which has many important advantages over the traditional discrete wavelet transform: shift invariance, implicit measure of local phase, and directional selectivity. In this paper, we apply the decomposition to the full spatio-temporal volume and use it for the reconstruction of dynamic (spatio-temporal) PET data.

Instead of using traditional wavelet thresholding schemes we introduce a locally defined and empirically-determined Cross Scale regularisation technique. We show that wavelet based regularisation has the potential to produce superior reconstructions and examine the effect various levels of boundary enhancement have on the overall images.

We demonstrate that wavelet-based spatio-temporally regularised reconstructions have superior performance over conventional Gaussian smoothing in simulated and clinical experiments. We find that our method outperforms conventional methods in terms of signal-to-noise ratio (SNR) and Mean Square Error (MSE), and removes the need to post-smooth the reconstruction.

1 Introduction

Positron Emission Tomography (PET) is a functional medical imaging modality which is able to record accurate pharmacokinetic information. When a radiotracer such as ^{18}F-FDG is administered to the patient, the reconstruction of the detected projection data enables the visualisation of a tracer distribution in-vivo. Dynamic PET typically involves detecting and independently reconstructing a contiguous sequence of scans ("frames"), which can range in duration from a few seconds to many minutes. The choice of the specific frame duration is usually difficult to justify, with short frames having higher temporal resolution and long frames having higher spatial resolution. The majority of clinical PET scans

---

* We are thankful to Anthonin Reilhac for the use of PET-SORTEO; Siemens Molecular Imaging for providing clinical data; and the Department for Business Enterprise and Regulatory Reform for their financial assistance.

which have been performed to date are static in nature. However, in this work we show the potential improvements in image quality that are possible when the goal of dynamic imaging is explicitly incorporated into the reconstruction.

The main motivating factor of Dynamic PET over simple Static images is that abnormal physiology provides clinicians far more information than abnormal anatomy alone. This is particularly true for cancer radiotherapy treatment plans, where there is growing evidence that PET is able to visualise a patient's responsiveness to treatment before anatomical changes are apparent. Detecting early responses to treatment enables clinicians to modify treatment plans as required, reducing the patient's discomfort and improving their survival chance.

True signal recovery from noisy estimates is a classical signal analysis problem. Many attempts have been made to reduce the noise inherent in dynamic PET using various regularisation techniques. One idea is to apply Gaussian temporal filtering to smooth the Time Activity Curve (TAC) estimates. Another is the method of Nichols et al, which estimate TACs using B-Spline temporal basis functions [1]. Reader et al. proposed using a specific compartmental model [2]. Kamasak et al. [3] extended the idea of Carson and Lange [4] of directly estimating kinetic parameters from the projection data, but require that that compartmental model is known a priori. Various data-driven reconstruction methods have also been previously explored in the literature, such as PCA [5] and the KL transform [6].

Wavelet denoising has also been a popular topic in PET recently, with there being many attempts to remove noise from both the projection data as well as the reconstructed images. Shidhara et al. provides a good summary of a number of these methods with emphasis on how their application affects pharmacokinetic parameter estimates [7]. Lee et al. [8] utilises Robust Wavelet Shrinkage, Bhatia et al. [9] remodelled the FBP algorithm in the wavelet domain and Verhaeghe et al. recently proposed a reconstruction algorithm using E-Spline wavelet-like temporal basis functions [10].

The method we present explicitly incorporates a modified spatio-temporal wavelet regularisation procedure directly into the reconstruction algorithm. The method decomposes the spatio-temporal activity estimate into the complex wavelet domain and empirically regularises the reconstruction. The Dual Tree – Complex Wavelet Transform (DT-CWT) [11] is used due to its many superior properties. We show that our method results in improved dynamic PET reconstructions when tested on simulated data and leads to less noisy and visually improved images for clinical colorectal data.

2 Method

2.1 Image Reconstruction

The forward projection model of dynamic PET for a matrix of F temporal I-dimensional detected projection data vectors $\mathbf{Y} \sim \text{Poisson}\left\{\hat{\mathbf{Y}}\right\}$ can be written as:

$$\hat{\mathbf{Y}} = \mathbf{PX} + \mathbf{R} + \mathbf{S} \tag{1}$$

where $\mathbf{X}$ is the $J \times F$ spatio-temporal image activity matrix used to represent the dynamic radioactivity distributions; $\mathbf{P}$ is the forward projection matrix representing the probability that an emission from the jth spatial basis function is detected by the ith Line of Response (LOR); and $\mathbf{R}$ and $\mathbf{S}$ are the Randoms and Scatter contribution vectors to the expected data.

Substituting Equation (1) into the Log-Likelihood function of a Poisson process, differentiating and then rearranging gives the conventional ML-EM algorithm [12] for reconstructing the spatio-temporal tracer distribution $\mathbf{X}$:

$$\mathbf{X}^{k+1}(t) = \frac{\mathbf{X}^k(t)}{\mathbf{P}^T \mathbf{1}} \mathbf{P}^T \frac{\mathbf{Y}(t)}{\mathbf{P}\mathbf{X}^k(t) + \mathbf{R}(t) + \mathbf{S}(t)}, \qquad (2)$$

where the product and division of vectors are understood to be carried out element-wise (as in [2]), $\mathbf{1}$ represents a vector of $1's$, and each temporal frame $t = 1, \cdots, F$ is reconstructed independently.

We modify the above algorithm to include spatio-temporal regularity between neighbouring voxels and temporal frames with the aim of preserving boundaries. After a single independent update of each of the F images using Equation (2), the reconstruction volume is decomposed, denoised and then recomposed using the multi-resolution complex wavelet transform. The overall regularised algorithm therefore becomes:

$$\mathbf{X}^{k+1}(t) = \frac{\tilde{\mathbf{X}}^k(t)}{\mathbf{P}^T \mathbf{1}} \mathbf{P}^T \frac{\mathbf{Y}(t)}{\mathbf{P}\tilde{\mathbf{X}}^k(t) + \mathbf{R}(t) + \mathbf{S}(t)} \qquad (3)$$

$$\tilde{\mathbf{X}}^{k+1}(t) = \mathbf{W}\left(\mu\left(\mathbf{W}^{-1}\left(\mathbf{X}^{k+1}\right)\right)\right) \qquad (4)$$

where $\mathbf{X}^k$ is the current reconstruction estimate for all time frames obtained from Equation (3), $\mathbf{W}$ and $\mathbf{W}^{-1}$ are the DT-CWT forward and inverse multi-resolution complex wavelet transforms, and μ is the denoising operator.

2.2 DT-CWT Cross Scale Regularisation

Gaussian Smoothing (GS) can be thought of as low-pass filtering in the frequency domain. Any high-frequency structures are assumed to be noise and smoothed regardless of their relative magnitudes. Wavelets on the other hand decompose signals into multi-resolution representations, based on scaled and translated "mother" wavelet functions. Compactly supported wavelets with large coefficients indicate jumps in signal value, whilst small absolute valued coefficients indicate mostly noise. This encodes important information at every resolution level in the coefficients on that level which have the largest absolute values. Keeping only these coefficients will result in less noisy reconstructions while ensuring edges remain sharp.

The Dual Tree – Complex Wavelet Transform (DT-CWT) of Kingsbury, which is documented in [11], is an efficient implementation of the complex-valued wavelet transform which has many advantageous properties over the traditional

Dyadic Discrete Wavelet Transform (DWT). For our work it can be considered a "black-box" which decomposes spatio-temporal volumes into multi-resolution complex coefficients. For a 1D signal, the complex valued wavelet coefficients are calculated by applying two separate standard DWT decompositions to the signal (with separate bio-orthogonal filters), with one tree containing the real coefficients and the other tree containing the imaginary coefficients.

The DT-CWT decomposition is shift invariant, directionally selective with strong orientation at multiple angles, has a measure of local phase[1] and is minimally redundant.[2] In this paper we use the advantageous properties of the DT-CWT and introduce a novel spatio-temporally varying denoising method aimed at being not only level dependent, but also adaptive to both varying signal and noise levels. We choose to use 3 decomposition levels and *near-symmetric* filters.

Conventional wavelet denoising methods usually consist of thresholding or shrinking wavelet coefficients with the aim of removing noise regardless of the signal's frequency content. The choice of particular threshold method and threshold value is in practice still an active area of research, and strongly influences the resulting images. Cross scale regularisation notes that edge information propagates across multiple frequencies, enabling an empirical level-dependent denoising scheme based on the boundary information from coarser levels.

Let F_w^l denote the multi-resolution complex wavelet decomposition for level l and directional sub-band w. Then, for each directional sub-band independently, and working from the second coarsest level to the finest, we pointwise multiply $|F_w^l|$ by the locally normalised coefficients of the next coursest level (performing interpolation where necessary):

$$M_l^{\text{new}} = |F_w^l| \cdot \frac{|F_w^{l+1}|}{(1-\alpha) \max\{|\{F_w^{l+1} \in N^3\}|\}}, \qquad (5)$$

where N^3 is proportional to an eighth of the size of the current decomposition level and α is the boundary enhancement term used to amplify dominant coefficients. The use of an enhancement factor is somewhat ad hoc but its aim (and advantage) is to encourage sharper edges between regional boundaries[3]. Finally, we use the phase of the original complex wavelet coefficients to convert the new wavelet magnitudes back into the complex domain.

The denoising scheme proposed here is an extension to the conventional cross-scale method. It is able to account for the spatially varying noise levels found in PET reconstruction by working with local maximums, enabling boundaries for regions of any activity to be sharpened.

---

[1] It is well known that phase carries significant visual information and therefore should not be corrupted during the denoising process.

[2] TI-DWT of Coifman and Donoho is also shift-invariant but at the cost of being maximally redundant.

[3] We note that choosing α to be too large may result in imaging artefacts being produced due to the possible over amplification and dampening of voxel values either side of a boundary and hence we encourage erring on the side of caution when choosing the value.

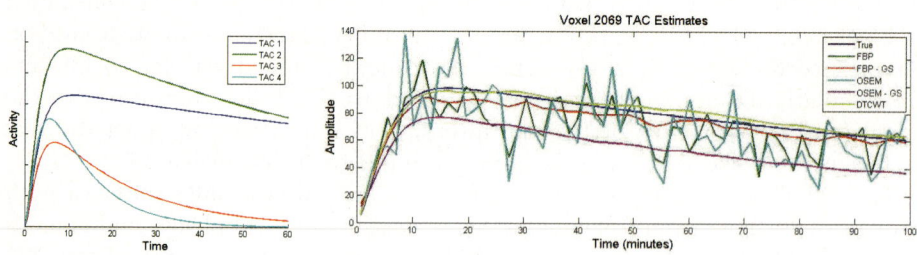

(a) Biologically plausible TACs (b) Example TACs estimates for the various reconstruction algorithms.

Fig. 1. Simulation TACs and reconstruction TAC estimates

3 Results and Discussion

The proposed DT-CWT denoising algorithm was assessed using both highly realistic 3D+t PET-SORTEO simulation data and clinical colorectal data. We compared our method to conventional FBP and OSEM, and a method which uses Gaussian Smoothing (GS) as opposed to Wavelet denoising. Many alternative reconstruction algorithms have previously been proposed but their clinical significance is less tried and tested. GS denotes the convolution of the current estimate with a spatio-temporal Gaussian kernel of size $\sigma = 1$.

3.1 PET-SORTEO Simulated 3D+t PET Data

The PET-SORTEO Monte Carlo-based simulator [13] is used to generate realistic dPET data based on the NCAT phantom. The biologically plausible TACs shown in Figure 1(a) taken from [2] were assigned to the four regions of the NCAT phantom shown in Figure 2. TAC 1 was assigned to the background, TAC 2 to the round anomalous region within the liver, TAC 3 to the liver and TAC4 to the round anomalous region in background.

Sixty four temporal frames each 93.75 seconds in duration were generated to produce sinograms of size $144 \times 288 \times 239$ covering the whole 1 hour 40 minute scan acquisition. A total of approximately 4.3 million events were recorded along the central slice through the phantom for which we show results. Randoms and Scatter events were not included in this simulation as, in the ideal case, they would be perfectly accounted for by the Randoms and Scatter matrices R and S respectively. Attenuation was also not simulated because it is assumed that this would be accounted for in practice using one of a variety of correction techniques. Images of size 64×64 were produced for reconstruction algorithms.

We compare the conventional reconstruction algorithms with our new method, after 10 iterations (8 subsets). Figure 1(b) shows (typical) example voxel TAC estimates for the different algorithms compared. We see that the un-regularised FBP and OSEM algorithms have greatly varying activity curves compared to

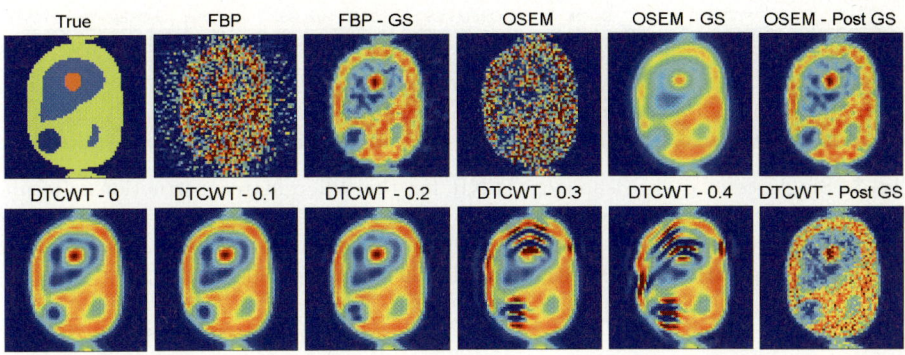

Fig. 2. Single central slice of frame 20 for different reconstructions. Top row: true image, FBP, FBP with post-Gaussian smoothing, OSEM, OSEM with inter-iteration GS and OSEM with post-GS. Bottom row: DT-CWT methods for enhancement levels 0, 0.1, 0.2, 0.3 and 0.4, and OSEM with post- DT-CWT denoising.

Table 1. Comparison of reconstruction algorithms: MSE and SNR

	MSE	ROI 1	ROI 2	ROI 3	ROI 4
FBP	66.35	3.511	4.767	-4.6114	-4.4709
FBP-GS	15.11	11.3985	11.5186	5.4651	**4.1076**
OSEM	52.67	2.3062	3.1173	-2.6621	-3.3012
OSEM-GS	13.79	11.5342	8.3733	4.0789	0.99131
OSEM- Post GS	12.48	11.6388	11.225	6.1949	**3.5224**
DT-CWT (0)	**10.02**	**11.6642**	**11.8975**	6.2744	2.9651
DT-CWT (0.1)	**10.04**	**11.6567**	**11.8726**	**6.3042**	3.0846
DT-CWT (0.2)	10.87	11.5011	11.7983	6.3400	2.7726
DT-CWT (0.3)	14.17	10.9838	9.0917	4.7827	1.3988
DT-CWT (0.4)	22.51	9.8971	4.3427	2.9892	0.54596
OSEM- Post DT-CWT	11.31	10.3631	9.6655	5.2576	2.8127

the regularise TACs. We note that the new method provides the best estimate out of all the algorithms, being not only lower in bias but temporally smoother.

Figure 2 shows the reconstructions of frame 20 for both conventional and our DT-CWT algorithms with five levels of enhancement. All of the regularised and smoothed images have reduced noise. Significant speckling remains for post reconstruction smoothing, however. The DT-CWT for small enhancement levels produces less noisy images with sharper edges between regions of interest. As expected, artefacts are introduced for large enhancement levels.

The quantitative accuracy of the reconstructions are compared by using the Mean Square Error (MSE) and Temporal Signal to Noise Ratio (TSNR) measures, taken from Verhaeghe et al [10]. Table 1 shows that the new method results in lower MSE than the conventional algorithms. Even though MSE is known not to be the best quantitative measure for medical imaging, it encourages further investigation. The average temporal SNR of each region shows that for the first

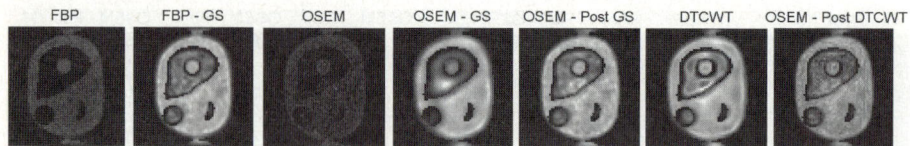

Fig. 3. Single central slice showing TSNR for the different reconstructions. Results shown for FBP (with and without post-GS), OSEM (with and without inter-iteration and post-GS), our DT-CWT method (with an enhancement level of 0.1) and OSEM with a single operation of post-reconstruction DT-CWT denoising.

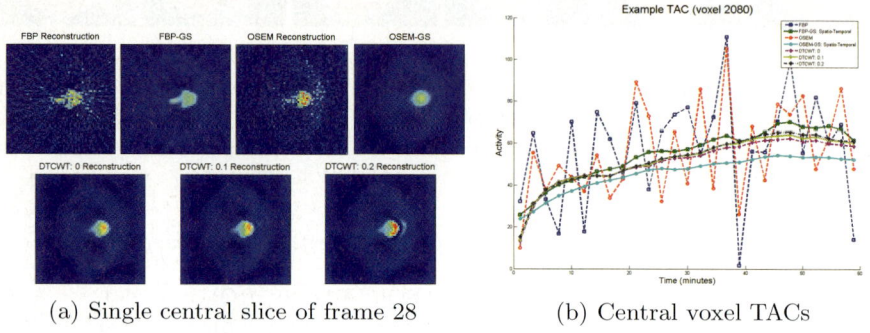

(a) Single central slice of frame 28   (b) Central voxel TACs

Fig. 4. FBP, FBP with post-GS, OSEM, OSEM with inter-iteration GS, and DT-CWT methods with enhancement levels 0, 0.1 and 0.2

three regions the new method out-performs the conventional methods. FBP with post-Gaussian smoothing results in larger TSNR for the last region, which we suspect is caused by slight biasing due to the region's proximity to the phantom's exterior. Figure 3 shows the TSNR values of each voxel in the 2D slice. We see that our DT-CWT with a boundary enhancement of 0.1 results in superior SNR around region edges than the OSEM-GS method and less speckling than post-Gaussian smoothing.

3.2 Clinical 3D+t Colorectal PET Data

To aid the validation process for the above new DT-CWT dynamic PET reconstruction technique we apply the algorithms to clinical colorectal data. A total of 321 million events where recorded for a 60 minute acquisition, acquired from Siemens Molecular Imaging. These events were then histogrammed into twenty eight equal duration contiguous sinograms of size $336 \times 336 \times 313$. Results are again shown for the 64×64 central slice reconstruction.

Figure 4(a) shows the reconstructions of the final frame (128 seconds of data) for the DT-CWT method with three levels of enhancement, FBP with and without post-Gaussian smoothing, and conventional OSEM with and without inter-iteration Gaussian smoothing. It appears that the DT-CWT method significantly reduces noise due to the spatio-temporal regularisation, but without overly blurring boundary edges seen in the OSEM-GS image. An enhancement greater than zero again appears to lead to sharper images, but it needs to be small enough not to introduce artefacts. Figure 4(b) compares the TACs obtained by the various methods, demonstrating again that noise is reduced by the DT-CWT method.

4 Conclusion

A novel approach to dynamic PET iterative reconstruction is proposed which ensures consistency between neighbouring voxels and frames using DT-CWT. The method regularises the reconstruction process using spatio-temporal wavelet denoising. The Cross-Scale Regularisation method is examined and shown to lead to better results than Gaussian smoothing for our experiments. Results are shown for simulated and clinical dPET data and imply that wavelet regularisation enables superior quantitative reconstructions.

References

1. Nichols, T., Qi, J., Asma, E., Leahy, R.: Spatiotemporal Reconstruction of List Mode PET Data. Trans. Med. Imag. 23(4), 396–404 (2002)
2. Reader, A.J., Matthews, J.C., Sureau, F.C., Comtat, C., Trebossen, R., Buvat, I.: Iterative Kinetic Parameter Estimation within Fully 4D PET Image Reconstruction. IEEE Nuc. Sci. Symp. Conf. 3, 1752–1756 (2006)
3. Kamasak, M.E., Bouman, C.A., et al.: Direct Reconstruction of Kinetic Parameter Images from Dynamic PET Data. IEEE Tran. Med. Imag. 24(5), 636–650 (2005)
4. Carson, R., Lange, K.: The EM Parametric Image Reconstruction Algorithm. J. Am. Stat. Assoc. 80, 20–22 (1985)
5. Kao, C.M., Yap, J.T., Mukherjee, J., Wernick, M.N.: Image Reconstruction for Dynamic PET Based on Low-Order Approximation and Restoration of the Sinogram. IEEE Transactions on Medical Imaging 16(6), 738–749 (1997)
6. Wernick, M.N., Infusino, E.J., Milosevic, M.: Fast Spatio-Temporal Image Reconstruction for Dynamic PET. IEEE Trans. on Med. Imag. 18(3), 185–195 (1999)
7. Shidahara, M., Ikoma, Y., Kershaw, J., Kimura, Y., Naganawa, M., Watabe, H.: PET Kinetic Analysis: Wavelet Denoising of Dynamic PET Data with Application to Parametric Imaging. Ann. Nucl. Med. 21, 379–386 (2007)
8. Lee, N.Y., Choi, Y.: A Modified OSEM Algorithm for PET Reconstruction using Wavelet Processing. Comp. Meth. Prog. Biomed. 80(3), 236–245 (2005)
9. Bhatia, M., Karl, W.C., Willsky, A.S.: A Wavelet-based Method for Multiscale Tomographic Reconstruction. IEEE Trans. Med. Imag. 15(1), 92–101 (1996)
10. Verhaeghe, J., Ville, D.V., Khalidov, I., d'Asseler, Y., Lemahieu, I., Unser, M.: Dynamic PET Reconstruction Using Wavelet Regularization With Adapted Basis Functions. MedImg. 27(7), 943–959 (2008)
11. Selesnick, I.W., Baraniuk, R.G., Kingsbury, N.G.: The Dual-Tree Complex Wavelet Transform. IEEE Signal Processing Magazine 22(6), 123–151 (2005)
12. Shepp, L., et al.: Maximum Likelihood Reconstruction for Emission Tomography. Tran. Med. Imag. 1(2), 113–122 (1982)
13. Reilhac, A., Lartizien, C., et al.: PET-SORTEO: A Monte Carlo-based Simulator with High Count Rate Capabilities. IEEE Trans. Nuc. Sci. 51(1), 46–52 (2004)

Evaluation of q-Space Sampling Strategies for the Diffusion Magnetic Resonance Imaging*

Haz-Edine Assemlal, David Tschumperlé, and Luc Brun

GREYC (CNRS UMR 6072), 6 Bd Maréchal Juin, 14050 Caen Cedex, France

Abstract. We address the problem of efficient sampling of the diffusion space for the Diffusion Magnetic Resonance Imaging (dMRI) modality. While recent scanner improvements enable the acquisition of more and more detailed images, it is still unclear which q-space sampling strategy gives the best performance. We evaluate several q-space sampling distributions by an approach based on the approximation of the MR signal by a series expansion of Spherical Harmonics and Laguerre-Gaussian functions. With the help of synthetic experiments, we identify a subset of sampling distributions which leads to the best reconstructed data.

1 Introduction

The random Brownian motion of the water molecules is constrained by the microstructure of the brain white matter. The Diffusion Magnetic Resonance Imaging (dMRI) modality captures this local average displacement in each voxel using the pulse gradient spin echo sequence [1] and thus indirectly leads to images of the brain architecture. These images provide useful information to diagnose early stages of stroke and other brain diseases [2]. However, this average molecular displacement is not directly measured. Indeed, as the diffusion gradient pulse duration δ is negligible compared to the diffusion time Δ, the normalized MR signal E defined in the q-space is related to the average displacement Probability Density Function (PDF) P by the *Fourier transform* [3]

$$P(\mathbf{p}) = \int_{\mathbf{q} \in \mathbb{R}^3} E(\mathbf{q}) \exp(-2\pi i \mathbf{q}^T \mathbf{p}) d\mathbf{q}, \quad \text{with } E(\mathbf{q}) = \frac{S(\mathbf{q})}{S_0}, \quad (1)$$

where $\mathbf{p}$ is the displacement vector and $\mathbf{q}$ stands for the diffusion wave-vector of the q-space. The symbols $S(\mathbf{q})$ and S_0 respectively denote the diffusion signal at gradient $\mathbf{q}$ and the baseline image at $\mathbf{q} = 0$.

Eq.(1) naturally suggests one should sample the whole q-space and use the Fourier transform to numerically estimate the PDF. This technique, known as Diffusion Spectrum Imaging (DSI) [4], is not clinically feasible mainly because of the long acquisition duration required to retrieve the whole set of needed q-space coefficients. As a result of DSI constraints, High Angular Resolution Diffusion Imaging (HARDI) [5] has come as an interesting alternative and proposes to

---

* We are thankful to Cyceron for providing data and the fruitful technical discussions.

sample the signal on a single sphere of the q-space. Most of the methods of the literature working on HARDI images [6,7,8,9] consider a single shell acquisition and have thus to assume strong priors on the radial behavior of the signal, classically a *mono*-exponential decay for instance.

Sampling schemes on several spheres in the q-space have been only proposed very recently [9,10,11,12,13,14]. Since the number of samples still remains too low for computing the Fourier transform, proposed methods rather consider computed tomography technique [13] or approximations of the MR signal radial attenuation by multi-exponential functions [9,11]. Note that even if these methods use a larger set of data, they are still using *a-priori* models of the radial behavior of the input signal. In section 2, we first overview the mathematical background of one previous diffusion features estimation method introduced in [15,16]. Then, we review several q-space sampling strategies proposed so far in the literature and detail the evaluation procedure of the experiments in section 3. We conclude on the results in section 4.

2 Spherical Polar Fourier Expansion

To be as self-contained as possible, we briefly overview our previous estimation method introduced in [15,16] based on the Spherical Polar Fourier (SPF) expansions. In order to be able to reconstruct the PDF from Eq.(1) even with few samples, we seek to build a basis in which the acquired signal is sparse.

Let E be the normalized MR signal attenuation. We propose to express it as a series in a spherical orthonormal basis named Spherical Polar Fourier (SPF) [17]:

$$E(\mathbf{q}) = \frac{S(\mathbf{q})}{S(0)} = \sum_{n=0}^{\infty} \sum_{l=0}^{\infty} \sum_{m=-l}^{l} a_{nlm} R_n(||\mathbf{q}||) y_l^m \left(\frac{\mathbf{q}}{||\mathbf{q}||} \right), \quad (2)$$

where a_{nlm} are the expansion coefficients, y_l^m are the real Spherical Harmonics functions (SH), and R_n is an orthonormal radial basis function.

The angular part of the signal E then is classically reconstructed by the complex SH Y_l^m which form an orthonormal basis for functions defined on the single sphere. They have been widely used in diffusion MRI [18]. Indeed, as the diffusion signal exhibits real and symmetric properties, the use of a subset of this complex basis restrained to real and symmetric SH y_l^m strenghten the robustness of the estimated reconstruction to signal noise and reduces the number of required coefficients [18].

Meanwhile, the radial part of the signal E is reconstructed in our approach [15,16] by the elementary radial functions R_n. A sparse representation of the radial signal should approximate it in a few radial order N. Based on these observations, we propose to estimate the radial part of E using the normalized generalized Gaussian-Laguerre polynomials R_n:

$$R_n(||\mathbf{q}||) = \left[\frac{2}{\gamma^{3/2}} \frac{n!}{\Gamma(n+3/2)} \right]^{1/2} \exp\left(-\frac{||\mathbf{q}||^2}{2\gamma} \right) L_n^{1/2} \left(\frac{||\mathbf{q}||^2}{\gamma} \right), \quad (3)$$

where γ denotes the scale factor and $L_n^{(\alpha)}$ are the generalized Laguerre polynomials. The Gaussian decay arises from the normalization of the Laguerre polynomials in spherical coordinates.

The SPF forms an orthonormal basis where a low order truncation assumes a radial Gaussian behavior as in [9,11] and a high order truncation provides model-free estimations. Besides, the square error between a function and its expansion in SPF to order $n <= N$ and $l <= L$ converges to zero as N and L go to infinity. We fit the signal to the SPF by a damped least square minimization procedure. The best fitting coefficients a_{nlm} are thus given by a regularized Moore-Penrose pseudo-inverse scheme:

$$\mathbf{A} = \arg\min_{\mathbf{A}} ||\mathbf{E} - \mathbf{M}\mathbf{A}||^2 + \lambda_l ||\mathbf{L}||^2 + \lambda_n ||\mathbf{N}||^2 = (\mathbf{M}_{reg})^{-1} \mathbf{M}^T \mathbf{E} \quad (4)$$

where $\mathbf{M} = (R_n(||\mathbf{q}_j||) y_l^m(\frac{\mathbf{q}_j}{||\mathbf{q}_j||}))_{nlm \times j \in \mathbb{N}^3 \times \mathbb{N}}$ denotes the SPF basis matrix, $\mathbf{M}_{reg} = \mathbf{M}^T\mathbf{M} + \lambda_n \mathbf{N}^T\mathbf{N} + \lambda_l \mathbf{L}^T\mathbf{L}$ and $\mathbf{E}, \mathbf{A}$ respectively denote the vectors $(E(\mathbf{q}_1), \dots, E(\mathbf{q}_{ns}))^T$ and $(a_{000}, \dots, a_{NLL})^T$. Since the matrix $\mathbf{M}_{reg}$ is likely to be ill-conditioned because of the highly reduced number of samples, we use regularization matrices $\mathbf{L}$ and $\mathbf{N}$ with entries $l^2(l+1)^2$ and $n^2(n+1)$ along their diagonal. They penalizes high variations of the angular and radial parts of SPF in the estimation under the assumption that they are likely to capture signal noise. The symbols λ_l and λ_n respectively denote angular and radial regularization weights.

3 Material and Methods

The number of data samples is limited because of the restricted acquisition. So the sampling scheme is actually something critical and should be chosen wisely. Indeed, given a fixed number of samples (clinical constraint), which repartition of the q-space samples is the best ? Which radial order truncation N should be chosen to fit Gaussian or bi-Gaussian MR datasets ? All these questions about the acquisition protocol are the focus of the following experiments.

3.1 q-Space Sampling

Let $n_s \in \mathbb{N}$ be the total number of samples and $n_b \in \mathbb{N}$ the number of sampling sphere. Let f be the number of samples on one sphere $x \in [1, n_b]$ so that

$$f_x(\eta) = \frac{q_x^\eta}{\sum_{i=1}^{n_b} q_i^\eta} n_s, \quad \text{and} \quad q_i(\beta) = \left(\frac{i-1}{n_b - 1}\right)^\beta (q_{max} - q_{min}) + q_{min} \quad (5)$$

where $q_i \in [q_{min}, q_{max}]$ refers to the radius of the i-th sphere. For simplicity sakes, the radii are considered as uniformly distributed ($\beta = 1$) between $[q_{min}, q_{max}] = [1, 30]\,\mathrm{cm}^{-1}$. The sampling points on each sphere should be as evenly spread as possible and are thus computed by electrostatic energy minimization as proposed in [14]. The spheres which possess very few samples are

Table 1. Overview of the different considered strategies for the q-space sampling. From a fixed number of total samples $n_s = 300$ and spheres n_b, the parameter η sets the spherical repartition of samples in the q-space as described by Eq.(5). The radii of the spheres are uniformly distributed ($\beta = 1$).

	$\eta = -2$	$\eta = -1$	$\eta = 0$	$\eta = 1$	$\eta = 2$	$\eta = 3$
$n_b = 2$						
$n_b = 5$						
$n_b = 10$						

randomly rotated to capture more signal ($f_x(\eta) \leq 6$ in our experiments). Overall, $f(\eta = 0)$ corresponds to a constant number of samples on each sphere as described in [13,15,19]. $f(\eta = 2)$ corresponds to a uniform spherical sampling as introduced in [11,12].

3.2 Data Processing

The following multi-exponential model was used to generate the considered synthetic data,

$$E(\mathbf{q}) = E(q \cdot \mathbf{u}) = \sum_{k=1}^{N_f} f_k \exp\left(-\frac{(q-m_k)^2 \mathbf{u}^T \mathbf{D}_k \mathbf{u}}{2\sigma^2}\right) \quad (6)$$

where $\sum_{k=1}^{N_f} f_k = 1$ and $||\mathbf{u}|| = 1$. The symbol N_f stands for the number of fibers, m_k is the mean diffusion and $\mathbf{D}_k$ is a 3×3 symmetric definite positive matrix defining the diffusion anisotropy for the k-th fiber. The scale factor γ was calculated on the data samples using the Apparent Diffusion Coefficient (ADC) with a linear least square fit so that $\gamma = (2\,\text{ADC})^{-1}$. Thus the decay of the SPF basis eigenfunctions at order $n = 0$ have the same scale as the sampled data. For a single fiber configuration as in Fig.1b, $\text{diag}(\mathbf{D}_k) = [1.5; 0.2; 0.2]\,\text{mm}^2\text{s}^{-1}$ and $\sigma = 5$.

In Fig.2, we determine which truncation order is sufficient to capture the standard data pattern presented in Fig.1. The normalized error of the power spectrum between the original and reconstructed data is expressed as

$$\text{Normalized Error} = \frac{\sum_{i=1}^{n_s} E[\mathbf{q}_i]^2 - \sum_{n=0}^{N} \sum_{l=0}^{L} \sum_{m=-l}^{l} a_{n,l,m}^2}{\sum_{i=1}^{n_s} E[\mathbf{q}_i]^2} \quad (7)$$

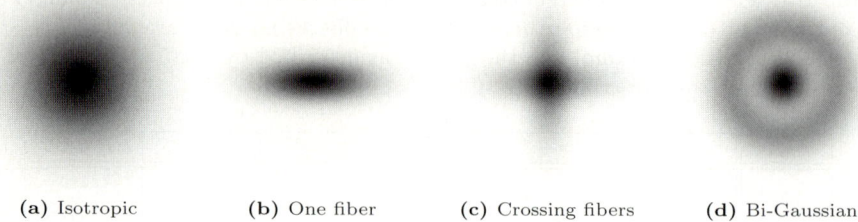

(a) Isotropic **(b)** One fiber **(c)** Crossing fibers **(d)** Bi-Gaussian

Fig. 1. Some standard pattern of q-space local diffusion data in the human brain white matter. Data are centered on a volumic image of size $64 \times 64 \times 64$.

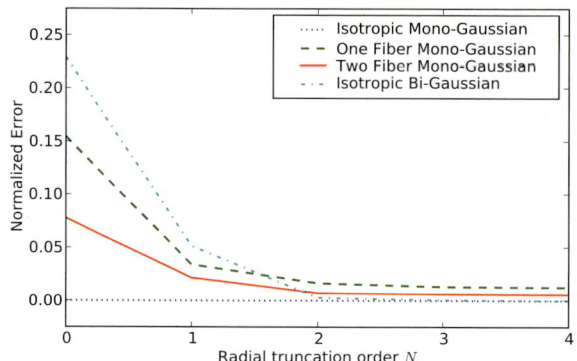

Fig. 2. Influence of radial truncation order N on the normalized error between the power spectrum of the original data and its reconstruction in the proposed basis. The number of samples is $n_s = 64^3$. The angular truncation order is $L = 4$.

The condition number C is an interesting index as it relates the correspondence between the sampling distribution and the reconstruction basis, *independently of the data*. It measures how numerically well-conditioned the regularized matrix $\mathbf{M}_{reg}$ from Eq.(4) is,

$$C = ||\mathbf{M}_{reg}||_\infty ||\mathbf{M}_{reg}^{-1}||_\infty \tag{8}$$

Fig.3 shows a comparison between several sampling strategies, which were generated according to Eq.(5). This figure illustrates the evolution of the reconstruction quality along with the number of sampling spheres n_b and the repartition of samples η on each sphere. Only the crossing fibers data configuration is illustrated in this experience as we found no significant differences with other data configuration. Fig.4 illustrates for the same experiment qualitative results for good and bad reconstruction. Fig.5 shows the comparison of two sampling schemes: non-uniform and uniform sampling of the q-space, respectively $\eta = 0$ and $\eta = 2$. The case $f(\eta = 2)$ corresponds to a uniform sampling considering spherical coordinates. $n_s = 300$, $n_b \in [1, 10]$ and the angular truncation order is set to $L = 4$.

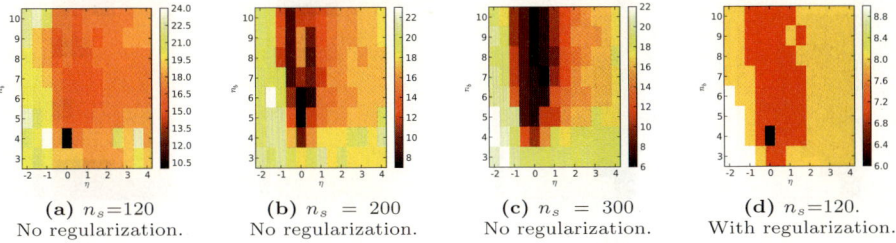

(a) n_s=120. No regularization. (b) $n_s = 200$. No regularization. (c) $n_s = 300$. No regularization. (d) n_s=120. With regularization.

Fig. 3. Condition number C evolution with the sampling distribution η and the number of sampling sphere n_b. The lower C is, the more stable the reconstruction is. The symbol n_s denotes the total number of samples. Angular truncation order is $L = 4$. Radial truncation order is $N = 3$, consequently $n_b \geq 3$ (120 coefficients). (d) Radial and angular regularization weights: $\lambda_n = 10^{-4}$, $\lambda_l = 10^{-6}$. Data simulates crossing fibers diffusion signal Fig.1c.

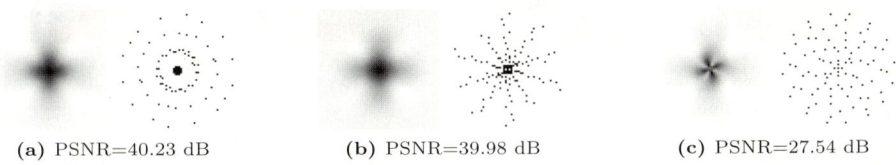

(a) PSNR=40.23 dB (b) PSNR=39.98 dB (c) PSNR=27.54 dB

Fig. 4. Example of some sampling distributions and their respective reconstruction

4 Results and Discussion

Fig.2 illustrates that a reasonably good radial truncation order N depends on the MR data pattern (*c.f.* Fig.1). Nonetheless, in all our experiments with standard data configurations in the brain white matter, the convergence to the data truth is achieved with N = 3. Concerning the sampling distribution η, the results of Fig.3 indicate that the best sampling distribution is $\eta \in [-1, 2]$, especially in the case of a small number of total samples (*c.f.* Fig.3(a-c)). This result is in accordance with the propositions already found in literature [11,12,15,19]. Therefore, Fig.5 shows a deeper comparison of two sampling $\eta = 0$ and $\eta = 2$. Fig.5(a) shows the evolution of C the condition number along with the number of sampling sphere n_b and the radial truncation order N. As expected, C is very high when $N > n_b$ and leads to very unstable results. When $N \leq n_b$, the condition number increases slowly along with increasing values of N and is quite constant along variations of n_b. Results obtained using the non-uniform sampling exhibit more monotonous evolutions than with the uniform sampling.

Fig.5(b) and (c) illustrate the PSNR (Peak Signal to Noise Ratio) evolution of the reconstruction of a Gaussian mixture MR signal. Although the maximum of the PSNR for all sampling protocols are quite the same (≈ 40) (*c.f.* Fig.3), it is clear that the non-uniform sampling protocol ($\eta = 0$) is more robust to wrong values of N and n_b. Besides, the robustness to wrong values of the scale

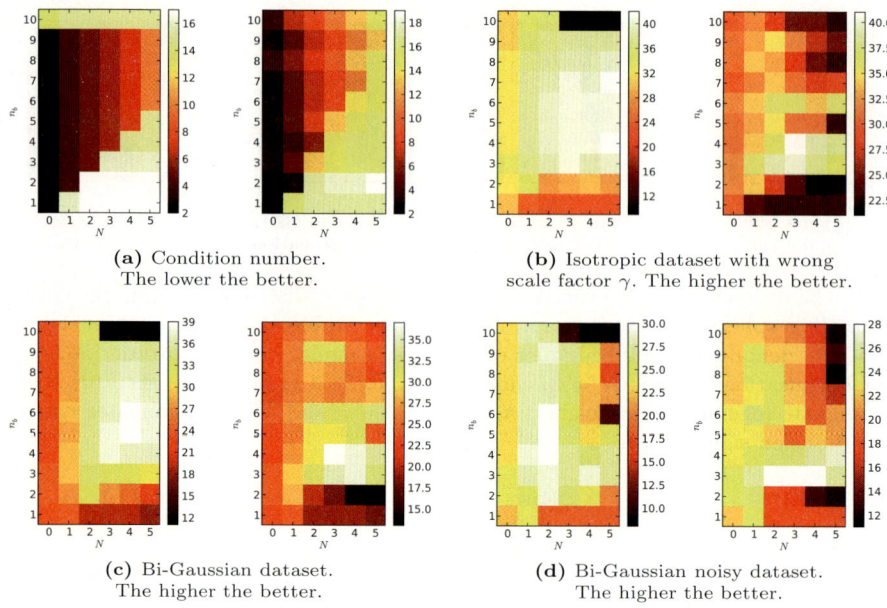

Fig. 5. Comparison of uniform ($\eta = 2$) vs non-uniform ($\eta = 0$) sampling (respectively left and right image) on Gaussian and bi-Gaussian isotropic datasets. N stands for the radial truncation in the SPF basis and n_b is the number of sampling sphere in the q-space. (b) Isotropic data with $\sigma^2 = 25$ (Fig.1a), with erroneous scale factor $\gamma = 5\sigma^2$. (d) The input data are noised with Rician noise (PSNR=18.9 dB).

factor γ is illustrated by the lines of Fig.5b. Indeed, the first order $N = 0$ of the SPF basis has a Gaussian decay and should entirely capture an isotropic Gaussian data (c.f. Fig.2). In Fig.5b, we set an arbitrary erroneous scale factor value γ not adapted to the signal decay σ so that $\gamma/\sigma^2 = 5$. The signal is reconstructed for $N \geq 3$ in accordance to Fig.2. Once again, Fig.5b shows that the non-uniform sampling protocol is the most robust to wrong values of γ. Finally, Fig.5d shows the results on a bi-Gaussian noisy dataset, estimated using our damped linear least square method Eq.(4). Besides the lower PSNR average compared to Fig.5c, it is remarkable that best results of Fig.5d were also obtained from lower radial truncation order N than Fig.5c. Indeed, a reconstruction using high N can significantly capture more noise than using lower N.

Out of the results, the non-uniform sampling protocol ($\eta = 0$) gives better global results than the uniform protocol ($\eta = 2$). The best reconstructions are obtained for $N \approx 3$ and $n_b \approx 4$. It confirms that a better reconstruction of the low q-space frequencies of the MR signal leads to a better reconstruction of the whole signal since low frequencies really carry the greatest part of the MR signal. Note that in contrast to our conclusion, Jones et al. in [14] interestingly observed in the restricted case of DTI with 2 spheres that more samples in the outer sphere gives the best results. This result might be explained by the strong restrictions of DTI to capture a Gaussian signal. Nonetheless, it is important to stress that the optimal parameters in this work are for the SPF basis.

5 Conclusion

In this paper, we proposed a unifying diffusion estimation formalism able to study the effect of several sampling schemes already proposed in the literature. We evaluated the influence of these schemes on the quality of the reconstruction for different shapes of diffusion signal. Out of the results, our findings indicate it is preferable to favour a high density of samples with low diffusion gradients rather than high diffusion gradients. We successfully identified a subset of sampling schemes which gives the best performances in adequacy with realistic clinical constraints.

References

1. Stejskal, E., Tanner, J.: Spin diffusion measurements: spin echoes in the presence of a time-dependent field gradient. Journal of Chemical Physics 42, 288–292 (1965)
2. LeBihan, D., Breton, E., Lallemand, D., et al.: MR imaging of intravoxel incoherent motions: Application to diffusion and perfusion in neurologic disorders. Radiology, 401–407 (1986)
3. Callaghan, P.: Principles of Nuclear Magnetic Resonance Microscopy. Oxford University Press, Oxford (1991)
4. Wedeen, V., Reese, T., Tuch, D., et al.: Mapping fiber orientation spectra in cerebral white matter with fourier transform diffusion MRI. In: ISMRM, vol. 82 (2000)
5. Tuch, D., Weisskoff, R., Belliveau, J., Wedeen, V.: High angular resolution diffusion imaging of the human brain, p. 321 (1999)
6. Tuch, D.: Q-ball imaging. Magn. Reson. Med. 52, 1358–1372 (2004)
7. Yablonskiy, D.A., Bretthorst, G.L., Ackerman, J.J.: Statistical model for diffusion attenuated MR signal. Magn. Reson. Med. 50, 664–669 (2003)
8. Liu, C., Bammer, R., Acar, B., Moseley, M.: Characterizing non-gaussian diffusion by using generalized diffusion tensors. Magn. Reson. Med. 51, 924–937 (2004)
9. Özarslan, E., Sherperd, T.M., Vemuri, B.C., et al.: Resolution of complex tissue microarchitecture using the diffusion orientation transform (dot). Neuroimage 31, 1086–1103 (2006)
10. Cercignani, M., Alexander, D.: Optimal acquisition schemes for in vivo quantitative magnetization transfer MRI. Magn. Reson. Med. 56, 803–810 (2006)
11. Assaf, Y., Basser, P.J.: Composite hindered and restricted model of diffusion (charmed) MR imaging of the human brain. Neuroimage 27, 48–58 (2005)
12. Wu, Y.C., Alexander, A.L.: Hybrid diffusion imaging. Neuroimage 36 (2007)
13. Pickalov, V., Basser, P.J.: 3D tomographic reconstruction of the average propagator from mri data. ISBI (2006)
14. Jones, D.K., Horsfield, M.A., Simmons, A.: Optimal strategies for measuring diffusion in anisotropic systems by magnetic resonance imaging. Magnetic Resonance in Medicine 42(3), 515–525 (1999)

15. Assemlal, H.E., Tschumperlé, D., Brun, L.: Efficient computation of pdf-based characteristics from diffusion MR signal. In: Metaxas, D., Axel, L., Fichtinger, G., Székely, G. (eds.) MICCAI 2008, Part II. LNCS, vol. 5242, pp. 70–78. Springer, Heidelberg (2008)
16. Assemlal, H.E., Tschumperlé, D., Brun, L.: Robust variational estimation of pdf functions from diffusion MR signal. In: CDMRI, MICCAI Workshop (2008)
17. Ritchie, D.W.: High-order analytic translation matrix elements for real-space six-dimensional polar fourier correlations. J. Appl. Cryst. 38, 808–818 (2005)
18. Frank, L.: Characterization of anisotropy in high angular resolution diffusion-weighted MRI. Magn. Reson. Med. 47, 1083–1099 (2002)
19. Khachaturian, M., Wisco, J., Tuch, D.: Boosting the sampling efficiency of q-ball imaging using multiple wavevector fusion. Magn. Reson. Med. 57, 289–296 (2007)

On the Blurring of the Funk–Radon Transform in Q–Ball Imaging

Antonio Tristán-Vega[1], Santiago Aja-Fernández[1], and Carl-Fredrik Westin[2]

[1] Laboratory of Image Processing, University of Valladolid, Spain
[2] Laboratory of Mathematics in Imaging, Harvard Medical School, Boston, MA
atriveg@lpi.tel.uva.es, sanaja@tel.uva.es, westin@bwh.harvard.edu

Abstract. One known issue in Q–Ball imaging is the blurring in the radial integral defining the Orientation Distribution Function of fiber bundles, due to the computation of the Funk–Radon Transform (FRT). Three novel techniques to overcome this problem are presented, all of them based upon different assumptions about the behavior of the attenuation signal outside the sphere densely sampled from HARDI data sets. A systematic study with synthetic data has been carried out to show that the FRT blurring is not as important as the error introduced by some unrealistic assumptions, and only one of the three techniques (the one with the less restrictive assumption) improves the accuracy of Q–Balls.

1 Introduction

High Angular Resolution Diffusion Imaging (HARDI) allows the characterization of complex tissue microarchitectures beyond one single fiber bundle per image voxel. Therefore it has become a very interesting topic in the recent literature [1,2,3,4]. Among the existing techniques, Q–Balls [5,6] have gained especial interest [7,8] for being fast and easy to estimate [9], and not needing further assumptions on the behavior of the diffusion signal outside the sampled sphere.

This technique is based on the integration of the attenuation signal in the equators of the sphere, estimating the Orientation Distribution Function (ODF) as the radial projection of the probability density along the corresponding axis. This is the so–called Funk–Radon Transform (FRT), whose main problem is that it is only an approximation of the radial integral defining the ODF. The error in the estimation of this integral produce the angular blurring of the ODF [6]. On the other hand, a recent study [8] has shown that the Diffusion Orientation Transform (DOT), as introduced in [3], may outperform Q–Balls in some situations, even when it is based upon the unrealistic assumption that the attenuation signal shows a mono–exponential decay. Based on this result, we propose three novel techniques to overcome FRT blurring from assumptions related to the one in [3]. They are tested with a systematical methodology similar to [8]. As a result we conclude, **first**, that the error (blurring) due to the FRT has less impact than the error introduced by the aforementioned assumption on the attenuation signal. **Secondly**, since such an assumption produces very accurate results with the DOT using very similar numeric schemes, the problem with Q–Balls relies on the estimation of the ODF instead of any other orientation information.

2 Theory

2.1 Characterization of Water Diffusion in the White Matter

Under the assumption of narrow pulses, the probability density for the displacement of water molecules to a position $\mathbf{R}$ for one single fiber bundle is related to the attenuation signal by the Stejskal–Tanner equation [10]:

$$P(\mathbf{R}) = \frac{1}{\sqrt{(4\pi^2\tau)^3|\mathcal{D}|}} \exp\left(\frac{-\mathbf{R}^T \mathcal{D}^{-1} \mathbf{R}}{4\tau}\right) \Leftrightarrow E(\mathbf{q}) = \exp\left(-b\mathbf{g}^T \mathcal{D}\mathbf{g}\right), \quad (1)$$

where $\mathbf{q} = q\mathbf{g}$, $\|\mathbf{g}\| = 1$, $b = 4\pi^2 \tau q^2$ is the magnitude of the sensitizing gradients, τ is the effective diffusion time and the positive–definite matrix $\mathcal{D}$ is the diffusion tensor. For complex micro–architectures the Gaussian model in eq. (1) no longer holds and $P(\mathbf{R})$ can be computed in terms of the Fourier transform of $E(\mathbf{q})$ [11]:

$$P(\mathbf{R}) = \mathfrak{F}\{E(\mathbf{q})\}(\mathbf{R}) = \iiint_{\mathbb{R}^3} E(\mathbf{q}) \exp(-2\pi i \mathbf{q}^T \mathbf{R}) d\mathbf{q}, \quad (2)$$

where the expresion of $E(\mathbf{q})$ in eq. (1) has to be substituted by:

$$E(\mathbf{q}) = \exp\left(-4\pi^2 \tau q^2 D(q, \mathbf{g})\right) < 1, \quad (3)$$

where $D(q, \mathbf{g})$ is a positive function, the Apparent Diffusion Coefficient (ADC), defined for each spatial direction $\mathbf{g}$. In general the ADC depends on q, but for the tensor model $D(q, \mathbf{g}) = \mathbf{g}^T \mathcal{D} \mathbf{g}$ and this is not the case; the diffusion process may be characterized then by the sampling of the attenuation signal $E(\mathbf{q})$ in a sphere of a given radius q_0, $E(q_0 \mathbf{g})$. The DOT (see [3]) relies on the over–simplified assumption that the ADC does not depend on q, $D(q, \mathbf{g}) = D(\mathbf{g})$.

2.2 The Orientation Distribution Function

Although the sampling of $E(q_0 \mathbf{g})$ for a given q_0 does not completely characterize the diffusion process, it is often enough to infer not the detailed behavior of $P(\mathbf{R})$, but only its underlying orientation information, associated to the presence of fiber bundles in these same directions. The ODF is defined in [5,6] as:

$$\Psi(\mathbf{r}) \equiv \Psi(\theta, \phi) = \int_0^\infty P(R\mathbf{r}) dR = \frac{1}{2} \int_{-\infty}^\infty P(R\mathbf{r}) dR, \quad (4)$$

where $R = \|\mathbf{R}\|$ and $\mathbf{r} = [\sin\theta\cos\phi, \sin\theta\sin\phi, \cos\theta]^T$. Although the ODF is not a true probability density (see [5]) it provides useful orientation information, as has been widely reported [7,8]. From eqs. (2) and (4) it follows:

$$2\Psi(\mathbf{r}) = \int_{-\infty}^\infty \iiint_{\mathbb{R}^3} E(\mathbf{q}) e^{-2\pi R i \mathbf{q}^T \mathbf{r}} d\mathbf{q} dR = \iiint_{\mathbb{R}^3} E(\mathbf{q}) \int_{-\infty}^\infty e^{-2\pi R i \mathbf{q}^T \mathbf{r}} dR d\mathbf{q}$$

$$= \iiint_{\mathbb{R}^3} E(\mathbf{q}) \delta(\mathbf{q}^T \mathbf{r}) d\mathbf{q} = \iint_{\langle \mathbf{r} \rangle^\perp} E(\mathbf{s}) d\mathbf{s}, \quad (5)$$

where $\langle \mathbf{r} \rangle^\perp$ is the orthogonal set to the span of $\mathbf{r}$, i.e., the ODF at direction $\mathbf{r}$ may be computed as the integral of $E(\mathbf{q})$ in the plane perpendicular to $\mathbf{r}$.

2.3 The Funk–Radon Transform

For a given $\mathbf{r}$ the computation of the ODF $\Psi(\mathbf{r})$ requires to integrate $E(\mathbf{q})$ in the plane perpendicular to $\mathbf{r}$, but HARDI techniques allow only to characterize $E(\mathbf{q})$ in a circumference of radius q_0 inside this plane. The principle of Q-Ball imaging is to reduce the integral in eq. (5) to the integral in the circumference $S_\mathbf{r} \equiv \{\mathbf{q} | \mathbf{q}^T\mathbf{r} = 0, \|\mathbf{q}\| = q_0\} \subset \langle \mathbf{r}\rangle^\perp$ to compute the FRT of $E(q_0\mathbf{g})$ as [5]:

$$\mathcal{G}\{E(q_0\mathbf{g})\}(\mathbf{r}) \stackrel{\Delta}{=} \oint_{S_\mathbf{r}} E(q_0\mathbf{g})q_0 d\mathbf{g} \propto \int_{-\infty}^{\infty}\int_0^{\infty}\int_0^{2\pi} P(\rho,\varphi,R)J_0(2\pi q_0\rho)\rho d\varphi d\rho dR$$

$$\simeq \int_{-\infty}^{\infty} P(R\mathbf{r})dR = 2\Psi(\mathbf{r}), \qquad (6)$$

where (ρ,φ,R) are the coordinates of a cylindrical system with the z axis aligned with $\mathbf{r}$: the FRT is proportional to the integral of $P(\mathbf{R})$ not along $\mathbf{r}$ but inside a tube along $\mathbf{r}$ which has the shape of a Bessel function J_0. Q–Balls obviate the need to characterize the whole $E(\mathbf{q})$ (they take into account its value only for q_0) at the expense of blurring the radial integral of $P(\mathbf{R})$. It is commonly assumed that this is the main drawback of Q–Ball imaging.

2.4 Beyond the Funk–Radon Transform

Given the nice results of DOT when assuming that the ADC is constant with q [3], even better than Q–Balls in certain situations [8], our aim is to use this same assumption to reduce the blurring due to the computation of the FRT.

Artificial Increase of the b-Value. Increasing the value of q_0 reduces the width of the Bessel kernel J_0 and therefore the blurring [5]. Assuming that $D(q, \mathbf{g}) \simeq D(q', \mathbf{g})$ for similar values of q and from eq. (3):

$$E(q_0'\mathbf{g}) = \exp\left(-4\pi^2\tau q_0'^2 D(q_0', \mathbf{g})\right)$$
$$\simeq \exp\left(-4\pi^2\tau q_0'^2 D(q_0, \mathbf{g})\right) = E(q_0\mathbf{g})^{q_0'^2/q_0^2} = E(q_0\mathbf{g})^\xi, \qquad (7)$$

and so we will refer to **Q–Balls–ξ** as the FRT of $E(q_0\mathbf{g})^\xi$, $\xi > 1$.

Integration in the Whole Orthogonal Plane to $\mathbf{r}$. If we now assume that $D(q, \mathbf{g}) \simeq D(\mathbf{g})$ for all q, the integral in eq. (5) may be explicitly computed. Using the auxiliar cylindrical coordinates (ρ,φ,R) introduced above:

$$2\Psi(\mathbf{r}) = \int_0^{2\pi}\int_0^{\infty} E(\rho,\varphi,0)\rho d\rho d\varphi \simeq \int_0^{2\pi}\int_0^{\infty} \exp(-4\pi^2\tau\rho^2 D(\mathbf{g}(\varphi)))\rho d\rho d\varphi$$

$$= \int_0^{2\pi} \frac{1}{8\pi^2\tau D(\mathbf{g}(\varphi))} d\varphi \Rightarrow \Psi(\mathbf{r}) \simeq \mathcal{G}\left\{\frac{1}{16\pi^2\tau}D^{-1}(q_0\mathbf{g})\right\}(\mathbf{r}), \qquad (8)$$

so we will refer to **Q–Balls–ADC** as the FRT of the inverse of the ADC.

Application of Stokes' Theorem. Instead of the integral in all the plain orthogonal to $\mathbf{r}$, we may compute the integral in the circle Ω inside $S_\mathbf{r}$ ($S_\mathbf{r} \equiv \partial \Omega$); since $E(\mathbf{q})$ shows in general an exponential decay, the error commited in this way will be small. Using once again the cylindrical coordinates system with $\mathbf{e}_z \equiv \mathbf{r}$, this approximation may be identified with the flux integral:

$$2\Psi(\mathbf{r}) \simeq \iint_\Omega E(\rho, \varphi, 0) dA = \iint_\Omega E(\rho, \varphi, 0) \mathbf{e}_z \cdot d\mathbf{A}$$

$$= \oint_{S_\mathbf{r}} F_\varphi(q_0, \varphi, 0) \mathbf{e}_\varphi d\mathbf{l} = \int_0^{2\pi} F_\varphi(q_0, \varphi, 0) q_0 d\varphi, \qquad (9)$$

for some $\mathbf{F}(\rho, \varphi, z) = F_\varphi(\rho, \varphi, z) \mathbf{e}_\varphi$ such that $\nabla \times \mathbf{F} = E_\rho \mathbf{e}_\rho + E_\varphi \mathbf{e}_\varphi + E \mathbf{e}_z$, by virtue of Stokes' theorem (note that E_ρ and E_φ are irrelevant since they do not contribute to the flux integral). Given the expression of the curl in cylindrical coordinates, F_φ and E must be related in the way:

$$\frac{1}{\rho} \frac{\partial \rho F_\varphi(\rho, \varphi, z)}{\partial \rho} = \exp\left(-4\pi^2 \tau \rho^2 D(\rho, \varphi, z)\right) \simeq \exp\left(-4\pi^2 \tau \rho^2 D(q_0, \varphi, z)\right)$$

$$\Rightarrow F_\varphi(\rho, \varphi, z) \simeq \frac{-\exp\left(-4\pi^2 \tau \rho^2 D(q_0, \varphi, z)\right)}{8\pi^2 \tau \rho D(q_0, \varphi, z)} + \frac{\Theta(\varphi, z)}{\rho}, \qquad (10)$$

where $\Theta(\varphi, z)$ is a constant with respect to ρ: $\mathbf{F}$ needs to be non–singular at $\rho = 0$ for Stokes' theorem to apply, so we must choose $\Theta(\varphi, z) = (8\pi^2 \tau D(\varphi, z))^{-1}$. This is only a mathematical artifact, and has no other meaning in terms of the assumptions made. From eqs. (9) and (10) we define **Q–Balls–Stokes** as:

$$2\Psi(\mathbf{r}) \simeq \int_0^{2\pi} q_0 F_\varphi(q_0, \varphi, 0) d\varphi \simeq \int_0^{2\pi} \frac{1 - E(q_0, \varphi, 0)}{8\pi^2 \tau D(q_0, \varphi, 0)} d\varphi \propto \mathcal{G}\left\{\frac{1 - E(q_0 \mathbf{g})}{D(q_0 \mathbf{g})}\right\}(\mathbf{r}). \qquad (11)$$

Note that in eq. (10) we need to assume that the ADC is constant only in a local sense (in a differential environment of q_0), since we only need to define $\mathbf{F}$ for q_0. It is worth to compare this with Q–Balls–ξ, where D should be constant in a range of values of q (the larger ξ, the wider the range) and with Q–Balls–ADC, where the ADC should be constant for all q. We may highly relax the assumption of constant ADC at the expense of neglecting the integral outside Ω.

3 Methods

3.1 Practical Computation of the Estimators

The three proposed estimators based on Q–Balls (Q–Balls–ξ, Q–Balls–ADC and Q–Balls–Stokes) may be computed as the FRT of a given 3–D function (see above); therefore, we use in all cases the method and parameters suggested in [9] to find the Spherical Harmonics (SH) expansion of the corresponding signal and then to analitically compute its FRT. Note that we have obviated all the constants relating the FRT with the estimators; this is not an issue since, as suggested in [5], we normalize the resulting ODF so that their minimum is 0 and they sum to 1. For the DOT, we use the parametric implementation in [3] with $R_0 = 12\mu$m (a larger R_0 makes the DOT too sensitive to noise).

3.2 Assessment of the Accuracy Resolving Fiber Crossings

A DWI signal has been generated from a synthetic architecture comprising two crossing fiber directions in a known angle. The error between local maxima of the ODF and the ground–truth directions has been measured whenever the two fibers have been correctly detected. This methodology has been extensively used in the related literature [1,2,3,4,5,6,8,9]. In [3,8] the diffusion signal is generated with a model based on isotropic diffusion inside a bounded cylinder; however, we prefer to use the more standard methodology of multi–tensor approaches (a linear combination of eq. (1)) for three reasons:

1. The multi–tensor approach has been extensively validated, see [1,2,4,5,6,9].
2. According to our experience, both approaches perform very similar.
3. The bounded cylinder is a simplified model for the diffusion inside a neural axon, which typically has a diameter of about 5μm. Comparing this to the voxel size (1–2 mm.), it is easy to appreciate that one single voxel describes not the microscopic diffusion inside a nervous cell but the macroscopic behavior given by several hundreds or more nervous fibers. This yields a mixture of independent and (roughly) identically distributed bounded cylinder statistics, and therefore a mixture of Gaussians is a more correct model.

3.3 Setting Up of the Experiments

We use a similar methodology to that of [8]. For several combinations of b values (b = 1500, 2500 and 3500mm/s) and gradient directions (N_g = 61 and 121) we measure the angular error commited in the estimation of the local maxima of two fiber bundles (matched to realistic biological parameters). We use order $L = 6$ in the SH expansion in all cases. For the noisy scenarios, we corrupt the diffusion signal with Rician noise adding a complex Gaussian noise with standard deviation σ and computing its envelope. Noise power is parameterized by the Peak Signal to Noise Ratio (PSNR), defined as the quotient between the value of the baseline and σ. Results are an average for 100 Montecarlo trials, and in this case we consider that a given estimator is able to find the two fibers if they are detected in more than the 50% of the trials.

4 Results and Discussion

In Fig. 1 the results without noise contamination are shown. **First**, note that the results are consistent with those previously reported in [8]: increasing the b value or the number of gradient directions improves the capability detection for all estimators, and the angular error is decreased as well. For a given configuration, Q–Balls perform worse than DOT, which is the same as saying that Q–Balls need a greater b value or more gradient directions to achieve an accuracy similar to DOT [8]. **Second**, if we compare traditional Q–Balls with the estimators based on a constant (at least in a range of b values) ADC (i.e., Q–Balls–ξ and Q–Balls–ADC), regular Q–Balls perform better in all cases: although assuming a constant

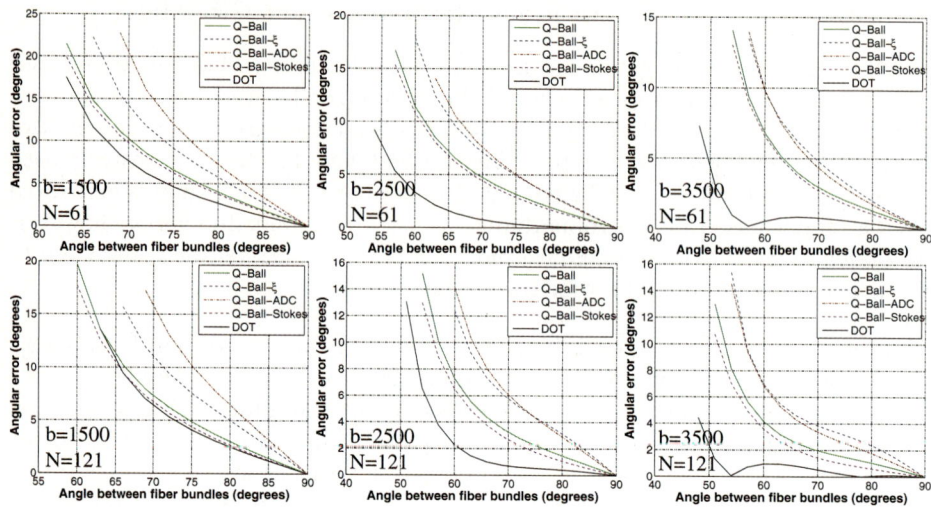

Fig. 1. Angular error in the recovering of two fiber bundles vs. the original angle between their directions, for the six configurations tested and for all estimators. The diffusion signals have not been contaminated with Rician noise.

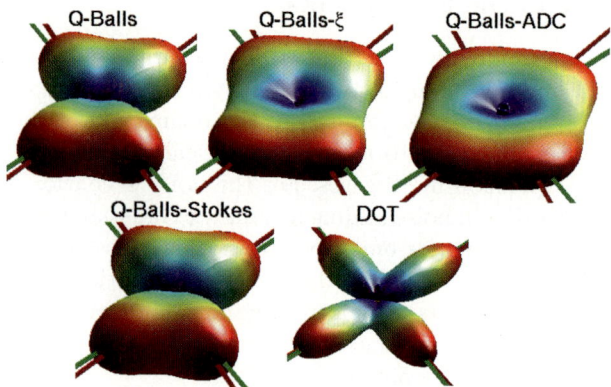

Fig. 2. 3–D plot of the orientation functions (ODF for Q–Balls based estimators and $P(R_0 \mathbf{r})$ for DOT), for $b = 3500$, $N_g = 121$ and an angle of $60°$. Red axis represent local maxima of the estimators, and green axis the ground–truth directions.

ADC allows to reduce (for Q–Balls–ξ) or completely eliminate (for Q–Balls–ADC) the blurring due to the FRT, the error introduced by this oversimplified assumption does not compensate its benefit. Note that Q–Balls–ADC perform worse than Q–Balls–ξ except for very high b–values (when they perform very similar), so the more restrictive the assumption the worse the accuracy. **Third,** Q–Balls–Stokes perform better than regular Q–Balls in all cases (and even better than DOT for $b = 1500$ and 121 gradient directions), although the improvement

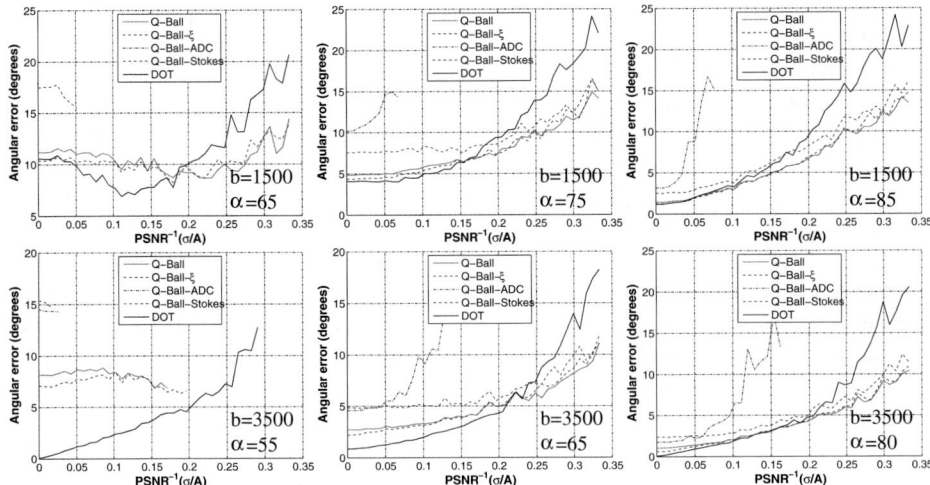

Fig. 3. Angular error vs. the inverse of the PSNR, for $N_g = 121$, and different b values and crossing angles, for all estimators

is quite subtle; in this case, the constant ADC assumption is needed only in a local (differential) sense, which is far more realistic. For Q–Balls–Stokes, the error due to the assumption has to be added to the error due to the integration inside $S_\mathbf{r}$ and not the whole orthogonal plane to $\mathbf{r}$, but they still improve the performance of Q–Balls. For illustrative purposes, we show in Fig. 2 a 3–D plot of the orientation functions given by each estimator: DOT is able to yield well defined lobs, meanwhile Q–Balls based estimators produce wider lobs and therefore a higher uncertainty in the location of fiber directions. Q–Balls–Stokes yield a very similar ODF to Q–Balls, but for Q–Balls–ξ and Q–Balls–ADC the lobs are even more blurred; once again, we may **conclude** that the constant ADC assumption introduces a high error in the estimation of the ODF which does not compensate the reduction of the FRT blurring, unless the assumption is applied in a local sense.

To test the behavior in the presence of noise, we vary the noise power σ and study the angular error (see Fig. 3). **First**, note that in general regular Q–Balls are still better than Q–Balls–ξ and Q–Balls–ADC, and Q–Balls–Stokes better than Q–Balls. **Second**, Q–Balls and Q–Balls–Stokes are more stable to noise than DOT: its accuracy is worsened in the presence of noise, but not as much as DOT accuracy does. **Third**, note that Q–Balls and Q–Balls–Stokes may be preferable to DOT for very noisy scenarios and large angles of crossing or low b values; this issue has been previously reported for regular Q–Balls in [8].

5 Conclusion

One of the benefits of Q–Ball estimation of fiber populations is that it does not require to make any assumption on the behavior of the diffusion signal;

this advantage carries out the drawback of the blurring in the radial integral defining the ODF, driving to broadened lobes in the orientation information. This drawback may be palliated by including some sort of assumptions. However, we have shown that the mono–exponential decay model in general introduces an important error, more important than the blurring inherent to Q–Balls. The same model has been successfully used in the DOT, which has been shown to be more accurate than Q–Balls in general. Since the implementations used here for both of them use the same numerical scheme (based on the SH expansion of the attenuation signal, compare [9] and [3]), the reason for this difference has to be in the orientation function Q–Balls estimate, which is, the ODF: the ODF is more sensible than the probability profile $P(R_0 \mathbf{r})$ computed with the DOT. On the other hand, we have introduced a new technique, Q–Balls–Stokes, to improve the accuracy of regular Q–Balls; although its benefit is quite subtle, it outperforms Q–Balls in all cases, and even may outperform, for noisy scenarios with low b values (or high crossing angles), the DOT.

Acknowledgments. Work partially funded by grant numbers TEC2007–67073/TCM from the CICyT (Spain) and NIH R01 MH074794, NIH P41 RR13218.

References

1. Descoteaux, M., Angelino, E., Fitzgibbons, S., Deriche, R.: Apparent Diffusion Profile estimation from High Angular Resolution Diffusion Images: estimation and applications. Magn. Res. in Medicine 56(2), 395–410 (2006)
2. Jansons, K.M., Alexander, D.C.: Persistent Angular Structures: new insights from diffusion magnetic resonance imaging data. Inverse Problems 19, 1031–1046 (2003)
3. Özarslan, E., Sepherd, T.M., Vemuri, B.C., Blackband, S.J., Mareci, T.H.: Resolution of complex tissue microarchitecture using the Diffusion Orientation Transform (DOT). Neuroimage 31, 1086–1103 (2006)
4. Tournier, J.D., Calamante, F., Connelly, A.: Robust determination of the fibre orientation distribution in diffusion MRI: Non–negativity constrained super–resolved spherical deconvolution. Neuroimage 35, 1459–1472 (2007)
5. Tuch, D.S., Reese, T.G., Wiegell, M.R., Wedeen, V.J.: Diffusion MRI of complex neural architecture. Neuron 40, 885–895 (2003)
6. Tuch, D.S.: Q–Ball imaging. Magn. Res. in Medicine 52, 1358–1372 (2004)
7. Campbell, J.S., Siddiqi, K., Rymar, V.V., Sadikot, A.F., Pike, G.B.: Flow-based fiber tracking with diffusion tensor and Q-ball data: Validation and comparison to principal diffusion direction techniques. Neuroimage 27(4), 725–736 (2005)
8. Prčkovska, V., Roebroeck, A., Pullens, W., Vilanova, A., ter Haar Romeny, B.: Optimal acquisition schemes in High Angular Resolution Diffusion Weighted Imaging. In: Metaxas, D., Axel, L., Fichtinger, G., Székely, G. (eds.) MICCAI 2008, Part II. LNCS, vol. 5242, pp. 9–17. Springer, Heidelberg (2008)
9. Descoteaux, M., Angelino, E., Fitzgibbons, S., Deriche, R.: Regularized, fast, and robust analytical Q-Ball imaging. Magn. Res. in Medicine 58, 497–510 (2007)
10. Stejskal, E.O., Tanner, J.E.: Spin diffusion measurements: Spin echoes in the presence of a time-dependent field gradient. J. of Chem. Phys. 42, 288–292 (1965)
11. Callaghan, P.T.: Principles of Nuclear Magnetic Resonance Microscopy. Clarendon Press, Oxford (1991)

Multiple Q-Shell ODF Reconstruction in Q-Ball Imaging

Iman Aganj[1], Christophe Lenglet[1,2], Guillermo Sapiro[1], Essa Yacoub[2], Kamil Ugurbil[2], and Noam Harel[2]

[1] Department of Electrical and Computer Engineering, University of Minnesota, USA
[2] Center for Magnetic Resonance Research, University of Minnesota, USA
{iman,clenglet,guille,yaco0006,ugurb001,harel002}@umn.edu

Abstract. Q-ball imaging (QBI) is a high angular resolution diffusion imaging (HARDI) technique which has been proven very successful in resolving multiple intravoxel fiber orientations in MR images. The standard computation of the orientation distribution function (ODF, the probability of diffusion in a given direction) from q-ball uses linear radial projection, neglecting the change in the volume element along the ray, thereby resulting in distributions different from the *true* ODFs. A new technique has been recently proposed that, by considering the solid angle factor, uses the mathematically correct definition of the ODF and results in a dimensionless and normalized ODF expression from a single q-shell. In this paper, we extend this technique in order to exploit HARDI data from multiple q-shells. We consider the more flexible multi-exponential model for the diffusion signal, and show how to efficiently compute the ODFs in constant solid angle. We describe our method and demonstrate its improved performance on both artificial and real HARDI data.

1 Introduction

Diffusion-weighted magnetic resonance imaging (DWMRI) provides valuable information about the fiber architecture of neural tissue by measuring the diffusion of water molecules in three-dimensional (3D) space. The diffusion function may be measured by using the model-free diffusion spectrum imaging (DSI) [1], which is the direct Fourier inversion of the diffusion signal. This technique is however time intensive, as it measures the diffusion signal on a 3D Cartesian lattice. Thus, an alternative approach based on sampling on one or multiple spherical shells has been proposed, referred to as high angular resolution diffusion imaging (HARDI) [2].

While the 3D probability density function (PDF) of the diffusion is helpful in studying the tissue microstructure, the orientation distribution function (ODF) – the marginal probability of diffusion in a given direction – is the quantity of interest for mapping the orientation architecture of the tissue. Q-ball imaging (QBI), [3], is a widely used ODF reconstruction scheme for HARDI, based on a spherical tomographic inversion called the Funk-Radon transform. This technique's simplicity and its ability to resolve intravoxel fiber orientations have made it popular for fiber tracking and characterizing white matter architecture. Moreover, a few works have suggested exploiting data from multiple q-shells to benefit from the high signal-to-noise ratio (SNR) and high angular contrast-to-noise ratio (CNR) of the data acquired at respectively low and high b-values, [3]–[5]. Using multiple q-shells also allows us to employ richer models for the diffusion signal, as discussed in this paper.

Nonetheless, with the exception of our previous paper [6] and a very recent parallel and independent work [7] (the differences will be detailed in Sec. 2.2), the definition of the ODF used in QBI has been different from the actual marginal PDF of diffusion in a constant solid angle. It has been computed as a linear radial projection of the PDF, which does not take into account the quadratic growth of the volume element with respect to its distance from the origin (see Sec. 2.1 for details). This inaccurate formulation generally distorts the ODF, and has created the need for post-processing such as manual normalization and sharpening [8].

We recently proposed, [6], a new ODF expression for QBI which is derived from the proper definition of the ODF in constant solid angle. We showed that the computed ODF is inherently normalized and dimensionless, producing without any post-processing, sharp ODFs with improved resolution of multiple fiber orientations. In this paper, we extend this work by deriving a general formulation for multiple q-shell QBI. We demonstrate the improvement achieved by considering the information from multiple q-shells, and using richer multi-exponential models.

In Sec. 2 we describe the foundation of our mathematical derivation, along with a brief version of the proof, and also provide an implementation scheme. Experimental results are presented in Sec. 3, along with a brief discussion.

2 ODF Computation in Solid Angle: Multiple q-Shell Formulation

2.1 General ODF Definition

The PDF of the diffusion of water molecules, $P(\vec{r})$, gives the displacement probability $P(\vec{r})dv$ of a molecule, initially placed at the origin, to be in the infinitesimal volume dv located at $\vec{r}$ after a certain amount of time. We assume this function to be symmetric (i.e. $P(-\vec{r}) = P(\vec{r})$), which is a quite common assumption in DWMRI. The PDF is represented in the standard spherical coordinates, (r, θ, ϕ), with the displacement vector $\vec{r} = r\hat{u}$ and the unit direction vector $\hat{u}(\theta, \phi) = (\sin\theta\cos\phi, \sin\theta\sin\phi, \cos\theta)^T$. The volume element in this case is $dv = r^2 dr d\Omega$ with $d\Omega = \sin\theta\, d\theta d\phi$ being the infinitesimal solid angle element.

We denote by $ODF(\hat{u})d\Omega$ the probability of diffusion in the direction $\hat{u}$ through the solid angle $d\Omega$, which is computed by integrating the displacement probabilities, i.e., $P(\vec{r})dv = P(r\hat{u})r^2 dr d\Omega$, for all magnitude r, while keeping $\hat{u}$ constant:

$$ODF(\hat{u}) = \int_0^\infty P(r\hat{u})r^2 dr \qquad (1)$$

The above definition, which is normalized and dimensionless, is the integral of the probability values in a cone of "very small" constant solid angle. This correct definition was used for instance by the authors of [1] in DSI, where $P(\vec{r})$ was first computed from the diffusion data via Fourier inversion and then integrated to calculate the ODF. However to the best of our knowledge, the expression for ODF reconstruction so far used in QBI [3], (except for our previous work [6] and a very recent parallel and independent paper [7], both for single q-shell) is different from Eq. (1), in the sense that the integral is not weighted by the important (and mathematically correct) factor r^2. Without including this factor, the radial projection gives an artificial weight to $P(\vec{r})$ which is, respectively, too large and too small for points close to and far from the origin. Moreover, the ODF will not be necessarily normalized or dimensionless, and manual normalization will be required.

Next we derive a closed-form ODF expression in *multiple* q-shell QBI using the *correct r^2-weighted* integral.

2.2 Q-Ball Imaging ODF Reconstruction

In this section, we derive the ODF expression in multiple q-shell QBI, and present a brief proof of the derivation.

Let $E(\vec{q})$ be the 3D Fourier transform function of $P(\vec{r})$. Theoretically, we know that $E(0) = 1$, since the zero frequency of a PDF is its integral over the entire space, yielding 1. In addition, we have the values of $E(\vec{q})$ measured on M different q-balls, i.e., the frequencies with constant norm $|\vec{q}| = q_i$, $i = 1, \ldots, M$, as $\tilde{E}_i(\hat{u}) := E(q_i \hat{u}) = \frac{S_i(\hat{u})}{S_0}$, where $S_i(\hat{u})$ is the HARDI signal on the ith q-ball and S_0 is the base-line image.

Our mathematical derivation is based on the following two relatively simple yet fundamental facts from Fourier analysis:

- The Fourier transform of $P(\vec{r})|\vec{r}|^2$ is $-\nabla^2 E(\vec{q})$, where ∇^2 is the Laplacian operator.
- For a symmetric function $f: \mathbb{R}^3 \to \mathbb{R}$ with the 3D Fourier transform function $F(\vec{q})$, and for the arbitrary unit vector $\hat{u}$, we have that $\int_0^\infty f(r\hat{u})dr = \frac{1}{8\pi^2} \iint_{\hat{u}^\perp} F(\vec{q})d^2\vec{q}$, with $\hat{u}^\perp$ being the plane perpendicular to $\hat{u}$.

Combining these statements with Eq. (1) leads to

$$ODF(\hat{u}) = -\frac{1}{8\pi^2} \iint_{\hat{u}^\perp} \nabla^2 E(\vec{q}) d^2\vec{q}$$

Now, without loss of generality, we choose our coordinates such that $\hat{z} = \hat{u}$, thus making $\hat{u}^\perp$ the q_x-q_y plane. We then use the following expansion for the Laplacian in spherical coordinates, (q, θ, ϕ):

$$\nabla^2 E = \frac{1}{q}\frac{\partial^2}{\partial q^2}(qE) + \frac{1}{q^2}\nabla_b^2 E$$

where ∇_b^2 is the Laplace-Beltrami operator, which is defined independently of the radial component q, as $\nabla_b^2 E = \frac{1}{\sin\theta}\frac{\partial}{\partial\theta}\left(\sin\theta \frac{\partial E}{\partial\theta}\right) + \frac{1}{\sin^2\theta}\frac{\partial^2 E}{\partial\phi^2}$. The surface integral on the q_x-q_y plane is computed by fixing $\theta = \frac{\pi}{2}$ and using the expression $d^2\vec{q} = qdqd\phi$

$$ODF(\hat{z}) = -\frac{1}{8\pi^2} \int_0^{2\pi} \int_0^\infty \nabla^2 E(\vec{q}) q dq d\phi$$

$$= -\frac{1}{8\pi^2} \int_0^{2\pi} \int_0^\infty \left(\frac{1}{q}\frac{\partial^2}{\partial q^2}(qE) + \frac{1}{q^2}\nabla_b^2 E\right) q dq \, d\phi$$

The integral of the first term can be seen to be constant and independent of $E(\vec{q})$,

$$\int_0^{2\pi} \int_0^{\infty} \left(\frac{1}{q}\frac{\partial^2}{\partial q^2}(qE)\right) q\,dq\,d\phi = -2\pi E(0) = -2\pi$$

Therefore,

$$ODF(\hat{z}) = \frac{1}{4\pi} - \frac{1}{8\pi^2} \int_0^{2\pi} \int_0^{\infty} \frac{1}{q} \nabla_b^2 E(\vec{q})\,dq\,d\phi$$

while $\theta = \frac{\pi}{2}$ is kept constant in the integration.

To compute the integral of the second term, the values of $E(\vec{q})$ are required in the entire q-space, which are in general – except for the time-consuming DSI modality – not available. Thus, we need to approximate $E(\vec{q})$ from the values measured on the q-balls. In this work, we consider the following radial multi-exponential model [9],

$$E(q\hat{u}) \cong \sum_{k=1}^{N} \lambda_k(\hat{u})\alpha_k(\hat{u})^{q^2}$$

with the constraints

$$0 < \alpha_k(\hat{u}), \lambda_k(\hat{u}) < 1$$

$$\sum_{k=1}^{N} \lambda_k(\hat{u}) = 1 \qquad (2)$$

where Eq. (2) comes from the fact that $E(0) = 1$.[1] Once the values of λ_k and α_k are estimated (see Sec. 2.3), they can be used in the following ODF expression, which is obtained by a few more steps of calculation,

$$ODF(\hat{z}) = \frac{1}{4\pi} + \frac{1}{16\pi^2} \int_0^{2\pi} \nabla_b^2 \sum_{k=1}^{N} \lambda_k(\hat{u})\ln(-\ln\alpha_k(\hat{u}))\,d\phi$$

Finally, rewriting the expression independent of the choice of the axes, the following analytical formula can be derived for the ODF:

$$ODF(\hat{u}) = \frac{1}{4\pi} + \frac{1}{16\pi^2} FRT\left\{\nabla_b^2 \sum_{k=1}^{N} \lambda_k(\hat{u})\ln(-\ln\alpha_k(\hat{u}))\right\} \qquad (3)$$

where $FRT\{f(\hat{u})\} := \iint_{\hat{u}^\perp} f(\vec{w})\delta(|\vec{w}| - 1)d^2\vec{w}$ is the Funk-Radon transform [3].

The above ODF expression is dimensionless and intrinsically normalized, since the integrals of the first and second terms over the sphere are respectively 1 and 0. This is in contrast to the (single q-shell) ODF formulas used in original QBI, i.e., $\frac{1}{Z}FRT\{\tilde{E}_1(\hat{u})\}$, and also in [7], where a normalization factor Z is needed. Additional differences can be observed in the approach presented here and in [6], compared to

---

[1] This is in fact an additional advantage of this model over the original QBI model for single q-shell, i.e. $E(q\hat{u}) \cong E(q_1\hat{u})\delta(q - q_1)$, where $E(0)$ was assumed to be zero.

[7]. As demonstrated here, integration of the radial part of the Laplacian on the plane always results in a constant without requiring any model for the diffusion signal. Yet, [7] uses the Bessel approximation of the Dirac delta function which yields a variable (sometimes negative) term. As for the integral of the tangential term of the Laplacian, we use the exponential model that is particularly consistent with $E(0) = 1$, in contrast to [7] that assumes the tangential term to be zero outside the q-ball, leading to an expression similar to Laplacian-Beltrami sharpening.

2.3 Parameter Estimation

In order to approximate the diffusion signal in a direction $\hat{u}$ by a weighted sum of N exponentials, we need to estimate the $2N$ parameters $\lambda_k(\hat{u})$ and $\alpha_k(\hat{u})$, for $k = 1, \ldots, N$. We continue this subsection considering a fixed direction, and therefore drop the notation $(\hat{u})$. To estimate the aforementioned parameters, at least $2N - 1$ independent equations – besides Eq. (2) – are required, which can be obtained from the HARDI signals measured on M q-balls, for $M \geq 2N - 1$. Numerical optimization approaches such as the trust region algorithm, [10], may be employed to solve this non-linear system in the most general case. Here, however, we discuss two special cases with closed-form analytical solutions.

The mono-exponential assumption ($N = 1$) requires measurement on at least $M = 1$ q-ball. As it has been shown in [6], $M = 1$ leads to $\lambda_1 = 1$ and $\alpha_1 = \tilde{E}_1^{\frac{1}{q_1^2}}$.[2] Furthermore, if measured values are provided on more than one q-balls and the mono-exponential model is still desired, one can fit the best exponential by computing the average Apparent Diffusion Coefficient ($ADC := -\frac{1}{b}\ln\frac{S}{S_0}$) across all the q-shells.

Another practical case of great interest arises when we consider the richer bi-exponential model ($N = 2$, see for example [11]) to reconstruct the ODFs from (at least) $M = 3$ q-shells. Parameterizing the problem in terms of b-values, $b_i = \tau q_i^2$, and choosing the physical units such that the diffusion time $\tau = 1$ (see also Footnote 2), we obtain (for $M = 3$) the following system of equations for each direction:

$$\lambda \alpha^{b_i} + (1-\lambda)\beta^{b_i} = \tilde{E}_i \quad , \quad i = 1,2,3$$
$$0 < \alpha, \beta, \lambda < 1$$

An analytical solution can be derived for the particular and reasonable case when the sequence $0, b_1, b_2, b_3$ is an arithmetic progress.[3] We describe this solution here, along with some regularization that guarantees the parameters to remain within the correct range.[4] Without loss of generality, let us assume $\alpha \geq \beta$, and also choose the physical units such that $b_1 = 1$, $b_2 = 2$, and $b_3 = 3$. Then,

---

[2] Note that if the set $\{a_k(\hat{u})\}$ is a solution, then $\{a_k(\hat{u})^\gamma\}$ for a constant γ can be shown to result in the same computed ODF. Therefore, since in the mono-exponential case $\gamma := q_1^2$ is a constant, $a_1(\hat{u}) = \tilde{E}_1(\hat{u})$ is also a correct solution.
[3] The sequence $x_1, x_2, \ldots, x_i, \ldots$ is an arithmetic progress if $x_i - x_{i-1}$ is constant.
[4] Recall that the three parameters can also be computed in the general case following optimization techniques such as those in [10]. The proposed ODF model is general, and it becomes only simpler when the data is acquired at an arithmetic sequence of b-values.

$$\lambda \alpha^i + (1-\lambda)\beta^i = \tilde{E}_i \quad , \quad i = 1,2,3$$

We first define and calculate the following two quantities:

$$A := \frac{\alpha + \beta}{2} = \frac{\tilde{E}_3 - \tilde{E}_1 \tilde{E}_2}{2(\tilde{E}_2 - \tilde{E}_1^2)} \quad , \quad B := \frac{\alpha - \beta}{2} = \sqrt{\left(\frac{\tilde{E}_3 - \tilde{E}_1 \tilde{E}_2}{2(\tilde{E}_2 - \tilde{E}_1^2)}\right)^2 - \frac{\tilde{E}_1 \tilde{E}_3 - \tilde{E}_2^2}{\tilde{E}_2 - \tilde{E}_1^2}}$$

The parameters are afterward computed as follows:

$$\alpha = A + B \quad , \quad \beta = A - B \quad , \quad \lambda = \frac{1}{2} + \frac{\tilde{E}_1 - A}{2B}$$

However, we still need to ensure that they are real and in the correct ranges. One can verify that these conditions are satisfied by enforcing the following constraints:

$$0 < \tilde{E}_3 < \tilde{E}_2 < \tilde{E}_1 < 1 \quad , \quad \tilde{E}_1^2 < \tilde{E}_2 \quad , \quad \tilde{E}_2^2 < \tilde{E}_1 \tilde{E}_3$$

$$\tilde{E}_3 - \tilde{E}_1 \tilde{E}_2 < \tilde{E}_2 - \tilde{E}_1^2 + \tilde{E}_1 \tilde{E}_3 - \tilde{E}_2^2$$

Thus, we can obtain the optimal values of α, β, and λ, by initially projecting $\tilde{E}_i$s onto the subspace defined by these inequalities,[5] and then computing the parameters.

2.4 Implementation

Our implementation of the ODF reconstruction from the estimated values of $\lambda_k(\hat{u})$ and $a_k(\hat{u})$ makes use of the spherical harmonic (SH) basis, $Y_l^m(\hat{u})$, which is common for the analysis of HARDI data. The steps taken here to numerically compute Eq. (3) are similar to those described in [8]. Particularly, we use the real and symmetric *modified SH* basis introduced in [8], where SH functions are indexed by a single parameter j corresponding to l_j and m_j. We adopt a minimum least square scheme to compute a set of modified SH coefficients, c_j, such that $\sum_{k=1}^{N} \lambda_k(\hat{u}) \ln(-\ln a_k(\hat{u})) \approx \sum_{j=1}^{R} c_j Y_j(\hat{u})$, where $R = (L+1)(L+2)/2$, with L being the order of the SH basis (we chose L= 4 throughout our experiments). Next, since the SH elements are eigenfunctions of the Laplace-Beltrami operator, we compute $\nabla_b^2 \sum_{k=1}^{N} \lambda_k(\hat{u}) \ln(-\ln a_k(\hat{u}))$ by multiplying the coefficients c_j by their corresponding eigenvalues, $-l_j(l_j + 1)$. Then, as suggested in [8], the Funk-Radon transform is computed by multiplying the coefficients by $2\pi P_{l_j}(0)$, where $P_l(\cdot)$ is the Legendre polynomial of degree l, with $P_l(0) = (-1)^{\frac{l}{2}} \frac{1 \times 3 \times \cdots \times (l-1)}{2 \times 4 \times \cdots \times l}$ for even l. Finally, given that $Y_1(\hat{u}) = \frac{1}{2\sqrt{\pi}}$, the SH coefficients of the ODF are derived as

$$c_j' = \begin{cases} \dfrac{1}{2\sqrt{\pi}} & j = 1 \\ -\dfrac{1}{8\pi}(-1)^{\frac{l_j}{2}} \dfrac{1 \times 3 \times \cdots \times (l_j + 1)}{2 \times 4 \times \cdots \times (l_j - 2)} c_j & j > 1 \end{cases}$$

---

[5] Note that such projection is usually necessary, because the bi-exponential assumption may not be accurate and the data may be noisy. Moreover, using a small separating margin of $\delta = 0.01{\sim}0.1$ in the inequalities makes the ODFs in practice more stable.

The implementation of the proposed formula for the true ODF is as straightforward as the one introduced in [8] for the original ODF formula.

3 Results and Discussion

To demonstrate the advantages of exploiting multiple q-shells in QBI, we first show the experimental results on an artificial example which consists of large diffusion values in two orthogonal directions. We synthesized diffusion images by sampling the sum of two exponentials, $E(\vec{q}) = (|\sin\phi|^{q^2/2} + |\cos\phi|^{q^2/2})/2$, on seven q-shells ($b = q^2 = 1, 2, ..., 7$) and in 76 directions, uniformly distributed on the hemisphere. Figure 1 illustrates the ODFs reconstructed from single q-shells for different b-values, three q-shells with mono-exponential model, and three q-shells with bi-exponential model. As can be observed, for the data acquired at low b-values ($b = 1, 2, 3$), the bi-exponential model using three q-shells is the only method correctly resolving the horizontal and vertical ODF peaks, corresponding to the strong ADC values in those directions ($\phi = 0°, 90°, 180°, 270°$). It should be noted, however, that the drawback of such a more general model is its lesser robustness to noise, as low order models are often more robust (e.g., computing the average of a signal is more robust than estimating the actual signal). ODFs are shown as they are; no min-max normalization is used in any of the figures. Dark red represents negative values.

We also tested our method on the real HARDI dataset introduced in [12]. An anesthetized young Macaca mulatta monkey was scanned using a 7T MR scanner (Siemens) equipped with a head gradient coil (80mT/m G-maximum, 200mT/m/ms) with a diffusion weighted spin-echo EPI sequence. Diffusion images were acquired (twice during the same session, and then averaged) over 100 directions uniformly distributed on the sphere. We used three b-values of 1000, 2000, and 3000 s/mm², TR/TE of 4600/65 ms, and the voxel size of 1×1×1 mm³. The ODFs were reconstructed from the three q-shells using both mono-exponential and bi-exponential methods, and also from the single q-shells individually. Figure 2 depicts the results on a coronal slice through the centrum semiovale area, superimposed on the fractional anisotropy (FA) map. Note how using the bi-exponential method allows for more clear recovery of certain fiber bundles, such as callosal radiations and corticospinal tract, and better resolution of crossing areas (see outlined regions in Fig. 2). Figure 2 (top, right) is the only subfigure illustrating results by the original QBI (without r^2).

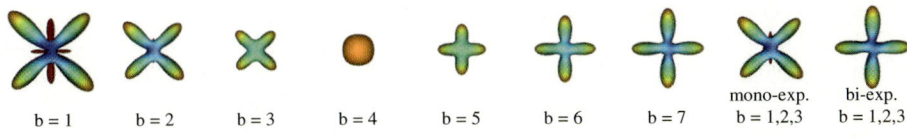

Fig. 1. Results of the ODF reconstruction on synthetic data. Note how the bi-exponential model correctly resolves the maxima of the ODF from low b-values.

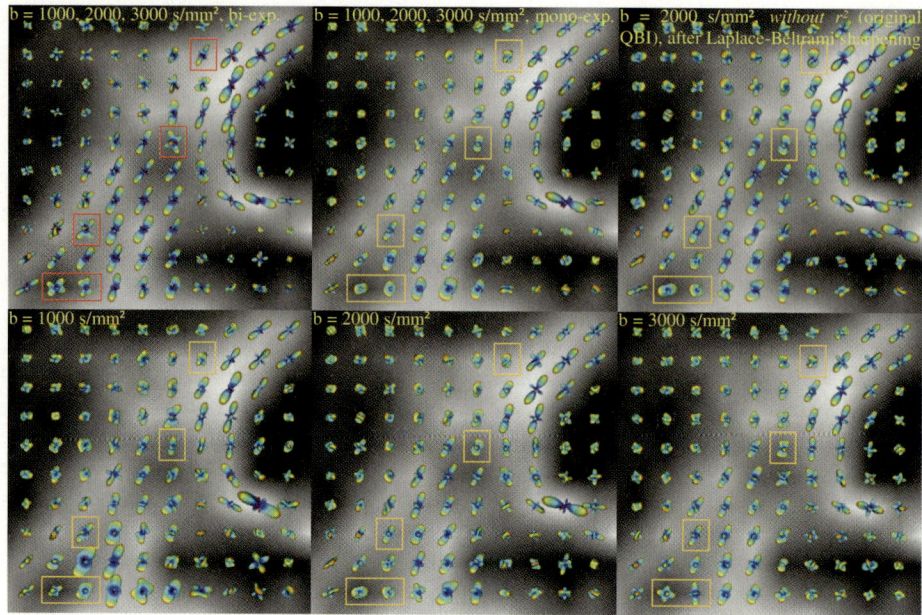

Fig. 2. Reconstructed ODFs from the real brain data, shown on the FA map. The bi-exponential model ODFs (top, left) have been scaled down 1.5 times for better comparison. All the ODFs except those in (top, right) have been reconstructed considering the factor r^2.

Acknowledgments. This work was partly supported by NIH, NSF, the Keck Foundation, ONR, NGA, ARO, and DARPA.

References

1. Wedeen, V., Hagmann, P., Tseng, W., Reese, T., Weisskoff, R.: Mapping complex tissue architecture with diffusion spectrum magnetic resonance imaging. Magnetic Resonance in Medicine 54(6), 1377–1386 (2005)
2. Tuch, D., Reese, T., Wiegell, M., Makris, N., Belliveau, J., Wedeen, V.: High angular resolution diffusion imaging reveals intravoxel white matter fiber heterogeneity. Magnetic Resonance in Medicine 48(4), 577–582 (2002)
3. Tuch, D.: Q-ball imaging. Magnetic Resonance in Medicine 52(6), 1358–1372 (2004)
4. Khachaturian, M.H., Wisco, J.J., Tuch, D.S.: Boosting the sampling efficiency of q-ball imaging using multiple wavevector fusion. Magn. Res. Med. 57(2), 289–296 (2007)
5. Wu, Y.C., Field, A.S., Alexander, A.L.: Computation of diffusion function measures in q-space using magnetic resonance hybrid diffusion imaging. IEEE Trans. on Medical Imaging 27(6), 858–865 (2008)
6. Aganj, I., Lenglet, C., Sapiro, G.: ODF reconstruction in q-ball imaging with solid angle consideration. In: Proc. 6th Intl. Symp. on Biomedical Imaging, Boston (2009)
7. Tristán-Vega, A., Westin, C., Aja-Fernández, S.: Estimation of fiber orientation probability density functions in high angular resolution diffusion imaging. NeuroImage 47(2), 623–650 (2009)

8. Descoteaux, M., Angelino, E., Fitzgibbons, S., Deriche, R.: Regularized, fast, and robust analytical q-ball imaging. Magnetic Resonance in Medicine 58(2), 497–510 (2007)
9. Özarslan, E., Shepherd, T., Vemuri, B., Blackband, S., Mareci, T.: Resolution of complex tissue microarchitecture using the diffusion orientation transform (DOT). NeuroImage 31, 1086–1103 (2006)
10. Branch, M.A., Coleman, T.F., Li, Y.: A subspace, interior, and conjugate gradient method for large-scale bound-constrained minimization problems. SIAM J. on Scientific Computing 21(1), 1–23 (1999)
11. Yeh, C.H., Cho, K.H., Lin, H.C., Wang, J.J., Lin, C.P.: Reduced encoding diffusion spectrum imaging implemented with a bi-Gaussian model. IEEE Trans. on Medical Imaging 27(10), 1415–1424 (2008)
12. Lenglet, C., Yacoub, E., Ghose, G., Adriany, G., Krüger, G., Sapiro, G., Ugurbil, K., Harel, N.: High resolution diffusion MRI on in-vivo monkey brains at 7T. In: Proc. 14th Annual Meeting of the Organization for Human Brain Mapping, San Francisco (2009)

Lossless Online Ensemble Learning (LOEL) and Its Application to Subcortical Segmentation*

Jonathan H. Morra, Zhuowen Tu, Arthur W. Toga, and Paul M. Thompson

Laboratory of Neuro Imaging, UCLA School of Medicine, Los Angeles, CA, USA

Abstract. In this paper, we study the classification problem in the situation where large volumes of training data become available sequentially (online learning). In medical imaging, this is typical, e.g., a 3D brain MRI dataset may be gradually collected from a patient population, and not all of the data is available when the analysis begins. First, we describe two common ensemble learning algorithms, AdaBoost and bagging, and their corresponding online learning versions. We then show why each is ineffective for segmenting a gradually increasing set of medical images. Instead, we introduce a new ensemble learning algorithm, termed Lossless Online Ensemble Learning (LOEL). This algorithm is lossless in the online case, compared to its batch mode. LOEL outperformed online-AdaBoost and online-bagging when validated on a standardized dataset; it also performed better when used to segment the hippocampus from brain MRI scans of patients with Alzheimer's Disease and matched healthy subjects. Among those tested, LOEL largely outperformed the alternative online learning algorithms and gave excellent error metrics that were consistent between the online and offline case; it also accurately distinguished AD subjects from healthy controls based on automated measures of hippocampal volume.

1 Introduction

The fields of data mining and biomedical engineering have recently seen a vast increase in the amount of available data. Ongoing medical imaging studies commonly analyze images from hundreds or even thousands of patients, sometimes scanned at multiple time-points. Many brain MRI studies focus on one particular brain region (hippocampus, caudate, etc.), and a first step in studying these structures is finding them on brain MRI, using a classification or segmentation algorithm. Boosting [1] and bagging [2] algorithms and their extensions have shown great promise for effective classification of voxels in images [3,4,5], but it is not always straightforward to create a training dataset for the algorithm

---

* This work was funded by the National Institutes of Health through the NIH Roadmap for Medical Research, Grant U54 RR021813 entitled Center for Computational Biology (CCB), the National Institute for Biomedical Imaging and Bioengineering, the National Center for Research Resources, National Institute on Aging, the National Library of Medicine, and the National Institute for Child Health and Development (EB01651, RR019771, HD050735, AG016570, LM05639).

to learn which features are relevant for classification. In studies where data acquisition is ongoing (such as the Alzheimer's Disease Neuroimaging Initiative, ADNI [6], which scans 800 subjects every 6 months for 3 years), one may wish to begin to use a segmenter after each set of scans becomes available; in other applications, one may not have access to all previous scans used to train the algorithm in the past, or have time to retrain. In either case, an online algorithm is desirable. In imaging studies, the set of relevant features for classification may lie in a very high-dimensional space, so the algorithm must be able to use this information in a reasonable amount of time. Ensemble learning methods (such as bagging and boosting) are good candidate classifiers for combining information from thousands of potentially useful features: they combine weak classifiers - which individually may perform only slightly better than chance - to create a strong classifier that outperforms all of the component classifiers. These learning algorithms can be very effective for image segmentation as they can "select" important features, and overlook unimportant ones.

In such a situation, training data may arrive as a sequence of image sets, e.g., 100 volumes at a time. For example, in multi-site drug trials or longitudinal studies such as ADNI [6], it is vital to begin data analysis as soon as possible, while benefiting from the increasing pool of available scans. The original formulations of boosting and bagging required all training data to be available before training could begin; this is known as batch learning. The recently-developed online versions of bagging and boosting [7] have drawbacks because the algorithm focuses on updating the weights based on the sampled data each time, to simulate the batch training mode on a fixed set of weak learners. By just focusing on updating the weights (in boosting), and selecting the training samples (in bagging), these methods overlook the need to select appropriate features automatically, which is vital in image segmentation applications.

In this paper, we first use Oza's versions of online boosting and online bagging and then introduce our new algorithm, LOEL, which extends the idea of online learning to medical image segmentation. LOEL is lossless and outperforms both boosting and bagging in the online case, and is comparable to both in the offline case.

2 Methods

2.1 Problem and Previous Work

When segmenting brain structures in 3D MRI scans, one seeks to assign each voxel to one or more regions of interest (ROI). Here we focus on the two-class case and, without loss of generality, we will study the segmentation of the hippocampus, a structure that degenerates in Alzheimer's disease and is a target of interest in ongoing drug trials. Let $X = (x_1 \cdots x_N)$ be all the voxels in the manually labeled testing set and $Y = (y_1 \cdots y_N)$ be the ground truth labels for each x_n, such that $y_n \in [-1, 1]$. From discriminative learning point of view, we seek a classifier to minimize the error $e = \sum_i |y_i - F(X_{N_i})|$ where X_{N_i} is an image patch centered at voxel i. An ensemble learner essentially combines the outputs of weak learners, which can be based upon a feature pool. Each weak learner h_n, which takes in X and outputs Y, pushes the overall solution towards the optimal solution. Combining these weak learners is the function of the specific ensemble algorithm. For instance in AdaBoost $F(X_{N_i}) = \sum \alpha_j h(X_{N_i})$, and in bagging $F(X_{N_i}) = \sum h(X_{N_i})$.

2.2 Background

To optimally combine a set of different weak learners from a feature pool, most ensemble methods either re-weight or iteratively modify the training data presented to each weak learner, bias the weak learners in some way, or both. Boosting (and its variants) can create a highly effective ensemble classifier as it keeps updating a weight w_i over the training examples in X to force weak learners to focus on difficult examples. While this is effective, it is not the only way to perturb the data. Bagging repeatedly resamples the training data, with replacement. After each resampling, a weak learner is created based on the resampled data, and the average prediction over all weak learners defines the strong learner. This resampling provides enough variation in the data to make each weak learner $h_n(X)$ different enough to contribute to the classification problem. Random forests [8] both resample the data and limit the search space from which to construct each $h_n(X)$. This provides randomization on both the dataset and the feature space. Even the extreme case of randomization has shown success, where extremely randomized trees [9] allow only one feature for each split of the tree and randomize the cut point of that feature.

2.3 Online Learning

First, we must use weak learners that can take advantage of sequentially presented training data. Unless the base learning algorithm can use data presented online, online ensemble learning becomes very difficult. For this paper, we will use both decision stumps and a modified 1-deep decision tree (explained later) that are both lossless in the online case. To coax an ensemble method into an online mode, the weak learner selection method must be changed.

To adapt bagging for online training, we use Oza's method [7] to sample the training data with replacement as more training data become available. In offline bagging, each sample is presented to each weak learner from 0 to N times, where N is fixed before learning. The number of times, K, that a sample is presented to each weak learner, may be modeled as a binomial distribution $P(K = k) = \binom{N}{k} \left(\frac{1}{N}\right)^k \left(1 - \frac{1}{N}\right)^{N-k}$. In the online case, we can view $N \to \infty$, and then the binomial distribution tends to a Poisson distribution with mean 1, $P(K = k) = \exp(-1)/k!$. Given a set of weak learners, running bagging in the online case is therefore equivalent to batch bagging. The online bagging algorithm is described in Fig. 1.

For online boosting, the algorithm is slightly more complicated. Again, we follow Oza's idea [7], which switches the roles of feature selecting and example gathering. Once a set of weak learners is obtained, the "difficulty" of an example

> Given a set of weak learners H and a new example $(\boldsymbol{x}, y)$
> For each weak learner $h_n \in H, n \in 1, \cdots, N$
> - Set $p = rand(0,1)$
> - while $p > e^{-1}$
>   - Update classifier h_n with example $(\boldsymbol{x}, y)$
>   - $p = p * rand(0,1)$

Fig. 1. The online bagging training procedure from Oza [7]

> Initialize $\lambda_n^{sc} = 0, \lambda_n^{sw} = 0$ before seeing any training examples.
> Given a set of weak learners H and a new example $(\boldsymbol{x}, y)$, set $\lambda = 1$
> For each weak learner $h_n \in H, n = 1, \cdots, N$
> - Update h_n with example $(\boldsymbol{x}, y)$ and weight λ
>   if $y = h_n(\boldsymbol{x})$ else
>   - $\lambda_n^{sc} = \lambda_n^{sc} + \lambda$ • $\lambda_n^{sw} = \lambda_n^{sw} + \lambda$
>   - $\epsilon_n = \frac{\lambda_n^{sc}}{\lambda_n^{sc} + \lambda_n^{sw}}$ • $\epsilon_n = \frac{\lambda_n^{sc}}{\lambda_n^{sc} + \lambda_n^{sw}}$
>   - $\lambda = \lambda \frac{1}{2(1-\epsilon_n)}$ • $\lambda \frac{1}{2\epsilon_n}$

Fig. 2. The online boosting training procedure. λ_n^{sc} keeps track of the correctly classified examples, and λ_n^{sw} keeps track of the incorrectly classified examples per weak learner. λ attempts to model the weights w from batch AdaBoost.

is estimated by having each weak learner classify it, and then updating the weak learner and its weight based on the difficulty of that example. Online boosting is described in Fig. 2.

By Oza's own admission, the online boosting algorithm is not lossless compared to its batch mode; an online learning algorithm is lossless if it returns a model identical to that of the corresponding batch algorithm trained on the same examples. This can best be seen by example. Assume that weak learner n sees an example and correctly classifies it. That example's weight will decrease when weak learner $n+1$ classifies it. Based on its decreased weight weak learner $n+1$ may or may not classify it correctly. Then another example is presented to weak learner n, and it is updated such that it no longer correctly classifies the previously seen example. This means that the weight assigned for the previous example was incorrect, and it should have been assigned a higher weight when given to weak learner $n+1$ (and all $m > (n+1)$ weak learners). In addition to this drawback, online boosting does not lend itself to feature selection. Although Grabner [10] has shown a way to induce online boosting into feature selection, it still suffers a drawback in that it is lossy versus its batch mode. Additionally, Fern [11] has produced an online ensemble learning method based on Arc-x4, however it too suffers from the inability to generate new weak learners.

2.4 LOEL

The two main drawbacks of online bagging (no feature selection) and online boosting (it is lossy) make them less than ideal for online ensemble learning. We

> Given a pool of weak learners **H** and a new example (x, y)
> For each weak learner $h_n \in \mathbf{H}, n = 1, \cdots, N$
> • Update h_n with example (x, y)
> For $t = 1 \cdots T$
> • Create a new feature pool, $\mathbf{H_{sm}}$, of size S by random sampling from **H**
>   For $s = 1 \cdots S$
>   • Randomize the parameters of h_s
>   • $\epsilon_s = error(h_s)$
> • Add $h^* = argmin_{\mathbf{H_{sm}}} \epsilon_s$ to the model

Fig. 3. The LOEL training procedure. Test data are classified using an unweighted vote of each h^*. For all experiments in this paper, we set $size(\mathbf{H_{sm}}) = 0.3 size(\mathbf{H})$.

overcame these limitations with the Lossless Online Ensemble Learning (LOEL) algorithm (Fig. 3).

The first for loop in LOEL is the weak learner updating loop, where the next example is added to all weak learners without weighting. Any weak learner can be used with LOEL, so long as it (1) is lossless, and (2) has a compact way of storing examples that is independent of the number of examples seen. An example of the second caveat is the decision stump. By storing two histograms of the data already seen (a histogram of the positive data, and a histogram of the negative data), each weak learner can keep track of the examples it has seen, independently of the total number of examples. By transforming these histograms into cumulative distribution functions, the error for a threshold can be estimated quickly, and in order to randomize the parameters, we just randomly choose a cut point.

Because each example is given exactly once to each weak learner, perturbations must be made on the weak learners themselves to differentiate between each run of the interior loop of Fig. 3. These perturbations were borrowed from both random forests (restricting the weak learner space) and from extremely randomized trees (randomizing the parameters of each weak learner) and as such should prove effective in LOEL.

Following the logic of Breimann [8], we can show that as more weak learners are added to the classifier we are fitting a more effective model. If $I(h_n(X) = Y)$ is an indicator function, then $margin_N(X, Y) = \sum_{n=1}^{N} I(h_n(X) = Y) - I(h_n(X) \neq Y)$ The margin is the confidence in each sample; increasing margin means a sample is more likely in a given class. We can then define the optimal classifier as $Y_N^* = P(margin_N(X, Y) < 0)$ In LOEL, $h_n(X) = h_n^{s,p}$ where s is the size of the resampled feature pool, and p are the randomized parameters. Then, following the law of large numbers $P_{X,Y}(P(h^{s,p}(X) = Y) - P(h^{s,p}(X) \neq Y) < 0)$.

LOEL is provably lossless as it is very similar to its batch version. The only difference between batch and online modes is the existence of the first loop in Fig. 3. So long as the weak learners conform to the specifications above, the construction of the weak learners will be no different in batch versus online modes. In fact, in online learning, the model that is output at each iteration is not even used when the next training example is presented, the compact representation of the whole weak learner pool is instead stored and updated.

This is in contrast to the online bagging and boosting methods where the model itself is updated. By having access to the entire feature pool and all examples already seen, LOEL can select weak learners that minimize the error over all weak learners and all examples.

3 Results

3.1 Tests on Standardized Data

We first compared AdaBoost, bagging, and LOEL in the offline case on a standard dataset from the UCI machine learning repository (archive.ics.uci.edu/ml/). We chose to use the breast cancer data because it presented a medical imaging two-class classification test. For this dataset we only aimed to show that LOEL is as effective as both AdaBoost and bagging in the offline case. We will reserve the online case to the full hippocampal segmentation task.

Fig. 4 shows how testing error varies as the number of weak learners grows. The error is defined as the number of incorrect examples divided by the total number of examples. For this test, we defined a weak learner as a decision stump, and randomly chose half the data set for training and half for testing. All three methods perform well on this data, with LOEL best at minimizing the testing error.

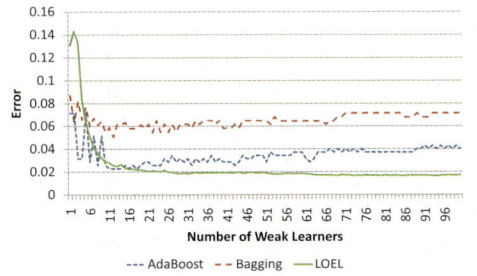

Fig. 4. Effects of varying the number of weak learners as a function of the testing error on a standard breast cancer dataset. LOEL outperforms both AdaBoost and bagging when minimizing error on the test set.

3.2 Hippocampal Segmentation

To apply LOEL to a real imaging problem, we segmented the hippocampus in a dataset from a study of Alzheimer's disease (AD) which significantly affects the morphology of the hippocampus [12]. This dataset includes 3D T1-weighted brain MRI scans of individuals in three diagnostic groups: AD, mild cognitive impairment (MCI), and healthy elderly controls. All subjects were scanned on a 1.5 Tesla Siemens scanner, with a standard high-resolution spoiled gradient echo (SPGR) pulse sequence with a TR (repetition time) of 28 ms, TE (echo time) of 6 ms, 220mm field of view, 256x192 matrix, and slice thickness of 1.5mm. For training we used 20 subjects in a variety of disease states (AD, MCI, or Normals).

Given the ground truth segmentation (A) and an automated segmentation (B), both represented as binary sets, we define the following error metrics; $d(a,b)$ is the Euclidean distance between 2 points, a and b:
- Precision = $\frac{A \cap B}{B}$
- Relative Overlap = $\frac{A \cap B}{A \cup B}$
- Recall = $\frac{A \cap B}{A}$
- Mean = $\text{avg}_{a \in A}(\min_{b \in B}(d(a,b)))$

Fig. 5. Error metrics used to validate hippocampal segmentations

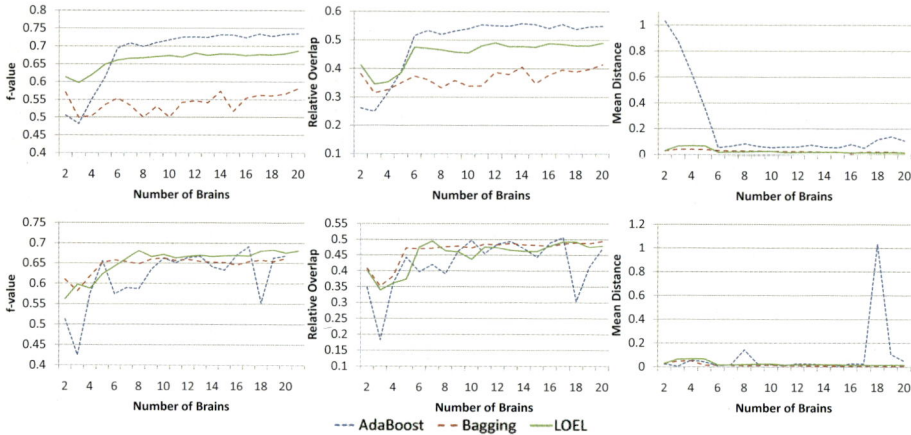

Fig. 6. Hippocampal segmentation errors as a function of the number of training brains. Offline training is the upper row and online, the lower row. The f-value is the average of precision and recall. In the offline case, all three methods show improvement as more training data is added. AdaBoost is not as effective in the offline case at minimizing the mean distance. In the online case, both bagging and LOEL show similar trends in each category. However, for bagging, this can be attributed to always choosing the prior feature. Since the prior improves as more brains are added the error metrics also tend to improve. The volatility of online AdaBoost arises from the fact that it is lossy.

For testing we used an independent set of 80 subjects (40 AD, 40 Normals). To assess segmentation accuracy, we present results that varied the number of training brains while testing on all 80 subjects. For the tests in this section, we slightly changed our weak learner formulation. Instead of a weak learner being a decision stump, it is instead a 1-deep modified decision tree. Some of our features are based on a "prior" image, which we define as the pointwise average of all the available training masks, which takes values in the range [0,1]. The features based on this image are so strong that they tend to overpower the other features. To provide more balance, we define the first level of the decision tree to be "is the prior less than 0.2." This gives other features more prominence during the construction of weak learners. This formulation of the weak learners still follows the rules set out by the LOEL requirements because the root node is hardcoded. Instead of storing a positive and negative histogram per weak learner, we store

Table 1. This table shows *p*-values comparing the mean hippocampal volume of 40 AD vs. 40 normal subjects. Online bagging was not effective because every subject had the exact same hippocampal volume. Both AdaBoost and LOEL correctly distinguish AD from normal, but as shown by Fig. 6, AdaBoost is too volatile in the online case. Without the ability to make such a well known differentiation, a segmentation is not accurate enough for real use.

	AdaBoost	Bagging	LOEL
Offline	0.00023	0.034	0.028
Online	0.022	NA	0.0027

4 histograms, a positive and negative histogram for examples in which the prior is less than 0.2 and the same for examples in which the prior is greater than 0.2.

Fig. 6 shows our results in both the offline and online cases. In the offline case, all three methods are effective after 6 or 7 brains have been used for training. In the online case, AdaBoost is quite volatile, whereas both bagging and LOEL gradually improve with more training brains. Bagging and LOEL are close in the online case, but error metrics only tell half the story. Because the prior is such a good feature, by just choosing the prior for each weak learner, bagging is able to keep up with LOEL. Table 1 shows results of a 2-sample *t*-test comparing the mean hippocampal volume of AD to normal subjects. Each algorithm correctly differentiates AD from normal in the offline case, but LOEL and AdaBoost are the only algorithms that also do so in the online case. Bagging is just returning the prior as it cannot make any distinction between brains in the online case. AdaBoost can distinguish AD from normal, but the error metrics show that online AdaBoost is too volatile to be effective.

4 Conclusion

In this paper we developed a new ensemble learning method that is lossless in the online case. While this algorithm is not better than boosting or bagging in the offline case, it outperformed both of them in the online case. In the future, we hope to apply LOEL to more classification tasks to see if it generalizes well to other imaging problems and other domains.

References

1. Freund, Y., Schapire, R.: A decision-theoretic generalization of on-line learning and an application to boosting. Journal of Computer Sys. Sci. 55, 119–139 (1997)
2. Breiman, L.: Bagging predictors. Machine Learning 24(2), 123–140 (1996)
3. Morra, J., Tu, Z., Apostolova, L., et al.: Mapping hippocampal degeneration in 400 subjects with a novel automated segmentation approach. In: ISBI, May 2008, pp. 336–339 (2008)
4. Tu, Z., Narr, K., Dollar, P., et al.: Brain anatomical structure parsing by hybrid discriminative/generative models. IEEE TMI (2008)

5. Rohlfing, T., Maurer, C.R.: Multi-classifier framework for atlas-based image segmentation. Pattern Recognition Letters 26(13), 2070–2079 (2005)
6. Jack, C., Bernstein, M., Fox, N., et al.: The Alzheimer's Disease Neuroimaging Initiative (ADNI): The MR imaging protocol. Journal of MRI 27(4), 685–691 (2008)
7. Oza, N.: Online bagging and boosting. IEEE Systems, Man, and Cybernetics 3, 2340–2345 (2005)
8. Breiman, L.: Random forests. Machine Learning 45(1), 5–32 (2001)
9. Geurts, P., Ernst, D., Wehenkel, L.: Extremely randomized trees. Machine Learning 63(1), 3–42 (2005)
10. Grabner, H., Bischof, H.: On-line boosting and vision. In: CVPR, vol. 1, pp. 260–267 (2006)
11. Fern, A., Givan, R.: Online ensemble learning: An empirical study. In: Proceedings of the Seventeenth International Conference on Machine Learning, pp. 279–286. Morgan Kaufmann, San Francisco (2000)
12. Becker, J., Davis, S., Hayashi, K., et al.: 3D patterns of hippocampal atrophy in mild cognitive impairment. Archives of Neurology 63(1), 97–101 (2006)

Improved Maximum a Posteriori Cortical Segmentation by Iterative Relaxation of Priors

Manuel Jorge Cardoso[1], Matthew J. Clarkson[1,2], Gerard R. Ridgway[1,2], Marc Modat[1], Nick C. Fox[2], and Sebastien Ourselin[1,2]

[1] Centre for Medical Image Computing (CMIC), University College London, UK
[2] Dementia Research Centre (DRC), University College London, UK

Abstract. Thickness measurements of the cerebral cortex can aid diagnosis and provide valuable information about the temporal evolution of several diseases such as Alzheimer's, Huntington's, Schizophrenia, as well as normal ageing. The presence of deep sulci and 'collapsed gyri' (caused by the loss of tissue in patients with neurodegenerative diseases) complicates the tissue segmentation due to partial volume (PV) effects and limited resolution of MRI. We extend existing work to improve the segmentation and thickness estimation in a single framework. We model the PV effect using a maximum a posteriori approach with novel iterative modification of the prior information to enhance deep sulci and gyri delineation. We use a voxel based approach to estimate thickness using the Laplace equation within a Lagrangian-Eulerian framework leading to sub-voxel accuracy. Experiments performed on a new digital phantom and on clinical Alzheimer's disease MR images show improvements in both accuracy and robustness of the thickness measurements, as well as a reduction of errors in deep sulci and collapsed gyri.

1 Introduction

Automatic thickness measurements of the cerebral cortex from magnetic resonance imaging (MRI) can aid diagnosis and provide valuable information about the temporal evolution of several diseases. Several surface [1] and voxel-based [2,3,4] approaches have been proposed. Although surface based approaches allow easier inter-subject thickness comparisons they are computationally very demanding, often requiring laborious manual interaction at several stages. In contrast, voxel based approaches are much more computationally efficient but are also more prone to noise and partial volume (PV) effects. The presence of PV effect in collapsed grey matter folds leads to the existence of PV-corrupted deep sulci and collapsed gyri, the latter mainly caused by the loss of white matter in patients with neurodegenerative diseases.

Several methods have been used to segment the brain into its different structures. Expectation-Maximisation (EM) based algorithms proposed by Wells et al. [5], Van Leemput et al. [6] and Ashburner and Friston [7] are among the most popular and accurate [8]. Prior information about the brain anatomy is generally used to initialise and locally constrain EM based segmentation algorithms,

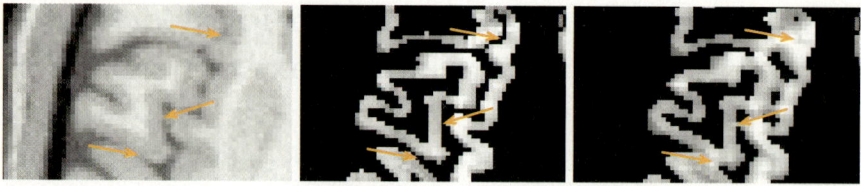

Fig. 1. BrainWeb thickness measurements: Left) BrainWeb image (noise 3%, INU 20%); Centre) Proposed method; Right) MAP with MRF but without the proposed improvements. The orange arrows point to areas of improved delineation with the proposed method.

increasing the robustness to noise. However, in some cases, due to intensity non-uniformity (INU), PV and noise, the local difference in intensity is insufficient to provide a correct segmentation of fine structures. The use of priors may also cause problems in areas that have some degree of natural variability, as the prior information used is representative of a normal population and not of the particular subject under study. All these problems lead to an incorrect delineation of collapsed grey matter folds, resulting in incorrect thickness estimates. Acosta et al.[4], used information derived from an Euclidean distance tranform to modify the cost function of a Markov Random Field (MRF) and added a post processing step to solve this problem. However, the use of an *ad-hoc* mask produced by a distance-ordered homotopic thinning (DOHT) algorithm that binarily unassigns voxels from the thickness calculation may lead to an erratic solution. Hutton et al.[2] used a mathematical morphology based layering method to detect deep sulci, without taking the PV effect or the intensity of the voxels into account, resulting in a loss of accuracy. Additionally, both approaches are only concerned with improvements in the delineation of deep sulci. However, incorrect thickness estimates can also result from loss of tissue in the gyri, which together with PV effects and structural readjustments can lead to a collapsed gyri.

We propose a unified Maximum a Posteriori (MAP) based framework that iteratively changes the priors, improving the PV classification and the delineation of deep sulci and gyri (Fig.1). Both the solution of the EM algorithm and the information derived from the Euclidean distance are used to locally modify the priors and the weighting of the MRF, enabling the detection of small variations in intensity while maintaining robustness of noise. Because of the MRF, the thickness of the PV layer is reduced, making it more in line with the theoretical anatomical limit. This obviates the need for an empirical threshold or distance to stop the search for the correct border within the PV classified area. After the convergence of the MAP algorithm, the cortical thickness is computed using an Eulerian-Lagrangian approach, as in Acosta et al. [4].

2 Method

2.1 Intensity Model and MRF Regularization

Starting from the image model developed by Van Leemput et al.[6], let $y = \{y_1, y_2, ..., y_n\}$, denote the intensities of an MR image of size n. Let $z = \{z_1, z_2, ... z_n\}$

denote the tissue type to which voxel i belongs. For K tissue types, let $z_i = e_k$ for some k, $1 \leq k \leq K$ where e_k is a unit vector with the kth component equal to one and all the other components equal to zero.

Additionally, consider that a bias field can be represented as a linear combination $\sum_j c_j \phi_j$ of J smoothly varying basis functions $\phi_j(x)$, with $1 \leq j \leq J$ and x denotes the spatial position, and $C = \{c_1, c_2, ..., c_j\}$ denote the bias field parameters. Let $\Phi_y = \{\theta_1, \theta_2, ..., \theta_K, C\}$ represent the overall model parameters. Due to the multiplicative nature of the MR bias field, log-transformed intensities are used, making the bias field additive. Now suppose that the intensity of the voxels that belong to class k are log-normal distributed with mean μ_k and variance σ_k^2 grouped in $\theta_k = \{\mu_k, \sigma_k^2\}$. The probability density that voxel i with intensity y_i belongs to class k is then

$$f(y_i \mid z_i = e_k, \Phi_y) = G_{\sigma_k}\left(y_i - \mu_k - \sum_j c_j \phi_j(x_i)\right) \qquad (1)$$

where $G_{\sigma_k}()$ denotes a zero-mean normal distribution with variance σ_k^2.

By applying the EM algorithm, the Maximum Likelihood (ML) of the model parameter Φ_y provides the following equations:

$$p_{ik}^{(m+1)} = \frac{f(y_i \mid z_i = e_k, \Phi_y^{(m)}) f(z_i = e_i)}{\sum_{j=1}^{K} f(y_i \mid z_i = e_k, \Phi_y^{(m)}) f(z_i = e_i)} \qquad (2)$$

$$\mu_k^{(m+1)} = \frac{\sum_{i=1}^{n} p_{ik}^{(m+1)} \left(y_i - \sum_{j=1}^{J} c_j^{(m)} \phi_j(x_i)\right)}{\sum_{i=1}^{n} p_{ik}^{(m+1)}} \qquad (3)$$

$$\left(\sigma_k^{(m+1)}\right)^2 = \frac{\sum_{i=1}^{n} p_{ik}^{(m+1)} \left(y_i - \mu_k^{(m+1)} - \sum_{j=1}^{J} c_j^{(m)} \phi_j(x_i)\right)^2}{\sum_{i=1}^{n} p_{ik}^{(m+1)}} \qquad (4)$$

where m denotes the number of iterations. The estimation of $c_j^{(m+1)}$ is provided by Van Leemput et al. [6].

Instead of a ML type approach, we adapted the model to a MAP approach by incorporating prior probability information derived from digital brain atlas. These atlases are brought into correspondence using an affine registration [9] followed by a free-form non-rigid registration algorithm [10]. The prior probability is introduced as a weight $\pi_{ik} = \{\pi_{i1}, \pi_{i2}, \pi_{i3}\}$, where π_{i1}, π_{i2} and π_{i3} contain the digital atlas prior probability of white matter (WM), grey matter (GM) and cerebrospinal fluid (CSF) respectively and are integrated in equation 1 as

$$f(y_i \mid z_i = e_k, \Phi_y) = \pi_{ik} \, G_{\sigma_k}\left(y_i - \mu_k - \sum_j c_j \phi_j(x_i)\right) \qquad (5)$$

Equations 2, 3 and 4 remain valid and the initial values for p_{ik}^0, μ_k^0 and σ_k^0 are given by their equations with $c_j^{(0)} = 0$ and $f(y_i \mid z_i = e_k, \Phi_y^0) = \pi_{ik}$.

Unfortunately, the intensity model alone only works in relatively ideal conditions because it only classifies the voxels of the image based on the intensity and the initial prior information. Therefore, the model has to be made more robust to noise by including spatial constraints derived from the anatomical properties of the tissues. This is achieved by the use of an MRF that assumes the probability that voxel i belongs to tissue k depends on its neighbours. Using the same approximation as described in [6], Equation 2 will now be

$$p_{ik}^{(m+1)} = \frac{f(y_i \mid z_i = e_k, \Phi_y^{(m+1)}) f(z_i = e_k \mid p_{\mathcal{N}_i}^{(m)} \Phi_z^{(m)})}{\sum_{j=1}^{K} f(y_i \mid z_i = e_k, \Phi_y^{(m+1)}) f(z_i = e_k \mid p_{\mathcal{N}_i}^{(m)} \Phi_z^{(m)})} \quad (6)$$

with,

$$f(z_i = e_k \mid p_{\mathcal{N}_i}^{(m)} \Phi_z^{(m)}) = \frac{e^{-\beta U_{\mathrm{mrf}}(z_i \mid p_{\mathcal{N}_i}^{(m)}, \Phi_z^{(m)})}}{\sum_{j=1}^{K} e^{-\beta U_{\mathrm{mrf}}(z_i \mid p_{\mathcal{N}_i}^{(m)}, \Phi_z^{(m)})}} \quad (7)$$

where $U_{\mathrm{mrf}}(z_i \mid p_{\mathcal{N}_i}, \Phi_z)$ is an energy function dependant on the parameters $\Phi_z = \{G, H\}$. G and H are $K \times K$ matrixes that control the energy of the transition between classes, and $p_{\mathcal{N}_i}$ is the value of p in the 6 nearest neighbours $\mathcal{N}_i = \{i^n, i^s, i^e, i^w, i^t, i^b\}$. At this stage β is constant and equal to 1. Please refer to Van Leemput et al. [6] for the estimation of $U_{\mathrm{mrf}}(z_i \mid p_{\mathcal{N}_i}, \Phi_z)$.

2.2 Prior Probability Relaxation

The EM algorithm is known to converge to a local optimum. In a MAP approach, the prior probability drives the EM algorithm to a sensible solution, making it more robust to noise and INU. However, in areas with high anatomical variability, the MAP approach can lead to an erroneous solution because the prior probability might be too low to allow the EM to converge to the expected solution. It can also bias the segmentation towards the template, possibly overshadowing some anatomical differences. We propose a method where the prior probability is changed iteratively at each convergence of the EM algorithm, in an anatomically coherent way. As our model parameters become closer to the true solution, we are able to locally relax our prior probability without loosing robustness to noise, INU and PV.

Initially we model the problem with 3 classes, {WM, GM, CSF}. The prior probability of WM, GM and CSF are derived from an anatomical brain atlas and non-brain structures are removed. After the convergence of the EM algorithm, the model parameters Φ_y are closer to the true solution, even though the structures in areas with low prior probability might not converge to the correct solution. Once the model parameters are closer to the true solution, the priors are relaxed by letting neighbouring classes share prior probability. The updated prior probability after the first convergence of the EM algorithm will be

$$\pi_{ik} = \left\{ p_{i1} + \alpha\, p_{i2},\ p_{i2} + \alpha\, (p_{i1} + p_{i3}),\ p_{i3} + \alpha\, p_{i2} \right\} \Big/ \Pi_i \quad (8)$$

where α is a pre-specified parameter that controls the percentage of prior probability sharing (set to 0.2 here) and Π_i is a normalisation constant ensuring $\sum_{k=1}^{K} \pi_{ik} = 1$.

After the second convergence of the EM algorithm, we use the values of p_{ik}, μ_k, σ_k to initialise a 5 class model, that considers 3 pure tissue classes and 2 mixture classes {WM, GM, CSF ,WM/GM, GM/CSF}. All the classes are modelled as Gaussian mixtures in the same framework as before. The prior probability, average and variance for the 5 class model are denoted as π_{ik}^*, μ_k^* and $(\sigma_k^2)^*$, where the superscript * is used to indicate that they belong to the 5 class model. They are initialised as

$$\pi_{ik}^* = \left\{ p_{i1},\ p_{i2},\ p_{i3},\ \sqrt{p_{i1}^* p_{i2}},\ \sqrt{p_{i2}^* p_{i3}} \right\} / \Pi_i \qquad (9)$$

$$\mu_k^* = \left\{ \mu_1,\ \mu_2,\ \mu_3,\ \Gamma_{1/2}\ \mu_1 + (1 - \Gamma_{1/2})\ \mu_2,\ \Gamma_{2/3}\ \mu_2 + (1 - \Gamma_{2/3})\ \mu_3 \right\} \qquad (10)$$

$$(\sigma_k^2)^* = \left\{ \sigma_1^2,\ \sigma_2^2,\ \sigma_3^2,\ \Gamma_{1/2}^2\ \sigma_1^2 + (1 - \Gamma_{1/2}^2)\ \sigma_2^2,\ \Gamma_{1/2}^2\ \sigma_2^2 + (1 - \Gamma_{1/2}^2)\ \sigma_3^2 \right\} \qquad (11)$$

where Π_i is a normalisation constant over k and $\Gamma_{j/k}$ is the average of the fractional content (FC) between classes j and k, excluding values of FC outside [0,1], where FC is defined as $FC = (\mu_j - \bar{y}_i)/(\mu_j - \mu_k)$ and $\bar{y}_i = y_i - \sum_j c_j \phi_j(x_i)$ is the INU corrected intensity. This new stage of the EM algorithm is initialised with $c_j^* = c_j$ and $f(y_i \mid z_i = e_k, \Phi_y) = \pi_{ik}^*$.

2.3 Deep Sulci and Gyri Delineation

After the EM algorithm converges again, due to the presence of the MRF, fine structures such as deep sulci and gyri might not be correctly segmented. In Van Leemput et al.[6], the *super-* and *sub-diagonal* of the matrices G and H are constrained to be equal to the diagonal itself, i.e., $G_{(i,i)} = G_{(i,i+1)} = G_{(i,i-1)}$ and $H_{(i,i)} = H_{(i,i+1)} = H_{(i,i-1)}$. This type of constraint helps the detection of fine structures, however it globally makes the segmentation less robust to noise. To overcome this limitation, we propose a method to locally weight the MRF algorithm and relax the prior probability. This way, the MRF can still be robust to noise and simultaneously allow the segmentation and correct labelling of fine structures. In a similar way to [4], we use the information derived from a Euclidian distance transform to estimate the location of deep sulci and gyri and change the priors and the weighting of the MRF only in those locations. The functions ω_i^{gyri}, ω_i^{sulci} that are used to relax the priors are defined as follows:

$$\omega_i^{\text{gyri}} = log\left(p_i^* {}_{\text{GM}_{0.5}} (1 - \|\nabla E_i^{\text{CSF}+}\| (1 - p_i^* {}_{\text{CSF}} - p_{i\text{GM/CSF}}^*)) + 1 \right) \Big/ \Omega^{\text{gyri}} \qquad (12)$$

$$\omega_i^{\text{sulci}} = log\left(p_i^* {}_{\text{GM}_{0.5}} (1 - \|\nabla E_i^{\text{WM}+}\| (1 - p_i^* {}_{\text{WM}} - p_i^* {}_{\text{WM/GM}})) + 1 \right) \Big/ \Omega^{\text{sulci}} \qquad (13)$$

where the Ω are normalisation factors, $E_i^{\text{WM}+}$ is the distance to the sum of WM and WM/GM labelled areas thresholded at 0.5 (and similarly for $E_i^{\text{CSF}+}$ with

CSF and GM/CSF), and $p^*_{GM_{0.5}}$ is p^*_{GM} also thresholded at 0.5. The weighting of the MRF is incorporated in Equation 7 by replacing β with a spatially-varying value

$$\beta_i = \left((1 - \omega_i^{\text{sulci}})\,(1 - \omega_i^{\text{gyri}})\right)/\Omega^\beta \tag{14}$$

The values of ω^{sulci} and ω^{gyri} vary between [0,1] and have a value of 1 near the centre of the sulci and the centre of the gyri respectively. In a same way, the value of β_i is normalized by Ω^β to lie between [0,1] and has a value of 0 near the centre of the sulci and gyri. The functions ω_i^{sulci} and ω_i^{gyri} are going to be used to iteratively relax π_{ik} to give more prior probability to the respective mixture classes in areas where deep sulci and gyri should exist. π_{ik} is updated as

$$\pi^*_{ik} = \left\{p_{i1},\ p_{i2},\ p_{i3},\ p_{i4} + \omega_i^{\text{gyri}} p_{i2},\ p_{i5} + \omega_i^{\text{sulci}} p_{i2}\right\}/\Pi_i \tag{15}$$

This last EM stage is iterated several times and every time the EM converges, ω_i^{sulci}, ω_i^{gyri}, β_i and π^*_{ik} are updated, and a new EM starts. The algorithm finishes when the change in p^*_{ik} at successive converged values of the EM algorithm is less than a predefined ε.

2.4 Thickness Calculation

The cortical thickness is then computed using a hybrid Lagrangian-Eulerian approach to solve the Laplace equation, as in [4]. This method takes into account the PV effect and greatly improves the thickness results. The final values of p_{ik} are used to create the labelled image, where each voxel is set to the most probable tissue. The grey matter fractional content image, used in the thickness calculation algorithm, is set to 1 for every voxel belonging to pure GM and set to the correspondent FC for voxels belonging to mixture classes.

3 Experiments and Results

We created a very high resolution phantom containing finger and sheet like collapsed sulci and gyri. The Euclidean thickness of the structure is constant and equal to 8. This leads to an average Laplace equation based thickness of 8.13 and a standard deviation of 0.15 measured in the high resolution phantom. We then use Fourier-resampling to reduce the resolution by a factor of 5, before adding complex Gaussian noise (either low or high level) and taking the magnitude, resulting in two low resolution Rician noise corrupted phantoms. To obtain artificial priors, the ground truth image was Gaussian filtered ($\sigma = 4\,mm$) to simulate the anatomical variability.

The results are shown in Fig.2. The average (standard deviation) thickness using the proposed method is 8.36 (0.44) and 8.76 (0.77) for the low and high noise phantom respectively. These values are in line with the expected value of 8.13(0.15). The MAP approach with the MRF but without the proposed improvements yields an average of 12.87 (2.98) and 12.49 (2.82) for the low and high noise phantom respectively, values of thickness much higher than expected

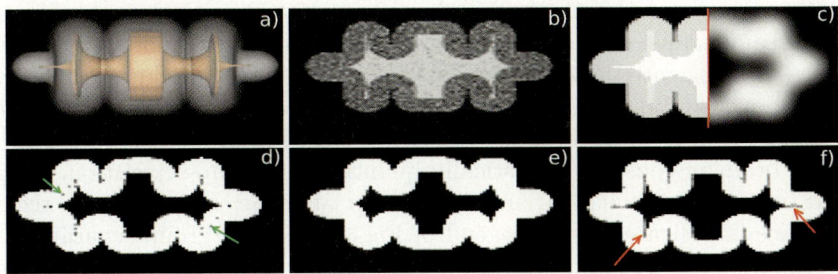

Fig. 2. Phantom segmentation for thickness: a) 3D model of the phantom, b) High noise phantom, c) True labels and GM prior used, d) ML without MRF, e) ML with MRF, f) Proposed method. The green arrows point to the presence of noise causing wrong thickness measurements. The red arrows point to the detected deep gyri.

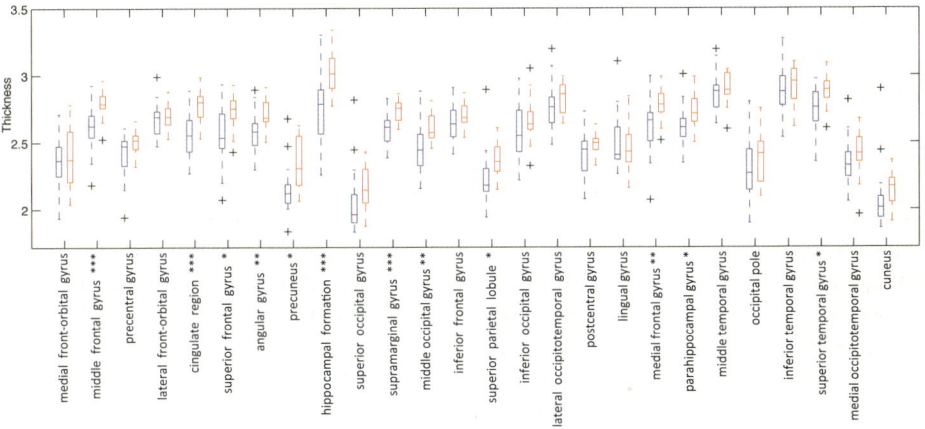

Fig. 3. Box plot of the distribution for all AAL regions over all patients (blue/left) and controls (red/right). The symbols *, ** and *** correspond to areas with a significance level of p<0.01, 0.001 and 0.0001 respectively.

due to the mis-detection of the deep sulci and gyri. Finally, the approach without either the MRF or the proposed improvements yielded an average of 12.11 (2.55) and 9.35 (3.1) for the low and high noise phantom respectively. The average thickness for the high noise phantom using this last technique is closer to the true value of 8 than for the the low noise phantom, but this is due to the noise introduced by the lack of MRF leading to a number of short paths to mis-segmented voxels.

Secondly we tested our method on real data, comprising 28 Alzheimer's disease (AD) patients and 17 age- and gender-matched controls. T1-weighted volumetric images were aquired on a 1.5 T Signa unit (GE Medical Systems, Milwaukee, WI) with 256x256 in-plane resolution, and 124 contiguous 1.5 mm coronal slices were acquired using a spoiled fast GRASS sequence (TR = 15 ms; TE = 5.4 ms; flip angle = 15; TI = 650 ms).

Further details of the protocol and subject characteristics can be found in [11]. The same transformation used to map the priors to the individual subjects was used to propagate the AAL template [12], and average thickness values were computed over 26 bilateral AAL regions. Fig.3 shows the distribution, at baseline, of values over patients and controls, illustrating group separation in the different brain regions. To statistically quantify the group-separation, we performed two-tailed unequal-variance two-group t-tests over all the AAL regions; significance is indicated in the legend of Fig.3. The best group separation was acheived in two of the regions (cingulate and hippocampal formation) known to be severely affected in AD.

4 Conclusions

We present an extension of previous work to improve the accuracy of cortical thickness measurements by refining and enhancing the segmentation of the cortex. The main contribution of this work lies in a method that iteratively relaxes and modifies the prior information in an anatomically coherent way to ameliorate the key problem of PV effect and reduce the bias towards the priors.

The method achieves better delineation of collapsed grey matter folds without loosing robustness to noise and intensity inhomogeneity. All segmentation steps (such as the transition from pure-tissue to PV model) are encompassed in a single framework, without *ad-hoc* post-processing. Quantitative analysis of a phantom using the proposed method demonstrated improvements in the accuracy and robustness of the thickness calculation when compared to other methods. Results on real data showed clinically-expected patterns of cortical thickness in AD, with highly significant group differences in several areas.

In the future, we plan to expand and improve our technique to study the temporal evolution of cortical thickness in neurodegenerative diseases.

References

1. Fischl, B., Dale, A.: Measuring the thickness of the human cerebral cortex from magnetic resonance images. PNAS 97, 11044–11049 (2000)
2. Hutton, C., Vita, E.D., Ashburner, J., Deichmann, R., Turner, R.: Voxel-based cortical thickness measurements in MRI. Neuroimage 40, 1701–1710 (2008)
3. Lohmann, G., Preul, C., Hund-Georgiadis, M.: Morphology-based cortical thickness estimation. In: IPMI 2003, pp. 89–100 (2003)
4. Acosta, O., Bourgeat, P., Fripp, J., Bonner, E., Ourselin, S., Salvado, O.: Automatic delineation of sulci and improved partial volume classification for accurate 3D voxel-based cortical thickness estimation from MR. In: Metaxas, D., Axel, L., Fichtinger, G., Székely, G. (eds.) MICCAI 2008, Part I. LNCS, vol. 5241, pp. 253–261. Springer, Heidelberg (2008)
5. Wells, M., Grimson, W.E.L., Kikinis, R., Jolesz, F.A.: Adaptive segmentation of MRI data. IEEE Transactions on Medical Imaging 15, 429–442 (1996)
6. Van Leemput, K., Maes, F., Vandermeulen, D., Suetens, P.: Automated model-based tissue classification of MR images of the brain. IEEE Transactions on Medical Imaging 18, 897–908 (1999)

7. Ashburner, J., Friston, K.: Unified segmentation. Neuroimage 26, 839–851 (2005)
8. Klauschen, F., Goldman, A., Barra, V., Meyer-Lindenberg, A., Lundervold, A.: Evaluation of automated brain MR image segmentation and volumetry methods. Human Brain Mapping 30, 1310–1327 (2009)
9. Smith, S., Jenkinson, M., Woolrich, M., Beckmann, C., Behrens, T., Bannister, P., DeLuca, M., Drobnjak, I., Flitney, D.: Advances in functional and structural MR image analysis and implementation as FSL. Neuroimage 23, 208–219 (2004)
10. Modat, M., Taylor, Z.A., Barnes, J., Hawkes, D.J., Fox, N.C., Ourselin, S.: Fast free-form deformation using the normalised mutual information gradient and graphics processing units. In: High-Performance MICCAI workshop (2008)
11. Schott, J., Price, S., Frost, C., Rossor, M., Fox, N.: Measuring atrophy in Alzheimer disease: a serial MRI study over 6 and 12 months. Neurology 65(1), 119–124 (2005)
12. Tzourio-Mazoyer, N., Landeau, B., Crivello, F., Etard, O., Delcroix, N., Mazoyer, B., Joliot, M.: Automated anatomical labeling of activations in SPM using a macroscopic anatomical parcellation of the MNI. Neuroimage 15, 273–289 (2002)

Anatomically Informed Bayesian Model Selection for fMRI Group Data Analysis

Merlin Keller[1,2,3], Marc Lavielle[2,5], Matthieu Perrot[1,4], and Alexis Roche[1]

[1] LNAO, Neurospin, CEA, F-91191 Gif-sur-Yvette, France
merlin.keller@cea.fr
[2] Department of Probability and Statistics, University of Paris Sud, France
[3] PARIETAL team, INRIA Saclay, France
[4] INSERM U.797, Orsay, France
[5] University René Descartes, Paris, France

Abstract. A new approach for fMRI group data analysis is introduced to overcome the limitations of standard voxel-based testing methods, such as Statistical Parametric Mapping (SPM). Using a Bayesian model selection framework, the functional network associated with a certain cognitive task is selected according to the posterior probabilities of mean region activations, given a pre-defined anatomical parcellation of the brain. This approach enables us to control a Bayesian risk that balances false positives and false negatives, unlike the SPM-like approach, which only controls false positives. On data from a mental calculation experiment, it detected the functional network known to be involved in number processing, whereas the SPM-like approach either swelled or missed the different activation regions.

1 Introduction

One of the goals of fMRI group studies is to identify the brain structures that are consistently involved in a given cognitive task across individuals. Mass univariate, or voxel-based, detection [1] is to date the most widely used approach to address such questions. It starts with normalizing individual images onto a common brain template using nonrigid image registration. Next, a t-statistic is computed in each voxel to locally assess mean group effects. The candidate regions are then defined as the connected components (clusters) of the resulting statistical map above an arbitrary threshold called the cluster-forming threshold.

To account for the multiple testing problem [2], only the clusters whose sizes exceed a critical value are reported. This critical size acts as a second threshold, and is generally tuned to control the probability of one or more clusters being detected by chance. Such statistical calibration is achieved in practice using either analytical approximations or resampling techniques [3]. For scientific reporting purposes, the detected clusters may finally be related to known anatomical regions based on expert knowledge, or using a digital brain atlas such as the Automated Atlas Label (AAL) [4], or the Cortical Sulci Atlas (CSA) [5].

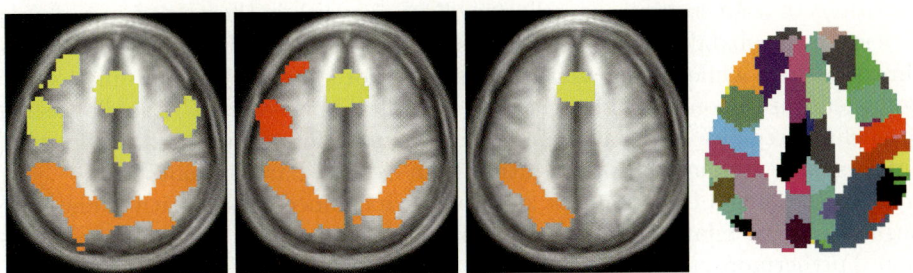

Fig. 1. Clusters detected at different cluster-forming thresholds by the SPM-like approach (axial slices $z = 37$mm in Talairach, with the subjects' mean anatomical image in the background). From left to right, the threshold is tuned to control the false positive rate (FPR) respectively at 10^{-2}, 10^{-3} and 10^{-4} uncorrected. Each cluster with corrected p-values less than 5% is represented with a specific color, showing how distinct functional regions are merged. Far right: the CSA atlas.

This approach, which we will refer to in the following as Statistical Parametric Mapping-like (SPM-like), is simple and widely applicable. However it suffers from the following drawbacks:

Arbitrary Cluster-Forming Threshold. The fact that a suprathreshold cluster is found significant by the cluster size test only implies that it contains *some* active voxels [3]. Low values of the cluster-forming threshold may result in merging functionally distinct regions, thus yielding poor localization power, while high values may result in missing active regions. This is illustrated in Figure 1 (the dataset and procedure are detailed in Section 3.2).

Exclusive Control of False Positives. False negative regions are not controlled, meaning that the absence of activations outside the detected clusters cannot be assessed. Consequently, there is no guarantee that the whole functional network can be recovered. This partly explains the poor reproducibility of group analyses across datasets [6].

Assumption of Perfect Match Between Individual Brains. Due to unavoidable intersubject registration errors, the observed activations are not well-localized, and possibly displaced across distinct functional regions, which may result in blurring the group activation map and creating unhandled false positives [7].

To date, these issues have been tackled separately. In [8], the SPM-like approach is extended to control false negatives using Bayesian inference, while [9] addresses the arbitrary threshold problem. Uncertainty on the localization of individual effects is accounted for in [10] by comparing high-level features extracted from the individual images and in [7] by extending the mass univariate model.

This paper introduces a new approach for fMRI group data analysis that jointly addresses all the above issues. Our method rests upon a Bayesian model selection framework in which models are functional networks, defined as binary partitions of a given brain parcellation. Each network is then rated in terms of a posterior probability. Because regions are defined beforehand, the method is threshold-free, while taking advantage of the prior knowledge about functionally homogeneous regions provided that the parcellation is sensible. A similar use of pre-defined regions with Bayesian modeling can be found in [11,12], while other authors have used spatial priors rather than explicit parcellations [13].

By controlling a Bayesian risk, our approach balances false positives and false negatives, with relative weights that may be tuned depending on the application. Furthermore, the generative model, described in Section 2.1, accounts for spatial uncertainty on the individual effects due to spatial normalization errors. Results of this procedure are presented on both simulated and real fMRI data in Section 3, and we conclude with a brief discussion in Section 4.

2 Method

2.1 Generative Model

After scanning several subjects during an fMRI experiment, individual datasets are processed separately so that, for each subject $i = 1, \ldots, n$, we are given an image of estimated effects $Y_i \in \mathbb{R}^p$, and an image of estimation variances $s_i^2 \in \mathbb{R}^p$, where p is the number of voxels in the search volume $V = \{v_k, k = 1, \ldots, p\} \subset \mathbb{R}^3$. Following [7], we extend the mass univariate model in [14] by relaxing the assumption that the individual images are perfectly aligned so that, at voxel k,

$$Y_i(v_k) = \mu(v_k + u_{ik}) + \varepsilon_{ik}. \quad (1)$$

Here, we note $Y_i(v_k) = Y_{ik}$ to emphasize that it is a spatial map; $\mu \in \mathbb{R}^p$ is the map of mean population effects; the vector u_{ik} is a hidden variable that models the subject-to-atlas registration error for subject i at voxel k; finally, the ε_{ik} are independently distributed Gaussian variables $\mathcal{N}(0, \sigma_I^2 + s_{ik}^2)$, where σ_I^2 is the between-subject variance and s_{ik}^2 the within-subject variance due to estimation errors in the effects. This generalizes the model in [14], which corresponds to the special case where the estimation variances s_{ik}^2 and the registration errors u_{ik} are neglected.

The displacements u_{ik} are modeled by a Karhunen-Loève expansion using elementary displacements w_{ib} in a limited number of fixed control points $\{v_{k_b}, b = 1, \ldots, B\}$. As is a common approach in deformable models, those control points are interpolated to the whole brain image using a radial basis function K,

$$u_{ik} = \sum_{b=1}^{B} K(v_k, v_{k_b}) w_{ib}, \quad (2)$$

where $K(v_k, v_{k_b}) = \exp-\{\|v_k - v_{k_b}\|^2/\gamma^2\}$, and γ controls the displacement field's smoothness. The w_{ib}'s are independent trivariate Gaussian variables with zero mean and common spherical covariance matrix $\sigma_S^2 \mathbf{I}_3$, where σ_S models the standard registration error.

2.2 Bayesian Model Selection Framework

Our approach to functional network selection is based on an *a priori* partition of the search volume into N regions of interest $V = V_1 \cup \ldots \cup V_N$, assumed to be homogeneous functional areas. Thus, throughout region V_j the population mean effects $\{\mu_k, v_k \in V_j\}$ are modeled as independent random variables with common distribution $\mathcal{N}(\eta_j, \sigma_j^2)$, where η_j is the regional mean effect and σ_j^2 the regional variance.

Based on the above model (1) and (2), our final task is to select the regions involved in the considered task. To this end, we define region V_j as being *involved* in the task if its regional mean effect is nonzero, *i.e.* $\eta_j \neq 0$, and *inactive* if $\eta_j = 0$. The functional network we wish to recover is thus represented in the following by the unknown binary label vector $\Gamma^* \in \{0,1\}^N$, such that $\Gamma_j^* = 1$ if $\eta_j \neq 0$ and $\Gamma_j^* = 0$ if $\eta_j = 0$. Adopting a Bayesian model selection viewpoint, we estimate Γ^* by selecting the most probable network given the data Y:

$$\hat{\Gamma}^* = \arg\max_{\Gamma} p(\Gamma|Y) \tag{3}$$

$$= \arg\max_{\Gamma} p\{\forall j, \Gamma_j = 1 : \eta_j \neq 0; \quad \forall j, \Gamma_j = 0 : \eta_j = 0|Y\}. \tag{4}$$

However, computing $p(\Gamma|Y)$ for all 2^N possible choices of Γ is intractable. To cut down computational complexity, we use the following independence approximation:

$$p(\Gamma|Y) \approx \prod_{\Gamma_j=1} p(\eta_j \neq 0|Y) \prod_{\Gamma_j=0} p(\eta_j = 0|Y). \tag{5}$$

It can be shown that (5) would be exact in absence of spatial uncertainty ($\sigma_S^2 = 0$, $u_{ik} \equiv 0$) and given the inter-subject variance σ_I^2. Using (5), the most probable network $\hat{\Gamma}^*$ is the one for which all regions j with $p(\eta_j \neq 0|Y) > 0.5$. are active.

2.3 Posterior Probability Computation

For all $j = 1, \ldots, N$, the posterior probabilities $P_j = p(\eta_j \neq 0|Y)$ and $p(\eta_j = 0|Y) = 1 - P_j$ are computed through their Bayes' factor:

$$\frac{P_j}{1-P_j} = \frac{p(Y|\eta_j \neq 0)}{p(Y|\eta_j = 0)}, \tag{6}$$

where $p(Y|\eta_j \neq 0) = \int_{(\eta_j, \sigma_j^2) \in \mathbb{R} \times \mathbb{R}^+} p(Y|\eta_j, \sigma_j^2) \pi(\eta_j, \sigma_j^2) d(\eta_j, \sigma_j^2)$ is the marginal likelihood in the model where region j is involved in the considered task and $p(Y|\eta_j = 0) = \int_{\sigma_j^2 \in \mathbb{R}^+} p(Y|\eta_j = 0, \sigma_j^2) \pi(\sigma_j^2) d(\sigma_j^2)$ the marginal likelihood in the model where region j is inactive, assuming a uniform prior $\pi(\eta_j \neq 0) = \pi(\eta_j = 0) = 0.5$ on the state of region j. The priors $\pi(\eta_j, \sigma_j^2)$ and $\pi(\sigma_j^2)$ are normal-inverse-Gamma and inverse-Gamma distributions, as in [7].

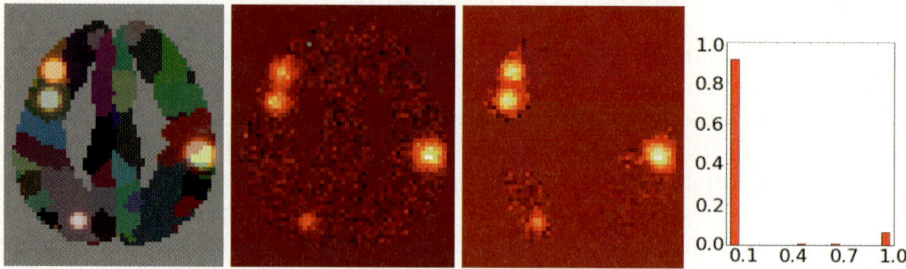

Fig. 2. Results on simulated data. From left to right: original activation pattern (with CSA atlas in the background), t-score map, posterior mean estimate $\hat{\mu} = \mathbb{E}(\mu|Y,\hat{\theta})$ of the mean population effect map μ and histogram of posterior probabilities P_j found by our approach.

Computing the marginal likelihoods $p(Y|\eta_j \neq 0)$ is non trivial, since it involves evaluating integrals on high dimensional spaces. Following [15], we use the basic marginal equality:

$$p(Y|\eta_j \neq 0) = \frac{p(Y|\theta_j, \eta_j \neq 0)\pi(\theta_j)}{\pi(\theta_j|Y, \eta_j \neq 0)}, \qquad (7)$$

valid for any value of the parameter $\theta_j = (\sigma_I^2, \sigma_S^2, \eta_j, \sigma_j^2)$, and apply it to the maximum *a posteriori* $\hat{\theta}_j$, which we estimate using a MCMC-SAEM algorithm [16]. The "null" likelihood $p(Y|\eta_j = 0)$ is computed in a similar fashion.

3 Results

3.1 Simulated Data

We designed an artificial activation map μ simulating the mean population effect defined in (1), based on the CSA atlas, which we used to analyze real fMRI data (see Section 3.2). To reflect realistic situations, we placed two activations in neighboring regions, one at the intersection of several regions, and a smaller one inside the largest atlas region (see Figure 2, far left).

$n = 40$ images were generated by warping this map according to the deformation model defined by (2), with one control point in each voxel, choosing $\gamma = 40$mm and $\sigma_S = 8$mm. Homoscedastic noise ε_{ik} was then added to each image according to the model in Section 2.1, with $\sigma_I^2 = 1$, and the s_{ik}^2's generated as independent chisquare variables.

We then applied our Bayesian model selection algorithm to this dataset, to recover the atlas regions $j = 1,\ldots,N$ with a nonzero regional mean activation η_j, still using the deformation model defined in (2), except this time control points were restricted to a regular grid with regular spacing equal to γ along each axis. We also used the SPM-like approach, described in Section 1. The cluster-forming threshold was tuned to control the voxel-level false positive rate

(FPR) at 10^{-3} uncorrected. Clusters with corrected p-values less than 5% in the cluster-size test were reported, and labeled according to their maximum statistic.

Results from this simulation study are illustrated in Figure 2. The posterior mean estimate $\hat{\mu}$ of the mean effect map μ is more contrasted than the t-score map, indicating a better fit of our model, which accounts for localization uncertainty. The histogram of posterior probabilities illustrates the discriminative power of our Bayesian model selection algorithm in separating involved from inactive regions, with more than 90% of the posterior probabilities P_j either above 0.9 or under 0.1. Furthermore, regions j with regional means η_j above 0.04, were all correctly reported as active and the regional means η_j were estimated with an average relative error $\epsilon = \frac{1}{N}\sum_j |\hat{\eta}_j - \eta_j|/\eta_j$ of 7%. In contrast, while at the chosen threshold the SPM-like method detected all activations, with corrected p-values smaller than 10^{-3} in the cluster-size test, neighboring active regions were merged in both the left and right hemispheres.

3.2 Real fMRI Data

We now present results of our method on a real fMRI dataset. We considered the activation maps of 38 subjects for a 'Calculation–Sentences' contrast, which subtracts activations due to audio or video instructions from the overall activations during the computation tasks. This contrast may thus reveal regions specifically involved in number processing. As in the simulation study, the data was analyzed using both the SPM-like approach and our model selection algorithm, based on the CSA atlas [5], derived from the anatomical images of 63 subjects and comprising 125 regions which correspond to subdivisions of cortical sulci.

As in the simulation study, the histogram of posterior probabilities suggests a good discriminative power, with over 80% of the posterior probabilities either above 0.9 or below 0.1. As shown in Figure 3 and Table 1, our method detected the bilateral intra-parietal and fronto-cingular networks known to be active during number processing [17], with posterior probabilities higher than 0.94 for all frontal regions and higher than 0.83 for all parietal regions. Interestingly, the

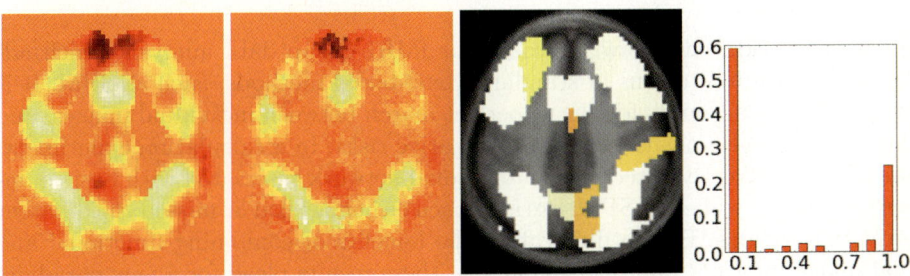

Fig. 3. Real fMRI data, number processing task. From left to right: classical t-score map, posterior mean estimate $\hat{\mu} = \mathbb{E}(\mu|Y,\hat{\theta})$ of the mean population effect map μ, map of posterior probabilities P_j, histogram of posterior probabilities.

Table 1. Number processing task, regions detected using the Bayesian model selection approach. Reported regions have a posterior probability of being involved in the task greater than 0.5, and constitute the most probable functional network given the data. $\hat{\eta}_j$ is the posterior estimate of the regional mean effect. Asterisks (*) mark regions that are found significant at 5% by the SPM-like approach (corrected cluster-level inference, cluster-forming threshold set to FPR = 10^{-3}), and correspond to the middle activation map in Figure 1.

Frontal lobe		
Sulcus/Fissure	P_j	$\hat{\eta}_j$
Left middle frontal	1.00	2.94
Right middle frontal*	1.00	3.17
Left superior frontal	0.94	2.11
Right superior frontal	1.00	1.93
Left middle precentral	1.00	4.11
Right middle precentral	1.00	1.98
Left inferior precentral	1.00	5.30
Right inferior precentral	0.97	2.69
Left anterior cingular	1.00	3.39
Right anterior cingular	1.00	4.15
Left inferior frontal*	1.00	4.38

Parietal lobe		
Sulcus/Fissure	P_j	$\hat{\eta}_j$
Left intra-parietal*	1.00	4.87
Right intra-parietal	1.00	3.03
Left precuneus	0.98	5.58
Right precuneus	0.85	3.84
Right inferior postcentral	0.88	2.30
Right parieto-occipital	0.83	1.30

Other		
Sulcus/Fissure	P_j	$\hat{\eta}_j$
Right callosal	0.79	1.99

bilateral precuneus sulci where also detected. Although not considered as part of the core numerical system, the precuneus has been linked to memory access and a wide range of high-level tasks [18]. In contrast, only three activated clusters were detected by the SPM-like approach at the chosen cluster-forming threshold. Each cluster contained over a thousand voxels, and extended over several atlas regions, hence merging several functionally distinct areas. Also, no activations were detected in the right frontal area. Using different thresholds could not solve these problems, as illustrated in Figure 1.

4 Discussion

We have introduced a new approach for fMRI group data analysis which addresses several limitations of standard voxel-based methods, such as SPM. It is threshold-free, accounts for the imperfect match between individual images, and controls both false positive and false negative risks. In a calculation experiment, our method correctly detected the functional network associated with basic number processing, while the SPM-like approach either swelled or missed the different activation regions. Beside illustrating the benefits of combining functional and anatomical information in neuroimaging, these results plead for a new paradigm for fMRI group data analysis.

Acknowledgments. Support was provided by the EC-funded IMAGEN project.

References

1. Friston, K.J.: 2. In: Human Brain Function, pp. 25–42. Academic Press, London (1997)
2. Nichols, T., Hayasaka, S.: Controlling the Familywise Error Rate in Functional Neuroimaging: A Comparative Review. Statistical Methods in Medical Research 12(5), 419–446 (2003)
3. Hayasaka, S., Nichols, T.: Validating Cluster Size Inference: Random Field and Permutation Methods. Neuroimage 20(4), 2343–2356 (2003)
4. Tzourio-Mazoyer, N., Landeau, B., Papathanassiou, D., Crivello, F., Etard, O., Delcroix, N., Mazoyer, B., Joliot, M.: Automated anatomical labeling of activations in SPM using a macroscopic anatomical parcellation of the MNI MRI single-subject brain. Neuroimage 15(1), 273–289 (2002)
5. Perrot, M., Rivière, D., Mangin, J.F.: Identifying cortical sulci from localizations, shape and local organization. In: 5th Proc. ISBI, Paris, France, pp. 420–423 (2008)
6. Thirion, B., Pinel, P., Mériaux, S., Roche, A., Dehaene, S., Poline, J.B.: Analysis of a large fMRI cohort: Statistical and methodological issues for group analyses. Neuroimage 35(1), 105–120 (2007)
7. Keller, M., Roche, A., Tucholka, A., Thirion, B.: Dealing with spatial normalization errors in fMRI group inference using hierarchical modeling. Statistica Sinica 18(4), 1357–1374 (2008)
8. Friston, K., Glaser, D.E., Henson, R.N.A., Kiebel, S., Phillips, C., Ashburner, J.: Classical and Bayesian inference in neuroimaging: Applications. Neuroimage 16(2), 484–512 (2002)
9. Smith, S.M., Nichols, T.E.: Threshold-free cluster enhancement: addressing problems of smoothing, threshold dependence and localisation in cluster inference. Neuroimage 44(1), 83–98 (2009)
10. Thirion, B., Tucholka, A., Keller, M., Pinel, P., Roche, A., Mangin, J.F., Poline, J.B.: High level group analysis of FMRI data based on Dirichlet process mixture models. In: Karssemeijer, N., Lelieveldt, B. (eds.) IPMI 2007. LNCS, vol. 4584, pp. 482–494. Springer, Heidelberg (2007)
11. Bowman, D.F., Caffo, B., Bassett, S.S., Kilts, C.: A bayesian hierarchical framework for spatial modeling of FMRIdata. Neuroimage 39(1), 146–156 (2008)
12. Makni, S., Idier, J., Vincent, T., Thirion, B., Dehaene-Lambertz, G., Ciuciu, P.: A fully Bayesian approach to the parcel-based detection-estimation of brain activity in fMRI. Neuroimage 41(3), 941–969 (2008)
13. Penny, W.D., Trujillo-Barreto, N., Friston, K.J.: Bayesian fMRI time series analysis with spatial priors. Neuroimage 23(2), 350–362 (2005)
14. Friston, K., Ashburner, J., Frith, C., Poline, J.B., Heather, J., Frackowiak, R.: Spatial registration and normalization of images. Hum. Brain Mapp. 3(3), 165–189 (1995)
15. Chib, S.: Marginal likelihood from the Gibbs output. J. Amer. Statist. Assoc. 90, 1313–1321 (1995)
16. Kuhn, E., Lavielle, M.: Coupling a stochastic approximation of EM with a MCMC procedure. ESAIM P&S 8, 115–131 (2004)
17. Pinel, P., Thirion, B., Mériaux, S., Jobert, A., Serres, J., Le Bihan, D., Poline, J.B., Dehaene, S.: Fast reproducible identification and large-scale databasing of individual functional cognitive networks. BMC Neurosci. 8(1), 91 (2007)
18. Cavanna, A.E., Trimble, M.R.: The precuneus: a review of its functional anatomy and behavioural correlates. Brain 129(3), 564–583 (2006)

A Computational Model of Cerebral Cortex Folding

Jingxin Nie[1], Gang Li[1], Lei Guo[1], and Tianming Liu[2]

[1] School of Automation, Northwestern Polytechnical University, Xi'an, China
[2] Department of Computer Science and Bioimaging Research Center,
The University of Georgia, Athens, GA, USA

Abstract. Folding of the human cerebral cortex has intrigued many people for many years. Quantitative description of cortical folding pattern and understanding of the underlying mechanisms have emerged as an important research goal. This paper presents a computational 3D geometric model of cerebral cortex folding that is initialized by MRI data of human fetus brain and deformed under the governance of partial differential equations modeling the cortical growth. The simulations of this 3D geometric model provide computational experiment support to the following hypotheses: 1) Mechanical constraints of the brain skull regulate the cortical folding process. 2) The cortical folding pattern is dependent on the global cell growth rate in the whole cortex. 3) The cortical folding pattern is dependent on relative degrees of tethering of different cortical areas and the initial geometry.

1 Introduction

Anatomy of the human cerebral cortex is extremely variable across individuals in terms of its size, shape and structure patterning [1]. The fact that folding pattern of the cortex is a good predictor of its function [2] has intrigued many people for many years [3~5]. Recently, understanding of the underlying folding mechanisms [3~5] and their computational simulations [4, 5] have emerged as important research goals. Though each human brain grows from a similar shape of neuronal tube in the very beginning, the major cortical folding variation develops after 8 months of fetus brain development. Since many neurodevelopmental processes are involved in this cortex folding development, including neuronal proliferation, migration and differentiation, glial cell proliferation, programmed cell death, axon development and synaptogenesis, how these processes interact with each other and dynamically accomplish the cortical folding is still largely unknown [6].

In the neuroscience community, several hypotheses have been proposed to explain the gyrification or folding of the cerebral cortex from different perspectives [3, 6]. Since the cortical area becomes almost three times larger than the cranial area in human brain after evolution, the mechanical constraint was firstly considered as the major factor that determined the cortical folding pattern [7]. Then, the areal difference, especially the cytoarchitectonic difference, which causes regional mechanical property variation, is considered as the direct reason that causes gyrification [7]. The axongenesis process, which might cause areal differentiation [3, 6], is also considered as an important factor that determines the folding pattern.

Due to the complexity of the neurobiology involved in gyrification of the cerebral cortex, computational modeling of such a process is very challenging. In the literature, there have been a couple of attempts to develop computational models to understand the cortex folding process. For example, in [4], the authors proposed a 2D continuum mechanics based model of growth to synthesize brain cortex shapes by using physical laws. Recently, a computational morphogenetic model was proposed to study the fundamental mechanisms of cortical folding in [5]. In this model, the 2D annular cortex and radial glial fibres were modeled by finite-elements and the growth of cortex was modeled as the expansion of finite elements. More recently, MRI and diffusion tensor imaging data were combined with finite element modeling techniques to generate biologically meaningful models of the cortical folding process [15].

In this paper, a 3D morphogenetic model is proposed to study the mechanisms of cortical gyrification. Since the human cortex can be considered as a highly convoluted thin shell [2], the triangulated surface of the developing cortex is adopted as its representation. The geometric model is driven by mechanical forces occurring in the growing brain for simulation of shape dynamics of the developing cortex. Parametric models for cerebral cortex are initialized by the structural fetus MRI data [8] from 22 to 36 week gestation. The morphogenetic model is deformed under the governance of partial differential equations. The mechanical forces and boundary conditions are guided by MRI data. After applying mechanical and growth properties of cortex on each triangular element, the time-varying system is solved by the Newmark scheme.

2 Methods

2.1 Materials and Pre-processing

T2 MRI data of fetus brain (SE sequence TR=1329.88ms and TE=88.256ms) [8] from 22 to 36 gestation weeks are used for the cortical surface reconstruction and folding model initialization. ITKSnap[9] is used to manually extract fetus brain from the structural MRI data and then the skull, cortex plate, white matter zone (including subplate and intermediate zones), ventricle zone, basal ganglia and thalami are distinguished from the brain regions (Figure 1a). The inner surface of the skull and outer surface of cortex plate are reconstructed from the volumes (Figure 1b).

2.2 Computational Model of Cortical Folding

The proposed computational model of folding of the human cerebral cortex is composed of four key components: 1) Deformable model of the cortex. This model provides a geometric representation of the cortex that can be deformed into dynamic shapes via mechanical forces. 2) Driving forces of the folding. The mechanical driving forces are inferred from the cortex growth model and deform the cortical surface under partial differential equations. 3) Geometric constraints. The growth of the cortex is constrained by the geometric constraints of the brain structures, as well as boundary conditions. 4) Model solvers. The numerical solution to the partial differential equations provides the dynamic evolution of the geometric surface model of the cortex. Figure 2 provides an overview of the proposed computational model.

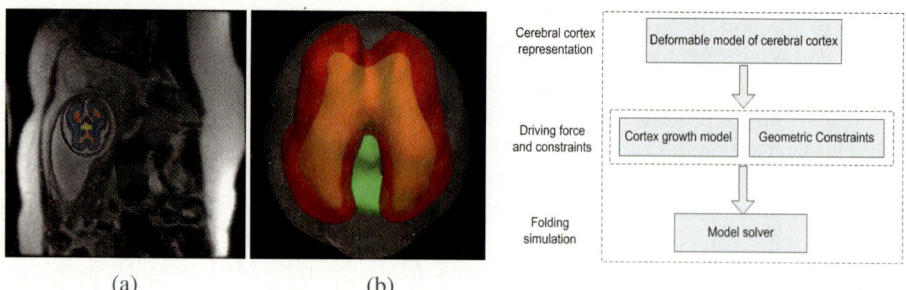

Fig. 1. Fetus brain structure reconstruction **Fig. 2.** Flowchart of the simulation model

2.2.1 Deformable Model

To model mechanical properties of the developing cortex, the elasto-plasticity model is adopted in our methods, akin to that in [5]. The elasticity property enforces the surface model to restore to the original shape and at the same time, the plasticity property tends to maintain the deformed shape permanently.

The developing cortex is represented as tens of thousands of triangle elements (21,136 in our experiments), each of which presents a small cortical region. During the development or growth of cortex, the elastic and plastic properties could be obtained from the deformed ($\mathbf{x}_c^i$) and reference ($\mathbf{x}_{c0}^i$) coordinates of the triangle corner i. The elastic force of each triangle element is defined along each edge of the triangle:

$$\mathbf{f}_{ce}^{i,j} = -\frac{K_c (l_{c0}^{i,j} - l_c^{i,j})}{l_{c0}^{i,j} l_c^{i,j}} (\mathbf{x}_c^i - \mathbf{x}_c^j), i, j \in \{1,2,3\}, i \neq j \qquad (1)$$

where i and j are the triangle vertex indices, $l_{c0}^{i,j} = \|\mathbf{x}_{c0}^i - \mathbf{x}_{c0}^j\|$ is the rest length of edge ij, and $l_c^{i,j}$ is the current distance between vertices i and j, K_c is the elastic constant. As plasticity plays an important role in soft tissue deformation, in our model, the plasticity of cortex is modeled as an adaptation of the reference configuration to the deformed configuration:

$$\frac{dl_{c0}^{i,j}}{dt} = -\frac{1}{\tau_{ce}} (l_c^{i,j} - l_{c0}^{i,j}), i, j \in \{1,2,3\}, i \neq j \qquad (2)$$

where τ_{ce} is the time constant for the plasticity, which is similar to that in [13].

Since the cortex is modeled as a zero thickness surface, the rigidity of cortex is introduced as bending energy [10]. As computing mean curvature on the triangulated surface is computationally expensive, the simplified version of bending stress is defined on each edge of the surface triangle:

$$\mathbf{f}_{be}^{i,j} = -\frac{K_b (l_{c0}^{p,q} - l_c^{p,q})}{l_{c0}^{p,q} l_c^{p,q}} (\mathbf{x}_c^p - \mathbf{x}_c^q), i, j \in edge\ \mathbf{e} \qquad (3)$$

where i and j are the two vertices of edge e, p and q are the two vertices that share the same triangle with edge e as illustrated, $l_{c0}^{p,q} = \|\mathbf{x}_{c0}^p - \mathbf{x}_{c0}^q\|$ is the rest distance between vertices p and q, $l_c^{p,q}$ is the current distance between vertices p and q, and K_b is the elastic constant. Also, the bending energy decreases with the plasticity of $l_c^{p,q}$:

$$\frac{dl_{c0}^{p,q}}{dt} = -\frac{1}{\tau_{cb}}(l_c^{p,q} - l_{c0}^{p,q}) \qquad (4)$$

where τ_{cb} is the time constant for the plasticity of bending energy.

2.2.2 Cortex Growth Model

Modeling the average size and number of neurons at the cellular level is still an open problem in the computational neuroscience field. Here, we adopt the classic logistic-growth function [11] to describe the growth of cortical tissues as that in [5]:

$$\frac{dA_{ti}}{dt} = A_{ti} m \left(1 - \frac{A_{ti}}{k}\right) \qquad (5)$$

where m is known as the Malthusian parameter, A_{ti} is the area of triangle ti and k is the carrying capacity of the system [11]. By changing the rest area of triangular element, the growth of cortex will generate mechanical stress that partly drives the deformation of the cerebral cortex surface.

2.2.3 Constraints

The development of cortex is limited by certain mechanical or boundary conditions such as cranial volume and self collision [7]. To prevent the cortex from developing into the skull or other brain tissues, a volumetric constraint model is maintained during the simulated folding of the cortex. Voxels from the skull, basal ganglia/thalami or ventricular zone are extracted from the scanned 3D MRI image and grouped into a new image as a mask, outside which volumes of other brain regions are set to zero. As a result, the cortex model can only be deformed in the zero value space.

Also, we applied similar techniques in [12] to prevent the self-intersection of deformed cortical surfaces. Specifically, current deformed cortex surface is rasterized to a volumetric model. When any vertex of the surface is being deformed to a new position $\mathbf{x}'$, the new position would be checked if it is inside the developing skull or other brain tissue volume, or it will cause its neighboring triangles to intersect with the other rasterized triangles. Otherwise, another new position $\tilde{\mathbf{x}}$ for this vertex will be found on the line from $\mathbf{x}'$ to the original position x, and it is the closest point to position $\mathbf{x}'$ that satisfies the constraints.

2.2.4 Model Solver

The proposed computational simulation system is formulated as a time-varying partial differential equation, which is commonly adopted in many deformable model approaches [10]. Specifically, the dynamics of each cortical surface vertex can be simply formulated as $\ddot{\mathbf{x}}_i = \mathbf{f}_i / m_i$, where $\ddot{\mathbf{x}}_i$ is the acceleration of the vertex i, $\mathbf{f}_i$ is the force that combines all forces affecting vertex i, and m_i is the mass of vertex i, which is usually defined as the sum of one thirds of the masses of all triangles around vertex i. By combining all equations on the cortical surface together, we have the discrete form of developing cerebral cortex as:

$$\ddot{\mathbf{x}} = \mathbf{M}^{-1}F(\mathbf{x}, \dot{\mathbf{x}}) \tag{6}$$

where $\mathbf{x}, \dot{\mathbf{x}}$ and $\ddot{\mathbf{x}}$ are the vertex's position, velocity and acceleration respectively, $\mathbf{M}$ is a $3n \times 3n$ (n is the number of vertices) diagonal mass matrix on vertices where $diag(\mathbf{M}) = (m_1, m_1, m_1, m_2, m_2, m_2, \ldots, m_n, m_n, m_n)$ and $F(\mathbf{x}, \dot{\mathbf{x}})$ is the net force vector that combines all forces on cortical surface vertices. The Newmark scheme, which is widely used for solving ODE (ordinary differential equation) integration problem, is adopted in our implementation.

3 Results

We simulated the computational model of cortical folding introduced in Section 2. The parameters in the deformable model and growth model were the same in both simulations with and without skull constraints, which were set as: $K_c = 1$, $\tau_{ce} = 1000$, $K_b = 5$, $\tau_{cb} = 1000$, $m = 0.002$, $k = 3$, $\Delta t = 0.05$. The folding development results of the 3D morphogenetic model are illustrated in Figure 3. Figure 3a and Figure 3b show the snapshots of cortex development at the iteration number 0, 40, 80, 120, 160 and 200 with and without skull constraints respectively. By visual evaluation, it is evident that reasonably realistic convolutions are generated during these simulations. To quantitatively evaluate the produced convolutions, we use the curvature as the measurement of cortical folding. Also, we use the total surface area of the developing cortex to measure its growth rate. The differences between the total area of cortex and the average absolute Gaussian curvature of the cortex surface are illustrated in Figure 4a and Figure 4b respectively. Figure 4a shows that the cortical surface area increases almost linearly with the simulation iteration numbers, irrespective of whether or not there is skull constraint. The results in Figure 4a indicate that the cortex increases its surface area and convolutes itself to reduce the fast growing internal tension with or without skull constraint. However, as shown in Figure 4b, it is intriguing that the increase in speed of average curvature in simulation with skull constraint is much higher than the one without skull constraint, meaning that cortex development with skull constraint is much more convoluted than that without skull constraint. This computational simulation result shows that the skull boundary condition is important in regulation of the cortical folding process.

The results in Figure 3 and Figure 4 also tell that the cortex growth pattern is quite different because of the skull constraint. Without skull constraint, the cortex expands with the similar shape of the initial cortex during the first 40 iterations, and then small shape changes appear during 40~80 iterations. After that, primary sulci rapidly develop during 80~160 iterations and then, secondary sulci develop between major sulci. In this model simulation, smaller tertiary gyri and sulci are not found to be developed. Since most of the primary sulci developed in this model simulation are long but not deep, the average absolute Gaussian curvature is slowly increased during the cortical development process. It is striking that the cortex growth pattern in the simulation with skull constraint is quite different, that is, the primary and secondary sulci are developed much earlier and faster, e.g., in the iteration 40~120. Also, smaller tertiary gyri and sulci are developed during last iterations (120~200). The sulci developed in this model simulation are deeper, compared to those simulations without skull constraint. Thus, the average absolute Gaussian curvature increases faster as shown in Figure 4b. The quite different cortical growths patterns, due to the existence of skull constraints or not, further demonstrate that mechanical constraints of the brain skull significantly regulate the cortical folding process.

The second experiment investigates the effect of global cell growth rate on the cortical folding process. The Malthusian parameter m in Eq. (5) models the cell growth

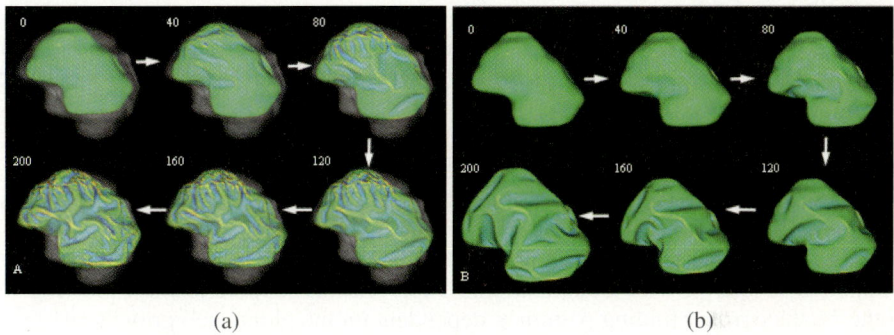

Fig. 3. Cortical development with or without skull constraints. (a) and (b) show the snapshots of cortex development at the iteration number 0, 40, 80, 120, 160 and 200 with or without skull constraints respectively. The parameters are set as: $K_c = 1$, $\tau_{ce} = 1000$, $K_b = 5$, $\tau_{cb} = 1000$, $m = 0.002$, $k = 3$. Mean curvature bar: -0.6 ▬▬▬ 0.8.

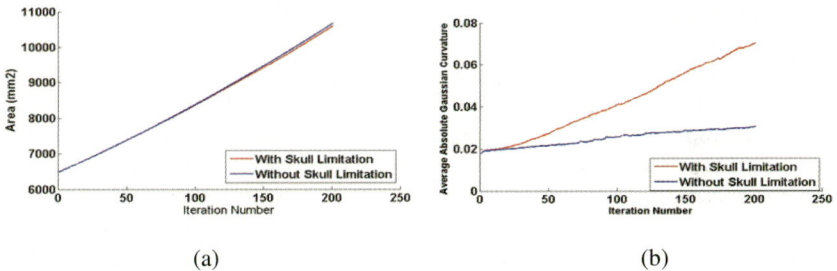

Fig. 4. The differences of the total area of cortex and the average absolute Gaussian curvature of the cortex surface during convolution development

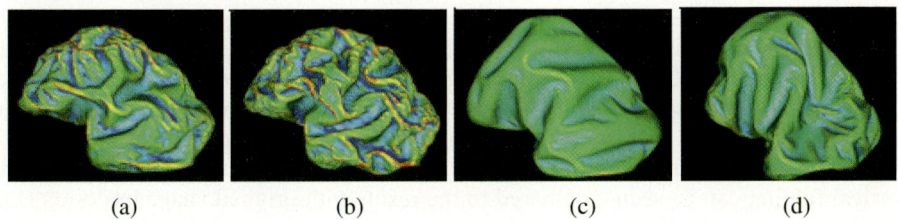

Fig. 5. (a) and (b) are simulations with skull constraints. (a) The parameters are set as those in Figure 3. (b) The parameter m is changed to 0.004. (c) and (c) are simulations without skull constraints. Parameters are the same as (a) and (b).

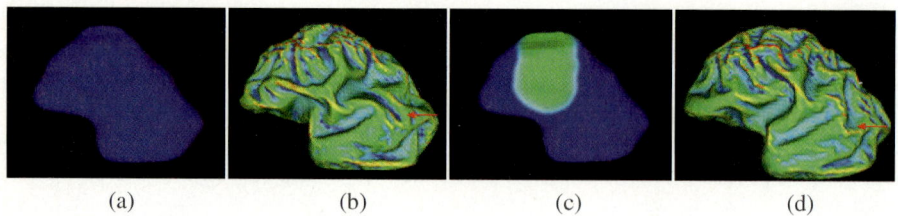

(a) (b) (c) (d)

Fig. 6. Effect of initial cortex shape on the development and distribution of convolution. Compared to the original cortex (a), the green region in (c) is deformed around 2mm inside. (b) and (d) are the results of 200 iterations of simulation. Other parameters are set the same as in Figure 5.

rate. When the growth parameter m is increased from 0.002 (Figure 5a) to 0.004 (Figure 5b), the cortical growth speed is almost doubled according Eq. (5). As a result, more deep sulci and smaller gyri can be found in the simulated folding, as shown in Figure 5b. Also, the average absolute mean curvature increased significantly from 0.31 to 0.35 in the cortex development simulation with the skull constraint. These simulation results provide computational experimental support to the following hypothesis: the cortical folding pattern is dependent on the global cell growth rate in the whole cortex. It is interesting that the effect of global cell growth rate on the cortical folding process is much less significant in the simulations without skull constraint, as shown in the Figure 5c and 5d. For example, even though the parameter m is increased to 0.004 from 0.002, the average absolute mean curvature only increased slightly. This result further demonstrates that the skull constraint is an important modulator of cortical folding pattern formation.

The computational results in this experiment demonstrate that overgrowth of the cortex will increase the cortical folding and convolution. This simulation result might provide theoretical clues to the following two independent studies: 1) In a MRI study of Autism, it was reported that the left frontal cortical folding is significantly increased in autism patient, but there is also a significant decrease in the frontal folding patterns with age in the autistic group [13]; and 2) It was reported that in Autism, the brain overgrows at the beginning of life and slows or arrests growth during early childhood [14]. In the future, it would be very interesting to combine our folding simulation studies with longitudinal MRI studies of Autistic brains and normal controls to further elucidate the relationship between brain growth and cortical folding in both Autism and normal neurodevelopment.

It was hypothezied that relative degrees of tethering of different cortical areas or initial geometry of cortex had significant influence on cortical folding pattern [7]. To examine this hypothesis, a small artificial deformation is applied to the originally reconstructed cortex surface as illustrated in Figure 6c. The green region is manually labeled and is deformed around 2mm towards the ventricular zone. The cortical folding simulation results in Figure 6b and 6d demonstrate that initial geometry of the cortex has significant influence on the resulted cortical folding pattern. However, if there is no skull constraint in the simulation, less influence of the intial geometry on cortical folding can be seen, compared to the result with original shape of cortex (figure not shown). It is also apparent from the results in Figure 6 that the local shape differences not only cause the folding pattern variation near the locally deformed region, but also influence the cortical folding pattern all over the cortex, as denoted by red arrows in Figure 6. This result demonstrates that cortical folding process is a global and system-level behaviour, but not a localized procedure, and provides computational experiment support to the idea that cortical folding process might be a minimization of global energy function [3].

4 Conclusion

We believe that the combination of computational simulation of cortex folding and in-vivo neuroimaging of fetus brain development will be very helpful to understand the mechanisms of cortical folding, as well as interactions between different mechanisms. Also, in the long term, the combination of computational modeling and neuroimaging might be helpful to understand the mechanisms of many neurological disorders that result in abnormal cortical folding.

References

1. Talairach, J., Tournoux, P.: Co-planar Stereotaxic Atlas of the Human Brain. Thieme, New York (1988)
2. Fischl, B., Rajendran, N., Busa, E., Augustinack, J., Hinds, O., Yeo, B.T., Mohlberg, H., Amunts, K., Zilles, K.: Cortical Folding Patterns and Predicting Cytoarchitecture. Cereb. Cortex 18(8), 1973–1980 (2008)
3. Van Essen, D.: A tension-based theory of morphogenesis and compact wiring in the central nervous system. Nature 385, 313–318 (1997)
4. Raghavan, R., Lawton, W., Ranjan, S.R., Viswanathan, R.R.: A continuum mechanics-based model for cortical Growth. J. Theor. Biol. 187, 285–296 (1997)
5. Toro, R., Burnod, Y.: A Morphogenetic Model of the Development of Cortical Convolutions. Cerebral Cortex 15, 1900–1913 (2005)
6. Rakic, P.: A Century of Progress in Corticoneurogenesis: From Silver Impregnation to Genetic Engineering. Cerebral Cortex 16, i3–i17 (2006)
7. Brown, M., Keynes, R., Lumsden, A.: The developing brain. Oxford University Press, Oxford (2002)
8. Beth Israel Deaconess Medical Center,
   http://radnet.bidmc.harvard.edu/fetalatlas/
9. Yushkevich, P.A., Piven, J., Hazlett, H.C., Smith, R.G., Ho, S., Gee, J.C., Gerig, G.: User-guided 3D active contour segmentation of anatomical structures: Significantly improved efficiency and reliability. Neuroimage 31, 1116–1128 (2006)
10. Terzopoulos, D., Platt, J., Barr, A., Fleischer, K.: Elastically Deformable Models. Computer Graphics 21, 205–214 (1987)
11. Murray, J.: Mathematical biology. Springer, Heidelberg (1993)
12. Fischl, B., Sereno, M.I., Dale, A.M.: Cortical surface-based analysis II: inflation, flattening and a surface-based coordinate system. Neuroimage 9, 195–207 (1999)
13. Hardan, A.Y., Jou, R.J., Keshavan, M.S., Varma, R., Minshew, N.J.: Increased frontal cortical folding in autism: a preliminary MRI study. Psychiatry Research: Neuroimaging 131, 263–268 (2004)
14. Courchesne, E., Pierce, K., Schumann, C.M., Redcay, E., Buckwalter, J.A., Kennedy, D.P., Morgan, J.: Mapping early brain development in autism. Neuron 56(2), 399–413 (2007)
15. Geng, G., Johnston, L.A., Yan, E., Britto, J.M., Smith, D.W., Walker, D.W., Egan, G.F.: Biomechanisms for Modelling Cerebral Cortical Folding. Medical Image Analysis (in press) (2009)

Tensor-Based Morphometry of Fibrous Structures with Application to Human Brain White Matter

Hui Zhang[1], Paul A. Yushkevich[1], Daniel Rueckert[2], and James C. Gee[1]

[1] Penn Image Computing and Science Laboratory (PICSL),
Department of Radiology, University of Pennsylvania, USA
[2] Department of Computing, Imperial College London, London, UK

Abstract. Tensor-based morphometry (TBM) is a powerful approach for examining shape changes in anatomy both across populations and in time. Our work extends the standard TBM for quantifying local volumetric changes to establish both rich and intuitive descriptors of shape changes in fibrous structures. It leverages the data from diffusion tensor imaging to determine local spatial configuration of fibrous structures and combines this information with spatial transformations derived from image registration to quantify fibrous structure-specific changes, such as local changes in fiber length and in thickness of fiber bundles. In this paper, we describe the theoretical framework of our approach in detail and illustrate its application to study brain white matter. Our results show that additional insights can be gained with the proposed analysis.

1 Introduction

Tensor-based morphometry (TBM) is one of the most popular deformation-based approaches for analyzing anatomy. It computes, for each voxel in the image domain, the spatial derivatives of the transformations that align a set of input subject images to a template of choice. These images can be acquired from different populations, enabling cross-sectional study of anatomical differences between populations. TBM can also be applied to study longitudinal changes in anatomy by examining the transformations that match images acquired sequentially of the same subjects. The standard TBM has primarily taken advantage of the determinant of the spatial derivative matrix (known as the Jacobian matrix) [1,2], which enables statistical mapping of local volumetric changes across populations and in time.

A well-understood weakness of using only the Jacobian determinant is that significant amount of information captured in the full matrix is being discarded. As a result, it will not be able to detect many patterns of differences that involve anisotropic changes along different spatial directions but result in no net volumetric changes. Recently, Lepore et al [3] proposed the generalized TBM as a solution to this problem. The generalized TBM extends the standard approach by applying multivariate statistics on the full deformation tensors which are derived from the Jacobian matrices and completely capture shape changes contained within them. The consistent gain in power to detect structural abnormalities makes the approach highly desirable for drug trials or computer-assisted diagnosis. However, the multivariate approach makes it difficult to interpret the detected abnormalities in anatomically intuitive terms.

In this paper, we propose a different approach for remedying the weakness of the standard TBM. The approach is specifically tailored for examining fibrous structures such as white matter and muscle. It is driven by the key observation that, for fibrous structures, the effect of transformation depends not only on the properties of the transformation itself but also on the configuration of the fibrous structure undergoing the warping. The proposed approach leverages the configuration information of the fibrous structures available from diffusion tensor imaging (DTI) and establishes both rich and intuitive descriptors of shape properties. Its ability to gain additional insights is demonstrated in an application to examine gender-related white matter differences in the aging population.

The paper is organized as follows: Section 2 describes the proposed approach in detail. Section 3 describes the application of the proposed approach to examine gender difference of white matter in the aging population. Section 4 summarizes the contribution and discusses future works.

2 Method

2.1 Tensor-Based Morphometry

In the TBM framework, given an input subject, we first establish the spatial correspondence between the subject and a template using a high-dimensional nonlinear image registration algorithm. The correspondence between the two images is captured by some diffeomorphic spatial transformation $\phi : \Omega \to \Omega$, where $\Omega \subseteq \mathbb{R}^n$ is the image domain ($n = 2$ for 2D and $n = 3$ for 3D). In particular, the Jacobian of the transformation, $J_\phi : x \mapsto D\phi(x)$, establishes a local affine transformation model that maps the local neighborhood around a point x in the template to the corresponding neighborhood around the point $\phi(x)$ in the subject, such that,

$$\phi(x + \epsilon) = \phi(x) + J_\phi(x)\epsilon + O(\|\epsilon\|^2),$$

with J_ϕ being a $n \times n$ matrix, the $(i,j)^{th}$ entry of which is $(D\phi)_{ij} := \partial \phi_i / \partial x_j$. Beause the determinant of the Jacobian matrix J_ϕ quantifies the volume change from mapping a local neighborhood in the template to the corresponding one in the subject, a map of local volumetric change can be produced by computing this quantity at each point in the image domain [1,2]. This approach is most commonly used in the TBM analysis, in part because the descriptive nature of the measure makes it easy to understand and to interpret. On the other hand, its inability to differentiate other patterns of shape changes that do not result in volume change has motivated active research in identifying alternative complementary measures.

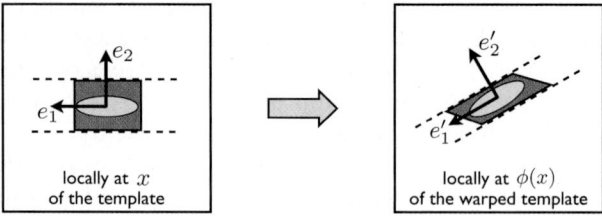

Fig. 1. The schematic illustrates the local behavior of warping some fibrous structure with the transformation ϕ. See the main text in Section 2.2 for the details.

2.2 Overview of the Proposed Framework

The proposed framework builds upon the standard TBM analysis by establishing a set of descriptors of shape changes that are natural and specific for fibrous structures. We observe that the fiber orientation information encoded in DTI can be leveraged to decompose the Jacobian matrix of a transformation into parts that can be interpreted in intuitive terms. This observation is illustrated in Fig. 1, which depicts, in the left panel, the local neighborhood around a point x in a DTI template, and in the right panel, the transformed version of this neighborhood using some transformation ϕ. The original neighborhood around x is represented using a shaded rectangle; its transformed version, which is centered around $\phi(x)$, is represented using a shaded parallelogram. The diffusion tensor at x and its warped version at $\phi(x)$ are shown as two lightly-shaded ellipses. The eigenvectors of each diffusion tensor form a natural local reference frame for its neighborhood: their primary eigenvectors, denoted by e_1 at x and e'_1 at $\phi(x)$, are parallel to the orientations of the underlying fiber bundles; their secondary eigenvectors, denoted by e_2 at x and e'_2 at $\phi(x)$, are perpendicular to the fiber orientations. The local trajectories of the underlying fiber bundles are depicted by the pairs of dashed curves, which shall not be interpreted as the fiber bundle boundaries. Observe that the effect of the Jacobian matrix J_ϕ on the transformation of the original neighborhood can be parsed into three steps: (1) rotating the rectangle such that e_1 and e_2 coincide with e'_1 and e'_2, respectively; (2) compressing the rectangle along e'_2, and (3) shearing the rectangle along e'_1. In other words, by factoring out some *appropriate* rotation matrix, the action of the remainder of J_ϕ can be interpreted intuitively in the *local* reference frame of the *warped* underlying fiber bundle.

It turns out that this kind of decomposition of the Jacobian matrix can be done in general for fibrous structures, provided the fiber orientation information is available. In this paper, we consider the particular scenario in which the fiber orientation is derived from DTI measurements. Specifically, given the diffusion tensor D at x, its eigenvectors $\{e_i\}_{1 \leq i \leq n}$, ordered in the descending order of the corresponding eigenvalues, form the basis of a natural local reference frame for the underlying fiber bundle; the rotation matrix that constitutes a change of basis from this local reference frame to the laboratory frame, which we will

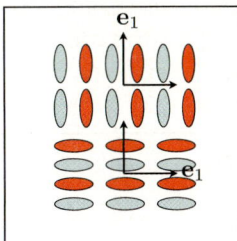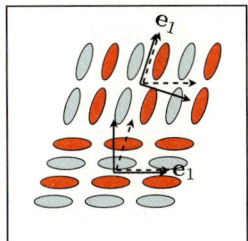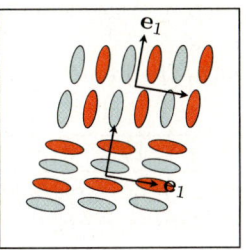

Fig. 2. Tensor reorientation strategies for recovering correct fiber configuration after warping with a horizontal shear transformation. From left to right, the image before warping, the warped image using the PPD strategy, the warped image using the FS strategy. Observe how the original fiber connectivity, indicated with identically colored ellipses, is intact when PPD is used but is severely disrupted when FS is used.

denote by Q, has e_i as its ith column. Similarly, the eigenvectors $\{e'_i\}_{1 \leq i \leq n}$ of the warped diffusion tensor D' at $\phi(x)$ form the basis of a natural local reference frame for the warped fiber bundle; the change-of-basis matrix from this local reference frame to the laboratory frame will be denoted as Q'. The appropriate rotation matrix that matches the local reference frame of D to the one of D' is then $Q'Q^{-1}$. Therefore, we can write the Jacobian matrix as

$$J_\phi = (Q'RQ'^{-1})(Q'Q^{-1}), \tag{1}$$

with R denotes the remainder of J_ϕ after factoring out the rotation $Q'Q^{-1}$ and being viewed in the local reference frame of D'. The following section describes the computation of R and shows that the structure of the matrix makes it particularly amenable to intuitive description of its action similar to the example given in Fig. 1.

2.3 Computation of the Residual Deformation and Its Structure

The key to computing R is in finding the tensor corresponding to the fiber bundle configuration after warping. This is known as the tensor reorientation problem, the solution to which has been established by the seminal work of Alexander et al. [4]. The authors proposed and validated a number of strategies for tensor reorientation, including the finite strain (FS) strategy and the preservation of principal direction (PPD) strategy. We choose to use the PPD strategy, summarized in Algorithm 1, because it preserves the connectivity of the underlying fiber bundle, crucial to the fidelity of warping. As illustrated in Fig. 2, the preservation of connectivity requires that the appropriate reorientation depends both on the warping transformation and the fiber configuration before warping, as done in the PPD strategy. In contrast, the FS strategy applies an identical reorientation to all tensors regardless of their fiber configurations, which evidently can disrupt fiber connectivity and thus represents only an approximation to PPD.

Given our choice of the reorientation strategy, the computation of the residual deformation viewed in the local frame of the warped tensor can now be summarized in Algorithm 2, which uses Equation (1) and the fact that Q' is orthogonal, i.e., $Q'^{-1} = Q'^{\mathrm{T}}$. The structure of the residual deformation is formally stated with Theorem 1.

Algorithm 1. PPD strategy for tensor reorientation

1: compute e'_1: $e'_1 = Je_1/\|Je_1\|$
2: compute e'_2: $e'_2 = n/\|n\|$, where $n = Je_2 - ((Je_2)^{\mathrm{T}} e'_1)e'_1$
3: compute e'_3: $e'_3 = e'_1 \times e'_2$

Algorithm 2. Compute the residual deformation R at a point x

1: compute the Jacobian matrix J at x
2: compute the matrix $Q = (e_1, e_2, e_3)$ with $\{e_i\}_{1 \leq i \leq 3}$ being the eigenvectors of the diffusion tensor D at x ordered in the descending order of the corresponding eigenvalues
3: compute the matrix $Q' = (e'_1, e'_2, e'_3)$ with $\{e'_i\}_{1 \leq i \leq 3}$ being derived from J and $\{e_i\}_{1 \leq i \leq 3}$ using the PPD strategy
4: compute the matrix $R = Q'^{\mathrm{T}} J Q$

Theorem 1. *The residual deformation R, computed using Algorithm 2, is an upper-triangular matrix with positive diagonal entries.*

Proof. First, we simplify and rewrite Equation (1) as

$$JQ = Q'R. \qquad (2)$$

Recall that, by defintion, $Q = (e_1, e_2, e_3)$. Hence we have $JQ = (Je_1, Je_2, Je_3)$. Here we use a different formulation of the PPD strategy that was pointed out by Cao et al [5]. They recognized that the PPD strategy, as described in Algorithm 1, is in fact equivalent to the application of the Gram-Schmidt orthonormalization procedure, which produces an orthonormal basis from a non-orthogonal but linearly-independent basis. In this case, the non-orthogonal but linearly-independent basis is composed of the vectors Je_1, Je_2, and Je_3. The orthonormal basis that the Gram-Schmidt procedure generates from this basis consists of precisely the vectors e'_1, e'_2, and e'_3. The procedure is summarized in Algorithm 3; its equivalence to Algorithm 1 can be readily verified.

Algorithm 3. Gram-Schmidt procedure applied to Je_1, Je_2, and Je_3

1: Initialize $v_i = Je_i$ for $1 \leq i \leq 3$
2: compute u_1: $u_1 = v_1$
3: compute u_2: $u_2 = v_2 - \mathrm{proj}_{u_1} v_2$, where $\mathrm{proj}_a b = (a^{\mathrm{T}} b)a/(a^{\mathrm{T}} a)$
4: compute u_3: $u_3 = v_3 - \mathrm{proj}_{u_1} v_3 - \mathrm{proj}_{u_2} v_3$
5: compute e'_1, e'_2, and e'_3: $e'_1 = u_1/\|u_1\|$, $e'_2 = u_2/\|u_2\|$, and $e'_3 = u_3/\|u_3\|$

The equivalence of Algorithms 1 and 3 is important because the Gram-Schmidt procedure can be further viewed as the QR-decomposition of matrices which *uniquely* decompose any invertible matrix A into an orthogonal matrix Q_A and an upper triangular matrix R_A with positive diagonal entries such that $A = Q_A R_A$ (See [6] for a proof). In particular, the column vectors of the orthogonal matrix Q_A are computed from applying the Gram-Schmidt procedure to the column vectors of the matrix A. In our case, JQ is the matrix to be decomposed with the QR-decomposition procedure. The matrix is clearly invertible since J is the Jacobian matrix of a diffeomorphic transformation and Q is an orthogonal matrix. By definition, Q', whose column vectors are e_1', e_2' and e_3', is precisely the orthogonal matrix computed from the QR-decomposition of JQ. From Equation (2) and the uniqueness of the QR-decomposition, it is evident that R is the upper-triangluar matrix with positive diagonal entries. □

An additional property of the proposed decomposition can be seen by rewriting Equation (1) as

$$J_\phi = (Q'Q^{-1})(QRQ^{-1}),$$

which reads that the effect of J_ϕ can also be seen as first applying the same residual deformation but viewed in the local reference frame of D, then applying the same rotation $Q'Q^{-1}$. In other words, the order in which the residual deformation and the rotation are applied does not change the output.

2.4 Intuitive Descriptors for White Matter Morphometry

To derive intuitive descriptors for white matter morphometry, we first observe that, in white matter, the primary eigenvector, e_1, has been shown to provide a good estimate to the orientation of the underlying axon fiber bundle [7]. On the other hand, the secondary and the tertiary eigenvectors, e_2 and e_3, can not be determined consistently or can be of any two orthogonal unit vectors lying in the plane perpendicular to e_1, because the secondary and tertiary eigenvalues are often very close to one another or can not be consistently differentiated due to noise. In this scenario, the residual deformation will take the following more general form:

$$R = \begin{pmatrix} s_1 & V^T \\ 0 & S_{23} \end{pmatrix},$$

where V is a 2-dimensional vector and S_{23} is a 2-by-2 matrix. It can be viewed as the QR-decomposition with the basis formed by e_1 and the subspace orthogonal to it, spanned by e_2 and e_3. Because $\det R = s_1 \times \det(S_{23})$, the structure of R enables us to decompose the determinant of Jacobian, $\det J = \det R$, into two components, s_1 and $\det S_{23}$. s_1 measures local changes along the eigenvector e_1, i.e., elongation or compression along the fiber bundle; $\det S_{23}$, referred to as s_{23} hereafter, measures local changes orthogonal to e_1, i.e., expansion or shrinkage in the cross-sectional area of the fiber bundle.

3 Application

To demonstrate the utility of the proposed analysis, we applied the analysis to study gender difference of white matter in the aging population. The subjects used in the present study were extracted from the IXI brain database (http://www.ixi.org.uk) developed jointly by Imperial College of Science Technology & Medicine and University College London. The IXI database consists of brain MR images from 550 normal subjects between the age of 20 and 80 years acquired at three sites and freely available for downloads. We selected a total of 35 subjects (16 males and 19 females) with the following criteria: 65 years or older, scanned at the same site, and with available DTI data of sufficient quality. To spatially normalize the data, we applied the approach described in [8] which simultaneously constructs a population-specific DTI template from the subject data and normalizes the subjects to the resulting template. The approach is based on high-dimensional tensor-based image registration and has been shown to outperform scalar-based registration.

After normalization, we applied both the standard TBM and the proposed approach to the Jacobian matrix fields computed from the spatial transformations mapping the subjects to the template. The standard voxel-based statistical mapping on the whole-brain white matter was then computed for the Jacobian determinant map, the maps of the two proposed descriptors. The white matter region is defined as the voxels with fractional anisotropy above 0.2. The voxels with significant differences between the gender groups were determined after FDR-based multiple comparison correction at the significance level $p_{FDR} < 0.05$.

The results are shown in Fig. 3, which clearly demonstrates that additional insights can be gained with the proposed approach. The two signifcant clusters

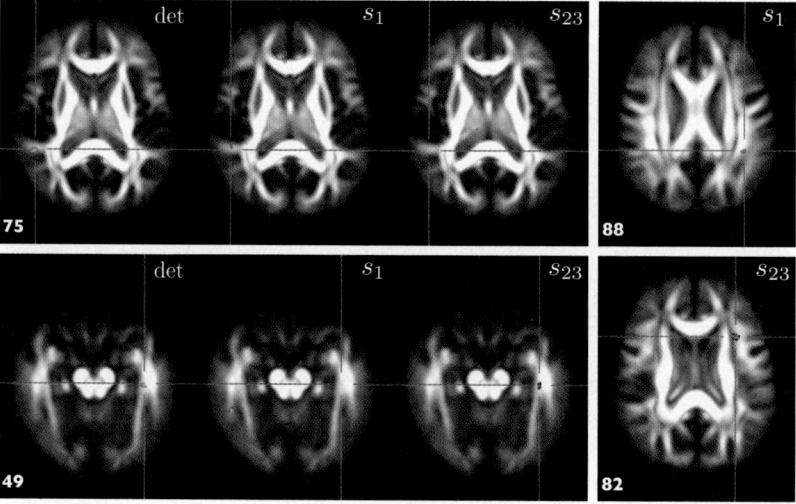

Fig. 3. Results of the voxel-based statistical mappings on the Jacobian determinant (det), s_1 and s_{23}. See Sec. 3 for the details

were identified with the standard TBM approach, shown on slice 49 and 75 respectively. The cluster on the slice 75 co-localizes with one of the clusters of s_1, suggesting that local volumetric change at the location can be attributed to local change along the fiber bundle. On the other hand, the cluster on the slice 49 co-localizes with one of the clusters of s_{23}, indicating that local volumetric change at the location can be attributed to local change in the cross-sectional area of the fiber bundle. Furthermore, additional clusters, such as the examples on the slices 82 and 88, were identified by s_1 and s_{23}. These group differences were otherwise not detected by the standard TBM alone.

4 Discussion

In summary, we have described a new approach for TBM tailored specifically for examining fibrous structures. The approach derives the information on fibrous structure configuration from DTI data and combines it with the transformations computed from image registration to elucidate shape and orientational changes specific to fibrous structures. The resulting descriptors are highly intuitive and specific. We note that additional orientational descriptors can also be determined from the rotation matrix $Q'Q^{-1}$, e.g., $e_1^T e_1'$ which measures the angle between e_1 and e_1'. Future works will examine the application of such orientational descriptors and apply this new theoretical framework to study cardiac laminar structures.

Acknowledgments. The authors gratefully acknowledge support of this work by the NIH via grants EB006266, NS045839, DA022897.

References

1. Freeborough, P.A., Fox, N.C.: Modeling brain deformations in Alzheimer disease by fluid registration of serial MR images. J. Comput. Assisted. Tomogr. 22 (1998)
2. Gee, J.C., Bajcsy, R.K.: Elastic matching: continuum mechanical and probabilistic analysis. In: Brain warping. Academic Press, San Diego (1999)
3. Lepore, N., Brun, C., Chou, Y.Y., Chiang, M.C., Dutton, R.A., Hayashi, K.M., Luders, E., Lopez, O.L., Aizenstein, H.J., Toga, A.W., Becker, J.T., Thompson, P.M.: Generalized tensor-based morphometry of HIV/AIDS using multivariate statistics on deformation tensors. IEEE TMI 27(1) (January 2008)
4. Alexander, D.C., Pierpaoli, C., Basser, P.J., Gee, J.C.: Spatial transformations of diffusion tensor magnetic resonance images. IEEE TMI 20(11) (2001)
5. Cao, Y., Miller, M., Mori, S., Winslow, R.L., Younes, L.: Diffeomorphic maching of diffusion tensor images. In: Proc. MMBIA (2006)
6. Gallier, J.: Geometric methods and applications, for computer science and engineering. In: Texts in applied mathematics. Springer, New York (2000)
7. Pajevic, S., Pierpaoli, C.: Color schemes to represent the orientation of anisotropic tissues from diffusion tensor data: application to white matter fiber tract mapping in the human brain. MRM 42 (1999)
8. Zhang, H., Avants, B.B., Yushkevich, P.A., Woo, J.H., Wang, S., McCluskey, L.F., Elman, L.B., Melhem, E.R., Gee, J.C.: High-dimensional spatial normalization of diffusion tensor images improves the detection of white matter differences in amyotrophic lateral sclerosis. IEEE TMI 26(11), 1585–1597 (2007)

A Fuzzy Region-Based Hidden Markov Model for Partial-Volume Classification in Brain MRI

Albert Huang[1], Rafeef Abugharbieh[1], and Roger Tam[2]

[1] Department of Electrical and Computer Engineering
{alberth,rafeef}@ece.ubc.ca
[2] Department of Radiology, The University of British Columbia, Vancouver, B.C., Canada
roger@msmri.medicine.ubc.ca

Abstract. We present a novel fuzzy region-based hidden Markov model (*fr*bHMM) for unsupervised partial-volume classification in brain magnetic resonance images (MRIs). The primary contribution is an efficient graphical representation of 3D image data in which irregularly-shaped image regions have memberships to a number of classes rather than one discrete class. Our model groups voxels into regions for efficient processing, but also refines the region boundaries to the voxel level for optimal accuracy. This strategy is most effective in data where partial-volume effects due to resolution-limited image acquisition result in intensity ambiguities. Our *fr*bHMM employs a forward-backward scheme for parameter estimation through iterative computation of region class likelihoods. We validate our proposed method on simulated and clinical brain MRIs of both normal and multiple sclerosis subjects. Quantitative results demonstrate the advantages of our fuzzy model over the discrete approach with significant improvements in classification accuracy (30% reduction in mean square error).

1 Introduction

Graphical models have long been successfully used in various signal processing and analysis applications such as speech recognition, computer vision, error correction coding, and genome analysis. Such models provide a graphical representation of probabilistic distributions by expressing complex computations for inference and learning as simpler graphical structures [1]. There exist two major classes of graphical models - directed and undirected. The directed graphical models, or Bayesian Networks (BN), specify a particular directionality on the links of the graphs, which are useful for conveying causal relationships between the underlying random variables. An example of BN is the hidden Markov model (HMM), which is commonly used to represent stochastic processes. On the other hand, undirected graphical models or Markov random fields (MRF) do not carry any directional implications but rather specify some constraints between the random variables. Both directed and undirected graphical models have been applied successfully in the context of brain tissue segmentation from magnetic resonance imaging (MRI) data, such that each of the image voxels represents an underlying hidden random variable of tissue class label, which cannot be observed directly but can be indirectly estimated given observations by inference.

Performing exact inference on a fully connected high dimensional graphical model is a daunting task. Regardless of whether the model is directed or undirected, the amount of computations is expensive if not intractable. For the directed representation, 2D/3D HMMs (causal MRF) have been proposed on a regular rectangular pixel lattice [2], but estimating the exact states requires exponential time thus a block-based approach [3] and an iterative approximation method [4] have been proposed to improve efficiency. However, modeling an image in such a way is odd as voxels do not typically bear causal orders. Recently, a more data-driven model [5] was proposed as a tree-structure extension of the iterative approximation method [4]. For the undirected representation, performing a maximum a posteriori (MAP) estimation on a hidden MRF (HMRF) is a computationally difficult problem [6]. In such cases, the optimal solutions were usually computed using some optimization techniques through local optimization or optimization on a relaxed problem [7-9].

For image segmentation tasks, the above mentioned estimation methods commonly provide a single discrete label to each image voxel. An alternative model subdivides the content of one voxel into numerous classes simultaneously, allowing for a more accurate modeling of a common physical imaging limitation, namely, partial volume effects. Discrete segmentations thus appear as a special case by assuming that no partial volume voxels exist, where all classes are null except for the hard estimate. One can intuitively infer the partial volumes from the class distributions of a discrete labeling process using techniques such as the classical forward-backward algorithm [10]. However, a more accurate model should simultaneously model all pixel likelihoods without assuming one single, particular true label class. Furthermore, classifications based on partial-volume models have shown to achieve improved accuracies in tissue volume measurements [11, 12]. A number of interesting works in this aspect have been done using graphical models. Bricq *et al.* [13] converted 3D scan data into a 1D chain. Such vectorization is not truly 3D as only a single fixed-ordering neighboring pixel is considered in the estimation process, and the scan order is predefined irrespective of the data. Others [12, 14] utilized fuzzy hidden MRFs to incorporate information from immediate neighbors. However, parameter estimation in such an undirected model is known to be difficult and time consuming. In contrast, estimation in a directed model is comparatively easy with the results achieved being generally similar to those of an undirected model [15]. Therefore, starting with a more natural, data-driven region-based HMM (rbHMM) that was proposed in [5], where the advantages of rotational invariance and increased efficiency were shown, we propose, in this paper, a novel partial-volume extension for brain tissue segmentation – henceforth referred to as fuzzy rbHMM or *fr*bHMM. We integrate the classical forward-backward scheme in the tree-structured parameter estimation algorithm and refine region boundaries to the voxel level resulting in a more accurate classification model for partial-volume effects. We present quantitative validation results demonstrating the advantages of modeling each voxel in brain MRI scans as mixtures of multiple classes as opposed to one single label in simulated as well as real clinical MR data of both normal and Multiple Sclerosis (MS) patient subjects.

2 Methods

We first briefly describe the discrete rbHMM of [5] and present our proposed extension for modeling partial volumes within a new fuzzy framework (hereafter referred to by *fr*bHMM). We then describe how the forward-backward algorithm is employed for estimating the 3D *fr*bHMM parameters and region class likelihoods, and how the classification resolution is improved by further refining image regions.

2.1 Region-Based Hidden Markov Model Overview

In [5], Huang *et al.* proposed a method where an image U is first divided into a set R of contiguous homogeneous local regions r_i, each of size $N_i = \|r_i\|$, where $1 \leq i \leq N_R$ and $N_R = \|R\|$ is the total number of regions. Each voxel with coordinates (x, y, z) belongs to a region r_i if the pixel is labeled as $L(x, y, z) = i$. The assumption was that each region would exhibit similar properties such as intensity or texture, and that by grouping them together using, e.g., a watershed transform or a normalized cut, the complexity and computational cost can be largely reduced. For grayscale images, e.g. MRI, such regional features f_i can be simply defined by the mean observed voxel intensities of r_i. The observed f_i represented noisy regions with true underlying discrete states s_i, which can then be optimally estimated in a MAP sense based on the three statistical model assumptions:

Assumption 1: The observations for the underlying model states $l \in \{1, 2, ..., N_s\}$, where N_s is the total number of given underlying states, follow Gaussian distributions with mean μ_l and variance σ_l^2, which are estimated from the observed samples..

Assumption 2: If s_i is known, then f_i is conditionally independent of other regions.

Assumption 3: The true underlying state s_i is governed by an irregular Markov mesh such that each region r_i has a set of spatially neighboring regions R_i'. The transitional probabilities are defined as $P(s_i = l \mid n_i) = \alpha_{n_i, l}$, where $n_i = \{(s_i'', f_i''): r_i'' \in R_i''\}$ is a set of states and features of some preceding neighbors R_i'', which is a subset of R_i' where states s_i'' are already known.

The primary advantages of this region-based modeling and its tree-structured parameter estimation scheme are increased efficiency over pixel-based methods and invariance to rotations that are commonly observed in medical images.

2.2 Proposed Fuzzy Region-Based Hidden Markov Model

Our main contribution here is the extension of rbHMM by introducing fuzzy states that allow each region to belong to multiple classes simultaneously. Rather than considering one single 'true' underlying state s_i, we now consider an underlying state vector $S_i = (t_{i,1}, t_{i,2}, ..., t_{i,Ns})$ such that $\sum_{l=1}^{Ns} t_{i,l} = 1$, $t_{i,l} \in [0,1]$ represents the proportion of the lth class in region r_i for $l = 1, ..., Ns$. The term $t_{i,l}$ can also be seen as the probability of labeling region r_i with label l given the model and observations. For discrete or crisp segmentation, $t_{i,l} = 0$ for all l in S_i except for the single element where $s_i = l$, then $t_{i,l} = 1$.

To compute the model parameters, K-means clustering is used as a simple way to initialize the state means and variances from the samples. The state probabilities $S_i = (t_{i,1}, t_{i,2}, ..., t_{i,Ns})$ for $1 \leq i \leq N_R$ are then calculated based on a Gaussian mixture assumption. The transition probabilities $\alpha_{n_i, l}$ are determined based on probability-weighted empirical frequencies given the constraint $\sum_{i=1}^{N_R} \alpha_{n_i, l} = 1$ for $1 \leq l \leq N_s$. Once these model parameters are initialized, the likelihoods, $t_{i,l}$, are computed using the forward-backward algorithm, which has been shown to be efficient in 1D [10]. Thus, similar to rbHMM, we iteratively construct a 3D Markov tree from a randomly selected region outwards by traversing all regions [5].

For each region, we substitute the global region index i with (b,k) such that r_i is the kth region on branch b; thus, $t_{i,l}$ can be represented as $t_{(b,k),l}$. For each of the tree branches formed, the forward-backward algorithm is applied to estimate the likelihood of class l by defining a forward term, $\zeta_{(b,k)}(l)$, and a backward term, $\eta_{(b,k)}(l)$:

$$\zeta_{(b,k)}(l) = P(\vec{f}_{(b,k)}, t_{(b,k),l} = 1 | \mu_l, \sigma_l^2) \qquad 1 \leq l \leq N_s \qquad (1)$$

$$\eta_{(b,k)}(l) = P(\vec{f}_{(b,k)} | t_{(b,k),l} = 1, \mu_l, \sigma_l^2) \qquad 1 \leq l \leq N_s \qquad (2)$$

where $\vec{f}_{(b,k)}$ is the set of the observed mean intensity features from the start of the tree branch to region $r_{(b,k)}$, and $\vec{f}_{(b,k)}$ is the set of the observed mean intensity features from region $r_{(b,k+1)}$ to the end of the branch. We can solve both terms at each region $i = (b,k)$ inductively by:

$$\zeta_{(b,k+1)}(l) = [\sum_{m=1}^{N_s} \zeta_{(b,k)}(m) \alpha_{n_i,l}] P(f_{(b,k+1)} | \mu_l, \sigma_l^2) \qquad \begin{array}{c} k=1,\ldots,length-1 \\ 1 \leq l \leq N_s \end{array} \qquad (3)$$

$$\eta_{(b,k)}(l) = \sum_{m=1}^{N_s} [\eta_{(b,k+1)}(m) \alpha_{n_i,l} P(f_{(b,k+1)} | \mu_m, \sigma_m^2)] \qquad \begin{array}{c} k=length-1,\ldots,1 \\ 1 \leq l \leq N_s \end{array} \qquad (4)$$

where *length* is the number of regions in the branch. The forward term is initialized as $\zeta_{(b,1)}(l)=P(f_{(b,0)} | \mu_l, \sigma_l^2)$ and the backward term is initialized as $\eta_{(b,length)}(l)=1/N_s$. The likelihood, $t_{i,l}$, is thus calculated based on both the forward and the backward terms as:

$$t_{i,l} = t_{(b,k),l} = [\zeta_{(b,k)}(l) \eta_{(b,k)}(l)] / \sum_{m=1}^{N_s} [\zeta_{(b,k)}(m) \eta_{(b,k)}(m)] \qquad (5)$$

Once all region likelihoods are found, the algorithm then re-evaluates the model parameters $[\mu_l, \sigma_l^2, \alpha_{n_i,l}]$ for each state $l \in \{1,2,\ldots,N_s\}$ using probability weighting, by assuming a linear model such that the estimated region class probabilities represent the underlying partial volumes. A new Markov tree is then constructed from a random region and the estimation process repeats. The convergence criterion is defined as a minimum mean absolute change or a maximum number of iterations reached.

While using watershed regions to divide the image into contiguous homogeneous regions as proposed by Huang et al. [5] works well for discrete classification, the fuzzy approach can benefit from further subdivision along the region boundaries. The boundary between two watershed regions represents an optimal sharp division based on intensity gradients, and in the discrete rbHMM framework provides an adequate level of detail because each region only receives one class label (Fig. 1a). However, in our proposed fuzzy rbHMM framework, a finer resolution around the region boundaries would allow for superior capturing of gradient changes due to partial volume effects (Fig. 1b). Thus, we first pre-segment an image using the watershed transform. Once the watershed regions are established, we refine them by assigning voxels around all region boundaries as individual regions so as to provide increased boundary resolution for the likelihood estimation procedure (Fig. 1c).

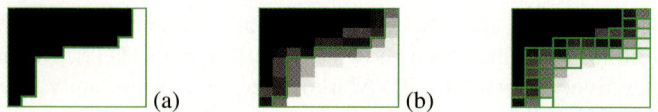

Fig. 1. Image (grayscale) and watershed subdivision (green) for (a) ideal and (b) partial-volume edges with two regions. By assigning boundary voxels as individual regions (c), we increase the resolution for subsequent estimations.

3 Results and Discussion

We tested our fuzzy partial-volume classification technique, $f$rbHMM, on 3D MR brain images and compared the performance to that of the discrete approach, rbHMM [5]. We first validated on simulated T1-weighted BrainWeb scans (181×217×181 dimensions, 1mm×1mm×1mm spacing, 0% noise) of normal and MS anatomical models to quantify our accuracy as the ground truths are available [16]. We then applied our method to real clinical 3DT1 MR scans (256×256×120 dimension, 0.837mm× 0.837mm×1.10mm spacing) of 18 relapse-remitting MS (RRMS) patients and 14 healthy controls from the UBC MRI Research Centre to demonstrate the robustness of the proposed method in maintaining control/subject measurements at reduced resolution, and therefore, increased partial-volume effects. We performed a 4-class segmentation - background, white matter (WM), gray matter (GM) and cerebrospinal fluid (CSF). For MS data, lesions cause errors in CSF and/or GM classification due to intensity overlap, but $f$rbHMM remains robust for WM and more importantly, does not show unexpected stability problem when model assumptions are violated. $f$rbHMM required approximately twice the runtime as rbHMM. Results of classification improve iteratively, but for the purpose of fair comparisons, both discrete and fuzzy estimations were run for 10 iterations.

3.1 Simulated Images

We examined the segmentation accuracies of both rbHMM and $f$rbHMM. Fig. 2 shows qualitative results obtained by both methods. For MS data, both methods classified periventricular lesions as GM; however, $f$rbHMM performed better than rbHMM in capturing the partial WM details of ambiguous regions (Fig. 2). Quantitatively, Table 1 shows that mean square errors (MSE) of the segmentation results. At the original resolution, $f$rbHMM achieved approximately 20% lower MSE for both WM and GM results. Analyzing the MSE gains of partial volume regions (0<probability<1) yielded similar performance. To simulate progressively reduced resolution, hence increased partial volumes, we performed smoothing by using a Gaussian kernel (7×7×7 dimension) with varying standard deviations to incorporate intensities within ±3mm. Again, $f$rbHMM was superior (about 40% MSE reduction).

3.2 Clinical Scans

Next, we tested both rbHMM and $f$rbHMM classification accuracy on high resolution 3DT1 scans of real clinical control (C) and subject (S) groups. With no ground truths available, in order to evaluate the robustness of the proposed $f$rbHMM approach with increased partial-volumes, we examined the WM volume fraction measurements

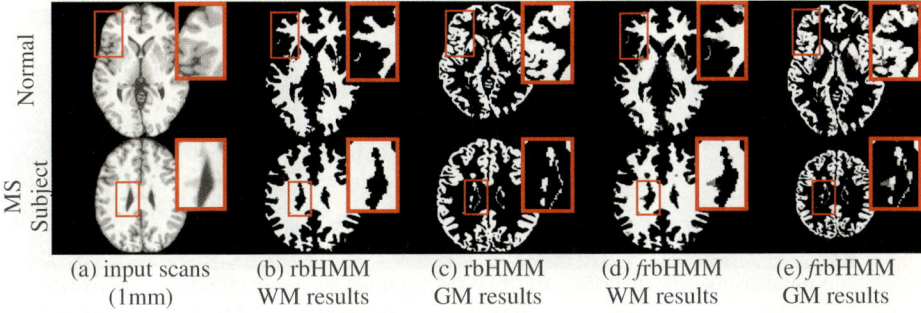

(a) input scans (1mm) (b) rbHMM WM results (c) rbHMM GM results (d) *fr*bHMM WM results (e) *fr*bHMM GM results

Fig. 2. Experimental results on simulated BrainWeb MRI scans. (*a*) Input T1-weighted scans at 1mm slice thickness, (*b-c*) results of discrete rbHMM, and (*d-e*) results of proposed *fr*bHMM.

Table 1. Quantitative MSE of simulated BrainWeb MRIs of normal and MS subject anatomical models. Classifications were performed using discrete and fuzzy rbHMMs, and results were compared to the discrete and fuzzy phantoms, respectively. The better performance for each comparison is highlighted in bold. Gain is defined as (rbHMM-*fr*bHMM)/rbHMM.

Data	Tissue	Original Scan			Gaussian kernel std. dev. = 1.0 voxel			Gaussian kernel std. dev. = 2.0 voxel		
		rbHMM	*fr*bHMM	% gain	rbHMM	*fr*bHMM	% gain	rbHMM	*fr*bHMM	% gain
Normal	WM	0.0089	**0.0069**	22.47	0.0217	**0.0133**	38.71	0.0352	**0.0213**	39.49
	GM	0.0149	**0.0119**	20.13	0.0364	**0.0213**	41.48	0.0572	**0.0345**	39.69
MS Subject	WM	0.0090	**0.0069**	23.33	0.0222	**0.0136**	38.74	0.0348	**0.0213**	38.79
	GM	0.0151	**0.0121**	19.87	0.0364	**0.0213**	41.48	0.0565	**0.0345**	38.94

(WMVF = $V_{WM} / V_{BRAIN} \times 100\%$, where V_{WM} and V_{BRAIN} are the WM and intradural volumes respectively). We targeted the WM as it is the largest tissue by volume and the pathological regions in patient scans are the most distinct in WM and thus can be readily excluded. We first demonstrate that both methods (rbHMM and *fr*bHMM) performed comparably in terms of the WMVF measure when using the high resolution scans. However, we then demonstrate how the proposed *fr*bHMM is far more robust when the image resolution is reduced.

Table 2 shows the average WMVF obtained by using the original (high resolution) scans. Both methods showed that the average WMVF in the controls were significantly ($p<0.05$) higher (+3.53% for discrete, +3.11% for fuzzy) than those of the

Table 2. Quantitative average WMVF measurement on high resolution clinical MRI data. Note that both the rbHMM and *fr*bHMM segmentation methods show consistent and significant differences between the control and the subject groups, while no significant differences were observed between the two methods for either group, which is expected in high resolution data.

	rbHMM	*fr*bHMM	Δ (methods)	*p*-Value
Controls (C)	42.57 (σ=1.66)	41.98 (σ=1.43)	0.58	0.33
Subjects (S)	39.03 (σ=2.82)	38.88 (σ=2.59)	0.15	0.87
Δ (groups)	3.53	3.11		
p-Value	<0.05	<0.05		

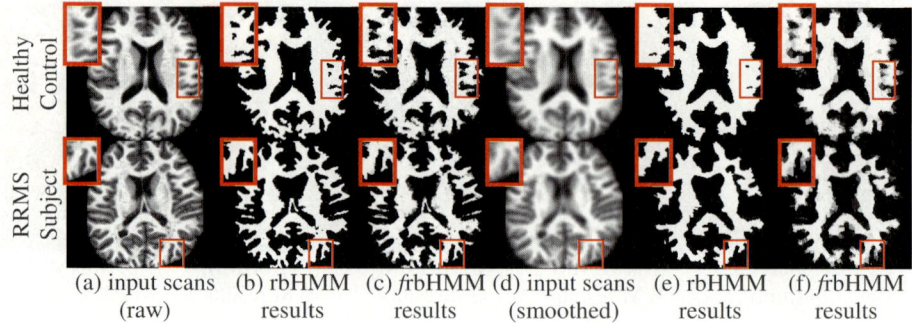

(a) input scans (raw) (b) rbHMM results (c) frbHMM results (d) input scans (smoothed) (e) rbHMM results (f) frbHMM results

Fig. 3. Example results on real clinical MRI scans. (*a-c*) Input 3DT1 scans at original resolution and results of discrete and fuzzy rbHMMs, (*d-f*) smoothed 3DT1 scans (kernel standard deviation=2.0 voxel) and results of discrete and fuzzy rbHMMs.

Table 3. Quantitative segmentation comparisons on real clinical data with escalated partial volume effects. Classifications were performed using discrete and fuzzy rbHMMs, and results were compared to the segmentations obtained based on the original high resolution scans. The superior performance is highlighted in bold. Gain is defined as (rbHMM-frbHMM)/rbHMM.

Metric	Gaussian kernel std. dev. = 1.0 voxel			Gaussian kernel std. dev. = 2.0 voxel		
	rbHMM	frbHMM	% gain	rbHMM	frbHMM	% gain
MSE (C)	0.0159 (σ=0.0018)	**0.0102** (σ=**0.0010**)	35.89 ($p<0.05$)	0.0250 (σ=0.0027)	**0.0179** (σ=**0.0022**)	28.40 ($p<0.05$)
MSE (S)	0.0155 (σ=0.0015)	**0.0100** (σ=**0.0008**)	35.48 ($p<0.05$)	0.0244 (σ=0.0022)	**0.0173** (σ=**0.0016**)	29.10 ($p<0.05$)
MSD (C)	11.37 (σ=6.33)	**2.29** (σ=**3.10**)	79.86 ($p<0.05$)	35.48 (σ=11.05)	**18.06** (σ=**10.30**)	49.10 ($p<0.05$)
MSD (S)	6.72 (σ=5.97)	**1.43** (σ=**1.75**)	78.72 ($p<0.05$)	22.71 (σ=13.74)	**8.55** (σ=**8.24**)	62.35 ($p<0.05$)

RRMS patients due to the presence of WM lesions and enlarged ventricles in MS patients. Comparing the two methods within groups, no significant evidence ($p \geq 0.05$) of differences in WMVF was observed demonstrating that both methods achieved similar performances on high resolution data.

Similar to the simulated scans case, we then progressively reduced the image resolutions by Gaussian smoothing. Fig. 3 shows the effects of such smoothing on the classifications of control and subject scans. Again, the proposed *frb*HMM classified ambiguous intensity regions (zoomed-in regions of Fig. 3) with greater accuracy than the discrete model. Quantitatively, Table 3 shows the average MSE (image-to-image comparison) and the mean square difference or MSD (WMVF comparison) of the control and subject groups. The proposed *frb*HMM consistently achieved significantly ($p<0.05$) lower MSE (approximately 30% improvement) and MSD for both groups.

4 Conclusions

We introduced a novel fuzzy 3D region-based hidden Markov model for modeling and estimation of partial volumes in image voxels within an unsupervised framework.

The paper's main contribution is a new *fuzzy* 3D HMM framework based on irregularly-shaped homogeneous regions with further spatial refinement at the region boundaries, where the contents of each region are assigned to multiple underlying classes simultaneously rather than assuming a single true discrete label. To compute the region class likelihoods, we employ a classical iterative forward-backward scheme. We evaluated the classification accuracy and robustness of our method under increased partial volume effects using both simulated and real clinical brain MRI data of healthy controls and MS subjects. Results showed the proposed *fr*bHMM approach to be consistently superior to the discrete rbHMM in labeling intensity-ambiguous regions, such as white matter with reduced signal due to pathology. Future work includes investigating the utility of our *fr*bHMM approach for quantifying the extent of white matter disease such as diffusedly-abnormal white matter (DAWM).

References

1. Bishop, C.M.: Pattern Recognition and Machine Learning, pp. 359–422. Springer, Heidelberg (2006)
2. Li, J., Najmi, A., Gray, R.M.: Image classification by a two dimensional hidden Markov model. IEEE Trans. Signal Proc. 48(2), 517–533 (2000)
3. Ibrahim, M., John, N., Kabuka, M., Younis, A.: Hidden Markov models-based 3D MRI brain segmentation. Image and Vision Computing 24, 1065–1079 (2006)
4. Joshi, D., Li, J., Wang, J.Z.: A comp. efficient approach to the estimation of two- and three-dimensional hidden Markov models. IEEE Trans. Image Proc. 15(7), 1871–1886 (2006)
5. Huang, A., Abugharbieh, R., Tam, R.: Image segmentation using an efficient rotationally invariant 3D region-based hidden Markov model. In: IEEE CVPR, Workshop on Mathematical Methods in Biomed. Image Analysis (MMBIA), Anchorage-Alaska, pp. 107–111 (2008)
6. Zhang, Y., Brady, M., Smith, S.: Segmentation of brain MR images through a hidden Markov random field model and the expectation-maximization algorithm. IEEE Trans. Med. Imag. 20(1), 45–57 (2001)
7. Besag, J.: On the statistical analysis of dirty pictures (with discussion). J. of Royal Statist. Soc., Ser.B 48(3), 259–302 (1986)
8. Komodakis, N., Tziritas, G., Paragios, N.: Fast, approximately optimal solutions for single and dynamic MRFs. In: IEEE CVPR, Minneapolis-Minnesota (2007)
9. Kolmogorov, V.: Convergent tree-reweighted message passing for energy minimization. IEEE Trans. Pattern Anal. Mach. Intell. 28(10), 1568–1583 (2006)
10. Rabiner, L.R.: An intro. to hidden Markov model. In: IEEE ASSP Magazine, pp. 4–16 (1986)
11. Santago, P., Gage, H.D.: Quantification of MR brain images by mixture density and partial volume modeling. IEEE Trans. Med. Imag. 12(3), 566–574 (1993)
12. Van Leemput, K.: A unifying framework for partial volume segmentation of brain MR images. IEEE Trans. Med. Imag. 22(1), 105–119 (2003)
13. Bricq, S., Collet, C., Armspach, J.P.: Unifying framework for multimodal brain MRI segmentation based on hidden Markov chains. Medical Image Analysis 12, 639–652 (2008)
14. Choi, H.S., Haynor, D.R., Kim, Y.: Partial volume tissue classification of multichannel magnetic resonance images – a mixel model. IEEE TMI 10(3), 395–407 (1991)
15. Domke, J., KArapurkar, A., Aloimonos, Y.: Who killed the directed model? In: CVPR (2008)
16. BrainWeb: Simulated Brain Database, http://www.bic.mni.mcgill.ca/brainweb/

Brain Connectivity Using Geodesics in HARDI

Mickaël Péchaud[1,2], Maxime Descoteaux[3], and Renaud Keriven[2]

[1] LIENS, École Normale Supérieure
[2] IMAGINE, Université Paris Est
[3] Neurospin, IFR 49 CEA Saclay, France

Abstract. We develop an algorithm for brain connectivity assessment using geodesics in HARDI (high angular resolution diffusion imaging). We propose to recast the problem of finding fibers bundles and connectivity maps to the calculation of shortest paths on a Riemannian manifold defined from fiber ODFs computed from HARDI measurements. Several experiments on real data show that our method is able to segment fibers bundles that are not easily recovered by other existing methods.

1 Introduction

Diffusion MRI and fiber tractography have gained importance in the medical imaging community for the last decade. Many new diffusion models and fiber tracking algorithms have recently appeared in the literature always seeking better brain connectivity assessment, in particular regarding complex fiber configuration such as crossing, branching or kissing fibers. Clinical applications are also asking for robust tractography methods, as they are the unique *in vivo* tool to study the integrity of brain connectivity.

The most commonly used model is the diffusion tensor (DT), which is only able to characterize one fiber compartment per voxel. Several alternatives have been proposed to overcome this limitation of DTI, mainly using high angular resolution diffusion imaging (HARDI). Several competing HARDI reconstruction technique exist in the literature, which all have their advantages and disadvantages. Nonetheless, the community seems to now agree that a sharp orientation distribution function (ODF), often called fiber ODF or fiber orientation density function (fODF) [1,2,3,4], able to discriminate low angle crossing fibers needs to be used for fiber tractography.

Three classes of algorithms exist: deterministic, probabilistic and geodesic. A large number of tractography algorithms have been developed for DTI, which are limited in regions of fiber crossings. While HARDI-based extensions of streamline deterministic [5,6,7,4] and probabilistic [8,9,10,11,12,13,4] tracking algorithms have flourished in the last few years (the list is not exhaustive), [14] was the only attempt to generalize DTI geodesic tracking [15,16] for HARDI measurements.

In this paper, we develop an algorithm for brain connectivity assessment using geodesics in HARDI. We propose to recast the problem of finding connectivity maps in the white matter to the calculation of shortest paths on a Riemannian manifold. This Riemannian manifold is defined from fiber ODFs computed from HARDI measurements.

2 Method

Firstly, let us provide some basics definitions about Riemannian manifolds.

Definitions. Let (M, g) be a Riemannian manifold i.e.

- M is a n-dimensional manifold
- for all $x \in M$, $g(x)$ is a symmetric positive definite $n \times n$ matrix inducing a metric $||y||_x \stackrel{\text{def.}}{=} \sqrt{y^T g^{-1}(x) y}$ over that manifold.

The *length* of a smooth curve $\gamma : [0,1] \to M$ is then defined as

$$\mathcal{L}(\gamma) \stackrel{\text{def.}}{=} \int_0^1 ||\gamma'(t)||_{\gamma(t)} dt \stackrel{\text{def.}}{=} \int_0^1 \sqrt{\gamma'(t)^T g^{-1}(\gamma(t)) \gamma'(t)} dt. \tag{1}$$

Given a set $\mathcal{A} \subset M$ of seeds points and a set $\mathcal{B} \subset M$ of ending points, a *geodesic* $\gamma^*(t) \subset M$ joining $\mathcal{A}$ to $\mathcal{B}$ is defined as a curve with minimal length between $\mathcal{A}$ and $\mathcal{B}$:

$$\gamma^*(\mathcal{A}, \mathcal{B}) \stackrel{\text{def.}}{=} \operatorname*{argmin}_{\gamma \in \pi(\mathcal{A}, \mathcal{B})} \mathcal{L}(\gamma), \tag{2}$$

where $\pi(\mathcal{A}, \mathcal{B})$ is the set of curves γ such that $\gamma(0) \in \mathcal{A}$ and $\gamma(1) \in \mathcal{B}$. The corresponding *geodesic distance* is $d(\mathcal{A}, \mathcal{B}) \stackrel{\text{def.}}{=} \mathcal{L}(\gamma^*(\mathcal{A}, \mathcal{B}))$.

Let us also define the *Euclidean length* of the curve γ

$$\mathcal{L}_{euc}(\gamma) \stackrel{\text{def.}}{=} \int_0^1 ||\gamma'(t)|| dt. \tag{3}$$

and

$$\mathcal{L}_{sq}(\gamma) \stackrel{\text{def.}}{=} \int_0^1 ||\gamma'(t)||_{\gamma(t)}^2 dt. \tag{4}$$

Following [15] if we interpret the metric induced by g as a "speed" over M, for any smooth curve γ, $\mathcal{L}(\gamma)/\mathcal{L}_{euc}(\gamma)$ can be thought of as the average of inverse speed along the curve, while $\sqrt{\mathcal{L}_{sq}(\gamma)/\mathcal{L}_{euc}(\gamma) - (\mathcal{L}(\gamma)/\mathcal{L}_{euc}(\gamma))^2}$ represents the standard deviation of this quantity.

Connectivity measures. Considering $\mathcal{A}$ and $\mathcal{B}$ two subset of M we define

$$\begin{aligned} \mathcal{C}(\mathcal{A}, \mathcal{B}) &\stackrel{\text{def.}}{=} \frac{\mathcal{L}(\gamma^*(\mathcal{A}, \mathcal{B}))}{\mathcal{L}_{euc}(\gamma^*(\mathcal{A}, \mathcal{B}))}, \quad \mathcal{C}_{max}(\mathcal{A}, \mathcal{B}) \stackrel{\text{def.}}{=} \max_{t \in [0..1]} ||(\gamma^*(\mathcal{A}, \mathcal{B}))'(t)||_{\gamma(t)} \\ \mathcal{C}_\sigma(\mathcal{A}, \mathcal{B}) &\stackrel{\text{def.}}{=} \sqrt{\left(\frac{\mathcal{L}(\gamma^*(\mathcal{A}, \mathcal{B}))}{\mathcal{L}_{euc}(\gamma^*(\mathcal{A}, \mathcal{B}))}\right)^2 - \frac{\mathcal{L}_{sq}(\gamma^*(\mathcal{A}, \mathcal{B}))}{\mathcal{L}_{euc}(\gamma^*(\mathcal{A}, \mathcal{B}))}} \end{aligned} \tag{5}$$

$\gamma^*(\mathcal{A}, \mathcal{B})$ being a geodesic between $\mathcal{A}$ and $\mathcal{B}$, $\mathcal{C}(\mathcal{A}, \mathcal{B})$, $\mathcal{C}_\sigma(\mathcal{A}, \mathcal{B})$ and $\mathcal{C}_{max}(\mathcal{A}, \mathcal{B})$ are respectively measures of average inverse speed, inverse speed standard deviation, and worst inverse speed to reach $\mathcal{B}$ from $\mathcal{A}$. They can thus be interpreted as three different connectivity measures between $\mathcal{A}$ and $\mathcal{B}$.

2.1 HARDI Riemannian Manifold

We now explain how we recast the fibers bundles tracking problem from HARDI data to the calculation of connectivity maps on a Riemannian manifold.

Let us denote $E \subset \mathbb{R}^3$ the white matter volume, $\mathcal{S} = \{e_{\theta,\varphi} \mid \theta \in [0, 2\pi), \varphi \in [0, \pi)\}$ the unit sphere and $M \stackrel{\text{def.}}{=} E \times \mathcal{S}$. Using such a 5-dimensional space can disambiguate crossing configurations since in such a space $(x, y, z, e_{\theta,\varphi})$ and $(x, y, z, e_{\theta',\varphi'})$ are completely different points. The idea was introduced [17], but the authors proposed to segment rather than track bundles using level-sets, which is time-consuming and less accurate.

At every point $(x, y, z) \in E$, we can compute the fODF $f_{xyz} : e_{\theta,\varphi} \in \mathcal{S} \to f_{xyz}(e_{\theta,\varphi}) \in \mathbb{R}^+$. The full data can thus be naturally modelled as a mapping f from M to $\mathbb{R}^+$: $f : (x, y, z, e_{\theta,\varphi}) \in M \mapsto f_{xyz\theta\varphi} \stackrel{\text{def.}}{=} f_{xyz}(e_{\theta,\varphi}) \in \mathbb{R}^+$.

Let us define the metric g at any point $(x, y, z, e_{\theta,\varphi})$ of M as

$$g_{xyz\theta\varphi} \stackrel{\text{def.}}{=} \begin{pmatrix} \overbrace{\rho(f_{xyz\theta\varphi}) \quad 0 \quad 0}^{E} & \overbrace{0 \quad 0}^{\mathcal{S}} \\ 0 \quad \rho(f_{xyz\theta\varphi}) \quad 0 & 0 \quad 0 \\ 0 \quad 0 \quad \rho(f_{xyz\theta\varphi}) & 0 \quad 0 \\ \hline 0 \quad 0 \quad 0 & \alpha \quad 0 \\ 0 \quad 0 \quad 0 & 0 \quad \alpha \end{pmatrix} = \begin{pmatrix} \rho(f_{xyz\theta\varphi})I_3 & 0 \\ 0 & \alpha I_2 \end{pmatrix}$$

where ρ is an increasing function from $\mathbb{R}^+$ to $\mathbb{R}^{+*}$ and α is a parameter controlling the speed on the angular space $\mathcal{S}$ w.r.t. the speed on the E volume. Such a metric "favors" paths going through areas of high diffusion.

Recasting the problem in the white matter volume, let us consider two points (x_1, y_1, z_1) and $(x_2, y_2, z_2) \in E$ between which one wishes to estimate the connectivity. Let us denote $\mathcal{A} = \{x_1, y_1, z_1, e_{\theta,\varphi} \mid e_{\theta,\varphi} \in \mathcal{S}\}$ and $\mathcal{B} = \{x_2, y_2, z_2, e_{\theta,\varphi} \mid e_{\theta,\varphi} \in \mathcal{S}\} \subset E \times \mathcal{S}$.

$\mathcal{C}(\mathcal{A}, \mathcal{B})$, $\mathcal{C}_\sigma(\mathcal{A}, \mathcal{B})$ and $\mathcal{C}_{max}(\mathcal{A}, \mathcal{B})$ are then natural measures of connectivity between (x_1, y_1, z_1) and (x_2, y_2, z_2). Furthermore, let us denote $\pi : E \times \mathcal{S} \to E$ the projection such that $\pi(x, y, z, e_{\theta,\varphi}) = (x, y, z)$. To the geodesic $\gamma^*(\mathcal{A}, \mathcal{B})$ in $E \times \mathcal{S}$ then corresponds a projected path $\pi(\gamma^*(\mathcal{A}, \mathcal{B}))$ in $E \subset \mathbb{R}^3$. Since $\gamma^*(\mathcal{A}, \mathcal{B})$ follows a high diffusion trajectory, $\pi(\gamma^*(\mathcal{A}, \mathcal{B}))$ is likely to follow an actual fiber bundle in the volume. With this point of view, α can be seen as a smoothing parameter of the angular variations of the fibers.

However, among the paths $\gamma : [0, 1] \to M$, one would like to favor the ones such that at every point t_0, $\pi(\gamma(t_0))$ follows the corresponding direction in $\mathcal{S}$: if we denote $(x_0, y_0, z_0, e_{\theta_0,\varphi_0}) \stackrel{\text{def.}}{=} \gamma(t_0)$, one would like to have

$$(\pi(\gamma)_x(t_0), \pi(\gamma)_y(t_0), \pi(\gamma)_z(t_0)) \approx \pm e_{\theta_0,\varphi_0} \|(\pi(\gamma)_x(t_0), \pi(\gamma)_y(t_0), \pi(\gamma)_z(t_0))\|$$

In order to encourage these paths, we propose the following approach : let us consider a point $(x, y, z, e_{\theta,\varphi})$. Instead of using an isotropic metric $\rho(f_{xyz\theta\varphi})I_3$ in the first three directions, one would like to favor propagation along the $e_{\theta,\varphi}$ direction. In order to do so, $\rho(f_{xyz\theta\varphi})I_3$ is replaced by the following matrix:

$$(R_{\theta,\varphi})^T \begin{pmatrix} \rho(f_{xyz\theta\varphi}) & 0 & 0 \\ 0 & min(\varepsilon, \rho(f_{xyz\theta\varphi})) & 0 \\ 0 & 0 & min(\varepsilon, \rho(f_{xyz\theta\varphi})) \end{pmatrix} R_{\theta,\varphi}$$

where $R_{\theta,\varphi}$ is a rotation which maps the first axis to the $e_{\theta,\varphi}$ direction, and ε is some constant. As long as $\rho(f_{xyz\theta\varphi}) > \varepsilon$, this tensor favors propagation in the $e_{\theta,\varphi}$ direction. However if $\rho(f_{xyz\theta\varphi}) \leqslant \varepsilon$ (i.e. if the diffusion is small at this point), this does not make sense, and we keep the isotropic tensor defined by $\rho(f_{xyz\theta\varphi})I_3$.

The choice of this metric is a natural way of handling the 5-dimensional HARDI data and to obtain connectivity maps and fibers. It ensures that (i) the full HARDI angular information is used, (ii) geodesics go through areas of high diffusion, (iii) geodesics travel in those areas in the correct directions and (iv) crossing configurations are disambiguated.

3 Implementation

3.1 Djikstra and Fast-Marching Algorithms

Two algorithms can be used to compute connectivity measures on discretized Riemannian manifolds (M, g). Assuming an initial seed $\mathcal{A} \subset M$, they both consist in successive evaluations of geodesic distances $d(\mathcal{A}, \{x\})$ and connectivity measures from each point $x \in M$ to $\mathcal{A}$. For one point x, $d(\mathcal{A}, \{x\})$ is iteratively evaluated from the $\{d(\mathcal{A}, \{y\})\}_{y \in N(x)}$, where $N(x)$ is the set of neighbors of x in the chosen discretization. This calculation is called *local update step*. Only this local update step differs between the two following methods.

- *Djikstra algorithm*–initially designed to compute distances and shortest paths in graphs–can be used to approximate connectivity maps and geodesics on Riemannian manifolds. While this algorithm is fast, paths are constrained to be on the edges on the discretization, which limits its accuracy.
- *Fast-Marching* algorithm [18,19] and its variants can be view as a refinement of Djikstra algorithm in which the paths are not constrained anymore. However, while being of same asymptotic complexity, it is much slower than Djikstra algorithm, and thus can not be directly applied to our problem.

In most tracking methods, connectivity measures are obtained explicitly from fibers computed from deterministic or probabilistic streamlines. However, in Djikstra and Fast-Marching algorithms, the connectivity measures are computed intrinsically *without* the actual computation of any fiber, although the geodesics – i.e. the fibers – can be retrieved from the output of the algorithm by performing a gradient descent on the distance map.

3.2 Our Implementation

For our problem, E was discretized as a subset of a 3-dimensional grid, at the HARDI measurement spatial definition. S was meshed in such a way that every vertex of the mesh corresponds to a direction of HARDI measurements. Furthermore, in order to achieve good precision, we chose to use a 26-neighborhood in the discretization of E. Since we are mainly interested in precision in the high diffusion directions, we propose to compute $d(\mathcal{A},\{x\})$ at each point by using Djikstra local update step. The Fast-Marching local update step is then only applied for neighbors near to the current $e_{\theta,\varphi}$ direction, and only if the diffusion is important enough (i.e. $\rho(f_{xyz\theta\varphi}) > \varepsilon$) at current point. This lead to significant speed-up ($\sim \times 50$ w.r.t the full Fast-Marching computation) of the method, while the precision in the fibers direction is preserved.

4 Experimental Results

4.1 Real HARDI Data

We use a human brain dataset obtained on a Siemens 3T Trio scanner, with isotropic resolution of $1.7mm^3$, 60 gradient directions, a $b = 1000$ s/mm^2, seven $b = 0$ s/mm^2 images, TE $= 100$ ms and TR $= 12$s, GRAPPA factor of 2 and a NEX of 3. The data is corrected to subject motion.

From these HARDI measurements, the fiber ODF was reconstructed. As mentioned in the introduction, several fiber ODF reconstruction algorithm exist [1,2,3,4]. Here, we used the analytical spherical deconvolution transform of the q-ball ODF using spherical harmonics [4]. We used an order 4 estimation with symmetric deconvolution fiber kernel estimated from the real data, resulting in a profile with FA $= 0.7$ and $[355, 355, 1390] \times 10^{-6}$mm^2/s.

The geodesic tracking is performed within a white matter mask was obtained from a minimum fractional anisotropy (FA) value of 0.1 and a maximum ADC value of 0.0015. These values were optimized to produce agreement with the white matter mask from the T1 anatomy. The mask was morphologically checked for holes in regions of low anisotropy due to crossing fibers.

4.2 Geodesic Connectivity Results

For each bundle except the Superior Longitudinal Fasciculus (SLF), experiments were carried out with $\rho(f) = ln(f)/ln(2)$, $\varepsilon = 1$ and $\alpha = 2$ after thresholding values of the fODF under 1 to avoid negative values. Our method however demonstrates robustness w.r.t the exact choice of these parameters. Since SLF has high curvature, we set angular speed $\alpha = 8$ in order to favor tracking of actual SLF rather than projections on the occipital cortex. Runtime was about 90min for each bundle. It can be further reduced by computing only some of the connectivity maps, or by computing them only on a subset of white matter. While results presented below show connectivity maps on the full maps, experiments show that the bundles can be retrieved by stopping the algorithm when 20% of the mask has been visited. The runtime is then reduced to about 14min.

Figure 1 shows connectivity measures and some geodesics obtained from different seeds manually placed into major fibers bundles, which agree with our knowledge of the white matter anatomy. Notice the correctness of the maps

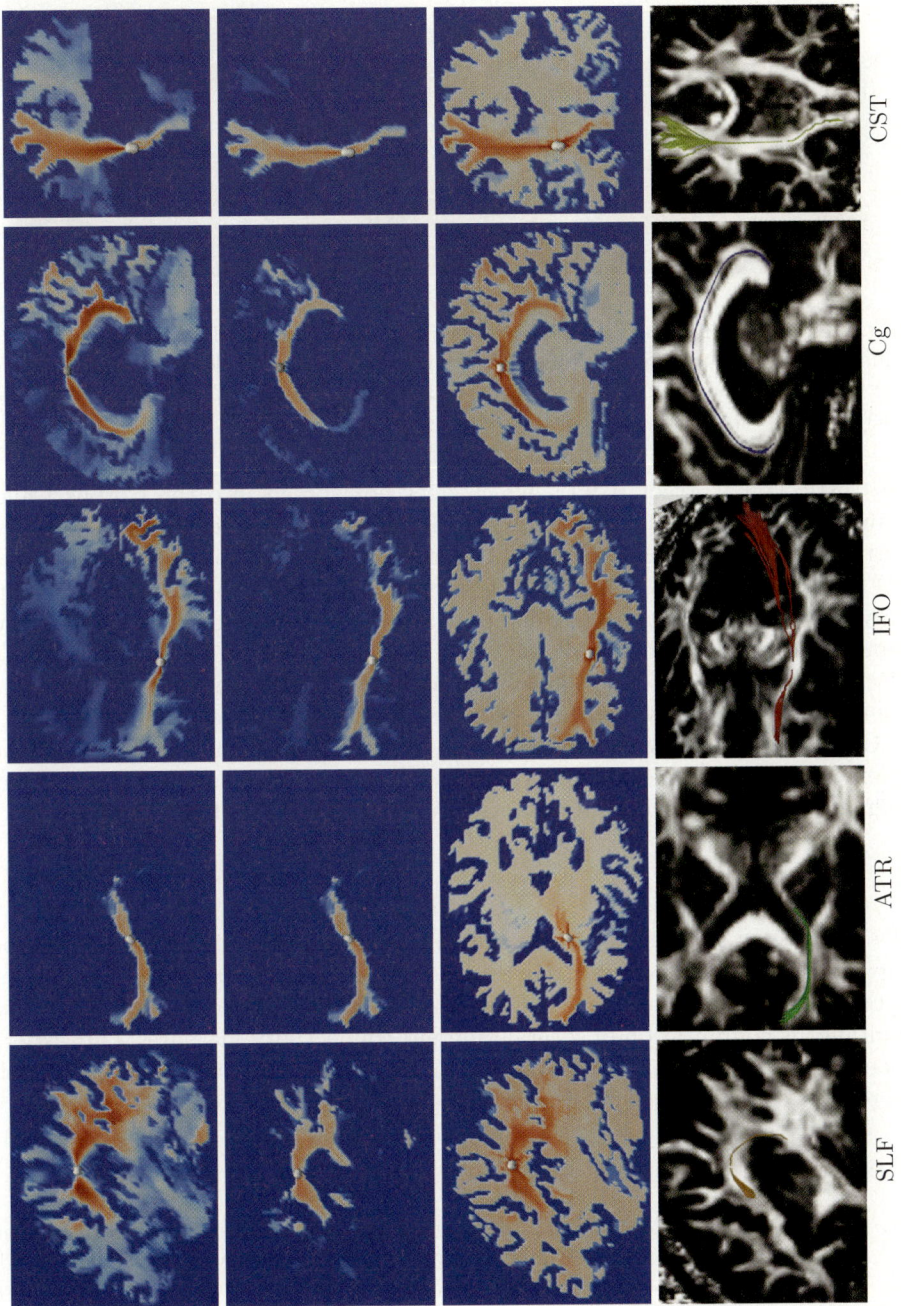

Fig. 1. Geodesic tracking results on five major fibers bundles. From left to right, $\mathcal{C}$, $\mathcal{C}_{max}$, $\mathcal{C}_{sigma}$ and some geodesics superimposed over the FA.

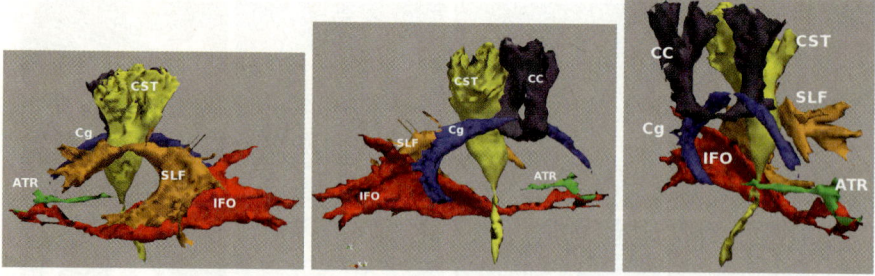

Fig. 2. Geodesic tracking results on major fibers bundles. We show isosurfaces of the connectivity measures of each bundle in a different color. In yellow, the CST; in blue, the Cg; in red, the IFO; in orange, the SLF; in green, the ATR; in dark blue, a small part of the CC projections to the superior cortex.

on Corticospinal Tract (CST), which does not spread into the Corpus Callosum (CC). Also, the Cingulum (Cg), which is a thin structure close to CC is correctly handled by our method. This clearly shows the advantage of using a 5D space: since fibers in Cg and CC are perpendicular, these two bundles are very distant in our 5D space, while they are extremely close in 3D. Other fibers bundles are also correctly retrieved, such as the Inferior Fronto-Occipital (IFO) fasciculus and the Anterior Thalamic Radiations (ATR). Furthermore, coherent results are obtained by the three proposed connectivity measures.

On figure 2 isosurfaces of the connectivity maps are shown for all the previous fibers bundles, as well as a small part of CC projections. Notice that CC is not segmented by our method. Rather, fibers are tracked from the given seed.

5 Conclusion

We presented a geodesic based tracking algorithm on HARDI data. Our method rapidly estimates connectivity maps inside a white matter mask from seed points, without the need for an explicit computation of fibers. Its versatility allows simultaneous computation of several different connectivity measures. Our experiments plead in favor of the use of a 5D space and show that our method is able to recover complex fiber bundles, which are often difficult to track.

References

1. Jansons, K.M., Alexander, D.C.: Persistent angular structure: new insights fom diffusion magnetic resonance imaging data. Inverse Problems 19, 1031–1046 (2003)
2. Tournier, J.D., Calamante, F., Connelly, A.: Robust determination of the fibre orientation distribution in diffusion MRI: Non-negativity constrained super-resolved spherical deconvolution. Neuroimage 35(4), 1459–1472 (2007)
3. Jian, B., Vemuri, B.C.: A unified computational framework for deconvolution to reconstruct multiple fibers from diffusion weighted MRI. IEEE Transactions on Medical Imaging 26(11), 1464–1471 (2007)

4. Descoteaux, M., Deriche, R., Knösche, T.R., Anwander, A.: Deterministic and probabilistic tractography based on complex fibre orientation distributions. IEEE Transactions in Medical Imaging 28(2), 269–286 (2009)
5. Kreher, B.W., Schneider, J.F., Mader, J., Martin, E., Hennig, J., Il'yasov, K.A.: Multitensor approach for analysis and tracking of complex fiber configurations. Magnetic Resonance in Medicine 54, 1216–1225 (2005)
6. Bergmann, Ø., Kindlmann, G., Peled, S., Westin, C.F.: Two-tensor fiber tractography. In: ISBI, Arlington, Virginia, USA, pp. 796–799 (2007)
7. Wedeen, V., Wang, R., Schmahmann, J., Benner, T., Tseng, W., Dai, G., Pandya, D., Hagmann, P., D'Arceuil, H., de Crespigny, A.: Diffusion spectrum magnetic resonance imaging (dsi) tractography of crossing fibers. Neuroimage 41(4), 1267–1277 (2008)
8. Parker, G.J.M., Alexander, D.C.: Probabilistic anatomical connectivity derived from the microscopic persistent angular structure of cerebral tissue. Philosophical Transactions of the Royal Society, Series B 360, 893–902 (2005)
9. Perrin, M., Poupon, C., Cointepas, Y., Rieul, B., Golestani, N., Pallier, C., Riviere, D., Constantinesco, A., Bihan, D.L., Mangin, J.F.: Fiber tracking in q-ball fields using regularized particle trajectories. In: Christensen, G.E., Sonka, M. (eds.) IPMI 2005. LNCS, vol. 3565, pp. 52–63. Springer, Heidelberg (2005)
10. Seunarine, K.K., Cook, P.A., Embleton, K., Parker, G.J.M., Alexander, D.C.: A general framework for multiple-fibre pico tractography. In: Medical Image Understanding and Analysis (2006)
11. Behrens, T.E.J., Johansen-Berg, H., Jbabdi, S., Rushworth, M.F.S., Woolrich, M.W.: Probabilistic diffusion tractography with multiple fibre orientations. what can we gain? Neuroimage 34(1), 144–155 (2007)
12. Savadjiev, P., Campbell, J.S.W., Descoteaux, M., Deriche, R., Pike, G.B., Siddiqi, K.: Labeling of ambiguous sub-voxel fibre bundle configurations in high angular resolution diffusion MRI. Neuroimage 41(1), 58–68 (2008)
13. Zhang, F., Hancock, E.R., Goodlett, C., Gerig, G.: Probabilistic white matter fiber tracking using particle filtering and von mises-fisher sampling. Medical Image Analysis 13(1), 5–18 (2008)
14. Melonakos, J., Mohan, V., Niethammer, M., Smith, K., Kubicki, M., Tannenbaum, A.: Finsler tractography for white matter connectivity analysis of the cingulum bundle. In: Ayache, N., Ourselin, S., Maeder, A. (eds.) MICCAI 2007, Part I. LNCS, vol. 4791, pp. 36–43. Springer, Heidelberg (2007)
15. Lenglet, C., Prados, E., Pons, J., Deriche, R., Faugeras, O.: Brain connectivity mapping using riemannian geometry, control theory and pdes. SIAM Journal on Imaging Sciences 2(2), 285–322 (2009)
16. Jbabdi, S., Bellec, P., Toro, R., Daunizeau, J., Pelegrini-Issac, M., Benali, H.: Accurate anisotropic fast marching for diffusion-based geodesic tractography. International Journal of Biomedical Imaging, 1–12 (2008)
17. Jonasson, L., Bresson, X., Hagmann, P., Thiran, J., Wedeen, V.: Representing Diffusion MRI in 5D Simplifies Regularization and Segmentation of White Matter Tracts. IEEE Transactions on Medical Imaging 26, 1547–1554 (2007)
18. Sethian, J.A.: Level Set Methods and Fast Marching Methods. Cambridge University Press, Cambridge (1999)
19. Deschamps, T., Cohen, L.: Fast extraction of minimal paths in 3D images and applications to virtual endoscopy. Medical Image Analysis 5(4), 281–299 (2001)

Functional Segmentation of fMRI Data Using Adaptive Non-negative Sparse PCA (ANSPCA)

Bernard Ng[1], Rafeef Abugharbieh[1], and Martin J. McKeown[2]

[1] Biomedical Signal and Image Computing Lab, Department of Electrical Engineering
[2] Department of Medicine (Neurology), Pacific Parkinson's Research Center
The University of British Columbia, Vancouver, BC, Canada
bernardn@ece.ubc.ca, rafeef@ece.ubc.ca,
mmckeown@interchange.ubc.ca

Abstract. We propose a novel method for functional segmentation of fMRI data that incorporates multiple functional attributes such as activation effects and functional connectivity, under a single framework. Similar to PCA, our method exploits the structure of the correlation matrix but with neighborhood information adaptively integrated to encourage detection of spatially contiguous clusters yet without falsely pooling non-active voxels near the functional boundaries. In addition, our method adaptively combines PCA and replicator dynamics, which we show to be equivalent to non-negative sparse PCA, based on the sparsity of the activation pattern. We validate our method quantitatively on synthetic data and demonstrate that it outperforms methods including replicator dynamics, PCA, Gaussian mixture models, and general linear models. Furthermore, when applied to real fMRI data, our method successfully segmented the Brodmann area 6 into its known functional sub-regions, whereas other conventional methods that we examined failed to attain such delineation.

1 Introduction

Segmentation of functional magnetic resonance imaging (fMRI) data has by far been dominated by univariate analysis approaches. These methods examine each voxel in isolation, thus voxel interactions are ignored. To account for spatial correlations, Descombes et al. proposed modeling fMRI data using Markov random fields (MRF) [1], whereas Woolrich et al. proposed using a spatio-temporal autoregressive model [2]. Due to computational complexity, only local spatial correlations are typically modeled. Another approach for functionally segmenting the brain relies on identifying voxels with temporal responses similar to a pre-selected seed region [3], which directly models the correlations between spatially disconnected voxels. However, pre-specifying a seed region can be difficult. To automatically identify seed regions, Golland et al. proposed using Gaussian mixture models (GMM) under a hierarchical framework [4], which alleviates the need to pre-define the number of clusters. Instead, expert knowledge is exploited to determine the necessary level of decomposition. The limitations to these seed-based approaches are that the detected clusters may not be spatially contiguous and the detected voxels may not necessarily pertain to task-related responses. To detect spatially contiguous clusters, Woolrich et al. proposed applying spatial mixture models on the activation statistics [5]. Similarly, Thirion et al. proposed using spectral clustering with activation statistics and physical distances between voxels as similarity metrics [6]. Using activation statistics encourages detection of task-related clusters, but unexpected responses will be neglected. Thus, jointly optimizing both functional connectivity and activation effects is desired.

To identify functional clusters without seeding, Friston et al. proposed using principal component analysis (PCA), which exploits the structure of the covariance matrix [7]. Thus, correlations between spatially disconnected voxels are also modeled. However, PCA often results in diffused weightings (i.e. spatial component maps with non-zero weights assigned to the majority of the voxels), which complicates cluster identification [8]. Another covariance-based method employing replicator dynamics was proposed by Lohmann et al. [9]. The authors noted that replicator dynamics has the interesting property of detecting clusters with *mutually* correlated voxels. This property, as we have shown previously [10], is in fact a result of the equivalence between replicator dynamics and non-negative sparse PCA. Thus, replicator dynamics can be used to handle the problem of diffused weightings in classical PCA. However, connections within a brain region tend to be dense [11], hence direct application of replicator dynamics may not be suitable for functional segmentation. A balance between diffused and sparse weightings is thus needed.

In this paper, we propose a new iterative method for functional segmentation of fMRI data that integrates the above desired characteristics, namely incorporation of activation effects, functional connectivity, neighborhood information, spatial continuity, and a balance between sparse and diffused weightings, under a single framework. Similar to PCA, the proposed method exploits the structure of the full correlation matrix, where correlations between spatially disconnected voxels are modeled. However, as opposed to computing voxel correlations in a pair-wise manner, our method incorporates neighborhood information into the correlation estimates. Employing a similar approach, Neumann et al. showed that incorporating neighborhood information encourages detection of spatially contiguous clusters, but may pool voxels near the functional boundaries into the clusters [12]. Therefore, we instead devise our method to *adaptively* incorporate neighborhood information based on activation dissimilarity, which we demonstrate in Section 3.4 to be an effective means of mitigating non-active voxels from being falsely pooled. To account for activation effects, we replace the diagonal of the correlation matrix (which is simply a set of ones) with the correlation between each voxel and the expected response. Voxels within the detected clusters will thus be highly correlated as well as activated. To draw a balance between diffused and sparse weightings, we propose combining the weight estimates from PCA and replicator dynamics in an iterative manner with the relative contributions adaptively adjusting to the sparsity of the activation pattern. We thus refer to this method as adaptive non-negative sparse PCA (ANSPCA).

2 Materials

After obtaining informed consent, fMRI data were collected from 10 Parkinson's disease (PD) patients on and off medication (4 men, 6 women, mean age 66 ± 8 years). Each subject used their right-hand to squeeze a bulb with sufficient pressure such that a horizontal bar shown on a screen was kept within an undulating pathway.

The pathway remained straight during baseline periods, and became sinusoidal at a frequency of 0.25 Hz, 0.5 Hz or 0.75 Hz during time of stimulus. Each run lasted 260s, alternating between baseline and stimulus of 20 s duration.

fMRI was performed on a Philips Gyroscan Intera 3.0 T scanner (Philips, Best, Netherlands) equipped with a head-coil. T2*-weighted images with blood oxygen level dependent (BOLD) contrast were acquired using an echo-planar (EPI) sequence with an echo time of 3.7 ms, a repetition time of 1985 ms, a flip angle of 90°, an in plane resolution of 128×128 pixels, and a pixel size of 1.9×1.9 mm. Each volume consisted of 36 axial slices of 3 mm thickness with a 1 mm gap. A 3D T1-weighted image consisting of 170 axial slices was further acquired to facilitate anatomical localization of activation. Each subject's fMRI data was pre-processed using Brain Voyager's (Brain Innovation B.V.) trilinear interpolation for 3D motion correction and sinc interpolation for slice timing correction. Further motion correction was performed using motion corrected independent component analysis (MCICA) [13]. The voxel time courses were high-pass filtered to account for temporal drifts and temporally whitened using an autoregressive AR1 model. No spatial warping or smoothing was performed. For testing our proposed method, we have selected Brodmann Area 6 (BA6), which is known to consist of multiple functional subdivisions, as the region of interest (ROI). Anatomical delineation of this ROI was performed by an expert based on anatomical landmarks and guided by a neurological atlas. The segmented ROIs were resliced at the fMRI resolution and used to extract the preprocessed voxel time courses within each ROI for subsequent analysis.

3 Methods

This section presents our new iterative method for functional segmentation of an ROI. A modified correlation matrix incorporating activation effects and neighborhood information is first estimated. ANSPCA is then applied to detect the most correlated *and* activated cluster. Subsequent clusters are detected by removing the previously identified voxels from the modified correlation matrix, and repeating the procedure.

3.1 Modified Correlation Matrix

Let N_i and N_j be the neighborhood of voxels i and j (including voxels i and j). We compute a modified correlation estimate between voxels i and j, $C(i,j)$, as follows:

$$C(i,j) = \begin{cases} corr(I_{N_i}(t), I_{N_j}(t)), & i \neq j \\ corr(I_{N_i}(t), ref(t)), & i = j \end{cases}, \quad (1)$$

$$I_{N_m}(t) = \sum_p w_{mp} I_p(t), \; w_{mp} = \exp(-|\Delta_{mp}| d_{mp}^2 / 2), \; st \; \sum_p w_{mp} = 1, \; p \in N_m \quad (2)$$

where the matrix $I_p(t)$ consists of voxel time courses belonging to N_m ($m \in \{i, j\}$) along the rows. d_{mp} is the Euclidean distance between voxels m and p. Δ_{mp} is the difference in activation statistics (t-values) between voxels m and p. The t-values are estimated by applying a general linear model (GLM) to each voxel with a column of ones and a box-car convolved with the hemodynamic response, *ref(t)*, as regressors.

We note that naively incorporating neighborhood information may pool voxels near functional boundaries into the clusters. Therefore, we have specifically designed w_{kp} to adaptively reduce the influence from neighboring voxels with dissimilar activation level, which we demonstrate in Section 3.4 to be an effective way of moderating non-active voxels from being mistakenly declared as part of a functional cluster.

3.2 Replicator Dynamics

Replicator dynamics is a well known concept that originated from theoretical biology for modeling the evolution of different species. In our context, each voxel corresponds to a species with its fitness measured by its correlations to other voxels. Let w_{RD} be a weight vector with the ith element representing the degree of which the ith voxel belongs to the most correlated cluster. w_{RD} can be estimated by [14]:

$$w_{RD}(k+1) = \frac{w_{RD}(k).*Cw_{RD}(k)}{w_{RD}^T(k)Cw_{RD}(k)}, \qquad (3)$$

where $.*$ represents element-wise product and k is the iteration number. Based on the fundamental theorem of natural selection [14], w_{RD} is guaranteed to converge provided C is real-value, non-negative, and symmetric. Since voxels belonging to the same cluster will presumably display positive correlations, we null out the negative elements to ensure C is non-negative [9]. Restricting C to be non-negative enforces w_{RD} to be non-negative. Also, (4) constrains the elements of w_{RD} to sum to one. Moreover, (4) maximizes the same objective function as PCA, i.e. $w_{RD}{}^T Cw_{RD}$. Thus, replicator dynamics is in fact a solution to the non-negative sparse PCA problem [8]:

$$\arg\max_{w_{RD}} w_{RD}^T Cw_{RD}, \quad st \quad \sum_i w_{RD}^i \leq K, w_{RD}^i \geq 0. \qquad (4)$$

Prior studies have noted that replicator dynamics has the desirable property of detecting clusters with mutually correlated voxels [9], [12]. This property can actually be explained by the fact that imposing sparsity given limited weights (i.e. $\sum w_{RD}{}^i = 1$) encourages weights to be assigned to mutually correlated voxels [10].

3.3 Adaptive Non-negative Sparse PCA

Let C be the modified correlation matrix as described in Section 3.1 and let w be a weight vector with the ith element corresponding to the degree of which the ith voxel belongs to the most correlated and activated cluster. To adaptively adjust the sparsity of w, we propose to iteratively estimate w as follows:

$$w(k) = \gamma \cdot w_{PCA}(k) + (1-\gamma) \cdot w_{RD}(k), \qquad (5)$$

$$w_{PCA}(k) = Cw(k-1), \quad st \quad \|w_{PCA}(k)\|_1 = 1 \qquad (6)$$

$$w_{RD}(k) = w(k-1).*Cw(k-1)/(w^T(k-1)Cw(k-1)) \qquad (7)$$

where $w_{PCA}(k)$ is the PCA estimate of $w(k)$ (i.e. using the Power method), but with $\|w_{PCA}(k)\|_1=1$ to ensure that $\|w(k)\|_1=1$ as required for computing $w_{RD}(k)$. γ is the percentage of activated voxels estimated as the number of voxels with t-values above a user-specified threshold over the total number of voxels in the ROI. The typical t-threshold of 1.96 is used. We note that the t-threshold only serves to estimate γ, and not to remove voxels with t-values below the threshold. In fact, voxels with t-values falling below the t-threshold but functionally connected to their neighbors can still be declared as part of a functional cluster. Using the percentage of activated voxels as γ is particularly suitable for drawing a balance between sparse weighting, $w_{RD}(k)$, and diffused weighting, $w_{PCA}(k)$, since a sparse activation pattern will result in a low percentage of activated voxels, which place greater influence from $w_{RD}(k)$ in estimating w and vice versa. To avoid bias, we initialize $w(0)$ to $1/N_r$, where N_r is the number of voxels within the ROI. Upon convergence, elements of w corresponding to the most correlated and activated cluster will rise above $1/N_r$, but the detected voxels may not form a spatially connected patch. Therefore, we perform connected component analysis to first group the detected voxels into spatially connected clusters. We then find the cluster with the highest $w^T C w$, remove the other clusters from C, and reapply the above procedure until no spatially disconnected clusters are detected. The resulting cluster upon convergence will thus consist of voxels that are highly activated, functionally connected, and spatially connected. To identify subsequent clusters, we remove only voxels in the previously detected functional clusters from C and repeat the procedure above.

3.4 Empirical Evaluations

To test our proposed method on data with ground truth, we generated 1,000 synthetic datasets with simulated activation patterns consisting of two clusters that were one voxel apart (Fig.1). Also, the signal intensity of the activated voxels was set to decrease as a function of their distances from cluster centroids. The time courses of the activated voxels in the larger cluster were generated by convolving a box-car function having the same stimulus timing as in our experiment with the hemodynamic response and adding Gaussian noise. The smaller cluster was generated in a similar manner but with the box-car delayed by 2 seconds.

For comparisons with the state-of-the-art, we also tested the following methods: replicator dynamics [9] with Pearson's correlation, PCA [7], GMM [4] assuming two clusters and background, and GLM with Gaussian spatial smoothing and a threshold estimated from Gaussian random field (GRF) theory for an uncorrected p-value of 0.05. For PCA, we renormalized the PCs such that $\|w_{PCA}\|_1 = 1$ and used the same threshold as ANSPCA (i.e. $1/N_r$). Also, only the first PC was used, since the second PC mainly detected non-active voxels (squares in Fig. 1b). Fig. 1 contains the synthetic data results with the average true positive rate (TP) and false positive rate (FP) indicated. We note that TP and FP are computed only based on whether the voxels are correctly labeled as active, and not based on the cluster labels.

Replicator dynamics (Fig. 1a) did not falsely declare any non-activated voxels as active (FP = 0.00), but many activated voxels were missed (TP = 0.15). In contrast, PCA (Fig. 1b) detected most of the activated voxels with its first PC (TP = 0.83), but also detected many non-active voxels (FP = 0.04). Neither of these methods was able to separate the two clusters. GMM behaved similarly to PCA with one of its mixtures encompassing both clusters, and the other mixture including mainly non-active voxels (Fig. 1c). Hence, a high FP of 0.13 with only a TP of 0.77 was obtained.

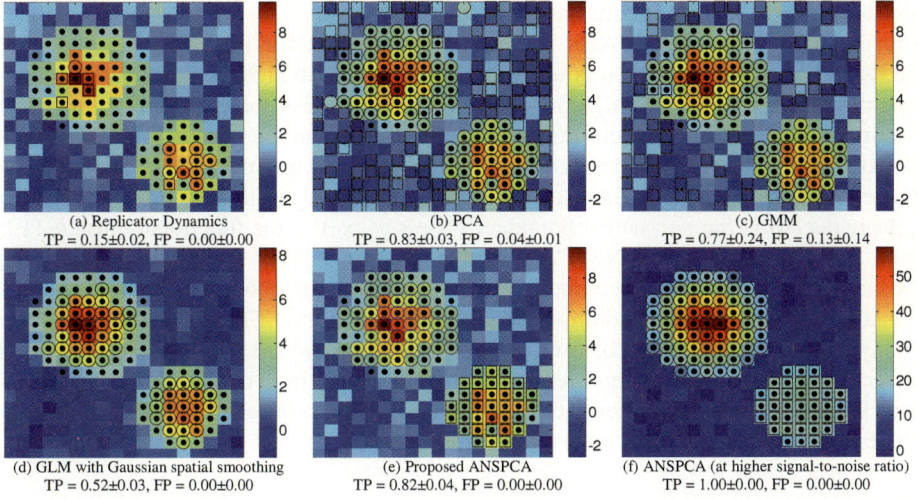

Fig. 1. Synthetic data results. t-map estimated using GLM with "dots" indicating the ground truth activated voxels. Voxels with a circle (square) correspond to the first (second) cluster detected. Note how ANSPCA was able to separate the two clusters and achieve a FP of 0.00.

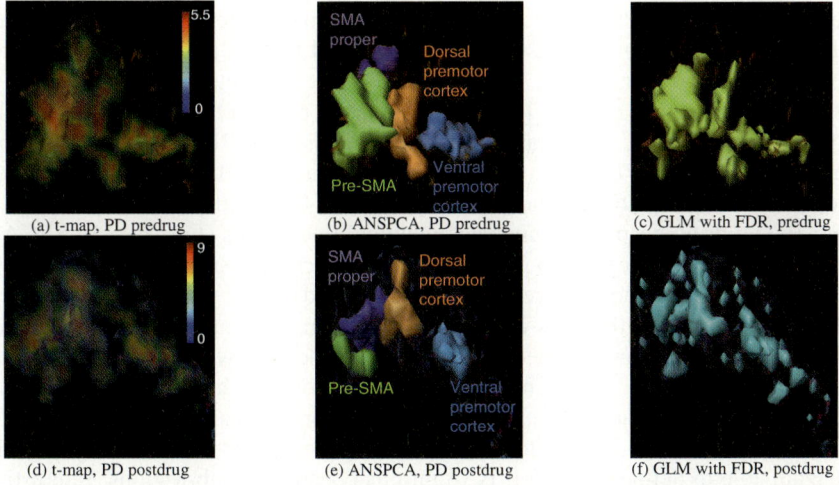

Fig. 2. Real fMRI data results. (a) & (d) Left BA6 t-map of a PD subject before and after medication. (b) & (e) Proposed ANSPCA segments the BA6 into its known sub-regions, whereas (c) & (f) GLM appears to over-divide the BA6.

GLM resulted in a FP of 0.00 with a TP of 0.52. Examining Fig. 1d, post-processing the voxels detected by GLM with connected component analysis could have separated the two clusters. Using ANSPCA, we were able to separate the two clusters as shown in Fig. 1e. Compared to PCA, with a mere decrease of 0.01 in TP, ANSPCA achieved a FP of 0.00 without any non-active voxels near the functional boundaries being falsely declared. Being able to incorporate neighborhood information without falsely pooling the non-active boundary voxels is especially important for functionally segmenting ROIs with unclear sub-region boundaries such as the BA6 [15]. We thus further tested our method by varying the signal-to-noise ratio (SNR). For the case shown in Fig. 1f, we increased the SNR, which presumably would increase the correlation between the active and non-active boundary voxels if their information is mistakenly pooled in the correlation estimates. This increase in correlation would result in a higher chance of falsely declaring the non-active boundary voxels as part of the functional clusters [12]. Yet, as shown in Fig. 1f, ANSPCA was able to attain a TP of 1 without including any of the non-active voxels. We note that by incorporating neighborhood information and functional connectivity in addition to activation effects, ANSPCA was able to detect many voxels with t-values below the t-threshold determined from GRF. Also, upon detecting the larger cluster and removing the corresponding voxels from C, ANSPCA was able to adapt to the sparser activation pattern without falsely declaring voxels near the functional boundaries as part of the second cluster.

4 Results and Discussion

Results obtained by applying ANSPCA on the BA6 are shown in Fig. 2. We only included the left BA6 results for an exemplar PD subject due to space limitation. Nevertheless, ANSPCA did correctly separate the SMA and PM in all subjects, although the SMA and PMd appeared partly joined in 3 subjects. For comparison, we applied replicator dynamics, PCA, GMM, and GLM to the data. However, except for GLM, the results obtained were similar to that in the synthetic data experiments with no spatially contiguous clusters identified. Thus, we only included the GLM results in favour of space. Also, the t-threshold estimated using GRF with Gaussian spatial smoothing of 8mm FWHM was found to be too stringent. Hence, we instead present the thresholded t-maps for an uncorrected p-value of 0.05 with FDR correction.

For PD predrug, despite the unclear functional boundaries (Fig. 2a), ANSPCA was able to delineate the left BA6 into its known functional sub-regions, namely pre-SMA, SMA proper, dorsal premotor cortex (PMd), and ventral premotor cortex (PMv) [15]. We argue that this delineation was attained by the additional functional connectivity information included in our proposed method, which was not modeled in the activation statistics. Also, incorporating neighborhood information enabled ANSPCA to detect PMd and PMv as two spatially contiguous clusters, whereas GLM over-divided PMd and PMv into multiple sub-regions. For PD postdrug, ANSPCA was again able to delineate the left BA6 into its constituent sub-regions. Interestingly, our results suggest that the extent of activation within the pre-SMA (Fig. 2b) reduced upon medication (Fig. 2e). This "focusing" effect conforms to prior findings in computational model studies, where increased dopamine level was found to be associated with more focused activation patterns. In contrast, GLM split the SMA proper into multiple pieces with islands of activation scattered across the BA6.

5 Conclusions

We proposed a novel method that integrates multiple functional attributes such as activation effects, functional connectivity, and neighborhood information under a single framework for functionally segmenting fMRI data. By adaptively combining PCA and replicator dynamics, our method facilitates functional segmentation of activation patterns with various degree of sparsity. Applying our method to synthetic data outperformed all other examined methods including replicator dynamics, PCA, GMM, and GLM. When applied to real data, the integration of the various functional attributes enabled our method to segment the BA6 into its constituent functional sub-regions, whereas other examined methods failed to attain such delineation.

References

1. Descombes, X., Kruggel, F., von Cramon, D.Y.: Spatio-Temporal fMRI Analysis Using Markov Random Fields. Trans. Med. Imaging 17, 1028–1039 (1998)
2. Woolrich, M.W., Jenkinson, M., Brady, J.M., Smith, S.M.: Fully Bayesian Spatio-temporal Modeling of fMRI Data. Trans. Med. Imaging 28, 213–231 (2004)
3. Biswal, B., Yetkin, F.Z., Haughton, V.M., Hyde, J.S.: Functional Connectivity in the Motor Cortex of Resting Human Brain Using Echo-planar MRI. Magn. Reson. Med. 34, 537–541 (1995)
4. Golland, P., Golland, Y., Malach, R.: Detection of Spatial Activation Patterns as Unsupervised Segmentation of fMRI Data. In: Ayache, N., Ourselin, S., Maeder, A. (eds.) MICCAI 2007, Part I. LNCS, vol. 4791, pp. 110–118. Springer, Heidelberg (2007)
5. Woolrich, M.W., Behrens, T.E., Beckmann, C.F., Smith, S.M.: Mixture Models with Adaptive Spatial Regularization for Segmentation with an Application to fMRI Data. Trans. Med. Imaging. 24, 1–11 (2005)
6. Thirion, B., Flandin, G., Pinel, P., Roche, A., Ciuciu, P., Poline, J.B.: Dealing with the Shortcomings of Spatial Normalization: Multi-subject Parcellation of fMRI Datasets. Hum. Brain Mapp. 27, 678–693 (2006)
7. Friston, K.J., Frith, C.D., Liddle, P.F., Frackowiak, R.S.: Functional Connectivity: The Principal Component Analysis of Large (PET) Data Sets. J. Cereb. Blood Flow Metab. 13, 5–14 (1993)
8. Zass, R., Shashua, A.: Nonnegative Sparse PCA. In: Advances in Neural Information Processing Systems, pp. 1561–1568 (2006)
9. Lohmann, G., Bohn, S.: Using Replicator Dynamics for Analyzing fMRI Data of the Human Brain. Trans. Med. Imaging. 21, 485–492 (2002)
10. Ng, B., Abugharbieh, R., McKeown, M.J.: Discovering Sparse Functional Brain Networks Using Group Replicator Dynamics (GRD). In: 21st Int. Conf. IPMI (accepted 2009)
11. Bassett, D.S., Bullmore, E.: Small-World Brain Networks. Neuroscientist 12, 512–523 (2006)
12. Neumann, J., von Cramon, D.Y., Forstmann, B.U., Zysset, S., Lohmann, G.: The Parcellation of Cortical Areas Using Replicator Dynamics in fMRI. Neuroimage 32, 208–219 (2006)
13. Liao, R., Krolik, J.L., McKeown, M.J.: An Information-theoretic Criterion for Intrasubject Alignment of fMRI Time Series: Motion Corrected Independent Component Analysis. Trans. Med. Imaging. 24(1), 29–44 (2005)
14. Schuster, P., Sigmund, K.: Replicator Dynamics. J. Theor. Biol. 100, 533–538 (1983)
15. Mayka, M.A., Corcos, D.M., Leurgans, S.E., Vaillancourt, D.E.: Three-dimensional Locations and Boundaries of Motor and Premotor Cortices as Defined by Functional Brain Imaging: A Meta-analysis. Neuroimage 31, 1452–1474 (2006)

Genetics of Anisotropy Asymmetry: Registration and Sample Size Effects

Neda Jahanshad[1,2], Agatha D. Lee[1], Natasha Leporé[1], Yi-Yu Chou[1], Caroline C. Brun[1], Marina Barysheva[1], Arthur W. Toga[1], Katie L. McMahon[3], Greig I. de Zubicaray[3], Margaret J. Wright[4], and Paul M. Thompson[1]

[1] Laboratory of Neuro Imaging, Department of Neurology, UCLA, CA USA
[2] Medical Imaging Informatics Group, Department of Radiology, UCLA, CA USA
[3] University of Queensland, fMRI Laboratory, Centre for MR, Brisbane, Australia
[4] Queensland Institute of Medical Research, Brisbane, Australia

Abstract. Brain asymmetry has been a topic of interest for neuroscientists for many years. The advent of diffusion tensor imaging (DTI) allows researchers to extend the study of asymmetry to a microscopic scale by examining fiber integrity differences across hemispheres rather than the macroscopic differences in shape or structure volumes. Even so, the power to detect these microarchitectural differences depends on the sample size and how the brain images are registered and how many subjects are studied. We fluidly registered 4 Tesla DTI scans from 180 healthy adult twins (45 identical and fraternal pairs) to a geometrically-centered population mean template. We computed voxelwise maps of significant asymmetries (left/right hemisphere differences) for common fiber anisotropy indices (FA, GA). Quantitative genetic models revealed that 47-62% of the variance in asymmetry was due to genetic differences in the population. We studied how these heritability estimates varied with the type of registration target (T1- or T2-weighted) and with sample size. All methods consistently found that genetic factors strongly determined the lateralization of fiber anisotropy, facilitating the quest for specific genes that might influence brain asymmetry and fiber integrity.

1 Introduction

Asymmetries in brain structure and function have been the topic of neuroimaging studies for many years. Anatomical asymmetries may help to reveal the origins of lateralized cognitive functions or behavioral traits, such as language and handedness, that may arise from partially genetic hemispheric differences during development [1]. Studies of brain asymmetry can also inform clinical research, as aberrant asymmetries have been hypothesized or detected in disorders such as schizophrenia, dyslexia, or hemiparesis, which may arise from a derailment in processes that establish normal brain lateralization and hemispheric specialization. Deformation-based morphometry studies have used the theory of random Gaussian vector fields to detect statistical departures from the normal level of brain asymmetry [2].

Many imaging studies have used MRI to study brain asymmetries, but very few have used DTI. In DTI, the MR signal attenuation due to water diffusion in direction k decreases according to the Stejskal-Tanner equation: $S_k(\mathbf{r}) = S_0(\mathbf{r})e^{-b_k D_k(\mathbf{r})}$ where $S_0(\mathbf{r})$ is the non-diffusion weighted baseline intensity, $D_k(\mathbf{r})$ is the apparent diffusion coefficient (ADC), and b_k is Le Bihan's factor; the fractional and geodesic anisotropy (FA and GA), calculated from a local tensor approximation for $D_k(\mathbf{r})$, are commonly used measures of fiber integrity; FA correlates highly with IQ (intelligence quotient) in normal subjects [3].

Previous DTI asymmetry studies have focused on specific tracts (e.g., the corticospinal tract [4], and the arcuate fasciculus involved in language processing [5,6]). Frontal and temporal white matter show left greater than right FA even in early infancy [7], suggesting greater myelination in the left hemisphere [7]. Frontal FA differences between the two hemispheres diminish as the brain develops, but temporal lobe asymmetries persist [8].

Studies of asymmetries in white matter characteristics may be confounded by the vast structural asymmetries present. In frontal and occipital regions, the natural petalia (torquing) of the brain shifts the right hemisphere structures anterior to their left hemisphere counterparts [1]. Men may have greater anatomical asymmetries than women [1], making it advantageous to reduce these pronounced macrostructural differences when gauging the level of microstructural asymmetry in a mixed-sex population.

Twin studies have long been used to determine genetically and environmentally influenced human traits. Monozygotic twins share all their genes while dizygotic twins share, on average, half. Estimates of the proportion of variance attributable to genes versus environment can be inferred by fitting structural equation models to data from both types of twins. Twin neuroimaging studies reveal that genetic factors strongly influence several aspects of brain structure, e.g., cortical thickness, and gray and white matter volumes [9], but twin studies using DTI are rare.

Here we created the first DTI-based maps of asymmetries (left/right hemisphere differences) in fiber characteristics (FA, GA) in a large twin population (N=180). We adjusted, as far as possible, for the known structural differences between hemispheres by aligning brains to a symmetrized minimal deformation target (MDT) created from all of the images.

The choice of registration target is known to affect the accuracy of region of interest (ROI) analyses [10], so we evaluated the effects of using different registration targets based on the separate structural MRI images, including (1) an MDT created by geometrically adjusting an individual subject's image, (2) a population-averaged MDT, and (3) a population-averaged MDT based on the non-diffusion-sensitized T2-weighted images collected as part of the DTI protocol. We then determined whether genetic factors influenced the residual asymmetries, and examined the stability of the estimates with respect to sample size and the choice of registration target.

2 Methods

2.1 Image Acquisition and Subject Information

Structural and diffusion tensor (DT) MRI scans were acquired from 180 subjects using a high magnetic field (4T) Bruker Medspec MRI scanner. T1-weighted images were collected using an inversion recovery rapid gradient echo sequence, with parameters: TI/TR/TE= 1500/2500/3.83 $msec$; flip angle=15 degrees; slice thickness = 0.9 mm, and 256x256x256 acquisition matrix. Diffusion-weighted images were also acquired using 30 gradients (27 diffusion-weighted images and 3 with no diffusion sensitization; i.e., T2- weighted images) with gradient directions uniformly distributed on the hemisphere. Parameters were: 23 cm FOV, TR/TE 6090/91.7ms, b-value =1132 s/mm^2, scan time: 3.05 minutes. Each 3D volume consisted of 21 5-mm thick axial slices with a 0.5mm gap and 1.8x1.8 mm^2 in-plane resolution. The subjects included 90 young adult monozygotic (MZ) twins and 90 dizygotic (DZ) same sex twins (45 pairs of each). All subjects were right-handed young adults (average age 24.37, stdev 1.936).

2.2 Creating Templates

To determine whether asymmetric differences are influenced by the template used for registration, several templates were created and compared. Three templates were created using the T1-weighted images to help adjust for the structural differences across subjects and hemispheres, and another template was created from the T2-weighted images acquired along with the diffusion weighted scans, which are in perfect register with the diffusion tensor data. T1-weighted structural MR images were edited to remove extracerebral tissues and were linearly registered to a symmetrical template. This symmetrical template was created by averaging a high-resolution single subject average scan, the Colin27 [11], with the same image reflected in the midsagittal plane. This centered each subjects midline within the image volume. All subjects images were linearly registered to the symmetrical template using FLIRT software http://fsl.fmrib.ox.ac.uk/fsl/flirt with 9-parameter registration and a correlation ratio cost function.

T1 Template 1(non-symmetric). One minimal deformation target (MDT) was created using only the original scan orientations, using non-linear fluid registration as described in [12,13]. This template was not symmetrical as all the images used to create it were of the original orientation. MDTs were created using the method proposed by Kochunov [14] (although alternative methods are possible): the N 3D vector fields fluidly registering a specific individual to all other subjects were averaged and applied to that subject, geometrically adjusting their anatomy, but retaining the image intensities and anatomical features of that specific subject. **T1 Template 2 (initial symmetrization).** Linearly aligned subject images were reflected over the midline to produce a mirrored set. Another MDT was then created from four independent (one per pair) monozygotic (MZ) twins and four independent dizygotic (DZ) twin image volumes randomly selected with their corresponding reflected images. These 16 image sets were then used to generate an MDT using fluid registration as described in [12,13]. The flipped images of the same brains were included during MDT construction to make it symmetric.

T1 Template 3 (symmetric population averaged MDT). A population-averaged MDT was created to further reduce the structural asymmetries. 8 separate MDTs were constructed as described above, each formed from 6 subjects and their corresponding images flipped over the midline. For 4 of these MDTs, the initial template image was in the original orientation while for the other 4, the template was in the flipped orientation. All 8 MDTs were then averaged together to produce the population averaged MDT, incorporating T1 information from 50 independent subjects.

T2 Template (symmetric population averaged MDT). Another population averaged MDT was constructed from the T2-weighted images, in the same manner as for the T1-weighted population MDT, with the same set of subjects. All subjects' images were first linearly aligned to a single subject image. This image of the single subject was aligned such that the midsagittal plane of the brain was centered. Another image was created by mirroring the result in the midsagittal plane. This flipped image was averaged with its original to create a symmetric template to linearly align all the T2-weighted scans and their mirror images before creating the MDT.

Structural T1 images from 100 subjects (25 MZ, 25 DZ pairs) were then fluidly registered to each of the 3 T1-weighted MDTs using a 3D Navier-Stokes-based fluid warping technique enforcing diffeomorphic mappings, using least squares intensity differences as a cost function [12,13]. T2-weighted images for each of the 180 subjects were registered to the T2-weighted MDT with the same technique. 3D deformation fields for all mappings were retained.

2.3 Anisotropy Asymmetry Maps

Diffusion tensors were computed from the diffusion-weighted images using Med-INRIA software http://www.sop.inria.fr/asclepios/software/MedINRIA.

Scalar images of anisotropy measures were created for each of the 180 subjects from the eigenvalues (λ_1, λ_2, λ_3) of the symmetric $3x3$ diffusion tensor. These included the fractional anisotropy (FA), geodesic anisotropy (GA) computed in the Log-Euclidean framework [15], hyperbolic tangent of the GA (tGA), to take values in the same range as FA, i.e., [0,1], and mean diffusivity (MD):

$$FA = \sqrt{\frac{3}{2}} \frac{\sqrt{(\lambda_1 - \hat{\lambda})^2 + (\lambda_2 - \hat{\lambda})^2 + (\lambda_3 - \hat{\lambda})^2}}{\sqrt{\lambda_1^2 + \lambda_2^2 + \lambda_3^2}}, \hat{\lambda} = MD = \frac{\lambda_1 + \lambda_2 + \lambda_3}{3} \quad (1)$$

$$GA(S) = \sqrt{Trace(\log S - <\log S> I)^2}, <\log S> = \frac{Trace(\log S)}{3} \quad (2)$$

Extra-cerebral tissue was manually deleted from one directional component of the diffusion tensors (D_{xx}) creating a mask that was then applied to the scalar anisotropy maps created for each subject. Once masked, these anisotropy images were then linearly aligned to the symmeterized templates and fluidly registered to each of the MDTs by applying the deformation fields described in Section 2.2.

Each aligned anisotropy map was then mirrored across midline, and the voxel-wise difference map between the original and flipped images was created. In this new map, the left side of the image represents the difference between the subjects right and left hemispheres; voxels on the other side of the image have the opposite sign. Maps were obtained of the percent difference between the resulting difference image and the average of the two mirror image orientations.

2.4 Calculating Genetic Contributions

Voxel-wise maps of the intra-class correlations (ICC) within MZ and DZ twins, r_{MZ} and r_{DZ} respectively, were derived as well as Falconer's heritability estimate, $h^2 = 2(r_{MZ} - r_{DZ})$ [16] for the asymmetry in FA, GA, tGA and MD.

Average measures of the anisotropy difference were examined in certain regions of interest (ROIs). We determined the genetic contribution to the asymmetries in each lobe of the brain. ROIs were traced for the four lobes (frontal, parietal, temporal, and occipital) in one hemisphere of each MDT and were flipped to define the same ROI in the opposite hemisphere. This ensured consistency between hemispheres and reduced errors due to manual labeling. For each anisotropy measure, covariances for the average ROI values in pairs of MZ and DZ twins were entered into a univariate structural equation model to estimate additive genetic (A), shared environmental (C) and unique environmental (E) components of the variance in asymmetry [17]. Mx modeling software http://www.vcu.edu/mx/ was used.

This form of structural equation modeling finds the maximum likelihood estimate (eq. 3) for Σ ($\alpha = 1$ for MZ and 0.5 for DZ) to estimate genetic versus environmental contributions to the variance, where S_g is the observed covariance matrix for each twin group g:

$$ML_g = N_g \{\ln|\Sigma_g| - ln|S_g| + tr(S_g \Sigma_g^{-1}) - 2m\}, \Sigma = \begin{bmatrix} a^2+c^2+e^2 & \alpha a^2+c^2 \\ \alpha a^2+c^2 & a^2+c^2+e^2 \end{bmatrix} \quad (3)$$

3 Results

Figure 1A shows the mean FA asymmetry as a percent difference between left and right hemispheres, relative to which genetic effects were determined. Frontal and temporal regions show high asymmetry ($\sim 25\%, p < 0.05$). Frontal FA is higher in the right hemisphere, while temporal FA is higher on the left. The asymmetries found in the temporal lobe correspond to language centers [1] consistent with [7,8]. The magnitude of the asymmetry difference is somewhat dependent on the number of subjects used in the study, but patterns are largely consistent. Figure 1B shows differences arising in ICC and Falconer's heritability estimates when using the T1-weighted population template for 100 subjects and the T2-weighted MDT for the different population sizes. Despite evidence for some subcortical effects, voxelwise maps are somewhat noisy even with N=180 subjects, partly

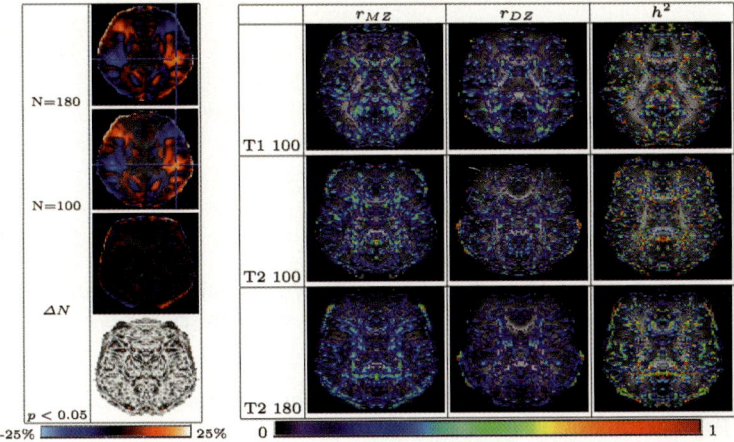

Fig. 1. A: The mean asymmetry in FA, in a sample of N=180 subjects, reaches 25% in frontal and temporal regions. The localization of results based on 180 vs only 100 subjects is largely consistent, as shown by the difference image and the image of the p-values. **B:** ICC and Falconer's h^2 maps for asymmetries in FA images. *Top:* FA results of 100 subjects mapped to the population-averaged T1 MDT; *Center:* results from 100 subjects mapped to population-averaged T2 MDT; *Bottom:* results from 180 subjects mapped to the T2 MDT

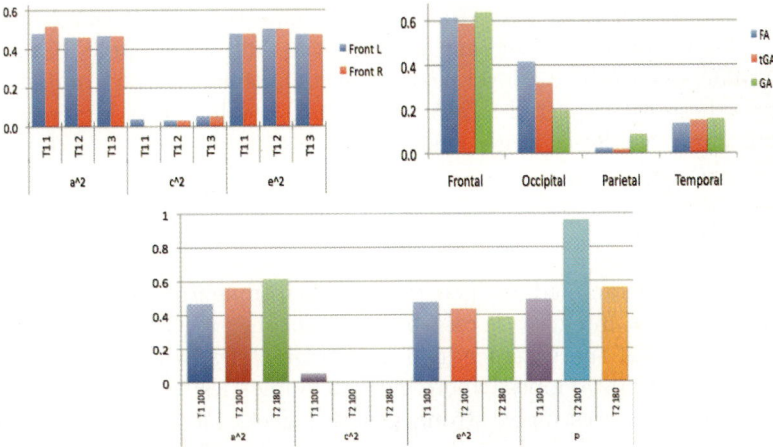

Fig. 2. A/C/E Genetic effects: *Top Left: Symmetrization Effects:*ACE results showing genetic and environmental contributions of template choice asymmetry in FA; *Top Right: Frontal Lobe FA* ACE results of using the population averaged T1 template (100 subjects) and T2 template (100 and 180 subjects) for FA asymmetry in the frontal lobe. p-values derived from χ^2 statistics show the ACE model fits well in all cases ($p > 0.05$); *Bottom: $N = 180$ Genetic Effects* genetic component of variance (A) determined from mapping 180 subjects to the T2-weighted MDT for all anisotropy measures, in each lobe. Genetic effects are greatest in lobes with the highest mean asymmetries (Fig. 1).

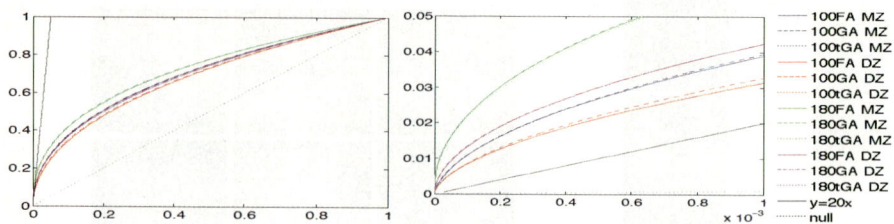

Fig. 3. CDF of significant p-values for anisotropy asymmetries mapped to the T2-weighted population MDT for 100 (left) and 180 subjects (right)

because h^2 is a difference in correlations. We therefore summarize FA asymmetry in lobar ROIs, to increase power for genetic analyses.

Figure 2 shows genetic (a^2) vs environmental (c^2, e^2) effects on FA asymmetry. Intriguingly, the asymmetry in frontal lobe mean FA was $\sim 50\%$ determined by genetic factors, with no evidence for a shared environmental effect ($c^2 \sim 0\%$). The e^2-term contains registration errors as well as unique effects, so there is some evidence that using 180 (vs 100) subjects, and using a T2 vs T1 template, more accurately captures the true genetic contributions to these asymmetries, as the e^2-term is slightly lower. In structural equation models, $p > 0.05$ denotes that the ACE model fits well. All models here yield a good fit.

Figure 3 plots the cumulative distribution function (cdf) of the p-values associated with the ICC against those that would be expected from a null distribution. As the cdf initially rises faster than 20 times the null, we are able to reasonably claim significance at the 5% level. For null distributions (i.e. no group difference detected), these are expected to fall along the x = y line, and larger deviations from that curve represent larger effect sizes.

4 Discussion

In this study, we examined the genetic and environmental contributions to the differences in fiber integrity across brain hemispheres. Genetic factors determined about half of the variance in these asymmetries, with greatest effects in the frontal and occipital lobes, where mean asymmetries were greatest (reaching 25%) (Fig. 1A). Interestingly, strong genetic effects (significant ACE models) were detectable for anisotropy indices (FA, GA). Results were stable when the images were fluidly registered to various different anatomical templates, including ones constructed to have hemispheric symmmetry. These results suggest that specific genetic factors determining hemispheric asymmetries in fiber architecture may be identifiable in very large samples.

Acknowledgments. Supported by grants from the NLM, NIH and NICHD.

References

1. Toga, A., Thompson, P.: Mapping brain asymmetry. Nat. Rev. Neurosci. 4(1) (2003)
2. Thirion, J.P., Prima, S., Subsol, G., Roberts, N.: Statistical analysis of normal and abnormal dissymmetry in volumetric medical images. Med. Im. Analy. 4(2) (2000)
3. Chiang, M., Barysheva, M., Lee, A., Madsen, S., Klunder, A., Toga, A., McMahon, K., de Zubicaray, G., Wright, M., Srivastava, A., Balov, N., Thompson, P.: Genetics of brain fiber architecture and intelligence. Journal of Neuroscience (2009)
4. Westerhausen, R., Huster, R.J., Kreuder, F., Wittling, W., Schweiger, E.: Corticospinal tract asymmetries at the level of the internal capsule: Is there an association with handedness? Neuroimage 37(2), 379–386 (2007)
5. de Jong, L., Kovacs, S., Bamps, S., Calenbergh, F.V., Sunaert, S., van Loon, J.: The arcuate fasciculus: a comparison between diffusion tensor tractography and anatomy using the fiber dissection technique. Surgical Neurology 71(1) (2009)
6. Rodrigo, S., Naggara, O., Oppenheim, C., Golestani, N., Poupon, C., Cointepas, Y., Mangin, J.F., Le Bihan, D., Meder, J.F.: Human subinsular asymmetry studied by diffusion tensor imaging and fiber tracking. AJNR 28(8), 1526–1531 (2007)
7. Dubois, J., Hertz-Pannier, L., Cachia, A., Le Bihan, D., Dehaene-Lambertz, G.: Structural asymmetries in the infant language and sensori-motor networks. Cerebral Cortex 19(2), 414–423 (2008)
8. Barnea-Goraly, N., Menon, V., Eckert, M., Tamm, L., Bammer, R., Karchemskiy, A., Dant, C.C., Reiss, A.L.: White matter development during childhood and adolescence: A cross-sectional diffusion tensor imaging study. Cereb. Cortex 15(12), 1848–1854 (2005)
9. Pfefferbaum, A., Sulluvan, E.V., Carmelli, D.: Genetic regulation of regional microstructure of the corpus callosum in late life. Neuroreport 12(8), 1677–1681 (2001)
10. Wang, Q., Seghers, D., D'Agostino, E., Maes, F., Vandermeulen, D., Suetens, P., Hammers, A.: Construction and validation of mean shape atlas templates for atlas-based brain image segmentation. In: Christensen, G.E., Sonka, M. (eds.) IPMI 2005. LNCS, vol. 3565, pp. 689–700. Springer, Heidelberg (2005)
11. Holmes, C.J., Hoge, R., Collins, L., Woods, R., Toga, A.W., Evans, A.C.: Enhancement of MR images using registration for signal averaging. J. Comput. Assist. Tomogr. 22(2), 324–333 (1998)
12. Leporé, N., Brun, C., Pennec, X., Chou, Y.Y., Lopez, O., Aizenstein, H., Becker, J., Toga, A., Thompson, P.: Mean template for tensor-based morphometry using deformation tensors. In: Ayache, N., Ourselin, S., Maeder, A. (eds.) MICCAI 2007, Part II. LNCS, vol. 4792, pp. 826–833. Springer, Heidelberg (2007)
13. Leporé, N., Chou, Y.Y., Lopez, O.L., Aizenstein, H.J., Becker, J.T., Toga, A.W., Thompson, P.M.: Fast 3D fluid registration of brain magnetic resonance images, vol. 6916. SPIE, San Diego (2008)
14. Kochunov, P., Lancaster, J., Thompson, P., Toga, A., Brewer, P., Hardies, J., Fox, P.: An optimized individual target brain in the Talairach coordinate system. Neuroimage 17(2), 922–927 (2002)
15. Arsigny, V., Fillard, P., Pennec, X., Ayache, N.: Log-Euclidean metrics for fast and simple calculus on diffusion tensors. MRM 56(2), 411–421 (2006)
16. Falconer, D., Macka, T.F.: Introduction to Quantitative Genetics, 4th edn. Addison Wesley Longman, Amsterdam (1995) (Pearson Education)
17. Rijsdijk, F.V., Sham, P.C.: Analytic approaches to twin data using structural equation models. Briefings in Bioinformatics 3(2), 119–133 (2002)

Extending Genetic Linkage Analysis to Diffusion Tensor Images to Map Single Gene Effects on Brain Fiber Architecture*

Ming-Chang Chiang[1], Christina Avedissian[1], Marina Barysheva[1], Arthur W. Toga[1], Katie L. McMahon[2], Greig I. de Zubicaray[2], Margaret J. Wright[3], and Paul M. Thompson[1]

[1] Laboratory of Neuro Imaging, Dept. of Neurology,
UCLA School of Medicine, Los Angeles, CA
[2] University of Queensland, Functional Magnetic Resonance Imaging Laboratory,
Centre for Magnetic Resonance, Brisbane, Australia
[3] Queensland Institute of Medical Research, Brisbane, Australia

Abstract. We extended genetic linkage analysis - an analysis widely used in quantitative genetics - to 3D images to analyze single gene effects on brain fiber architecture. We collected 4 Tesla diffusion tensor images (DTI) and genotype data from 258 healthy adult twins and their non-twin siblings. After high-dimensional fluid registration, at each voxel we estimated the genetic linkage between the single nucleotide polymorphism (SNP), Val66Met (dbSNP number rs6265), of the BDNF gene (brain-derived neurotrophic factor) with fractional anisotropy (FA) derived from each subject's DTI scan, by fitting structural equation models (SEM) from quantitative genetics. We also examined how image filtering affects the effect sizes for genetic linkage by examining how the overall significance of voxelwise effects varied with respect to full width at half maximum (FWHM) of the Gaussian smoothing applied to the FA images. Raw FA maps with no smoothing yielded the greatest sensitivity to detect gene effects, when corrected for multiple comparisons using the false discovery rate (FDR) procedure. The BDNF polymorphism significantly contributed to the variation in FA in the posterior cingulate gyrus, where it accounted for around 90-95% of the total variance in FA. Our study generated the first maps to visualize the effect of the BDNF gene on brain fiber integrity, suggesting that common genetic variants may strongly determine white matter integrity.

1 Introduction

Imaging genetics is a rapidly growing field that combines mathematical methods from image analysis and quantitative genetics to discover how specific genes influence the brain, cognition, and risk for disease. Although epidemiologists can relate genetic data to behavior in thousands of subjects, a more mechanistic understanding of these effects

---

* This work was funded in part by NIH grant R01 HD050735.

is likely to be gained by linking genetic variants to specific features in images (such as measures of fiber integrity) that are highly correlated with intellectual performance and risk for disease, and may explain the basis of the genetic effect. Mapping these effects in 3D may also focus on specific regions where the genetic influences are stronger than elsewhere. This may also increase sensitivity for detecting genetic linkage because millions of hypotheses (voxelwise statistics) are tested simultaneously throughout the brain, while false discovery rate methods can still control the false positive rate. Structural MRI studies in twins have shown that many aspects of brain structure are highly heritable, including cortical gray matter density and thickness [1]. More recently, the first genetic studies of 3D diffusion tensor images have revealed that fiber integrity is under strong genetic control, is correlated with intelligence quotient (IQ) and the same genes underlie both fiber integrity and IQ [2]. These initial studies fitted quantitative genetic models to separate additive genetic from common and unique environmental components of inter-subject variance in images, for measures of fiber integrity such as the fractional anisotropy (FA) and generalized FA in high-angular resolution diffusion images (HARDI; [3]). McIntosh et al. [4] first studied the association between FA and individual genes, identifying the T-allele in a single nucleotide locus (dbSNP number rs6994992) of the neuregulin 1 gene as being associated with reduced FA in the anterior limb of the internal capsule.

In this paper we extended the variance-component genetic linkage analysis method [5] to create voxel-level maps in fluidly registered DTI data from a population, to estimate the influences of a specific gene on fiber integrity in the brain. A common variant in the brain-derived neurotrophic factor (BDNF) gene was linked with the variation in FA, an accepted measure of fiber integrity. BDNF modulates synaptic plasticity in the hippocampus, and is crucially involved in memory acquisition and retention. We selected the most studied single nucleotide polymorphism (SNP) of the BDNF gene, Val66Met (dbSNP number rs6265), where valine (Val) is substituted by methionine (Met) at codon 66 in the 5′-proregion of the BDNF protein. This Val66Met SNP has been found to be associated with subjects' memory performance and memory-related hippocampal activation using functional MRI [6]. We acquired 4 Tesla diffusion tensor images from 258 twins and their non-twin siblings, and fitted structural equation models (SEM; [5]) at each voxel to estimate the contribution of the BDNF Val66Met SNP to the variance in FA. After multiple comparisons correction using FDR, we still found significant linkage between this common BDNF polymorphism and FA in the posterior cingulate gyrus. To inform future genetic linkage studies in image databases, we performed a post hoc (exploratory) test to see how the overall significance of voxelwise gene effects varied with respect to the size of the Gaussian filter kernel applied to the FA images.

2 Methods

2.1 Subject Description and Genotyping

258 subjects (110 males/148 females; age: 23.8±1.9 years, mean±SD), consisting of 39 monozygotic (MZ) twin pairs, 65 dizygotic (DZ) twin pairs, 1 set of DZ triplets, and 47 of their non-twin siblings, were recruited from 133 different nuclear families, as part of a 5-year research project evaluating healthy Australian twins using structural

and functional MRI and DTI. The genotype of the BDNF Val66Met polymorphism was determined using primer extension on the Sequenom Mass-Array system [7], with Val/Val identified in 174 subjects, Val/Met in 68 subjects, and Met/Met in 16 subjects. Information from a larger sample of subjects [7], which include all subjects in this study, has shown that the frequency of BDNF Val allele is 0.81, and that the genotype distribution follows Hardy-Weinberg equilibrium. This candidate gene was chosen based on prior reports that it explained variation in memory performance, task-related activation on fMRI, and its known molecular role as a key growth factor affecting brain development and plasticity [6].

2.2 Image Acquisition and Registration

All MR images were collected using a 4 Tesla Bruker Medspec MRI scanner. Diffusion-weighted scans were acquired using single-shot echo planar imaging with a twice-refocused spin echo sequence to reduce eddy-current induced distortions. Acquisition parameters were optimized to provide the best signal-to-noise ratio for estimation of diffusion tensors. Imaging parameters were: 21 axial slices (5 mm thick), FOV = 23 cm, TR/TE 6090/91.7 ms, 0.5 mm gap, with a 128×100 acquisition matrix. 30 images were acquired: 3 with no diffusion sensitization (i.e., T2-weighted images) and 27 diffusion-weighted (DW) images ($b = 1132$ s/mm^2) in which the gradient directions were evenly distributed on an imaginary hemisphere. The reconstruction matrix was 128×128, yielding a 1.8×1.8 mm^2 in-plane resolution. Total scan time was 3.05 minutes. We used the FMRIB software library (FSL, http://www.fmrib.ox.ac.uk/fsl/) for initial pre-processing of the diffusion images. For each subject, motion artifacts were corrected by linearly registering all the T2-weighted and DW images to one of the T2-weighted image (the "eddy_correct" command). Then the three T2-weighted images were averaged and stripped of non-brain tissues to yield a binary brain extraction mask (cerebellum included), using the Brain Extraction Tool (BET) [8], followed by expert manual editing if necessary. The masked T2-weighted image was then registered to the ICBM standardized brain template with a 9-parameter linear transformation using the software FLIRT [9]. The resulting transformation parameters were used to rotationally reorient the diffusion tensors (computed from DW images using the "DTIFIT" command) at each voxel. The tensor-valued images were linearly realigned based on trilinear interpolation of the log-transformed tensors, and resampled to isotropic voxel resolution (with dimensions: 128×128×93 voxels, resolution: 1.7×1.7×1.7 mm^3). The fractional anisotropy (FA) image derived from the affine-registered DT image was then fluidly registered to a randomly selected subject's FA image, based on maximizing the Jensen–Rényi divergence (JRD) of the joint intensity histogram [10]. Here we preferred direct fluid alignment of FA, due to the need for computational efficiency in 258 subjects, although we are exploring alternative more CPU-intensive methods we developed to fluidly align diffusion tensors using information theory [11].

2.3 Linkage between the BDNF Polymorphism and FA

We used structural equation modeling [5] to analyze the linkage between BDNF polymorphism and brain diffusion anisotropy, in which the total variance of FA at each voxel was attributed to the additive genetic variance of the BDNF polymorphism (σ_a^2; the variance due to the additive effect of the BDNF polymorphism), the residual genetic variance (σ_g^2; the variance due to all other genes on the genome), the variance of the shared family rearing environment (σ_c^2), and the individual unique (σ_e^2) environmental factors. We note that linkage does not necessarily mean that the genetic marker (e.g. the BDNF Val66Met polymorphism here) directly causes a difference in an image, but rather indicates that the genetic marker is close to the genes that influence the phenotype. Genes close to each other on the genome tend to be inherited together, so one can genotype a set of specific genes to identify which genetic marker an influential polymorphism is close to, and in that case the genotyped gene is said to be in *genetic linkage* with the trait – here the FA of the image.

Because of the known genetic similarity between relatives of different kinds, it is possible to write the covariance matrix of FA for the ith family, denoted by Φ_i, in terms of the different sources of variance being modeled (namely, σ_a^2, σ_g^2, σ_c^2, σ_e^2), as follows:

$$\Phi_{ijk} = \begin{cases} \sigma_a^2 + \sigma_g^2 + \sigma_c^2 + \sigma_e^2, \text{ if } j = k, \text{ or } j \text{ and } k \text{ are MZ twins} \\ \sigma_a^2 + \sigma_g^2 + \sigma_c^2, \text{ if } j \neq k, \text{ and } j \text{ and } k \text{ are MZ twins} \\ \pi_{ijk}\sigma_a^2 + 1/2\sigma_g^2 + \sigma_c^2, \text{ if } j \neq k, \text{ and } j \text{ and } k \text{ are not MZ twins,} \end{cases} \quad (1)$$

where π_{ijk} is the expected proportion of alleles that arose from the same ancestor allele, i.e., identical by descent (IBD), for subjects j and k. We estimated π_{ijk} using the Haseman-Elston method detailed in [12]. The structural equation model in Eq (1) was fitted using the maximum-likelihood method [5], given by

$$\log L = \sum_{i=1}^{N} -\frac{1}{2}\log|\Phi_i| - \frac{1}{2}y_i^T \Phi_i^{-1} y_i, \quad (2)$$

where the n_i-sample vector y_i is the FA value of all n_i subjects in family i, adjusted for the age and sex of each subject. N denotes the number of families. σ_a^2, σ_g^2, σ_c^2, and σ_e^2 were estimated using the Broyden-Fletcher-Goldfarb-Shanno (BFGS) method [13] to maximize log$L$ in Eq (2). The significance of the influences of the BDNF genetic variation (polymorphism) was determined by the difference between the log-likelihood of the full model that included σ_a^2, σ_g^2, σ_c^2, and σ_e^2 and the restricted model including σ_g^2, σ_c^2, and σ_e^2 only, denoted by logL_f for the full and logL_r for the restricted model. Minus two times this difference, or -2(logL_r - logL_f), is asymptotically distributed approximately as a chi-squared distribution with one degree of freedom. The resulting statistics were plotted at each point in the image to show the voxelwise significance of the genetic linkage between the BDNF gene and FA in all 258 subjects. The overall significance of the resulting statistical maps was assessed using the false discovery rate (FDR) method [14] to correct for multiple comparisons. By convention, a FDR value ≤ 0.05 was considered to be significant.

3 Results

Fig. 1 shows that 90-95% variance of FA (with no smoothing; see below) in the posterior cingulate gyrus and right frontal area was attributable to the genetic influences of

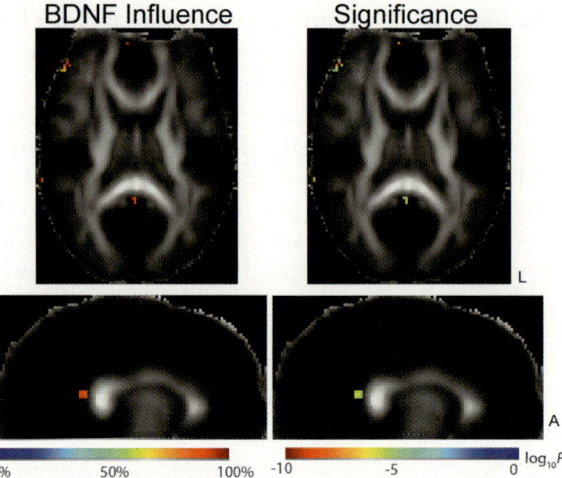

Fig. 1. Proportional contribution (*left upper and lower panels*) and its statistical significance (*right upper and lower panels*; the color scale is proportional to the decadic logarithm of the voxel *P*-value) of the BDNF polymorphism to the local variation in brain fiber integrity, measured by FA. The colored regions are the clusters composed of 26-connected voxels with *P*-values not greater than the threshold, computed by the FDR procedure that controls the expected false discovery rate to be no greater than 5%. For better visualization, only clusters with 10 or more voxels are displayed. The BDNF polymorphism significantly contributes to 90-95% variance of FA mainly in the posterior cingulate gyrus and in the right frontal area. L: left hemisphere. A: anterior.

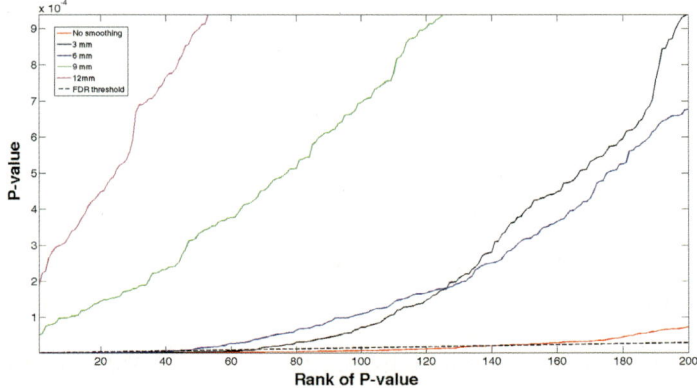

Fig. 2. Plot of the ordered voxel-level *P*-values showing the significance of the linkage between the BDNF polymorphism and FA smoothed using a 3D Gaussian kernel with different FWHM (in mm). The *P*-value was computed by comparing the log-likelihood of the full versus the restricted structural equation models. *P*-values are considered significant overall when they are not greater than the threshold where the individual curve intersects the dashed line y=0.05x/n, where n is the number of voxels within the brain-only mask; then the false discovery rate is controlled at no more than 5%.

the BDNF polymorphism. BDNF is known to be an important gene for long-term memory and learning, which may be enhanced by greater myelination and therefore axonal conduction speed in the cingulate gyrus, which is known to receive fibers from the subiculum of the hippocampus, which is involved in working memory.

To assess how different levels of smoothing influence the effect size of the linkage between the BDNF polymorphism and diffusion anisotropy, we also fitted the structural equation model [Eq (1)] with subjects' FA images (stripped of non-brain tissues) smoothed using a Gaussian filter with a full width at half maximum (FWHM) = 3, 6, 9, or 12 mm. Fig. 2 displays the voxel-level P-values of the significance for the FA-BDNF linkage, plotted against their rank. FA with no smoothing yielded the greatest number of FDR-significant voxels - defined as voxels where the P-value was not greater than the threshold that controlled the FDR at the level of 0.05, as also shown in Table 1. Even so, if we compared the smoothing effect based on the size of FDR-significant clusters, which were sets of connected (26-neighborhood) FDR-significant voxels, FA that was moderately smoothed (FWHM = 3 and 6 mm) yielded a single large cluster in the posterior cingulate gyrus, while FA with no smoothing yielded many tiny clusters that were one or two voxels in size (Table 1). As it is not legitimate to search over multiple filtered images to find effects, we report the unsmoothed data for purposes of statistical inference but we report the smoothed data as a *post hoc* assessment of the parameters that are likely to give best sensitivity in future analyses of independent (non-overlapping) data. Scale-space searches (i.e., over multiple filtered images) have been proposed in fMRI studies [15] although they are computationally intensive and can inflate type I error unless subjected to a global FDR procedure.

Table 1. The effect of FA smoothing on the detection of FA-BDNF linkage

	FWHM (mm)				
	0	3	6	9	12
Number of FDR-significant voxels	142	68	44	0	0
FDR-significant clusters*	1(18), 2(9), 3(5), 4(4), 5(1), 10(1), 11(1), 13(1), 16(1), 20(1)	1(1), 2(1), 7(1), 58(1)	44(1)		

*Listed based on their size in voxels (the number of clusters of each size is in parentheses).

4 Conclusion

In this paper we first visualized the linkage between the BDNF Val66Met polymorphism and brain fiber architecture by analyzing the FA images of a large sample of twins and non-twin siblings. We also compared the effects of different magnitudes of image smoothing, and found that using raw FA images with no smoothing was most sensitive for detecting the FA-BDNF linkage when the FDR method was used to correct for multiple comparisons across the whole brain. The practical importance of this paper is that by finding a common gene variant that affects fiber integrity, measured by FA, one could (1) study whether it is over-represented in the many common diseases where FA is reduced, to provide a more mechanistic understanding of the disease, (2) co-vary for (adjust) its effects in studies of FA to improve statistical power, (3) look at the trajectory of FA over time in relation to the BDNF variant subgroups, and discover how the gene acts to affect fiber integrity, and (4) see if the BNDF variant confers increased risk for other deficits than FA (e.g. structural or functional deficits in the same regions).

Brain fiber integrity measured by FA is highly heritable, and higher FA is associated with better intellectual performance [2]. Our results show that BDNF is one of the genes that influence the fiber architecture in the posterior cingulate region. Both BDNF and the cingulate gyrus have key roles in mediating cognitive function, and future studies will aim to evaluate the cross-trait linkage of BDNF to FA in this region and to the subjects' cognitive function and intellectual performance.

References

1. Thompson, P.M., Cannon, T.D., Narr, K.L., van Erp, T., Poutanen, V.P., Huttunen, M., Lonnqvist, J., Standertskjold-Nordenstam, C.G., Kaprio, J., Khaledy, M., Dail, R., Zoumalan, C.I., Toga, A.W.: Genetic influences on brain structure. Nat. Neurosci. 4, 1253–1258 (2001)
2. Chiang, M.C., Barysheva, M., Shattuck, D.W., Lee, A.D., Madsen, S.K., Avedissian, C., Klunder, A.D., Toga, A.W., McMahon, K.L., de Zubicaray, G.I., Wright, M.J., Srivastava, A., Balov, N., Thompson, P.M.: Genetics of brain fiber architecture and intellectual performance. J. Neurosci. 29, 2212–2224 (2009)
3. Chiang, M.C., Barysheva, M., Lee, A.D., Madsen, S., Klunder, A.D., Toga, A.W., McMahon, K.L., de Zubicaray, G.I., Meredith, M., Wright, M.J., Srivastava, A., Balov, N., Thompson, P.M.: Brain fiber architecture, genetics, and intelligence: a high angular resolution diffusion imaging (HARDI) study. In: Metaxas, D., Axel, L., Fichtinger, G., Székely, G. (eds.) MICCAI 2008, Part I. LNCS, vol. 5241, pp. 1060–1067. Springer, Heidelberg (2008)
4. McIntosh, A.M., Moorhead, T.W., Job, D., Lymer, G.K., Munoz Maniega, S., McKirdy, J., Sussmann, J.E., Baig, B.J., Bastin, M.E., Porteous, D., Evans, K.L., Johnstone, E.C., Lawrie, S.M., Hall, J.: The effects of a neuregulin 1 variant on white matter density and integrity. Mol. Psychiatry 13, 1054–1059 (2008)
5. Almasy, L., Blangero, J.: Multipoint quantitative-trait linkage analysis in general pedigrees. Am. J. Hum. Genet. 62, 1198–1211 (1998)
6. Hariri, A.R., Goldberg, T.E., Mattay, V.S., Kolachana, B.S., Callicott, J.H., Egan, M.F., Weinberger, D.R.: Brain-derived neurotrophic factor val66met polymorphism affects human memory-related hippocampal activity and predicts memory performance. J. Neurosci. 23, 6690–6694 (2003)
7. Hansell, N.K., James, M.R., Duffy, D.L., Birley, A.J., Luciano, M., Geffen, G.M., Wright, M.J., Montgomery, G.W., Martin, N.G.: Effect of the BDNF V166M polymorphism on working memory in healthy adolescents. Genes. Brain Behav. 6, 260–268 (2007)
8. Smith, S.M.: Fast robust automated brain extraction. Hum. Brain Mapp. 17, 143–155 (2002)
9. Jenkinson, M., Smith, S.: A global optimisation method for robust affine registration of brain images. Med. Image Anal. 5, 143–156 (2001)
10. Chiang, M.-C., Dutton, R.A., Hayashi, K.M., Lopez, O.L., Aizenstein, H.J., Toga, A.W., Becker, J.T., Thompson, P.M.: 3D pattern of brain atrophy in HIV/AIDS visualized using tensor-based morphometry. Neuroimage 34, 44–60 (2007)
11. Chiang, M.C., Leow, A.D., Klunder, A.D., Dutton, R.A., Barysheva, M., Rose, S.E., McMahon, K.L., de Zubicaray, G.I., Toga, A.W., Thompson, P.M.: Fluid registration of diffusion tensor images using information theory. IEEE Trans. Med. Imaging 27, 442–456 (2008)

12. Haseman, J.K., Elston, R.C.: The investigation of linkage between a quantitative trait and a marker locus. Behav. Genet. 2, 3–19 (1972)
13. Press, W.H., Teukolsky, S.A., Vetterling, W.T., Flannery, B.P.: Numerical recipes in C++. Cambridge Univ. Press, Cambridge (2002)
14. Benjamini, Y., Hochberg, Y.: Controlling the false discovery rate: a practical and powerful approach to multiple testing. Journal of the Royal Statistical Society. Series B (Methodological) 57, 289–300 (1995)
15. Siegmund, D.O., Worsley, K.J.: Testing for a signal with unknown location and scale in a stationary Gaussian random field. The Annals of Statistics 23, 608–639 (1995)

Vascular Territory Image Analysis Using Vessel Encoded Arterial Spin Labeling

Michael A. Chappell, Thomas W. Okell, Peter Jezzard, and Mark W. Woolrich

Oxford Centre for Functional MRI of the Brain, University of Oxford,
John Radcliffe Hospital, Headington, Oxford, OX4 3HD, UK
michael.chappell@clneuro.ox.ac.uk

Abstract. Arterial Spin Labeling (ASL) permits the non-invasive assessment of cerebral perfusion, by magnetically labeling all the blood flowing into the brain. Vessel encoded (VE) ASL extends this concept by introducing spatial modulations of the labeling procedure, resulting in different patterns of label applied to the blood from different vessels. Here a Bayesian inference solution to the analysis of VE-ASL is presented based on a description of the relative locations of labeled vessels and a probabilistic classification of brain tissue to vessel source. In simulation and on real data the method is shown to reliably determine vascular territories in the brain, including the case where the number of vessels exceeds the number of independent measurements.

1 Introduction

Arterial Spin Labeling (ASL) MRI is becoming an increasingly popular method for imaging cerebral blood flow (CBF), since it is both non-invasive and relatively rapid. ASL operates by labeling the water in blood magnetically via RF pulse inversion before entry to the brain and then imaging it as it passes into the capillaries. This 'tag' image is compared to a control image, taken in the absence of labeled blood, to remove the large static magnetization signal of the brain tissues.

More recently a number of methods have been proposed that use an ASL approach for Vascular Territory Imaging (VTI). The purpose of VTI is to identify the different regions of the brain that are supplied by individual feeding vessels. This type of imaging has a number of clinical applications, for example visualization of the vascular changes brought about by stroke or vascular stenosis. ASL based VTI can be achieved by making the ASL label spatially selective around individual vessels, for example [1, 2]. An alternative, but related, approach is Vessel Encoded (VE) ASL [3, 4]. In this method the strength of the inversion is modulated spatially across the labeling plane. A series of such images are collected each with different modulations chosen to uniquely encode each vessel's contribution.

VE-ASL is typically analyzed by assembling an encoding matrix that represents the effects of the different encoding steps on the vessels in the labeling plane. This matrix is then inverted to predict individual flow contributions in every brain voxel. In principle the encoding matrix is known *a priori* based on the experimental setup. However, due to head motion or imperfect alignment there may be some deviation in practice, leading to imperfect separation of vascular territories and inaccurate CBF estimates.

Here we present a Bayesian solution to the analysis for VE-ASL data. Using the sinusoidal form of [5] we derive the relationship between vessel location and encoding matrix. A generative model based on this encoding matrix and a probabilistic classification of each voxel to a source vessel was constructed, using the assumption that voxels are typically fed by a single vessel. This method provides a unified approach to the analysis of VE-ASL combining the effects of vessel location on the encoding matrix with the estimation of vascular territories and local blood within a single adaptive algorithm.

2 Methods

The tag-control differencing of traditional ASL can be represented in any voxel in matrix form **y=Ax**:

$$\mathbf{y} = \begin{bmatrix} y_1 \\ y_2 \end{bmatrix} \quad A = \begin{bmatrix} -1 & 1 \\ 1 & 1 \end{bmatrix} \quad \mathbf{x} = \begin{bmatrix} F \\ S \end{bmatrix}, \quad (1)$$

where **x** represents the sources of signal, F being the signal from the flowing blood and S being the static magnetization of the tissues; **y** is the vector of measured values, y_1 is the tag image ($y_1=S-F$) and $y2$ is the control ($y_2=S+F$). This concept can be extended to VE-ASL with multiple sources of blood whose selection depends upon the spatial encoding. For example a three vessel encoding might look like (R, L and B – the right and left carotid, and basilar arteries respectively):

$$\mathbf{y} = \begin{bmatrix} 1 & 1 & 1 & 1 \\ -1 & -1 & -1 & 1 \\ 1 & -1 & 0 & 1 \\ 1 & 1 & -1 & 1 \end{bmatrix} \begin{bmatrix} R \\ L \\ B \\ S \end{bmatrix}, \quad (2)$$

Note the structure of the encoding matrix: the top row produces the control image, the second the tag image and there are two encoded tag images; the final column must always be all unity values, since this dictates the contribution of the static magnetization of the tissues to the measured signal that appears in all images.

It is possible to find the contributions from each vessel in every brain voxel by matrix inversion: $\mathbf{x}=\mathbf{A}^{-1}\mathbf{y}$. In practice the encoding matrix will not be square, thus the matrix pseudo-inverse will be required. Hence this method provides a solution optimal according to a least-squares cost function.

To account for any encoding setup and allow for misalignment between vessel locations and spatial modulation of the tag, we derived a general encoding matrix based on the sinusoidal modulation assumption [4]. Each vessel encoded ASL image is the result of labeled blood arriving in the tissue from multiple source vessels. The extent of the inversion of the blood in each vessel is set by the spatial modulation of the applied tagging and is thus determined by the relative geometry between the vessel and the spatial modulation. The spatial modulation occurs across the tagging plane, although the variation in inversion is only prescribed in one direction at a time, for example modulation parallel to the x-axis. Each spatial modulation may thus be defined in terms of a modulation centre, (c_x, c_y), and a modulation angle, θ, relative to a

Cartesian axis placed in the tagging plane. Each vessel/source can be defined in terms of its location in the tagging plane, (x,y), relative to the same axes, as illustrated in Fig. 1. The inversion state of each vessel during the acquisition of a single encoded image is determined by its distance, d, from the modulation centre and the form of the spatial modulation, f: $m = f(d)$, where from Fig. 1:

$$d = \begin{cases} \sqrt{(x-c_x)^2 + (y-c_y)^2} \cos\left(\theta - \arctan\left(\frac{y-c_y}{x-c_x}\right)\right) & x - c_x > 0 \\ \sqrt{(x-c_x)^2 + (y-c_y)^2} \cos\left(\theta - \arctan\left(\frac{y-c_y}{x-c_x}\right) + \pi\right) & x - c_x < 0 \\ (y-c_y)\cos(\theta - \pi/2) & x - c_x = 0, y - c_y > 0 \\ (y-c_y)\cos(\theta + \pi/2) & x - c_x = 0, y - c_y < 0 \end{cases} \quad (3)$$

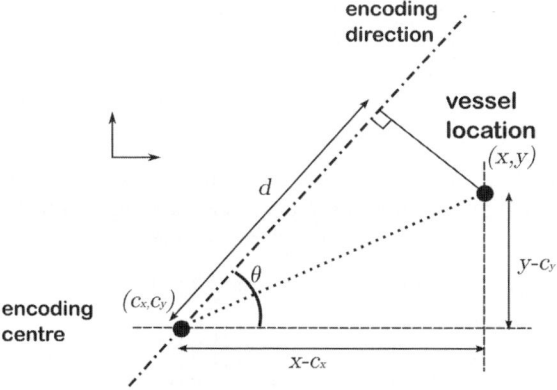

Fig. 1. The geometry for the spatial encoding of a vessel

The spatial encoding function may be approximated by a sinusoidal form [5] $m = \sin(\pi d / 2D)$, where D is the spatial scale along the encoding direction. This form represents the periodic nature of the actual encoding applied. In a vessel encoding experiment a number of encoded images will be acquired. Hence there will be a modulation value for each combination of vessel and modulation phase, i.e. for the ith encoded image and jth vessel $m_{ij} = f(\mathbf{x}_j, \mathbf{c}_i, \theta_i, D_i)$. This modulation value corresponds to an entry in a general encoding matrix:

$$\mathbf{E} = \begin{bmatrix} 1 & 1 & \cdots & 1 & 1 \\ -1 & -1 & \cdots & -1 & 1 \\ m_{11} & m_{12} & \cdots & m_{1M} & 1 \\ \vdots & \vdots & \ddots & \vdots & 1 \\ m_{N1} & m_{N2} & \cdots & m_{NM} & 1 \end{bmatrix} \quad (4)$$

This form of encoding matrix permits each voxel to be fed by every vessel. In practice vascular territories are relatively well defined, such that most vessels will only be sourced from a single vessel. This was incorporated into the forward model by way of a classification matrix, such that in voxel k the vector of signal intensities arising from the blood flow from vessel c was given by $\mathbf{s}_{k,c} = \mathbf{EP}_c\mathbf{f}_k$, where $\mathbf{f}_k = \begin{bmatrix} f_k & s_k \end{bmatrix}^T$ with flow, f_k, and static signal s_k, $\mathbf{E}$ is the encoding matrix based on vessel locations $\mathbf{x}_j \in \{\mathbf{X}: j=1,2,...,M\}$ (and known encoding setup) and $\mathbf{P}_c$ is the classification matrix that selects vessel c, which is a $(M+1)\times 2$ matrix with all elements set to zero except $P_{c,1}=1$ and $P_{M+1,2}=1$.

Assuming Gaussian noise the Likelihood was formed:

$$\Pr(\mathbf{Y}|\mathbf{F},\mathbf{X},\mathbf{q}=\kappa,\pi,\phi) = \prod_k \Pr(\mathbf{y}_k | q_k = \kappa_k, \mathbf{f}_k, \mathbf{X}, \phi_k),$$
$$\Pr(\mathbf{y}_k | \mathbf{f}_k, \mathbf{X}, q_k = \kappa_k, \pi_{\kappa_k}, \phi_k) = \left(\phi_k^{N/2}/(2\pi)^{N/2}\right) e^{-\frac{\phi_k}{2}(\mathbf{y}_k - \mathbf{s}_{k,\kappa_k})^T(\mathbf{y}_k - \mathbf{s}_{k,\kappa_k})}, \quad (5)$$

where $\mathbf{q}$ is the map of discrete class labels and κ is a specific configuration thereof, ϕ_k is the noise precision and π_c is the proportion of voxels belonging to vessel c. Application of Bayes' theorem gave the posterior distribution:

$$\Pr(\mathbf{F},\mathbf{X},\mathbf{q}=\kappa,\pi,\phi|\mathbf{Y}) \propto \Pr(\mathbf{Y}|\mathbf{F},\mathbf{X},\mathbf{q}=\kappa,\phi)\Pr(\mathbf{F},\mathbf{X},\phi)\Pr(\mathbf{q}=\kappa|\pi)\Pr(\pi), \quad (6)$$

where the following priors were chosen:

$$\Pr(\mathbf{F},\mathbf{X},\phi) = \Pr(\mathbf{F})\Pr(\mathbf{X})\Pr(\phi),$$
$$\Pr(\mathbf{F}) = Uniform, \quad \Pr(\phi) = \phi^{-1}, \quad \Pr(\mathbf{X}) = N(\mathbf{X}_0, 0.1), \quad (7)$$

where vessel locations were normalized to scale between -1 and 1 and $\mathbf{X}_0$ are the vessel locations estimated from the ideal encoding:

$$\Pr(q_k = c | \pi) = \pi_c, \text{ with } \sum \pi_c = 1, \quad \Pr(\pi_c) = Uniform(0,1). \quad (8)$$

For the purposes of inference we marginalized analytically over both the flow and class label in every voxel:

$$\Pr(\mathbf{X},\pi,\phi|\mathbf{Y}) \propto \prod_k \left[\phi_k^{-1} \sum_c \left\{\pi_c |\mathbf{P}_c^T \mathbf{E}^T \mathbf{E} \mathbf{P}_c| e^{-\frac{\phi}{2}\left(\mathbf{y}_k - \mathbf{EP}_c(\mathbf{P}_c^T \mathbf{E}^T \mathbf{EP}_c)^{-1}\mathbf{P}_c^T \mathbf{E}^T \mathbf{y}_k\right)}\right\}\right] \Pr(\mathbf{X})\Pr(\pi). \quad (9)$$

The resulting marginal distribution was inferred using Metropolis Hastings (MH) and point estimates for $\mathbf{X}$, π and ϕ were determined. These point estimates were then used to determine the flow in every voxel from each vessel.

3 Results

Analysis was performed on simulated data to establish the ability of the method to infer vessel locations and flow contributions from VE-ASL data. Four source vessels were defined with flow contributions as in Fig. 2 (top). To simplify the interpretation (and for comparison with real data later) the vessels were all assumed to lie on the x-axis with locations: -1.1, 0.9, -0.2, 0.1. The encoding setup reflected this restriction employing modulation only in the x-direction, as shown in Table 1.

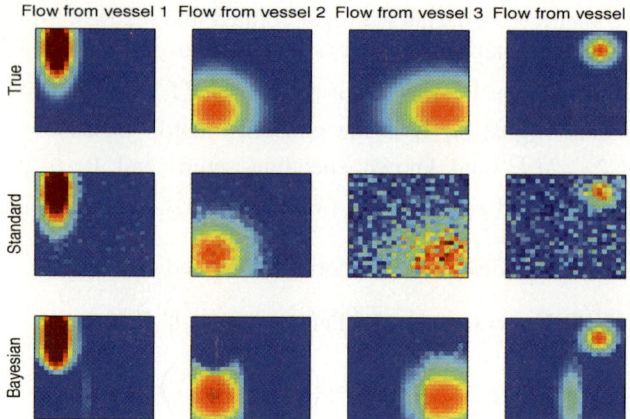

Fig. 2. Four-vessel simulation showing contributions to the flow from each vessel as separate columns. Top row: true simulated flow maps; middle row: results of standard matrix inversion analysis, using true vessel locations; bottom row: results of Bayesian classification model.

Table 1. Four vessel simulated data encoding setup

Cycle	c	θ°	D
1	(0,0)	0	1
2	(-0.5,0)	0	0.5
3	(0.5,0)	0	1

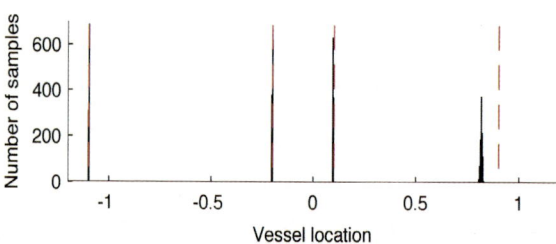

Fig. 3. MH samples for vessel locations, true locations superimposed (red dashed lines)

A standard analysis was performed using the correct vessel locations to form the encoding matrix, the individual flow maps are shown in Fig. 2 (middle row). The Bayesian analysis was initialized with 'ideal' vessel locations of -1, 1, -0.1, 0.1 and the resulting flow maps are shown in Fig. 2 (bottom row). The standard analysis was able to separate out the 4 vessel's contributions. However, the flow estimates were visibly noisy, a result of the encoding matrix being rank deficient, since the number of independent encodings is less than the number of sources. Unlike the standard analysis the Bayesian approach was also able to estimate the vessel locations, as shown in Fig. 3. It was able to give more accurate estimates of CBF and, for the majority of the voxels, correctly identify the main source vessel. There was some ambiguity in the contribution from vessels 3 and 4. The probabilistic classification was not able to fully model the substantial overlap between the territories of the simulated vessels because it sought to classify each voxel to a specific vessel source.

Table 2. Encoding setup for the first real dataset

Cycle	C	θ°	D
1a	(0,0)	0	1
1b	(0,0)	180	1
2a	(-0.5,0)	0	0.5
2b	(-0.5,0)	180	0.5

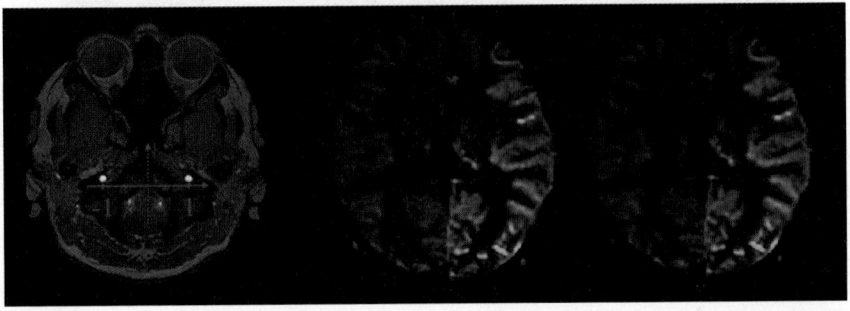

Fig. 4. Vessel encoding of the carotid and vertebral vessels. Angiographic image of the tagging plane (left) with encoding geometry imposed. Vascular territory map from the three-vessel analysis using standard matrix inversion (middle) and Bayesian method (right), intensity represents CBF, colour coding indicates dominant source vessel.

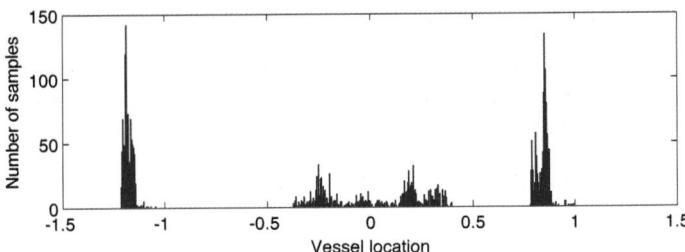

Fig. 5. MH samples for the estimation of vessel location for the first set of real data

The Bayesian analysis method was applied to a single slice of real vessel encoded data. This data was encoded following a similar one-dimensional setup to the simulated data used above, as shown in Table 2. Whilst four cycles were used to collect the data, there are only two truly independent cycles in this case.

The tagging plane for this subject is shown in Fig. 4 (left) and the encoding was arranged such that the vessels should fall at locations -1, 0, 1, the two vertebral arteries being regarded as a single vessel. The results of a standard analysis taking these vessel locations is shown in Fig. 4 (middle). The Bayesian classification analysis estimated a VTI map as in Fig. 4 (right), there was very good agreement between the estimated VTI images from both methods. The estimated locations for the Bayesian analysis are given in Fig. 5, they tend to imply a slight mis-alignment between the

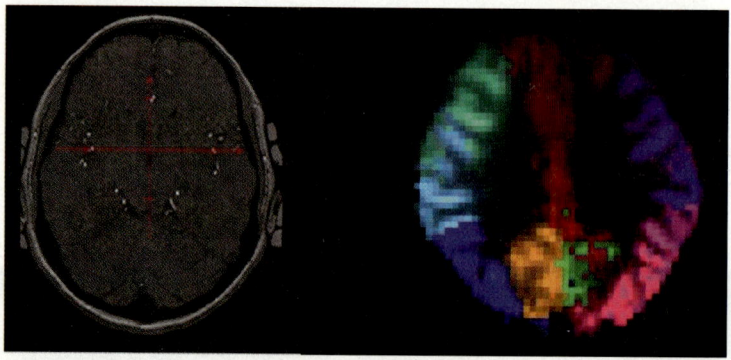

Fig. 6. Vessel encoding above the 'Circle of Willis'. Angiographic image of the tagging plane (left) with encoding geometry. Vascular territory map from the Bayesian analysis (right), intensity represents CBF, colour coding indicates dominant source vessel.

left-right encoding and the carotid arteries. The results also suggest that both the vertebral arteries feed the posterior territory, since there is a mode either side of zero in locations consistent with the vertebral locations in Fig. 4. This is consistent with the physiology since the two vertebral arteries merge to become the basilar above the tagging plane chosen here.

Finally the Bayesian method was applied to a more complex scenario when tagging above the Circle of Willis. The tagging plane is shown in Fig. 6 (left) and 12 encodings (6 independent) were collected, 4 left-right and 8 anterior-posterior. From the angiographic image 11 'vessels' were identified, where for practicality some very closely space vessels were merged. The Bayesian method was able to identify unique territories for 9 of the vessels, Fig. 6 (right), this is simply not possible using encoding matrix inversion. The two pairs of posterior vessels were not separable, implying that they were not uniquely tagged due to the thickness of the tagging region.

4 Discussion

A Bayesian approach to the analysis of VE-ASL data has been presented. Having defined the geometrical relationship between vessels in the tagging plane and the encoding geometry it is now possible to specify the correct encoding matrix for any dataset. Alongside this, within the Bayesian inference it is possible to account for subject movement or misalignment by determining the exact vessel locations from the data. The inference of vessel locations will also be correcting for disagreement between the assumed sinusoidal modulation of the tag and the true function achieved in practice. The true form can be determined theoretically [4] and could be incorporated into the model. It has been shown the modulation function itself will vary with the flow velocity in the tagged vessel and it would be possible to incorporate this effect within the model introducing a further 'flow speed' parameter.

The presented analysis approach uses a probabilistic classification between voxels and the source vessels permitting analysis of data that contains greater vessels than there are independent encodings. This classification approach makes the assumption that each voxel is fed by only single vessel. The 'soft' probabilistic form of the classification makes some allowance for mixing, as might be expected in the 'watershed regions' at the borders of the vascular territories. However, simulations suggest it is not very accurate at estimation in regions of extensive mixing. For example the posterior territory is fed by the basilar artery, which is the result of merging of the two vertebral arteries and was seen in the first real dataset (Fig. 4). The classification approach would be unable to accurately model this, though neither would the standard matrix inversion approach be appropriate in that situation. It would be feasible to extend the classification to permit two (or more) sources per voxel to more accurately assess mixing in 'watershed' regions. It is also possible to define a full 'partial-flow' model by removing the classification matrix, whilst it is only possible to infer with this model if the number of encoding cycles at least equals the number of vessels. If such data were available this would provide a true ability to analyze mixed vascular territories.

Acknowledgments. The authors thank Eric Wong for provision of VE-ASL data.

References

1. Davies, N.P., Jezzard, P.: Selective Arterial Spin Labeling (SASL): Perfusion Territory Mapping of Selected Feeding Arteries Tagged Using Two-Dimensional Radiofrequency Pulses. Magn. Reson. Med. 49, 1133–1142 (2003)
2. Hendrikse, J., van der Grond, J., Lu, H., van Zijl, P.C.M., Golay, X.: Flow Territory Mapping of the Cerebral Arteries with Regional Perfusion MRI. Stroke 35, 882–887 (2004)
3. Gunther, M.: Efficient Visualisation of Vascular Territories in the Human Brain by Cycled Arterial Spin Labeling MRI. Magn. Reson. Med. 56, 671–675 (2006)
4. Wong, E.C.: Vessel-Encoded Arterial Spin-Labeling Using Pseudocontinuous Tagging. Magn. Reson. Med. 58, 1086–1091 (2007)
5. Wong, E.C., Kansagra, A.: Mapping Middle Cerebral Artery Branch Territories with Vessel Encoded Pesudo-Continuous ASL: Sine/Cosine Tag Modulation and Data Clustering in Tagging Efficiency Space. In: Proc. ISMRM, Toronto (2008)

Predicting MGMT Methylation Status of Glioblastomas from MRI Texture

Ilya Levner[1,2,3], Sylvia Drabycz[4], Gloria Roldan[5,6,7,8], Paula De Robles[5,6,7,8], J. Gregory Cairncross[5,6,7,8], and Ross Mitchell[1,2,3,6,7,8]

[1] Department of Radiology, University of Calgary, Alberta, Canada
[2] Southern Alberta Cancer Research Institute, University of Calgary, Alberta, Canada
[3] Alberta Ingenuity Center for Machine Learning, Canada
[4] Department of Electrical and Computer Engineering, University of Calgary, Alberta, Canada
[5] Department of Oncology, Tom Baker Cancer Centre, Alberta Cancer Board, Canada
[6] Hotchkiss Brain Institute, Calgary, Alberta, Canada
[7] Department of Clinical Neurosciences, University of Calgary, Alberta Canada
[8] Clark Smith Brain Tumor Centre, Southern Alberta Cancer Research Institute, Canada

Abstract. In glioblastoma (GBM), promoter methylation of the DNA repair gene MGMT is associated with benefit from chemotherapy. Because MGMT promoter methylation status can not be determined in all cases, a surrogate for the methylation status would be a useful clinical tool. Correlation between methylation status and magnetic resonance imaging features has been reported suggesting that non-invasive MGMT promoter methylation status detection is possible. In this work, a retrospective analysis of T2, FLAIR and T1-post contrast MR images in patients with newly diagnosed GBM is performed using L1-regularized neural networks. Tumor texture, assessed quantitatively was utilized for predicting the MGMT promoter methylation status of a GBM in 59 patients. The texture features were extracted using a space-frequency texture analysis based on the S-transform and utilized by a neural network to predict the methylation status of a GBM. Blinded classification of MGMT promoter methylation status reached an average accuracy of **87.7%**, indicating that the proposed technique is accurate enough for clinical use.

1 Introduction

Glioblastoma multiforme (GBM) is the most common primary brain tumor in adults. Standard treatment now includes a DNA alkylating agent, Temozolomide (TMZ), which is the only known chemotherapeutic that prolongs survival [1]. Interestingly, the effectiveness of TMZ may be predictable; via a test for methylation of the O6-methylguanine-DNA methyltransferase (MGMT) gene promoter. Methylation of the MGMT promoter inhibits the repair of therapeutic DNA damage induced by TMZ thus rendering a drug-resistant cancer more sensitive to chemotherapy [2]. For unknown reasons, MGMT is silenced in 50% of newly diagnosed GBMs [3]. Therefore, a sensitive and specific test that reliably predicts the methylation status of a given GBM would be a helpful diagnostic alternative to the standard physical biopsy currently employed to diagnose the MGMT status of glioblastomas.

Recently Eoli et al., in [4], found significant correlations between MGMT promoter methylation status and magnetic resonance (MR) imaging features. Motivated by these findings, this research presents an automated method for predicting the methylation status of the GBM based on texture analysis of T2, FLAIR and T1-postcontrast MRI scans. In order to analyze the MR images, the proposed system utilizes the 2-dimensional discrete orthogonal S-transform[5] to extract texture features that are subsequently used by an ℓ_1-Regularized neural network to predict the methylation status of a given GBM. In a leave-one-out cross validation study, the proposed system achieved an average accuracy of 87.7%, high enough for use in clinical diagnosis.

1.1 Related Research

Image texture refers to the local characteristic pattern of image intensity that may be used to identify a tissue. Texture, by definition, also determines local spectral or frequency content in an image; in so far as changes in local texture will cause changes in the local spatial frequency. Aspects of texture in an MR image can thus be quantified by assessing the local spatial frequency content using a space-frequency transform: strong low frequencies appear as homogenous smooth regions, while strong high frequencies are seen as heterogeneous detailed regions.

Texture patterns have been shown to correlate with tissue histopathology in models of multiple sclerosis. In particular, Zhang et al.[6] characterized image texture in vivo using the polar S-Transform (pST) of histologically verified multiple sclerosis lesions within T2-weighted MRI. Both high and low frequency components, representing inflammation and demyelination, were significantly elevated in pathological regions compared to normal control tissue. Their work was one of the first studies to suggest that local spatial-frequency measures of image texture may provide a sensitive and precise indication of disease activity.

Likewise, in [7], researchers applied a variant of the S-transform similar to the pST in order to extract texture features from T2, FLAIR, and T1-postcontrast MR images of patients with oligodendrogliomas, a tumor related to GBM. Their study produced a highly accurate classifier capable detecting the co-deletion status of 1p and 19q chromosomes, a favorable genotype associated with slow-growing oligodendrogliomas. Unfortunately, none of the aforementioned S-Transform based techniques have produced classifiers with high enough accuracy for clinical use in predicting the methylation status of GBM's [8].

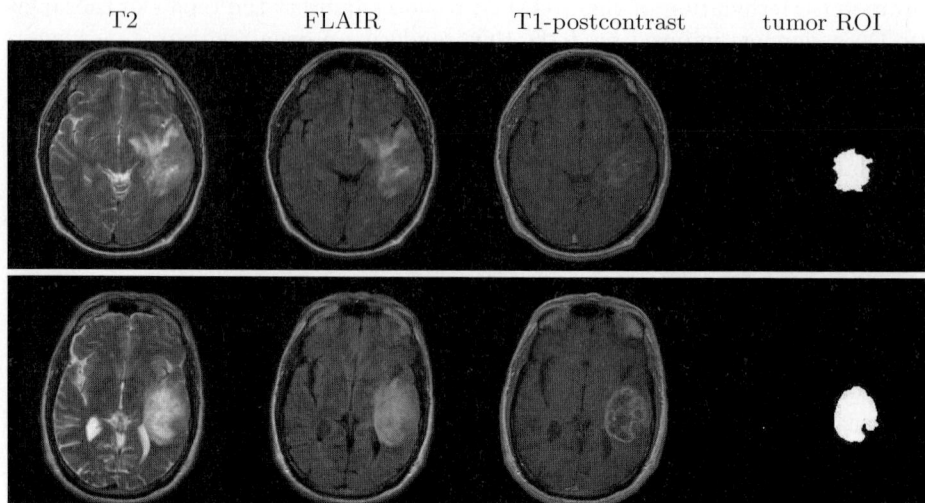

Fig. 1. Methylated (**Top**) versus Unmethylated (**Bottom**) tumor appearance. **Left-to-Right:** T2 image, FLAIR image, T1-postcontrast image, tumor ROI. The most prominent feature of a methylated tumor is the diffuse border visible in all three MRI modalities. In addition, unmethylated tumors tend to exhibit more extensive necrosis and are more likely to appear as ring enhancing within the T1-postcontrast image.

2   Texture Analysis and Classification

2.1   2D-DOST Feature Extraction

To quantify image texture within an ROI, the 2-dimensional variant discrete orthogonal S-transform (2D-DOST) was utilized. Recent results by Drabycz et. al. [5], indicates that the rotationally invariant DOST outperforms leading wavelet-based texture analysis methods. The spatial-frequency technique extracts texture features by decomposing an MR image into a set of images at various spatial frequencies. With 2D-DOST a local spatial frequency spectrum describing the amplitude of each frequency component in cycles per cm (cm^{-1}) from the lowest (the average of the entire image) to the highest (the fluctuations between neighboring pixels) is obtained for each pixel in the original image. The number of points in the spectrum is proportional to the image or ROI size.

Formally, let (i,j) index a discrete set of sites on a spatially regular $N \times M$ lattice:

$$S = \{(i,j) | 1 \leq i \leq N, 1 \leq j \leq M\} \tag{1}$$

The discrete 2-D Fourier transform (2D-FT) of a function $g(i,j)$ and its inverse, defined on lattice S are given by:

$$G(u,v) = \sum_{i=0}^{N-1} \sum_{j=0}^{M-1} g(i,j) e^{-(\sqrt{-1})2\pi(\frac{ui}{N} + \frac{vj}{M})} \tag{2}$$

$$g(i,j) = \frac{1}{NM} \sum_{u=0}^{N-1} \sum_{v=0}^{M-1} G(u,v) e^{(\sqrt{-1})2\pi(\frac{ui}{N}+\frac{vj}{M})} \tag{3}$$

The 2D-DOST of a $N \times N$ image g is calculated by partitioning the 2D-FT of the image, G, multiplying by the square root of the number of points in the partition, and performing an inverse 2D-FT. For given frequency orders $p_i, p_j > 1$ we extract the part of the Fourier spectrum where $m = 2^{p_i-1}$ to $2^{p_i}-1$ and $n = 2^{p_j-1}$ to $2^{p_j}-1$ and perform a circular shift by half of the bandwidth:

$$G_{p_i,p_j}\left[\frac{m}{N}, \frac{n}{N}\right] = \begin{cases} G\left[\frac{m+2^{p_i}}{N}, \frac{n+2^{p_j}}{N}\right], & \text{for } m = [-2^{p_i-2}, -1] \\ & n = [-2^{p_j-2}, -1] \\ G\left[\frac{m+2^{p_i-1}}{N}, \frac{n+2^{p_j-1}}{N}\right], & \text{for } m = [0, 2^{p_i-2}] \\ & n = [0, 2^{p_j-2}] \end{cases} \tag{4}$$

The 2D-DOST is then calculated by taking the 2D-FT of each scaled, shifted part of the Fourier spectrum:

$$D_{p_i,p_j}[i', j'] = \frac{1}{\sqrt{2^{p_i+p_j-2}}} \times \sum_{m=-2^{p_i-2}}^{2^{p_i-2}-1} \sum_{n=-2^{p_j-2}}^{2^{p_j-2}-1} G_{p_i,p_j}\left[\frac{m}{N}, \frac{n}{N}\right] e^{2\pi\left(\frac{mi'}{2^{p_i-1}}+\frac{nj'}{2^{p_j-1}}\right)} \tag{5}$$

Based on the 2D-DOST, a rotationally invariant spectrum, was created by averaging specific frequency orders together [5]. The process is depicted in Figure 2. The average spectrum from all pixels within the tumor volume was then calculated to obtain a single spectrum for each patient; pixels not within the tumor masks were excluded from analysis. Furthermore, slices where the visible tumor area was less than 50 mm^2 were excluded from analysis as well. To remove edge effects and other artifacts that might interfere with the analysis, the aforementioned texture extraction process was carried out on 16×16 pixel ROIs extracted from the binary mask of each tumor slice. Finally, the spectra were log-transformed and z-scaled (to zero mean and standard deviation of one) prior to application of neural networks in order to stabilize the variance.

2.2 Artificial Neural Networks

The standard 2-layer neural network [9] is defined by:

$$h_{\boldsymbol{\omega}}(\boldsymbol{x}) = \boldsymbol{W}_2 \tanh(\boldsymbol{W}_1\boldsymbol{x} + \boldsymbol{b}_1) + \boldsymbol{b}_2 \tag{6}$$

where $\boldsymbol{\omega} = \{\boldsymbol{W}_1, \boldsymbol{W}_2, \boldsymbol{b}_1, \boldsymbol{b}_2\}$ are the parameters to be learned based on a set of training pairs $\langle \boldsymbol{x}_k, \boldsymbol{y}_k \rangle_{k=1}^n$ with input vector $\boldsymbol{x} \in \mathbb{R}^d$ and $\boldsymbol{y}$ corresponding to the target output. In our case, $\boldsymbol{x}$ is the set of MRI texture coefficients extracted by the 2D-DOST and $y \in \{+1, -1\}$ indicates the methylation status of a given subject. The matrices $\boldsymbol{W}_1, \boldsymbol{W}_2$ connect the input layer to the hidden layer, and the hidden layer to the output layer (respectively). To prevent overfitting ℓ_1-regularization [10] is employed in conjunction with error minimization as follows:

$$E(\boldsymbol{y}, h_{\boldsymbol{\omega}}(\boldsymbol{x}), \lambda) = \|\boldsymbol{y} - h_{\boldsymbol{\omega}}(\boldsymbol{x})\|_{\ell_2} - \lambda\|\boldsymbol{\omega}\|_{\ell_1} \tag{7}$$

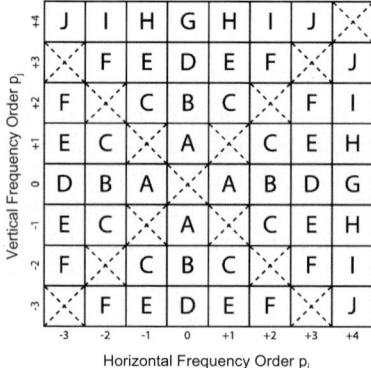

Fig. 2. Rotationally invariant features generated from 2D-DOST (N=8). Features marked with the same letter are averaged together to get a rotation invariant spectrum. The diagonal elements, where $|p_i| = |p_j|$, are excluded, since they tend to contain the majority of the noise and thus degrade classification performance.

where the ℓ_p-norm for vector $\boldsymbol{x}$ is defined as:

$$\|\boldsymbol{x}\|_{\ell_p} = \left(\sum_{i=1}^{d} |x(i)|^p \right)^{\frac{1}{p}} \qquad (8)$$

The stochastic weight updates are then defined by:

$$\boldsymbol{\delta}_j = \boldsymbol{W}_j - \eta \frac{\partial E_{mse}(\boldsymbol{y}, \boldsymbol{h}_\omega(\boldsymbol{x}))}{\partial \boldsymbol{W}_j} \qquad (9)$$

$$\boldsymbol{W}_j = sign(\boldsymbol{\delta}_j) \max(0, \boldsymbol{\delta}_j - \eta \lambda) \qquad (10)$$

where $j \in \{1, 2\}$, $\frac{\partial E_{mse}}{\partial \boldsymbol{W}_j}$ is the error gradient, η is the learning rate, λ is the regularization parameter, and the function $sign(\boldsymbol{A})$ returns ± 1 based on the sign of each matrix element in $\boldsymbol{A}$.

From a Bayesian point of view[10], ℓ_1-regularization induces a Laplacian prior over the weights. In contrast to weight decay (i.e., ℓ_2-regularization), ℓ_1-regularization, can drive the weights completely to zero, rather than simply make their magnitudes small and thus enables feature selection. If the ℓ_1-norm of jth column vector is zero (i.e., $\|\boldsymbol{W}(\cdot, j)\|_{\ell_1} = 0$), then the jth feature, $\boldsymbol{x}(j)$, is never used and can therefore be removed. Analogously, the width of the hidden layer can be controlled by letting ℓ_1-regularization prune unnecessary hidden nodes. Once again, if a given column vector is zero within weight matrix $\boldsymbol{W}_2$, the corresponding hidden unit is effectively ignored by the output layer.

3 Experimental Procedure

Patients with newly diagnosed GBM (astrocytoma grade IV, WHO classification) were identified and included in the study based on: (i) age (18 years or older), (ii) existence of preoperative T2, FLAIR and T1-post contrast MR images, and (iii) existence of paraffin embedded GBM tissue from the first surgery enabling the assessment of MGMT promoter status via MS-PCR [3].

3.1 MRI Signal Preprocessing

Because imaging parameters varied across the cohort, all images were re-sampled to ensure a common field-of-view (FOV) and pixel resolution. Images were cropped and/or zero-padded to achieve a 22cm FOV. The 2D Fourier transform of each image was cropped and/or zero-padded to achieve a consistent image resolution of 0.859 mm/pixel. The resulting processed images had a FOV=22cm and matrix size of 256x256. A rigid registration for all MR sequences on each case was performed by maximizing the normalized mutual information metric using in-house software. Each volume was converted from 16-bit integer to floating point values and normalized such that cerebrospinal fluid (CSF) in the anterior horn of the left ventricle (or right ventricle if the left was obscured) had an average value of: 1.0 for FLAIR, 5.0 for T2, and 2.0 for T1 post-contrast with a standard deviation of 0.1. Tumor boundaries, outlined on T1 post-contrast images using MIPAV [11], were utilized for creating the regions of interest (ROIs) demarcating the tumor regions. Figure 1 presents examples of the collected data.

Fifty-nine patients (39 men; 20 women) were included in the texture study, with median age 59 years (range 29-82) at the time of diagnosis. Thirty-one subjects had tumors that were methylated (53%). Median imaging parameters were as follows for T2, FLAIR and T1-post contrast: TR=4160/9004/500 ms, TE=102/105/14 ms, 19 slices; median inversion time for FLAIR = 2400 ms.

For each T2, FLAIR, and T1-postcontrast imaging modality, 10 rotationally invariant texture feature coefficients were computed using the 2D-DOST[1] The 30 features, after log-normalization and z-scaling, were presented to a neural network in a leave-one-out cross validation strategy (LOOCV). For all experiments the following parameters were kept constant: (i) Learning rate $\eta = 0.0005$, number of stochastic weight updates $= 10000$, (iii) number of hidden units $= 2$ (Note that preliminary experiments varied the number of hidden nodes. However, ℓ_1-regularization consistently pruned the network down to two nodes). The neural network's ability to predict GBM methylation status was evaluated using the following performance indicators: accuracy, sensitivity, specificity, positive, and negative predictive values. Two experiments were performed in this study. The first examined the effect of regularization on the network performance. The second experiment used regularization parameters corresponding to local maxima with respect to accuracy, in order to examine network stability. In each of the 10 trials, the learning parameters (ω from Equation 6) were randomly initialized prior to network training and subsequent texture feature classification.

---

[1] Since the Z-dimension of each voxel in our data was approximately 10 times the in-plane dimensions, the relatively straightforward generalization of 2D-DOST to 3 dimensions was not utilized.

Table 1. Neural network prediction as a function of the L1-regularization parameter, λ in Equation 10

L1-Regularization	Accuracy	Sensitivity	Specificity	PPV	NPV
0.0001	0.898	0.893	0.903	0.893	0.903
0.0005	**0.932**	**0.929**	**0.936**	**0.929**	**0.936**
0.001	0.915	0.897	0.933	0.929	0.903
0.005	0.898	0.867	0.931	0.929	0.871
0.01	0.898	0.867	0.931	0.929	0.871
0.1	**0.915**	**0.897**	**0.933**	**0.929**	**0.903**
0.2	0.848	0.828	0.867	0.857	0.839

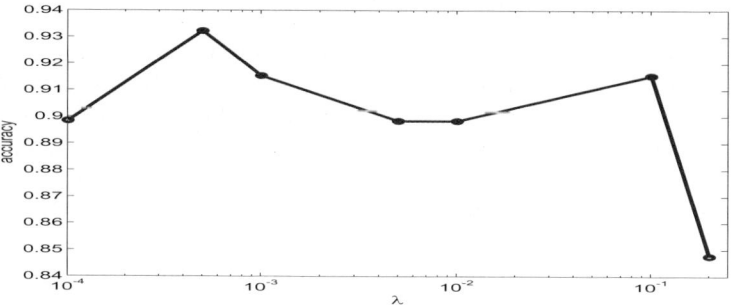

Fig. 3. Accuracy as a function of ℓ_1-Regularization parameter λ from Equation 10. Data taken from Table 1.

Table 2. Performance based on 10 random initializations of the network parameters. **Top:** Performance based on parameter $\lambda = 0.1$ in Equation 10. **Bottom:** Performance based on $\lambda = 0.0005$.

L1 = 0.1	Accuracy	Sensitivity	Specificity	PPV	NPV
Best Run	0.915	0.897	0.933	0.929	0.903
Worst Run	0.814	0.815	0.813	0.786	0.839
Mean	**0.877**	**0.854**	**0.900**	**0.893**	**0.862**
Standard deviation	0.042	0.039	0.047	0.053	0.036

L1 = 0.0005	Accuracy	Sensitivity	Specificity	PPV	NPV
Best Run	0.932	0.962	0.909	0.893	0.968
Worst Run	0.661	0.633	0.690	0.679	0.645
Mean	**0.812**	**0.814**	**0.812**	**0.789**	**0.833**
Standard deviation	0.071	0.089	0.058	0.059	0.088

3.2 Results

Table 1 shows the effect of regularization on network performance. Two local maxima exist at $\lambda = \{0.0005, 0.1\}$ with respective accuracy of 93.2% and 91.5% which can be clearly observed in Figure 3. In turn, Table 2 shows the average performance from 10 random initialization trials performed with the regularization parameters set to $\lambda = \{0.0005, 0.1\}$. Performance based on $\lambda = 0.1$ indicates this regularization setting is a more stable solution that achieves higher average score across all metrics, while also attaining a lower standard deviation than the $\lambda = 0.0005$ setting. With $\lambda = 0.1$, the average accuracy was 87.7%. The worst-case accuracy remained above 80%, an important threshold for clinical utility. The best-case accuracy was on par with that from physical biopsy ($\sim 90\%$).

4 Discussion

In this study, we sought to identify a quantitative texture pattern in MR images that is significantly associated with MGMT promoter methylation status. We hypothesized that textural features would correlate with MGMT status, providing a non-invasive imaging test for detection of MGMT promoter methylation in GBM. Using the 2D-DOST in conjunction with neural networks we were able to create a system for accurately predicting methylation status of a given GBM. Our system achieved an average accuracy of 87.7%. The worst-case accuracy remained above 80%, an important threshold for clinical utility. The best-case accuracy was on par with that from physical biopsy ($\sim 90\%$). We therefore conclude that our proposed virtual biopsy technique may complement traditional biopsies, particularly for patients in whom direct testing is inconclusive, or infeasible.

References

1. Stupp, R., Mason, W., van den Bent, M., Weller, M., Fisher, B., Taphoorn, M., Belanger, K., Brandes, A., Bogdahn, C.M.U., Curschmann, J., Janzer, R., Ludwin, S., Gorlia, T., Allgeier, A., Lacombe, D., Cairncross, J., Eisenhauer, E., Mirimanoff, R.: Radiotherapy plus concomitant and adjuvant temozolomide for glioblastoma. New England Journal of Medicine 352(10), 987–996 (2005)
2. Peter, H., Roger, S.: MGMT methylation status: the advent of stratified therapy in glioblastoma? Disease markers 23(1-2), 97–104 (2007)
3. Hegi, M., Diserens, A., Gorlia, T., Hamou, M., de Tribolet, N., et al.: MGMT gene silencing and benefit form temozolomide in glioblastoma. New England Journal of Medicine 352(10), 997–1003 (2005)
4. Eoli, M., Menghi, F., Bruzzone, M., Simone, T.D., Valletta, L., Pollo, B., Bissola, L., Silvani, A., Bianchessi, D., D'Incerti, L., Filippini, G., Broggi, G., Boiardi, A., Finocchiaro, G.: Methylation of o6-methylguanine dna methyltransferase and loss of heterozygosity on 19q and/or 17p are overlapping features of secondary glioblastomas with prolonged survival. Clinical Cancer Research 13(9), 2606–2613 (2007)
5. Drabycz, S., Stockwell, R.G., Mitchell, R.: Image texture characterization using the discrete orthonormal s-transform. Journal of Digital Imaging (2008), doi:10.1007/s10278-008-9138-8
6. Zhang, Y., Wells, J., Buist, R., Peeling, J., Yong, V.W., Mitchell, J.R.: A novel MRI texture analysis of demyelination and inflammation in relapsing-remitting experimental allergic encephalomyelitis. In: Larsen, R., Nielsen, M., Sporring, J. (eds.) MICCAI 2006. LNCS, vol. 4190, pp. 760–767. Springer, Heidelberg (2006)
7. Brown, R., Zlatescu, M., Sijben, A., Roldan, G., Easaw, J., Forsyth, P., Parney, I., Sevick, R., Yan, E., Demetrick, D., Schiff, D., Cairncross, G., Mitchell, R.: The use of magnetic resonance imaging to noninvasively detect genetic signatures in oligodendroglioma. Clinical Cancer Research 14, 2357–2362 (2008)

8. Drabycz, S.: Effcient S-Transform Techniques for Magnetic Resonance Imaging. PhD thesis, University of Calgary (2009)
9. Haykin, S.: Neural Networks: A Comprehensive Foundation. Macmillian College Pub. Co. (1994)
10. Williams, P.M.: Bayesian regularisation and pruning using a laplace prior. Neural Computation 7, 117–143 (1995)
11. McAuliffe, M.J., Lalonde, F.M., McGarry, D., Gandler, W., Csaky, K., Trus, B.L.: Medical image processing, analysis & visualization in clinical research. In: CBMS 2001: Proceedings of the Fourteenth IEEE Symposium on Computer-Based Medical Systems, Washington, DC, USA, p. 381. IEEE Computer Society, Los Alamitos (2001)

Tumor Invasion Margin on the Riemannian Space of Brain Fibers

Dana Cobzas[1], Parisa Mosayebi[1], Albert Murtha[2], and Martin Jagersand[1]

[1] Department of Computer Science, University of Alberta, Canada
[2] Department of Oncology, University of Alberta, Canada

Abstract. Gliomas are one of the most challenging tumors to treat or control locally. One of the main challenges is determining which areas of the apparently normal brain contain glioma cells, as gliomas are known to infiltrate for several centimeters beyond the clinically apparent lesion visualized on standard CT or MRI. To ensure that radiation treatment encompasses the whole tumour, including the cancerous cells not revealed by MRI, doctors treat a volume of brain extending 2cm out from the margin of the visible tumour. This expanded volume often includes healthy, non-cancerous brain tissue.

Knowing that glioma cells preferentially spread along nerve fibers, we propose the use of a geodesic distance on the Riemannian manifold of brain fibers to replace the Euclidean distance used in clinical practice and to correctly identify the tumor invasion margin. To compute the geodesic distance we use actual DTI data from patients with glioma and compare our predicted growth with follow-up MRI scans. Results show improvement in predicting the invasion margin when using the geodesic distance as opposed to the 2cm conventional Euclidean distance.

1 Introduction

Primary brain tumors are tumors which start from a glial cell in the nervous system. High grade variations of these tumors grow very fast often leading to a life-threatening condition. Current imaging techniques such as CT and MRI detect only the part of the tumor with a high concentration of tumor cells. The conventional medical practice is to perform maximally safe surgical resection and then irradiate the remaining tumor cells (visible and occult). The radiotherapy is conventionally applied to a margin of about 2cm around the visible tumor which is a very rough approximation of the probable location of tumor cells. This approach does not consider tumor growth dynamics in different brain tissues, thus it may result in killing some healthy cells while leaving alive cancerous cells in other areas. These cells may cause re-occurrence of the tumor later in time which limits the effectiveness of the therapy.

To improve the therapeutic outcome, more accurate prediction of the tumor invasion margin is necessary. Based on the generally accepted belief that glioma cells preferentially spread along nerve fibers [1], we propose here a new approach of computing the tumor invasion margin that makes use of a geodesic distance defined on a manifold of brain fibers. This formulation is very easily transferable to radiation therapy software by replacing the uniform (Euclidean) distance currently used to define the 2cm invasion margin (that will be radiated) with the geodesic distance.

Many efforts have been made to mathematically model the Glioma tumor growth. Following [2] these approaches are classified in three major categories: microscopic, mesoscopic and macroscopic. Micorscopic models describe the growth process in sub-cellular level, concentrating on activities that happen inside the tumor cell. Mesoscopic approaches focus on interactions between tumor cells and their surrounding tissue while macroscopic approaches focus on tissue level processes considering macroscopic quantities such as tumor volume and flow. As we are interested in modeling tumor invasion, we will restrict our discussion to macroscopic models.

Most models on macroscopic tumor growth use a reaction-diffusion term based on diffusion equation introduced by Murray [3]. Swanson et al. [4] used this term to generate a model assuming different motility of tumor cells in gray and white matter. They further enhanced their model to simulate the virtual gliomas [5]. However, this is an isotropic model which only simulates high grade glioma while low-grade gliomas exhibit complex shapes and are not well simulated by an isotropic model. More recent approaches use anisotropic diffusion along white matter fibers as given by the diffusion tensors (from Diffusion Tensor Images-DTI) to simulate more complex tumors. With limited availability of DTI data, existing techniques simulate growth based either on atlas tensors registered with the patient [6] or tensors from a healthy subject [7] unregistered with the patient. Recently a mechanical model of the mass effect was added to the reaction diffusion equation [6,8] resulting in a more physically plausible growth simulation.

In this paper, we introduce a novel model more directly driven by the particular patient DTI data to predict the tumor invasion margin using the geodesic distance defined on the Riemannian manifold of brain. The formulation of white matter as a Riemannian manifold was first introduced by O'Donnell et al. [9] and later formalized by Lenglet et al. [10]. They used this model for white matter connectivity mapping (tractography). Our geodesic growth model is concerned with predicting only the current tumor spread (invasion) that is not visible in the MRI images for better radiation therapy planning and therefore doesn't include mass effect. Konukoglu et. al [11] has previously used the diffusion equation to find tumor invasion margin but their method was tested only on synthetically grown tumors. Our geodesic model can more easily be incorporated into radiation planning software that already makes use of a distance (Euclidean) in defining the target region.

In addition to introducing the geodesic distance in the tumor growth concept, another contribution of the paper is the application of the method on actual patient specific DTI data. Furthermore, our method takes into account natural barriers to glioma growth such as the skull, the tentorium cerebelli and the falx cerebri. We tested our model on eight different patients by growing the tumor on the DWI scan of the patient and comparing the predicted distance with real growth shown on later MRI scans of the same patient. Comparative results of using geodesic distance show an improvement vs. uniform (Euclidean) distance.

2 Material and Methods

2.1 Tumor Invasion Using Geodesic Distance on Brain Fibers Manifold

The brain tumor infiltrating component can be mathematically modeled using anisotropic diffusion [7,6].

$$\frac{\partial c}{\partial t} = \nabla \cdot (D \nabla c) = \mathcal{L} c \qquad (1)$$

where c is the normalized concentration of tumor cells and D is the diffusion tensor of the tumor cells. Knowing that tumor diffusion is similar to water diffusion [1], D can be replaced with the diffusion tensor obtained from diffusion tensor imaging.

Tumor grows with different speed in white vs gray matter (with a factor of about $\alpha = 10$ [4]). While ideally this should be directly reflected by the diffusion tensors (DT) magnitude, due to noise and discretization problems and the fact that tumor might grow at a different speed than water diffusion, $D \neq DT$. One could estimate a function $D(x) = C(x)DT(x)$ where $C(x)$ is a matrix representing a spatial transform function. However $C(x)$ is intractable to estimate from limited data. Instead, after experimenting with real patient DTI data, we found that the linear weights $w(x) = \alpha FA(x)$ produce good results. FA represents the fractional anisotropy computed from tensor data.

The diffusion tensors in white matter are anisotropic, indicating the direction of fibers. As a consequence the anisotropic diffusion growth model would encourage diffusion of cancer cells along fibers [1]. We propose the use of a geodesic distance on the Riemannian manifold of white matter fibers to model the anisotropic tumor growth. O'Donnell et al [9] and Lenglet et al. [10] introduced the formulation of the white matter as a Riemannian manifold characterized by the infinitesimal anisotropic diffusion operator $\mathcal{L}$. They made the link between the diffusion tensor data D and the white matter manifold geometry and showed that the diffusion operator can be associated with a metric $G = D^{-1}$. This metric allows computation of geodesic path and distances between points on the brain and was previously used for fiber connectivity.

Geodesic Distance Calculation. Following [10], the distance Φ from a non-empty closed subset K is found by solving the eikonal equation on the 3-dimensional Riemannian manifold (M, g) (connected and complete)

$$\begin{cases} |\text{grad}\Phi| = 1 & \text{in} \quad M \backslash K \\ \Phi(x) = \Phi_0(x) & \text{for} \quad x \in K \end{cases} \qquad (2)$$

where $\Phi_0(x) = 0 \quad \forall x \in K$.

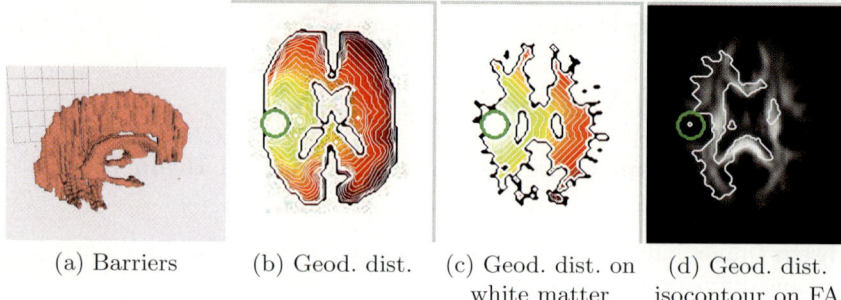

(a) Barriers   (b) Geod. dist.   (c) Geod. dist. on white matter   (d) Geod. dist. isocontour on FA

Fig. 1. The result of applying the geodesic distance model to a DTI atlas. Colors show the geodesic distance from the initial position.

Representing the distance function Φ as the zero levelset of a signed distance function Ψ, $\Psi(x,t) = 0 \Leftrightarrow t = \Phi(x)$, Equation 2 can be reformulated as finding Ψ the viscosity solution of

$$\begin{cases} \frac{\partial \Psi}{\partial t} + |\text{grad}\Psi| = 0 \ \forall t > 0 \\ \Psi(x,0) = \Psi_0(x) \end{cases} \quad (3)$$

where Ψ_0 is the signed distance function of Φ_0.

To numerically solve hyperbolic Hamilton-Jacobi Equation 3 we approximated the continuous flux $|\text{grad}\Psi|^2$ as [10]:

$$|\text{grad}\Psi|^2 = \sum_{i=1}^{3} g^{ii} \left(\max(D_{x_i}^- \Psi, 0)^2 + \min(D_{x_i}^+ \Psi, 0)^2 \right) + \sum_{i \neq j} g^{ij} \text{minmod}(D_{x_i}^+ \Psi, D_{x_i}^- \Psi) \text{minmod}(D_{x_j}^+ \Psi, D_{x_j}^- \Psi) \quad (4)$$

where $g_{i,j=1...3}^{ij}$ are components of the inverse matrix G^{-1}, $D_{x_i}^{\pm}\Psi$ are upwind approximation of the gradient of Ψ in x_i and $\text{minmod}(a,b) = \min(a,0) + \max(b,0)$.

Geodesic Distance for Tumor Growth Prediction. When using the geodesic distance in the context of growth prediction, we chose as the origin of the grwoth (subset K) the visible tumor margin. In addition, as the brain contains several obvious natural barriers to glioma growth such as the skull, ventricular system, the tentorium cerebelli and the falx cerebri, M is defined as the brain volume that doesn't contain those barriers. Fig. 1(a) shows an example of segmented barriers (ventricles, falx, tentorium). Fig. 1(b-d) shows examples of geodesic distance computed on the ICBM DTI-81 atlas [12]: (b) shows the geodesic distance computed with linear tensor weighting that originates from a sphere (green circle in the figure) until reaches the skull boundary. (c) shows the geodesic distance computed only in the white matter tensors instead of the whole brain tensors; (d) shows an isocontour of the geodesic distance aligned with FA values. Notice how the distance follows the fiber directions.

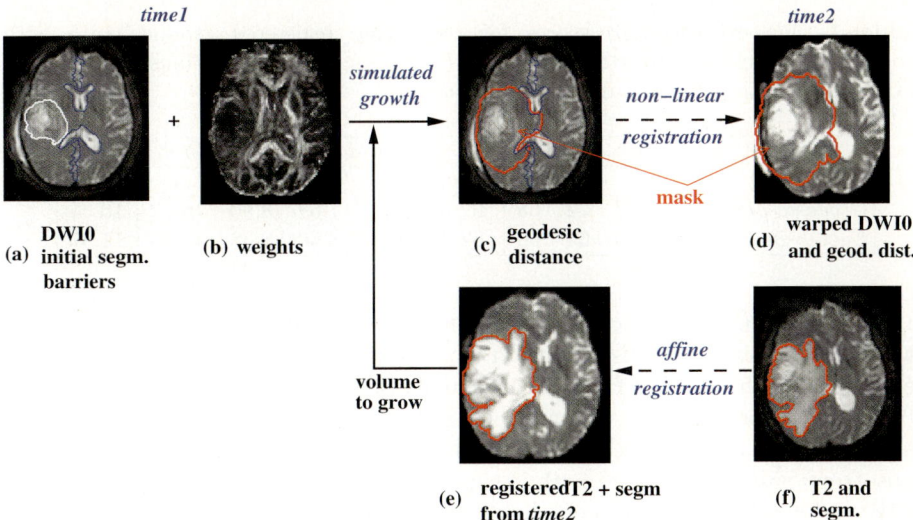

Fig. 2. Overview of validation system. Tumor growth is simulated on DTI data from *time1* and compared with the manual segmentation on data at *time2*.

2.2 Patients and Data

We used MRI and DTI data from clinical scans of patients with GBM.[1] Each patient has a pre-RT MRI scan. Follow-up DTI or MRI scans have been made after treatment at intervals of about 3-6 months. DTI data has a resolution of $128 \times 128 \times 60$ while MRI data has a resolution of $512 \times 512 \times 21$. Typically at least one or two DTI data is acquired after radiation and the rest of the scans are conventional MRI images (T2, T1, FLAIR). To minimize the effects of radiation treatment not accounted in our model, we use data from the first DTI scan acquired after radiation for estimating the diffusion-based invasion margin and compare our model with the actual growth observed in later MRI-T2 scans.

Both the tumor growth and the comparison is done based on segmentations of the high signal region adjacent to the gross tumor on MRI-T2 or DWI0 (the DWI scan with zero b-value similar to T2). This region contains tumor, associated edema and microscopic tumor cell infiltration. Segmentations are done using a semi-automatic tool developed in our lab. Growth barriers (ventricular system, falx cerebri and tentorium cerebelli) are manually delineated using the same software. An expert radiation oncologist validated all segmentations.

2.3 Data Processing and Validation Procedure

Fig. 2 shows an overview of the growth *validation* system. We grow the tumor from *time1* to approximately its size at *time2* and then compare the result of our model with the actual growth. This validation assumes that the visible growth

---

[1] The data collection protocol was approved by REB and the patients that have provided an informed consent.

Table 1. Jaccard (overlap) scores for comparing registered ground truth with geodesic and Euclidean growth. $\text{Jaccard}(A,B) = (A \cap B)/(A \cup B)$ $\text{Hausdroff}(A,B) = \max\left\{\sup_{a \in A} \inf_{b \in B} d(a,b), \sup_{b \in B} \inf_{a \in A} d(a,b)\right\}$.

	Jaccard score (%)					Hausdorff distance (mm)				
	1	2	3	4	mean	1	2	3	4	mean
Geodesic dist.	65	75	72	65	69.2	9.32	7.68	8.90	16.72	10.65
Euclidean dist.	59	65	64	60	62.0	10.02	8.60	9.38	17.49	11.37

in the subsequent times occurs over the invisible but already-infilterated regions at the initial time. We use the first or second DTI scan after treatment to generate growth starting from the manually segmented visible high signal on DWI0 (Fig. 2 (a) - edema, tumor swelling - *time1*). We extract diffusion tensors using ExploreDTI [13] that are then weighted (Fig. 2 (b)) based on the Fractional Anisotropy values. Tumor growth is simulated by iteratively solving Eq. 3.

We *validated* growth by comparing the results from the geodesic distance (Fig. 2 (c)) with manually segmented high signal on T2/DWI0 from later follow up scans (Fig. 2 (f) - *time2*). This comparison requires *registration*. We used affine registration of T2-MRI/DWI0 data from *time2* with the DTI (DWI0) data at *time1* to determine the approximate growth volume used as a stopping criterion for the geodesic distance simulation. We also used the same registration for visual comparisons (comparing (c) with (e) - see Fig. 3). For fair comparison between Euclidean and geodesic distance, we apply the same process also for the Euclidean distance instead of simply growing the tumor to the 2cm margin.

The linear registration doesn't take into account the mass effect as a consequence of tumor growth from *time1* to *time2*. This is easily noticed in Fig. 2 (e) which shows the result of affine registration: the growth affected ventricle shape in *time2* is incorrectly registered with data at *time1*. Therefore for numerical scores we applied non-linear registration of DWI0 data and the predicted geodesic growth from *time1* to T2-MRI data and segmented edema at *time2*. For correct non-linear registration we masked edema label (*time2*) and the generated growth label (*time1*). Those regions contain abnormalities and they cannot be taken into account for the registration score. Fig. 2 (d) shows the result of non-linear registration that can now be compared with (f). Now the shape of the ventricles correctly aligns on the space of *time2*. For both registrations we used FSL tools [14] (FLIRT for linear and FNIRT for non-linear registration).

3 Results

Our dataset includes 24 DWI but we could only use the 8 data that showed tumor growth after treatment. We applied the growth models with the data processing explained in Section 2.3 to each patient data. Fig. 3 (2) shows the comparative results of real growth with geodesic and Euclidean growth. The results show that where the tensor values are less noisy, the geodesic distance model can track the path of fibers and therefore matches tumor growth, as opposed to when using

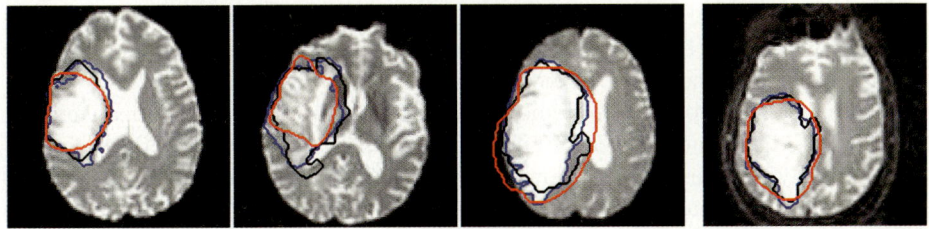

Fig. 3. (1) Comparative results on *time2* DWI0 corresponding to Table 1 Patient 1-4 (left-right). Blue line shows manual segmentation, black line shows simulated geodesic growth and red line shows simulated Euclidean growth.

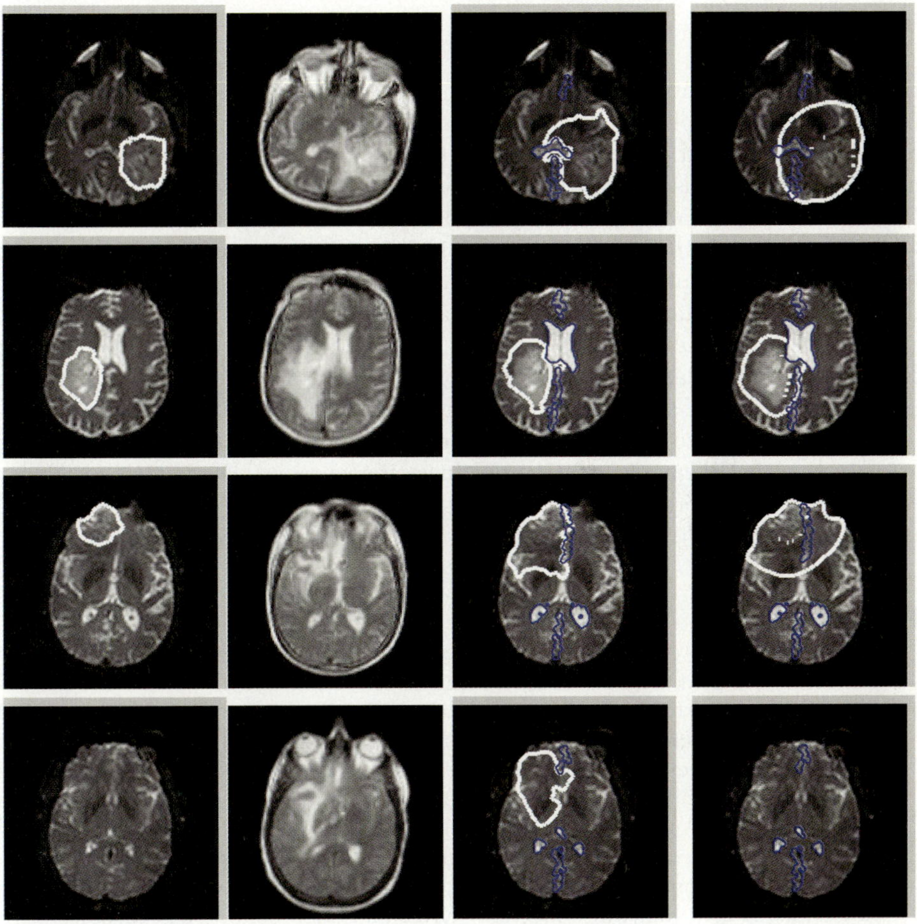

(a) Patient at *time1* (b) Patient at *time2* (c) Geod. dist. (d) Euclid. Dist.

Fig. 3. (2) Comparative results for different patients of Geodesic (c) and Euclidean (d) simulated growth starting from segmented tumor at *time1* (a) and linearly registered followed up scans at *time2* (MRI-T2 or DWI) (b). Barriers are shown in blue.

the Euclidean model. Notice how in the example from the last row of Fig. 3 the Euclidean distance has not reached the shown tumor slice while the geodesic distance correctly models the growth.

To numerically compare our model with the conventional Euclidean model, we calculated the Jaccard scores and Haudorff distances shown in Table 1. Corresponding visual results are shown in Fig. 3 (1). As mentioned in Section 2.3 for reducing the mass effect we applied non-linear registration to warp data from *time1* into the space of *time2*. Due to registration problems we could only calculate scores for 4 patients. Numerical results show an improvement of about 5-10% for simulated growth using the geodesic distance compared to the Euclidean distance. This difference correspond to millions of saved brain cells.

4 Discussion

In this paper, we introduced the use of geodesic distance on the Riemannian manifold of brain fibers to detect the glioma brain tumor invasion margin. The model was tested on several real patients data and a DTI atlas. In contrast to most of the previous works in this area, we used real tensors of the patients obtained by the standard clinical procedure instead or registered atlas tensors. Comparative results between real growth in follow up scans and simulated growth based on geodesic and Euclidean distance prove that the use of the geodesic distance could significantly improve radiation therapy treatment.

To further improve results on noisy clinical data we plan to apply better tensor extraction and regularization. Furthermore, although the non-linear registration used between *time1* and *time2* to numerically validate results solves the problem of mass effect to a good extent, it cannot solve it completely. Hence, the error in the non-linear registration produces inaccuracies. For better non-linear registration in the presence of mass effect we plan to incorporate a mechanical model into the registration (similar to [15]).

References

1. Kuroiwa, T., Ueki, M., Chen, Q., Suemasu, H., Taniguchi, I., Okeda, R.: Biomechanical characteristics of brain edema: the difference between vasogenic-type and cytotoxic-type edema. Acta Neurochir. Suppl. 60, 158–161 (1994)
2. Hatzikirou, H., Deutsch, A., Schaller, C., Simon, M., Swanson, K.: Mathematical modelling of glioblastoma tumor developement: A review. Mathematical Models and Methods in Applied Sciences 15(11), 1779–1794 (2005)
3. Murray, J.: Mathematical Biology. Springer, Heidelberg (1989)
4. Swanson, K., Alvord, E.J., Murray, J.: A quantitative model for differential motility of gliomas in grey and white matter. Cell Proliferation 33, 317–329 (2000)
5. Swanson, K., Alvord, E., Murray, J.: Virtual brain tumors (gliomas) enhance the reality of medical imaging and highlight inadequacies of current therapy. British Journal of Cancer 85, 14–18 (2002)

6. Clatz, O., Sermesant, M., Bondiau, P.Y., Delingette, H., Warfield, S.K., Malandain, G., Ayache, N.: Realistic simulation of the 3d growth of brain tumors in MR images coupling diffusion with mass effect. IEEE Transactions on Medical Imaging 24(10), 1334–1346 (2005)
7. Jbabdi, S., Mandonnet, E., Duffau, H., Capelle, L., Swanson, K., Pelegrini, M., Guillevin, R., Benali, H.: Simulation of anisotropic growth of low-grade gliomas using dif. tensor imag. Magnetic Resonance in Medicine 54, 616–624 (2005)
8. Hogea, C., Davatzikos, C., Biros, G.: Modeling glioma growth and mass effect in 3D MR images of the brain. In: Ayache, N., Ourselin, S., Maeder, A. (eds.) MICCAI 2007, Part I. LNCS, vol. 4791, pp. 642–650. Springer, Heidelberg (2007)
9. O'Donnell, L., Haker, S., Westin, C.-F.: New approaches to estimation of white matter connectivity in diffusion tensor MRI: Elliptic PDEs and geodesics in a tensor-warped space. In: Dohi, T., Kikinis, R. (eds.) MICCAI 2002. LNCS, vol. 2488, p. 459. Springer, Heidelberg (2002)
10. Lenglet, C., Deriche, R., Faugeras, O.: Inferring white matter geometry from diffusion tensor MRI: Applic. to connectivity mapping. In: MICCAI (2004)
11. Konukoğlu, E., Clatz, O., Bondiau, P.-Y., Delingette, H., Ayache, N.: Extrapolating tumor invasion margins for physiologically determined radiotherapy regions. In: Larsen, R., Nielsen, M., Sporring, J. (eds.) MICCAI 2006. LNCS, vol. 4190, pp. 338–346. Springer, Heidelberg (2006)
12. LONI: atlases, http://www.loni.ucla.edu/atlases/
13. ExploreDTI, http://www.exploredti.com/
14. FSL: tools, http://www.fmrib.ox.ac.uk/fsl/
15. Mohamed, A., Zacharaki, E., Shen, D., Davatzikos, C.: Deformable registration of brain tumor images via a statistical model of tumor-induced deformation. Medical Image Analysis 10(5), 752–763 (2006)

A Conditional Random Field Approach for Coupling Local Registration with Robust Tissue and Structure Segmentation

Benoit Scherrer[1,3], Florence Forbes[2,3], and Michel Dojat[1,3]

[1] INSERM, U836, Grenoble, F-38042, France
[2] INRIA, MISTIS, Grenoble, France
[3] Université Joseph Fourier, Grenoble, France

Abstract. We consider a general modelling strategy to handle in a unified way a number of tasks essential to MR brain scan analysis. Our approach is based on the explicit definition of a Conditional Random Field (CRF) model decomposed into components to be specified according to the targeted tasks. For a specific illustration, we define a CRF model that combines robust-to-noise and to nonuniformity Markovian tissue and structure segmentations with local affine atlas registration. The evaluation performed on both phantoms and real 3T images shows good results and, in particular, points out the gain in introducing registration as a model component. Besides, our modeling and estimation scheme provide general guidelines to deal with complex joint processes for medical image analysis.

1 Introduction

The analysis of MR brain scans is a complex task that requires several sources of information to be taken into account and combined. The analysis is frequently based on segmentations of tissues and of subcortical structures performed by human experts. For automatic segmentation, difficulties arise from the presence of various artifacts such as noise or intensity nonuniformities. For structures, the segmentation requires in addition the use of prior information usually encoded via a pre-registered atlas. Recently growing interest has been on tackling this complexity by combining different approaches. As an illustration, Yang *et al.* [1] propose to use a region based tissue classification approach followed by a watershed algorithm to label brain sulci while Yu *et al.* [2] combine a region-based bias field estimation and a level set method to segment the cortex. A step further the combinaison of methods is *coupling*, giving the possibility to introduce mutual interactions between components of a model. Such a coupling can be naturally expressed in a statistical framework via the definition of joint distributions. In this vein, Ashburner and Friston [3] couple a global statistical tissue segmentation approach with the estimation of a bias field and a global registration of an atlas of tissue probability maps. Another growing feature in the literature is to locally estimate model parameters on the image to better fit local image properties. For instance, Scherrer et al. [4] couple a *local* tissue segmentation approach with a structure segmentation approach; Pohl et al. [5] couple structure segmentation with the *local affine* registration of an atlas.

In this paper, we propose to go further towards coupling methods by constructing a *Conditional Random Field* (CRF) model that performs a number of essential tasks. We will focus on developing a statistical framework that allows 1) tissue segmentation using *local* Markov Random Field (MRF) models, 2) MRF segmentation of structures and 3) *local affine* registration of an atlas. All tasks are linked and completing each one of them can help in refining the others. The idea is to capture in a single model all the relationships that could be formalized between these tasks. Our basis toward a solution is similar to that in [4] with the major difference that therein a joint model was not explicitly given but defined through the specification of a number of compatible conditional MRF models. In this work, we specify directly a joint model from which the conditional models are derived. As a result, cooperation between tissues and structures is treated in a more symmetric way which results in new more consistent conditional models. In addition, interaction between the segmentation and registration steps is easily introduced. An explicit joint formulation has the advantage to provide a strategy to construct more consistent or complete models that are open to incorporation of new tasks. For estimation, we provide an appropriate variational EM framework allowing a Bayesian treatment of the parameters. The evaluation performed on both phantoms and real 3T brain scans shows good results and demonstrates the clear improvement provided by coupling the registration step to tissue and structure segmentation.

2 A CRF Approach to Segmentation and Registration

We consider a finite set V of N voxels on a regular 3D grid. Our tissue and structure segmentation task is recast into a missing data framework in which the observed data $\mathbf{y} = \{y_1, \ldots, y_N\}$ are the intensity values observed respectively at each voxel and the missing data $\mathbf{z} = (\mathbf{t}, \mathbf{s})$ is made of two sets: the tissue classes $\mathbf{t} = \{t_1, \ldots, t_N\}$ and the subcortical structure classes $\mathbf{s} = \{s_1, \ldots, s_N\}$. The t_is take their values in $\{e_1, e_2, e_3\}$ that represents the three tissues cephalo-spinal-fluid, grey matter and white matter. Each e_k is a 3-dimensional binary vector whose kth component is 1, all other components being 0. For the subcortical structure segmentation we consider L structures, the s_is taking their values in $\{e'_1, \ldots, e'_L, e'_{L+1}\}$ where e'_{L+1} corresponds to an additional background class. Tissues and structures are linked and we denote by T^{s_i} the tissue of structure s_i at voxel i. The model parameters $\theta = (\psi, \mathcal{R})$ include both the intensity distributions parameters ψ and the registration parameters $\mathcal{R}$. We consider them in a Bayesian framework as realizations of random variables that take their values in $\underline{\Theta} = \underline{\Psi} \times \underline{\mathcal{R}}$.

To capture interactions between the various fields $\mathbf{y}$, $\mathbf{t}$, $\mathbf{s}$ and θ we adopt a *conditional random field* approach which consists in specifying a conditional model $p(\mathbf{t}, \mathbf{s}, \theta | \mathbf{y})$. We define $p(\mathbf{t}, \mathbf{s}, \theta | \mathbf{y})$ as a Gibbs measure with energy function

$H(\mathbf{t},\mathbf{s},\theta|\mathbf{y})$ ie. $p(\mathbf{t},\mathbf{s},\theta|\mathbf{y}) \propto \exp(H(\mathbf{t},\mathbf{s},\theta|\mathbf{y}))$ where the energy is decomposed in the following terms. We denote by $g(y_i|t_i, s_i, \psi_i)$ positive functions of y_i and consider the decomposition:

$$H(\mathbf{t},\mathbf{s},\theta|\mathbf{y}) = H_T(\mathbf{t}) + H_S(\mathbf{s}) + H_{T,S}(\mathbf{t},\mathbf{s}) + H_{T,\mathcal{R}}(\mathbf{t},\mathcal{R}) + H_{S,\mathcal{R}}(\mathbf{s},\mathcal{R})$$
$$+ H_\Psi(\psi) + H_\mathcal{R}(\mathcal{R}) + \sum_{i \in V} \log g(y_i|t_i, s_i, \psi_i) \ . \quad (1)$$

A number of essential tasks. In what follows, we show how the terms in (1) can be specified so that the model performs the tasks listed below.

Robust-to-noise segmentation. Robust-to-noise segmentation is generally addressed via MRF modelling. It introduces local spatial dependencies between voxels, providing a labelling regularization. For tissue and structure segmentations, we use standard Potts models setting $H_T(\mathbf{t}) = \sum_{i \in V} \sum_{j \in \mathcal{N}(i)} \eta_T \langle t_i, t_j \rangle$ and $H_S(\mathbf{s}) = \sum_{i \in V} \sum_{j \in \mathcal{N}(i)} \eta_S \langle s_i, s_j \rangle$, where $\langle \cdot, \cdot \rangle$ denotes the scalar product, $\mathcal{N}(i)$ represents the voxels neighboring i and η_T and η_S are additional interaction strength parameters.

Local approach to deal with nonuniformity. Generally, tissue intensity models are estimated globally through the entire volume and then suffer from imperfections at a local level. We adopt as in [4] a local segmentation alternative. The principle is to locally compute the tissue models in various subvolumes of the initial volume. These models better reflect local intensity distributions and are likely to handle different sources of intensity nonuniformity. We consider intensity models that depend on the tissue class k but also on the voxel localization so that ψ decomposes into $\psi = \{\psi_i, i \in V\}$ where $\psi_i = {}^t(\psi_i^k, k = 1, 2, 3)$. Although possible in our Bayesian framework, this general setting results in too many parameters which could not be estimated accurately. The local approach [4] provides an intermediate efficient solution where the ψ_i's are first considered as constant over subvolumes. Let $\mathcal{C}$ be a regular cubic partitionning of the volume V in a number of nonoverlapping subvolumes $\{V_c, c \in \mathcal{C}\}$. We write $\psi = \{\psi_c, c \in \mathcal{C}\}$ where $\psi_c = {}^t(\psi_c^k, k = 1, 2, 3)$ is the common value of all ψ_i for $i \in V_c$. In addition to ensure consistency and spatial regularity between the local estimations of the ψ_c's we consider a MRF prior $p(\psi) \propto \exp(H_\Psi(\psi))$. The specific form of $H_\Psi(\psi)$ is the same as in [4]. When Gaussian intensity distributions are considered, it corresponds to assign *auto-normal* Markov priors to the mean parameters. Outside the issue of estimating ψ, having voxel dependent ψ_i's is not a problem. We easily go back to this case, from estimated ψ_c's, by using a cubic splines interpolation step.

Incorporating a priori knowledge via local affine atlas registration. The *a priori* knowledge required for structure segmentation is classically provided via a global non-rigid atlas registration. Most methods first register the prior information to the medical image and then segment the image based on that aligned information. Although reliable registration methods are available, it is still important, in the subsequent segmentation task, to overcome biases caused by commitment to the initial registration. Also segmentation results provide information that can be used for feedback on registration. Global registration approaches generally lead to a high dimensional minimization problem which is computationally greedy and subject to a high number of local optima. We rather choose a hierarchical local affine registration model as in [5]. We consider 1) a global affine transformation given by parameters $\mathcal{R}^G$, which describes the non structure-dependent deformations, and 2) one local affine structure-dependent deformation for each structure, defined in relation to $\mathcal{R}^G$ and capturing the residual structure-specific deformations. It follows $L+2$ affine transformation parameters $\mathcal{R} = (\mathcal{R}^G, \mathcal{R}_1^S, \ldots, \mathcal{R}_{L+1}^S)$ to be estimated. Interactions between labels and registration parameters are introduced through $H_{T,\mathcal{R}}(\mathbf{t}, \mathcal{R})$ and $H_{S,\mathcal{R}}(\mathbf{s}, \mathcal{R})$. Similarly to [5], the interaction between $\mathbf{S}$ and $\mathcal{R}$ is chosen so as to favor configurations for which the segmentation of a structure l is aligned on its prior atlas. We denote by $\zeta_S = \{\zeta_S^l, l = 1, \ldots, L+1\}$ the statistical atlas of the brain subcortical structures under consideration and by $\rho(\mathcal{R}^G, \mathcal{R}_l^S, i)$ the interpolation function assigning a position in the atlas space to the image space. We compute the spatial *a priori* distribution $f_S^l(\mathcal{R}, \cdot)$ of one structure l by $f_S^l(\mathcal{R}, i) = \frac{\zeta_S^l(\rho(\mathcal{R}^G, \mathcal{R}_l^S, i))}{\sum_{l'=1..L+1} \zeta_S^{l'}(\rho(\mathcal{R}^G, \mathcal{R}_{l'}^S, i))}$. The normalization across all structures is necessary as $\mathcal{R}_l^S$ are structure-dependent parameters and multiple voxels in the atlas space could be mapped to one location in the image space. Although some atlas are potentially available for tissues, in our setting we build f_T, the spatial *a priori* distribution of the $K = 3$ tissues, from the f_S^l's: $f_T^k(\mathcal{R}, i) = \sum_{l \ st. T^l = k} f_S^l(\mathcal{R}, i) + \frac{1}{K} f_S^{L+1}(\mathcal{R}, i)$. Agreement between structure segmentation and atlas is then favored by setting $H_{S,\mathcal{R}}(\mathbf{s}, \mathcal{R}) = \sum_{i \in V} \langle s_i, \log(f_S(\mathcal{R}, i) + \epsilon) \rangle$, with the vectorial notation $f_S = {}^t(f_S^1, \ldots, f_S^{L+1})$. The logarithm and a positive scalar ϵ are introduced respectively for homogeneity between probabilities and energies, and to ensure the existence of the logarithm. We choose $\epsilon = 1$, making in addition $H_{S,\mathcal{R}}(\mathbf{s}, \mathcal{R})$ positive, but the overall method does not seem sensitive to its exact value. Similarly, we define the interaction between $\mathbf{t}$ and $\mathcal{R}$ by $H_{T,\mathcal{R}}(\mathbf{t}, \mathcal{R}) = \sum_{i \in V} \langle t_i, \log(f_T(\mathcal{R}, i) + \epsilon) \rangle$. Then, the term $H_\mathcal{R}(\mathcal{R})$ can be used to introduce *a priori* knowledge to favor estimation of $\mathcal{R}$ close to some average registration parameters computed from a training data set if available. In our case, no such data set were available and we set $H_\mathcal{R}(\mathcal{R}) = 0$.

Cooperative tissue and structure segmentations. Tissues and structures are linked: a structure is made of a specific tissue and knowledge on structures locations provides information for tissue segmentation. Inducing cooperation between tissue and structure segmentations can be done through the term $H_{T,S}(\mathbf{t}, \mathbf{s})$. We set $H_{T,S}(\mathbf{t}, \mathbf{s}) = \sum_{i \in V} \langle t_i, e_{T^{s_i}} \rangle$, so as to favor situations for which the tissue T^{s_i} of structure s_i is the same as the tissue given by t_i. Cooperation between tissue and structure labels also appear via the energy data term $\sum_{i \in V} g(y_i | t_i, s_i, \psi_i)$. Considering Gaussian intensity distributions, we denote by $\mathcal{G}(\cdot | \mu, \lambda)$ the Gaussian distribution with mean μ and precision λ (*i.e.* the inverse of the variance). Denoting $\psi_i^k = \{\mu_i^k, \lambda_i^k\}$, we see ψ_i as a 3-dimensional vector, so that when $t_i = e_k$, then $\mathcal{G}(y_i | \langle t_i, \psi_i \rangle)$ denotes the Gaussian distribution with mean μ_i^k and precision λ_i^k. To account for both tissue and structure information, we set: $g(y_i | t_i, s_i, \psi_i) =$

$\mathcal{G}(y_i|\langle t_i,\psi_i\rangle)^{\frac{1+\langle s_i,e'_{L+1}\rangle}{2}} \mathcal{G}(y_i|\langle e_{T^{s_i}},\psi_i\rangle)^{\frac{1-\langle s_i,e'_{L+1}\rangle}{2}}$. When tissue and structure segmentations contain the same information at voxel i, ie. either $t_i = e_{T^{s_i}}$ or $s_i = e'_{L+1}$, then the expression of g above reduces to the usual $\mathcal{G}(y_i|\langle t_i,\psi_i\rangle)$. When this is not the case, the expression of g above leads to $\mathcal{G}(y_i|\langle t_i,\psi_i\rangle)^{1/2}\mathcal{G}(y_i|\langle e_{T^{s_i}},\psi_i\rangle)^{1/2}$ which is a more appropriate compromise.

3 A Bayesian EM Estimation Framework

We consider the EM algorithm and more specifically its *Maximization-Maximization* interpretation as a general estimation technique in the presence of missing data. Let $\mathcal{T}$ and $\mathcal{S}$ be respectively the spaces in which **t** and **s** take their values. We denote by $\mathcal{D}$ the set of probability distributions on $\mathcal{Z} = \mathcal{T} \times \mathcal{S}$. In a Bayesian framework, EM can be used to find Maximum A Posteriori (MAP) estimations (see *eg* [6]) and leads to the alternating maximization over $q \in \mathcal{D}$ and $\theta \in \Theta$ of the function defined by $F_{\text{MAP}}(q,\theta) = \sum_{\mathbf{z} \in \mathcal{Z}} \log p(\mathbf{y},\mathbf{z}|\theta)\, q(\mathbf{z}) + \log p(\theta) + I[q]$, where $I[q] = -\mathbb{E}_q[\log q(\mathbf{Z})]$ is the entropy of q ($\mathbb{E}_q$ denotes the expectation with regard to q and capital letters indicate random variables while small letters denote their realizations). However, the dependencies between the missing data usually make the optimization over $\mathcal{D}$ intractable. We then propose to use a Variational EM approach [7] in which the E-step is not performed exactly. The optimization is solved over a restricted class of probability distributions which factorize as $q(\mathbf{t},\mathbf{s}) = q_T(\mathbf{t})\, q_S(\mathbf{s})$ where q_T (resp. q_S) belongs to the set $\mathcal{D}_T$ (resp. $\mathcal{D}_S$) of probability distributions on $\mathcal{T}$ (resp. on $\mathcal{S}$). Further generalizing by dividing the approximate E-step into two stages, it follows a variant that falls in the modified Generalized Alternating Minimization (GAM) procedures family [8]. From the definition of F_{MAP}, we therefore derive a 3-steps algorithm. At iteration $r+1$, with current estimates denoted by $q_T^{(r)}$, $q_S^{(r)}$ and $\theta^{(r)}$, it consists of:

$$\textbf{E-T-step:}\quad q_T^{(r+1)} = \arg \max_{q_T \in \mathcal{D}_T} \mathbb{E}_{q_T}[\mathbb{E}_{q_S^{(r)}}[\log p(\mathbf{T}|\mathbf{S},\mathbf{y},\theta^{(r)})]] + I[q_T] \quad (2)$$

$$\textbf{E-S-step:}\quad q_S^{(r+1)} = \arg \max_{q_S \in \mathcal{D}_S} \mathbb{E}_{q_S}[\mathbb{E}_{q_T^{(r+1)}}[\log p(\mathbf{S}|\mathbf{T},\mathbf{y},\theta^{(r)})]] + I[q_S] \quad (3)$$

$$\textbf{M-step:}\quad \theta^{(r+1)} = \arg \max_{\theta \in \Theta} \mathbb{E}_{q_T^{(r+1)} q_S^{(r+1)}}[\log p(\theta|\mathbf{T},\mathbf{S},\mathbf{y})]. \quad (4)$$

Equations (2-4) show that for inference the specification of the three conditional distributions $p(\mathbf{t}|\mathbf{s},\mathbf{y},\theta)$, $p(\mathbf{s}|\mathbf{t},\mathbf{y},\theta)$ and $p(\theta|\mathbf{t},\mathbf{s},\mathbf{y})$ is sufficient. These models can be easily deduced from the conditional distribution $p(\mathbf{t},\mathbf{s},\theta|y)$ confirming that there is no need to define the complete joint model $p(\mathbf{t},\mathbf{s},\mathbf{y},\theta)$ and emphasizing the rational of using a CRF approach for segmentation purpose. Moreover, the model definition in (1) induces that the conditional models $p(\mathbf{t}|\mathbf{s},\mathbf{y},\theta)$ and $p(\mathbf{s}|\mathbf{t},\mathbf{y},\theta)$ are MRF with energy functions denoted by $H(\mathbf{t}|\mathbf{s},\mathbf{y},\theta)$ and $H(\mathbf{s}|\mathbf{t},\mathbf{y},\theta)$ obtained by omitting in expression (1) the terms that do not depend on **t**, resp. on **s**. The two-stage E-step (2) and (3) requires then to compute $H_T^{(r+1)}(\mathbf{t}) = \mathbb{E}_{q_S^{(r)}}[H(\mathbf{t}|\mathbf{S},\mathbf{y},\theta^{(r)})]$ and $H_S^{(r+1)}(\mathbf{s}) = \mathbb{E}_{q_T^{(r+1)}}[H(\mathbf{s}|\mathbf{T},\mathbf{y},\theta^{(r)})]$. Neglecting terms not depending on **t**, it comes:

$$H_T^{(r+1)}(\mathbf{t}) = \sum_{i \in V}\left[\langle t_i, \log(\tilde{f}_T^{(r)}(\mathcal{R}^{(r)},i)) \rangle + \sum_{j \in \mathcal{N}(i)} \eta_T \langle t_i,t_j \rangle + \log(g_{T_i}(y_i|t_i)) \right], \quad (5)$$

where $g_{T_i}(y_i|t_i) = \mathcal{G}(y_i|\langle t_i,\psi_i^{(r)}\rangle)^{\frac{1+q_{S_i}^{(r)}(e'_{L+1})}{2}}$ and $\tilde{f}_T^{(r)} = {}^t(\tilde{f}_T^{k(r)}, k = 1, 2, 3)$ with $\tilde{f}_T^{k(r)}$ defined by $\log(\tilde{f}_T^{k(r)}(\mathcal{R}, i)) = \log(f_T^k(\mathcal{R}, i) + \epsilon) + \sum_{l\ st.T^l=k} q_{S_i}^{(r)}(e'_l)$. In the latter expression, the term $\sum_{l\ st.T^l=k} q_{S_i}^{(r)}(e'_l)$ is the probability, given the current distribution $q_{S_i}^{(r)}$, that voxel i belongs to a structure whose tissue is k. Intuitively, the higher this probability the more favored is tissue k. Similarly,

$$H_S^{(r+1)}(\mathbf{s}) = \sum_{i\in V}\left[\langle s_i, \log(\tilde{f}_S^{(r)}(\mathcal{R}^{(r)}, i))\rangle + \sum_{j\in\mathcal{N}(i)} \eta_S\langle s_i, s_j\rangle + \log(g_{S_i}(y_i|s_i))\right], \quad (6)$$

where $g_{S_i}(y_i|s_i) = \left(\prod_{k=1}^3 \mathcal{G}(y_i|\psi_i^{k(r)})^{q_{T_i}^{(r+1)}(e_k)}\right)^{\frac{1+\langle s_i,e'_{L+1}\rangle}{2}} \mathcal{G}(y_i|\langle e_{T^{s_i}},\psi_i^{(r)}\rangle)^{\frac{1-\langle s_i,e'_{L+1}\rangle}{2}}$
and $\log \tilde{f}_S^{l(r)}(\mathcal{R}, i) = \log(f_S^l(\mathcal{R}, i) + \epsilon) + q_{T_i}^{(r+1)}(e_{T^l})(1 - \langle e'_l, e'_{L+1}\rangle)$ where the term $q_{T_i}^{(r+1)}(e_{T^l})(1 - \langle e'_l, e'_{L+1}\rangle)$ favors a structure whose tissue is T^l if l is a proper structure. We recognize in (5) and (6) the standard decomposition of a MRF model into three terms: an external field, a regularizing spatial term and a data term. Then, solving the current E-T and E-S steps is equivalent to solve the segmentation task for standard MRFs whose definition depends on the previous iteration. In this work we consider a Mean field like algorithm to actually compute $q_T^{(r+1)}$ and $q_S^{(r+1)}$ but any other MRF estimation strategy could be possible.

The independence of ψ and $\mathcal{R}$ then leads to a two-stage M-step **M-ψ** and **M-$\mathcal{R}$**. For the **M-ψ** step, the choice of a Markovian prior energy $H_\Psi(\psi)$ as in [4] requires the use of a Mean Field like approximation for the maximization. Similarly to [4], we update the $\psi_c^k = \{\mu_c^k, \lambda_c^k\}$'s with the values obtained at convergence of the following scheme ((ν) denotes the iteration number):

M-ψ :
$$\mu_c^{k(\nu+1)} = \frac{\lambda_c^{k(\nu)}\sum_{i\in V_c} a_{ik}y_i + \lambda_c^{0k}|\mathcal{N}(c)|^{-1}\sum_{c'\in\mathcal{N}(c)}\mu_{c'}^{k(\nu)}}{\lambda_c^{k(\nu)}\sum_{i\in V_c} a_{ik} + \lambda_c^{0k}}$$
$$\lambda_c^{k(\nu+1)} = \frac{\alpha_c^k + \sum_{i\in V_c} a_{ik}/2 - 1}{b_c^k + 1/2[\sum_{i\in V_c} a_{ik}(y_i - \mu_c^{k(\nu+1)})^2]},$$

where $\{\lambda_c^{0k}, \alpha_c^k, b_c^k, c\in\mathcal{C}\}$ are hyperparameters to be specified, $\mathcal{N}(c)$ denotes the indices of the subvolumes neighboring subvolume c, $|\mathcal{N}(c)|$ the number of them and $a_{ik} = \frac{1}{2}(q_{T_i}(e_k) + q_{T_i}(e_k)q_{S_i}(e'_{L+1}) + \sum_{l st.T^l=k} q_{S_i}(e'_l))$. The first term in a_{ik} is the probability for voxel i to belong to tissue k without any structure knowledge. The sum over k of the two other terms is one and they can be interpreted as the probability for i to belong to the tissue class k when information on structure segmentation is available. Parameter values per voxel are then computed by cubic splines interpolation between ψ_c and $\psi_{c'}$ for all $c'\in\mathcal{N}(c)$ so that smooth variations between neighboring subvolumes are ensured and the intensity nonuniformity is handled inside each subvolume. For the **M-$\mathcal{R}$** step, we get from (4), $\mathcal{R}^{(r+1)} = \arg\max_{\mathcal{R}\in\underline{\mathcal{R}}}\left(H(\mathcal{R}) + \mathbb{E}_{q_T^{(r+1)}}[H_{T,\mathcal{R}}(\mathbf{T},\mathcal{R})] + \mathbb{E}_{q_S^{(r+1)}}[H_{S,\mathcal{R}}(\mathbf{S},\mathcal{R})]\right)$. In practice, the global parameters $\mathcal{R}^G$ are determined in a pre-processing step using some standard intensity based method such as FLIRT[1]. For the other

---
[1] http://www.fmrib.ox.ac.uk/fsl/flirt/

transformations, we adopt a relaxation approach and update the 12 parameters defining each local affine transformation $\mathcal{R}_l^S$ by maximizing in turn:

$$\text{M-}\mathcal{R}: \quad \mathcal{R}_l^{S\,(r+1)} = \arg\max_{\mathcal{R}_l^S}\left(H(\mathcal{R}) + \sum_{i\in V}\sum_{k=1}^{3} q_{T_i}^{(r+1)}(e_k)\log\left(f_T^k(\mathcal{R},i)+\epsilon\right)\right.$$
$$\left.+ \sum_{i\in V}\sum_{i=1}^{L+1} q_{S_i}^{(r+1)}(e_l')\log\left(f_S^l(\mathcal{R},i)+\epsilon\right)\right).$$

There exists no simple expression and the optimization is performed numerically using a variant of the Powell algorithm.

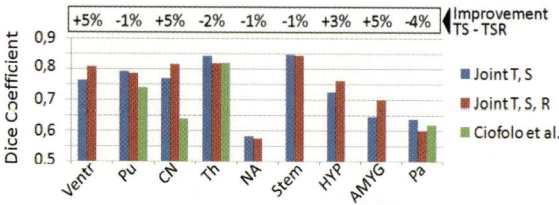

Fig. 1. Evaluation on IBSR v2 (9 right structures) and comparison with [9]

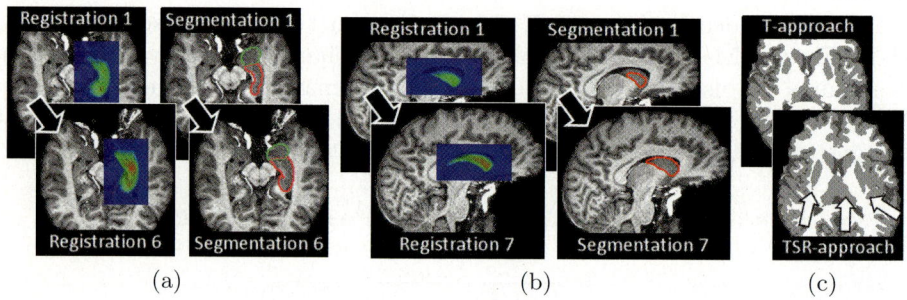

Fig. 2. (a) Evolution of hippocampus local affine registration and segmentation; (b) Evolution of the caudate atlas registration and segmentation after an artificial perturbation of the initial registration; (c) Tissue segmentations with T and TSR approaches

4 Evaluation

We chose to set parameters η_T and η_S to the inverse of a decreasing temperature as generally done. The precision parameters λ_c^{0k} were set to $N_c\lambda_g^k$ where N_c is the number of voxels in c and λ_g^k is a rough precision estimation for class k obtained by a standard global EM algorithm. The α_c^k's were set to $|\mathcal{N}(c)|$, b_c^k to $|\mathcal{N}(c)|/\lambda_g^k$ and the tissue subvolumes size to 20^3 voxels. The atlas used was the Harvard-Oxford subcortical probabilistic atlas. For a fair comparison, we first carried out tissue segmentation only. The results were equivalent to that in [4] and quantitatively comparable to the results from FAST and SPM5 for lower computational times. They showed robustness both to noise and to nonuniformities. We then rather focused on evaluating the coupling performance. We computed via STAPLE a 3-structure BrainWeb gold standard from three manual expert segmentations of the left caudate, left putamen and left thalamus. When combining tissue and structure segmentations (TS approach), the mean Dice metric over 8 experiments (phantoms with 3%, 5%, 7%, 9% of noise, and 20% or 40% of nonuniformity) was respectively 74%, 90% and 90% for the three structures (computational time: 25 min on a Pentium 2Ghz, 2Go RAM). When adding registration in the combination (TSR approach), it reached respectively 91%, 95% and 94% (computational time: 50 min), showing great improvement for the caudate whose atlas was initially badly registered. Comparatively, [4] reported respectively 74%, 85% and 91%. We then considered 18 images from the IBSR v2 database. The mean Dice metric for the 9 right structures (17 were segmented) is reported in Fig. 1). Most structure segmentations were improved by the introduction of registration in the coupling (mean improvement: +4.5% ; mean degradation: -1.2%). Then Fig. 2 shows the results for a real 3T brain scan. Fig. 2(a) illustrates how registration and structure segmentation improve with iterations while in Fig. 2(b), the initial caudate registration was perturbed artificially to point out the ability of our approach to correct the mis-alignment and recover a correct segmentation. Eventually, Fig. 2(c) shows that the final tissue segmentation is much better with the TSR approach.

5 Discussion

Our approach provides general guidelines to deal with complex joint processes. It is based on the initial specification of a joint probabilistic model decomposed into parts to account for various type of interactions. We used this strategy to integrate an atlas registration with a tissue and structure segmentation process. We proposed a model that captures several level of interactions 1) spatial dependencies between voxels for robustness to noise, 2) spatial dependencies between local intensity models to ensure their consistency, 3) relationships between tissue and structure labels and 4) relationships between labels and local affine atlas registration parameters. In addition to the inclusion of registration, we built on the approach in [4] by introducing new tissue and structure interaction terms. As a result of the joint approach, these new terms correspond to a more symmetric cooperation between tissues and structures. Besides, we obtained very good results that confirmed the benefits of allowing symmetric interactions and including registration as part of the model components rather than as a separate step. Further refinements include the introduction of an *a priori* $H(\mathcal{R})$ for the registration and the addition of a sulci lines segmentation process. We believe the use of training data as in [5] will facilitate registration parameters estimation and further improve the results. Also, interactions between sulci lines and tissue segmentation could reduce the over-regularization effect of MRF around sulci.

References

1. Yang, F., Kruggel, F.: Automatic segmentation of human brain sulci. Medical Image Analysis 12(4), 442–451 (2008)
2. Yu, Z.Q., Zhu, Y., Yang, J., Zhu, Y.M.: A hybrid region-boundary model for cerebral cortical segmentation in MRI. Comp. Med. Imag. and Graph 30(3), 197–208 (2006)
3. Ashburner, J., Friston, K.J.: Unified Segmentation. NeuroImage 26, 839–851 (2005)
4. Scherrer, B., Forbes, F., Garbay, C., Dojat, M.: Fully bayesian joint model for MR brain scan tissue and structure segmentation. In: Metaxas, D., Axel, L., Fichtinger, G., Székely, G. (eds.) MICCAI 2008, Part II. LNCS, vol. 5242, pp. 1066–1074. Springer, Heidelberg (2008)
5. Pohl, K.M., Fisher, J., Grimson, W.E.L., Kikinis, R., Wells, W.M.: A Bayesian model for joint segmentation and registration. NeuroImage 31(1), 228–239 (2006)
6. Gelman, A.: et al: Bayesian Data Analysis, 2nd edn. Chapman and Hall, Boca Raton (2004)
7. Jordan, M., Ghahramani, Z., Jaakkola, T., Saul, L.: An introduction to variational methods for graphical models. In: Learning in Graphical Models, pp. 105–162 (1998)
8. Byrne, W., Gunawardana, A.: Convergence theorems of Generalized Alternating Minimization Procedures. J. Machine Learning Research 6, 2049–2073 (2005)
9. Ciofolo, C., Barillot, C.: Shape analysis and fuzzy control for 3D competitive segmentation of brain structures with level sets. In: Leonardis, A., Bischof, H., Pinz, A. (eds.) ECCV 2006. LNCS, vol. 3951, pp. 458–470. Springer, Heidelberg (2006)

Robust Atlas-Based Brain Segmentation Using Multi-structure Confidence-Weighted Registration

Ali R. Khan[1], Moo K. Chung[2], and Mirza Faisal Beg[1]

[1] School of Engineering Science, Simon Fraser University, 8888 University Drive, Burnaby BC, V5A 1S6, Canada
akhanf@sfu.ca, mfbeg@ensc.sfu.ca
[2] Waisman Laboratory for Brain Imaging and Behavior, University of Wisconsin, Madison, WI 53706, USA
mkchung@wisc.edu

Abstract. We present a robust and accurate atlas-based brain segmentation method which uses multiple initial structure segmentations to simultaneously drive the image registration and achieve anatomically constrained correspondence. We also derive segmentation confidence maps (SCMs) from a given manually segmented training set; these characterize the accuracy of a given set of segmentations as compared to manual segmentations. We incorporate these in our cost term to weight the influence of initial segmentations in the multi-structure registration, such that low confidence regions are given lower weight in the registration. To account for correspondence errors in the underlying registration, we use a supervised atlas correction technique and present a method for correcting the atlas segmentation to account for possible errors in the underlying registration. We applied our multi-structure atlas-based segmentation and supervised atlas correction to segment the amygdala in a set of 23 autistic patients and controls using leave-one-out cross validation, achieving a Dice overlap score of 0.84. We also applied our method to eight subcortical structures in MRI from the Internet Brain Segmentation Repository, with results better or comparable to competing methods.

1 Introduction

Developing robust, automated tools for brain MR image registration and segmentation is challenging due to many factors including the high degree of neuroanatomical variability in both healthy controls and patients. Registration and segmentation of medical images can be aided by using expert-derived features, but this manual intervention step can become costly in very large studies and can also suffer from rater drift. Automated computation of such features can eliminate the need for manual intervention, however the reliability and accuracy of automatically generated features is also influenced by the variability in image quality and neuroanatomy, in addition to the systemic bias, if any, present in this automated method. Hence, using a small set of manually labeled training images, learning the accuracy of the automatically generated features can be used to improve the overall utility of these features.

We have extended the large deformation atlas-based brain MRI segmentation approach of [1], which used Freesurfer segmentation labels to initialize the region of interest (ROI) based registration, to instead use the Freesurfer labels as anatomical constraints simultaneously during registration. The main motivation for this is that the simultaneous usage of the automated segmentations as separate cost terms allows the overall MR image matching to help avoid local minima, while providing flexibility in setting weights for different channels to emphasize certain properties, such as larger weight for smaller structures, or smaller weight where the channel data is known to be less reliable. We accomplish this by using a multi-cost registration framework, with each additional data term utilizing the matching of one automatically-generated segmentation label.

Our approach is also similar in spirit to [2], which presented multi-channel registration with a few semi-automatically defined subcortical structures that were quality controlled and corrected manually prior to their use in the registration. However, instead of correcting the automated segmentations manually for each image, we attempt to learn the errors made by the automatic segmentation method using the segmentation confidence maps from a small set of manually labeled images, and account for these for segmentation of all other images in the database. To avoid computation of SCMs for each cohort atlas and to work with cohort datasets that do not have some manually segmented scans to construct the SCMs, we show how to transfer SCMs from another database atlas. We generate and apply the SCMs to weight the automated segmentations that are used as "features" in our atlas-based segmentation.

In single atlas propagation, errors or bias in the atlas segmentation, perhaps due to manual rater error, can also lead to the bias being propagated in all atlas-propagation derived segmentations. Furthermore, if the atlas contains anatomical variability, which the registration is not able to accommodate fully, then the propagated segmentations will also possess this template-dependent anatomical bias. To account for this additional source of variability, we present a supervised atlas correction procedure, which involves performing atlas-based segmentation on a manually labeled training set to learn the systematic bias present in the atlas, and correcting the atlas segmentation correspondingly. In this paper we describe our method for the generation of SCMs, multi-structure registration and supervised atlas correction, apply these techniques to two datasets, and compare our results with current brain segmentation methods.

2 Method and Materials

2.1 Brain MRI Datasets

The Internet Brain Segmentation Repository (IBSR) dataset consists of 18 T1-weighted MR scans, with some manually segmented structures. This is a public database used by many groups to test segmentation methods ([3,4,5,6,7]).

The amygdala dataset consisted of T1-weighted scans from 24 subjects (12/12 autism/control), aged 10-24 [8], along with manual segmentations.

2.2 Segmentation Confidence Maps

In using automated segmentations for registration, segmentation errors could result in correspondence errors. We wish to learn the errors that an automated segmentation method makes so that if a given region in an automated segmentation consistently exhibits lower accuracy, we would like to reduce its contribution to the registration. To this end we have defined a segmentation confidence map (SCM), α^j, for each anatomical structure, j, as the probability of accuracy:

$$\alpha^j(x) = P(f^j_{error}(x) < \epsilon), \qquad (1)$$

where $f^j_{error}(x)$ is the distribution of segmentation errors at spatial location x, and ϵ is a distance bound placed on the confidence map. To find $f^j_{error}(x)$, we require a map of segmentation errors between a manual gold standard, M^j, and an automated segmentation, A^j. Because correspondence between M^j and A^j is not known, we approximate this using the signed distance transforms of the binary segmentations, denoted as $DT(\cdot)$, to obtain the closest boundary distances between the manual and automated contours, so that:

$$f^j_{error}(x) \approx d^j_{M,A}(x) = \begin{cases} 0 & \text{if } M^j(x) = A^j(x), \\ (|DT_{M^j}(x)| + |DT_{A^j}(x)|)^2 & \text{if } M^j(x) \neq A^j(x). \end{cases}$$

We also used grayscale dilation followed by Gaussian smoothing ($\sigma = 1.0$) to widen the affected neighborhood. After computing this approximation for f^j_{error}, we can determine α^j by evaluating $P(f^j_{error}(x) < \epsilon)$ over a manually labeled training set.

Supervised Training/Learning. For a given small set of M training images A_k, we first compute error maps f^j_{error,A_k} for each structure j in each image A_k. To learn the combined confidence map, we then spatially transform these to a chosen template space, B, using the large deformation diffeomorphic metric mapping (LDDMM) transformation between individual automated segmentations, A_k^j and B^j. To compute the confidence map on B, we use the transformed error maps $f^j_{error,A_k} \circ \phi_{B^j,A_k^j}$, to generate sample histograms at each voxel using a $3 \times 3 \times M$ neighborhood. We used a distance bound, $\epsilon = 1$mm, and Equation 1 to compute α^j_B for each segmented structure j. Note that for computational reasons we computed confidence maps for each structure in each hemisphere separately, then combined them to create a confidence map relating to both hemispheres of a given structure. Figure 1 shows the SCM for the caudate nucleus in which the highest variability in automated segmentation is found to be around its tail. This is reasonable as the narrow caudate tail is where automated segmentation algorithms are likely to yield the highest variability.

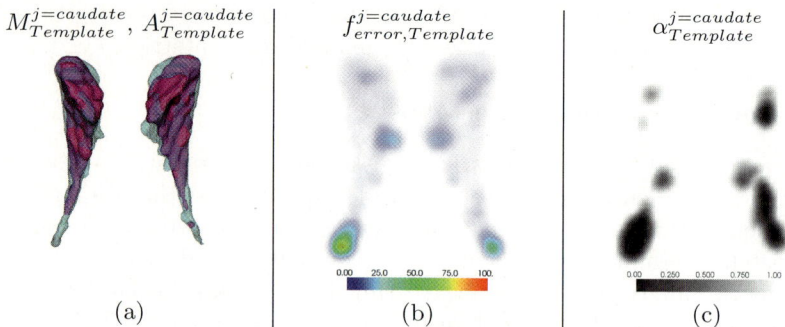

Fig. 1. Visualizations showing the generation of the segmentation confidence map (SCM) for the caudate nucleus: (a) manual (magenta) and initial automated (blue) segmentations for the template brain, (b) distance error map $f_{error,Template}^{j=caudate}$, (c) caudate SCM, $\alpha_{Template}^{j=caudate}$, computed using distance error maps from all images in the training set. Note that the SCM identifies regions of highest segmentation variability to be near the tail of the caudate.

Propagation to Cohort Atlas. If cohorts are structurally similar such as matched for age and pathological state, then the SCMs learned from one cohort can be propagated to the other cohort atlas. We propagate SCMs from one cohort atlas, α_B^j, to another, α_C^j, by spatially transforming the maps, defined on B, to the space of C using the LDDMM transformation between their automated segmentations, B^j and C^j. By performing this step for each structure, j, we can estimate the SCMs for any cohort atlas given a previously trained SCM.

2.3 Multi-structure Confidence-Weighted Registration

To introduce multiple structures into a diffeomorphic registration scheme, we extended the large deformation diffeomorphic metric mapping (LDDMM) [9] method to use multiple data terms, each weighted with a SCM. Let the pair A^{MR} and B^{MR} of brain ROI MR images be given to be registered, where B is the designated template, and let their N automated segmentations, $A^j, j \in [1, \ldots, N]$ and $B^j, j \in [1, \ldots, N]$ be available. The diffeomorphic transformation matching A and B is given by $\varphi = \phi_1 : \Omega \to \Omega$ such that $A(\phi_1^{-1}) \approx B$. This transformation ϕ_1^{-1} results from velocity $\dot{\phi}_t = v_t(\phi_t), v_t \in V, t \in [0,1]$ where V is a space of smooth vector fields on Ω. The energy for the extended confidence-weighted multi-structure registration to be minimized is therefore:

$$\int_0^1 \|v_t\|_V^2 dt + \|A^{MR}(\phi_1^{-1}) - B^{MR}\|_{L^2}^2 + \sum_{j=1}^N \|\sqrt{\alpha_B^j}\left(A^j(\phi_1^{-1}) - B^j\right)\|_{L^2}^2, \quad (2)$$

which uses the confidence map for a given structure, α_B^j to weight the mismatch $A^j(\phi_1^{-1}) - B^j$. Note that because the cost is computed in the coordinate frame of template B, the SCM need only be specified for B. Figure 2 shows the multi-structure registration images for the the left amygdala ROI registration, along with the corresponding SCMs.

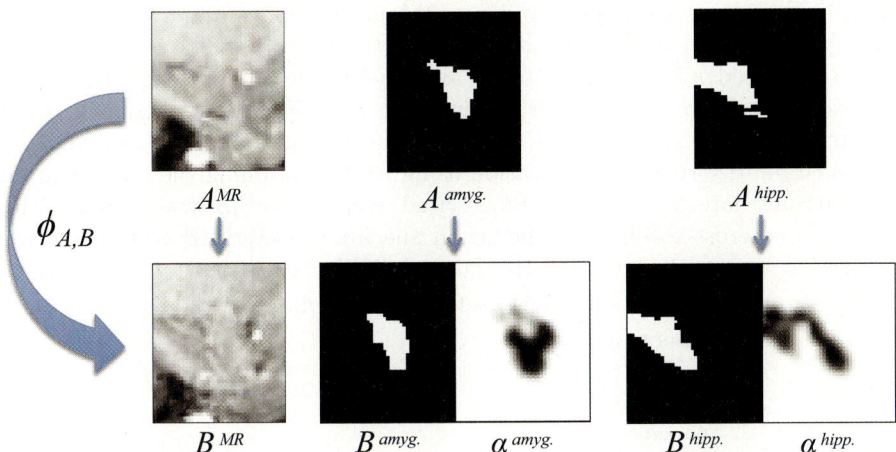

Fig. 2. Illustration of the multi-structure confidence-weighted registration for the left ROI in the amygdala segmentation, showing the MR images, initial segmentations, and SCMs. The multi-structure registration used the left hippocampus, amygdala and lateral ventricle along with the MRI images to find the optimal ROI transformation.

2.4 Supervised Atlas Correction

Suppose atlas-based segmentation between an atlas, A and a target image T gives an invertible transformation $\phi_{A,T}$ which transforms the atlas labels, A_M to T via $\phi_{A,T}(A_M)$. In the ideal case of perfect registration, if T_M are known target labels, then $\phi_{T,A}(T_M) = A_M$, but due to errors in registration and manual labeling, this is not observed. However, if, given the manually labelled target T_M, the atlas labels were 'corrected' to be $\phi_{T,A}(T_M)$, then label propagation would result in perfect segmentation correspondence. We use this insight to average the back-propagated labels, $\phi_{T,A}(T_M)$, for all images in a training set, and denote this as the 'corrected' atlas segmentation. The corrected segmentation accounts for both manual labeling inconsistencies and systematic correspondence errors, thus improving the overall label propagation.

2.5 Experimental Procedure

All brain MR images were processed with the Freesurfer image analysis suite (version 4.1.0), using the subcortical processing stream [10], which labels 37 volumetric structures; these segmentations were used as the initial automated segmentations for our method. In preparation for atlas-based ROI segmentation, the MR images underwent pre-processing including affine registration, definition of a bounding box for each hemisphere and histogram-based intensity normalization. Thus for each target image, a cropped region of interest (ROI) for each hemisphere, containing the structures to be segmented, was linearly aligned and intensity normalized to the corresponding ROI in the template MRI.

For the IBSR dataset, we used two disjoint sets for training and testing; nine brains were used to generate Freesurfer SCMs for the left and right caudate, putamen, pallidum, nucleus accumbens, thalamus, hippocampus, amygdala, and lateral ventricles, with the other nine used as the test data. The multi-structure registration used all eight structures along with the MRI to find the diffeomorphic transformation for each hemispheric ROI. For the amygdala dataset, we propagated the IBSR SCMs to an arbitrarily chosen control subject, and performed multi-structure registration using ROIs containing the hippocampus, amygdala and lateral ventricles. Supervised atlas correction was tested with a leave-one-out cross-validation scheme on the above described test data. Spatial overlap was measured with the Dice similarity coefficient, $DSC(A,M) = \frac{2V(A \cap M)}{V(A)+V(M)}$, where $V(A)$ and $V(M)$ refers to the volume of the automated and manual segmentations respectively.

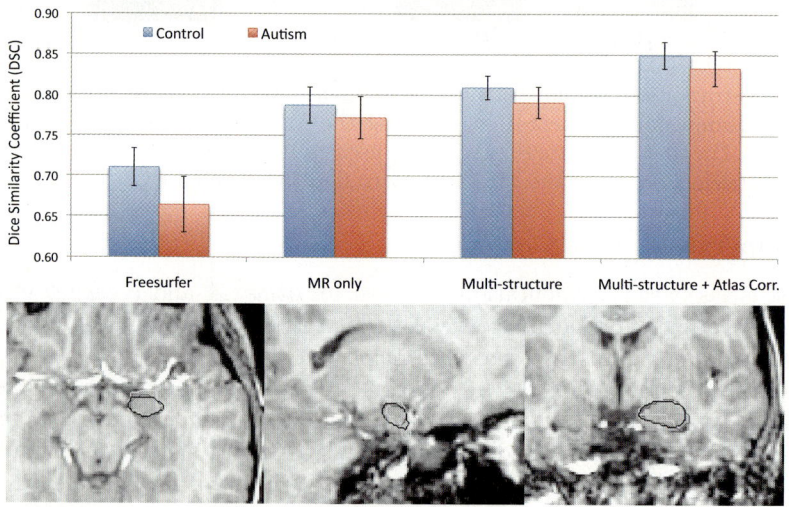

Fig. 3. Top: Mean DSC for the amygdala dataset, where the height of the error bars is equal to the standard deviation. Bottom: Representative axial (left), sagittal (center), and coronal (right) slices showing amygdala segmentations for the manual rater (pink), Freesurfer (yellow) and the multi-structure atlas-corrected method.

Table 1. Dice similarity coefficients for amygdala segmentation for our method and competing methods using various datasets, with standard deviations shown where available. Note that both methods in the first two rows use the same amygdala dataset.

Method	Cohort	Age range	DSC (L ; R)
Our method	healthy/autistic	13-23/10-24	0.85 ± 0.033 / 0.83 ± 0.043
Fischl et al. [10]	healthy/autistic	13-23/10-24	0.71 ± 0.047 / 0.66 ± 0.068
Pohl et al. [11]	schiz.+healthy	18-41	0.86 ± 0.028; 0.85 ± 0.030
Chupin et al. [12]	healthy/Alzheimer's	$< 35/66$-81	0.81 ± 0.04 / 0.76 ± 0.07
Heckemann et al. [13]	healthy	20-54	0.80 ; 0.81

Table 2. DSCs on the IBSR dataset, with **bold** entries denoting the highest performing for each structure, with standard deviation shown in parentheses where available

Method	Lat. Vent.	Caud.	Put.	Thal.	Pall.	Nuc. Acc.	Hipp.	Amyg.
Our method	**0.85** (0.06)	**0.83** (0.03)	**0.87** (0.02)	**0.89** (0.01)	0.72 (0.09)	**0.61** (0.10)	**0.76** (0.03)	0.66 (0.08)
Fischl et al. [10]	0.78 (0.07)	0.82 (0.05)	0.81 (0.02)	0.86 (0.02)	0.71 (0.13)	0.58 (0.08)	0.75 (0.02)	**0.68** (0.06)
Akselrod-Ballin et al. [3]	-	0.80	0.79	0.84	**0.74**	-	0.69	0.63
Gouttard et al. [4]	**0.85**	0.76	0.78	-	0.72	-	0.67	0.64
Joshi et al. [5]	-	0.54	0.49	0.60	-	-	0.41	-
Ciofolo et al. [6]	-	0.65	0.70	0.77	0.58	-	-	-
Zhou et al. [7]	-	0.80 (0.08)	0.81 (0.06)	0.84 (0.06)	-	-	0.70 (0.11)	0.64 (0.15)
Shen et al. [14] (in [5])	-	0.54	0.45	0.74	-	-	0.30	-
Woods et al. [15] (in [5])	-	0.40	0.36	0.65	-	-	0.50	-

3 Results

Spatial overlaps for the amygdala dataset are shown in top row of Figure 3, with the multi-structure segmentation outperforming the Freesurfer segmentations used in the multi-structure registration, and the supervised atlas correction further improving the results. For all methods performance is better for the control subjects, with the highest mean DSC being 0.85 and 0.83 for control and autism subjects respectively. Bottom panel shows representative MRI slices of an autism subject, with manual and our automated (multi-structure, atlas-corrected) segmentation outlines. Table 1 compares the amygdala DSCs to competing methods, and Table 2 summarizes results on the IBSR database.

4 Conclusions and Discussions

As evident in Table 1, performance of our amygdala segmentations compares very favorably among the current state-of-the-art methods; only the method in [11], which performs hierarchical parcellation of the brain, reports slightly higher but comparable numbers. Multiple atlas propagation and fusion is used in [13] with good results, a technique that can also be applied with the proposed method to further improve performance at the cost of additional registrations. The best results for the IBSR database, shown in Table 2, are emphasized in bold, with our method showing the highest spatial overlap for the majority of structures (lateral ventricles, caudate, putamen, thalamus, nucleus accumbens, and hippocampus), and within 0.02 of the highest for the pallidum and amygdala.

Supervised training in this setting, used in both the SCM generation and atlas correction steps, can be problematic if differences exist between the training set and the test set, such as manual segmentation protocols, scanner differences, or pathological differences. For the supervised atlas correction these differences could lead to degraded performance, since errors in the corrected segmentation would correspond directly with final segmentation errors, which is why we chose to use cross-validation on the test data for this purpose. For the SCM generation, however, we did use a single training set for both the IBSR and amygdala segmentation; satisfactory results were obtained likely because the Freesurfer segmentations had consistent bias or errors for both datasets. We plan to further study the consistency and applicability of SCMs generated from different training sets. To conclude, we have proposed a novel two-fold strategy for improving performance of atlas-based brain segmentation using multi-structure confidence-weighted registration, and supervised atlas-correction. Results show promise for improved segmentation of many subcortical structures, including the amygdala, with performance better than or comparable to the leading current methods.

References

1. Khan, A.R., Wang, L., Beg, M.F.: Freesurfer-initiated fully-automated subcortical brain segmentation in MRI using large deformation diffeomorphic metric mapping. Neuroimage 41(3), 735–746 (2008)
2. Magnotta, V.A., Bockholt, H.J., Johnson, H.J., Christensen, G.E., Andreasen, N.C.: Subcortical, cerebellar, and magnetic resonance based consistent brain image registration. Neuroimage 19(2 Pt 1), 233–245 (2003)
3. Akselrod-Ballin, A., Galun, M., Gomori, J.M., Brandt, A., Basri, R.: Prior knowledge driven multiscale segmentation of brain MRI. Medical image computing and computer-assisted intervention 10(Pt 2), 118–126 (2007)
4. Gouttard, S., Styner, M., Joshi, S., Smith, R., Hazlett, H., Gerig, G.: Subcortical structure segmentation using probabilistic atlas priors. In: Proceedings of SPIE, vol. 6512, p. 65122J (2007)
5. Joshi, A., Shattuck, D., Thompson, P., Leahy, R.: Surface-constrained volumetric brain registration using harmonic mappings. IEEE Transactions on Medical Imaging 26(12), 1657–1669 (2007)
6. Ciofolo, C., Barillot, C.: Brain segmentation with competitive level sets and fuzzy control. Information processing in medical imaging 19, 333–344 (2005)
7. Zhou, J., Rajapakse, J.: Segmentation of subcortical brain structures using fuzzy templates. Neuroimage 28(4), 915–924 (2005)
8. Nacewicz, B.M., Dalton, K.M., Johnstone, T., Long, M.T., McAuliff, E.M., Oakes, T.R., Alexander, A.L., Davidson, R.J.: Amygdala volume and nonverbal social impairment in adolescent and adult males with autism. Archives of general psychiatry 63(12), 1417–1428 (2006)
9. Beg, M.F., Miller, M.I., Trouvé, A., Younes, L.: Computing large deformation metric mappings via geodesic flows of diffeomorphisms. International Journal of Computer Vision 61(2), 139–157 (2005)
10. Fischl, B., Salat, D., Busa, E., Albert, M., Dieterich, M., Haselgrove, C., van der Kouwe, A., Killiany, R., Kennedy, D., Klaveness, S.: Whole brain segmentation automated labeling of neuroanatomical structures in the human brain. Neuron 33(3), 341–355 (2002)
11. Pohl, K.M., Bouix, S., Nakamura, M., Rohlfing, T., McCarley, R.W., Kikinis, R., Grimson, W.E.L., Shenton, M.E., Wells, W.M.: A hierarchical algorithm for MR brain image parcellation. IEEE Transactions on Medical Imaging 26(9), 1201–1212 (2007)

12. Chupin, M., Mukuna-Bantumbakulu, A., Hasboun, D., Bardinet, E., Baillet, S., Kinkingnéhun, S., Lemieux, L., Dubois, B., Garnero, L.: Anatomically constrained region deformation for the automated segmentation of the hippocampus and the amygdala: method and validation on controls and patients with Alzheimer's disease. Neuroimage 34(3), 996–1019 (2007)
13. Heckemann, R., Hajnal, J., Aljabar, P., Rueckert, D., Hammers, A.: Automatic anatomical brain MRI segmentation combining label propagation and decision fusion. Neuroimage 33(1), 115–126 (2006)
14. Shen, D., Davatzikos, C.: Hammer: hierarchical attribute matching mechanism for elastic registration. IEEE Transactions on Medical Imaging 21(11), 1421–1439 (2002)
15. Woods, R.P., Grafton, S.T., Holmes, C.J., Cherry, S.R., Mazziotta, J.C.: Automated image registration: I. general methods and intrasubject, intramodality validation. Journal of Computer Assisted Tomography 22(1), 139–152 (1998)

Discriminative, Semantic Segmentation of Brain Tissue in MR Images

Zhao Yi[1], Antonio Criminisi[2], Jamie Shotton[2], and Andrew Blake[2]

[1] University of California, Los Angeles, USA
zyi@ucla.edu
[2] Microsoft Research Cambridge, UK
{antcrim,jamie.shotton,ablake}@microsoft.com

Abstract. A new algorithm is presented for the automatic segmentation and classification of brain tissue from 3D MR scans. It uses discriminative Random Decision Forest classification and takes into account partial volume effects. This is combined with correction of intensities for the MR bias field, in conjunction with a learned model of spatial context, to achieve accurate voxel-wise classification. Our quantitative validation, carried out on existing labelled datasets, demonstrates improved results over the state of the art, especially for the cerebro-spinal fluid class which is the most difficult to label accurately.

1 Introduction

This paper introduces a new, supervised technique for the classification of 3D MR scans of the brain. The ultimate goal is to assign a class label to each brain voxel from the following set: white matter, grey matter and cerebro-spinal fluid. Such automatic analysis is of practical interest to many clinical applications related to early detection and treatment of schizophrenia [1], epilepsy [2] and Alzheimer's [3]. Automatic segmentation of brain tissue is a challenging problem, owing to acquisition noise, non-uniformities in the MR magnetic field, the complex anatomy of the brain, limited resolution and partial volume effects.

In order to address these problems we propose an algorithm in three steps: 1) bias field correction using polynomials of optimal degree; 2) learned models for automatic tissue classification/segmentation; and 3) partial volume estimation. Model training accounts for much of the accuracy of our technique, and is utilized as much as possible, not only in the segmentation process, but also during bias field correction and partial volume estimation. The tissue classification step is achieved via randomized decision trees [4,5], an efficient, state-of-the-art discriminative classification technique.

Previous Work. The substantial existing literature on this topic may be roughly grouped into the following four different sets:

Clustering algorithms. Representative work in this area includes the use of K-means [6], mean-shift [7], and expectation-maximization (EM) [8,9,10]. Their limitation is that the cluster geometry and the number of clusters have to be known, where parametric forms such as Gaussian or Gaussian mixtures are commonly assumed but without taking into consideration existing domain knowledge.

Atlas-based approaches. Segmentation is reduced to a template matching problem, where labels are transferred from a prelabeled atlas to the subject volume via registration techniques [2,3,11]. However, registration itself is challenging, especially for the human cortex due to the high variability of the cortical shape and the location of sulci and gyri across individuals.

Deformable models. Relying on curve propagation, deformable models minimize a certain energy associated with the curve to partition the image domain, like active contours [12] and level sets [13,14]. Those techniques typically suffer from problems with initialization and local minima.

Supervised learning. Surprisingly, supervised learning has received relatively little attention in brain tissue segmentation. In [2] the intensity distribution of each class at every location is modeled as a Gaussian, with spatial information encoded globally via a probabilistic atlas and locally via an anisotropic non-stationary Markov random field. This Gaussian assumption, however, is restrictive to inter-subject variability and image distortions. The work in [15] learns a multi-class discriminative appearance model by a probabilistic boosting tree together with a generative active shape model for each subcortical structure. It works well for regular subcortical structures, but is not suitable for the brain tissue segmentation task which involves highly convoluted cortical surfaces.

2 Discriminative Brain Tissue Segmentation

Given the observed MR brain volume $I : \Omega \subset \mathbb{R}^3 \mapsto \mathbb{R}^+$ our goal is to assign to each voxel a class label from the following set: white matter (WM), gray matter (GM), and cerebro-spinal fluid (CSF). This task is formulated as a maximum-a-posteriori (MAP) classification problem, whose output is the label map $L^\star$: $\Omega \mapsto \{$CSF, GM, WM$\}$ such that

$$L^\star = \arg\max_L \log P(L|I) = \arg\max_L \log P(I|L) + \log P(L). \qquad (1)$$

Under the simplistic but common assumption that voxel intensities are mutually independent given their labels, the data likelihood in (1) can be rewritten as

$$\log P(I|L) = \sum_{\mathbf{x} \in \Omega} \log P(I(\mathbf{x})|L(\mathbf{x})). \qquad (2)$$

The label prior in (1) can be decomposed into two terms in the Markov Random Field framework, i.e.

$$\log P(L) = \sum_{\mathbf{x} \in \Omega} \log U(L(\mathbf{x})) + \sum_{\mathbf{x},\mathbf{y}} V(L(\mathbf{x}), L(\mathbf{y})), \qquad (3)$$

where U is the unary location prior, and V imposes spatial smoothness between neighboring labels (not considered yet). The following sections describe details of how to model $P(I(\mathbf{x})|L(\mathbf{x}))$ as well as $U(L(\mathbf{x}))$. We start by looking at the likelihood $P(I(\mathbf{x})|L(\mathbf{x}))$ and how it is affected by the magnetic bias field.

2.1 Bias Field Correction

Owing to the bias field induced by the MR scanner, the observed intensity of voxels is a corrupted version of the true intensity of the underlying tissue. In order to model the likelihood $P(I(\mathbf{x})|L(\mathbf{x}))$, we need to recover the true intensity of each voxel by estimating the bias field and correcting for it.

Let $\bar{I}$ denote the true intensity, b the bias field, and n the random noise. Here a multiplicative bias with i.i.d. Gaussian noise is assumed, i.e., $I(\mathbf{x}) = b(\mathbf{x}) \cdot \bar{I}(\mathbf{x}) + n(\mathbf{x})$. This MR image formation model has been used frequently [16,17] as it is simple and known to be consistent with the inhomogeneous sensitivity of the reception coil. Since the bias field is smoothly varying in space, we adopt a low-order polynomial model: $b(\mathbf{x}) = \boldsymbol{\lambda} \cdot \boldsymbol{\Gamma}^n(\mathbf{x})$, where $\boldsymbol{\lambda}$ is the coefficient vector, $n \in \{0, 1, 2, \ldots\}$ is the order of polynomial, and $\boldsymbol{\Gamma}^n$ is the base polynomial vector. For example, $\boldsymbol{\Gamma}^1(\mathbf{x}) = (x, y, 1)^T$, $\boldsymbol{\Gamma}^2(\mathbf{x}) = (x^2, xy, x, y^2, y, 1)^T$. As MR acquisition is done sequentially, it is reasonable to assume that $\boldsymbol{\lambda}$ is different slice by slice. Thus, our bias model holds for every individual slice and $\boldsymbol{\Gamma}^n$ is applied to (x, y) only (not to the third dimension).

On the other hand, we can assume that the true intensity of each voxel depends only on the underlying tissue label $\bar{I}(\mathbf{x}) = \mu_{L(\mathbf{x})}$, where $\mu \in \{\mu_{\text{CSF}}, \mu_{\text{GM}}, \mu_{\text{WM}}\}$ is the tissue intensity for label $L(\mathbf{x})$, and have uniform values throughout the volume. Given the values of n, I and $\boldsymbol{\Gamma}^n$, if L were known then iterative least squares fitting could be applied to determine the optimal solution of $\boldsymbol{\lambda}$ for each slice and $\mu_{\text{CSF}}, \mu_{\text{GM}}, \mu_{\text{WM}}$ for every volume. In practice, however, a ground-truth labeling for L is not available but probabilistic tissue labeling may be used to tackle the problem. Let $q_{\text{CSF}}(\mathbf{x}), q_{\text{GM}}(\mathbf{x}), q_{\text{WM}}(\mathbf{x})$ denote the probabilities of the voxel $\mathbf{x}$ belonging to each tissue. The expected value of the true intensity in this case is a weighted sum of all tissue intensities and our intensity model changes to

$$\bar{I}(\mathbf{x}) = \sum_{L \in \{\text{CSF}, \text{GM}, \text{WM}\}} q_L(\mathbf{x}) \mu_L. \qquad (4)$$

The same iterative fitting procedure can be applied as before. The optimal degree of the polynomial is obtained on the validation set by performing model selection using T-tests for successive degrees ($n = 0, \cdots, 4$). The Jaccard index $\text{JAC}(L, S) = |L \cap S| / |L \cup S|$ is used to measure the accuracy of the output label map L given the manual segmentation S. We obtain P values on WM and GM less than 5% between n and $n - 1$ when $n \leq 3$, and greater than 5% when $n > 3$. P values on CSF are always greater than 5% indicating no statistically significant difference between degrees. This is because dark CSF regions are insensitive to multiplicative bias. Thus we choose $n = 3$ for accuracy.

2.2 Maximum a Posteriori (MAP) Classification

In brain MR images, the (bias-corrected) intensity of a given tissue is approximately uniform, and the spatial assignment of different tissues is constrained by the underlying anatomy. Thus, it makes sense to use both intensity and location features as the basis of our tissue models. In the Bayesian formalism (1) we use intensity as a likelihood and location as a prior (see Fig. 1).

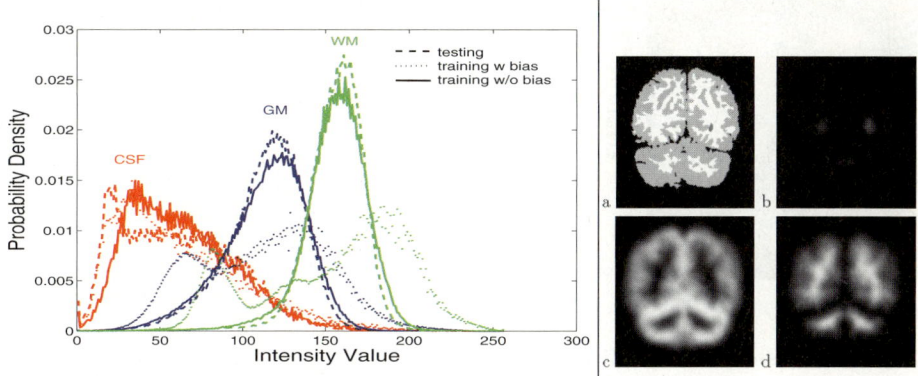

Fig. 1. MAP Classification Model: (left) Tissue intensity likelihood. The improved alignment of the training/testing distributions is an indication of the benefit of bias field correction (best viewed in color). **(right)** Probabilistic atlas example. **(a)** reference brain segmentation; **(b-d)** CSF/GM/WM probability maps.

Our intensity models are multi-modal and non-parametric since they take the form of simple histograms. This overcomes the unimodal limitations of single Gaussian [11,17] and the inefficiencies of EM-based Gaussian mixtures [8,9,10], without loss of accuracy. Location information is also exploited by constructing a probabilistic atlas from our own training set. We randomly select a reference volume from the training set, and then affinely register all other volumes to the chosen one. The atlas is obtained by averaging and Gaussian smoothing the label maps of the registered brain volumes. Our model so far has incorporated intensity information and location prior. Next we show how to incorporate further features such as gradient, texture, and context in our discriminative framework.

2.3 Tissue Classification via Random Decision Forests

A random decision forest [4] is a collection of T deterministic decision trees which differ from each other due to random repartitions of training data. This is known to aid generalization accuracy — intuitively, where one tree fails the others do well. Furthermore, a decision forest provides posterior probabilities for labels, as opposed to hard labellings, by pooling votes across the population of trees.

Training. During training, each point $\mathbf{x}$ is associated with a known class label $L(\mathbf{x}) = \{$ GM, WM, CSF $\}$, and is pushed through each of the trees starting at the root. Each tree node applies a binary test of the form: $f(\mathbf{x}; \boldsymbol{\theta}) > \tau$ and sends the data to one of its two child nodes accordingly. $f(\cdot)$ is a function characterized by its parameters $\boldsymbol{\theta}$ and applied to the voxel $\mathbf{x}$. τ is a threshold. For now it suffices to say that f computes certain visual features on the point at hand. At training time the parameters $\boldsymbol{\theta}, \tau$ of each node and the tree structure are all optimized by minimizing the data information gain. Randomness in the trees arises from noise being injected in the selection of the optimal node parameters. During

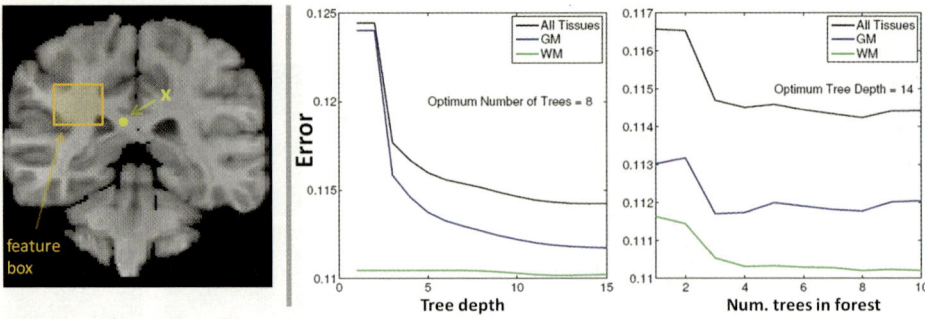

Fig. 2. Decision forests filters and results: (left) A shape filter used to provide context for the point **x** is computed from the feature box shown. (**middle-right**) Classification error — total (black), GM (blue), and WM (green) — as a function of the tree depth and the number of trees in the forest (best viewed in color).

training the leaf nodes update and store the empirical distributions over classes $P_{l_t(\mathbf{x})}(L(\mathbf{x}) = c)$, where l_t indexes the leaf node in the tth tree.

Testing. During testing each point **x** is pushed through each tree until it reaches a leaf node. The same input point **x** will end up in different leaf nodes, with different posterior probabilities. The output of the forest, for the point **x** is defined simply as the mean of all such posteriors: $P(L(\mathbf{x}) = c) = \sum_{t=1}^{T} P_{l_t(\mathbf{x})}(L(\mathbf{x}) = c) / T$. Now, a Maximum Likelihood classification for each voxel is obtained as: $c^\star = \arg\max_c P(L(\mathbf{x}) = c)$. Spatial prior could now be incorporated as before (1) but a more effective approach is described below.

Context-rich visual features. Here we use "shape filters" similar to the ones used in [5]; but applied to the 3D volume and without the need for "textonization". Fig. 2(left) illustrates these concepts on a 2D slice. For each voxel **x** a feature box F of random size and shape is selected at a random displacement from **x**. The size of the feature box is selected between 1 and 30 voxels. The feature response is then defined as $f(\mathbf{x}; F) = \sum_{\mathbf{q} \in F} C_i(\mathbf{q})$ where C_i indicates different "channels". In particular, here we make use of the following five image channels: the raw intensities $C_1(\mathbf{x}) = I(\mathbf{x})$, the image gradient $C_2(\mathbf{x}) = |\nabla I(\mathbf{x})|$, the atlas-based probabilities $C_3(\mathbf{x}) = P(L(\mathbf{x}))$, the intensity likelihood $C_4(\mathbf{x}) = P(I(\mathbf{x})|L(\mathbf{x}))$ from the trained histograms, and the label posterior $C_5(\mathbf{x}) = P(L(\mathbf{x})|I(\mathbf{x}))$ output of the MAP classifier from Sect. 2.2. The ability of our features to look at a large distance from the center pixel **x** yields context-rich information. As illustrated in Fig. 2(middle-right), increasing the tree depth or the forest size tends to decrease the decision forest classification error.

2.4 Modeling Partial Volume Effects

The limited image resolution causes many voxels to contain material from multiple tissues, which is the main reason of misclassification. The goal of this section is to locate such partial voxels $\Omega_m \subset \Omega$ in the image, as well as estimating the mixing fraction $\alpha : \Omega_m \mapsto [0,1]$.

Modeling mixed tissue classes. Here we assume that partial voxels contain at most two different tissue types and we adopt a mixture model to capture the mixing effect as follows: $I(\mathbf{x}) = \alpha(\mathbf{x})I_1 + (1 - \alpha(\mathbf{x}))I_2$, where I_1, I_2 are the underlying tissue intensities and α the mixing factor. When considering partial volume effects, the tissue classification problem is modified by extending the set of class labels to the following: { CSF, GM, WM, CSF/GM, GM/WM } (the transition CSF/WM is ignored here as it occurs rarely in practice [17]). Since partial voxels usually occur at tissue boundaries, we identify them by labelling the voxels at each side of the boundaries as partial. Then we learn the models for the CSF/GM and GM/WM mixtures directly, via the same method described before for pure tissue modeling. This technique proves to work better than modeling the mixed tissues by mixing the models of the pure tissues (see Fig. 4d,e for comparison).

Mixing fraction estimation. Using the models described above we can now assign one of the five class labels to each voxel. Then, we estimate the mixing fraction α by maximum-likelihood: $\alpha^\star(\mathbf{x}) = \arg\max_{\alpha \in [0,1]} \log P(I(\mathbf{x})|\alpha)$. Since we conservatively consider both sides of the tissue boundaries to be partial voxels, the built partial volume classifier tends to underestimate pure voxels. Thresholding the mixing fraction, so that partial voxels with $\alpha(\boldsymbol{x}) \leq \delta$ or $\alpha(\boldsymbol{x}) \geq 1 - \delta$ are relabeled as pure, marginally improves labelling accuracy. This threshold is also learned from the validation set, and in practice we found $\delta = 0.1$ to work well.

3 Results and Validation

Our approach is validated on the Internet Brain Segmentation Repository[1], where 20 normal subjects of T1-weighted brain MR images with expert segmentation are available. The volume size is around $256 \times 256 \times 60$, with voxel resolution $1mm \times 1mm \times 3mm$. We compute voxel-wise classification accuracy and the associated standard error by running our measurements on different random training-validation-testing splits. In each run the forest classifier is employed for discriminative optimization. Our results are compared to the state-of-the-art in Fig. 3. We achieve nearly 40% improvement on CSF, 5% on GM, and parity on WM, compared with the best methods. Note that our results are close to the "ideal" score obtained by human experts (last row).

Next, we demonstrate how the test paradigm may further be improved by taking into account partial volume effects. In Fig. 4d we show the confusion matrix results of partial volume classification, and show that, relative to our own results of pure tissue classification, error can be reduced if partial voxels are labelled in datasets. We propose that this is the way brain tissue labelling algorithms should be evaluated in the future.

[1] http://www.cma.mgh.harvard.edu/ibsr/

Method	CSF	GM	WM
Adaptive MAP	0.069	0.564	0.567
Biased MAP	0.071	0.558	0.562
Fuzzy c-means	0.048	0.473	0.567
Maximum-a-posteriori (MAP)	0.071	0.550	0.554
Maximum-likelihood	0.062	0.535	0.551
Tree-Structure k-means	0.049	0.477	0.571
MPM-MAP [11]	0.227	0.662	0.683
BSE/BFC/PVC [17]	—	0.595	0.664
Constrained GMM [8]	—	0.680	0.660
Spatial-varying GMM [9]	—	0.768	0.734
Coupled surface [14]	—	0.701	—
FSL [10]	—	0.756^2	—
SPM [18]	—	0.790^2	—
MAP with histograms	**0.549 ± 0.017**	**0.814 ± 0.004**	**0.710 ± 0.005**
Decision Forest Classifier	**0.614 ± 0.015**	**0.838 ± 0.006**	**0.731 ± 0.007**
Inter-rater consistency	—	0.876	0.882

Fig. 3. Comparison of our approaches with the state of the art. Mean and std. error of Jaccard indices are obtained from repeated random runs. We are targeting CSF/GM/WM segmentation only, but note that [17] also classifies the background.

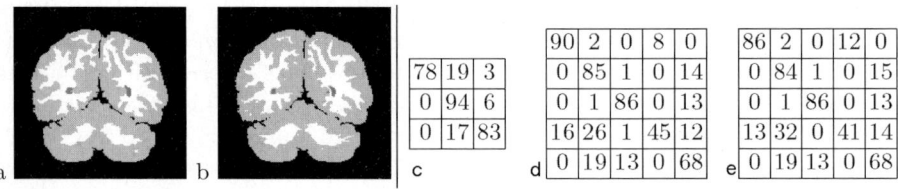

Fig. 4. Segmentation results: **(a)** Ground-truth with black-gray-white corresponding to CSF-GM-WM; **(b)** Label map obtained by our approach. **(c-e)** Confusion matrices (in %) for tissue classification. **(c)** without partial volume classification; **(d)** modeling partial voxels by direct histogram learning; **(e)** modeling partial voxels by uniform mixture of pure voxels. Matrix rows (top-bottom) correspond to ground-truth, while columns (left-right) are our labelling, both in CSF, GM, WM, CSF/GM, GM/WM order. (d) yields best results, i.e., maximal overlap averaged on 3 pure tissue classes.

4 Conclusions

We have proposed a learning-based method combining bias field correction, histogram tissue likelihood, and atlas based prior, with a decision forest classifier that uses context, to achieve substantial improvements on tissue labelling of brain MR images. Performance obtained is now very close to that of expert practitioners. We also showed that further improvements could be obtained in classification error performance by taking account of partial volume effect, and this suggests a modified test paradigm for future studies.

---

[2] Dice index reported by [19], different from Jaccard index we use in Fig. 3. By definition, Dice > Jaccard. Thus for a fair comparison we also present here the mean Dice indices of our approach: CSF 0.699, GM 0.900, WM 0.831.

References

1. Styner, M., et al.: Morphometric analysis of lateral ventricles in schizophrenia and healthy controls regarding genetic and disease-specific factors. In: Proc. National Academy of Science, pp. 4872–4877 (2005)
2. Fischl, B., et al.: Whole brain segmentation: automated labeling of neuroanatomical structures in the human brain. NeuroImage 33, 341–355 (2002)
3. Maintz, J., Viergever, M.: A survey of medical image registration. Medical Image Analysis 2, 1–37 (1996)
4. Amit, Y., Geman, D.: Shape quantization and recognition with randomized trees. Neural Computation 9, 1545–1588 (1997)
5. Shotton, J., Winn, J., Rother, J., Criminisi, A.: Textonboost: joint appearance, shape, and context modeling for multi-class object recognition and segmentation. In: Eur. Conf. Computer Vision, pp. 1–15 (2006)
6. Pham, D., Prince, J.: Adaptive fuzzy segmentation of magnetic resonance images. IEEE Trans. Medical Imaging 18, 737–752 (1999)
7. Ramon, J., Veronica, M., Oscar, Y.: Data-driven brain MRI segmentation supported on edge confidence and a priori tissue information. IEEE Trans. Medical Imaging 25, 74–83 (2006)
8. Greenspan, H., Rurf, A., Goldberger, J.: Constrained Gaussian mixture model framework for automatic segmentation of MR brain images. IEEE Trans. Medical Imaging 25, 1233–1245 (2006)
9. Peng, Z., Wee, W., Lee, J.: Automatic segmentation of MR brain images using spatial-varying Gaussian mixture and Markov random field approach. In: Proc. Conf. Computer Vision and Pattern Recognition Workshop, pp. 80–87 (2006)
10. Zhang, Y., Brady, M., Smith, S.: Segmentation of brain MR images through a hidden Markov model and the expectation-maximization algorithm. IEEE Trans. Medical Imaging 20, 45–57 (2001)
11. Marroquin, J., Vemuri, B., Botello, S., Calderon, F., Fernandez-Bouzas, A.: An accurate and efficient Bayesian method for automatic segmentation of brain MRI. IEEE Trans. Medical Imaging 21, 934–945 (2002)
12. McInerney, T., Terzopoulos, D.: Deformable models in medical image analysis. Medical Image Analysis 1, 91–108 (1996)
13. Yang, J., Staib, L., Duncan, J.: Neighbor-constrained segmentation with level set based 3D deformable models. IEEE Trans. Medical Imaging 23, 940–948 (2004)
14. Zeng, X., Staib, L., Schultz, R., Duncan, J.: Segmentation and measurement of the cortex from 3D MR images using coupled-surface propagation. IEEE Trans. Medical Imaging 17, 74–86 (1998)
15. Tu, Z., et al.: Brain anatomical structure segmentation by hybrid discriminative/generative models. IEEE Trans. Medical Imaging 27, 495–508 (2008)
16. Vovk, U., Pernus, F., Likar, B.: A review of methods for correction of intensity inhomogeneity in MRI. IEEE Trans. Medical Imaging 3, 405–421 (2007)
17. Shattuck, D., Sandor-Leahy, S., Schaper, K., Rottenberg, D., Leahy, R.: Magnetic resonance image tissue classification using a partial volume model. NeuroImage 13, 856–876 (2001)
18. Ashburner, J., Friston, K.: Multimodal image coregistration and partitioning - a unified framework. NeuroImage 6, 209–217 (1997)
19. Tsang, O., et al.: Comparison of tissue segmentation algorithms in neuroimage analysis software tools. In: IEEE Engineering in Medicine and Biology Society, pp. 3924–3928 (2008)

Use of Simulated Atrophy for Performance Analysis of Brain Atrophy Estimation Approaches*

Swati Sharma[1,2], Vincent Noblet[2], François Rousseau[2], Fabrice Heitz[2], Lucien Rumbach[1,3], and Jean-Paul Armspach[1]

[1] LINC-IPB (UMR CNRS-UDS 7191), Strasbourg, France
swati.sharma@linc.u-strasbg.fr
[2] LSIIT (UMR CNRS-UDS 7005), Strasbourg, France
[3] Centre Hospitalier Universitaire, Besançon, France

Abstract. In this paper, we study the performance of popular brain atrophy estimation algorithms using a simulated gold standard. The availability of a gold standard facilitates a sound evaluation of the measures of atrophy estimation, which is otherwise complicated. Firstly, we propose an approach for the construction of a gold standard. It involves the simulation of a realistic brain tissue loss based on the estimation of a topology preserving B-spline based deformation fields. Using this gold standard, we present an evaluation of three standard brain atrophy estimation methods (SIENA, SIENAX and BSI) in the presence of bias field inhomogeneity and noise. The effect of brain lesion load on the measured atrophy is also evaluated. Our experiments demonstrate that SIENA, SIENAX and BSI show a deterioration in their performance in the presence of bias field inhomogeneity and noise. The observed mean absolute errors in the measured Percentage of Brain Volume Change (PBVC) are 0.35% ± 0.38, 2.03% ± 1.46 and 0.91% ± 0.80 for SIENA, SIENAX and BSI, respectively, for simulated whole brain atrophies in the range 0 − 1%.

1 Introduction

The last decade has seen the emergence of sophisticated image processing techniques, based on Magnetic Resonance Imaging (MRI) acquisitions, for assessing the brain volume. The associated ease of use and portability of these methods has attracted the attention of the medical community in a large way. This has led to an increasing interest in the use of the brain atrophy measurements as a reliable index of disease progression since brain atrophy is a common feature of many neuro-degenerative diseases such as Multiple Sclerosis (MS)[1], Alzheimer's disease (AD) and Dementia. Although, the existing approaches for

---

* We are thankful to Alsace Region and ARSEP for supporting this study. We also thank Dr. Evan Fletcher (University of California, Davis) for his support on the BSI software.

measuring atrophy are sensitive and reproducible, their accuracy and reliability are affected by a number of factors. For instance, non-destructive biologic factors such as inflammation, edema, steroid therapy, dehydration, alcohol consumption and normal aging may contribute to a change in the brain volume. MRI artefacts including motion artefacts, sequence variations, bias field inhomogeneity, noise and others may influence the brain atrophy measurements. Other sources of error are more method specific and include inaccuracies in registration and segmentation of images. Since these tools are being increasingly used as a marker of disease evolution in many pathologies, their validation is a key problem. However, in the real scenario, the non-availability of the ground truth complicates the evaluation and comparison of these techniques. In this paper, we address the problem of creation of a gold standard. We propose a topology preserving non-rigid registration based framework for simulating brain images with a known realistic atrophy. Using these simulations as a gold standard, an evaluation of the performance of three popular atrophy estimation methods ("Structural Image Evaluation, using Normalization, of Atrophy" (SIENA) [2], for cross-sectional studies (SIENAX) [3] and "Boundary Shift Integral" (BSI) [4]), on the basis of their robustness to bias field inhomogeneity and noise is presented. Influence of brain lesion load on the atrophy measurements is also investigated.

2 Proposed Approach for Atrophy Simulation

Designing methods that simulate realistic atrophy is of great importance for the evaluation of atrophy measurement techniques, since it is a way of generating ground truth data. In the literature, several approaches have been proposed for simulating brain atrophy. In [5], Karacali et al. have proposed a Jacobian-based method where deformation fields are estimated in order to induce the desired volume variations in the regions of interest. An additional penalization term is also considered in order to prevent the *corner Jacobians* from being negative in order to ensure that the estimated deformation field preserves topology. However, the penalization term cannot rigorously guarantee topology preservation and restricts the simulation of large atrophies in one go. Pieperhoff et al. have recently presented a similar approach relying on "Local Volume Ratio (LVR)" [6] instead of the Jacobian. Unfortunately, none of these methods address the problem of enforcing skull invariance, which is a desirable property for the simulation of realistic brain atrophy. The bio-mechanical-based approach proposed by Camara et al. [7] relies on a bio-mechanical model for simulating brain tissue deformation, using a finite-element approach. Their framework also incorporates the skull invariance constraint.

Here, we present an alternative to the methods discussed above. The proposed approach estimates a deformation field that preserves topology so that the Jacobian is at each voxel, as close as possible to the desired local level of atrophy. Contrary to Karacali et al. [5] who consider the sum of squared differences between the Jacobian of the transformation and the desired level of atrophy, we consider the logarithm of the Jacobian so that dilations ($1 < J < +\infty$) and contractions ($0 < J < 1$) have a similar influence on the objective function. Besides, additional constraints are introduced in order to ensure that the skull remains invariant by the estimated transformation. The proposed approach is detailed in the following section.

2.1 Optimization Problem

We consider a B-spline based multi-resolution deformable model (For details see [8]). Let $s \triangleq [x,y,z]^t \in \Omega \subset \mathbb{R}^3$. Let $\Omega_J \subset \Omega$ be the area where the desired simulated atrophy level $J(s)$ (the value of the Jacobian at each voxel $s \in \Omega_J$) is user-specified. For estimating the corresponding deformation field u, we consider the following objective function:

$$E_{u,J,\lambda} = \int_{\Omega_J} |\log(J_u(s)) - \log(J(s))|^2 \, ds + \lambda \, C \int_{\Omega} E_{Reg}(u(s)) \, ds, \quad (1)$$

where J_u stands for the Jacobian of u, E_{reg} is a regularization term that ensures that the estimated transformation is smooth, λ is the weight of the regularization term and C is a scaling factor computed at the beginning of each scale [9]. Among the many regularization terms proposed in the literature, we choose the membrane energy. We guarantee exact topology preservation by maintaining the positivity of the Jacobian in the continuous domain. As opposed to Karcali *et. al*, who need an additional term for topology preservation, we directly solve the following constrained optimization problem.

$$\hat{u} = \arg \min_{0 < J_u(s) < +\infty} E_{u,J,\lambda}. \quad (2)$$

The procedure for solving this optimization problem is quite involved and is detailed in [8]. We use the Levenberg-Marquardt optimization procedure in order to improve the convergence rate. In our framework, we invoke the skull invariance constraint by optimizing those B-spline parameters that do not affect the skull, while setting the other parameters to zero. Finally, to obtain the warped image, it is more convenient to consider the backward transformation so that standard interpolation techniques can be used for the regularly sampled data.

3 Experimental Results

3.1 Simulation of Atrophy

In this section, we study the performance of the proposed atrophy simulation algorithm. First, we investigate the influence of considering the logarithm of the Jacobian in the objective function (*Log*-norm) instead of the standard sum of squared differences (L_2-norm). Fig. 1 highlights the fact that using the L_2 norm leads to nearly the same dispersion of Jacobian values, whatever be the simulated atrophy rate, whereas the *Log*-norm shows a constant relative dispersion, which is more consistent. A quantitative analysis of the ability of the proposed

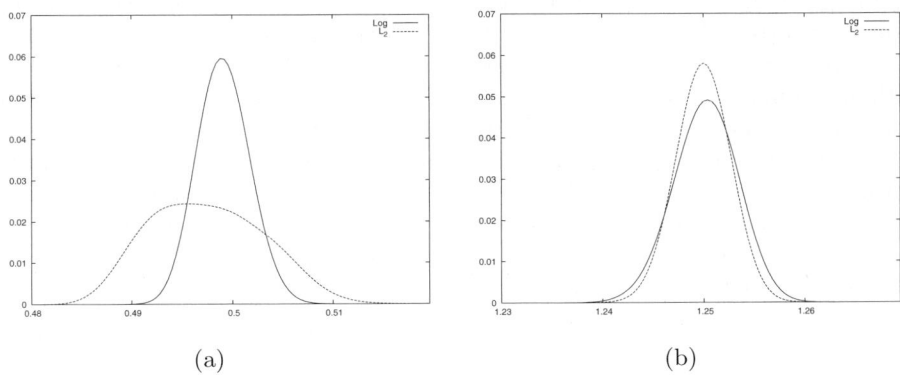

Fig. 1. Jacobian distributions obtained by simulating uniform (a) atrophy of 50% and (b) hypertrophy of 25%

Table 1. Influence of considering the skull constraint on the mean and standard deviation of Jacobian values of the simulated deformation fields

Desired Atrophy	Without skull constraint	With skull constraint
10%(J=0.9)	0.9017 ± 0.0021	0.9032 ± 0.0115
20%(J=0.8)	0.8015 ± 0.0021	0.8019 ± 0.0202
40%(J=0.6)	0.6008 ± 0.0018	0.6025 ± 0.0797
50%(J=0.5)	0.5005 ± 0.0017	0.5140 ± 0.2088

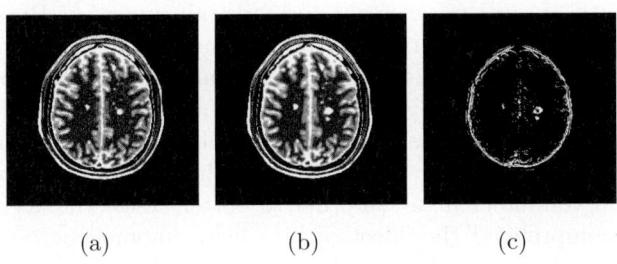

Fig. 2. Simulation of brain atrophy with an increase in MS lesion load: a) Original BrainWeb image with moderate lesions (b) Image with 10% of global atrophy and 100% of MS lesion increase (c) Difference between images (a) and (b)

algorithm for simulating the desired atrophy has also been performed (see Table 1). Simulations have been performed by considering a uniform atrophy over gray and white matter using the Brainweb[1] image. It can be seen that, on the average, the desired atrophy is well achieved without and with the skull constraint. Note that the proposed simulation algorithm can easily achieve very high atrophy, contrary to the method proposed in [5], which requires the estimation

---

[1] http://www.bic.mni.mcgill.ca/brainweb/

of a large atrophy in an incremental way. For example, it is possible to simulate a uniform atrophy of 99.9%($J = 0.001$), without the skull constraint, with an obtained average Jacobian value of 0.00106 ± 0.000716. Such an atrophy rate, although unrealistic, highlights the ability of the proposed method to produce an accurate solution for low Jacobian values. The proposed simulation framework is also versatile and can be used for simulating a more complicated pattern of atrophy. For instance, it can be used for simulating a global brain atrophy and a change in a given pathological area such as multiple sclerosis lesion evolution or tumor growth, simultaneously. In Fig. 2, we present a simulation of 10% of global brain atrophy and 100% of MS lesion volume increase using an image with "Moderate" lesion load from the BrainWeb MS database.

3.2 Evaluation of SIENA, SIENAX and BSI

In this paper, we use the SIENA and SIENAX implementations available as a part of the FMRIB Software Library (FSL) version 4.1[2]. We use the BSI implementation developed by Imaging of Dementia and Ageing lab, University of California, Davis[3]. While the implementations of SIENA and SIENAX are completely automated, the implementation of BSI requires manual intervention for obtaining a gray-white matter mask, in order to define the brain boundaries on which the boundary shift integral is calculated. This problem is automatically alleviated in our case since the gray-white matter mask of the baseline image is available (with BrainWeb). We refer the reader to [2], [3] and [4] for a complete description of SIENA, SIENAX and BSI algorithms, respectively.

Our evaluation framework consists of the simulation of a number of atrophies (uniform over the brain) on a single normal brain image of BrainWeb. These simulations are a simplified version of the atrophy that occurs in reality but are adequate for the purpose of evaluation of the atrophy estimation approaches. The results are illustrated by simulating brain atrophy ranging between 0-1% (step size 0.1%) and 1-10% (step size 1%). Although, the brain atrophy range of 0-1% is more relevant to neuro-degenerative pathologies, we also present results for larger brain volume changes, in order to better assess the accuracy of these methods. To comprehend the effect of bias field inhomogeneity and noise, we create three sets of images. The baseline image as well as the atrophied images are degraded (a) using different intensity non-uniformity (INU) fields (20% INU) available with the BrainWeb database (b) by adding Gaussian noise to all the brain scans such that a signal to noise ratio (SNR) of 15dB is achieved (c) bias field inhomogeneity followed by noise using the same parameters as in (a) and (b). Fig. 3(a-d) shows the PBVC between any two brain scan pairs, $B1$ and $B2$, such that the simulated atrophy on brain $B1$ is less than that of $B2$ (for the simulated atrophy ranges of 0-1% and 1-10%). Fig. 3 compares the methods under consideration with respect to the ground truth, for (a) the noise-free case and for observations degraded with (b) bias field inhomogeneity (c) noise (d)

---
[2] http://www.fmrib.ox.ac.uk/fsl/fsl/list.html
[3] http://neuroscience.ucdavis.edu/idealab/software/index.php

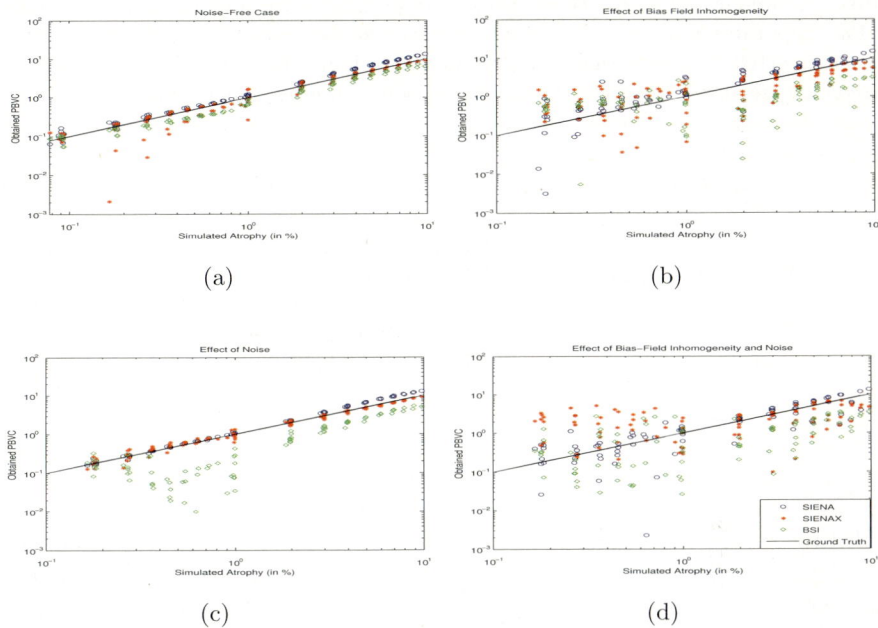

Fig. 3. Comparison of absolute errors in the estimated by SIENA, SIENAX and BSI with the ground truth for (a) noise-free observations and those degraded by (b) bias field inhomogeneity (c) noise (d) bias field inhomogeneity and noise

both bias field inhomogeneity and noise. In these figures, the absolute error in the estimated PBVC with reference to the ground truth is shown. Fig. 3(a) shows that SIENA overestimates the atrophy, while BSI underestimates it for large atrophy values when no artefact has been added. For low atrophy values (less than 1%), SIENA, SIENAX and BSI show a similar performance in terms of the error in PBVC measured with respect to the ground truth. As can be seen from Fig. 3(d), the introduction of bias field inhomogeneity and noise leads to a visible increase in the errors for all the three methods. A prominent reason for this is the incorrect extraction of brain, when using BET, due to the addition of bias field inhomogeneity, mostly at the brain boundaries. In our observation, the addition of noise over bias field inhomogeneity leads to a significant change in the brain extraction as compared to the brain extraction performed when only bias field inhomogeneity is added (Fig. 3(b)). However, for the observations that are degraded with Gaussian noise only, we do not observe any gross errors in the extraction of the brain. Brain extraction is crucial for SIENAX because the segmentation performed on the brain area is directly related to the calculation of the brain volume. Although, SIENA uses a combined brain mask from the two examinations for the evaluation of the brain volume change, it can be seen that non-brain areas are included in the calculations if they are included in one of the examinations. This is the reason for the degradation of the performance of SIENA. In our experiments on BSI, a bias field correction, available with

Table 2. Summary of results discussed in section 3.2 for the simulated atrophy range $0-1\%$. This table illustrates the mean error in the estimated PBVC (in percentage) for various artefacts. Note that, for presence of lesions, the error represents the non-desired change that is observed when comparisons are done using different versions of the same brain with varying lesion load.

Artefact	SIENA	SIENAX	BSI
Noise-free	0.0615 ± 0.0407	0.0874 ± 0.0759	0.1072 ± 0.0899
Bias Field Inhomogeneity	0.2940 ± 0.4343	0.8420 ± 0.7502	1.0412 ± 0.3827
Noise	0.0292 ± 0.0226	0.0673 ± 0.0433	0.4400 ± 0.1082
Bias Field Inhomogeneity and Noise	0.3492 ± 0.3812	2.0277 ± 1.4622	0.9131 ± 0.7993
Presence of Lesions	0.0941 ± 0.0772	0.2359 ± 0.2089	-

the implementation of BSI, is applied after the registration step. Since the bias field correction step comes after the brain extraction and registration steps are performed, the error in these steps possibly propagate to the end. We note that, for BSI too, brain extraction is an important step since the final result depends on getting a good mask of the brain. Our experiments also suggest that an improper extraction of the boundary of the brain leads to a mis-calculation of the boundary shift integral. Also, the effect of addition of Gaussian noise only (Fig. 3(c)), does not have a significant effect on the measurements of SIENA and SIENAX but has an impact on the BSI measurements due to the use of intensity values directly in the calculation of the boundary shift integral.

To determine the effect of presence of lesions on atrophy, SIENA and SIENAX algorithms are run between "normal" brain and images with "mild", "moderate", "severe" lesion loads available with BrainWeb. In all these cases, no additional atrophy is simulated. Hence, it is expected that the atrophy estimated between these cases is close to zero. The deviations from zero atrophy represent the change in the estimated atrophy due to the presence of lesions. We observe that lesions can lead to a significant non-desired change of up to 0.2% when comparing a normal brain with the same brain with lesions using SIENA. SIENAX is more affected by the presence of lesions when a normal brain is compared with the same brain with lesions (maximum PBVC is $\sim 0.42\%$). Since a gray-white matter mask delineating the brain boundaries is provided to BSI for carrying out its calculations, the presence of lesions is not expected to have any effect on atrophy estimation. Hence, BSI is not tested here. Table 2 summarizes the results corresponding to various sources of error discussed in this section. We would also like to bring to the knowledge of the reader that Smith et al. [10] report the overall mean absolute error of SIENA and BSI to be $\sim 0.2\%$ which differs significantly from the results presented here (See Table 2). Smith et al. used incremental atrophy summation with first-last differencing for performing this evaluation [10]. Their calculation of mean absolute error is not based on a ground truth as is the case for our evaluation framework.

4 Conclusions

In this paper, we proposed a topology preserving scheme for simulating atrophy using a B-spline based deformation model to create a gold standard for the comparison of atrophy estimation approaches. Additional constraints were introduced in order to ensure that the skull remains invariant in the simulated image and the estimated transformation is smooth. Our experiments showed that the proposed simulation algorithm can achieve the desired atrophy with accuracy. Using the simulated gold standard, we assessed the performance of three freely available algorithms (SIENA, SIENAX and BSI). Our analysis procedure consisted of simulation of atrophies on a single BrainWeb image in the presence of bias field inhomogeneity and noise. The experiments showed that, SIENA is the best performer with respect to the error in the estimated PBVC in the noise-free case as well as when the images are degraded with bias field inhomogeneity and noise. Bias field inhomogeneity and noise were responsible for incorrect brain extraction which considerably affected the accuracy of all the methods. Mean errors of $0.35\% \pm 0.38$, $2.03\% \pm 1.46$ and $0.91\% \pm 0.80$ were observed in the estimated atrophy by SIENA, SIENAX and BSI, respectively. The observed errors were also significantly larger as compared to Smith et al. [10] who reported the overall mean absolute error for SIENA and BSI as $\sim 0.2\%$. The tests that we performed also indicated that SIENA and BSI estimated longitudinal atrophy more accurately than SIENAX in a real scenario, where the images are corrupted with bias field inhomogeneity and noise. Since SIENAX has been developed for cross-sectional studies, its results should be cautiously interpreted when used in longitudinal studies. To conclude, the errors that we observed in our experiments were comparable to the whole brain annual atrophy rates $(0.5 - 2.8\%)$ that have been reported for various pathologies. This highlights the need for the development of more robust methods capable of measuring atrophy accurately.

References

1. Simon, J.H.: Brain atrophy in multiple sclerosis: What we know and would like to know. Multiple sclerosis (Houndmills, Basingstoke, England) 12(6), 679–687 (2006)
2. Smith, S.M., De Stefano, N., Jenkinson, M., Matthews, P.M.: Normalized accurate measurement of longitudinal brain change. J. Comput. Assist. Tomogr. 25(3), 466–475 (2001)
3. Smith, S.M., Zhang, Y., Jenkinson, M., Chen, J., Matthews, P.M., Federico, A., De Stefano, N.: Accurate, robust and automated longitudinal and cross-sectional brain change analysis. Neuroimage 17(1), 479–489 (2002)
4. Freeborough, P.A., Fox, N.C.: The boundary shift integral: An accurate and robust measure of cerebral volume changes from registered repeat MRI. IEEE Trans. Med. Imaging 16, 623–629 (1997)
5. Karacali, B., Davatzikos, C.: Simulation of tissue atrophy using a topology preserving transformation model. IEEE Trans. Med. Imaging 25(5), 649–652 (2006)

6. Pieperhoff, P., Sudmeyer, M., Homke, L., Zilles, K., Schnitzler, A., Amunts, K.: Detection of structural changes of the human brain in longitudinally acquired MR images by deformation field morphometry: Methodological analysis, validation and application. Neuroimage 43(2), 269–287 (2008)
7. Camara, O., Schweiger, M., Scahill, R., Crum, W., Sneller, B., Schnabel, J., Ridgway, G., Cash, D., Hill, D., Fox, N.: Phenomenological model of diffuse global and regional atrophy using finite-element methods. IEEE Trans. Med. Imaging 25(11), 1417–1430 (2006)
8. Noblet, V., Heinrich, C., Heitz, F., Armspach, J.P.: 3-D deformable image registration: a topology preservation scheme based on hierarchical deformation models and interval analysis optimization. IEEE Trans. Image Process 14(5), 553–566 (2005)
9. Noblet, V., Heinrich, C., Heitz, F., Armspach, J.P.: Retrospective evaluation of a topology preserving non-rigid registration method. Med. Image Anal. 10(3), 366–384 (2006)
10. Smith, S.M., Rao, A., De Stefano, N., Jenkinson, M., Schott, J.M., Matthews, P.M., Fox, N.C.: Longitudinal and cross-sectional analysis of atrophy in Alzheimer's disease: Cross validation of BSI, SIENA and SIENAX. Neuroimage 36, 1200–1206 (2007)

Fast and Robust 3-D MRI Brain Structure Segmentation*

Michael Wels[1,4], Yefeng Zheng[2], Gustavo Carneiro[3,**], Martin Huber[4], Joachim Hornegger[1], and Dorin Comaniciu[2]

[1] Chair of Pattern Recognition, Department of Computer Science, University Erlangen-Nuremberg, Germany
michael.wels@informatik.uni-erlangen.de
[2] Integrated Data Systems, Siemens Corporate Research, Princeton, NJ, USA
[3] Institute for Systems and Robotics, Electrical and Computer Engineering Department, Technical University of Lisbon, Portugal
[4] Siemens CT SE5 SCR2, Erlangen, Germany

Abstract. We present a novel method for the automatic detection and segmentation of (sub-)cortical gray matter structures in 3-D magnetic resonance images of the human brain. Essentially, the method is a top-down segmentation approach based on the recently introduced concept of Marginal Space Learning (MSL). We show that MSL naturally decomposes the parameter space of anatomy shapes along decreasing levels of geometrical abstraction into subspaces of increasing dimensionality by exploiting parameter invariance. At each level of abstraction, i.e., in each subspace, we build strong discriminative models from annotated training data, and use these models to narrow the range of possible solutions until a final shape can be inferred. Contextual information is introduced into the system by representing candidate shape parameters with high-dimensional vectors of 3-D generalized Haar features and steerable features derived from the observed volume intensities. Our system allows us to detect and segment 8 (sub-)cortical gray matter structures in T1-weighted 3-D MR brain scans from a variety of different scanners in on average 13.9 sec., which is faster than most of the approaches in the literature. In order to ensure comparability of the achieved results and to validate robustness, we evaluate our method on two publicly available gold standard databases consisting of several T1-weighted 3-D brain MR scans from different scanners and sites. The proposed method achieves an accuracy better than most state-of-the-art approaches using standardized distance and overlap metrics.

1 Introduction

Currently, many scientific questions in neurology, like the revelation of mechanisms affecting generative or degenerative processes in brain development, require quantitative volumetric analysis of (sub-)cortical gray matter structures

---

* This work was partially funded by the Health-e-Child project (IST 2004-027749).
** G. Carneiro contributed to this work when he was with the Integrated Data Systems Department of Siemens Corporate Research.

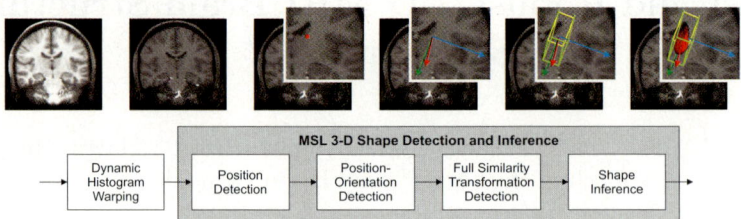

Fig. 1. The processing pipeline of the proposed 3-D shape detection and inference method. Each image (detection and delineation of the left caudate) schematically represents the input and/or output of individual processing steps. Please view in color.

in large populations of patients and healthy controls. For instance, atrophy in the presence of Alzheimer's disease considerably affects morphology of the hippocampus. In addition, 3-D segmentation of various deep gray matter structures facilitates image-based surgical planning, therapy monitoring, and the generation of patient-specific geometrical models from imaging data for further processing. As a result of unclear boundaries, shape complexity, and different anatomical definitions, precise manual delineation is usually time consuming and user dependent. Moreover, typical artifacts present in MR imaging (Rician noise, partial volume effects, and intra-/inter-scan intensity non-uniformities) challenge the consistency of manual delineations. Therefore, a system for the automatic detection and segmentation of (sub-)cortical gray matter structures not only has the potential to increase segmentation consistency, but also has the capability of facilitating large-scale neuromorphological studies.

We propose a fully automatic method for the detection and delineation of the following eight (sub-)cortical gray matter structures: the left and right caudate nucleus, hippocampus, globus pallidus, and putamen. Our method consists of two major steps: 1) we standardize the observed MR intensities by non-rigidly aligning their histogram to a template histogram by means of Dynamic Histogram Warping (DHW) [1]; and 2) for each (sub-)cortical structure of interest we detect and infer its position, orientation, scale, and shape in an extended Marginal Space Learning (MSL) framework [2], which explicitly integrates shape inference into the overall MSL formulation. The overall system block diagram is depicted in Fig. 1.

In contrast to other methods [3–5] where a partly manually initialized nine parameter registration is part of the approaches we do not require the input volumes to be spatially normalized. In some cases [3, 4], the feature pools used for discriminative model generation are enriched with features explicitly encoding normalized location. In accordance with this observation, the approaches are only evaluated on spatially normalized data sets from one type of MR scanner that are not publicly available [4, 5]. Nevertheless, Morra et al. [3] report state-of-the-art results on data sets that have not been subject to spatial normalization. Apart from that, the mentioned methods make use of machine learning in a similar manner as we do, but follow a bottom up approach ascending from the lowest level of abstraction, i.e., the level of individual voxels, to the level of complete anatomical entities.

Alignment of a probabilistic atlas by means of an affine registration also plays an important role in further approaches [6, 7]. While sometimes [6] quantitative evaluation is only carried out on simulated data, the method of Akselrod-Ballin et al. [7] is trained and evaluated on only one publicly available dataset that has been subject to a specific preprocessing including intensity standardization. By generating observation or discriminative models based on intensity values without explicitly allowing for inter-scan intensity variations [3–5, 7] the resulting models are at the risk of being over-adapted to specific contrast-characteristics of the data at hand.

2 Methods

2.1 Combined 3-D Shape Detection and Shape Inference

For combined 3-D rigid anatomy detection and shape inference we use a method based on the concept of Marginal Space Learning (MSL) [2]. We estimate the structure of interest's center $\boldsymbol{c} = (c_1, c_2, c_3) \in \mathbb{R}^3$, orientation $\boldsymbol{\theta} = (\theta_1, \theta_2, \theta_3) \in [-\pi, \pi] \times [-\pi/2, \pi/2] \times [-\pi, \pi]$ represented as Euler angles in $z - x - z$ convention, scale $\boldsymbol{s} = (s_1, s_2, s_3) \in \{\, \boldsymbol{s} \in \mathbb{R}^3 \,|\, s_i > 0, i = 1, 2, 3 \,\}$, and shape $\boldsymbol{X} = (\boldsymbol{x}_1, \ldots, \boldsymbol{x}_n) \in \mathbb{R}^{3 \times n}$. The latter consists of canonically sampled 3-D points on the surface of an object to be segmented. Note that $\boldsymbol{\theta}$ is relative to $\boldsymbol{c}$, $\boldsymbol{s}$ is relative to $\boldsymbol{c}$ and $\boldsymbol{\theta}$, and $\boldsymbol{X}$ is relative to $\boldsymbol{c}$, $\boldsymbol{\theta}$, and $\boldsymbol{s}$. Let $\mathcal{V} = \{\, 1, 2, \ldots, N \,\}$, $N \in \mathbb{N}$, be a set of indices to image voxels, $\boldsymbol{Y} = (y_v)_{v \in \mathcal{V}}$, $y_v \in \{-1, 1\}$, a binary segmentation of the image voxels into object and non-object voxels, and f be a function with $\boldsymbol{Y} = f(\boldsymbol{I}, \boldsymbol{\Theta})$ that provides a binary segmentation of volume $\boldsymbol{I}$ using segmentation parameters $\boldsymbol{\Theta} = (\boldsymbol{c}, \boldsymbol{\theta}, \boldsymbol{s}, \boldsymbol{X})$. Let $\boldsymbol{Z} = (z_{\boldsymbol{\Theta}})$ be a family of high-dimensional feature vectors extracted from a given input volume $\boldsymbol{I} = (i_v)_{v \in \mathcal{V}}$ and associated with different discretized configurations of $\boldsymbol{\Theta}$. In our context $\boldsymbol{Z}$ includes voxel-wise context encoding 3-D generalized Haar features [8] to characterize possible object centers and steerable features [2] that are capable of representing hypothetical orientations and optionally scaling relative to a given object center or shape surface point. These features were chosen for our method because of their fast computation and effective representation [2].

We search for the optimal parameter vector

$$\boldsymbol{\Theta}^* = \arg\max_{\boldsymbol{\Theta}} p(y = 1 | \boldsymbol{\Theta}, \boldsymbol{I}, \boldsymbol{M}^{(\boldsymbol{\Theta})}) = \arg\max_{\boldsymbol{\Theta}} p(y = 1 | \boldsymbol{Z}, \boldsymbol{M}^{(\boldsymbol{\Theta})}) \quad (1)$$

maximizing the posterior probability of the presence, i.e., $y = 1$, of a sought anatomy given the discriminative model $\boldsymbol{M}^{(\boldsymbol{\Theta})}$ and the features $\boldsymbol{Z}$ extracted from the input volume $\boldsymbol{I}$ using a certain set of values for the parameters $\boldsymbol{\Theta}$.

Let $\pi^{(\boldsymbol{c})}(\boldsymbol{Z})$, $\pi^{(\boldsymbol{c}, \boldsymbol{\theta})}(\boldsymbol{Z})$, $\pi^{(\boldsymbol{c}, \boldsymbol{\theta}, \boldsymbol{s})}(\boldsymbol{Z})$, $\pi^{(\boldsymbol{c}, \boldsymbol{\theta}, \boldsymbol{s}, \boldsymbol{X})}(\boldsymbol{Z})$ denote the vectors of components of $\boldsymbol{Z}$ associated with individual groups of elements $(\boldsymbol{c})$, $(\boldsymbol{c}, \boldsymbol{\theta})$, $(\boldsymbol{c}, \boldsymbol{\theta}, \boldsymbol{s})$, and $(\boldsymbol{c}, \boldsymbol{\theta}, \boldsymbol{s}, \boldsymbol{X})$ of the parameter vector $\boldsymbol{\Theta}$. The MSL method avoids exhaustively searching the high-dimensional parameter space spanned by all the possible $\boldsymbol{\Theta}$ by exploiting the fact that ideally for any discriminative model for center detection with parameters $\boldsymbol{M}^{(\boldsymbol{c})}$ working on a restricted amount of possible features

$$c^* = \arg\max_{c} p(y = 1|\pi^{(c)}(Z), M^{(c)}) \tag{2}$$

holds, as the object center c is invariant under relative reorientation, relative rescaling, and relative shape positioning. Similarly, we have

$$\theta^* = \arg\max_{\theta} p(y = 1|\pi^{(c^*,\theta)}(Z), M^{(c,\theta)}) \tag{3}$$

for combined position-orientation detection with model parameters $M^{(c,\theta)}$ where only features $\pi^{(c^*,\theta)}(Z)$ with $c = c^*$ are considered. This is due to the fact that position and orientation are invariant under relative rescaling and relative shape positioning. Analogous considerations yield

$$s^* = \arg\max_{s} p(y = 1|\pi^{(c^*,\theta^*,s)}(Z), M^{(c,\theta,s)}) \tag{4}$$

for the object's scaling, and

$$X^* = \arg\max_{X} p(y = 1|\pi^{(c^*,\theta^*,s^*,X)}(Z), M^{(c,\theta,s,x)}, M^{(c,\theta,s,X)}) \tag{5}$$

for the object's shape where $M^{(c,\theta,s,x)}$ are the parameters of a local shape model with respect to individual surface points x and parameters $M^{(c,\theta,s,X)}$ represent a global shape model. Equations (2)–(5) naturally establish a chain of discriminative models exploiting search space parameter invariance for combined 3-D shape detection and shape inference. It allows us to apply different discriminative models descending along geometrical abstraction as, in our framework, the object center c alone is the most abstract and the complete set of parameters Θ is the least abstract shape representation. Therefore, MSL establishes a hierarchical decomposition of the search space along decreasing levels of geometrical abstraction with increasing dimensionality of the considered parameter subspace.

2.2 3-D Shape Detection: Similarity Transformation Estimation

Let $\mathcal{Z}$ be the set of annotated image volumes in their transformed feature representation as mentioned above. We will refer to $\mathcal{Z}$ as the training data. In order to find the first parts of the optimal parameter vector Θ^* describing a nine parameter similarity transformation, i.e., c^*, θ^*, and s^*, we have to learn discriminative models $p(y = 1|\pi^{(c^*)}(Z))$, $p(y = 1|\pi^{(c^*,\theta)}(Z))$, and $p(y = 1|\pi^{(c^*,\theta^*,s)}(Z))$. Following the concept of MSL [2] we generate a set of positive and negative training examples $\mathcal{C} = \{(\pi^{(c)}(Z), y) \,|\, Z \in \mathcal{Z}\}$ to train a probabilistic boosting tree (PBT) model [9] for position detection. The feature vectors $\pi^{(c)}(Z)$ consist of 3-D generalized Haar features [8] encoding voxel context of candidate object centers based on observed intensity values. Decreasing the level of geometric abstraction we analogously train a PBT model for combined position-orientation detection based on an extended set of training examples $\mathcal{P} = \{(\pi^{(c,\theta)}(Z), y) \,|\, Z \in \mathcal{Z}\}$ where $\pi^{(c,\theta)}(Z)$, associated with (c, θ) and an image volume, is made of steerable features [2]. They allow varying orientation and scaling to be encoded in terms of aligned and scaled intensity sampling patterns. In accordance with this scheme, steerable features are also used to finally train a PBT for full nine parameter similarity transformation detection based on $\mathcal{S} = \{(\pi^{(c,\theta,s)}(Z), y) \,|\, Z \in \mathcal{Z}\}$ where $\pi^{(c,\theta,s)}(Z)$ is derived from (c, θ, s) and the associated image volume.

Table 1. Average segmentation accuracy (left and right structures grouped together) for IBSR 18 of models trained from mutually exclusive training and test data. Except for the Dice coefficient $(2 \cdot TP/(2 \cdot TP + FP + FN)$ where TP, FP, and FN denote the number of true positive, false positive, and false negative voxels, respectively) see [13] on details on the used accuracy metrics.

Structure	Overlap Err. [%]	Dice Coeff. [%]	Volume Diff. [%]	Abs. Dist. [mm]	RMS Dist. [mm]	Max. Dist. [mm]
Caudate nucleus	32.42 ± 6.14	80.49 ± 4.51	9.57 ± 8.45	0.67 ± 0.17	1.10 ± 0.23	7.76 ± 1.82
Hippocampus	41.96 ± 4.69	73.34 ± 3.73	21.14 ± 17.29	0.91 ± 0.15	1.33 ± 0.21	6.34 ± 1.63
Globus pallidus	39.72 ± 7.05	74.97 ± 5.88	20.97 ± 12.38	0.79 ± 0.24	1.24 ± 0.37	5.53 ± 1.63
Putamen	29.82 ± 5.20	82.37 ± 3.65	13.76 ± 7.59	0.72 ± 0.20	1.15 ± 0.28	6.60 ± 1.85

2.3 3-D Shape Inference under Global Shape Constraints

For the final object shape we further decompose

$$\pi^{(c,\theta,s,X)}(Z) = \left(\pi^{(c,\theta,s,x_i)}(Z)\right)_{i=1,\ldots,n}$$

where $\pi^{(c,\theta,s,x_i)}(Z)$ are the features associated with an image volume and individual relatively aligned candidate points (c, θ, s, x_i) for the surface of the object of interest. In order to apply discriminative modeling we assume the x_i and correspondingly $\pi^{(c,\theta,s,x_i)}(Z)$ to be independently and identically distributed (i.i.d.) and approximate

$$X^* = \arg\max_X p(y=1|\pi^{(c^*,\theta^*,s^*,X)}(Z), M^{(c,\theta,s,x)}, M^{(c,\theta,s,X)})$$

$$\approx \arg\max_X \left[\prod_{i=1}^n p(y_i=1|\pi^{(c^*,\theta^*,s^*,x_i)}(Z), M^{(c,\theta,s,x)})\right] p(X|c^*,\theta^*,s^*, M^{(c,\theta,s,X)}) \quad (6)$$

in an iterative manner. The term $p(y_i = 1|\pi^{(c,\theta,s,x_i)}(Z))$ describes the probability that the relatively aligned point (c, θ, s, x_i) is part of the shape to be inferred, i.e., lies on its surface, and $p(X|c^*, \theta^*, s^*, M^{(c,\theta,s,X)})$ is a global shape model [10]. We estimate $p(y = 1|\pi^{(c,\theta,s,x_i)}(Z))$ with a PBT model [9] using steerable features [2] trained on $\mathcal{X} = \{(\pi_{c,\theta,s,x_i}(Z), y) | i = 1, \ldots, n; Z \in \mathcal{Z}\}$. An iterative approach for (6) is suitable as, in practice, $X \in \mathbb{R}^{3 \times n}$ only varies around the mean shape positioned relatively to the (c^*, θ^*, s^*) detected before at time $t = 0$ and the previous most likely anatomy shape in each iteration $t = 1, \ldots, T$.

3 Material and Experimental Setting

For training and quantitative evaluation of our system there were four sets of T1-weighted MRI scans available. The first one is a subset of the "Designed Database of MR Brain Images of Healthy Volunteers"[1] [11] (DDHV) containing

---

[1] The database was collected and made available by the CASILab at the University of North Carolina, Chapel Hill. The images were distributed by the MIDAS Data Server at Kitware, Inc. (insight-journal.org/midas). The authors would like to thank Martin Styner, Clement Vachet, and Paul Pandea for helping to preprocess parts of the data.

20 scans. The associated ground-truth annotations were manually recovered from automatically generated segmentations [12] of the structures of interest. The second collection of 18 MRI scans was provided by the Center of Morphometric Analysis at the Massachusetts General Hospital and is publicly available on the Internet Brain Segmentation Repository[2] (IBSR 18). The scans are accompanied by detailed ground-truth annotations including the (sub-)cortical structures of interest in this paper.[3] A subset[4] of the data provided by the NIH MRI Study of Normal Brain Development[5] consisting of 10 pediatric data sets states another collection (NIH) of annotated MR scans used for model generation. They have been manually annotated by the authors for training purposes. Additionally, we use data provided by the ongoing "3-D Segmentation in the Clinic: A Grand Challenge" competition[6] [13] for training and evaluation of the proposed method. The collection consists of several volumetric T1-weighted MR brain scans of varying spatial resolution and size from multiple sources (MICCAI'07 training/testing). The vast majority of data (29 scans) has been provided by the Psychiatry Neuroimaging Laboratory (PNL) at the Brigham and Women's Hospital (BWH), Boston. The other 20 data sets arose from a pediatric study, a Parkinson's Disease study, and a test/re-test study carried out at the University of North Carolina's (UNC) Neuroimaging Laboratory (NIAL), Chapel Hill. A predefined evaluation protocol is carried out fully automatically after uploading the testing fraction of the data to the Cause'07 file server. We refer to Heimann et al. [13] for details on the used evaluation measures and scoring system.

All the images were re-oriented to a uniform orientation ("RAI"; right-to-left, anterior-to-posterior, inferior-to-superior) and resampled to isotropic voxel spacing ($1.0 \times 1.0 \times 1.0$ mm^3) for processing. For increasing the amount of training data we exploited natural brain symmetry and therefore doubled the size of any training data set used for model generation by mirroring all the data sets with respect to the mid-sagittal plane. Throughout all our experiments we ensured that training and testing data are mutually exclusive: We trained on DDHV,

---

[2] www.cma.mgh.harvard.edu/ibsr

[3] We corrected the ground-truth annotations for the left and the right caudate in the IBSR 18 data set to better meet the protocol applied by the "3-D Segmentation in the Clinic: A Grand Challenge" competition where the caudate is grouped with the nucleus accumbens in the delineations [13, 14].

[4] The following 10 data sets were used: defaced_native_100{2,3,7}_V{1,2}_t1w_r2, defaced_native_100{1,4,8}_V2_t1w_r2, and defaced_native_1005_V2_t1w_r2.

[5] The NIH MRI Study of Normal Brain Development is a multi-site, longitudinal study of typically developing children, from ages newborn through young adulthood, conducted by the Brain Development Cooperative Group and supported by the NICHD, the NIDA, the NIMH, and the NINDS (Contract #s N01-HD02-3343, N01-MH9-0002, and N01-NS-9-2314, -2315, -2316, -2317, -2319 and -2320). A listing of the participating sites and a complete listing of the study investigators can be found at www.bic.mni.mcgill.ca/nihpd/info/participating_centers.html. This manuscript reflects the views of the authors and may not reflect the opinions or views of the NIH.

[6] www.cause07.org

Table 2. Average left/right caudate segmentation accuracy for the MICCAI'07 testing data set. The complete results can be found at www.cause07.org ("Segmentation Team"). As of 03/10/2009 our method ranks number 2 in the overall ranking list.

Cases	Overlap Err. [%]	Score	Volume Diff. [%]	Score	Abs. Dist. [mm]	Score	RMS Dist. [mm]	Score	Max. Dist. [mm]	Score	Total Score
Average UNC Ped	27.31	82.82	7.24	86.70	0.65	76.08	1.29	76.99	10.73	68.44	78.21
Average UNC Eld	34.48	78.31	10.73	81.18	0.73	72.82	1.31	76.59	11.57	65.96	74.97
Average BWH PNL	31.72	80.05	-16.54	70.20	0.65	76.08	1.26	77.56	11.19	67.09	74.20
Average All	31.38	80.27	-5.91	75.92	0.66	75.40	1.27	77.24	11.17	67.14	75.19

NIH, and IBSR 18 1-9 to evaluate on IBSR 18 10-18 and on DDHV, NIH, and IBSR 18 10-18 to evaluate on IBSR 18 1-9. We trained on DDHV, NIH, IBSR 18, and MICCAI'07 training to evaluate on MICCAI'07 testing.

As pointed out by Heimann et al. [13] there are differences in the annotation protocols used for annotating the caudate nuclei in data sets originating from the BWH and the UNC. In the former the "tail" of the caudate is continued much further dorsally. We therefore decided to detect it as a separate structure that can be attached to the caudate if required. We did not try to automatically determine the annotation protocol used from the imaging data itself as this may lead to over-fitted systems.

As our real discriminative models are not ideal as assumed for theoretical considerations we keep the top 100 candidates after position detection and the top 25 candidates after position-orientation detection for further processing steps in order to make the full similarity transformation detection more robust. For shape inference we use $T = 3$ iterations.

In an optimized and parallelized C++ implementation of our segmentation method it takes on average 13.9 sec. to detect and segment 8 (sub-)cortical structures in an MRI volume on a Fujitsu Siemens notebook equipped with an Intel Core 2 Duo CPU (2.20 GHz) and 3 GB of memory. Intensity standardization takes 1–2 sec. Our method is therefore faster than other state-of-the-art approaches whose timing is 50 sec. for 8 structures [5], 60 sec. for 1 structure [3], and 8 min. for 8 structures [4].

4 Experimental Results

As can be seen from Table 1 in terms of the Dice coefficient our method achieves better results (80%,73%,75%,82%) for the segmentation of the caudate nuclei, hippocampi, globi pallidi, and putamina on the same IBSR 18 data set than the methods of Akselrod-Ballin et al. [7] (80%, 69%, 74%, 79%) and Gouttard et al. [12] (76%,67%,71%,78%) except for the caudate nuclei in comparison to the method of Akselrod-Ballin et al. [7], where we reach a comparable accuracy. It also reaches a higher score for the caudate nuclei and putamina on IBSR 18 than the method of Bazin and Pham [14] (78%,81%), which does not address segmentation of the hippocampi and globi pallidi.

The overall average score in Table 2 shows that for segmenting the caudate nuclei our method performs better than the methods of Morra et al. [3] (73.38), Bazin and Pham [14] (64.73) and Tu et al. [4] (59.71). All the mentioned methods were evaluated on the same MICCAI'07 testing data set.

5 Conclusions

In this paper we integrated shape inference into the overall MSL methodology from the theoretical point of view. We showed that MSL decomposes the parameter space of anatomy shapes along decreasing levels of geometrical abstraction into subspaces of increasing dimensionality and applied MSL to the difficult problem of (sub-)cortical gray matter structure detection and shape inference. In an evaluation on publicly available gold standard databases our method works equally fast, robust, and accurate at a state-of-the-art level.

References

1. Cox, I.J., Hingorani, S.L.: Dynamic histogram warping of image pairs for constant image brightness. In: Proc. ICIP, Washington, D.C., USA, pp. 366–369 (1995)
2. Zheng, Y., Barbu, A., Georgescu, B., Scheuering, M., Comaniciu, D.: Four-chamber heart modeling and automatic segmentation for 3D cardiac CT volumes using marginal space learning and steerable features. IEEE T. Med. Imag. 27(11), 1668–1681 (2008)
3. Morra, J.H., Tu, Z., Apostolova, L.G., Green, A.E., Toga, A.W., Thompson, P.M.: Automatic subcortical segmentation using a contextual model. In: Metaxas, D., Axel, L., Fichtinger, G., Székely, G. (eds.) MICCAI 2008, Part I. LNCS, vol. 5241, pp. 194–201. Springer, Heidelberg (2008)
4. Tu, Z., Narr, K.L., Dollár, P., Dinov, I., Thompson, P.M., Toga, A.W.: Brain anatomical structure segmentation by hybrid discriminative/generative models. IEEE T. Med. Imag. 27(4), 495–508 (2008)
5. Corso, J.J., Tu, Z., Yuille, A.L., Toga, A.W.: Segmentation of sub-cortical structures by the graph-shifts algorithm. In: Karssemeijer, N., Lelieveldt, B. (eds.) IPMI 2007. LNCS, vol. 4584, pp. 183–197. Springer, Heidelberg (2007)
6. Scherrer, B., Forbes, F., Garbay, C., Dojat, M.: Fully bayesian joint model for MR brain scan tissue and structure segmentation. In: Metaxas, D., Axel, L., Fichtinger, G., Székely, G. (eds.) MICCAI 2008, Part II. LNCS, vol. 5242, pp. 1066–1074. Springer, Heidelberg (2008)
7. Akselrod-Ballin, A., Galun, M., Gomori, J.M.J., Brandt, A., Basri, R.: Prior knowledge driven multiscale segmentation of brain MRI. In: Ayache, N., Ourselin, S., Maeder, A. (eds.) MICCAI 2007, Part II. LNCS, vol. 4792, pp. 118–126. Springer, Heidelberg (2007)
8. Tu, Z., Zhou, X.S., Barbu, A., Bogoni, L., Comaniciu, D.: Probabilistic 3D polyp detection in CT images: The role of sample alignment. In: Proc. CVPR, New York, USA, pp. 1544–1551 (2006)
9. Tu, Z.: Probabilistic boosting-tree: Learning discriminative models for classification, recognition, and clustering. In: Proc. ICCV, Beijing, China, pp. 1589–1596 (2005)

10. Cootes, T.F., Taylor, C.J., Cooper, D.H., Graham, J.: Active shape models—their training and application. Comp. Vis. Image Understand. 61(1), 38–59 (1995)
11. Bullitt, E., Zeng, D., Gerig, G., Aylward, S., Joshi, S., Smith, J.K., Lin, W., Ewend, M.G.: Vessel tortuosity and brain tumor malignancy: A blinded study. Acad. Radiol. 12(10), 1232–1240 (2005)
12. Gouttard, S., Styner, M., Joshi, S., Smith, R.G., Cody, H., Gerig, G.: Subcortical structure segmentation using probabilistic atlas priors. In: Proc. SPIE Med. Imag., San Diego, CA, USA, pp. 65122J-1–11 (2007)
13. Heimann, T., Styner, M., van Ginneken, B.: Workshop on 3D segmentation in the clinic: A grand challenge. In: Heimann, T., Styner, M., van Ginneken, B. (eds.) 3D Segmentation in the Clinic: A Grand Challenge, pp. 7–15 (2007)
14. Bazin, P.L., Pham, D.L.: Homeomorphic brain image segmentation with topological and statistical atlases. Med. Image Anal. 12(5), 616–625 (2008)

Multiple Sclerosis Lesion Segmentation Using an Automatic Multimodal Graph Cuts

Daniel García-Lorenzo[1,2,3,*], Jeremy Lecoeur[1,2,3], Douglas L. Arnold[4], D. Louis Collins[4], and Christian Barillot[1,2,3]

[1] INRIA, VisAGeS Unit/Project, IRISA, Rennes, France
[2] University of Rennes I, CNRS IRISA, Rennes, France
[3] INSERM, U746 Unit/Project, IRISA, Rennes, France
[4] Montreal Neurological Institute, McGill University, Montreal, Canada

Abstract. Graph Cuts have been shown as a powerful interactive segmentation technique in several medical domains. We propose to automate the Graph Cuts in order to automatically segment Multiple Sclerosis (MS) lesions in MRI. We replace the manual interaction with a robust EM-based approach in order to discriminate between MS lesions and the Normal Appearing Brain Tissues (NABT). Evaluation is performed in synthetic and real images showing good agreement between the automatic segmentation and the target segmentation. We compare our algorithm with the state of the art techniques and with several manual segmentations. An advantage of our algorithm over previously published ones is the possibility to semi-automatically improve the segmentation due to the Graph Cuts interactive feature.

1 Introduction

Multiple Sclerosis (MS) is a chronic demyelienating disease that affects the central nervous system. Magnetic Resonance Imaging (MRI) has been proven as a very useful technique to study MS.

Manual segmentation of MS lesions is often performed in clinical trials. However, it is a lengthy process which shows high intra- and inter-rater variability [1]. Automatic segmentation methods have been developed to deal with these limitations [2,3], but in clinical studies these segmentations are often revised by an expert and manually edited when necessary.

Graph Cuts is a recently developed technique for interactive segmentation which has been successfully employed in different medical domains such as organ segmentation [4], healthy brain MRI [5], and pathological brain MRI [6]. It is based on both regional and contour information and always reaches the global minimum of its cost function [4]. The user has to select some seeds in both the "object" and the "background" in order to perform the segmentation. The result can be refined interactively by adding new seeds.

---

[*] We are thankful to ARSEP (Association pour la Recherche en Sclérose en Plaques) and UEB (Université Européenne de Bretagne) for funding.

In this paper, we propose to automate the Graph Cuts algorithm to segment MS lesions using several MR sequences. The initialization for Graph Cuts is given by a Finite Gaussian Mixture Model (FGMM) estimated by robust version of the Expectation-Maximization (EM) algorithm [7]. An advantage of our method over other automated methods is the possibility for an expert to easily refine the segmentation as the original semi-automatic Graph Cuts.

2 Method

In the following sections, we group all the MR sequences to a unique multidimensional image of dimension m equal to the number of sequences. In our case $m = 3$: T1-w, T2-w and PD-w. We assume that all the MR sequences of the same patient are previously registered in the same space, intensity inhomogeneity correction has been performed and the brain has been extracted.

We explain the general framework of the Graph Cuts, and the choices required for boundary information (the Spectral Gradient) and for regional information (an EM-based approach).

2.1 Graph Cuts

The segmentation can be described by a flow graph $\mathcal{G} = \langle \mathcal{V}, \mathcal{E} \rangle$ which represents the image [4]. In the graph $\mathcal{G}$, each voxel of the image corresponds to a node. The node set $\mathcal{V}$ also contains two particular nodes called terminal nodes - also known as "source" and "sink" - which respectively represents the classes "object" and "background". Nodes are connected with undirected edges $\mathcal{E}$.

We define $\mathcal{P}$ as the set containing all the nodes p of the brain and $\mathcal{N}$ as the set containing all the connection between two nodes $\{p, q\}$. Segmentation is represented by V, where V_p can be either "object" or "background". The energy $E(V)$ is then minimize by the Graph Cuts:

$$E(\mathrm{V}) = \alpha \cdot \sum_{p \in \mathcal{P}} R_p(V_p) + \sum_{\substack{\{p,q\} \in \mathcal{N} \\ V_p \neq V_q}} B_{\{p,q\}} \qquad (1)$$

The regional term $R_p(\cdot)$ expresses how the voxel p fits into given models of the object and background. In the graph, this relation is expressed by the connection of all the nodes to the source and sink nodes, called t-links, with weights, W_{SO}^p and W_{SI}^p respectively.

The boundary term $B_{\{p,q\}}$ reflects the similarity of the voxels p and q. Neighboring nodes are connected in the graph, n-links, with weight $B_{\{p,q\}}$. Their values are close to zero when the existence of a contour between p and q is very likely and large otherwise. The coefficient α is used to adjust the importance of the region and boundary terms.

This graph representation enables us to employ the Boykov-Kolmogorov graph minimization method [4] which is able to efficiently find the global minimum of the energy function (1).

2.2 The Spectral Gradient

The boundary weights $B_{\{p,q\}}$ are usually computed by an edge detection technique such as local intensity gradient. In our case, we choose the Spectral Gradient previously employed for multi-sequence MRI brain segmentation [6].

The objective is to consider our three MR sequences as an RGB color image and use an invariant color-edge detector [6]. This detector is based on a physical property of color, the spectral intensity e, and its derivatives with respect to the light wavelength λ, e_λ and $e_{\lambda\lambda}$, that are simple to compute [8].

For the graph, the detector is discretized, giving the following boundary term [6]:

$$B_{\{p,q\}} = \exp\left(-\frac{(\varepsilon(p) - \varepsilon(q))^2 + (\varepsilon_\lambda(p) - \varepsilon_\lambda(q))^2}{2\sigma^2}\right) \cdot \frac{1}{dist(p,q)} \quad (2)$$

where σ is a smoothing parameter (in our experiments $\sigma = 1$), and

$$\varepsilon = \frac{1}{e} \cdot \frac{\partial e}{\partial \lambda} = \frac{e_\lambda}{e} \quad \text{and} \quad \varepsilon_\lambda = \frac{\partial \varepsilon}{\partial \lambda} = \frac{e \cdot e_{\lambda\lambda} - e_\lambda^2}{e^2} \quad (3)$$

2.3 Automatic Calculation of the Sink and the Source

In semi-automatic frameworks, the weights $R_p(\mathcal{B})$ and $R_p(\mathcal{O})$ for the voxel p are usually defined this way:

$$R_p(\mathcal{B}) = \begin{cases} \infty \\ 0 \\ \alpha \cdot -\ln P(I_p|\mathcal{O}) \end{cases} \quad R_p(\mathcal{O}) = \begin{cases} 0 & \text{if } p \in \mathcal{B} \\ \infty & \text{if } p \in \mathcal{O} \\ \alpha \cdot -\ln P(I_p|\mathcal{B}) & \text{elsewhere} \end{cases} \quad (4)$$

The point sets $\mathcal{B}$ and $\mathcal{O}$ are the seeds of the background and the object respectively. The probability $P(I_p|\mathcal{B})$ reflects how the intensity vector I_p of voxel p fits into the intensity model estimated from $\mathcal{B}$. Most authors assume seeds follow a Gaussian distribution[5,6,4].

Our objective is to eliminate the dependence on the selection of seeds to create a fully automated method. Therefore we need to remove all the dependencies to the point sets $\mathcal{B}$ and $\mathcal{O}$. We propose to replace $P(I_p|\mathcal{B})$ and $P(I_p|\mathcal{O})$ in (4) with weights W_{SI} and W_{SO} described below. We keep the rest of (4) the same to allow posterior interaction of an expert to refine the segmentation if not satisfied with the automatic one.

Although the nature of the MRI noise is usually Rician [9], brain image intensities in MRI have been successfully modeled as a 3-class Multivariate FGMM in healthy subjects [10] and in MS patients [2,3]. These three classes correspond to Cerebrospinal Fluid (CSF), Grey Matter (GM) and White Matter (WM). On the contrary, MS lesions are usually considered not as a new class but as outliers from this 3-class NABT model [2,3].

First, we estimate the NABT model using a robust EM [7] which computes the trimmed likelihood in order to avoid outliers and has been successfully used in MS patients [3,11]. This algorithm has a parameter h, the rejection ratio, which adjusts the number of voxels that are not taken into account in the M-step in order to be robust to outliers. In our experiments h is fixed to 10% of the voxels, this value is large enough to avoid errors in estimation due to the MS lesions, veins, or registration and brain extraction errors.

Once the NABT model is estimated, we compute the Mahalanobis distance of each voxel p to each class i.

$$d^i_{Mahalanobis}(p) = \sqrt{(p-\mu_i)^T \Sigma_i^{-1}(p-\mu_i)}. \qquad (5)$$

where μ_i is the mean vector and Σ_i is the covariance matrix of the class i.

The Mahalanobis distance follows a χ^2_m distribution with m degrees of freedom when the data follow an m-dimension Gaussian law. This characteristic allows to obtain the *p-value* for each voxel, the probability the voxel does not fit into the model. We only consider the class with the lowest *p-value* for each voxel. Voxels with high *p-value* are more likely to be outliers than the others.

Sink: NABT voxels. Voxels that follow the model should have a weight with a high value. Therefore we assign $W_{SI} = 1.0 - p\text{-}value$

Source: MS lesions. Outliers, voxels with high *p-value*, are normally MS lesions but they can also occur due to veins or registration and skull-stripping errors. To select MS lesions from other outliers we apply a priori knowledge about the intensity of the lesions.

MS lesions are usually described as "hyperintense" compared to the WM in T2-w and PD-w images, we choose a fuzzy logic approach to model this experts' knowledge. Figure 2 describes the fuzzy function associated to "hyperintense" using the previously computed NABT model information. For each sequence, T2-w and PD-w, we obtain the fuzzy weights, W_{PD} and W_{T2}. We merge this information with the *p-value* using the fuzzy AND operator:

$$W_{SO}^{fuzzy} = \text{AND}\{W_{PD}, W_{T2}, p\text{-}value\} \qquad (6)$$

One post-processing step is performed after Graph Cuts. As many false positives occur due to artifacts in the external CSF, all lesions detected neighboring the brain border are removed from the segmentation.

3 Evaluation

We test our algorithm (GC) in two different situations. At first, we use synthetic images to evaluate the impact of different levels of noise and inhomogeneity. Then MR images of ten MS patients are segmented and compared with the manual segmentation delineated by several experts.

The evaluation measure is the Dice Similarity Coefficient (DSC) [12], widely employed for image segmentation evaluation. DSC values range from 0.0 to 1.0 where a value higher than 0.7 is usually considered good agreement.

3.1 Data

Synthetic Images. Brainweb MRI simulator [13] allows the creation of synthetic MR volumes (T1-w, T2-w and PD) of an MS patient controlling some acquisition parameters as slice thickness, noise and field inhomogeneity. Three different phantoms are available with different lesion loads: mild, moderate and severe.

We perform the automatic segmentation varying the noise level (1%, 3%, 5%, 7% and 9%) and the intensity inhomogeneity (0%, 20% and 40%) for the three available phantoms. The ground truth is available, the evaluation is done comparing the results of our algorithm with this ground truth using the DSC. In these synthetic images, no errors due to registration or brain extraction exist, which means that the total number of outliers will be significantly reduced. For this reason we set h, the parameter of the robust EM, to 5% instead of 10%.

Real Images. Real images in our experiments consist of MR volumes (T1-w, T2-w and PD) of 10 patients with MS. All the images undergo the same preprocessing workflow: intensity inhomogeneity correction [14], intra-subject multimodal registration [15] and brain extraction [16].

Each patient image is manually segmented by 5 experts. A silver standard is built considering the consensus of 3 out of 5 experts to define a lesion voxel. Our algorithm and the EMS software [2] are compared with the silver standard using DSC. To have an idea of the common agreement among experts we compute the average inter-rater DSC (IRDSC). For each pair of experts we compute the DSC and for each patient, all the DSC values are averaged to the IRDSC. The common agreement is good if IRDSC is above 0.7.

STAPLE algorithm [17] was designed to study the performance of different raters when the ground truth is not available. The idea is to compute the sensibility and specificity of each rater while estimating the most probable true segmentation. We use the ITK[1] implementation to compute STAPLE among the 5 raters and our method. We did not include EMS algorithm because it is also an EM-based approach and it could bias the STAPLE results.

3.2 Results

Synthetic Images. Fig. 1 sums up the results for the three phantoms and variations in noise and inhomogeneity. The performance of the algorithm decreases significantly for high levels of noise (7% and 9%) and for low levels (1%), showing DSC values over 0.7 for 3% and 5%. On the contrary, the intensity inhomogeneity slightly affects the performance of the segmentation. Mild phantom (left figure) shows lower DSC scores, this is reasonable because errors affect more the DSC when the target region is smaller.

Real Images. Results are shown in Table 1 and Figure 4. Globally we conclude that our algorithm performs a better segmentation than EMS. Our algorithm obtains better scores for 7 out of 10 patients compared to EMS. Patients (3, 4, 6 and

---

[1] http://www.itk.org

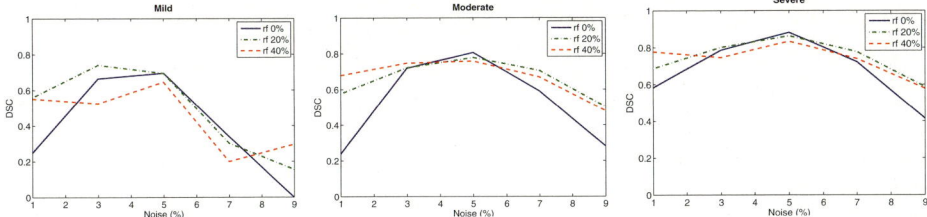

Fig. 1. From left to right: DSC values from mild, moderate and severe phantoms for different values of noise and inhomogeneity (rf)

Table 1. Total lesion load (TLL), the inter-rater DSC (IRDSC), the DSC for EMS software and the DSC for our method (GC)

	TLL(ml)	IRDSC	EMS	GC
Patient 1	33.9	0.77	0.67	0.75
Patient 2	2.8	0.70	0.61	0.75
Patient 3	1.4	0.60	0.42	0.38
Patient 4	1.0	0.61	0.41	0.46
Patient 5	20.0	0.81	0.80	0.86
Patient 6	2.7	0.51	0.48	0.40
Patient 7	6.0	0.69	0.72	0.71
Patient 8	6.2	0.61	0.69	0.72
Patient 9	1.2	0.64	0.35	0.50
Patient 10	47.7	0.81	0.71	0.73
Average		0.68	0.59	0.63

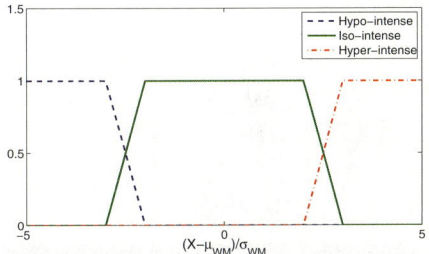

Fig. 2. Fuzzy membership functions for: hypo-intensity, hyper-intensity and iso-intensity. For each voxel we can assign its fuzzy value using these functions.

9) with low lesion loads ($< 2.7ml$) obtain poor scores for both algorithms as well as low experts agreement (IRDSC < 0.65). This can be partially explain because DSC decreases more a for small TLL. For the rest of the patients our DSC is always higher than 0.7 showing a good agreement with the target segmentation.

As described before, STAPLE gives the specificity and sensibility for each expert as presented in Figure 3. We can observe that the sensibility of our Graph Cuts algorithm is higher than three experts but with a slightly lower specificity.

4 Discussion

In this paper, we have proposed an automatic algorithm for the MS lesion segmentation for multi-sequence MRI. Experiments with synthetic images have shown good agreement with the ground truth for all levels of inhomogeneity and standard levels of noise. For very noisy images, a noise reduction preprocessing step might be necessary. The evaluation in real images demonstrates a good agreement of our segmentation with a group of experts while shows a better segmentation than state of the art algorithm EMS.

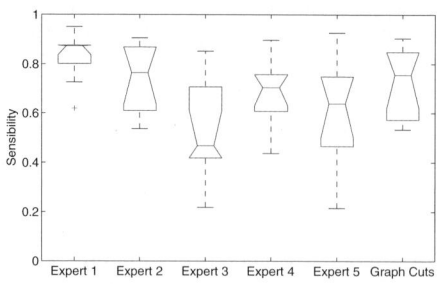
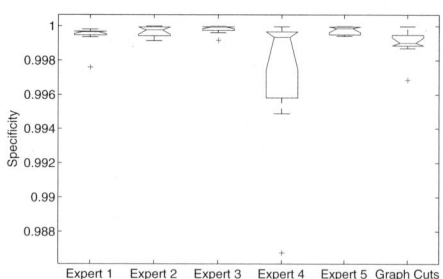

Fig. 3. Sensibility (left) and Specificity (right) boxplots for the different experts and the automatic segmentation. Specificity values are very high because the size of the lesions is very small compared to the size of the brain. However, small variations of specificity greatly modifies the DSC value.

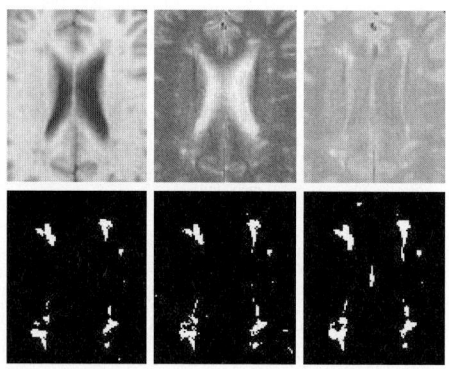

Fig. 4. Top, from left to right: T1-w, T2-w and PD images of patient 8. Bottom, from left to right: Consensus, EMS and Graph Cuts segmentations.

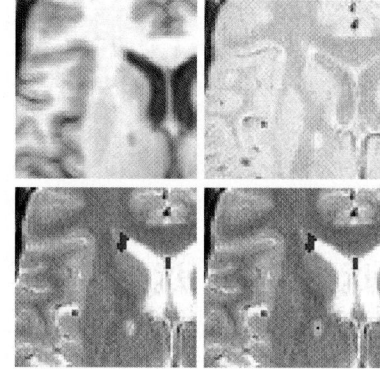

Fig. 5. Top, left to right: T1-w, and PD images of patient 4. Bottom, left to right: automatic solution and semi-automatic solution (*Red*: source seed, *Green*: Graph Cut solution, *Blue*: automatic segmentation).

Fully automated methods are often revised by an expert in clinical trial to verify their validity and edited when necessary. In Figure 5, we can observe an example of semi-automatic edition of our automatic segmentation. When a lesion is missed, a user can add a seed, in this case a source seed, and the Graph Cuts is recomputed in few seconds.

References

1. Grimaud, J., Lai, M., Thorpe, J., Adeleine, P., Wang, L., Barker, G.J., Plummer, D.L., Tofts, P.S., McDonald, W.I., Miller, D.H.: Quantification of MRI lesion load in multiple sclerosis: a comparison of three computer-assisted techniques. MR Imaging 14(5), 495–505 (1996)

2. Van Leemput, K., Maes, F., Vandermeulen, D., Colchester, A., Suetens, P.: Automated segmentation of multiple sclerosis lesions by model outlier detection. IEEE TMI 20(8), 677–688 (2001)
3. Aït-Ali, L.S., Prima, S., Hellier, P., Carsin, B., Edan, G., Barillot, C.: STREM: A robust multidimensional parametric method to segment MS lesions in MRI. MICCAI 8(Pt 1), 409–416 (2005)
4. Boykov, Y., Funka-Lea, G.: Graph cuts and efficient N-D images segmentation. International Journal of Computer Vision 70(2), 109–131 (2006)
5. Song, Z., Tustison, N., Avants, B., Gee, J.: Adaptative graph cuts with tissue priors for brain MRI segmentation. In: IEEE ISBI, pp. 762–765 (2006)
6. Lecoeur, J., Morissey, S., Ferré, J.C., Arnold, D., Collins, D., Barillot, C.: Multiple sclerosis lesions segmentation using spectral gradient and graph cuts. In: MIAMS Workshop, September 2008, pp. 92–103 (2008)
7. Neykov, N., Filzmoser, P., Dimova, R., Neytchev, P.: Robust fitting of mixtures using the trimmed likelihood estimator. Comput. Stat. & Data Analysis 52(1), 299–308 (2007)
8. Geusebroek, J.M., van den Boomgaard, R., Smeulders, A., Dev, A.: Color and scale: The spatial structure of color images. In: Vernon, D. (ed.) ECCV 2000. LNCS, vol. 1842, pp. 331–341. Springer, Heidelberg (2000)
9. Dietrich, O., Raya, J.G., Reeder, S.B., Ingrisch, M., Reiser, M.F., Schoenberg, S.O.: Influence of multichannel combination, parallel imaging and other reconstruction techniques on MRI noise characteristics. MRI 26(6), 754–762 (2008)
10. Schroeter, P., Vesin, J.M., Langenberger, T., Meuli, R.: Robust parameter estimation of intensity distributions for brain magnetic resonance images. IEEE TMI 17(2), 172–186 (1998)
11. García-Lorenzo, D., Prima, S., Collins, D.L., Arnold, D.L., Morrissey, S.P., Barillot, C.: Combining Robust Expectation Maximization and Mean Shift algorithms for Multiple Sclerosis Brain Segmentation. In: MIAMS Workshop, September 2008, pp. 82–91 (2008)
12. Zijdenbos, A., Dawant, B., Margolin, R., Palmer, A.: Morphometric analysis of white matter lesions in MR images: method and validation. IEEE TMI 13(4), 716–724 (1994)
13. Collins, D., Zijdenbos, A., Kollokian, V., Sled, J., Kabani, N., Holmes, C., Evans, A.: Design and construction of a realistic digital brain phantom. IEEE TMI 17(3), 463–468 (1998)
14. Sled, J.G., Zijdenbos, A.P., Evans, A.C.: A nonparametric method for automatic correction of intensity nonuniformity in MRI data. IEEE TMI 17(1), 87–97 (1998)
15. Collins, D., Neelin, P., Peters, T.M., Evans, A.C.: Automatic 3D Intersubject Registration of MR Volumetric Data in Standardized Talairach Space. JCAT 18, 192–205 (1994)
16. Smith, S.M.: Fast robust automated brain extraction. Hum. Brain Mapp. 17(3), 143–155 (2002)
17. Warfield, S., Zou, K., Wells, W.: Simultaneous truth and performance level estimation (STAPLE): an algorithm for the validation of image segmentation. IEEE TMI 23(7), 903–921 (2004)

Towards Accurate, Automatic Segmentation of the Hippocampus and Amygdala from MRI

D. Louis Collins[1,2] and Jens C. Pruessner[1,3]

[1] McConnell Brain Imaging Center, Montreal Neurological Institute
[2] Department Biomedical Engineering
[3] Douglas Hospital Research Center, Department of Psychology
McGill University, Montreal, Canada
{louis.collins,jens.pruessner}@mcgill.ca

Abstract. We describe progress towards fully automatic segmentation of the hippocampus (HC) and amygdala (AG) in human subjects from MRI data. Three methods are described and tested with a set of MRIs from 80 young normal controls, using manual labeling of the HC and AG as a gold standard. The methods include: 1) our ANIMAL atlas-based method that uses non-linear registration to a pre-labeled non-linear average template (ICBM152). HC and AG labels, defined on the template are mapped through the inverse transformation to segment these structures on the subject's MRI; 2) template-based segmentation, where we select the most similar MRI from the set of 80 labeled datasets to use as a template in the standard ANIMAL segmentation scheme; 3) label fusion methods where we combine segmentations from the 'n' most similar templates. The label fusion technique yields the best results with median kappas of 0.886 and 0.826 for HC and AG, respectively.

1 Introduction

The hippocampus (HC) is a part of the brain located in the medial aspect of the temporal lobe and is part of the limbic system. The HC plays an important role in general and spatial memory in humans and animals, integrating external with internal signals to form a cohesive and unified spatial and temporal orientation of oneself in the environment. HC dysfunction and neurodegeneration has been described in a variety of mental diagnoses, including Alzheimer's disease (AD) [1], Posttraumatic Stress Disorder [2], Major Depression [3], Schizophrenia [4, 5], and epilepsy [6]. The amygdala (AG) lies adjacent to the HC in the medial temporal lobe, is also part of the limbic system, and is most significantly associated with emotional memory and its regulation. Structural variations of the AG are now being discussed as implicated in mental diagnoses like Schizophrenia and anxiety disorders, and more and more studies now employ volume assessment of the HC and AG from MRI in their protocols [7]. Since HC and AG volumes can be important markers of neurodegeneration and can provide a useful outcome measure in clinical trials of new therapies for diseases such as AD, there is significant interest in developing robust, automated methods for segmenting the both the HC and AG.

Table 1. Methods survey

Author	Method summary	HC kappa
Hogan JDI;2000,**13**(2-1):217-8	landmark + fluid reg.	0.75
Kelemen TMI,1999.**18**(10):828-39	PCA constrained elastic registration	0.75 (HC+AG complex)
Klemencic JIST,2004,48(2):166-171	Appearance based	0.800
Fischl Neuron,2002. **33**(3):341-55.	classification +MRF	0.79-0.86
Khan NI, 2008;**41**(3):735-46.	LDDMM	0.77
Morey NI, Dec 2008;	FreeSurfacer	0.82
Morey NI, Dec 2008;	FSL/FIRST	0.79
Morra NI,2008;**43**(1):59-68	Auto context model + adaboost	0.835-0.859
Pohl TMI, 2007;**26**(9):1201-12	Hierarchical EM	0.808(l)-0.813(r)
Van der Lijn NI,2008;**43**(4): 708-20.	A priori + graph cuts	0.852(l)-0.864(r)
Heckemann NI,2006;33(1):115-26	b-spline + label fusion	0.81(l) – 0.83(r)
Aljabar NI, 2008;**43**(2):225-35.	b-spline + label fusion	0.84
Gousias NI, 2008;**40**(2):672-84	b-spline + label fusion,	0.88
Chupin NI, 2007;34(3):996-1019	seeding + morphology region growing	0.87 (young) ; 0.86 (AD subj)
Barnes NI, 2008;40(4):1655-71	Template library + linear reg + threshold	0.87 (controls); 0.86 (AD subj)

JDI=Journal Digital Imaging, NI=NeuroImage, TMI=IEEE Trans Medical Imaging, JIST=Journal of Imaging Science and Technology.

Manual segmentation of the HC and AG is considered the gold standard for volumetric assessment [8-11]. While it is possible to define a protocol that results in low inter- and intra-rater variability, the procedures remain time-consuming (30-60min per HC) and thus difficult to apply in studies involving large numbers (100s) of subjects. Automatic methods for segmentation require no manual intervention, and thus do not suffer from the problems of inter- and intra-observer variability. Most model-based automatic segmentation methods use one of (i) deformable models [12], (ii) appearance-based models [13, 14] or (iii) atlas-based techniques to identify the structure(s) of interest [15-17].

Since a model or template derived from a single individual will be biased in some way for all subjects to be segmented, Barnes et al. developed an efficient 'template library' HC segmentation method where the most similar brain from a group of 55 pre-labeled subjects was selected for the template atlas for registration-based segmentation [18]. Heckemann also developed a segmentation method that took advantage of a library of 30 pre-labeled subjects [19]. Instead of selecting the best template, they used a spline-based non-linear registration technique [20] with each template to generate 30 segmentations for a given subject. Label fusion techniques [21] were then used to combine the segmentations into a single consistent label set for the subject. Since this procedure required considerable computational effort, Aljabar et al. optimized the technique by selecting the 'n' most appropriate atlases from the library using normalized mutual information [22]. Recently, Chupin et al. reported on an ingenious Markovian model region growing procedure that uses morphometric and topological constraints with anatomical rules to identify HC-specific landmarks segment the HC and AG [23, 24]. At present, the work of Barnes [18], Chupin [23] and Gousias [25] yield the best published segmentation results for hippocampus (see Table 1 for a methods survey).

The goal of the current manuscript is to describe our recently developed fully automatic segmentation protocol for the HC and AG in human subjects from MRI data. The method combines atlas-based segmentation with a template library and label fusion. The main contributions are threefold: 1) instead of a b-spline technique, we use the publicly available ANIMAL non-linear registration algorithm for the atlas-based segmentation method [15, 26]; 2) we compare the technique to two other methods (the standard ANIMAL and a Barnes-like template library technique); and 3) when validated with manual labels from 80 subjects, the results are better than previously published automatic techniques.

2 Methods

The T1-weighted (T1w) MRI data (sagittal acquisition, 140-160 contiguous 1mm thick slices, TR=18 ms, TE=10 ms, flip angle 30°, rectangular field of view of 256mm SI and 204mm AP) used in this study come from a group of 152 young, neurologically healthy individuals acquired on a 1.5T Philips Gyroscan in the context of the International Consortium for Brain Mapping (ICBM) project [27]. The local Ethics Committee approved the study and informed consent was obtained from all participants. Eighty subjects (from the 152) were selected to limit the number of manually segmented HC and AG and so that the male (n=39) and female (n=41) groups were comparable in age (mean age 25.09 ± 4.9 years), handedness and years of education.

For the three procedures described below, the original T1w MRI data were pre-processed. First, each MRI volume was corrected for image intensity non-uniformity using a method that estimates a multiplicative bias field that maximizes the intensity histogram entropy [28]. Next, each dataset was stereotaxically transformed using an affine transformation into the Talairach-like MNI coordinate system [29] and resampled onto a $1mm^3$ isotropic grid using a tri-linear kernel.

HC and AG and labels were manually defined using the protocol defined in [8] where intra-class reliability coefficients (ICC) were reported of 0.900 and 0.925 for inter- (4 raters) and intra-rater (5 repeats) reliability, respectively, for the HC and 0.835 and 0.930 (respectively) for the AG in these 80 young normal controls.

2.1 Segmentation Procedures

Three segmentation procedures were employed in the experiments presented below. The first is based on the publicly available ANIMAL segmentation method and uses an average template [15, 26]. The second uses ANIMAL with the best single subject template selected from a template library (like Barnes [18]). The third uses ANIMAL with the best n templates selected from a template library and combines the n segmentations with label fusion. These three methods are described in greater depth below.

The ANIMAL technique with an average template. (*ANIMAL*) [15, 26] is an atlas-based segmentation method that uses non-linear registration to a pre-labeled average template to achieve segmentation (Fig. 1). The template labels are mapped through the inverse of subject-template registration to identify the structures of interest in the subject's MRI. To estimate the required non-linear transformation, the ANIMAL algorithm attempts to match image grey-level intensity features in local neighbourhoods in a hierarchical fashion by maximizing the cross-correlation of intensities between the subject and template images. The procedure begins by estimating the deformations required to match blurred versions of the subject and template data. The result is a dense deformation field, where a displacement vector is stored at each node of the field that best matches the local neighbourhoods. This deformation field is subsampled and used as input to the next iteration of the procedure, where the blurring is reduced and the estimation of the deformation field is refined. Labels, defined on the template, are mapped though the inverse of the recovered transformation to identify the HC and AG on the subject. Since the non-linear registration is imperfect, it is possible that CSF voxels might be included in the label set. A simple thresholding rule (0.4 * median intensity of HC label) is used to eliminate CSF.

The ANIMAL technique with a template library (*A+best template*). Even though the average template used by ANIMAL represents the average anatomy, it might not be optimal to segment certain individual subjects. We therefore investigated a second method, inspired by the work of Barnes et al. [18]. We used the 80 labeled MRI volumes described above as a template library. In order to achieve segmentation, the best template for a given subject is selected from the remaining 79 templates in the database in a leave-one-out fashion. The best template is selected using normalized mutual information between the subject to be segmented and each of the potential templates. Instead of using only linear transformations like Barnes [18], in our approach the selected template was used with non-linear registration in the ANIMAL segmentation procedure described above. The advantage of this technique is that the template that is most similar to the subject is used, and thus the non-linear deformations (required to match subject-to-template) are minimized, resulting in good segmentation. The computational cost of this method is slightly higher than the ANIMAL method since it requires evaluation of the normalized mutual information metric with each potential template.

The ANIMAL technique with a template library and label fusion (*A+fusion*). One of the disadvantages of the method described above is that it is possible that the single template selected may not be optimal for segmentation of the given subject and that errors in the non-linear estimation between subject and template may result in errors in segmentation. For these reasons, we consider combining multiple segmentations to minimize errors and maximize consistency between segmentations. To do so, the best n templates for a given subject are selected from the remaining 79 templates in the database using normalized mutual information. Each template is then used to produce an independent segmentation of the subject using the ANIMAL procedure. The result is n different segmentations and the issue becomes how to combine the segmentations to achieve a single consistent labeling of the subject. Following the work of Rofhling et al. [21], Heckemann et al. [19] and Aljabar et al. [22], we use label fusion. At each voxel, a voting strategy is used; the label with the most votes from the n templates is assigned to the voxel. To avoid bias, a random selection is used when two or more labels tie in the voting scheme.

Before applying the label fusion method, the optimum number of templates n must be determined. To do so, we applied the technique with $n=2..20$ and examined the graph to see how K and S change with n (Fig. 2). Since both kappa and similarity increase with the number of labels fused, but appear to plateau after $n=11$, we decided to use $n=11$ for the label fusion procedure.

The computation cost of this method is much greater than the first two methods. Not only is normalized mutual information estimated for each potential template, but n non-linear registrations must be computed to achieve the final segmentation. The main differences between our work and those cited above are in the choice of non-linear registration scheme (i.e., ANIMAL vs. b-splines) and in the improved results for HC and AG presented below.

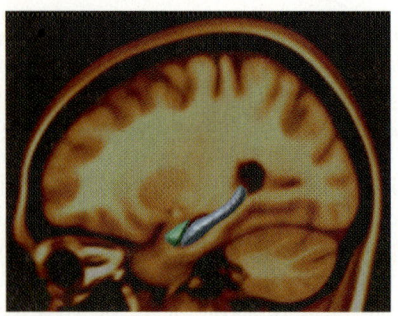

Fig. 1. Sagittal image of ICBM152 nonlinear average template with model HC (blue) + AG (green)

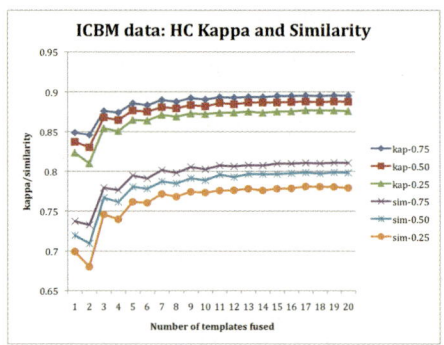

Fig. 2. Kappa (kap-) and Similarity (sim-) plotted (lower quartile (0.25), median (0.50), upper quartile (0.75)) against the number of templates fused

3 Experiments and Results

Each of the methods was applied to segment the HC and AG (left and right sides) in the set of 80 MRI volumes. Figure 3 shows the segmentation results on 2 subjects. For each of the methods, the HC and AG automatic labels were compared to the gold standard manual labels using Dice's Kappa [$\mathbf{K} = 2 * (V(M \cap A)) / (V(M) + V(A))$]; Jaccard Similarity [$\mathbf{S} = (V(M \cap A)) / (V(M \cup A))$] and Normalized volume difference [$\mathbf{D} = 2 * abs (V(M) - V(A))/(V(M) + V(A))$]; where M is the set of manually labeled voxels, A is the set of automatically labeled voxels, $\cap$ is the set intersection operator, where $\cup$ is the set union operator, abs($\bullet$) is the absolute volume and V($\bullet$) is the volume operator. **K** and **S** take on a value between 0 and 1.0, with 1.0 indicating perfect agreement. The values of **S** are always less than **K**. **D** takes on positive values. Values closer to 0.0 are better. The relationships between manual and automatic structure volumes are reported as Pearson's product-moment correlation (r). Tables 2 & 3 summarize the quantitative results for HC, and AG, respectively.

Table 2. Hippocampus segmentation results (median and inter-quartile range)

	A + ICBM152	A + best template	A + fusion
K	0.864 (0.844-0.874)	0.837 (0.823-0.849)	**0.886** (0.874-0.893)
S	0.761 (0.729-0.776)	0.720 (0.670-0.738)	**0.796** (0.795-0.808)
D	5.5% (2.4%-10.1%)	6.5% (3.3%-11.1%)	**4.9%** (2.7%-8.3%)
r	0.666	0.757	**0.834**

Table 3. Amygdala segmentation results (median and inter-quartile range)

	A + ICBM152	A + best template	A + fusion
K	0.821 (0.784-0.842)	0.769 (0.736-0.794)	**0.826** (0.799-0.856)
S	0.696 (0.546-0.727)	0.625 (0.582-0.658)	**0.703** (0.665-0.748)
D	9.1% (4.3%-17.4%)	12.2% (5.6%-22.0%)	**9.0%** (4.6%-15.6%)
r	0.605	0.405	**0.566**

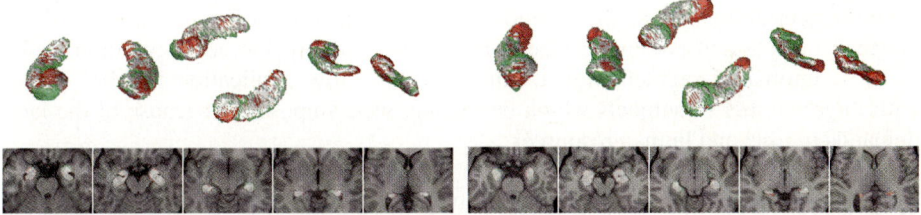

Fig. 3. Example fusion segmentation results for two subjects. White indicates agreement between manual and automatic segmentation, red=false positive and green=false negatives. (note: HC and AG are segmented separately, but are presented here together for simplicity) left: K_{HC}=0.89,0.89; K_{AG}=0.82,0.81; right: K_{HC}=0.85,0.85; K_{AG}=0.76,0.82.

Table 4. Volume results

	HC (cc^3)	compared to manual	AG (cc^3)	compared to manual
Manual	3.177	-	1.121	-
A + ICBM152	3.188	p=0.670	1.067	p<0.001
A + template	3.226	p=0.038	1.178	p=0.001
A + fusion	3.195	p=0.328	1.144	p=0.092

Table 4 compares the automatic and manual volumes of the segmented structures. The best template method overestimates the true HC volume (p=0.038), while the other techniques are unbiased. The standard ANIMAL technique underestimates the true AG volume (p<0.001), while the best template method overestimates its volume (p=0.001). The fusion technique is unbiased.

4 Discussion and Conclusion

We have presented and compared three methods for automatic segmentation of the HC and AG from MRI of the human brain. The procedures use registration of a subject's MRI to a pre-labeled volume to achieve segmentation. The label fusion approach improves on the other two methods because it combines information from multiple sources (i.e., multiple templates) to identify the HC and AG on the subjects. The fusion of multiple automatic label sets enables the procedure to eliminate inconsistent segmentations that may cause errors in the template library approach where only one template is used.

It is difficult to compare segmentation results between different published methods. The quality of the MRI data, the anatomical definition of the structure, the quality of the manual gold standard, the particular population studied and the different metrics reported make it difficult to compare results. However, with these caveats in mind, we have shown that ANIMAL non-linear registration atlas-based segmentation, combined with a template library and label fusion can achieve high levels of accuracy with a median kappa of 0.887 and similarity of 0.798 for HC (0.826 and 0.796, respectively for AG). These values are as high or higher than other previously published automatic techniques in the literature (see Table 1).

The label fusion technique was demonstrated to be robust and accurate and yields better results compared to the previous literature in terms of kappa and similarity between manual and automatic labels. In summary, the recent advances in precision in fully automated segmentation techniques will allow application in MRI studies with large number of subjects which previously were impossible because of the large demands in time and human resources.

References

1. Jack Jr., C.R., Petersen, R.C., Xu, Y., O'Brien, P.C., Smith, G.E., Ivnik, R.J., Boeve, B.F., Tangalos, E.G., Kokmen, E.: Rates of hippocampal atrophy correlate with change in clinical status in aging and AD. Neurology 55, 484–489 (2000)
2. Bremner, J.D., Randall, P., Scott, T.M., Bronen, R.A., Seibyl, J.P., Southwick, S.M., Delaney, R.C., McCarthy, G., Charney, D.S., Innis, R.B.: MRI-based measurement of hippocampal volume in patients with combat-related posttraumatic stress disorder. Am. J. Psychiatry 152, 973–981 (1995)
3. Bremner, J.D., Narayan, M., Anderson, E.R., Staib, L.H., Miller, H.L., Charney, D.S.: Hippocampal volume reduction in major depression. Am. J. Psychiatry 157, 115–118 (2000)
4. Tanskanen, P., Veijola, J.M., Piippo, U.K., Haapea, M., Miettunen, J.A., Pyhtinen, J., Bullmore, E.T., Jones, P.B., Isohanni, M.K.: Hippocampus and amygdala volumes in schizophrenia and other psychoses in the Northern Finland 1966 birth cohort. Schizophr. Res. 75, 283–294 (2005)
5. Buss, C., Lord, C., Wadiwalla, M., Hellhammer, D.H., Lupien, S.J., Meaney, M.J., Pruessner, J.C.: Maternal care modulates the relationship between prenatal risk and hippocampal volume in women but not in men. J. Neurosci. 27, 2592–2595 (2007)
6. Bernasconi, N., Duchesne, S., Janke, A., Collins, D.L., Bernasconi, A.: Voxel-based statistical analysis of grey matter and white matter in patients with unilateral temporal lobe epilepsy. In: Human Brain Mapping Conference (2003)
7. Berretta, S., Pantazopoulos, H., Lange, N.: Neuron numbers and volume of the amygdala in subjects diagnosed with bipolar disorder or schizophrenia. Biol. Psychiatry 62, 884–893 (2007)

8. Pruessner, J.C., Li, L.M., Serles, W., Pruessner, M., Collins, D.L., Kabani, N., Lupien, S., Evans, A.C.: Volumetry of hippocampus and amygdala with high-resolution MRI and three-dimensional analysis software: minimizing the discrepancies between laboratories. Cereb. Cortex. 10, 433–442 (2000)
9. Matsuoka, Y., Mori, E., Inagaki, M., Kozaki, Y., Nakano, T., Wenner, M., Uchitomi, Y.: Manual tracing guideline for volumetry of hippocampus and amygdala with high-resolution MRI. No To Shinkei 55, 690–697 (2003)
10. Bonilha, L., Kobayashi, E., Cendes, F., Li, L.M.: Protocol for volumetric segmentation of medial temporal structures using high-resolution 3-D magnetic resonance imaging. Hum. Brain Mapp. 22, 145–154 (2004)
11. McHugh, T.L., Saykin, A.J., Wishart, H.A., Flashman, L.A., Cleavinger, H.B., Rabin, L.A., Mamourian, A.C., Shen, L.: Hippocampal volume and shape analysis in an older adult population. Clin. Neuropsychol. 21, 130–145 (2007)
12. Ghanei, A., Soltanian-Zadeh, H., Windham, J.P.: Segmentation of the hippocampus from brain MRI using deformable contours. Comput. Med. Imaging Graph 22, 203–216 (1998)
13. Duchesne, S., Pruessner, J., Collins, D.L.: Appearance-based segmentation of medial temporal lobe structures. Neuroimage 17, 515–531 (2002)
14. Kelmencic, J., Pluim, J.P.W., Viergever, M., Schnack, H.G., Valencic, V.: Non-rigid regisgration based on active apearance models for 3D medical image segmentation. Journal of Imaging Science and technology 48, 166–171 (2004)
15. Collins, D.L., Holmes, C.J., PEters, T.M., Evans, A.C.: Automatic 3D model-based neuroanatomical segmentation. Human Brain Mapping 3, 190–208 (1995)
16. Csernansky, J.G., Joshi, S., Wang, L., Haller, J.W., Gado, M., Miller, J.P., Grenander, U., Miller, M.I.: Hippocampal morphometry in schizophrenia by high dimensional brain mapping. Proc. Natl. Acad. Sci. U S A 95, 11406–11411 (1998)
17. Shen, D., Moffat, S., Resnick, S.M., Davatzikos, C.: Measuring size and shape of the hippocampus in MR images using a deformable shape model. Neuroimage 15, 422–434 (2002)
18. Barnes, J., Foster, J., Boyes, R.G., Pepple, T., Moore, E.K., Schott, J.M., Frost, C., Scahill, R.I., Fox, N.C.: A comparison of methods for the automated calculation of volumes and atrophy rates in the hippocampus. Neuroimage 40, 1655–1671 (2008)
19. Heckemann, R.A., Hajnal, J.V., Aljabar, P., Rueckert, D., Hammers, A.: Automatic anatomical brain MRI segmentation combining label propagation and decision fusion. Neuroimage 33, 115–126 (2006)
20. Rueckert, D., Sonoda, L.I., Hayes, C., Hill, D.L., Leach, M.O., Hawkes, D.J.: Nonrigid registration using free-form deformations: application to breast MR images. IEEE Trans. Med. Imaging 18, 712–721 (1999)
21. Rohlfing, T., Brandt, R., Menzel, R., Maurer Jr., C.R.: Evaluation of atlas selection strategies for atlas-based image segmentation with application to confocal microscopy images of bee brains. Neuroimage 21, 1428–1442 (2004)
22. Aljabar, P., Heckemann, R., Hammers, A., Hajnal, J.V., Rueckert, D.: Classifier selection strategies for label fusion using large atlas databases. Med. Image Comput. Comput. Assist. Interv. Int. Conf. Med. Image. Comput. Comput. Assist. Interv. 10, 523–531 (2007)
23. Chupin, M., Mukuna-Bantumbakulu, A.R., Hasboun, D., Bardinet, E., Baillet, S., Kinkingnehun, S., Lemieux, L., Dubois, B., Garnero, L.: Anatomically constrained region deformation for the automated segmentation of the hippocampus and the amygdala: Method and validation on controls and patients with Alzheimer's disease. Neuroimage 34, 996–1019 (2007)

24. Colliot, O., Chetelat, G., Chupin, M., Desgranges, B., Magnin, B., Benali, H., Dubois, B., Garnero, L., Eustache, F., Lehericy, S.: Discrimination between Alzheimer disease, mild cognitive impairment, and normal aging by using automated segmentation of the hippocampus. Radiology 248, 194–201 (2008)
25. Gousias, I.S., Rueckert, D., Heckemann, R.A., Dyet, L.E., Boardman, J.P., Edwards, A.D., Hammers, A.: Automatic segmentation of brain MRIs of 2-year-olds into 83 regions of interest. Neuroimage 40, 672–684 (2008)
26. Collins, D.L., Evans, A.C.: ANIMAL: validation and applications of nonlinear registration-based segmentation. International Journal of Pattern Recognition and Artificial Intelligence 11, 1271 (1997)
27. Mazziotta, J.C., Toga, A.W., Evans, A., Fox, P., Lancaster, J.: A probabilistic atlas of the human brain: theory and rationale for its development. The International Consortium for Brain Mapping (ICBM). Neuroimage 2, 89–101 (1995)
28. Sled, J.G., Zijdenbos, A.P., Evans, A.C.: A nonparametric method for automatic correction of intensity nonuniformity in MRI data. IEEE Trans. Med. Imaging 17, 87–97 (1998)
29. Collins, D.L., Neelin, P., Peters, T.M., Evans, A.C.: Automatic 3D intersubject registration of MR volumetric data in standardized Talairach space. J. Comput. Assist. Tomogr. 18, 192–205 (1994)

An Object-Based Method for Rician Noise Estimation in MR Images

Pierrick Coupé[1], José V. Manjón[2], Elias Gedamu[1], Douglas Arnold[1], Montserrat Robles[2], and D. Louis Collins[1]

[1] McConnell Brain Imaging Centre, Montréal Neurological Institute, McGill University, 3801 University Street, Montréal, Canada H3A 2B4
[2] Biomedical Informatics Group (IBIME), ITACA Institute, Universidad Politécnica de Valencia, Camino de Vera, s/n. 46022 Valencia, Spain

Abstract. The estimation of the noise level in MR images is used to assess the consistency of statistical analysis or as an input parameter in some image processing techniques. Most of the existing Rician noise estimation methods are based on background statistics, and as such are sensitive to ghosting artifacts. In this paper, a new object-based method is proposed. This method is based on the adaptation of the Median Absolute Deviation (MAD) estimator in the wavelet domain for Rician noise. The adaptation for Rician noise is performed by using only the wavelet coefficients corresponding to the object and by correcting the estimation with an iterative scheme based on the SNR of the image. A quantitative validation on synthetic phantom with artefacts is presented and a new validation framework is proposed to perform quantitative validation on real data. The results show the accuracy and the robustness of the proposed method.

1 Introduction

In MR image analysis, the estimation of the noise level in an image is a mandatory step that must be addressed to assess the quality of the analysis and the consistency of the image processing technique. The noise variance is also an important measure for many image processing techniques such as denoising [1, 2] or registration. Furthermore, procedures that employ statistical analysis techniques, such as functional MR imaging or voxel-based morphometry, often base their conclusions on assumptions about the underlying noise characteristics. Usually, the real and imaginary parts of the MR complex raw data are considered corrupted by white additive Gaussian noise, where the noise variance is assumed to be the same in both parts (real and imaginary) [3, 4]. By taking the magnitude of the complex data, the noise is transformed into Rician noise [3, 4, 5, 6, 7]. Conventionally, the Rician noise is i) described by a Rayleigh distribution in the background [3, 4, 6, 7] (i.e. the signal of air in the background is considered to be zero), and ii) approximated by Gaussian noise in the foreground when Signal Noise Ratio (SNR) is high enough ($> 3dB$ [1]). These models for background and foreground noise distribution have been used in the majority of noise estimation methods [8, 6, 7]. However, the Rayleigh model of the background can fail when ghosting artefacts are present (i.e. non-zero signal) [6], and the Gaussian approximation of foreground is no longer valid for images with low SNR [6]. Some automatic techniques have been proposed [8, 6, 7]. Usually, these methods use the histogram of the background and some properties of the Rayleigh distribution. Recently, a new noise Rician variance estimation method based on maximum likelihood (ML) estimation from a partial histogram was presented by Sijbers [6]. More recently, Aja et al. [7] presented a set of new methods for noise estimation based on local statistics. In this paper, an adaptation of the Median Absolute Deviation (MAD) estimator in the wavelet domain is proposed for Rician noise. This robust and efficient estimator has been proposed by Donoho [9] for Gaussian noise and since has been widely used in image processing. We propose to adapt this operator for Rician noise by using only the wavelet coefficients corresponding to the object and then iteratively correcting the MAD estimation with an analytical scheme based on the SNR of the image [5].

2 Noise in MR Images

As mentioned previously, the distribution of noise can be modeled with a Rician distribution [3, 4, 6, 10]:

$$p(m) = \frac{m}{\sigma_n^2} exp(-\frac{m^2 + A^2}{2\sigma_n^2}) I_0(\frac{Am}{\sigma_n^2}). \tag{1}$$

where σ_n is the standard deviation of Gaussian noise in the complex domain, A is the amplitude of the signal without noise, m is the value in the magnitude image and I_0 is the zeroth order modified Bessel function. This model is used by the majority of the noise estimation methods [8, 6, 7]. Most of these methods can be classified as: i) methods that use background areas to estimate the noise variance and ii) methods that use the image object itself.

- **For the background-based methods**, where the signal is usually considered as zero in background (i.e. SNR = $0dB$), the Rician distribution is a Rayleigh distribution [6]:

$$p(m) = \frac{m}{\sigma_n^2} exp(-\frac{m^2}{2\sigma_n^2}). \tag{2}$$

Based on the properties of the Rayleigh distribution, the mean $\bar{m}_b$ and the variance σ_b^2 of the noise in the background can be related to σ_n:

$$\bar{m}_b = \sqrt{\frac{\pi}{2}} \sigma_n \tag{3}$$

$$\sigma_b^2 = \frac{4-\pi}{2} \sigma_n^2 \tag{4}$$

The assumption that SNR = $0dB$ in the background may not be valid in the presence of ghosting artefacts [6], while the Rayleigh distribution assumption

can be corrupted by using reconstruction filters [11, 10], by the suppression of the signal by the scanner [10, 11] or by zero-padding in the Fourier domain [11]. Finally, the noise level in the background may not be representative of the noise level inside the tissue [10, 11].
- **For the object-based methods with high SNR** (i.e. SNR $> 3dB$) [4,1], the Rician distribution can be well approximated using a Gaussian distribution:

$$p(m) \approx \frac{1}{2\pi\sigma_n^2} exp(-\frac{(m^2 - \sqrt{A^2 + \sigma_n^2})^2}{2\sigma_n^2}). \qquad (5)$$

This approximation enables us to use all the classical methods proposed for Gaussian noise estimation. Nevertheless, for low SNR, this approximation is no longer valid [4, 1, 6].

3 Proposed Method

In order to relax the assumptions performed by background-based methods (i.e. no signal in the background) and the object-based methods (Gaussian noise approximation), we propose an adaptation of the MAD estimator in wavelet domain [9] for Rician noise.

MAD Estimator. By using the usual notation for 3D wavelet decomposition: LLL denotes the low sub-band containing the feature information whereas LHH, LHL, LLH, HLL, HLH, HHL and HHH denote the high sub-bands containing the detailed information. The highest sub-band HHH is essentially composed of coefficients that correspond to the noise [9]. The fact that the highest sub-band HHH is mainly composed of the coefficients corresponding to the noise has been used by Donoho [9] to propose a robust estimation of noise variance. Based on the MAD estimator, this method enables the estimation of the noise variance in presence of Gaussian noise:

$$\hat{\sigma} = \frac{median(|y_i|)}{0.6745} \qquad (6)$$

where y_i are the wavelet coefficients of the HHH sub-band and $\hat{\sigma}$ the estimation of noise. As long as the y_i coefficients corresponding to the object are considered and the SNR is high enough, the Gaussian approximation of Rician noise leads to $\hat{\sigma}_n = \hat{\sigma}$.

Rician Adaptation. To obtain an unbiased estimation of σ_n for all SNR values, we propose to use the correction procedure introduced by Koay *et al* [5]. This analytical correction is based on an iterative estimation of the SNR in presence of Rician noise. In our case, the estimation $\hat{\sigma}$, obtained using the MAD estimator on the object, is used to initialize the procedure:

$$\hat{\sigma}_n = \sqrt{\hat{\sigma}^2/\xi(\theta)} \qquad (7)$$

where θ is the SNR value and ξ is the correction factor, which is expressed as:

$$\xi(\theta) = 2 + \theta^2 - \frac{\pi}{8} \times exp\left(-\frac{\theta^2}{2}\right)\left((2+\theta^2)I_0\left(\frac{\theta^2}{4}\right) + \theta^2 I_1\left(\frac{\theta^2}{4}\right)\right)^2 \quad (8)$$

where I_1 is the first order modified Bessel function. The correction factor is iteratively applied until convergence of the procedure or when a given number of iterations t is achieved. The distance $|\theta_t - \theta_{t-1}|$ can be used as stopping criterion. The resulting iterative correction scheme can be written as:

$$\theta_t = \sqrt{\xi(\theta_{t-1})\left(1 + \frac{\overline{m}_o}{\hat{\sigma}}\right) - 2} \quad (9)$$

where $\overline{m}_o$ is the mean signal of the object and $\hat{\sigma}$ the first estimation from MAD estimator. The correction factor $\xi(\theta_t)$ from the last iteration is finally used in Eq. 7.

Object Extraction. The first approximation, $\hat{\sigma}_n \approx \hat{\sigma}$, is solely based on the wavelet coefficients corresponding to the object. To extract the object we take advantage of the wavelet transform. Since the noise information is mainly contained in the highest sub-bands, the LLL sub-band contains a less noisy version of the image which can be used to facilitate the segmentation procedure. At the first level of decomposition, the size of LLL and HHH are identical. Thus, at this level of decomposition, we proposed to segment the object in the LLL sub-band and to use the obtained mask to extract the y_i coefficients corresponding to the object in the HHH sub-band. The segmentation is performed using a simple K-means (k=2) classification. For image with a low level of noise, the MAD estimation tends to be spoiled since the HHH sub-band is mainly composed of information corresponding to the high gradient areas (i.e. edges) of the image. To further increase the accuracy of the estimation at low noise levels, voxels with the highest local gradient are excluded from the estimation (i.e. removed from the segmented mask). Accordingly, we eliminate all those voxels whose the local gradient magnitude is higher than the median local gradient magnitude in the LLL sub-band.

4 Experiment on Synthetic Data

Materials. To evaluate the different methods, synthetic T1-weighted MR data with 20% of inhomogeneity from the Brainweb database [12] was corrupted with different levels of Rician noise (2 to 15%). In this paper, 2% of noise is equivalent to $\mathcal{N}(0, \nu\frac{2}{100})$, where ν is set to 255. As shown in [7], the size of the background has an impact on the accuracy of the background-based methods. Smaller backgrounds lead to more difficult estimations. In order to perfrom a fair comparison, zero padding of the Brainweb volume of $181 \times 217 \times 181$ voxels was performed to obtain a volume of $256 \times 217 \times 256$ voxels. Moreover, ghosting artefacts were implemented by using a repeated filtered version of the original image. First, the image is low-pass filtered with two gaussian kernels of different size ($3 \times 3 \times 3$ and $5 \times 5 \times 5$). Then, the absolute difference of the two filtered images is added to the original image with a half field of view offset (see Fig. 1, left).

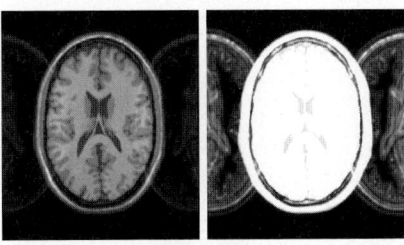 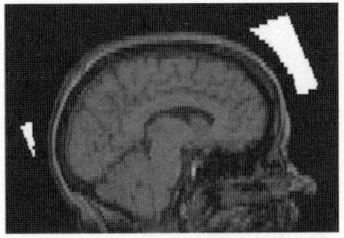

Fig. 1. Left: Simulated ghosting artefacts on brainweb with 20% inhomogeneity and the same image with saturation of the contrast to highlight the ghosting artefacts. Right: Noise regions of interest obtained with automated quality control software tool [13].

Compared Methods. For the experiments, we compared the following methods:

- the background-based method proposed by Sijbers [6]; denoted as "ML". The Sijbers method was applied using a histogram with 1000 bins.
- the two background-based methods based on local statistics proposed in [7]; denoted as LMB for the Local Means in Background and LVB for Local Variances in Background. The size of the local neighborhoods and the number of bins were $5 \times 5 \times 5$ voxels and 1000 bins respectively.
- the object-based method based on local variances proposed in [7]; denoted as LVO for Local Variances in Object. A local neighborhood of $3 \times 3 \times 3$ voxels was used.
- the classical MAD estimator estimated on the object [9]. The object was segmented in the wavelet domain without removing high gradient areas.
- the proposed robust MAD for Rician noise estimated on the object and denoted as RMAD.

Quality Measure. To estimate the accuracy of the different methods, the ratio between the estimated standard deviation $\hat{\sigma}_n$ and the applied standard deviation σ_n is computed for all the levels of noise. Moreover, the Mean Absolute Error over all the levels of noise is also used. The error for a given level of noise is computed as:

$$error = 1 - \frac{\sigma_n}{\hat{\sigma}_n} \qquad (10)$$

All the experiments were repeated 10 times, each with a new instantiation of noise, for each noise level and the average results are presented.

Results. Fig. 2 shows the results on the phantom with inhomogeneity and ghosting artefacts. Compared to the MAD estimator, the ability of the RMAD method to correctly estimate the higher levels of noise (i.e. where the Gaussian assumption failed) can be attributed to the SNR based correction factor. Moreover, the RMAD provided better estimations of the noise at low level by removing the high gradients before the MAD computation. As expected, the background-based methods are impacted by the ghosting artefacts. In fact, the assumption of zero signal in

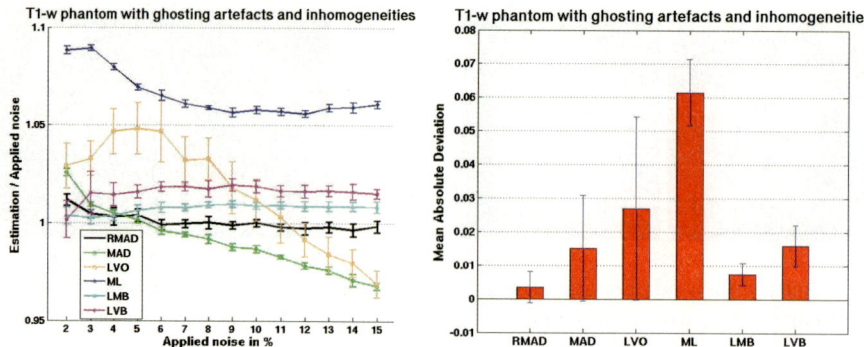

Fig. 2. Left: ratio of estimated vs. applied noise level, for the all noise levels applied to the synthetic image, for the 6 techniques compared. Note that RMAD (black line) estimation is closest to 1.0 for almost all noise levels.

the background is spoiled. All these methods tend to overestimate the noise level, especially the ML method. The LMB method obtained very good results. Finally, the RMAD method obtained the best result.

5 Experiments on Clinical Data

Material. The dataset used for the experiment is composed of 23 T1-w MR volumes of $256 \times 256 \times 56$ voxels. These data were acquired with a 1.5T Genesis Signa GE Medical system and an 1 channel head coil. The parameters of the sequence were: TR = 30ms, TE = 9ms, FOV=250 mm and bandwidth=122 kHz.

Background Extraction. In order to estimate the noise level in the real images, we used a region-based approach that is similar to the manual selection procedure usually used in the clinical environment. The noise region of interest (ROI) used to calculate the noise level was obtained by using the automated quality control (aQC) software tool described in [13]. Based on the registration of each subject with a template of ROIs (see Fig. 1, right), the AQc software provides ROIs associated with noise regions. To determine the noise level, we used the region anterior to the head which contains less artefacts [13].

Bronze Standard. In our study, we have chosen to use the assumption that the noise level for a given sequence on the same scanner should be constant. Based on this idea, the noise regions extracted from the background of MR images are used to estimated an average level of noise over all the data from a same site. To estimate this average level of noise, the properties of the second-order moment of a Rician distribution are used. The Bronze standard can be computed from the mean of the squared values extracted from backgrounds of all the data d:

$$\hat{\sigma}_n = \sqrt{\frac{\overline{\hat{M}_b^2}}{2}}, \hat{M}_b^2 = (\hat{m}_b^2(1), ..., \hat{m}_b^2(D)) \qquad (11)$$

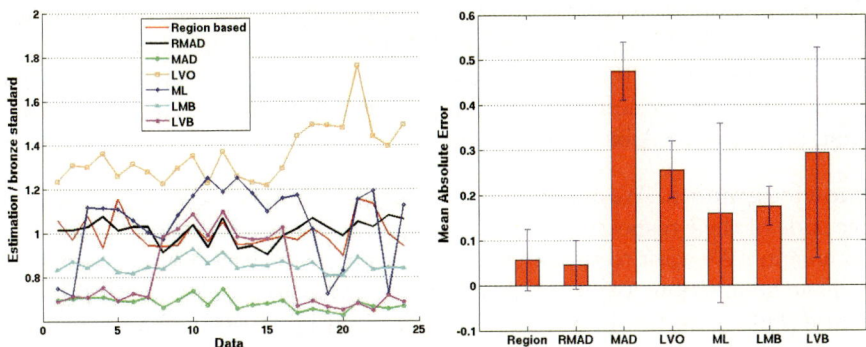

Fig. 3. Left: results of the compared methods for all the data. Right: mean absolute error over all the data.

where $\hat{m}_b^2(d)$ is the vector containing the squared value of noise extracted from the background of data d and $\hat{M}_b^2$ is the concatenation of the squared signal from all the data. Based on the same approach, the estimation of the noise level for a given data d is obtained with the region-based method by using the mean of the squared values extracted from the background of d.

Results. Fig. 3 shows the results obtained for site 1. For all the data, RMAD method provided a consistant estimation of the noise relative to the Bronze standard (small error) in a robust manner (small variance of error). The stability of the proposed method leads to a smaller error than the region-based method that was used to build the bronze standard. As assessed by experiments on synthetic phantom, the MAD estimator computed on the object tends to underestimate the noise level whereas the LVO method leads to an overestimation of the noise level. The LVB method appears to follow the MAD estimation and the RMAD estimation according to the data under process. The LMB method estimated in the background is a robust and stable estimator but leads to a slight underestimation. Finally, the ML method provided a good mean absolute error but was accomplished with a high variability.

6 Conclusion

In this paper, a new method based on the robust MAD estimator for Rician noise has been proposed and several state-of-the-art methods for Rician noise estimation in MR image have been compared. Experiments on synthetic data with simulated inhomogeneity and ghosting artefacts showed the efficiency of the proposed object-based approach compared to the background-based approaches. Experiments on real data have shown that the proposed RMAD method obtained the best result in terms of accuracy and robustness. The background-based methods had the highest variability except the LMB method which provided a robust noise estimation. These results show that the background in real data is spoiled by artefacts, thus violating the assumption of no signal in background. Finally, the proposed approach can be applied to situations where no background is present such as fetal imaging or images where the background is artificially set to zero by the scanner [10]. Moreover, the proposed approach can be potentially adapted to work with non stationary noise such as those attributed to parallel imaging (i.e. GRAPPA or SENSE).

Acknowledgments. We are grateful to Dr. Sijbers and Dr. Aja for providing the source code of their respective Rician noise estimation methods and for their useful comments. We want to thank Dr Levesque for the fruitfully discussions about MR image acquisition. We would like to thank NeuroRx Research for providing the data. This work has been partially supported by the Canadian Intitutes of Health Research Industry Cda (CECR)-Gevas-OE016 and by the Spanish Health Institute Carlos III through the RETICS Combiomed, RD07/0067/2001.

References

1. Nowak, R.: Wavelet-based rician noise removal for magnetic resonance imaging. IEEE TIP 8(10), 1408–1419 (1999)
2. Coupé, P., Yger, P., Prima, S., Hellier, P., Kervrann, C., Barillot, C.: An Optimized Blockwise NonLocal Means Denoising Filter for 3-D Magnetic Resonance Images. IEEE Transactions on Medical Imaging 27(4), 425–441 (2008)
3. Henkelman, R.M.: Measurement of signal intensities in the presence of noise in MR images. Medical Physics 12(2), 232–233 (1985)
4. Gudbjartsson, H., Patz, S.: The Rician distribution of noisy MRI data. Magnetic Resonance in Medicine 34, 910–914 (1995)
5. Koay, C.G., Basser, P.J.: Analytically exact correction scheme for signal extraction from noisy magnitude MR signals. Journal of Magnetic Resonance 179(2), 317–322 (2006)
6. Sijbers, J., Poot, D., den Dekker, A.J., Pintjens, W.: Automatic estimation of the noise variance from the histogram of a magnetic resonance image. Physics in Medicine and Biology 52(5), 1335–1348 (2007)
7. Aja-Fernandez, S., Alberola-Lopez, C., Westin, C.F.: Noise and signal estimation in magnitude MRI and Rician distributed images: a LMMSE approach. IEEE TIP 17(8), 1383–1398 (2008)
8. Sijbers, J., den Dekker, A., Audekerke, J.V., Verhoye, M., Dyck, D.V.: Estimation of the noise in magnitude MR images. Magnetic Resonance Imaging 16(1), 87–90 (1998)
9. Donoho, D.: De-noising by Soft-Thresholding. IEEE TIT 41(3), 613–627 (1995)
10. Dietrich, O., Raya, J.G., Reeder, S.B., Ingrisch, M., Reiser, M.F., Schoenberg, S.O.: Influence of multichannel combination, parallel imaging and other reconstruction techniques on MRI noise characteristics. Magnetic Resonance Imaging 26(6), 754–762 (2008)
11. Landman, B., Bazin, P.L., Prince, J.: Diffusion Tensor Estimation by Maximizing Rician Likelihood. In: ICCV 2007, pp. 1–8 (2007)
12. Collins, D., Zijdenbos, A., Kollokian, V., Sled, J., Kabani, N., Holmes, C., Evans, A.: Design and construction of a realistic digital brain phantom. IEEE TMI 17(3), 463–468 (1998)
13. Gedamu, E.L., Collins, D.L., Arnold, D.L.: Automated quality control of brain MR images. Journal of Magnetic Resonance Imaging 28(2), 308–319 (2008)

Cell Segmentation Using Front Vector Flow Guided Active Contours

Fuhai Li, Xiaobo Zhou*, Hong Zhao, and Stephen T.C. Wong

Center for Biotechnology and Informatics, The Methodist Hospital Research Institute and Department of Radiology, The Methodist Hospital, Weill Cornell Medical College, Houston, TX 77030, U.S.A.
{fli,xzhou,hzhao,stwong}@tmhs.org

Abstract. Phase-contrast microscopy is a common approach for studying the dynamics of cell behaviors, such as cell migration. Cell segmentation is the basis of quantitative analysis of the immense cellular images. However, the complicated cell morphological appearance in phase-contrast microscopy images challenges the existing segmentation methods. This paper proposes a new cell segmentation method for cancer cell migration studies using phase-contrast images. Instead of segmenting cells directly based on commonly used low-level features, e.g. intensity and gradient, we first identify the leading protrusions, a high level feature, of cancer cells. Based on the identified cell leading protrusions, we introduce a front vector flow guided active contour, which guides the initial cell boundaries to the real boundaries. The experimental validation on a set of breast cancer cell images shows that the proposed method demonstrates fast, stable, and accurate segmentation for breast cancer cells with wide range of sizes and shapes.

1 Introduction

Cell migration plays pivotal roles in cancer cell scattering, tissue invasion, and metastasis. Metastasis is a major cause of morbidity and mortality in most of cancer patients [1]. For breast cancer, five-year relative survival in local invasive breast cancer patients is 98.1%, whereas it is only 26% in patients with distant metastases in USA [2]. These dismal prognoses can be partly explained by the fact that a large majority of the drugs used today to treat cancer are pro-apoptotic, but migrating cells involved in metastases are known to show a decreased proliferation rate and are thus less sensitive to such chemotherapy. Thus the anti-migration drugs hold great promise for both anti-metastasis therapy and increasing the efficacy of the existing pro-apoptotic anti-cancer drugs. Phase-contrast microscopy is a common tool for study of dynamic behaviors of a population of cells under different treatments [3]. However, the complicated cell morphological appearance and the low signal to noise ratio (SNR) of the phase-contrast images, as seen in Figure 1, challenge the existing segmentation methods, new segmentation methods are needed.

---

* Corresponding author.

Although a number of cell segmentation methods have been proposed, cell segmentation remains an open problem [4]. For example, thresholding methods [5] cannot accurately separate cells from background because regions inside cells often have similar intensity as the background in the phase-contrast image. Voronoi based methods can only estimate the rough regions of cells [6]. Watershed methods assume that the edges (watersheds) have the maximum intensity (or maximum gradient) between two cells [7]; however, it is not always true. Graph cut based methods are robust to weak boundaries. Nevertheless, they require closed boundaries [8]. Active contours has two kinds of methods: region based [9] and edge based [10]. The region based active contours are robust to the initial boundaries and fast, but they always require that the intensity of objects is homogenous and different with background [9]. The edge based active contours are sensitive to the initial boundaries and a set of parameters. The evolution of contours may stop before reaching the real boundaries or pass through the real boundaries, without good initial boundaries or well-tuned parameters.

The limitation of above methods, which do the segmentation directly based on low-level features, e.g. intensity and gradient, is that they all assume the edges or regions inside objects have simple, distinct features, e.g. large gradient or homogenous intensity. In practice, we cannot distinct the real boundaries with other features by assuming clear cut gradient or homogenous intensity information. In this paper, we propose to segment cancer cells in phase-contrast images by introducing a high-level feature, fronts (leading protrusions), as seen in Figure 1. We identify the cell fronts first and then introduce the front vector flow to direct the active contours unambiguously to where the real boundaries are. We name this method as front vector flow guided active contour.

2 Methods

2.1 Problem Description

We provide two representative phase contrast cell images of living breast cancer cells MDA-MB231 in the column-(a) of Figure 1. We can see that 1) the cell centers have two distinct regions with lower (dark region) and higher intensity (bright region), 2) the leading protrusions of cells is far away from the cell centers and has non-closed arc shape, see the ridge-like structures, 3) the regions between the cell centers and leading protrusions have similar intensity as the background. The first property enables us to detect the cell bodies easily by detecting the two regions, which can be used as the initial boundaries of cells. However, the second and third properties make the segmentation very challenging. For example, the evolution of cell boundaries using edge-based active contours [10] will stop near the cell centers due to the rapid intensity variation, or easily go outside the cells due to the non-closed leading protrusions and the regions that have homogenous intensity as the background. To deal with these challenges, we proposed the following method of front vector flow guided active contour.

2.2 Front Vector Flow Guided Active Contour

The proposed front vector flow guided active contour method consists of the following steps: 1) cell center detection, 2) front (leading protrusions) detection, and 3) contour evolution following the front vector flow.

A. Cell center detection. To detect the cell center, we first detect the dark and bright regions inside cells respectively, and then combine the detection results together, as seen in Figure 1. In this paper, we make use of the multi-scale representation to detect the bright regions [11]. Specifically, we filter the original image using a series of Laplacian of Gaussian (LoG) filters with different scales, i.e., the σs of Gaussians. Then the maximum intensity projection (MIP) image of the filtered image is generated, and we use a three-class fuzzy c-means clustering [12] method to detect the bright regions accurately, as seen in the column-(b) of Figure 1. Since a dark region can be viewed as a bright region in the complemented cell image, we can detect it using the same method, as seen in the column-(c) of Figure 1. Finally, we employ the convex hull operation to obtain the cell center, as seen in the column-(d) of Figure 1.

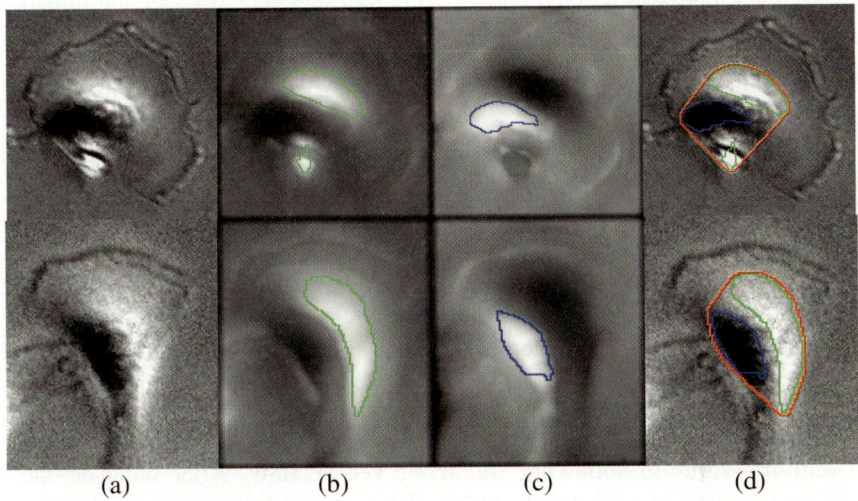

(a) (b) (c) (d)

Fig. 1. Two representative MDA-MB231 breast cancer cell images (column-(a)), the MIP images of the multi-scale LoG filtered original images for bright region detection (column-(b)), the MIP images of the multi-scale LoG filtered complemented images for dark region detection (column-(c)), and the cell body detection results (column-(d)). The green, blue and red curves imposed on the cell images indicate the boundaries of the detected bright regions, dark regions and cell centers respectively.

B. Front detection. The first stage of cell migration consists of initial cell polarization caused by localized actin polymerization to form filaments, and this is followed by the extension of cytoplasmic protrusions. The quantitative analysis of the cytoplasmic protrusion formation, disappearance, and variation is important for studies of cell migration. Considering the ridge shape of fronts, we detect the cell fronts using the curvilinear structure detectors [13, 14].

For a 1D ridge profile, $f(x) = c$ if $|x| \leq b$, and $f(x) = 0$ otherwise, we can detect the center point of $f(x)$ using the criterion: $k'(x,\sigma) = 0$, and $k''(x,\sigma) << 0$, where

$k'(x,\sigma) = c\sqrt{\sigma}(g(x+b,\sigma) - g(x-b,\sigma))$, $k''(x,\sigma) = c\sigma(g'(x+b,\sigma) - g'(x-b,\sigma))$, and $g(x,\sigma)$, $g'(x,\sigma)$ represent the Gaussian density function and its derivative respectively. For ridge profiles with different width, we can use a series of scales (multi-scale) to let $k''(x,\sigma)$ reaches its maximum value. In discrete case, a point x_n is labeled as center point, if $t = -\sqrt{\sigma_n^*} \times k'(x_n,\sigma_n^*)/k''(x_n,\sigma_n^*) \in [-\frac{1}{2}, \frac{1}{2}]$, and $|k''(x,\sigma_n^*)|$ is larger than a given threshold, where $\sigma_n^* = \arg\min_\sigma \{k''(x_n,\sigma)\}$.

It is straightforward to extend the method to 2D space because the cross-section of the 2D ridge profile in direction perpendicular to ridge center line is a 1D ridge profile. The eigenvector, (n_x, n_y), which corresponds to the minimum eigen-value, $\lambda_{x,y}$, of the Hessian matrix at a given point (x, y), indicates the cross-section direction at that point. In a 2D discrete case, a point is labeled as a center point if $|\lambda_{x,y}|$ is larger than a given threshold, and the following equation holds:

$$(tn_x, tn_y) \in [-1/2, 1/2] \times [-1/2, 1/2] \tag{1}$$

where $t = -\dfrac{k_x(\sigma_{x,y}^*)n_x + k_y(\sigma_{x,y}^*)n_y}{k_{xx}(\sigma_{x,y}^*)n_x^2 + 2k_{xy}(\sigma_{x,y}^*)n_x n_y + k_{yy}(\sigma_{x,y}^*)n_y^2}$, k_x, k_y, k_{xx}, k_{xy} and k_{yy} are the normalized partial derivatives of 2D cellular images convolved with 2D Gaussian kernels, and $\sigma_{x,y}^* = \arg\min_\sigma \lambda_{x,y}(x,y;\sigma)$. To remove the false center points, the hysteresis thresholding technique is employed, and then a link process links the broken center lines together [14]. The detected cell front is represented by a binary image, as seen in Figure 2-(e).

C. Contour evolution following the front vector flow. After obtained the cell centers and fronts, we still cannot obtain the accurate cell boundaries because the regions that locate between cell centers and the fronts are missed. To obtain the accurate boundaries, we propose to evolve the initial cell boundaries (the boundaries of the cell centers) to the real boundaries following the front vector flow.

We calculate the front vector flow as in the following:

$$\hat{\mathbf{V}}_{\mathbf{fvf}} = \min_{\mathbf{V}} \iint \mu(u_x^2 + u_y^2 + v_x^2 + v_y^2) + |\nabla I_f|^2 |\mathbf{V} - \nabla I_f| dxdy, \tag{2}$$

where, I_f represents the detected cell front image; $\nabla I_f = \left\langle \dfrac{\partial}{\partial x} I_f, \dfrac{\partial}{\partial y} I_f \right\rangle$ denotes the gradient of the detected front image; and $\mathbf{V} = \langle u(x,y), v(x,y) \rangle$ is the front vector flow. Figure 2 illustrates the relationship between the gradient and the front vector flow. As we can see, the front vector flow extends the gradient vector to a large region and converges to the detected front [15], as seen in Figure 2-(b), (c), (f), and (g). This motivates us to evolve the initial cell boundaries along with the front vector flow to reach the real boundaries. A problem is posed that the front vector flow may attract initial cell boundaries of different cells to one front. To avoid this, we associate each front with its corresponding cell uniquely using the convex property (arc shape) of the fronts, as seen in Figure 2(d). The red arrow, which is obtained by linking the midpoints of the front and the chord linking two endpoints of the front points, points to the corresponding cell. Thus we can find the corresponding cell along the direction of the red arrow, and evolve its initial boundary following the front vector flow of the front.

The contour evolution process along with front vector flow can be easily implemented under the active contour (level set) framework. The mathematical evolution equation is as follows.

$$\frac{d}{dt}\psi = -\left(\hat{\mathbf{V}}_{\mathbf{fvf}} \cdot \nabla \psi\right) + \beta \kappa |\nabla \psi|, \quad (3)$$

where ψ denotes the level set function, κ is the curvature, and β is the parameter that controls the smoothness of the boundary. This equation is straightforward and robust because the only parameter β, which controls the smoothness of the contour, will not influence the evolution much.

$$\kappa = div\left(\frac{\nabla \psi}{|\nabla \psi|}\right) = \frac{\psi_{xx}\psi_y^2 - 2\psi_x\psi_{xy}\psi_y + \psi_x^2\psi_{yy}}{\left(\psi_x^2 + \psi_y^2\right)^{3/2}}, \quad (4)$$

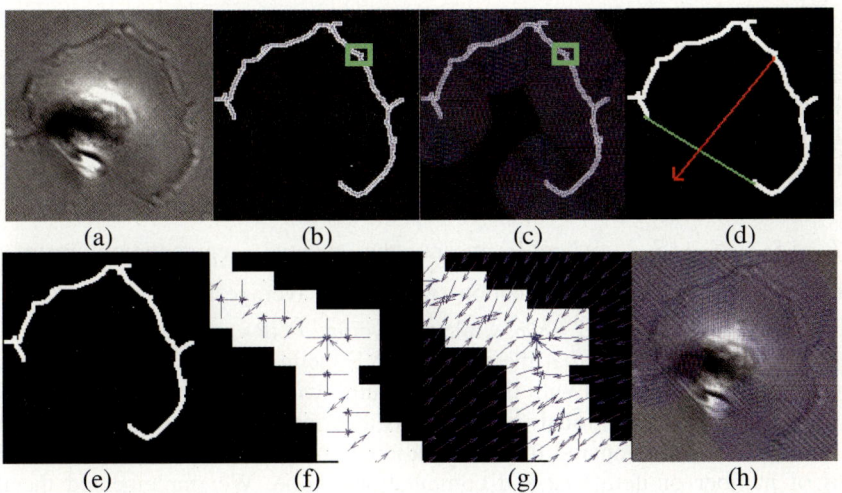

Fig. 2. An illustration of the front vector flow. (a) Original cell image, (e) detected front image, (b) gradient vectors, (c) front vector flow, (f) zoom in image of the green square in (b), (g) zoom in image of the green square in (c), (d) the red arrow, which is obtained by linking the midpoints of the front and the chord linking two endpoints of the front, points to the corresponding cell center, and (h) the front vector flow was imposed on the original cell image. The blue arrows represent the gradient vectors.

3 Experiments and Results

The MDA-MB231 breast cancer cell line was grown in Dulbecco's Modified Eagle's Medium (DMEM) containing 10% fetal bovine serum. Cell cultures were maintained in a humidified incubator at 37C, with 5% CO2. Images of cells were acquired in phase contrast mode of a FluoView™ FV1000 laser scanning confocal microscope (Olympus) using a 20x objective. We selected 50 cells and manually segmented them as the ground truth. To validate the performance of the proposed front vector flow guided (FVF) active contour method, we compared it with two kinds of widely used active contours: edge-based geodesic active contour (GAC) [10], region based Chan and Vese active contour (CV) [9], and the manually analyzed ground truth. The goal of the comparison is merely to show the robustness of the proposed method, which can handle the intensity variation and prevent the contour from leaking. GAC and CV are two widely used methods, which have been tested in certain phase contrast images. Therefore, we chose them for comparison. Both GAC and CV methods could be adapted by incorporating the front detection. However, it is not trivial, and instead we propose the new method that is straightforward and fast. In this validation, the active contour (level set) evolution equation of GAC and CV are as: $\frac{d}{dt}\psi = \alpha(\nabla g \cdot \nabla \psi) + g(\kappa + c)|\nabla \psi|$, $\frac{d}{dt}\psi = \delta_\varepsilon(\psi)\left[\mu \cdot \kappa - \nu - \lambda_1(I - c_1)^2 + \lambda_2(I - c_2)^2\right]$.

Table 1 lists the detailed parameters settings of the three methods (GAC, CV, and FVF). Figure 3 shows the comparison among GAC, CV, FVF and manual segmentation results. The boundaries of cell centers, as seen in Figure 1-(d), were used as the initial boundaries, and the stopping criterion is setting a maximum iteration number. As we can see, the edge leaks outside of cells in the results of GAC due to the non-closed cell fronts. The CV method works like a threshold method that only separates the bright regions from the background and dark regions. Whereas, the proposed FVF method delineates the cell boundaries accurately compared with the ground truth. To quantitatively analyze the accuracy of the segmentation, we employed following two error measures: false positive rate, $FPR = (S_A - S_M)/S_M$, and false negative rate, $FNR = (S_M - S_A)/S_M$, where S_M means the manual segmentation result and S_A means the automated segmentation results. The average FPRs of GAC, CV and FVF are as: 27.8%, 0%, and 7.8%, while the average FNRs are as: 15.6%, 63.5%, and 6.7%. The results indicate that the propose FVF method demonstrates accurate segmentation results compared with the ground truth, while the GAC and CV results are not reliable. The computational complexity is also important for segmentation methods. In Table 2, we compared the computational complexity of the three methods in terms of number of iterations and computational time. We implemented the three methods in Matlab (version 2007), and the comparison were did on a standard desktop PC (Intel core 2, 1.86 GHz). The CV method is the fastest, and the FVF method has similar complexity as the CV method. However, the computational complexity of the GAC method increased rapidly. In conclusion, the proposed FVF method is fast, stable, and accurate compared with the GAC and CV methods.

Table 1. Parameters settings of the GAC, CV and FVF active contours

	Parameter setting
GAC	$dt = 0.05$, $c = 1$, $\alpha = 0.2$
CV	$dt = 0.1$, $\lambda_1 = 1$, $\lambda_2 = 1$, $\mu = 0$, $v = -65$
FVF	$dt = 0.1$, $\beta = 1$

Table 2. Computational complexity comparison in terms of number of iteration and time

	GAC		CV		FVF	
	Img1	Img2	Img1	Img2	Img1	Img2
# of iteration	400	400	400	400	40	40
time (seconds)	240	210	11	8	18	11

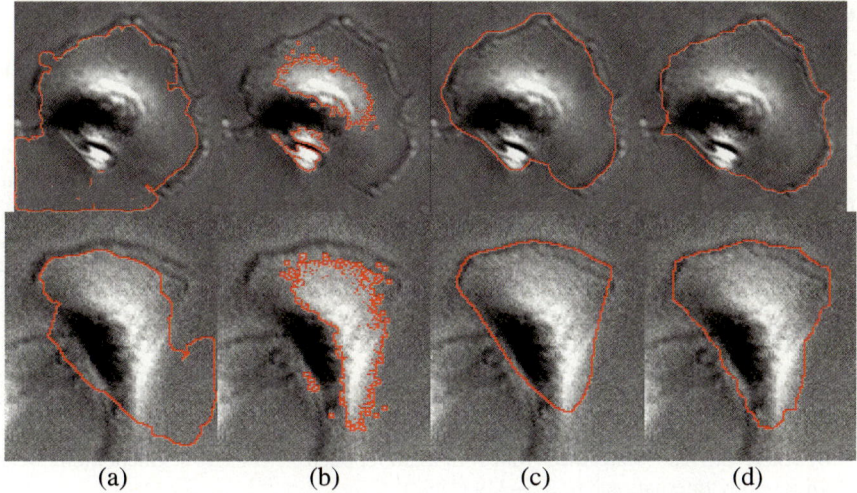

(a) (b) (c) (d)

Fig. 3. Comparison of segmentation results. (a) Segmentation results of GAC, (b) segmentation results of CV, (c) segmentation results of FVF, and (d) manual segmentation results.

4 Discussion and Conclusions

In this paper, we propose a new method for segmenting breast cancer cell images obtained by phase-contrast microscopy. The segmentation method takes advantage of the prior knowledge that the leading protrusion in cancer cells is a distinct high-level feature of cell boundaries compared to the commonly used low-level features such as edge gradient or cell intensity. Thus we propose to identify the protrusions first, which tell the segmentation algorithms clearly where the real boundaries are, and then introduce the front vector flow and implement the cell segmentation in the framework of active contour. The initial cell boundaries, which are obtained after the cell center detection, are attracted to the real edges following the front vector flow. The proposed method deals with the aforementioned challenges existing in the phase-contrast images well. The algorithm is fast, stable, and accurate compared with the manually segmented ground truth and is used to segment large amounts of breast cancer cells in the phase-contrast images of our high content screening studies. One limitation of the proposed method is the requirement of the accurate boundary detection results. It may fail when the noise or inaccurate boundary detection results exist. To improve the proposed method, we may integrate the edge detection and vector flow into active contour methods.

Although designed for breast cancer cells in phase contrast images, it is possible to generalize the proposed algorithm, including the cell center detection, front detection, and contour evolution, to other applications. For example, the center detection and front detection can be generalized to the blob and ridge structure detection in other biomedical images, e.g. nuclei and neurite images. For the contour evolution, it can be customized to other applications where part of boundaries of objects can be identified. In the future work, we will extend the proposed segmentation method for tracking live cancer cells in phase-contrast image movies.

References

1. Birchmeier, C., Birchmeier, W., Gherardi, E., Vande Woude, G.F.: Met, metastasis, motility and more. Nat. Rev. Mol. Cell Biol. 4, 915–925 (2003)
2. American Cancer Society, http://www.cancer.org
3. Wang, M., Zhou, X., Li, F., Huckins, J., King, R.W., Wong, S.T.: Novel cell segmentation and online SVM for cell cycle phase identification in automated microscopy. Bioinformatics 24, 94–101 (2008)
4. Adiga, U., Malladi, R., Fernandez-Gonzalez, R., de Solorzano, C.O.: High-throughput analysis of multispectral images of breast cancer tissue. IEEE Transactions on Image Processing 15, 1057–7149 (2006)
5. Sahoo, P., Soltani, S., Wong, A., Chen, Y.: A survey of Thresholding Techniques. Computer Vision Graphics Image Processing 41, 233–260 (1988)
6. Jones, T.R., Carpenter, A., Golland, P.: Voronoi-based segmentation of cells on image manifolds. In: Liu, Y., Jiang, T.-Z., Zhang, C. (eds.) CVBIA 2005. LNCS, vol. 3765, pp. 535–543. Springer, Heidelberg (2005)
7. Beucher, S.: The watershed transformation applied to image segmentation. Scanning Microscopy International 6, 299–314 (1992)
8. Shi, J., Malik, J.: Normalized cuts and image segmentation. IEEE Transactions on Pattern Analysis and Machine Intellegence 22, 888–905 (2000)
9. Chan, T., Vese, L.: Active contours without edges. IEEE Transactions on Image Processing 10, 266–277 (2001)
10. Casselles, V., Kimmel, R., Sapiro, G.: Geodesic Active Contours. International Journal of Computer Vision 22, 61–79 (1997)
11. Bai, W., Zhou, X., Ji, L., Cheng, J., Wong, S.T.: Automatic dendritic spine analysis in two-photon laser scanning microscopy images. Cytometry A 71, 818–826 (2007)
12. Dunn, J.C.: A Fuzzy Relative of the ISODATA Process and Its Use in Detecting Compact Well-Separated Clusters. Journal of Cybernetics 3, 32–57 (1973)
13. Steger, C.: An unbiased detector of curvilinear structures. IEEE Transactions on Pattern Analysis and Machine Intellegence 20, 113–125 (1998)
14. Xiong, G., Zhou, X., Degterev, A., Ji, L., Wong, S.T.C.: Automated Neurite Labeling and Analysis in Fluorescence Microscopy Images. Cytometry Part A 69A, 494–505 (2006)
15. Xu, C., Prince, J.L.: Snakes, shapes, and gradient vector flow. IEEE Transactions on Image Processing 7, 359–369 (1998)

Segmentation and Classification of Cell Cycle Phases in Fluorescence Imaging*

Ilker Ersoy[1], Filiz Bunyak[1], Vadim Chagin[2,3], M. Christina Cardoso[2], and Kannappan Palaniappan[1]

[1] Department of Computer Science, University of Missouri Columbia, USA
[2] Department of Biology, Technische Universität Darmstadt, Germany
[3] Institute of Cytology, Russian Academy of Sciences, St. Petersburg, Russia

Abstract. Current chemical biology methods for studying spatiotemporal correlation between biochemical networks and cell cycle phase progression in live-cells typically use fluorescence-based imaging of fusion proteins. Stable cell lines expressing fluorescently tagged protein GFP-PCNA produce rich, dynamically varying sub-cellular foci patterns characterizing the cell cycle phases, including the progress during the S-phase. Variable fluorescence patterns, drastic changes in SNR, shape and position changes and abundance of touching cells require sophisticated algorithms for reliable automatic segmentation and cell cycle classification. We extend the recently proposed graph partitioning active contours (GPAC) for fluorescence-based nucleus segmentation using regional density functions and dramatically improve its efficiency, making it scalable for high content microscopy imaging. We utilize surface shape properties of GFP-PCNA intensity field to obtain descriptors of foci patterns and perform automated cell cycle phase classification, and give quantitative performance by comparing our results to manually labeled data.

1 Introduction

The spatial distribution and temporal dynamics of proteins within living cells are being quantitatively studied using a variety of microscopy imaging modalities to understand the interaction between sub-cellular processes and cell behavior. The current method for live-cell visualization and tracking of proteins is to use translational fusion with fluorescent proteins. The analysis of cell cycle dependent changes is only now becoming feasible with the discovery of suitable markers that allow identification of cell cycle phases in proliferating cells [1]. Current experimental techniques use fusion proteins in combination with fluorescence time-lapse microscopy to mark sub-cellular structures in the nucleus to identify the cell cycle phase. Several cell cycle labeling approaches are being pursued including RFP-Ligase for localizing DNA methyltransferase, GFP-PCNA (proliferating cell nuclear antigen fused to green fluorescent protein) where PCNA is involved in DNA replication and repair, and YFP-RAD18 to

---

* Research partially supported by the US NIH NIBIB award R33-EB00573 (KP).

label postreplication repair of damaged DNA or immunostaining these endogenous proteins to characterize all cell cycle phases [1,2,3]. The focus of this paper is on fluorescent labeling using GFP-PCNA which enables cell cycle phases to be distinguished by characteristic patterns of GFP-PCNA at different points of cell cycle: M-phase or mitosis, followed by G1-phase, early, mid and late S-phases, and G2-phase (Figure 1). GFP-PCNA produces a complex distribution of foci patterns in different stages of the S-phase, but is fairly homogenous during G1- and G2-phases, and very diluted during M-phase. In order to identify cell cycle phases, individual nuclei need to be detected, segmented and classified. Cell segmentation, classification and tracking require robust and sophisticated algorithms in order to deal with noise, shape changes, texture and touching cells [4,5,6,7,8]. In this paper we describe a novel technique for fluorescent nuclei detection and segmentation using a fast implementation of multi-phase graph partitioning active contours (fastGPAC). Fluorescent particles corresponding to the localization of GFP-PCNA have characteristic distributions that we utilize to train a support vector machine to classify the segmented nuclei into four cell phases and three sub-phases in S-phase.

2 Methods

2.1 Segmentation Using FastGPAC

To segment HeLa cell nuclei we use level set-based multi-phase fast graph partitioning active contours (FastGPAC) which is our novel efficient implementation of graph partitioning active contours (GPAC). FastGPAC reduces the $O(N^4)$ computational complexity and memory requirements of the original GPAC algorithm [9,10] to $O(N^2)$ computational complexity and $O(n \times L)$ constant memory where $N \times N$ is the image size, L is number of histogram bins, and n is the number of phases. Graph partitioning active contours (GPAC) is introduced in [9,10] as a new powerful curve evolution framework. GPAC can be implemented using explicit snake-based or implicit level set-based active contours. Level set-based implementation where a curve $\mathcal{C}$ is represented implicitly via zero-level curve of a Lipschitz function $\phi\ \mathcal{C} = \{(x,y)|\phi(x,y) = 0\}$, provide advantages such as eliminating the need to reparameterize the curve and automatic handling of topology changes [11]. The variational cost function that minimizes pairwise dissimilarity within regions is written as [10]:

$$E_{WR} = \iint_\Omega \iint_\Omega w(p_1,p_2) H(\phi(p_1)) H(\phi(p_2)) dp_1 dp_2 \\ + \iint_\Omega \iint_\Omega w(p_1,p_2) \Big(1 - H(\phi(p_1))\Big)\Big(1 - H(\phi(p_2))\Big) dp_1 dp_2 \quad (1)$$

where Ω is the whole image domain, $w()$ is a pixel-to-pixel dissimilarity measure, H is the heaviside function, an indicator function for the points inside $R_i(\mathcal{C})$, and outside $R_o(\mathcal{C})$ of the curve ($H(\phi)$) and $(1 - H(\phi))$ respectively. Curve evolution equation is obtained with steepest descent minimization. The complete curve evolution equation (with regularization term, normalization factors α and β, and weights $\lambda_{1,2}$ and μ) is [10]:

$$\frac{\partial \phi(p_2)}{\partial t} = \delta(\phi(p_2))\Big[\lambda_2 \beta \iint_\Omega w(p_1,p_2)\Big(1 - H(\phi(p_1))\Big)dp_1 \\ -\lambda_1 \alpha \iint_\Omega w(p_1,p_2)H(\phi(p_1))dp_1 + \mu \operatorname{div}\Big(\frac{\nabla \phi(p_2)}{|\nabla \phi(p_2)|}\Big)\Big] \quad (2)$$

which is discretized as:

$$\frac{\Delta \phi(p_2)}{\Delta t} = \delta_\epsilon(\phi(p_2))\Big[\lambda_2 \beta \sum_{p_1 \in R_o(\mathcal{C})} w(p_1,p_2) - \lambda_1 \alpha \sum_{p_1 \in R_i(\mathcal{C})} w(p_1,p_2) + \mu \mathcal{K}\Big] \quad (3)$$

While powerful in terms of region description, heavy computational and memory requirements prevent GPAC's direct application to large images. Our FastGPAC approach reduces both computational and memory requirements of the *original* GPAC, without approximations such as dissimilarity computation at block or superpixel level [9,10], and makes segmentation of large images with GPAC approach possible. The bottleneck in the original GPAC is the computation of the 2-D regional (inside and outside) sums in Eq. 3, $\sum_{p_1 \in R_o(\mathcal{C})} w(p_1,p_2)$ and $\sum_{p_1 \in R_i(\mathcal{C})} w(p_1,p_2)$. To speed the process in [9], dissimilarities of every image point to every image point are pre-computed and stored in a $N^2 \times N^2$ lookup table W for an $N \times N$ image. But this $O(N^4)$ table quickly becomes impractical for large images (i.e. over a terabyte of memory for a 1024×1024 grayscale image). FastGPAC speeds up 2-D regional sum computations by maintaining two histograms $\mathbf{h}_i$ and $\mathbf{h}_o$ for regions $R_i(\mathcal{C})$, $R_o(\mathcal{C})$. When $w(p_1,p_2)$ does not incorporate spatial distance between points p_1 and p_2, $w(p_1,p_2)$ can be rewritten as $w(p_1,p_2) \equiv D(F(p_1), F(p_2))$ where $F(p)$ is a feature extracted from the point $p(x,y)$, and D is a similarity/dissimilarity measure defined on F (i.e. for $w(p_1,p_2) = |I(p_1) - I(p_2)|$, $F(p)$ is grayscale intensity $I(p)$ and D is L_1 metric.)

GPAC Region Sum Theorem. For cases where $w(p_1,p_2)$ does not incorporate spatial distance, the 2-D regional sums, $\sum_{p_1 \in R_r} w(p_1,p_2)$ (for $R_r = R_i$ and $R_r = R_o$) can be reduced to 1-D sums independent of the size or shape of the regions $R_i(\mathcal{C})$ and $R_o(\mathcal{C})$.

$$\sum_{p_1 \in R_r} w(p_1,p_2) \equiv \sum_{j=0}^{L-1} h_r(j) D(F(p_2), j) \quad (4)$$

where $\mathbf{h}_r$ is the histogram of the feature F in region R_r, $D()$ is a (dis)similarity measure, L is number of bins in $\mathbf{h}_r$ and $h_r(j) = \sum_{p \in R_r \wedge F(p)=j} 1$ is the jth bin of h_r corresponding to the number of points $p \in R_r$ whose features $F(p)$ are in j^{th} bin $(F(p) \in j)$.

Proof. This equality is derived by grouping the points p into feature class bins $F(p) \in j$, and by separating the original sum into two sums as follows:

$$\sum_{p_1 \in R_r} w(p_1, p_2) \equiv \sum_{p_1 \in R_r} D(F(p_1), F(p_2))$$

$$= \sum_{j=0}^{L-1} \sum_{p_1 \in R_r \wedge F(p_1) \in j} (D(F(p_2), j) \times 1) = \sum_{j=0}^{L-1} D(F(p_2), j) \times \underbrace{\sum_{p_1 \in R_r \wedge F(p_1) \in j} 1}_{h_r(j)} \quad (5)$$

Using the GPAC region sum theorem, FastGPAC transforms GPAC curve evolution Eq. 3 into:

$$\frac{\Delta \phi(p_2)}{\Delta t} = \delta_\epsilon(\phi(p_2)) \Big[\lambda_2 \beta \sum_{j=0}^{L-1} h_o(j) D(F(p_2), j) - \lambda_1 \alpha \sum_{j=0}^{L-1} h_i(j) D(F(p_2), j) + \mu \mathcal{K} \Big]$$

$$= \delta_\epsilon(\phi(p_2)) \Big[\sum_{j=0}^{L-1} [\lambda_2 \beta \ h_o(j) - \lambda_1 \alpha \ h_i(j)] D(F(p_2), j) + \mu \mathcal{K} \Big] \quad (6)$$

This transformation reduces N^4 pairwise dissimilarity computations (from each pixel to each pixel) to $N^2 2L$ dissimilarity computations (from each pixel to each of the L histogram bins) where L is constant and $L << N^2$. In our application, appearance of the nuclei changes during the different phases of the cell cycle. Use of two-phase schemes risk false misses, particularly during mitosis when signal-to-noise ratio drops near to background levels. Due to this, we use 4-phase segmentation. In [10], GPAC is extended to multi-phase in a way similar to Vese and Chan's multi-phase extension [12]. As in the case of 2-phase GPAC, each sum in the multi-phase GPAC is transformed to its efficient form using the GPAC regional sum theorem.

2.2 Cell Cycle Phase Classification

In order to classify detected nuclei into one of the six classes (M, G1, S (early, mid, late) and G2), we utilize the characteristic appearance of GFP-PCNA in fluorescent nuclei images. As shown in Figure 1, different phases are manifested by a rich textural information that can be captured by using the histograms of intensity as well as intensity surface curvature. We do not use 2-D geometric features of the cells in order to make the feature vector robust to changes in the shape of nuclei. Our choice of feature vector (64 bins of intensity histogram and 64 bins of intensity surface curvature histogram) captures the characteristic texture information of each class without more elaborated feature vector computations such as [13, 14, 7]. Shape-based properties of the intensity surface can be utilized for blob and ridge analysis [6]. The GFP-PCNA in nucleus produces spikes and blob-like patterns hence the utilization of blob detection methods to obtain a texture signature is theoretically sound. Ridges and blobs can be defined as local extrema of principal curvatures of the instensity surface. Principal curvatures and directions of a hypersurface L correspond to the eigenvalues

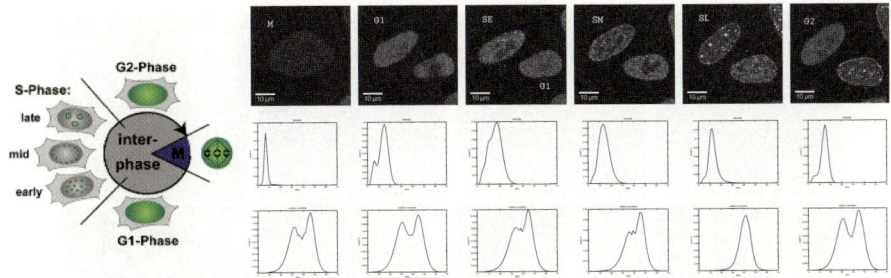

Fig. 1. GFP-PCNA fluorescence-based patterns during six periods of cell cycle and corresponding signatures. Left to right: M phase, G1 phase, early, mid, late S phases and G2 phase. Top to bottom: sample cell image, intensity histogram signature, surface curvature histogram signature.

$\kappa_1 \geq \ldots \geq \kappa_{n-1}$ and eigenvectors $\xi_1 \geq \ldots \geq \xi_{n-1}$ of the shape operator matrix on the tangent space W. In 2-D case, W is given as a function of the first and second fundamental forms. Since computation of principal curvatures is expensive, mean curvature $H = \frac{1}{2}(\kappa_1 + \kappa_2) = \frac{1}{2}trace(W)$ is often used to classify surface patches ($H < 0$: peak, ridge, or saddle ridge; $H = 0$: flat or minimal surface; $H > 0$: pit, valley, or saddle valley). In generalization of local extrema for real-valued functions of a vector variable, a point x_0 is classified as maximum if $\nabla L(x_0) = 0$ (critical point) and $\mathcal{H}(L(x_0))$ is negative definite (all eigenvalues $\lambda_i < 0$) where $\mathcal{H}$ is the Hessian matrix:

$$\mathcal{H} = \begin{bmatrix} L_{xx} & L_{xy} \\ L_{xy} & L_{yy} \end{bmatrix} \tag{7}$$

For critical points ($\nabla L(x_0) = 0$), eigenvalues λ_i and eigenvectors v_i of the Hessian matrix correspond to principal curvatures κ_i and principal directions ξ_i respectively. We utilize the histograms of $\lambda_1(\mathcal{H})$ ($|\lambda_1| > |\lambda_2|$) and intensity to obtain a characteristic signature for each cell cycle phase. By binning the intensity and surface curvature histograms into 64 bins we obtain a 128-D feature vector. Figure 1 shows the average signatures of each class. We train a support vector machine [15] with a test set of nucleus images for each of the six classes using these signatures as described in the following section.

3 Experimental Results

Genetically modified human HeLa Kyoto cell lines were generated and validated to stably express the fused protein green fluorescent protein-tagged proliferating cell nuclear antigen (GFP-PCNA). The first step involved creating HeLa Kyoto lines containing a stably integrated Flp-recombination site (FRT). This was followed by site-specific integration of a construct containing the human EF1α promoter to drive expression of the fusion gene, in this case GFP-PCNA, and a blasticidin resistance marker gene used for selection of the transgenic cells flanked by FRT sites. This strategy allows the Flp recombinase mediated integration of DNA into a specific site in the genome and a reliable and homogeneous

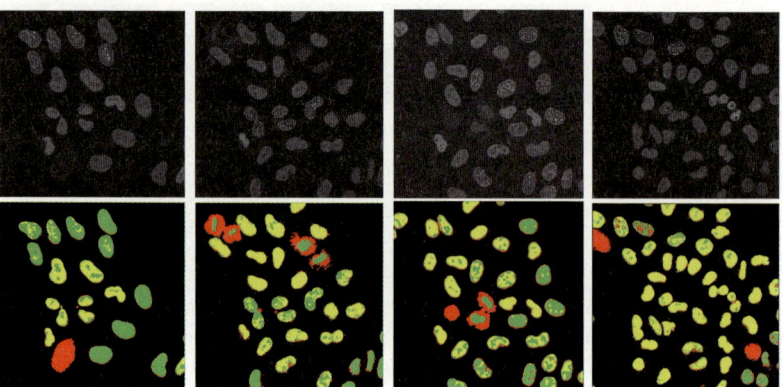

Fig. 2. Sample FastGPAC segmentation results for four sample frames. Top: Original frames, bottom: Recolored level set masks.

level of the fluorescent protein in every cell. Live cell analysis was performed by plating the cells on chambered glass coverslips before microscopy. The chambered glass coverslip was mounted onto the microscope stage and maintained in a humidified atmosphere of 5% CO_2 at 37°C on a microscope incubation system. For time lapse analysis, images were acquired with a Zeiss LSM 510 Meta laser scanning confocal microscope using the 488 nm laser line of an Argon ion laser at low power every 15 minutes. The image sequence has 174 1024×1024 frames. Figure 2 shows sample segmentation results for four frames using 4-phase level set FastGPAC method. When the 4-phase segmentation masks are recolored as in 2nd row (black-red-green-yellow in the order of increasing average phase intensity), some observations on the color scheme can be made i.e. just before mitosis, nuclei appear as solid red blobs (fluorescent intensity fades), just after mitosis daughter nuclei appear as red blobs with green centers. Since original GPAC requires terabyte size memory for 1024×1024 images, 220×160 regions are cropped and segmented for comparison. FastGPAC segments cropped images in 2.2 CPU seconds, original GPAC spends 415 CPU seconds ($189\times$ speedup). The actual completion time of original GPAC is longer due to extensive memory swaps. For the classification task, colored masks are binarized into foreground and background using a rule-based scheme to avoid merging of neighboring nuclei. 100 frames are labeled by an expert in the art to provide ground truth for quantification of the classification performance. A total of 1543 cells are chosen for training and testing. For each cell, a 128-D feature vector is derived from the intensity and surface curvature histograms. The feature vectors are used in 5-fold cross validation to obtain five runs for classifier performance training and testing. Each run of training is also performed in five folds to obtain the best parameters for SVM. Table 1 shows the average percentage confusion matrices of the proposed classification approach and of the Wndchrm method in [14] when applied to our data set for classification of four phases and three sub-phases in S-phase (columns do not add up to 100% due to rounding). Top 30% of the

Table 1. Average confusion matrix for 6 classes. Left: Wndchrm, right: proposed approach.

	M	G1	SE	SM	SL	G2	M	G1	SE	SM	SL	G2
M	90	1	1	0	0	0	95	1	0	0	0	1
G1	6	90	6	3	1	18	5	97	7	7	0	17
SE	1	2	80	12	1	0	0	0	90	16	0	0
SM	0	0	13	65	8	0	0	0	2	69	1	0
SL	0	0	1	20	90	1	0	0	0	9	98	0
G2	3	7	0	0	0	81	0	2	0	0	1	83

Table 2. Average confusion matrix for 4 classes. Left: Wndchrm, right: proposed approach.

	M	G1	S	G2	M	G1	S	G2
M	90	1	0	0	95	1	0	1
G1	6	90	3	18	5	97	4	17
S	1	2	97	1	0	0	96	0
G2	3	7	0	81	0	2	0	83

ranked 1025-D feature vector in [14] is used for classification as the best result. Proposed approach exceeds the accuracy of Wndchrm in all classes. As expected, separating G1 from G2 without resorting to temporal constraints is a challenge. Similarly the mid S-phase is highly confused since there are no clear cut boundaries between SE-SM and SM-SL. The proposed feature vector provides good performance in capturing the textural characteristics of the GFP-PCNA in nuclei. The computation of our feature vector for 1543 cells takes about 3 minutes, whereas the running time of Wndchrm on our data set is about 5 hours. The overall average accuracy of our classification approach is 92.3%, the same of Wndchrm is 86.4% where (worst case, best case) accuracies are (90.3%, 94.5%) for our approach and (84.9%, 87.5%) for Wndchrm. Table 2 shows the average percentage confusion matrices for the 4-phase classification.

4 Conclusions

The proteins of interest in fluorescence-based imaging are involved in basic cellular processes such as DNA repair and replication. PCNA is a key component of the DNA replication machinery. GFP-PCNA-based cell cycle analysis is more precise since PCNA is directly linked to the DNA replication, and provides higher resolution as well as information about the progress of S-phase through patterns of different sized foci. The imaging noise, lower SNR in some phases, complex textural patterns, significant shape changes during cell division and large data volumes require the development of a multiclass region-based segmentation algorithm with topological flexibility. We extended the recently proposed multiphase GPAC algorithm for fluorescence-based cell nucleus segmentation by incorporating density functions to capture the variability of regions for reliable and accurate segmentation. GPAC has not been previously applied to large biomedical segmentation applications due to extensive memory (on the order of terabytes) and computational requirements for large images. We derive a FastGPAC algorithm that requires constant memory and is highly scalable for high content screening time-lapse microscopy images. Preliminary results indicate that the multi-phase implementation is able to accurately segment nuclei of proliferating cells imaged for more than 40 hours. We also use a support vector machine to classify segmented nuclei into one of the four phases and three sub-phases. Quantitative results show highly accurate cell phase classification using intensity and surface curvature histograms without the need for elaborated feature extraction schemes that are computationally expensive. Future work includes improving the confusion of phases and incorporating these results into our multi-object multi-hypothesis tracker [4] to enforce temporal constraints and provide accurate lineage construction.

References

1. Easwaran, H., Leonhardt, H., Cardoso, M.: Cell cycle markers for live cell analyses. Cell Cycle 4(3), 453–455 (2005)
2. Sporbert, A., Gahl, A., Ankerhold, R., Leonhardt, H., Cardoso, M.: DNA polymerase clamp shows little turnover at established replication sites but sequential de novo assembly at adjacent origin clusters. Molecular Cell 10(6), 1355–1365 (2002)
3. Leonhardt, H., Rahn, H.-P., Weinzierl, P., Sporbert, A., Cremer, T., Zink, D., Cardoso, M.: Dynamics of DNA replication factories in living cells. J. Cell Biology 149(2), 271–280 (2000)
4. Bunyak, F., Palaniappan, K., Nath, S., Baskin, T., Dong, G.: Quantitative cell motility for *in vitro* wound healing using level set-based active contour tracking. In: Proc. IEEE Int. Symp. Biomedical Imaging, April 2006, pp. 1040–1043 (2006)
5. Nath, S.K., Palaniappan, K., Bunyak, F.: Cell segmentation using coupled level sets and graph-vertex coloring. In: Larsen, R., Nielsen, M., Sporring, J. (eds.) MICCAI 2006. LNCS, vol. 4190, pp. 101–108. Springer, Heidelberg (2006)
6. Ersoy, I., Bunyak, F., Palaniappan, K., Sun, M., Forgacs, G.: Cell spreading analysis with directed edge profile-guided level set active contours. In: Metaxas, D., Axel, L., Fichtinger, G., Székely, G. (eds.) MICCAI 2008, Part I. LNCS, vol. 5241, pp. 376–383. Springer, Heidelberg (2008)
7. Wang, M., Zhou, X., Li, F., Huckins, J., King, R.W., Wong, S.T.: Novel cell segmentation and online SVM for cell cycle phase identification in automated microscopy. Bioinformatics 24(1), 94–101 (2008)
8. Padfield, D., Rittscher, J., Thomas, N., Roysam, B.: Spatio-temporal cell cycle phase analysis using level sets and fast marching methods. Medical Image Analysis 13(1), 143–155 (2009)
9. Sumengen, B., Manjunath, B.: Graph partitioning active contours (GPAC) for image segmentation. IEEE Trans. Patt. Anal. Mach. Intell., 509–521 (April 2006)
10. Bertelli, L., Sumengen, B., Manjunath, B., Gibou, F.: A variational framework for multi-region pairwise similarity-based image segmentation. IEEE Trans. Patt. Anal. Mach. Intell., 1400–1414 (August 2008)
11. Sethian, J.: Level set methods and fast marching methods, 2nd edn. Cambridge Univ. Press, Cambridge (1999)
12. Vese, L., Chan, T.: A multiphase level set framework for image segmentation using the Mumford and Shah model. Int. J. Computer Vision 50(3), 271–293 (2002)
13. Boland, M.V., Murphy, R.F.: A neural network classifier capable of recognizing the patterns of all major subcellular structures in fluorescence microscope images of HeLa cells. Bioinformatics 17(12), 1213–1223 (2001)
14. Shamir, L., Orlov, N., Eckley, D.M., Macura, T., Johnston, J., Goldberg, I.: Wndchrm - An open source utility for biological image analysis. Source Code for Biology and Medicine 3(1) (2008)
15. Chang, C.C., Lin, C.J.: LIBSVM: A library for support vector machines (2001), http://www.csie.ntu.edu.tw/~cjlin/libsvm

Steerable Features for Statistical 3D Dendrite Detection

Germán González[1,*], François Aguet[2], François Fleuret[1,3,**], Michael Unser[2], and Pascal Fua[1]

[1] Computer Vision Lab, Ecole Polytechnique Fédérale de Lausanne, Switzerland
german.gonzalez@epfl.ch
[2] Biomedical Imaging Group, Ecole Polytechnique Fédérale de Lausanne, Switzerland
[3] Idiap Research Institute, Martigny, Switzerland

Abstract. Most state-of-the-art algorithms for filament detection in 3–D image-stacks rely on computing the Hessian matrix around individual pixels and labeling these pixels according to its eigenvalues. This approach, while very effective for clean data in which linear structures are nearly cylindrical, loses its effectiveness in the presence of noisy data and irregular structures.

In this paper, we show that using steerable filters to create rotationally invariant features that include higher-order derivatives and training a classifier based on these features lets us handle such irregular structures. This can be done reliably and at acceptable computational cost and yields better results than state-of-the-art methods.

1 Introduction

Most state-of-the-art approaches to filament detection in 3–D image-stacks rely on computing the Hessian matrix around individual voxels and labeling these voxels according to its eigenvalues. Some are optimized for ideal tubular structures, while others use statistical-learning techniques to improve detection results.

In this paper, we will show that the second-order derivatives used to compute the Hessian matrix do not provide a local description that is powerful enough to account for the fact that dendrites, such as those depicted by Fig. 1, are far from being regular tubular structures, which can drastically impact performance. To effectively account for such irregularities, one must use higher-order derivatives.

To this end, we rely on 3–D steerable filters [1] to create rotationally invariant features that include derivatives of order 2 to 4 that we use as input to a classifier trained to recognize voxels belonging to potentially irregular dendrites. Because the training data encompasses the deviations from the ideal model, the resulting algorithm has the potential to be more robust than traditional ones and can be trained to detect not only simple linear-structures but also junctions and crossings.

---

[*] This work was funded in part by the Swiss National Science Foundation.
[**] Supported by the Swiss National Science Foundation under the National Centre of Competence in Research (NCCR) on Interactive Multimodal Information Management (IM2).

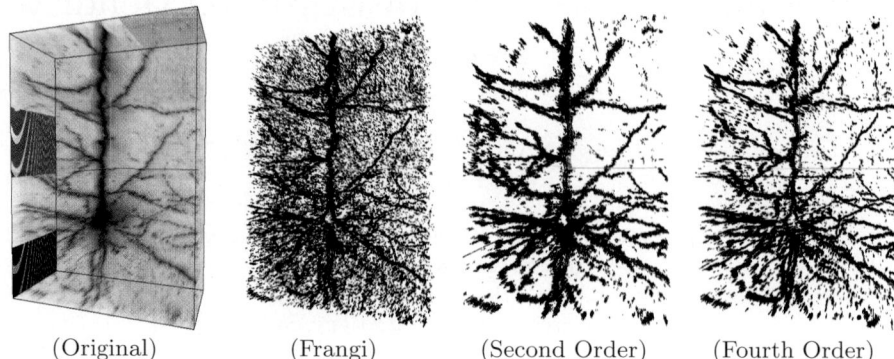

(Original)   (Frangi)   (Second Order)   (Fourth Order)

Fig. 1. Original image stack and its segmentation result for a false positive rate of 10^{-2} for three different methods: Frangi's non-linear relationship on the eigenvalues of the hessian [2], our methodology with second order features, and our methodology with fourth order features. As it will be demonstrated later, the fourth order method outperforms the other two ones.

Most automated approaches to finding linear structures in image stacks assume them to be locally tubular and model them as generalized cylinders. The most popular one involves computing the Hessian matrix at individual voxels by convolution with Gaussian derivatives and relying on the eigenvalues of the Hessian to classify voxels as filament-like or not [3,2,4]. The Hessians can be modified to create an oriented filter in the direction of minimum variance, which should correspond to the direction of any existing filament [5,1]. To find filaments of various widths, these methods perform the computation using a range of variances for the Gaussian masks and select the most discriminant one. The fact that intensity changes inside and outside the filaments has also been explicitly exploited by locally convolving the image with differential kernels [6], finding parallel edges [7], and fitting *superellipsoids* or cylinders to the linear structure based on its surface integral [8,9].

All these methods, however, assume image regularities that are present in high-quality images but not necessarily in noisier ones. Furthermore, they often require careful parameter tuning, which may change from one data-set to the next. As a result, probabilistic approaches able to learn whether a voxel belongs to a filament or not have begun to be employed. Instead of assuming the filaments to be cylinders, they aim at learning their appearance from the data. In [10], the eigenvalues of the structure tensor, are represented by a mixture model whose parameters are estimated via E-M. Support Vector Machines that operate on the Hessian's eigenvalues have also been used to discriminate between filament and non-filament voxels [11].

The latter approach [11] is closest to ours in that it also relies on the statistical learning paradigm. However, its ability to generalize is limited by the fact that it still relies on the eigenvalues of the Hessian and therefore on second order derivatives, whereas using higher-order derivatives gives us access to a much richer descriptor.

As shown in Fig. 2, our method outperforms one of the very best Hessian-based methods [2]. Interestingly, this stops being true if we limit it to using only second-order derivatives as opposed to fourth-order ones and our results actually become worse. In other words, these higher-order derivatives are required to take full advantage of the statistical-learning framework that has been advocated in the literature [10,11]. Furthermore, steerable filters provide a very effective framework to do this robustly. We view this observation as the main contribution of the paper.

2 Method

To demonstrate that higher-order derivatives provide better descriptive power at an acceptable computational cost, we rely on 3–D steerable filters [1] to create rotationally invariant feature vectors that can be used to classify voxels as being part of a dendrite or not. In practice, to achieve rotation invariance, we compute a local orientation and use it to steer the filters and to create the feature vectors corresponding to a reference orientation. In other words, we rotate the feature vectors to a reference orientation.

In the remainder of this section, we first recall the basic theory of steerable filters. We then show how we use them to create feature vectors given a local orientation estimate. Finally, we discuss how we use these feature vectors to train the classifier we use at run time to detect filament-like voxels.

2.1 Steerable Filters in 2–D and 3–D

Steerable filters were introduced as an efficient means to compute filters that can be rotated to any orientation for a small computational cost [12]. In three dimensions, steerable filter based detection of a feature g in a volume f at a given orientation and position $\mathbf{u} = (x, y, z)$, is formulated as:

$$r = f(\mathbf{u}) * g(\mathbf{R}^{\theta,\phi}\mathbf{u}), \quad g(\mathbf{R}^{\theta,\phi}\mathbf{u}) = \sum_l b_l(\theta, \phi) g_l(\mathbf{u}), \quad (1)$$

where θ and ϕ parameterize the orientation of the feature template in spherical coordinates, $\mathbf{R}_{\theta,\phi}$ is the 3–D rotation matrix, and r is the response. The functions $b(\theta, \phi)$ are trigonometric polynomials that interpolate the templates $g_l(\mathbf{u})$. This decomposition decouples the rotation of the filters from the convolution in Eq. (1), which makes the estimation computationally efficient.

The best known class of such filters, and the ones used in this paper, are Gaussian derivatives and their linear combinations [13]. To preserve the separability of the resulting kernels, we limit ourselves to diagonal covariance matrices. Let G^σ denote the isotropic Gaussian kernel of variance σ centered at the origin. Let $G^\sigma_{m,n,p}$ denote it m^{th} derivative with respect to x, n^{th} derivative with respect to y and p^{th} derivative with respect to z.

$$\forall \mathbf{u} \in \mathbb{R}^3, \ G^\sigma(\mathbf{u}) = \frac{1}{(2\pi\sigma^2)^{3/2}} \exp\left(-\frac{\|\mathbf{u}\|^2}{2\sigma^2}\right), \ G^\sigma_{m,n,p} = \frac{\partial^{m+n+p} G^\sigma}{\partial x^m \partial y^n \partial z^p}. \quad (2)$$

The rotation equations for a filter that is formed by a linear combination of Gaussian derivatives is:

$$b_{m,n,p}(\theta,\phi) = \sum_{i=0}^{m}\sum_{k=0}^{n}\sum_{q=0}^{p}\sum_{j=0}^{i}\sum_{l=0}^{k} \frac{m!n!p!(-1)^{i-j+p-q}}{(m-i)!(i-j)!j!(n-k)!(k-l)!l!(p-q)!q!}$$
$$\cos(\theta)^{m-i+j+k-l}\cos(\phi)^{m-i+n-k+q}\sin(\theta)^{i-j+n-k+l}\sin(\phi)^{j+l+p-q}$$
$$a_{m-i+n-k+p-q,\,i-j+k-l,\,j+l+q} \quad (3)$$

where $a_{m,n,p}$ is the coefficient that multiplies $G^\sigma_{m,n,k}$ at the reference orientation.

2.2 Feature Vectors

We take the features vectors to be the convolution of the volume f with the set of templates $G^\sigma_{m,n,p}$ of normalized energy,

$$v_\sigma(f,\mathbf{u}) = \left(f * \left[\frac{G^\sigma_{1,0,0}}{E_{1,0,0}}, \frac{G^\sigma_{0,1,0}}{E_{0,1,0}}, \frac{G^\sigma_{0,0,1}}{E_{0,0,1}} \frac{G^\sigma_{2,0,0}}{E_{2,0,0}} \cdots \frac{G^\sigma_{0,0,M}}{E_{0,0,M}} \right] \right)(\mathbf{u}), \quad (4)$$

where $E_{i,j,k}$ is the energy of the $G^\sigma_{i,j,k}$ function. These feature vector are equivalent to a steerable filter, and therefore can be steered to any orientation using Eq. (3).

2.3 Training and Detection

During a training phase, we use ground truth data for which the orientation is provided to train an SVM classifier. Then, to classify a voxel at run-time, we compute the local orientation to rotate the feature vectors to the reference orientation. Finally, the classifier is used to output the likelihood of the voxel belonging to the neuron.

The training data consists of quadruplets that include a 3–D location $\mathbf{u}$ in an image stack, two orientation angles θ and ϕ, and a single bit indicating whether it is a positive or negative sample. Formally, the training set can be written as

$$\mathcal{S} = \{(\mathbf{u}_1,\theta_1,\phi_1,1),\ldots,(\mathbf{u}_N,\theta_N,\phi_N,1),$$
$$(\mathbf{u}_{N+1},\theta_{N+1},\phi_{N+1},0),\ldots,(\mathbf{u}_{2N},\theta_{2N},\phi_{2N},0)\} \quad (5)$$

where the first N quadruplets represent the positive samples and the following N the negative ones.

The positive samples are taken from ground truth data. Negative samples are taken from two populations. The first one includes points closer than a given radius to the dendrites but not belonging to them, the second one are points taken at random in the whole volume, but not belonging to the neuron. The local orientation of negative points is given by the same algorithm as the one used during detection, which in our case is the steerable filters optimized using Canny criteria for filament detection of [1].

For each of the training points, the feature vector is computed and rotated back from its labeled orientation. Let $v^{\theta,\phi}$ be the feature vector rotated by angles θ and ϕ. The set of samples used for training is

$$\mathcal{V} = \{(v_1^{-\theta_1,-\phi_1}, 1), \ldots, (v_N^{-\theta_N,-\phi_N}, 1), (v_{N+1}^{-\theta_{N+1},-\phi_{N+1}}, 0), \ldots, (v_{2N}^{-\theta_{2N},-\phi_{2N}}, 0)\} \ . \tag{6}$$

After training an SVM, the detection score for a voxel $\mathbf{u}$ at orientation θ, ϕ becomes

$$\Psi : \mathbb{R}^D \to \mathbb{R}, \quad \psi(\mathbf{u}, \theta, \phi) = \sum_{n=0}^{N} a_n \, \kappa\left(v_n, v^{-\theta,-\phi}(\mathbf{u})\right) + b \ , \tag{7}$$

where κ is the standard Gaussian kernel, the variance ν of which is obtained by minimizing the error on a validation set.

At run-time, to classify a voxel as belonging to a filament or not, we need to estimate the orientation of that filament if it exists. In standard Hessian methods, this is done by computation the eigenvectors of the Hessian matrix. However, there is no obvious method to do the same using our feature vectors. To derive the orientations we need, we therefore use a modified linear Hessian method that relies on second-order steerable filters optimized according to the Canny criterion [1]. We have found empirically that the orientations it returns allow us to achieve better performance than when using other methods.

3 Results

In this section, we show that using fourth order steerable features allow us to detect dendrites more accurately in brightfield microscopy images than second order methods. We compare our method to both [2], which we believe to be one of the best Hessian-based methods, and to our own algorithm constrained to use only second-order derivatives. The ROC curve of Fig. 2 summarizes our findings.

The dataset used for these comparisons consists of two image stacks of neurons imaged using standard brightfield microscopy and the associated ground truth data. The first is used for training and validation and the second for testing. Fig. 1(Original) is a 3–D minimum intensity projection of the test stack. Cross-sections in the XY and XZ planes are shown in Figs. 3 and 4. In Fig. 4, please note the cone of shadow cast by the dendrites, which causes problems to second order filament detectors.

In the remainder of this section, we first describe implementation details of the training and detection procedures, and offer a more in-depth analysis of our results.

3.1 Training and Detection

For training we used as positive samples 2500 hand-labeled voxels and their associated orientations, and 2500 more for validation purposes. In addition, we collected 1250 negative samples around the neuron and 1250 chosen at random,

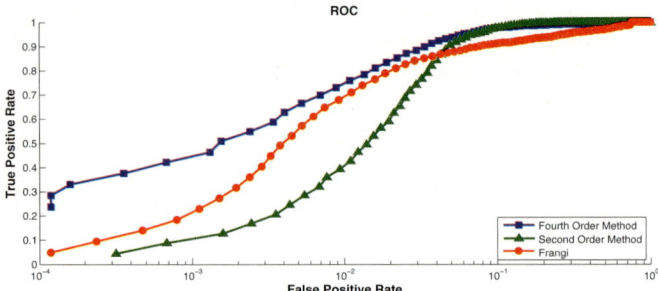

Fig. 2. ROC curve for several methods. The presented method of order four outperforms the method of Frangi [2] and our algorithm constrained to second order features. The improvement is due to the use of fourth order features, which allows us to emcompass a higher frequency signals. Please not the logarithmic scale in the false positive rate.

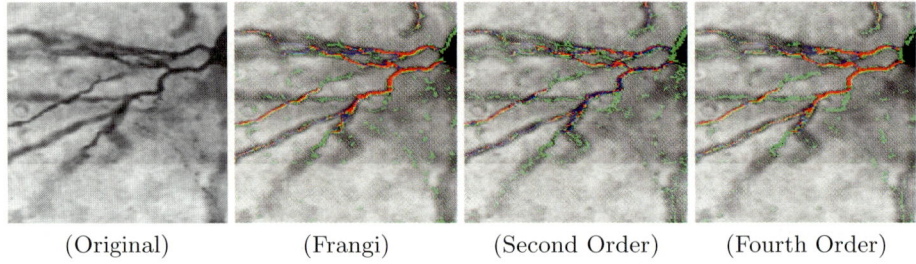

(Original) (Frangi) (Second Order) (Fourth Order)

Fig. 3. Detail of one of the images in the stack. We compare our detector using features of order four and two against that of Frangi [2]. In red we show true positives, in green false positives and in blue false negatives. The false positive rate is fixed to 10^{-2}. Our second-order detector fails to detect some filaments and is more sensitive to the shadow casted by the dendrites. However, our fourth order filter outperforms the second order Hessian-based method of Frangi. False positives for our method are clustered around the true dendrite locations, and the true positive rate is incremented from 67.7% to 74.5%.

but not belonging to the dendrites. The orientation of the negative samples is taken from the output of the orientation predictor [1], using same scale as the one used to compute the feature vectors. We use the method of [1] to compute the orientation as it is a more elongated template than the Hessian and provides a more accurate orientation estimation. During detection, the orientation is estimated using the same method as for assigning orientation to negative points.

3.2 Discussion

The ROC curve of Fig. 2 indicates that our fourth order filter outperform the second order methods over the entire range of false positive rates. This comes from the fact that fourth order derivatives can encompass higher frequency

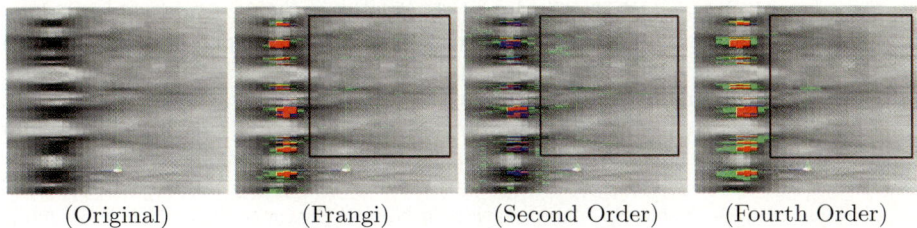

(Original) (Frangi) (Second Order) (Fourth Order)

Fig. 4. Detail of the YZ projection of several filaments in parallel. As in Fig. 3, we show true positives in red, false positives in green and false negatives in blue. Our method produces ellipsoids centered in the true filament but bigger in size. This is due to uncertainties in the training data. Frangi's method [2] detects the real dendrites accurately but produces many false-positives away from them. Our second order method responds mainly to the shadow of the dendrite in this cross-section. Please note the noise in the different images highlighted by the rectangles.

signals. For example, this is what explains that our fourth order method avoids confusion between the cone of shadow of the signal and the actual dendrite in the difficult case of Fig. 4.

Our features are linear combinations of SVM kernel functions evaluated at the support vectors. As we are using Gaussian kernels, these functions are smooth. By contrast, [2] uses ratios between features. This creates a sharper detection profile that makes the method more discriminative at low false positive rates than ours when using only second-order derivatives.

4 Conclusion

In this paper we have presented an approach to detecting dendrites in 3–D image stacks that outperforms state-of-the-art Hessian based methods in brightfield image stacks. The performance gain is due to the use of a rich feature set made of higher-order image derivatives. At the heart of our implementation are steerable filters that let us rotate the feature vectors to a reference orientation and train a classifier to recognize which ones correspond to dendrite voxels.

This approach is very generic because, instead of postulating *a priori* models for the filaments we are looking for, our algorithm can learn specific appearance models for each new situation. In future work, we will therefore extend our approach to other imaging modalities in which the filaments break the perfectly tubular structure assumption.

References

1. Aguet, F., Jacob, M., Unser, M.: Three-dimensional feature detection using optimal steerable filters. In: Proceedings of the 2005 IEEE International Conference on Image Processing (ICIP 2005), Genova, Italy, September 11-14, vol. II, pp. 1158–1161 (2005)

2. Frangi, A.F., Niessen, W.J., Vincken, K.L., Viergever, M.A.: Multiscale vessel enhancement filtering. In: Wells, W.M., Colchester, A.C.F., Delp, S.L. (eds.) MICCAI 1998. LNCS, vol. 1496, pp. 130–137. Springer, Heidelberg (1998)
3. Sato, Y., Nakajima, S., Atsumi, H., Koller, T., Gerig, G., Yoshida, S., Kikinis, R.: 3d multi-scale line filter for segmentation and visualization of curvilinear structures in medical images. Medical Image Analysis 2, 143–168 (1998)
4. Streekstra, G., van Pelt, J.: Analysis of tubular structures in three-dimensional confocal images. Network: Computation in Neural Systems 13(3), 381–395 (2002)
5. Meijering, E., Jacob, M., Sarria, J.C.F., Steiner, P., Hirling, H., Unser, M.: Design and validation of a tool for neurite tracing and analysis in fluorescence microscopy images. Cytometry Part A 58A(2), 167–176 (2004)
6. Al-Kofahi, K., Lasek, S., Szarowski, D., Pace, C., Nagy, G., Turner, J., Roysam, B.: Rapid automated three-dimensional tracing of neurons from confocal image stacks. IEEE Transactions on Information Technology in Biomedicine (2002)
7. Dima, A., Scholz, M., Obermayer, K.: Automatic segmentation and skeletonization of neurons from confocal microscopy images based on the 3-d wavelet transform. IEEE Transactions on Image Processing 11(7), 790–801 (2002)
8. Tyrrell, J., di Tomaso, E., Fuja, D., Tong, R., Kozak, K., Jain, R., Roysam, B.: Robust 3D modeling of vasculature imagery using superellipsoids. Medical Imaging 26(2), 223–237 (2007)
9. Schmitt, S., Evers, J.F., Duch, C., Scholz, M., Obermayer, K.: New methods for the computer-assisted 3D reconstruction of neurons from confocal image stacks. NeuroImage 23, 1283–1298 (2004)
10. Agam, G., Wu, C.: Probabilistic modeling-based vessel enhancement in thoracic ct scans. In: CVPR 2005: Proceedings of the 2005 IEEE Computer Society Conference on Computer Vision and Pattern Recognition (CVPR 2005), Washington, DC, USA, vol. 2, pp. 684–689. IEEE Computer Society, Los Alamitos (2005)
11. Santamaría-Pang, A., Colbert, C.M., Saggau, P., Kakadiaris, I.A.: Automatic centerline extraction of irregular tubular structures using probability volumes from multiphoton imaging. In: Ayache, N., Ourselin, S., Maeder, A. (eds.) MICCAI 2007, Part II. LNCS, vol. 4792, pp. 486–494. Springer, Heidelberg (2007)
12. Freeman, W., Adelson, E.: The design and use of steerable filters. Pattern Analysis and Machine Intelligence 13, 891–906 (1991)
13. Jacob, M., Unser, M.: Design of steerable filters for feature detection using canny-like criteria. Pattern Analysis and Machine Intelligence 26(8), 1007–1019 (2004)

Graph-Based Pancreatic Islet Segmentation for Early Type 2 Diabetes Mellitus on Histopathological Tissue

Xenofon Floros[1,4,5], Thomas J. Fuchs[1,4,5], Markus P. Rechsteiner[2,5], Giatgen Spinas[3,5], Holger Moch[2,5], and Joachim M. Buhmann[1,5]

[1] Department of Computer Science, ETH Zurich, Switzerland
{xenofon.floros,thomas.fuchs}@inf.ethz.ch
[2] Institute of Pathology, University Hospital Zurich, University Zurich
[3] Division of Endocrinology and Diabetes, University Hospital Zurich
[4] Life Science Zurich PhD Program on Systems Biology of Complex Diseases
[5] Competence Centre for Systems Physiology and Metabolic Diseases, Zurich

Abstract. It is estimated that in 2010 more than 220 million people will be affected by type 2 diabetes mellitus (T2DM). Early evidence indicates that specific markers for alpha and beta cells in pancreatic islets of Langerhans can be used for early T2DM diagnosis. Currently, the analysis of such histological tissues is manually performed by trained pathologists using a light microscope. To objectify classification results and to reduce the processing time of histological tissues, an automated computational pathology framework for segmentation of pancreatic islets from histopathological fluorescence images is proposed. Due to high variability in the staining intensities for alpha and beta cells, classical medical imaging approaches fail in this scenario.

The main contribution of this paper consists of a novel graph-based segmentation approach based on cell nuclei detection with randomized tree ensembles. The algorithm is trained via a cross validation scheme on a ground truth set of islet images manually segmented by 4 expert pathologists. Test errors obtained from the cross validation procedure demonstrate that the graph-based computational pathology analysis proposed is performing competitively to the expert pathologists while outperforming a baseline morphological approach.

1 Introduction

The computational pathology framework presented in this work aims at automated segmentation of type 2 diabetes mellitus (T2DM) islets. T2DM is a chronically progressive disease which is characterized by hyperglycaemia, insulin resistance, and insulin deficiency. Taken together, these factors lead to organ failure and the increased risk for cardiovascular diseases [1]. It is estimated that by 2010 there will be more than 220 million patients suffering from T2DM [2]. Thus, the search for diagnostic and treatment of this disease is pushing forward at tremendous speed not only in academia but in pharmaceutical industry as well.

Currently, the diagnosis of T2DM includes the measurement of Hemoglobin (Hb) A1c (normal: 4-6%, metabolic syndrome: 6-7%, T2DM: > 7%) which reflects the blood sugar levels [3]. As hyperglycaemia is a marker for the progressed disease status most of the patients are diagnosed as T2DM when the disease has already manifested. Therefore, the search for early T2DM and pre-diabetic markers is of urgent need. From mouse and rat models it is known that the pancreatic islets of Langerhans, which consists of beta cells for insulin production, increase in size to compensate the additional demand for insulin to maintain normoglycaemic blood levels [4]. The same situation seems to be true in humans as summarized in [5], hence indicating that pancreatic islet features could be used as early T2DM markers.

Motivation: New targets for T2DM prediction, prevention, and treatment generated by the available in vitro and in vivo animal models need to be quantitatively analyzed by high-throughput screening and later verified in human tissue. Therefore a computational pathology approach is necessary to be adopted. The aim of an automated analysis pipeline is first the detection of cell nuclei and second the segmentation of human pancreatic islets based on specific staining for α and β-cells. The robust segmentation of islets is the basis for further quantification of biomarkers regarding T2DM in human patients. Having correctly isolated the islets, it is possible to extract features (e.g. area of the islet) and test their ability to differentiate early T2DM patients and control cases.

Automated analysis of fluorescence images of human tissue poses two main difficulties which are going to be addressed in this work. (i) The 3D structure of the tissue leads to the problem that cell nuclei are not always perfectly cut in their maximum dimension producing numerous cutting artifacts. It has to be noted that this does not happen in applications with cell cultures or on blood smears for which the large majority of image processing tools in this field is developed. This problem is addressed in the presented work by training a robust classifier for object detection in contrary to using morphological or watershed based approaches. (ii) Variations in the production process of the histological slices can lead to areas of different thickness within one section. This preprocessing artifact produces not only blurred regions in the image but also illumination variation which are even worsened by variations in the fluorescent staining process. These problems are tackled by first using illumination invariant features for the classifier, second by employing clustering for the α and β-cell classification and third by facilitating a graph-based approach for the islet detection.

Tissue Preparation and Imaging: Human pancreatic tissue from either autopsies or biopsies were formalin fixed and paraffin embedded. Sections were cut at a thickness of 2 μm and stored at 4° Celsius till use.

For immunofluorescence, sections were deparaffinized and stained with antibodies specific for α and β-cells. Furthermore DAPI staining (DAKO, Carpenteria, CA) was used to label the cell nuclei. Fluorescence pictures were taken with a resolution of $1376 \times 1032 \times 3$ pixels and 20x magnification. Raw unedited material was used in the analysis (Figure 1).

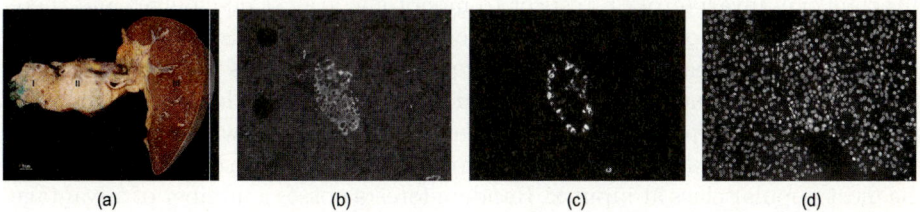

Fig. 1. Human pancreatic tissue: Primary tissue is taken from either whole pancreas from autopsies (I: normal pancreas, II: adenocarcinoma, III: spleen)(a) or biopsy resectates. Sections from fixed and embedded tissue blocks are stained with specific antibodies for β-cells (b), α-cells (c) and DAPI (d). Pictures b-d were taken with a magnification of 20x.

Problem Formulation: From a computational viewpoint the input to the pipeline consists of three fluorescence images: (i) DAPI-Channel $\rightarrow I_D$ (staining specific for cell nuclei detection), (ii) Alpha-Channel $\rightarrow I_\alpha$ (staining specific for α-cells) and (iii) Beta-Channel $\rightarrow I_\beta$ (staining specific for β-cells).

The output of the algorithm is the segmented area that the pancreatic islet of interest occupies. Prior information from expert pathologists is incorporated in order to guide the search for a meaningful extraction of the islet area. The domain knowledge can be summarized in two main hypotheses:

$\mathcal{H}_1$: *The islets are defined as an area with high density of α and β-cells*, with the α-cells being more specific in specifying the islet area.

$\mathcal{H}_2$: *There is only one islet of interest per image.* In most of the images additional structures are observed, such as smaller islets, disrupted islets or outliers due to staining failures. The main goal is to extract only the dominant islet in each image while excluding artefacts.

The distinct steps of the computational pathology pipeline are described in detail in Section 2.

2 Methods

(2.1) Cell Nuclei Detection: Cell nuclei on DAPI stained images, I_D, are detected by following the approach in [6] which showed excellent results on histopathological tissue with immunohistochemical staining. To generate a set of positive and negative training patches of size 65×65, a domain expert labeled two images from different patients. In addition to the selected cell nuclei their rotated and flipped counterparts were added to the positive training set. The negative class was down sampled to have a balanced training set. In total 1214 positive and 1214 negative samples were used for training.

For each of these samples a feature vector of length 281 was generated consisting of local binary patterns (LBP) [7] and a histogram of gray scale values. A great advantage of LBPs for this application is that they are illumination invariant, i.e. invariant with respect to monotonic gray scale-changes and therefore no gray-scale normalization or histogram equalization is needed.

Based on these features a random forests classifier [8] was learned to differentiate between cell nuclei and background. A random forest classifier consists of a collection of tree-structured classifiers $\{h(\mathbf{x}, \Theta_k), k = 1, \ldots\}$ where $\{\Theta_k\}$ are independent identically distributed random vectors and each tree casts a unit vote for the most popular class at input $\mathbf{x}$. Random forests posses a number of advantages over classical boosting approaches to object detection as described in [8] and [6]. One of them is the internal out of bag (OOB) error which provides an unbiased estimate of the generalization error. For this application it is shown (supplement Figure 1) that the classifier converges to an OOB error of about 3% after 25 trees.

Finally, to detect the nuclei we classified each pixel of the DAPI test images to generate an accumulator map with a probability at each pixel for being a cell nucleus or not. After non maxima suppression the detections within a range of 20 pixels were clustered to one final hit which is approximately the size of an average nucleus. The output of this step consists of a list of the coordinates of all detected cell-nuclei, $\mathbf{x_i} \in \mathbf{R}^2$, $i = 1, \ldots, N$.

(2.2) Cell Nuclei Classification: The two channels accounting for the staining of α and β cells, I_α and I_β respectively, are segmented into background and staining using k-means clustering (with k = 2 classes) on the intensity histograms. In order to classify each detected nucleus from step (2.1), a neighborhood of 10×10 pixels at the nucleus center is considered. The nucleus is classified based on a majority voting scheme of the segmented binary pixels in the patch of each channel I_α, I_β. If there is strong evidence provided from the segmented staining of channel I_α (I_β) then the nucleus is classified as α-cell (β-cell), otherwise we characterize it as "normal" cell. Thus, tuples of coordinates plus labels for all detected cells of the previous step are obtained : $(\mathbf{x_i}, y_i)$, $y_i = \{\alpha, \beta, n\}$ This approach mimics the workflow of the pathologists by first detecting all cell nuclei and then classifying them to their respective classes based on the intensity of the class-specific staining around each nuclei.

(2.3) Graph Construction: Based on the main hypothesis $\mathcal{H}_1$, a neighborhood graph on the identified α and β-cells is constructed, in such a way that clusters of cells correspond to connected components of the graph. Regions of the image with high cell density will be represented by a unique connected component in the graph. This construction is motivated in [9], where theoretical aspects of clustering with nearest-neighbor (NN) graphs are explored. In general this task can be solved either by constructing a knn graph or an ϵ-neighborhood graph. Empirical results showed that for this specific task of islet detection, the latter graph performed better, mainly because $\epsilon \in \mathbf{R}^+$ allows for more flexible structures.

Hence, given the set V of α and β-cells detected in the previous steps the ϵ-neighborhood graph $G = G_{eps}(V, \epsilon)$ is constructed, such that two nodes $\mathbf{x_i}, \mathbf{x_j}$ are connected with an edge iff $||\mathbf{x_i} - \mathbf{x_j}||_2 \leq \epsilon$. The euclidean distance is an intuitive choice for this problem setting, because it captures the local structure of cell proximities in the images.

(2.4) Islet Selection and Segmentation: Given the constructed graph G_{eps}, clusters of α and β-cells are identified by isolating the connected components of the graph. Under the hypotheses $\mathcal{H}_1$ and $\mathcal{H}_2$, the largest cluster corresponds to the islet of interest. Therefore the largest connected component G^{islet} of graph G is extracted, as a first crude approximation of the islet area. This first approximation depends on the parameter ϵ of the graph construction, and can be viewed as the computational equivalent of an expert focusing in the densely stained regions of the image trying to get a first impression of the islet location. Furthermore, it acts on the nuclei level and not on the staining intensities, thus resulting in higher robustness.

Based on the crude estimation of the islet boundaries, an active contour scheme is employed, in order to refine the detected islet area. The basic idea in active contours, [10], is to evolve a curve, subject to constraints based on the given image, in order to detect objects in the image. In the proposed pipeline, we apply the model described in [11], which does not use an edge-detector to stop the evolving curve in the boundary, hence does not depend on the gradient of the image. Furthermore it is shown to be quite effective under the presence of noise and does not require any preprocessing (e.g. smoothing) of the initial image [11]. As motivated above, we initialize the curve on the convex hull of G^{islet} and apply it on the superposition of the two stained channels $I_\alpha + I_\beta$ in order to refine the boundary of the islet. The active contour model used, is governed by two parameters, (s, r), with $s \in \mathbf{R}^+$ controlling the smoothness of the active contour and $r \in \mathbf{N}$ the number of iterations. The proposed initialization of the active contour is beneficial in two ways: (i) Active contours schemes are known to be sensitive in the curve initialization. A meaningful initialization is provided, tailored to the specific problem and (ii) starting close to the islet boundary also reduces the computation time needed.

The algorithm outputs a binary mask, I^{seg}_{islet} (of the same size as the input channels), which corresponds to the detected area of the human islet. The whole pipeline is governed by a tuple of parameters $\theta = (\epsilon, s, r)$. Based on this segmentation it is possible to automatically extract all biologically meaningful features that can be used as predictive markers for early T2DM, e.g. islet area, staining intensities, fractions of α and β-cells in the islet. Furthermore, the automatically extracted segmentation results are compared with manually segmented islets from expert pathologists in order to assess the algorithm performance against an objective ground truth.

Baseline method: According to our knowledge, there are no published approaches to the specific problem of pancreatic islet segmentation on histopathological tissue. The absence of a competing method was partially compensated by the construction of a baseline morphological approach which also exploits the prior knowledge on the islet segmentation, captured by hypotheses $\mathcal{H}_1$ and $\mathcal{H}_1$. The steps of the baseline method can be summarized as follows: (i) smooth the input staining $I_1 = I_\alpha + I_\beta$ using a gaussian filter, (ii) globally threshold I_1 to obtain a coarse segmentation, thus $I_2 = I_1 \geq t$, (iii) remove small holes by calculating the closing of $I_2 \rightarrow I_3$, (iv) extract the biggest contiguous region from I_3 and return this as the detected islet I_{islet}^{seg}. An alternative version has an extra step (v) where in addition an active contour is initialized with I_{islet}^{seg} as in step (2.5) of the proposed pipeline. Similarly to the proposed approach the main parameters form a tuple $\theta = (t, s, r)$.

Statistical Evaluation: Given the binary mask of the algorithmic segmentation (I_{islet}^{seg}) and the manually segmented islet from the expert pathologist (I_{islet}^{man}) the cell nuclei agreement between the two masks is calculated. For example, $TP = \#cells \in \{I_{islet}^{seg} \wedge I_{islet}^{man}\}$, $FP = \#cells \in \{I_{islet}^{seg} \wedge \neg I_{islet}^{man}\}$ etc. From the error counts we extract common evaluation metrics, such as Precision ($P = \frac{TP}{TP+FP}$), Recall ($R = \frac{TP}{TP+FN}$) and F-measure ($F = 2 \times \frac{P \times R}{P+R}$).

3 Results

The training set consists of 18 triplets of images (three stained channels) corresponding to two patients with T2DM and one control case. Four expert pathologists independently segmented the islet of interest for each of the images in the training set. For each one of the 18 training cases we calculated the consensus over the 4 experts, thus obtaining a consensus ground truth. This enables us to compare the performance of the algorithm against a "consensus" expert, but also to estimate the intra-pathologist labeling agreement.

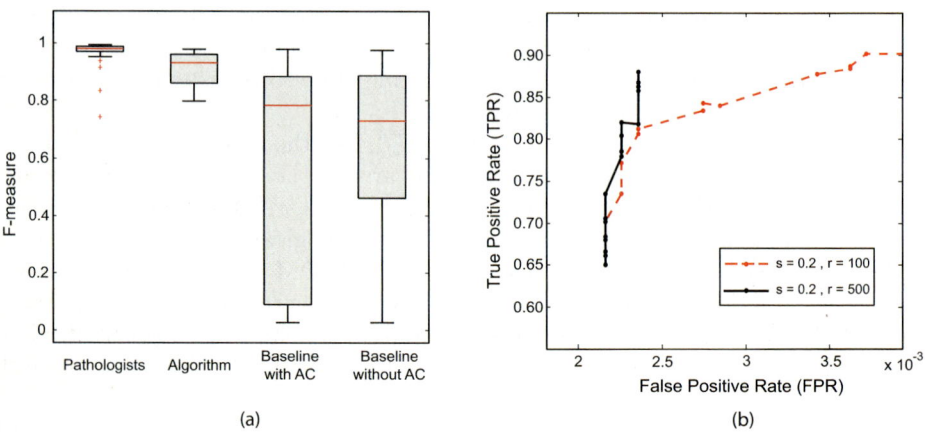

Fig. 2. (a) F-measure box plots (from left to right: pathologists, proposed algorithm, baseline with active contours (AC) and baseline without AC). The proposed pipeline performs comparably to the pathologists in terms of F-measure when compared to the expert consensus. Furthermore, the test error variance is low. Both baseline methods fail to achieve consistent segmentations as they perform well in some instances, but fail to segment properly a large number of cases in each cross validation fold. (b) ROC curves for parameter ϵ of the graph construction, keeping s fixed and equal to 0.2 and setting r equal to 100 (dashed line) and 500 iterations (continuous line).

A cross validation scheme was employed to compare the algorithmic approaches to the gold standard, i.e. the consensus of the pathologists. More specifically, a 3-fold cross validation is used, where in each fold the algorithm is trained on 12 cases (choosing the parameter values that minimize the error) and then the generalization performance is tested on the other 6 that are left aside as a validation set. For the pathologists, each one of them is compared against the consensus segmentations. It has to be noted that since the pathologists' segmentations are considered as the gold standard, the computational pathology approaches cannot perform better than the experts. The results are depicted in Figure 2(a).

Regarding the individual experts' annotations we observe that they are very close to the consensus ground truth (with an average F-measure of 0.97) and exhibit quite low variance. Such a high performance is expected since by construction the ground truth labels are computed by averaging the individual ones. The proposed algorithm performs comparably to the pathologists (with an average F-measure of 0.92 across folds) keeping also the variance in a reasonable range. On the other hand both baseline methods (with and without the active contour module) are outperformed by the graph-based segmentation in terms of the F-measure. Furthermore, we observe that the baseline segmentations exhibit high variance, which indicates also a tendency to generalize poorly to new data.

In Figure 2(b) a specific instance of a ROC curve is plotted to evaluate the performance of the proposed algorithm with respect to parameter ϵ which controls the graph construction and thus the initial key step of islet segmentation. More specifically parameter s, which controls the smoothness of the boundary, is kept fixed and for two values of parameter r, the number of iterations the active contour is updated ($r = 100, 500$), the true positive rate (TPR) is plotted against the false positive rate (FPR) over a wide range of parameter ϵ. At a first glance a complex behavior is observed for the large number of iterations in the active contour evolution ($r = 500$). For increasing values of ϵ, vertical ascents are observed in the plot where FPR stays the same and TPR increases. Furthermore, for some sequential increases of ϵ the FPR increases while TPR decreases, a behavior which is not usually observed in ROC curves. Both phenomena can be explained if we keep in mind that parameter ϵ does not directly affect the final segmentation, since the active contour based boundary refinement is applied in between. Increasing ϵ adds more nodes to the graph, thus increasing the initialization area. However if the active contour algorithm performs an adequate number of iterations it will dominate and converge to the islet, hence filtering out the false positive cells. A more balanced behavior is observed for a smaller number of iterations, where for increasing values of ϵ, in most of the times, both TPR and FPR are increased.

4 Conclusion

The computational pathology system presented in this work is able to, objectively and automatically, estimate the boundaries of human pancreatic islets.

The whole pipeline is transparent, modular and based on explicit hypotheses describing the domain knowledge. To the best of our knowledge this is the first framework that successfully tackles this specific segmentation problem. Cross validation results indicate that the algorithm performs competitively to human experts. Having a reliable pipeline to detect and isolate pancreatic islets from human histological tissue, enables researchers to test specific hypotheses regarding T2DM. We are convinced that the proposed framework can be the basis for further research regarding T2DM and that it can significantly assist the search for diagnostic and therapeutic markers.

Acknowledgments. This work has been partially supported by the Competence Center for Systems Physiology and Metabolic Diseases (CC-SPMD) of ETH Zurich.

References

1. Kasuga, M.: Insulin resistance and pancreatic beta cell failure. J. Clin. Invest. 116(7), 1756–1760 (2006)
2. Zimmet, P., Alberti, K.G., Shaw, J.: Global and societal implications of the diabetes epidemic. Nature 414(6865), 782–787 (2001)
3. Vijan, S., Stevens, D.L., Herman, W.H., Funnell, M.M., Standiford, C.J.: Screening, prevention, counseling, and treatment for the complications of type ii diabetes mellitus. Putting evidence into practice. J. Gen. Intern. Med. 12(9), 567–580 (1997)
4. Maedler, K., Schumann, D.M., Schulthess, F., Oberholzer, J., Bosco, D., Berney, T., Donath, M.Y.: Aging correlates with decreased beta-cell proliferative capacity and enhanced sensitivity to apoptosis: a potential role for fas and pancreatic duodenal homeobox-1. Diabetes 55(9), 2455–2462 (2006)
5. Bonner-Weir, S., O'Brien, T.D.: Islets in type 2 diabetes: in honor of dr. robert c. turner. Diabetes 57(11), 2899–2904 (2008)
6. Fuchs, T.J., Wild, P.J., Moch, H., Buhmann, J.M.: Computational pathology analysis of tissue microarrays predicts survival of renal clear cell carcinoma patients. In: Metaxas, D., Axel, L., Fichtinger, G., Székely, G. (eds.) MICCAI 2008, Part II. LNCS, vol. 5242, pp. 1–8. Springer, Heidelberg (2008)
7. Ahonen, T., Hadid, A., Pietikäinen, M.: Face recognition with local binary patterns. In: Pajdla, T., Matas, J(G.) (eds.) ECCV 2004. LNCS, vol. 3021, pp. 469–481. Springer, Heidelberg (2004)
8. Breiman, L.: Random forests. Machine Learning 45, 5–32 (2001)
9. Maier, M., Hein, M., von Luxburg, U.: Cluster identification in nearest-neighbor graphs. In: Hutter, M., Servedio, R.A., Takimoto, E. (eds.) ALT 2007. LNCS (LNAI), vol. 4754, pp. 196–210. Springer, Heidelberg (2007)
10. Kass, M., Witkin, A., Terzopoulos, D.: Snakes: Active contour models. International Journal of Computer Vision 1(4), 321–331 (1988)
11. Chan, T.F., Vese, L.A.: Active contours without edges. IEEE Transactions on Image Processing 10(2), 266–277 (2001)

Detection of Spatially Correlated Objects in $3D$ Images Using Appearance Models and Coupled Active Contours

Kishore Mosaliganti, Arnaud Gelas, Alexandre Gouaillard, Ramil Noche, Nikolaus Obholzer, and Sean Megason

Department of Systems Biology, Harvard Medical School, Boston, MA - 02115, USA
kishore@hms.harvard.edu

Abstract. We consider the problem of segmenting $3D$ images that contain a dense collection of spatially correlated objects, such as fluorescent labeled cells in tissue. Our approach involves an initial modeling phase followed by a data-fitting segmentation phase. In the first phase, cell shape (membrane bound) is modeled implicitly using a parametric distribution of correlation function estimates. The nucleus is modeled for its shape as well as image intensity distribution inspired from the physics of its image formation. In the second phase, we solve the segmentation problem using a variational level-set strategy with coupled active contours to minimize a novel energy functional. We demonstrate the utility of our approach on multispectral fluorescence microscopy images.

1 Introduction

Researchers in embryogenesis and cancer rely on automated segmentation of cells to understand the complex processes of tissue morphogenesis. Cell segmentation involves uniquely identifying fluorescent marked cells and organelles, such as nuclei, that are spatially correlated but whose position, number, and geometry must be determined [1]. The problem is complicated by individual variations in intensity, geometry, relative orientation and overlapping boundaries (Fig. 1).

A new aspect of the segmentation problem relates to fusing information of related structures present in multiple imaging channels. Current microscopes support high resolution imaging of as many as 32 separate channels containing information on uniquely tagged organelles. High throughput time-lapse imaging coupled with image analysis is now viewed as a tool to understand embryonic development by tracking every single cell to its ultimate fate. Therefore, segmentation tools must also be generic tracking solutions, possibly in a real-time environment coupled to the imaging.

The presence of millions of cells in dynamic imagery calls for the usage of models to drive the segmentation process. The models may be biologically inspired (packing, spatial distributions, mixing fractions, *etc.*), geometrical (shape, size, symmetry), or based on the physics of image formation (point spread function of the optics) [1]. Volumetric representations of objects, such as active contours, provide a natural mechanism to integrate multiple models elegantly into a segmentation exercise [2,3].

In this paper, we develop a novel fitting energy functional based on our proposed geometric and image formation models. By representing a cell as a pair (membrane +

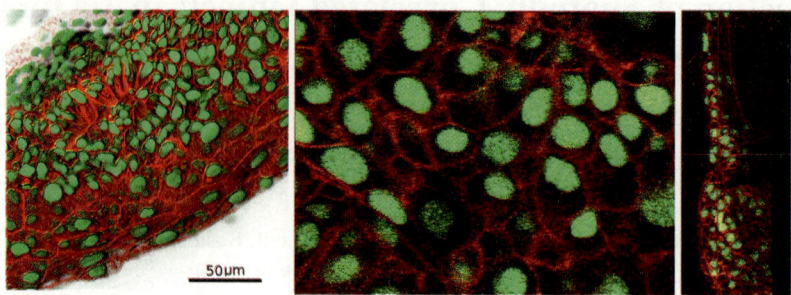

Fig. 1. Left: A 3D view of the zebrafish hind-brain showing a dense collection of cells. The cell membranes are marked in red, and nuclei are in green colors. Middle: A zoomed $x-y$ image plane showing arrangement details of nuclei within membranes. Right: An $x-z$ section showing poor structural resolution of the membranes along the z-axis.

nucleus) of active contours, we invoke the variational level-set methodology to obtain segmentations. We also employ spatial data structures to scale our methods to large datasets of the zebrafish embryogenesis process containing millions of cells. For the rest of this paper, we describe the proposed theory simultaneously with appropriate related work for the sake of clarity.

2 Theory and Computational Models

For notational convenience, let $I_m : \Omega \to [0, 255]$ and $I_n : \Omega \to [0, 255]$ denote the observed membrane and nuclear images. We assume that there are M observed cells (membrane bound with nucleus). For a cell i, the membrane is defined on $\psi_i \subset \Omega$ and the nucleus is defined on $\phi_i \subseteq \psi_i$. The background in I_m and I_n are defined as $\psi_{out} = \Omega - \bigcup_{i=1}^{M} \psi_i$ and $\phi_{out} = \Omega - \bigcup_{i=1}^{M} \phi_i$ respectively. Finally, let $\mathcal{N}_{\mu,\Sigma}$ denote a Gaussian distribution with mean μ and standard deviation Σ.

Brief Overview: The membrane intensity volume is sampled with 2-point correlation functions to produce a "correlation" image (Sec. 2.1). This correlation image is modeled as mixture of 3D spatial Gaussian functions. Additionally, the nucleus is modeled for its geometric shape as well as its intensity profile. The nucleus is given by a Gaussian shape function with constant intensity distribution within. An energy function is set up to fit the observed image data to these models, and its minimization leads to optimal settings of model parameters.

2.1 Appearance Models

Correlation Functions for cell shape: Membrane data is generated by tagging a fluorescent marker to point samples on cell surfaces. During imaging, the point spread function marks the membranes as thin, wispy foam structures. The data inherently has a poor SNR, creates bias fields in dense locations, and contains missing foam segments. Poor optical slicing resolution along the z-axis creates discontinuities in the structure

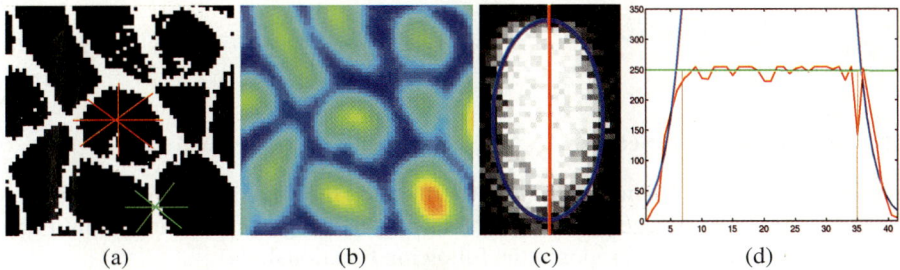

Fig. 2. (a) A thresholded image of the cell membrane showing the pcf sampling at a cell center (red) and on the periphery (green) of a cell. (b) The corresponding 2-pcf feature image is shown in the presence of binarization noise. (c) A typical nucleus with oblong shape (blue). (d) Plots of the intensity profile along a *1D* cross-section are shown with a constant intensity and Gaussian function fits indicated in green and blue, respectively.

thereby preventing the usage of explicit geometric models to fit intensity data. A more viable option is to implicitly model the 2-point correlation function (2-pcf) of the membrane volume [4]. Note that the membrane structure is located in the catchment basin of the 2-pcf image whose estimation is first described. Assume the presence of two materials in the image I_m, say, *0* (background) and *1* (membranes) as shown in Fig. 2(a). Any line segment when placed in the image has its end-points located in four different configurations, namely $\{(0,0), (0,1), (1,0), (1,1)\}$. The 2-pcf $P_{i,j}^k : \Omega \to [0,1]$ at any point $p \in \Omega$ measures the correlation of the end-points of a line segment of given length k with end-point in configuration (i,j). The following properties hold true: (i) $\sum_{i,j} P_{i,j}^k = 1$, (ii) $P_{01}^k = P_{10}^k$, (iii) $P_{00}^k + P_{01}^k = f_0$ and (iv) $P_{10}^k + P_{11}^k = f_1$, where parameters f_0 and f_1 represent the volume fractions of the individual phases. The 2-pcfs are computationally estimated by sampling the neighborhood of a point $x \in \Omega$ with randomly oriented line segments of constant length k and noting the frequencies of different configurations. We are interested in configurations where both end-points lie on the membrane, i.e. (1,1). In Fig. 2(b), the pcf $P_{1,1}^4$ is shown as an image. The value of k is chosen to be equal to the average diameter of cells (4 μm) in this specific case.

Cell model: Let C_i represent the ith cell with attributes of peak intensity a_i, location $\mu_i \in \Omega$, and its domain Σ_i. Assuming that 2-pcf values fit a mixture model of Gaussian cell functions, for $p \in \psi_i$ we write $C_i(p) = a_i \mathcal{N}_{\mu_i, \Sigma_i}(p)$ and 0 elsewhere.

Nucleus shape and distribution: The nucleus has a convex geometric shape containing a fluorescent marker tagged to DNA proteins (Fig. 2(c)). Ideally, the marker is uniformly distributed within. During imaging, the point spread function (PSF, say $\mathscr{P}$) of the instrument combines light sources from neighboring voxels to produce a blurred image that is computationally equivalent to a convolution operation $I * \mathscr{P}$. The nucleus boundaries have an intensity gradient while retaining a constant intensity profile well within (Figs. 2(c)-(d)).

Nucleus model: Suppose $g(.)$ is a thresholded image of the gradient magnitude image as given in Eq. 1. Let $N_i(p)$ denote the intensity profile of the ith nucleus given by the piecewise sum of a constant intensity region (c_i) with a Gaussian function at boundaries.

$$g(p) = \begin{cases} 1 & \text{if } |G_\sigma * I(p)| > \Gamma, \\ 0 & \text{else}. \end{cases} \quad N_i(p) = g(p) a_i \mathcal{N}_{\mu_i, \Sigma_i}(p) + (1 - g(p)) c_i \quad (1)$$

2.2 Variational Level Sets

Related Work: In [5], Mumford and Shah formulated the image segmentation problem as follows: given an image I, find a contour S which segments the image into non-overlapping regions. They proposed the following functional:

$$F^{MS}(u, S) = \int_\Omega (u - I)^2 dp + \int_{\Omega \setminus S} |\nabla u|^2 dp + \mu |S| \quad (2)$$

where S is a contour that segments the original image I and u is a piecewise smooth approximation of I. The first term computes the difference in intensities between u and I while the second term ensures the smoothness of u everywhere except on the contour S. The last term is a regularization for selectively obtaining smooth contours of S with a user-defined weight μ. In practice, it is difficult to minimize this functional since there are no bounds on shape/topology of the unknown contour S of lower dimension and the non-convexity of the functional. Later, Chan and Vese [2] proposed an energy that is a piece-wise constant (PC) approximation of their functional:

$$F^{CV}(S, c_1, c_2) = \lambda_1 \int_{\phi_{in}} |I - c_0|^2 dp + \lambda_2 \int_{\phi_{out}} |I - c_1|^2 dp + \mu |S| \quad (3)$$

where ϕ_{in}/ϕ_{out} are regions inside/outside of contour S, and c_0 and c_1 are two scalar constants that approximate the image intensities. The first two terms are often referred to as global binary fitting energy terms that seek to separate an image into two regions of constant image intensities. The last term is a regularization for selectively obtaining smooth contours. In an orthogonal development, Vese and Chan [6] extended their single level-set model to a multiphase model for segmenting multiple objects in images. This extension is applied in our work as well.

The piecewise smooth (PS) models such as [6] have overcome the difficulties of the PC models in the presence of smooth intensity variations. These models assume that the intensity function can be approximated by smooth functions inside and outside the contours and therefore, can correct intensity inhomogeneities [7]. These models do not capture spatial intensity distributions that characterize geometric image objects (for e.g. biological cells), which is of our interest.

Proposed active contour models: Based on our appearance models in Secs. 2.1 and 2.2, we define the following energy functions:

$$\begin{aligned} \mathscr{F}_m(S, \alpha_m, \mu_m, \Sigma_m) &= \lambda_{1,m} \sum_{i=1}^M \int_{\psi_i} |C_i - P_{11}^k|^2 dp + \lambda_{2,m} \int_{\psi_{out}} |P|^2 dp + \mu_{1,m} |S| \\ \mathscr{F}_n(S, \alpha_n, \mu_n, \Sigma_n, c) &= \lambda_{1,m} \sum_{i=1}^M \int_{\phi_i} |N_i - I_n|^2 dp + \lambda_{2,m} \int_{\phi_{out}} |I_n|^2 dp + \mu_{2,m} |S| \end{aligned} \quad (4)$$

where λ's, and μ's are positive user-defined weights and $(\alpha_\mathbf{m}, \mu_m, \Sigma_m, c)$ are vectors of model parameters for each cell/nuclei. In both equations, the first term is a summation across all cells that measures the fit of the model to observed data inside the contour. The second term fits the observed background to 0 outside the contours. *Note*: The rest of the analysis will neglect λ's, and μ's ($= 1$) and consider the case when $M = 1$.

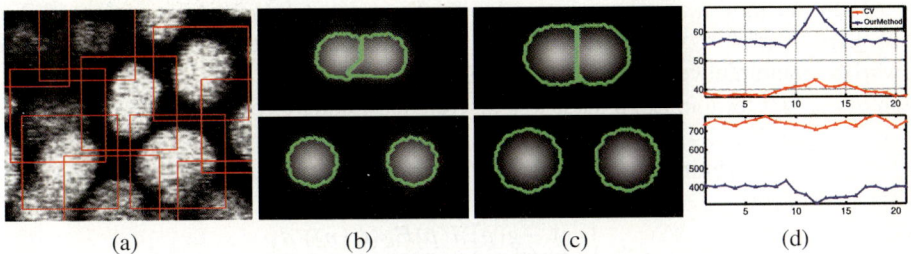

Fig. 3. (a) Rectangular regions of 2× cell diameter placed around cells to optimize calculations and limit memory usage. (b) Gaussian blob tracking using the CV method. (c) Gaussian blob tracking using the proposed method. (d) Comparisons of mean intensities (top) and observed blob sizes (bottom) across 21 time-points. Changes observed in CV method (blue) as compared to our method (red) during collision.

In level-set methods, a contour $S \subset \Omega$ is represented by the zero level-set of a Lipschitz function $\phi : \Omega \to \Re$. Using level-sets and Eq. 1, the above energy functionals are expanded as:

$$\mathscr{F}_m(\phi_m, \alpha_m, \mu_m, \Sigma_m) = \int_\Omega |\alpha_m \mathscr{N}_{\mu_m, \Sigma_m} - P_{11}^k|^2 H(\phi_m) dp + \int_\Omega |P|^2 \tilde{H}(\phi_m) dp$$
$$+ \int_\Omega \delta(\phi_m) |\nabla \phi_m| dp + O(\phi_m, \phi_n) \quad (5)$$

$$\mathscr{F}_n(\phi_n, \alpha_n, \mu_n, \Sigma_n, c) = \int_\Omega g|\alpha_n \mathscr{N}_{\mu_n, \Sigma_n} - I_n|^2 H(\phi_n) dp + \int_\Omega (1-g)|c - I_n|^2 H(\phi_n) dp$$
$$+ \int_\Omega |I_n|^2 \tilde{H}(\phi_n) dp + \int_\Omega \delta(\phi_n) |\nabla \phi_n| dp + O(\phi_m, \phi_n) \quad (6)$$

where H is the Heaviside function, and $\tilde{H}(.) = 1 - H(.)$. In order to encourage the nucleus (ϕ_n) to remain coupled within the membrane (ϕ_m), we add the *overlap term* $O(\phi_m, \phi_n) = v \int_\Omega H(\phi_n) \tilde{H}(\phi_m) dp$ to both energies. Note that when the nucleus is fully within the membrane, this term vanishes and is maximized when it does not overlap. We gain considerable synergy by fusing two separate image channels. In order to ensure the stable evolution of the level-set functions in both energy functions, we add the distance regularizing term to penalize its deviation from a signed distance function by Li *et al.* [8]. The deviation is characterized by the following integral $D(\phi) = \int_\Omega \frac{1}{2}(|\nabla \phi(p)| - 1)^2$. Since Eq. 5 is a particular case of Eq. 6 when $g(.) = 0$, we discuss the latter solution alone. This is a novel feature of our method in that it applies uniformly to both nuclei as well as membrane segmentation.

$$H_\varepsilon(x) = \frac{1}{2}\left(1 + \frac{2}{\pi} arctan(\frac{x}{\varepsilon})\right) \qquad \delta_\varepsilon(x) = \frac{1}{\pi} \frac{\varepsilon}{\varepsilon^2 + x^2} \qquad \frac{\partial \phi}{\partial t} = -\frac{\partial \mathscr{F}}{\partial \phi} \quad (7)$$

As in [2], the Heaviside and Delta functions in Eqs. 5-6 are approximated as in Eq. 7. The minimization of energy is done by a Maximum Expectation procedure. For fixed parameters (α, μ, Σ, c), we first solve the level-set evolution equation as the gradient descent equation where $\frac{\partial \mathscr{F}}{\partial \phi}$ is the the first order functional derivative of the energy

$\mathscr{F}$. Then the minimizing parameters (α, μ, Σ, c) are determined for a given ϕ. Let $\alpha N_{\mu,\Sigma}(p) = e^{m \cdot u'(p)}$ where $p = (x,y,z)$, m is the coefficient vector, and $u(p)$ is the trivariate monomial vector of order 2, i.e. $u(p) = \{x^i y^j z^k;\ i+j+k \leqslant 2\}$. The minimization of the first term in Eq. 6 leads to a discrete least-squares problem:

$$m^\star = \arg\min_{m} \sum_{p \in \Omega_{in}} g(p) \left(\ln(I(p)) - m \cdot u^t(p)\right)^2 = \left(M^t \cdot M\right)^{-1} \cdot M^t \cdot y \qquad (8)$$

$$c = \frac{\int_\Omega (1 - g(p)) I(p) H_\varepsilon(\phi(p))\ dp}{\int_\Omega (1 - g(p)) H_\varepsilon(\phi(p))\ dp} \qquad (9)$$

where M is a matrix of size $10 \times n$ with $M_{ij} = u_i(p_j)$ (n is the number of pixels in set $\{p \in \Omega_{in} | g(p) \neq 0\}$); y is a vector of size n with $y_i = \ln(I(p_i))$. At each iteration in the level-set evolution, we solve a linear system via a Singular Value Decomposition to compute the coefficients $m^\star$. The constant intensity minimizer c is determined as a weighted average of pixel intensities as in Eq. 9. The multiphase case ($M > 1$) is solved as in [3] where each nucleus/cell is represented by a unique level-set function.

3 Results and Discussion

The proposed method for detecting deformable correlated objects in 3D multichannel intensity images was quantitatively assessed with both synthetic and real fluorescence microscopy data. In all our experiments, for the sake of objectivity, we set $\lambda_i = 1$, $\mu_i = 100$, $\Gamma = 45$, and $\sigma = 3$ uniformly across all cells. Our goals are three-fold:

(1) Effectiveness of models: We show superior segmentation accuracies compared to the multiphase Chan-Vese (CV) algorithm [2,6] that is devoid of any underlying models. This shows that our models effectively represent underlying structures. First, we track a pair of isotropic Gaussian blobs ($\alpha = 100$, $\Sigma = 10$ pixel units) over 21 time-points as they collide (center separation of 15 pixel units at $t = 11$) and move apart. We show two time-points when they are closest and farthest apart for the CV and our method (Figs. 3(b) and (c)). The CV algorithm segments cells until the closest point where the cell contours do not represent the object shape truly. Our method recognizes the underlying Gaussian distribution and effectively fits the parameters even during close contact. Note that the CV algorithm neglects the Gaussian tails. In Fig. 3(c), we show plots of the mean intensity and sizes of the objects across time-points. Our algorithm (in blue) respects the underlying Gaussian distribution and shape and hence maintains a consistent size (larger) and mean (lower) across all time-points. Fig. 4(a) shows a 2D cellular microstructure constructed by modeling membranes using weighted Voronoi diagrams [9]. The nucleus model consists of randomly oriented and normally varying elliptic shapes and intensities (150 ± 75). The images ($500 \times 500 \times 100$) are convolved with an experimentally determined PSF ($0.15\mu m \times 0.15\mu m \times 0.75\mu m$) and degraded with Poisson ($\mu = p_i$) and Gaussian noise ($0, p_i$) where p_i is the pixel intensity. The CV method responds to absolute intensity values alone and spreads to neighboring cell regions leading to their shrinkage (Fig. 4(b)). In Fig. 5, we tabulate the Dice metric computed on nuclei and membrane segmentations separately for five phantom images (ground-truth) with

Detection of Spatially Correlated Objects in 3D Images   647

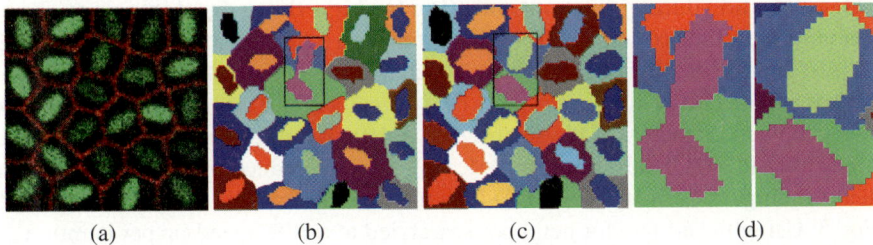

Fig. 4. (a) Phantom cell constructed from foam models, our proposed nucleus model and noise. (b) CV segmentation with enlarged cell boundaries. (c) Segmentation with the proposed method respects underlying intensity and shape distributions. (d) An instance of coupling benefits.

their with increasing noise levels. We apply $\{0.5, 0.75, 1, 1.5, 2\}$ multiplicative factors to p_i for setting the mean and variance in our noise models. The Dice metric on two segmentations A and B measures the ratio of their intersection $(A \cap B)$ to their union $(A \cup B)$. The result of our method is shown in Fig. 4(c).

Fig. 5 shows the output of our algorithm on zebrafish spinal cells (Fig. 2(a)). These datasets have pixel dimensions of $1024 \times 1024 \times 100$, pixel spacings of $0.2 \times 0.2 \times 1 \mu m^3$, file-size of $143MB$, and contain 7896 detected cells. The algorithm took 63 minutes to execute, excluding the pcf calculations for the membrane channel. We devised a novel way to validate our result using special staining protocols. While the entire membrane channel was fluorescent tagged, only a few random nuclei (48) were selectively tagged. This allowed us to segment cells using the membrane channel, and the nuclei were estimated by setting the nucleo-cytoplasmic ratio to 0.7. In the spinal cells, cells are mostly spherical with a centric-nucleus. The estimated nuclei were compared with the scattered nuclei by an expert on the basis of correspondence (42 matches), total number of cells found, visual inspection, and the volume distributions (not shown) observed. The incorrect matches resulted from boundary cells with partial/broken membranes and over-segmented large cells.

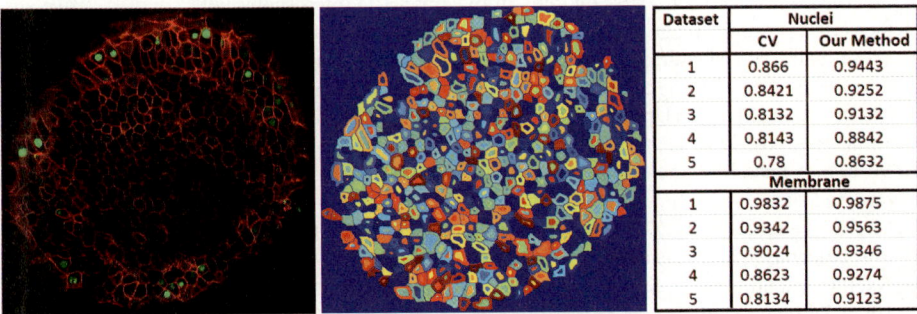

Dataset	Nuclei	
	CV	Our Method
1	0.866	0.9443
2	0.8421	0.9252
3	0.8132	0.9132
4	0.8143	0.8842
5	0.78	0.8632
	Membrane	
1	0.9832	0.9875
2	0.9342	0.9563
3	0.9024	0.9346
4	0.8623	0.9274
5	0.8134	0.9123

Fig. 5. Left: A 2D optical slice of zebrafish spinal cells with membranes and a few random nuclei. Middle: Segmentation of the membranes with estimated nuclei. Right: Dice metric computed on five phantom datasets for the nuclei and membrane segmentations separately.

(2) Memory and running time optimization for high-throughput imaging: The per iteration running time ($O(M^2|\Omega|)$) is a linear function of the number of cells (M), image size ($|\Omega|$) and the number of neighbors to each cell (potentially M). Two level-sets per cell were evolved on Ω limiting it to $\sim 10-25$ cells in our real datasets. Using ROIs of twice the cell diameter (of physical size $S = 4\mu m$ radius as shown in Fig. 3(a)) and kd-trees to hold ROI centroid locations leads to drastic reductions in peak memory as well as running time ($O(M|S|\log(M))$). The method was scalable to 7896 detected cells in Fig. 5. Using the kd-tree for neighbor search led to a 38% speed-up per iteration.

(3) Synergy by coupling: In multichannel data, the coupling mechanism leads to better segmentations in the presence of noise. In Fig. 4(d), we show a single zoomed instance where superior segmentations result from using the membrane as well as the nucleus.

4 Summary

In this work, we formulated models that are convenient and intuitive for the practitioner, namely the existence of a spatial intensity distribution correlated with shape and combined them with cell morphology. We have presented a computationally optimized framework for cell segmentation using variational active contours. A unique feature of our method is the synergistic coupling of nuclear and membrane segmentation problems into a single formulation. We successfully segment $3D + t$ confocal data on zebrafish embryogenesis and provide comparisons with a well-known segmentation method.

References

1. Khairy, K., Reynaud, E., Stelzer, E.: Detection of deformable objects in 3D images using markov-chain monte carlo and spherical harmonics. In: Metaxas, D., Axel, L., Fichtinger, G., Székely, G. (eds.) MICCAI 2008, Part II. LNCS, vol. 5242, pp. 1075–1082. Springer, Heidelberg (2008)
2. Chan, T., Vese, L.: An active contour model without edges. In: Scale-Space Theories in Comp. Vision, pp. 141–151 (1999)
3. Dufour, A., Shinin, V., Tajbakhsh, S., Guillon-Aghion, N., Olivo-Marin, J., Zimmer, C.: Segmenting and tracking fluorescent cells in dynamic 3-D microscopy with coupled active surfaces. IEEE Trans. Image Process 14, 1396–1410 (2008)
4. Mosaliganti, K., Machiraju, R., Leone, G.: Tensor classification of N-point correlation function features for histology tissue segmentation. Medical Image Analysis 13(1) (2009)
5. Mumford, D., Shah, J.: Optimal approximations by piecewise smooth functions and associated variational problems. Comm. on Pure and App. Math. 42(5), 577–685 (1989)
6. Vese, L., Chan, T.: A multiphase level set framework for image segmentation using the mumford and shah model. Intl. Journal of Comp. Vision 50, 271–293 (2002)
7. Li, C., Huang, R., Ding, Z., Gatenby, C., Metaxas, D., Gore, J.: A variational level set approach to segmentation and bias correction of images with intensity inhomogeneity. In: Metaxas, D., Axel, L., Fichtinger, G., Székely, G. (eds.) MICCAI 2008, Part II. LNCS, vol. 5242, pp. 1083–1091. Springer, Heidelberg (2008)
8. Li, C., Xu, C., Gui, C., Fox, M.D.: Level set evolution without re-initialization: A new variational formulation. In: Comp. Vision and Pattern Recogn., pp. 430–436 (2005)
9. Redenbach, C.: Microstructure models for cellular materials. Computational Materials Science 44(4), 1397–1407 (2009)

Intra-retinal Layer Segmentation in Optical Coherence Tomography Using an Active Contour Approach

Azadeh Yazdanpanah[1], Ghassan Hamarneh[2], Benjamin Smith[2], and Marinko Sarunic[1]

[1] School of Engineering Science,
[2] Medical Image Analysis Lab, School of Computing Science,
Simon Fraser University, Canada
{aya18,hamarneh,brsmith,msarunic}@sfu.ca

Abstract. Optical coherence tomography (OCT) is a non-invasive, depth resolved imaging modality that has become a prominent ophthalmic diagnostic technique. We present an automatic segmentation algorithm to detect intra-retinal layers in OCT images acquired from rodent models of retinal degeneration. We adapt Chan–Vese's energy-minimizing active contours without edges for OCT images, which suffer from low contrast and are highly corrupted by noise. We adopt a multi-phase framework with a circular shape prior in order to model the boundaries of retinal layers and estimate the shape parameters using least squares. We use a contextual scheme to balance the weight of different terms in the energy functional. The results from various synthetic experiments and segmentation results on 20 OCT images from four rats are presented, demonstrating the strength of our method to detect the desired retinal layers with sufficient accuracy and average Dice similarity coefficient of 0.85, specifically 0.94 for the the ganglion cell layer, which is the relevant layer for glaucoma diagnosis.

1 Introduction

Optical coherence tomography (OCT) is a novel non-invasive imaging modality which provides depth resolved structural information of a sample. The resolution in OCT systems approaches that of histology; the lateral resolution is typically 10-20μm and the axial resolution is typically $\sim$4μm [1].

OCT is a powerful tool for ophthalmic imaging and can be used to visualize the retinal cell layers to detect and monitor a variety of retinal diseases, including degeneration (thinning) of the retinal nerve cells layers due to glaucoma. OCT can be also adapted for imaging rodent eyes in order to complement medical research and gene therapy to combat retinal degeneration [2]. Fig. 1 shows a schematic of a rat's eye and a typical OCT depth profile of rodent retinal cell layers acquired *in vivo*. In this work, we developed an algorithm to automatically delineate the six retinal layers indicated in the figure in order to track glaucomatous degeneration.

Manual OCT segmentation is tedious, time-consuming, and suffers from inter- and intra-rater variability. Automated segmentation, on the other hand, holds the potential to reduce the time and effort required to delineate the retinal layers and also to provide repeatable, quantitative results. Several automated approaches have been employed in OCT segmentation [4,5]. They mostly rely on pixel-level, edge detection algorithms

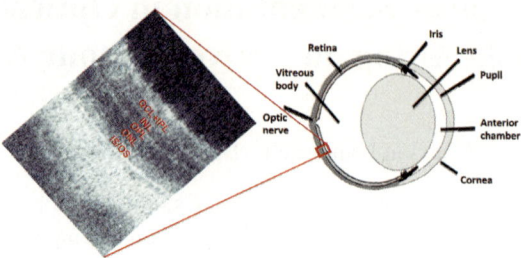

Fig. 1. A schematic anatomy of a rat's eye (right) is shown along with a typical OCT image (left) presenting a horizontal retinal cross-section with the labels indicating the retinal layers. The red box on the eye ball corresponds to the region which the image is taken from. The retina is divided into the inner and outer retina (IR and OR respectively). IR consists of the retinal nerve fiber layer, the inner ganglion cell layer (GCL), the inner plexiform layer (IPL), and the inner nuclear layer (INL). OR encompasses the outer plexiform layer (OPL), the outer nuclear layer (ONL), and the inner (IS) and outer (OS) segment photoreceptor layers [3].

such as the Canny-edge detector. Since OCT images are highly corrupted by speckle noise, some pre-processing steps are usually performed to reduce the effect of noise. The de-noising procedure, however, affects the sharpness of the edges which subsequently reduces the segmentation performance. Also, the conventional algorithms in OCT segmentation do not consider the intensity inhomogeneity in the image which can lead to inaccurate segments and inability to detect all layers. The predominant source of this artifact is the blood vessels on the topmost retinal layer which absorb light strongly, reducing the backscattered optical intensity of the underlying retinal tissue.

In this work, we propose a new method based on Chan–Vese active contour without edges [6] to address the segmentation of intra-retinal layers in OCT images. To the best of our knowledge, we are the first to segment OCT data using a multi-phase, level-set Mumford–Shah model that incorporates a shape prior based on expert anatomical knowledge of the retinal layers, avoiding the need for training. Our approach has four main features. First, it can segment all intra-retinal layers due to the multi-phase property of the algorithm. Second, we incorporate a shape prior term that enables the algorithm to accurately segment retinal layers, even where the region-based information is missing, such as in inhomogeneous regions. Third, our method is region-based and performs well on noisy OCT images. Finally, our algorithm is robust and avoids the re-initialization problem that is associated with the level set approach.

To achieve the needed accuracy and robustness for our application, we employ temporally and spatially adaptive (i.e. contextual) weights. We include concentric circles as a shape prior which mimic the true retinal layer structures and estimate the shape parameter using least squares. The methodology of our work is described in detail in Section 2. We apply the algorithm to 20 retinal OCT images acquired for both eyes of four rats. To evaluate the segmentation method, in Section 3, we measure the similarity between the automated segmentation with the ground truth manual segmentation using the Dice similarity coefficient (DSC). We conclude this paper in Section 4, with directions for future work to further automate our approach.

2 Methods

Our objective is to segment a given OCT image, $I : \Omega \longrightarrow \mathbb{R}$, defined on the image domain, into R disjoint sub-regions which accurately label the retinal layers. The decomposition of the image I, will be modeled using the level set framework as a set of $R-1$ signed distance functions (SDFs), ϕ. Further details of this representation are provided in Section 2.1. To determine a segmentation, we developed an automatic, variational algorithm, that minimizes the following specific energy functional:

$$E(\phi) = \lambda_I E_I(\phi) + \lambda_S E_S(\phi) + \lambda_R E_R(\phi) \qquad (1)$$

Each term of the energy functional captures a separate aspect of the problem. E_I, incorporates region-based information derived from the image. E_S incorporates the prior shape knowledge of the anatomy of retinal layers. E_R is a regularizing term which keeps region boundaries smooth and encourages each ϕ to be a SDF. Positive valued parameters, λ_I, λ_S, and λ_R, weight the different terms.

2.1 Region-Based Energy Term

The first term of equation (1) follows the work of Chan et al. [6] and encourages each region of the segmentation to have an approximately constant intensity. The intensity of the ith sub-region will be approximated by the constant μ_i, and the spatial extent will be represented by a characteristic function χ_i.

$$E_I = \sum_{i=1}^{R} \int_{\Omega} (I - \mu_i)^2 \chi_i \, dxdy \qquad (2)$$

By definition, each characteristic function takes the value 1 inside the region, and 0 outside. Following the approach of Mansouri et al. [7], each χ_i is represented using the level set method as a function of $R-1$ SDFs, ϕ. Simply, χ_i is the region inside the zero contour (zero level set) of the ith SDF, and outside all previous SDFs. The final region, χ_R is the region outside the zero contours of all SDFs. Using this partitioning, we guarantee unambiguous segmentation of R regions using $(R-1)$ SDFs. The characteristic function for the ith region is defined as follows, using the Heaviside step function, H, and delta function, δ [8]:

$$\chi_i = H(\phi_i)^{1-\delta(R-i)} \left[\prod_{k=1}^{i-1} (1 - H(\phi_k)) \right] \qquad (3)$$

2.2 Shape Prior Energy Term

OCT images may not always be piecewise constant. Intensity inhomogeneity may exist in regions due to the "shadows" of blood vessels on the topmost retinal layer. To compensate for these intensity inhomogeneities, we incorporated a shape prior term. Based on prior knowledge of retinal anatomy, a circular shape prior is used to model the retinal layer boundaries, and assists the algorithm when region-based information is insufficient to segment a layer accurately. In our model, each circular prior will share a common center point, but has a unique radius. The squared distance from a point, (x,y), to the shape prior constraining the ith boundary, can be defined as:

$$D_i(x,y) = [(x-c_x)^2 + (y-c_y)^2 - r_i^2]^2 \tag{4}$$

where (c_x, c_y) is the common center of the concentric layers, and r_i is the radius of the circular prior of the interface between the ith and the $(i+1)^{th}$ layer.

For each SDF ϕ_i, a shape constraint encourages the region boundary (the zero contour) to lie on a circle, minimizing the squared distance of the zero contour to the prior. Consequently, the shape term in the energy functional is:

$$E_S = \sum_{i=1}^{R-1} \int_\Omega D_i(x,y) \delta(\phi_i(x,y)) |\nabla \phi_i(x,y)| \, dxdy \tag{5}$$

The term, $\delta(\phi_i(x,y))|\nabla \phi_i(x,y)|$, selects out the zero contour of ϕ_i. This causes the shape term to have a non-zero value only on the region boundaries, and the term E_S is minimized when ϕ_i lies exactly on the circular shape.

The shape parameters, c_x, c_y and r_i for E_S are defined using a least square fit, with ϕ_i and μ_i held fixed. For this purpose, the parameter vector $\theta = [c_x \; c_y \; \tau_1 \; \tau_2 \; \cdots \; \tau_{R-1}]^T$ (where $\tau_i = r_i^2 - c_x^2 - c_y^2$) is estimated such that the error ε in $b = \Psi\theta + \varepsilon$ is minimized, where b and Ψ are determined by points (x,y) lying on $R-1$ boundaries.

2.3 Regularization Energy Term

Regularization terms were added to keep the boundary of the segmented layers smooth [6], and ϕ_i as a SDF. Smooth boundaries are encouraged by adding a contour length term, and ϕ_i can be kept close to a SDF by adding the penalty term of Chunming et al. [9]:

$$E_R = \sum_{i=1}^{R-1} \int_\Omega \delta(\phi_i(x,y))|\nabla \phi_i(x,y)| + \frac{1}{2}(|\nabla \phi_i(x,y)| - 1)^2 \, dxdy \tag{6}$$

2.4 Minimization of the Energy Functional

By substituting the energy terms defined by (2), (5), and (6) in (1), and re-arranging slightly, the minimization problem associated with our model is defined as:

$$\inf_{\mu_i, \phi_i} E = \int_\Omega \left\{ \lambda_I \sum_{i=1}^{R} [(I - \mu_i)^2 \chi_i] + \sum_{i=1}^{R-1} \left[A_i(x,y) \delta(\phi_i) |\nabla \phi_i| + \frac{1}{2}(|\nabla \phi_i| - 1)^2 \right] \right\} dxdy \tag{7}$$

where $A_i(x,y) = \lambda_R + \lambda_S D_i(x,y)$.

To minimize this function, we followed the approach of Chan et al. [6] and performed an alternating minimization. First, we hold the SDFs fixed, and solve for the unknown intensities μ_i:

$$\mu_i = \frac{\int_\Omega I(x,y) \chi_i \, dxdy}{\int_\Omega \chi_i \, dxdy} \tag{8}$$

Next, holding the intensities fixed, we use the Euler–Lagrange equation with respect to ϕ_i, and parameterize the descent direction using an artificial time t:

$$\frac{\partial \phi_j}{\partial t} = -\lambda_I \sum_{i=1}^{R}(I-\mu_i)^2 \frac{\partial \chi_i}{\partial \phi_j} + \left[\nabla A_j \cdot \frac{\nabla \phi_j}{|\nabla \phi_j|} + A_j \operatorname{div}\left(\frac{\nabla \phi_j}{|\nabla \phi_j|}\right)\right]\delta(\phi_j) + \triangle \phi_j - \operatorname{div}\left(\frac{\nabla \phi_j}{|\nabla \phi_j|}\right) \quad (9)$$

where

$$\frac{\partial \chi_i}{\partial \phi_j} = \begin{cases} (-H(\phi_i))^{1-\delta(i-j)}\delta(\phi_j)\prod_{k=1}^{i-1}(1-H(\phi_k))^{1-\delta(k-j)} & i \neq R, j \leq i \\ -\delta(\phi_j)\prod_{k=1}^{i-1}(1-H(\phi_k))^{1-\delta(k-j)} & i = R, j \leq i \\ 0 & i \neq R, \forall j > i \end{cases} \quad (10)$$

Note that in practice, we must use regularized versions of H and δ to obtain a well–defined descent direction. The regularization of Chan et. al [6] was used:

$$H_\varepsilon(z) = \frac{1}{2}\left(1 + \frac{2}{\pi}\arctan\left(\frac{z}{\varepsilon}\right)\right), \quad \delta_\varepsilon(z) = \frac{1}{\pi}\frac{\varepsilon}{\varepsilon^2 + z^2} \quad (11)$$

2.5 An Adaptive Weighting of Energy Terms

Choosing "good" weights for energy terms in segmentation is an open problem, and finding the correct tradeoff that results in a desirable segmentation is usually treated empirically. In this work, we automatically adapt the weights both temporally and spatially, i.e. the weights change with iteration number and along the spatial dimensions. Intuitively, in early iterations, the region-based term should be more dominant, allowing the curve freedom to evolve toward the boundary of each layer. As the algorithm progresses, the shape term becomes more important to assist the algorithm when image information is insufficient to segment the image. Therefore, we define λ_I and λ_S in terms of the nth iteration as mentioned in [10]:

$$\lambda_I(n) = \lambda_I(1) - \frac{n(\lambda_I(1) - \lambda_I(N))}{N}, \quad \lambda_S(n) = \lambda_S(1) + \frac{\lambda_S(N) - \lambda_S(1)}{\cosh[8(\frac{n\pi}{N} - 1)]} \quad (12)$$

where N is the total number of iterations.

We also want the shape term to have a greater effect where intensity information is missing, as in the inhomogeneous regions. Therefore, contextual information must be utilized. By choosing the weight of the shape term proportional to the inverse of the image gradient magnitude, we employ a spatially adaptive λ_S in each iteration. As a result, the shape term has a higher weight than region-based term, for pixels on weak edges. This also has the beneficial effect that image pixels with higher gradient (strong edges) have a stronger influence when solving for shape prior parameters. More plainly, the least squares fitting of the shape prior parameters is weighted by image gradient.

3 Results

3.1 Data Acquisition

Images used in this study were acquired using a custom spectrometer based Fourier domain (FD)OCT system. The FDOCT system operated at a central wavelength of 826nm

and had an axial resolution of $\sim 4\mu m$ (in air). Non-invasive OCT imaging was performed on four wistar strain albino rats. One eye on each rat underwent an axotomy procedure (severing the optic nerve), the other eye was maintained as a control in order to monitor retinal degeneration. The axotomy procedure is an accelerated model of glaucoma and causes the retinal nerve fiber layer to thin as the ganglion cells die. Each eye was imaged four times over a period of two weeks using OCT. All animal imaging procedures were performed under protocols compliant to the Canadian Council on Animal Care with the approval of the University Animal Care Committee at SFU.

3.2 Validation

To qualitatively evaluate the performance of our approach, we compared the segmentation resulting from our method and from two other approaches, using the ground truth manual expert delineations on 20 OCT images. We refer to our method as the active contour without edge with shape constraint and contextual weights (ACWOE-SW). The two other approaches are the classical Chan–Vese's active contour (ACWOE) and the ACWOE with shape constraint only (ACWOE-S). For each method, the parameters were chosen to give the best results. Based on our experience, the initial and final values for λ_I and λ_S were set as follows: $\lambda_I(1) = 1$, $\lambda_I(N) = 0.5$, $\lambda_S(1) = 0$, and $\lambda_S(N) = 1$. λ_R was set to 0.1×255^2. For all layers, the initial curve was estimated based on three points selected close to the interface of each layer. The same initialization was used for the three methods in all our experiments. Maximum of $N = 100$ iterations were used which guaranteed convergence in all our experiments. Fig. 2 shows an example of the segmented results (red contours) for each method for a typical OCT retinal image along with the expert ground truth segmentation. As shown, ACWOE-SW detects all 6 interfaces between the retinal layer properly, revealing the performance of this model on the images with intensity inhomogeneity. Even very thin layers, such as INL and OPL, which are difficult to distinguish by eye, are segmented by the algorithm. In contrast, ACWOE failed to segment the IPL, INL, and OPL layers due to the intensity inhomogeneity and low contrast of the image. ACWOE-S shows better segmentation than ACWOE, but it still has poor performance in inhomogeneous regions.

To provide a quantitative evaluation of our approach, we measured the area similarity between the manual and automated segmentation using DSC $\in [0, 1]$; more accurate segmentations correspond to higher DSC values. The average and standard deviation of DSC for the different retinal layers for all images is summarized for our method

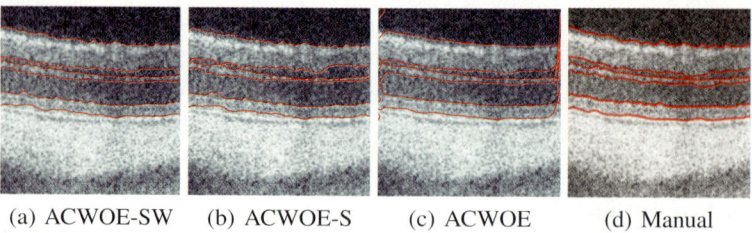

(a) ACWOE-SW   (b) ACWOE-S   (c) ACWOE   (d) Manual

Fig. 2. Segmentation results for an OCT retinal image

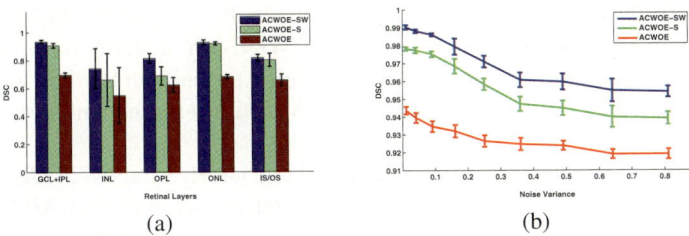

Fig. 3. (a) Segmentation results for different retinal layers. (b) DSC for different noise levels in the synthetic data; the image intensity is normalized to range from 0 to 1.

(ACWOE-SW) as: GCL+IPL (0.94 ± 0.012), INL (0.74 ± 0.143), OPL (0.82 ± 0.034), ONL (0.93 ± 0.018), and IS/OS (0.82 ± 0.023). Fig. 3(a) provides a quantitative comparison between the DSC of ACWOE-SW for the 20 images versus ACWOE-S, and ACWOE for different retinal layers. Our method is superior to the other approaches for all the examined layers.

3.3 Noise Tolerance

In order to evaluate the robustness of our algorithm to noise, controlled synthetic retinal OCT-like images were created with a known ground truth segmentation but corrupted with varying degrees of additive white Gaussian noise. As shown in Fig. 3(b), the DSC performance results reveal that adding a shape constraint to the energy functional makes the algorithm more accurate than standard ACWOE, while remaining robust in the presence of noise.

4 Discussion and Conclusion

We developed an automatic iterative algorithm to segment low contrast OCT images of rodent retinal layers. We used a multi-phase framework with a circular shape prior. We have demonstrated that our approach is able to accurately segment all of the intra-retinal layers, even given their small size and similar texture. Our approach also shows an improved performance in regions with intensity inhomogeneity due to the inclusion of shape prior constraint. We also introduced a contextual scheme to balance the weight of different terms in the energy functional which makes the algorithm even more robust when the image information is not sufficient to accurately detect layers. In addition, ACWOE-SW is more accurate in comparison with other active contours in the presence of noise. To demonstrate the robustness and performance of the algorithm, we applied it to both synthetic data and retina images from rats. The experimental results showed that we could classify the desired retinal layers. However, due to the various applications of OCT in diagnosis of retina diseases, we need a fully automatic segmentation algorithm which is more acceptable in clinical applications. Therefore, in future work, we will make the algorithm independent of the user by eliminating the dependency on the position of the initial curve by adopting convex functionals. We also need to apply our algorithm on a larger database from rats and assess the sensitivity of the algorithm with respect to the parameters and initial curve. Finally, we plan to expand our algorithm to human OCT images. Migrating our ACWOE-SW method to segment human retina images will require changing the shape prior to incorporate the foveal pit, but otherwise is anticipated to provide similarly high accuracy segmentation results.

Acknowledgments. The authors would like to thank Dr. H. Saragovi at McGill University for providing the axotomy rats. We also acknowledge support from MSFHR Career Investigator Award to MVS and grant support from NSERC/CIHR CHRP (MVS) and NSERC (GH).

References

1. Fercher, A.F., Drexler, W., Hitzenberger, C.K., Lasser, T.: Optical coherence tomography–principles and applications. Reports on progress in physics 66, 239–303 (2003)
2. Walsh, A., Sadda, S.R.: Optical coherence tomography in the diagnosis of retinal vascular disease. In: Retinal Vascular Disease, pp. 205–227. Springer, Heidelberg (2007)
3. Baroni, M., Diciotti, S., Evangelisti, A., Fortunato, P., Torre, A.L.: Texture classification of retinal layers in optical coherence tomography. In: 11th Mediterranean Conference on Medical and Biomedical Engineering and Computing, pp. 847–850 (2007)
4. Fernández, D.C., Salinas, H.M., Puliafito, C.A.: Automated detection of retinal layer structures on optical coherence tomography images. Opt. Express 13(25), 10200–10216 (2005)
5. Bagci, A.M., Shahidi, M., Ansari, R., Blair, M., Blair, N.P., Zelkha, R.: Thickness profiles of retinal layers by optical coherence tomography image segmentation. American Journal of Ophthalmology 146(5), 679–687 (2008)
6. Chan, T., Vese, L.: Active contours without edges. IEEE Trans. on Image Processing 10(2), 266–277 (2001)
7. Mansouri, A.R., Mitiche, A., Vázquez, C.: Multiregion competition: A level set extension of region competition to multiple region image partitioning. Computer Vision and Image Understanding 101(3), 137–150 (2006)
8. Smith, B., Saad, A., Hamarneh, G., Moeller, T.: Recovery of dynamic PET regions via simultaenous segmentation and deconvolution. In: MICCAI Workshop on Analysis of Functional Medical Image Data (MICCAI functional), pp. 33–40 (2008)
9. Li, C., Xu, C., Gui, C., Fox, M.: Level set evolution without re-initialization: a new variational formulation. In: IEEE Computer Society Conference on Computer Vision and Pattern Recognition (CVPR), pp. 430–436 (2005)
10. Pluempitiwiriyawej, C., Moura, J., Wu, Y.J.L., Ho, C.: STACS: new active contour scheme for cardiac MR image segmentation. IEEE Trans. on Medical Imaging 24(5), 593–603 (2005)

Mapping Tissue Optical Attenuation to Identify Cancer Using Optical Coherence Tomography

Robert A. McLaughlin[1], Loretta Scolaro[1], Peter Robbins[2], Christobel Saunders[3,4], Steven L. Jacques[5], and David D. Sampson[1]

[1] Optical+Biomedical Engineering Laboratory, Uni. Western Australia, WA, Australia
robertm@ee.uwa.edu.au
[2] PathWest QEII Medical Centre, WA, Australia
[3] Sir Charles Gairdner Hospital, WA, Australia
[4] School of Surgery, Uni. Western Australia, WA, Australia
[5] Biomedical Engineering/Dermatology, Oregon Health & Science University, OR, USA

Abstract. The lymphatic system is a common route for the spread of cancer and the identification of lymph node metastases is a key task during cancer surgery. This paper demonstrates the use of optical coherence tomography to construct parametric images of lymph nodes. It describes a method to automatically estimate the optical attenuation coefficient of tissue. By mapping the optical attenuation coefficient at each location in the scan, it is possible to construct a parametric image indicating variations in tissue type. The algorithm is applied to *ex vivo* samples of human axillary lymph nodes and validated against a histological gold standard. Results are shown illustrating the variation in optical properties between cancerous and healthy tissue.

1 Introduction

Cancer is the second most common cause of death worldwide, accounting for 12.5% of all mortality [1]. During cancer surgery, a critical task is to assess the spread (metastasis) of the cancer. The lymphatic system is a common route for metastasis. It is typically assessed by excising lymph nodes near the tumor and performing histo-pathological analysis. However, this results in the unnecessary excision of many healthy, uninvolved lymph nodes and can result in chronic disruption to the lymphatic system. For example, in breast cancer surgery, approximately 26% of patients undergoing local lymph node removal (axillary clearance) will suffer lymphedema.

Optical coherence tomography (OCT) [2] is a high-resolution imaging modality. It is conceptually similar to ultrasound, but uses reflections of low-power, near-infrared light instead of sound waves. It is capable of imaging tissue with a resolution of approximately 10 microns, and has the potential to assess lymph node involvement in cancer *in vivo* [3]. However, the signal values in an OCT data set are not determined absolutely by the tissue. They are also a function of many imaging and experimental parameters, including tissue depth, power and incident angle of the light source, imaging optics, and the effects of overlying tissue, including shadowing and refraction. For this reason, it is difficult to differentiate between image features due to the optical properties of a particular tissue type, and those due to imaging artifacts.

In this paper, we describe a method to differentiate tissues with differing optical properties in an OCT scan. Results are presented visually, as a parametric image in which intensity indicates the relative optical attenuation coefficient at a particular location. To the best of our knowledge, this is the first time that a parameterized OCT image has been generated in this manner. We present results from both phantom data, and cancerous and non-cancerous human lymph nodes.

2 Methods

2.1 Optical Properties of Tissue

OCT acquires images of tissue structure by detecting the coherence-gated backscattering of near infrared light. However, tissue is an optically turbid media and the signal attenuates and spreads with increasing depth, limiting the imaging depth of OCT to approximately 2-3mm. In OCT image formation, a focused light source is directed onto a particular location on the tissue and a depth scan is acquired in the z direction. Using terminology borrowed from ultrasound, this one-dimensional scan is referred to as an A-scan. A three-dimensional data volume is constructed by acquiring a sequence of A-scans at different x,y locations over the area to be scanned.

Attenuation of the OCT signal can be modeled using Beer's Law. The signal intensity $I(z)$ at a depth z can be expressed as follows [4]:

$$I(z) = I_0 e^{-\mu z} R(z) e^{-\mu z} = I_0 e^{-2\mu z} R(z) \qquad (1)$$

where I_0 is the incident intensity, $R(z)$ is the depth-dependent reflectivity, and μ is the observed attenuation coefficient of the tissue. The factor of 2 arises because the light must both travel into the tissue and return to the detector. The attenuation coefficient μ is affected by both scattering and absorption [5,6], parameterized by the scattering coefficient μ_s and absorption coefficient μ_a.

Scattering refers to the lossless redirection of light due to a local change in refractive index. For example, this may be due to interaction with structures such as cell membranes, collagen fibrils or cell nuclei [7]. The angular distribution of scattering may be modeled with a Henyey-Greenstein function, parameterized by an anisotropy factor g [8]. Let θ be the deviation in angle of light after a scattering event. Then g is defined as the expected value of $\cos\theta$. A value of $g \approx 1$ indicates forward scattering events in which light will continue in roughly the same direction. A value of $g \approx 0$ indicates an isotropic scattering function, where the angle of scatter is equally likely in all directions. Tissue is typically strongly forward scattering, with values of g in the range 0.85 to 0.97 [9].

The observed attenuation coefficient μ may be modeled by the following equation:

$$\mu = 2[a(g)\mu_s + \mu_a]G \qquad (2)$$

where:

$$a(g) = 1 - e^{\frac{(1-g)^m}{n}} \qquad (3)$$

with $m = 0.6651$ and $n = 0.1555$ [10]. The factor $a(g)$ modifies μ_s to represent the effectiveness of scatter in image formation and ranges from 1 at low g, to 0 at $g=1$. For $g = 0.97$, $a(g) \approx 0.46$ and μ_s is half as effective in preventing photons from reaching the coherence gate. For $g = 0.85$, $a(g) \approx 0.84$. For the 1325 nm central wavelength of light used in this report, the ratio of wavelength to scattering particle size in the tissue is greater than for visible or shorter near-infrared wavelengths. Hence, the value of g is likely to be about 0.4-0.6. Therefore, $a(g)$ is probably greater than 0.95. The factor G is the extra photon path length as photons are delivered obliquely toward a focus. With the low numerical aperture used in OCT this factor is approximately unity.

For near infrared light in tissue, scattering is the dominant attenuation mechanism [11], and the scattering coefficient μ_s is typically a factor of 10-100 times larger than the attenuation coefficient μ_a [12]. For the 1325 nm wavelength used in the experiments of this report, μ_a for pure water is 0.149 mm^{-1}. The value of μ_s for tissues at 1325 nm is in the 5-10 mm^{-1} range. Thus, the absorption can be neglected, and since $G \approx 1$, the equation for attenuation may be approximated by:

$$\mu \approx 2a(g)\mu_s \qquad (4)$$

Assuming that a single A-scan intersects only a single type of tissue, the attenuation parameter μ may be used to characterize a tissue. By taking the logarithm of the OCT signal values along a single A-scan, μ can be extracted from the slope of the line of best fit. We calculate this slope for each x,y location in the data set, deriving a 2D map $\mu(x,y)$. This μ is then represented visually as a 2D parametric image of the tissue in which the $\mu(x,y)$ is indicative of tissue type.

3 Experiment

Phantom and human *ex vivo* tissue samples were scanned with a swept-source OCT system (Thorlabs, New Jersey, USA) with a central wavelength of 1325nm and a spectral bandwidth of 100nm. The transverse resolution was 15µm and axial resolution was 12µm in air.

3.1 Phantom Experiment

Two imaging phantoms [13] were prepared to mimic the optical properties of tissue. Titanium oxide powder (Sigma Aldrich, St. Louis, USA), with an average particle size of 5µm, was mixed into a base material of room temperature vulcanizing (RTV) silicone (Wacker, Munich, Germany). Different quantities of titanium oxide were used to vary the optical properties of the phantoms, with the second phantom containing three times the concentration of the first. Both phantoms were scanned using OCT and the relative attenuation coefficient was estimated by finding the slope of the line of best fit to the log intensity values along an A-scan.

3.2 Human Tissue Experiment

Three human breast lymph nodes were taken from patients undergoing axillary clearance. Fresh excised lymph tissue was dissected into 2mm slices and a 3D-OCT scan of the fresh tissue was acquired. Each sample underwent subsequent histological analysis using Haematoxylin and Eosin (H&E) staining, and revealed the first node to be healthy, the second node to contain a well defined cluster of metastasis, and the third node to contain diffuse malignant cells intermingled throughout the tissue.

3.3 Tissue Image Pre-processing

During OCT scanning of the lymph node samples, the tissue was laid on a glass slide and immersed in a small quantity of glycerol to match the refractive index of the glass in order to reduce signals from the glass-air-tissue interfaces. However, tissue samples typically do not sit flat upon the glass slide, resulting in small glycerol-filled gaps between the tissue and glass. Unfortunately, this confounds the process of automatically estimating the attenuation coefficient. In order to characterize the tissue within an A-scan, it is necessary to identify where in the A-scan the light enters the tissue. Measurements prior to this position are not indicative of the tissue. The position within the A-scan will be dependent upon the size of any gap between the glass slide and the tissue. Identifying this position manually is impractical for a typical OCT acquisition comprising over a million A-scans.

Simple image processing techniques were utilized to automatically identify the point within each A-scan where the light entered the tissue. Note that each A-scan comprises a large peak of reflectivity early in the A-scan, corresponding to the change in refractive index as the light passes from air into the glass slide. This corresponds to a local maximum in the derivative of the intensity of the A-scan and was automatically identified for all A-scans in the acquisition, defining a set of points on the glass surface (plus a number of outliers). A 2D plane was robustly fitted to this point set and the intersection of the plane with each A-scan was taken as specifying the air-glass interface. Having extracted the location of the glass slide, the start of the tissue was found by averaging A-scan values within a moving window, and identifying the location at which the value exceeded a threshold. The attenuation co-efficient was then calculated by computing the slope of the line of the best fit for the log of the A-scan values, from the start of the tissue and extending over an optical path length of 0.5mm.

4 Results

Figure 1 shows representative A-scans from the two phantoms. The log of the reflectivity values are plotted against image depth. The line of best fit is superimposed upon each A-scan, and its slope is indicative of the concentration of titanium oxide powder. Note that signal attenuation is more gradual in the first phantom (Fig. 1, left) and markedly increased in the second (Fig. 1, right) with three times the concentration of titanium oxide. Fluctuations in the signals are characteristic of the speckle present in OCT, noted to be less in the phantom with a higher concentration of titanium oxide.

Figures 2-4 show parameterized OCT images of human lymph nodes with corresponding H&E histology. The intensity at each pixel in the parameterized OCT image is indicative of the attenuation coefficient for an A-scan that extends perpendicular to the image and into the sample, calculated over an optical path length of 0.5mm. Fig. 2

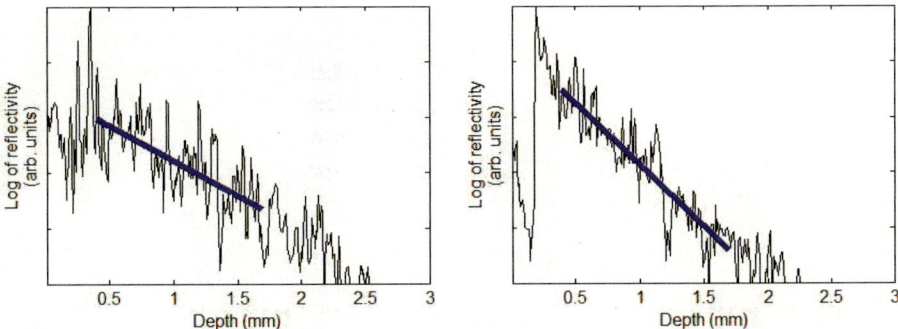

Fig. 1. A-scans from two phantom objects, with line of best fit showing attenuation due to scatter. Left: Phantom 1 (low concentration of TiO_2 in silicon). Right: Phantom 2 (high concentration of TiO_2 in silicon).

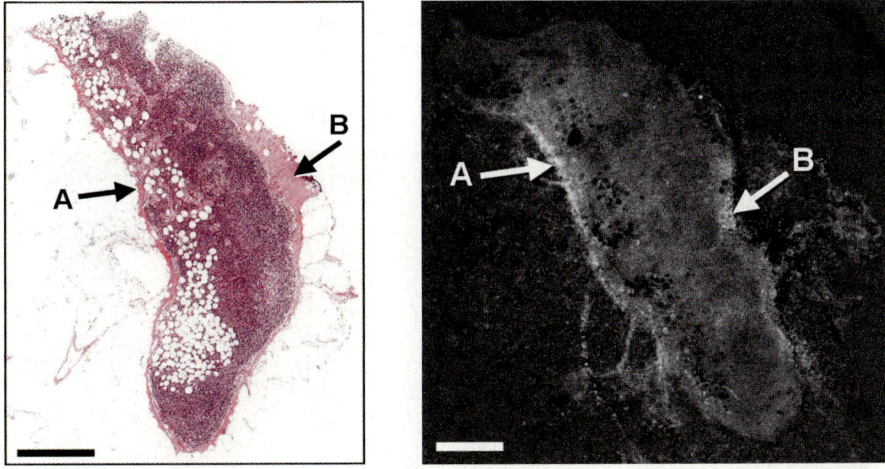

Fig. 2. Reactive, normal (uninvolved) axillary lymph node. Left: H&E histology; Right: Parameterized OCT image. (A, B): Stroma (bright areas). Scale bar = 1mm.

shows a reactive, benign (i.e., uninvolved) lymph node. The sample comprises primarily of the cortex of the lymph node, bounded by the fibrous stromal tissue of the lymph node capsule. Stroma was observed to have a higher attenuation coefficient than cortex, presenting as bright areas in the image (labeled A, B).

Figure 3 shows an involved lymph node, containing a well delineated cluster of metastatic malignant cells (labeled A), visible in both the parameterized OCT image and histology. The outer cortical regions of the lymph node (labeled B, C) appear as dark areas in the parameterized OCT image (low scatter). Lighter areas typically correspond to sinuses extending through the paracortex and medulla of the node.

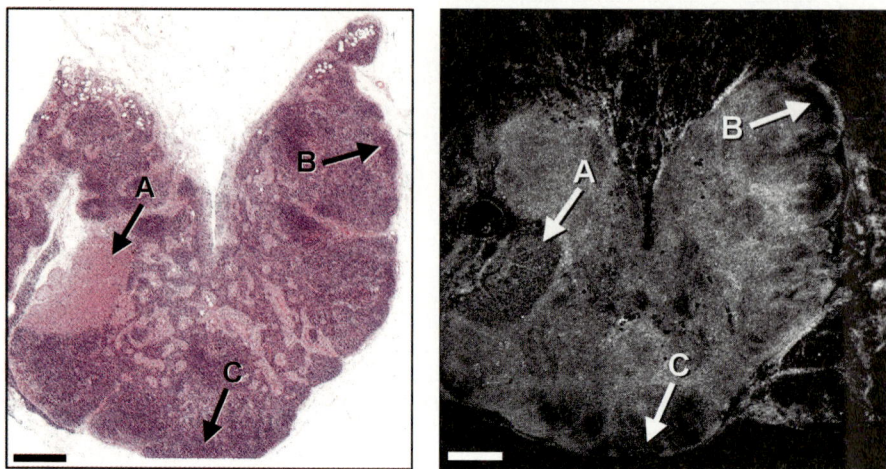

Fig. 3. Involved (malignant) axillary lymph node with well defined deposits of metastatic breast cancer. Left: H&E histology; Right: Parameterized OCT image. (A) Metastasis; (B, C): Lymph cortex (dark areas). Scale bar = 1mm.

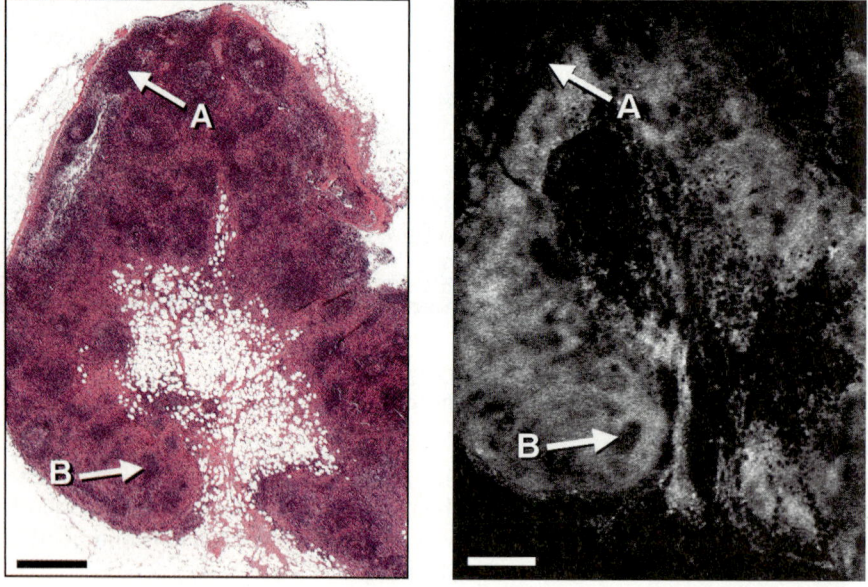

Fig. 4. Involved (malignant) axillary lymph node, with diffuse involvement of the node tissue by metastatic breast cancer cells. Left: H&E histology; Right: Parameterized OCT image. (A, B): Residual areas of healthy cortex (dark areas). Scale bar = 1mm.

Figure 4 shows an involved lymph node in which the metastatic malignant cells are distributed in a diffuse fashion within the nodal lymphoid tissue. Rather than forming discrete aggregates, the metastatic malignant cells in this example are diffusely intermingled amongst the normal cells native to the lymph node. Malignant areas (i.e., those containing the metastatic breast cancer cells) typically have a higher attenuation coefficient (light areas) than the residual uninvolved lymph cortex. Two example dark areas corresponding to residual cortex are labeled A, B.

5 Discussion

The results presented here demonstrate the potential of OCT to differentiate tissue types based on estimates of the tissue's attenuation coefficient. Cancerous areas were visibly distinguishable from surrounding non-cancerous tissue. Stroma tissue was seen to be highly scattering, in agreement with previously reported results [4].

The estimation of such optical properties from OCT presents a useful contrast mechanism. Importantly, it removes some of the variability based on the image acquisition settings. However, the current implementation is based on significant assumptions. The technique assumes that each A-scan samples only a single tissue type. In complex biological structures, this may not be the case and image segmentation techniques will be required to identify regions of homogeneous tissue, such that the attenuation coefficient of each tissue may be calculated separately. The current implementation also utilizes signal attenuation as the single parameter for image contrast. Other authors have used different techniques to separately estimate the effects of the scattering coefficient μ_s and anisotropy g of scattering [10]. We note that more complex models are possible, accounting for the heterogeneity of size, shape, and density of the scatterers in biological tissue [14] and speckle noise [15], and may provide more sophisticated quantitative measures for tissue differentiation.

6 Conclusion

This paper has presented preliminary results for a new form of parameterized OCT image, in which the intensity of each pixel is indicative of the tissue's attenuation coefficient across an A-scan. The results demonstrate the potential of such a parameterized image to distinguish between cancerous and non-cancerous tissue. Future work will utilize segmentation techniques to account for heterogeneity in tissue type within individual A-scans.

References

1. Garcia, M., Jemal, A., Ward, E.M., Center, M.M., Hao, Y., Siegel, R.L., Thun, M.J.: Global Cancer Facts & Figures 2007. American Cancer Society, Atlanta (2007)
2. Bouma, B.E., Tearney, G.J.: Handbook of Optical Coherence Tomography. Marcel Dekker Inc., USA (2002)
3. Luo, W., Nguyen, F.T., Zysk, A.M., Ralston, T.S., Brockenbrough, J., Marks, D.L., Oldenburg, A.L., Boppart, S.A.: Optical Biopsy of Lymph Node Morphology using Optical Coherence Tomography. Technol. Cancer Res. T 4(5), 539–547 (2005)

4. Collier, T., Follen, M., Malpica, A., Richards-Kortum, R.: Sources of Scattering in Cervical Tissue: Determination of the Scattering Coefficient by Confocal Microscopy. Appl. Optics 44, 2072–2081 (2005)
5. Van Gemert, M.J.C., Jacques, S.L., Sterenborg, H.J.C.M., Star, W.M.: Skin Optics. IEEE Trans. Biomed. Eng. 36, 1146–1154 (1989)
6. Simpson, C.R., Kohl, M., Essenpreis, M., Cope, M.: Near-infrared Optical Properties of Ex vivo Human Skin and Subcutaneous Tissues Measured using the Monte Carlo Inversion Technique. Phys. Med. Biol. 43, 2465–2478 (1998)
7. Wang, L.V., Wu, H.: Biomedical Optics. Wiley Interscience, Malden (2007)
8. Yoon, G., Welch, A., Motamedi, M., van Gemert, M.: Development and Application of Three-dimensional Light Distribution Model for Laser Irradiated Tissue. IEEE J. Quantum Elect. 23, 1721–1733 (1987)
9. Key, H., Davies, E.R., Jackson, P.C., Wells, P.N.T.: Optical Attenuation Characteristics of Breast Tissues at Visible and Near-infrared Wavelengths. Phys. Med. Biol. 36, 579–590 (1991)
10. Samatham, R., Jacques, S.L., Campagnola, P.: Optical Properties of Mutant Versus Wild-type Mouse Skin Measured by Reflectance-mode Confocal Scanning Laser Microscopy (rCSLM). J. Biomed. Opt. 13, 041309-1–041309-7 (2008)
11. Collier, T., Arifler, D., Malpica, A., Follen, M., Richards-Kortum, R.: Determination of Epithelial Tissue Scattering Coefficient Using Confocal Microscopy. IEEE J. Sel. Top. Quant. Elect. 9, 307–313 (2003)
12. Qu, J., MacAulay, C., Lam, S., Palcic, B.: Optical Properties of Normal and Carcinomatous Bronchial Tissue. Appl. Optics 33, 7397–7405 (1994)
13. Pogue, B.W., Patterson, M.S.: Review of Tissue Simulating Phantoms for Optical Spectroscopy, Imaging and Dosimetry. J. Biomed. Opt. 11(4), 041102-1–041102-16 (2006)
14. Schmitt, J.M., Knüttel, A.: Model of Optical Coherence Tomography of Heterogeneous Tissue. J. Opt. Soc. Am. A 14, 1231–1242 (1997)
15. Schmitt, J.M., Xiang, S.H., Yung, K.M.: Speckle in Optical Coherence Tomography. J. Biomed. Opt. 4(1), 95–105 (1999)

Analysis of MR Images of Mice in Preclinical Treatment Monitoring of Polycystic Kidney Disease

Stathis Hadjidemetriou[1], Wilfried Reichardt[1], Martin Buechert[2], Juergen Hennig[1], and Dominik von Elverfeldt[1]

[1] University Hospital Freiburg, Dept. of Diagnostic Radiology, Medical Physics, Hugstetter Street 55, 79106 Freiburg, Germany
efstathios.hadjidemetriou@uniklinik-freiburg.de
[2] Magnetic Resonance Development and Application Center, Hugstetter Street 55, 79106 Freiburg, Germany

Abstract. A common cause of kidney failure is autosomal dominant polycystic kidney disease (ADPKD). It is characterized by the growth of cysts in the kidneys and hence the growth of the entire kidneys with eventual failure in most cases by age 50. No preventive treatment for this condition is available. Preclinical drug treatment studies use an in vivo mouse model of the condition. The analysis of mice imaging data for such studies typically requires extensive manual interaction, which is subjective and not reproducible. In this work both untreated and treated mice have been imaged with a high field, $9.4T$, MRI animal scanner and a reliable algorithm for the automated segmentation of the mouse kidneys has been developed. The algorithm first detects the region of interest (ROI) in the image surrounding the kidneys. A parameterized geometric shape for a kidney is registered to the ROI of each kidney. The registered shapes are incorporated as priors to the graph cuts algorithm used to extract the kidneys. The accuracy of the automated segmentation has been demonstrated by comparing it with a manual segmentation. The processing results are also consistent with the literature for previous techniques.

1 Introduction

In autosomal dominant polycystic kidney disease (ADPKD), cysts progressively enlarge and accumulate fluid as well as possibly blood. The cysts disrupt the renal parenchyma and increase the total volume of the kidneys significantly. This eventually leads to end stage renal disease in most cases by age 50. No approved treatment for this condition is available, although clinical trials are performed with compounds known to slow its progression [1]. Early stages of ADPKD are asymptomatic, which has made the assessment of disease progression more difficult and has also hindered the development of medical treatments. The early kidney enlargement, however, associated with the disease progression can be assessed with imaging.

Preclinical drug treatment studies involve models of ADPKD in mice. The imaging of mouse kidneys has been performed in vivo primarily with X-ray micro-CT [2] and MRI [3,4,5]. Typically, the analysis of the images has been performed with extensive manual annotation [4,5]. This is time consuming due to the large number of mice involved in preclinical trials, subjective, and not reproducible. There have been attempts to restrict the manual interaction to the initialization of an automated segmentation. In CT images axial contours of kidneys were represented with a deformable model [2]. In MRI the largest coronal contours of kidneys were represented with splines or as the shortest path between annotated points [3]. MRI allows the repeated and accurate imaging of the kidneys without the use of a contrast agent, and thus the possibility of additional kidney complications. More generally, images of healthy human kidneys from MRI and CT have been processed with a variety of algorithms such as level sets [6] and graph cuts [7], often combined with a shape prior. A sufficiently validated and automated method for the volumetric quantification of polycystic kidneys from MR images and for the monitoring of treatment has not been evident in the literature.

In this work mouse models of ADPKD have been imaged with a high resolution MRI animal scanner. The image region of interest (ROI) surrounding the kidneys is localized and processed to restore intensity uniformity. Subsequently, a prior superspheroid shape [8] is registered to the ROI of each kidney. The registered shape is incorporated into the graph cuts algorithm, which provides the kidneys [9]. The automated processing has analyzed images of a preclinical trial for two compounds. The accuracy of the automated segmentation has been demonstrated by comparing it with a manual one by a medical expert. The processing results are also in agreement with those obtained with previous more interactive or invasive techniques, that these compounds slow the progression of ADPKD in rodent models [1].

2 Methods

2.1 Mouse Model of ADPKD, Treatment, and Image Acquisition

Twelve female mice bearing the *pcy/pcy* genotype were used as a model of ADPKD. All experiments were performed in accordance with the local animal care commission. The mice were distributed into three groups of four. The first group was treated with intraperitonial application of $5mg/kg/day$ of rapamycin. A similar treatment was applied to a second group with vasopressin-2-receptor antagonist SR121463 (Sanofi-Aventis). Both of these compounds have been shown to slow the rate of cystogenesis in mice and are currently on clinical trials [1]. The third group was untreated and was used as control. The imaging began four weeks after the initiation of the treatment and was repeated every two weeks for a total of four time points.

The imaging was performed with a $9.4Tesla$ small bore MRI animal scanner, Bruker Biospin. The coil was a cylindrical quadrature birdcage resonator with an inner diameter of $38mm$. To reduce motion artifacts the mice were anesthetized and the scan was performed with cardiac gating to also reduce blood flow artifacts. The acquisition was a fluid-sensitive T2-weighted spin echo RARE sequence ($TR/TE_{eff}/FA : 3000ms/36ms/180°$). The mice were placed horizontally on the $x-y$ plane along the coil axis, y. The field of view was coronal of $30 \times 30mm^2$ with a matrix size of 256×256 and a resolution of $0.12 \times 0.12mm^2$. The slice thickness Δz was $0.5mm$ without slice spacing. A sufficient number of slices, on average twenty-five, were included to ensure a complete coverage of both kidneys. The acquisition provided image $I(\mathbf{x}) \to \Re$, where $\mathbf{x} = (x, y, z)$. The middle coronal slices of four representative images are shown in the left column of figure 1.

2.2 Localization of the Image Region Surrounding the Kidneys

The images are first processed to extract the foreground. The contribution of the noise in the background to the histogram $\mathcal{H}$ is a Rayleigh distribution $\mathcal{R}$ with low signal to noise ratio [10]. It is fitted with its intensity of maximum density as well as its full width half maximum and subtracted from the image histogram to give $\mathcal{H} - \mathcal{R}$. The highest intensity, i, for which $\mathcal{R}(i) > \mathcal{H}(i) - \mathcal{R}(i)$ provides the upper bound of the intensity range of the background. That range is backprojected to the image and the corresponding voxels are set to zero. The largest connected component over the remaining non-zero image provides the foreground I_f.

The foregroung image in form $I_{f,b} = (I_f > 0)$ provides a binary representation of the mouse body. The eigenvector $\mathbf{e}$ in $I_{f,b}(\mathbf{x})$ corresponding to the largest eigenvalue passes from the spatial mean of $I_{f,b}$, $\mathcal{O}$, along direction (θ_e, ϕ_e), where θ_e is the rotation angle on the $x-y$ plane with the x axis, and ϕ_e is the rotation angle with the z axis. The eigenvector $\mathbf{e}$ together with vector $(0,0,1)$ provide the midsagittal plane, which lies approximately between the two kidneys. The image I_f is also processed with a uniform spherical filter of radius ρ centered on the midsagittal plane, where ρ is the kidney's axial radius. The point on that plane with maximum response is the point between the two kidneys, μ.

The shape of the kidneys is represented geometrically with a superspheroid, $f(\mathbf{x}) = \left|\sqrt{(x^2+z^2)/a^2}\right|^n + |y/b|^n - 1$ [8]. The shape axis y is initialized parallel to the eigenvector $\mathbf{e}$, with rotation $R(\theta_e, \phi_e)$. It is also initialized with $\rho = a < b$ to give a prolate superspheroid elongated along the mouse body axis. The exponent is set to $n = 2.25$ to represent the flat anterior and posterior ends of the kidneys compared to those of a prolate spheroid. The next step is a rough estimation of the center points of the two kidneys c'_s, where s stands for the side that can be left, c'_l, or right, c'_r. They are initially set to distance ρ from μ normal to the midsagittal plane. The location of each is varied to maximize $\sum I_f(\mathbf{x})$ in their interior $\{\mathbf{x} : f(\mathbf{x}) < 0\}$. This is performed with gradient descent and gives an improved estimate of the kidney centers, c_l and c_r.

Subsequently, the fit of the prior shape is refined for each kidney by varying four $\mathbf{m} = (m_1, m_2, m_3, m_4)$ of the parameters of the geometric shape. The first, m_1, is an overall scale that affects both a and b identically. The second, m_2, affects the eccentricity b/a along the body axis y. The third, m_3, is the z coordinate of the center of the superspheroid. The last, m_4, is a rotation of angle θ, $R_{(\theta,0)}$, on the $x-y$ plane around the spatial mean of $I_{f,b}$, $\mathcal{O}$. The superspheroid instances during registration are given by:

$$f(\mathbf{x}', \mathbf{m}) = \left|\sqrt{\frac{x'^2 + (z' - m_3)^2}{m_1^2 a^2}}\right|^n + \left|\frac{y'}{m_1 m_2 b}\right|^n - 1, \qquad (1)$$

where $n = 2.25$, and $(x', y', z') = R_{(\theta_e + m_4, \phi_e)}(x, y, z)$. The shape provided by equation (1) is converted to a binary image, $I_{shape,\mathbf{m}}(\mathbf{x}) = (f(\mathbf{x}, \mathbf{m}) < 0)$. The union of the spheres centered around c_l and c_r, each of radius 4ρ provides the region of interest, I_{ROI}, which is further processed for the extraction of the kidneys. Some examples of I_{ROI} are shown in the second column of figure 1. The fitting is performed over the ROI of $I_{f,b}(\mathbf{x})$ in the side around the midsagittal plane in which the kidney to be modeled lies, $I_{ROI,b,s}(\mathbf{x}) = I_{f,b}(\mathbf{x}) \times I_{ROI}(\mathbf{x}) \times I_s(\mathbf{x})$, where $\times$ is voxelwise multiplication and $s = \{l, r\}$.

The cost function for the shape fitting is the L_1 or equivalently the L_2 norm of the difference between the binary shape image $I_{shape,\mathbf{m}}$ and the binary ROI for each kidney $I_{ROI,b,s}$, $min_\mathbf{m} \|I_{shape,\mathbf{m}}(\mathbf{x} - c_s) - I_{ROI,b,s}(\mathbf{x})\|_1$. The minimization of the cost is performed with gradient descent. The intermediate coronal slices of the ROI of four representative images and the computed kidney shapes are shown in the second and third columns of figure 1, respectively.

2.3 Segmentation of the Kidneys from an Image

The region of interest I_{ROI} is processed for kidney segmentation. It is denoised with median filtering and processed to restore intensity uniformity [11]. Subsequently, the isotropic self-co-occurrence statistics of radius u in the region of interest are analyzed with Otsu's algorithm to obtain an intensity τ. The voxels in intensity range $[0, \alpha_1 \tau]$, where $0 < \alpha_1 < 1$ are set to background seeds and the voxels in intensity range $[\alpha_2 \tau, max_\mathbf{x} I(\mathbf{x})]$, where $1 < \alpha_2$ are set to foreground seeds. The classification of the voxels with intensities in the intermediate range $(\alpha_1 \tau, \alpha_2 \tau)$ is ambiguous. The registered prior kidney shape cancels foreground seeds for which $I_{shape,\mathbf{m}}(\mathbf{x}) = 0$ and sets their classification to ambiguous.

The ambiguities are resolved locally with the graph cuts algorithm [9]. The image is represented as an undirected and weighted graph $\mathcal{G}(\mathcal{V}, \mathcal{E})$ [9]. The image voxels together with two bounding nodes s and t are the nodes $\mathcal{V}$ of the graph. A neighborhood edge $\{p, q\}$ is included in the graph between the node corresponding to every voxel p and the node corresponding to voxel q if $q \in \mathcal{N}_p$, where $\mathcal{N}_p$ is the 26-connected neighborhood of node p. Boundary edges are established from every node p to both s and t to give $\{p, s\}$ and $\{p, t\}$. The edges are assigned weights, which simulate flow capacities [9]. A subset of edges $\mathcal{C} \in \mathcal{E}$ is called an s/t-cut if the bounding nodes are completely separated in the induced graph $\mathcal{G}_\mathcal{C} = (\mathcal{V}, \mathcal{E} - \mathcal{C})$. The bounding node in $\mathcal{G}_\mathcal{C}$ to which a node p remains connected to determines its classification as foreground if $\{p, s\} \in \mathcal{G}_\mathcal{C}$ and as background if $\{p, t\} \in \mathcal{G}_\mathcal{C}$. The cost $|\mathcal{C}|$ of a cut is the sum of all edge weights in $\mathcal{C}$. The cut of globally minimum cost is provided by the equivalent maximum flow solution from s to t.

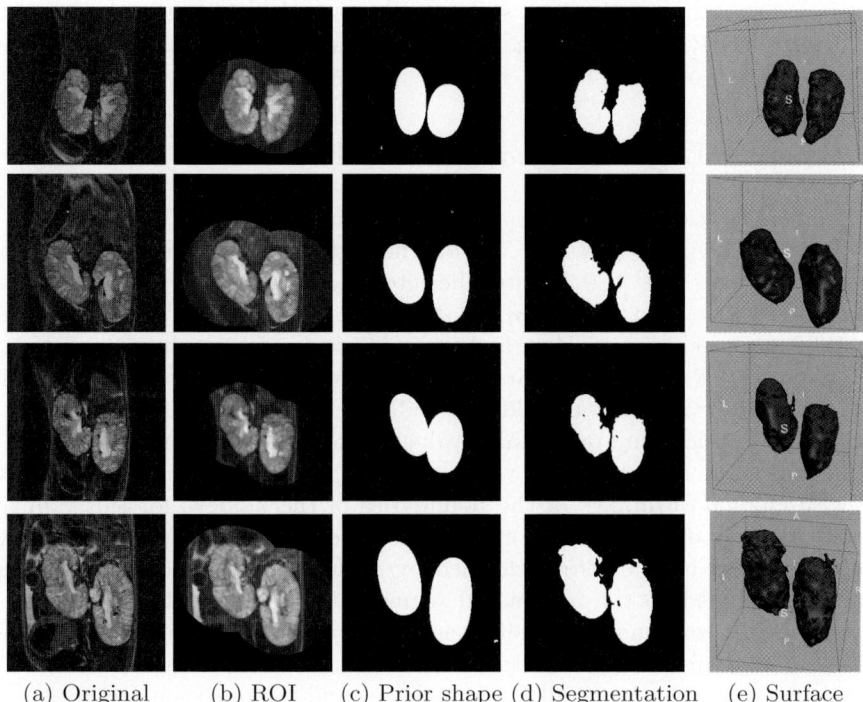

(a) Original (b) ROI (c) Prior shape (d) Segmentation (e) Surface

Fig. 1. The processing of four representative images shown along the rows. The middle coronal slices of the original images are in the left, next to them are the regions of interest, in the third column are the prior shapes, and in the fourth column are the segmented kidneys. In the fifth column is a rendering of the segmentation surfaces.

The edge weights are positive. The total weight of neighborhood edge $\{p,q\} \in \mathcal{N}$, $V_{T,pq}$, is a product of factors that depend on I_{ROI} and I_{shape}. The weight derived from I_{ROI} depends on the intensity difference between adjacent voxels $V_{1,pq} = \exp\left(-(I_{ROI}(\mathbf{x}_p) - I_{ROI}(\mathbf{x}_q))^2/\sigma^2\right)$, where σ is a fraction β of the dynamic range, $\sigma = \beta(max_\mathbf{x} I_{ROI}(\mathbf{x}) - min_\mathbf{x} I_{ROI}(\mathbf{x}))$. The anisotropic spatial resolution is represented by factor $V_{2,pq} = 1/d_{pq}$, where $d_{pq} = ||\mathbf{x}_p - \mathbf{x}_q||_2$. The shape boundary provided by ∇I_{shape} is smoothed with a Gaussian filter of standard deviation equal to ρ. Subsequently, its dynamic range is rescaled with γ and reversed to give $\Phi(\mathbf{x}) = 1 - \gamma \nabla I_{shape}(\mathbf{x}) * G(\rho)$ as well as the shape edge weight $V_{3,pq} = (\Phi(\mathbf{x}_p) + \Phi(\mathbf{x}_q))/2$ [12]. The product:

$$V_{T,pq} = \exp\left(-\frac{(I_{ROI}(\mathbf{x}_p) - I_{ROI}(\mathbf{x}_q))^2}{\sigma^2}\right)\left(\frac{1}{d_{pq}}\right)\left(\frac{\Phi(\mathbf{x}_p) + \Phi(\mathbf{x}_q)}{2}\right) \quad (2)$$

gives the total weight of edge $\{p,q\} \in \mathcal{N}$.

The weights to the bounding nodes are selected so that the minimum s/t cut preserves the classification of the seed nodes as well as includes neighborhood edges and thus segments the image. Some representative images and the corresponding segmentations are shown in the second and fourth columns of figure 1, respectively. A surface rendering of the kidney segmentations is shown in the fifth column of figure 1.

3 Results: Data Analysis and Evaluation

The implementation is in $C++$ and uses the ITK library [13]. The radius of the self-co-occurrences was $u = 3mm$. The intensity range that provided the background seeds was $[0, 0.3\tau]$ and the intensity range that provided the foreground seeds was $[1.2\tau, max_\mathbf{x} I_{ROI}(\mathbf{x})]$, that is, $\alpha_1 = 0.3$ and $\alpha_2 = 1.2$. A value of $\beta = 1/32$ was used for σ in $V_{1,pq}$ and the value of γ enforced the dynamic range of $V_{3,pq}$ to be $[0.7, 1.0]$. These parameters were kept constant for the processing of all 48 images. Only the axial kidney radius ρ varied with the input image. It is sufficient to select an approximate value for it by observation.

The automatic segmentations were compared with the region enclosed within slicewise manual outlinings of the boundaries of the kidneys for thirty images of both treated and untreated mice out of the total of 48 images analyzed. The manual outlinings were performed by a medical expert (M.D.), who is a co-author, blinded to the automated segmentations of the kidney regions. In the comparison an image is classified as kidney volume correctly detected, TP, kidney volume missed by the detection, FN, and volume falsely detected, FP. These values provide the recall $RE = \frac{TP}{TP+FN}$, and the precision $PR = \frac{TP}{TP+FP}$. A score of 1.0 for recall indicates completeness and a score of 1.0 for precision indicates exactness. The average and standard deviation of the precision were $PR = 94.1 \pm 1.5\%$, and those of the recall were $RE = 94.6 \pm 1.8\%$. In both cases the high mean values of the criteria and their low standard deviations indicate a high quality detection.

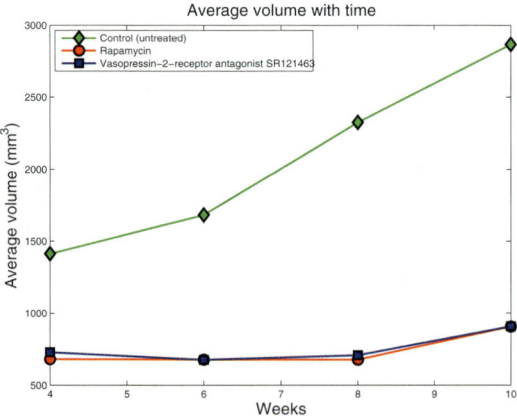

Fig. 2. The average automatically extracted volume of both kidneys over the 48 images as a function of time for the three groups of mice. As expected, the untreated, control, group in green shows a much greater increase in kidney volume.

In figure 2 are the average values of the automatically extracted volume of both kidneys for the 48 images within every group along the number of weeks after initiation of treatment. As expected, the group of untreated, control, mice shows a large increase in kidney volume. The mice treated with either compound show very limited increase in kidney volume. The processing was performed on an AMD 2GHz CPU. The average and standard deviation of the computation time were $57 \pm 29 min$. They were dominated by the varying time duration of the registrations of the prior shape to the two kidneys.

4 Discussion

The spinal cord does not constrain the locations of the kidneys in mice, and thus their relative distance can vary. The kidneys are also connected to the urinary tract and are in contact with fat, the liver, and other organs that can have similar intensities. This necessitates the use of a robust model for mice body anatomy and for the delineation of the kidney boundaries. This is sufficiently represented with the localizations and the registrations of the superspheroids and their use as priors in the graph cuts algorithm. The graph cuts criterion provides segmentations with tight boundaries and penalizes leaking to neighboring anatomic structures.

A manual outlining of the kidneys was performed for thirty images by a medical expert. The enclosed region was used for a volume based validation of the detected kidneys, which demonstrated the high quality of the processing. The surfaces of the detected regions and the manual outlinings could also be compared with measures such as the mean surface distance and the Hausdorff distance. The validation could be repeated with a manual segmentation by a different expert. The parameters of the algorithm were set to accommodate image characteristics such as contrast to noise ratio and resolution. Their settings are also a trade-off between computational requirements and performance. A sensitivity analysis with respect to the parameters of the algorithm would further demonstrate its robustness.

The processing results are in agreement with the effects established with previous techniques, that the two compounds prevent cystogenesis in mice [1]. Previous techniques often involve sacrificing the mice and thus do not allow the monitoring at multiple time points that MRI permits. Micro-CT as well as some MRI acquisition protocols involve the administration of a contrast agent. These agents can cause interfering kidney complications, particularly in mice with compromised kidney function such as those used in this study. The MR acquisitions in this work were performed without the administration of a contrast agent. The processing has been shown to be sufficiently robust to the resulting lower contrast. The method described can analyze MR images of mice in preclinical trials for ADPKD in a non-invasive, reliable, reproducible, and automated manner.

References

1. Walz, G.: Therapeutic approaches in autosomal dominant polycystic kidney disease (ADPKD): is there light at the end of the tunnel? Nephrol. Dial Transplant. 21(7), 1752–1757 (2006)

2. Gleason, S., Sarraf, H., Abidi, M., Karakashian, O., Morandi, F.: A new deformable model for analysis of X-ray CT images in preclinical studies of mice for polycystic kidney disease. IEEE Trans. on Medical Imaging 21(10), 1302–1309 (2002)
3. Fei, B., Flask, C., Wang, H., Pi, A., Wilson, D., Shillingford, J., Murcia, N., Weimbs, T., Duerk, J.: Image segmentation, registration and visualization of serial MR images for therapeutic assessment of polycystic kidney disease in transgenic mice. In: Proc. of IEEE-EMBS, pp. 467–469 (2005)
4. Wallace, D., Hou, Y., Huang, Z., Nivens, E., Savinkova, L., Yamaguchi, T., Bilgen, M.: Tracking kidney volume in mice with polycystic kidney disease by magnetic resonance imaging. Kidney International 73, 778–781 (2008)
5. Reichardt, W., Romaker, D., Becker, A., Buechert, M., Walz, G., Elverfeldt, D.: Monitoring kidney and renal cyst volumes applying MR approaches on a rapamycin treated mouse model of ADPKD. In: MAGMA (2008)
6. Abdelmunim, H., Farag, A., Miller, W., AboelGhar, M.: A kidney segmentation approach from DCE-MRI using level sets. In: Proc. of IEEE CVPR Workshops, pp. 1–6 (2008)
7. Ali, A., Farag, A., Baz, A.: Graph cuts framework for kidney segmentation with prior shape constraints. In: Ayache, N., Ourselin, S., Maeder, A. (eds.) MICCAI 2007, Part I. LNCS, vol. 4791, pp. 384–392. Springer, Heidelberg (2007)
8. Gielis, J.: A generic geometric transformation that unifies a wide range of natural and abstract shapes. American Journal of Botany 90(3), 333–338 (2003)
9. Boykov, Y., Lea, G.: Graph cuts and efficient N-D image segmentation. International Journal of Computer Vision 70(2), 109–131 (2006)
10. Gudbjartsson, H., Patz, S.: The Rician distribution of noisy MRI data. Magnetic Resonance in Medicine 34, 910–914 (1995)
11. Hadjidemetriou, S., Studholme, C., Mueller, S., Weiner, M., Schuff, N.: Restoration of MRI data for intensity non-uniformities using local high order intensity statistics. Medical Image Analysis 13(1), 36–48 (2009)
12. Freedman, D., Zhang, T.: Interactive graph cut based segmentation with shape priors. In: Proc. of CVPR, pp. 755–762 (2005)
13. The Insight Segmentation and Registration Toolkit, http://www.itk.org

Actin Filament Tracking Based on Particle Filters and Stretching Open Active Contour Models

Hongsheng Li[1], Tian Shen[1], Dimitrios Vavylonis[2], and Xiaolei Huang[1]

[1] Department of Computer Science & Engineering, Lehigh University, USA
[2] Department of Physics, Lehigh University, USA

Abstract. We introduce a novel algorithm for actin filament tracking and elongation measurement. Particle Filters (PF) and Stretching Open Active Contours (SOAC) work cooperatively to simplify the modeling of PF in a one-dimensional state space while naturally integrating filament body constraints to tip estimation. Our algorithm reduces the PF state spaces to one-dimensional spaces by tracking filament bodies using SOAC and probabilistically estimating tip locations along the curve length of SOACs. Experimental evaluation on TIRFM image sequences with very low SNRs demonstrates the accuracy and robustness of this approach.

1 Introduction

Actin proteins are present in all eukaryotic cells. Their ability to polymerize into long filaments underlies basic processes of cell life such as cell motility, cytokinesis during cell division, and endocytosis. The kinetics of polymerization of individual actin filaments *in vitro* have been studied extensively using Total Internal Reflection Fluorescence Microscopy (TIRFM) [1], [2], [3] (Fig. 1(a) and 1(c)). In these experiments, actin filaments are attached to a glass slide by surface tethers that act as pivot points that can be used as fiducial markers to help distinguish the elongation of each end [1], [2], [3]. Two basic features of actin kinetics that can be extracted from TIRFM are (i) the average rate of filament elongation at each end, and (ii) the fluctuations in the average rate. Both of these two numbers depend in a unique way on the details of the microscopic mechanism of monomer addition to the ends of the filament [1], [2].

In [4], we presented the stretching open active contours (SOAC) for filament segmentation and tracking. This automated method allowed simultaneous measurements of multiple filaments. Related methods have been applied to tracking microtubule (MT) filaments. Hadjidemetriou *et al.* [5] minimized an image-based energy function to segment MTs at each time step using consecutive level sets method. Saban *et al.* [6] automatically detected tips in the first frame and then proceeded to track each tip separately by searching for the closest match in subsequent frames. However, the above methods did not utilize temporal coherency of the motion or the growth of filaments.

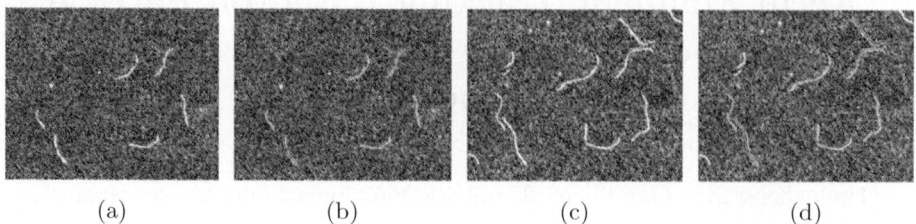

(a) (b) (c) (d)

Fig. 1. An example of actin filament tracking using the proposed method

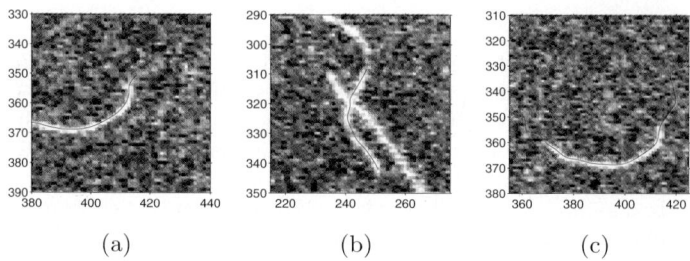

(a) (b) (c)

Fig. 2. Problems observed in our previous method [4]: (a) An "over-grown" active contour because of the low SNR near the tip, and (b) an "under-grown" active contour because of the intensity gap on filament body. (c) An over-grown active contour covering both tips of a filament. (Best viewed in color.)

Particle Filter (PF) based methods have also been proposed to track MTs. In [7], PFs were utilized to track the tips of polymerizing microtubules. In these images, MTs were labeled by plus-end tracking proteins that associate with the tips but not with the body of growing MTs. Without using supporting information from the MT body, Markov Random Fields were employed to model the joint transition model of multiple tips; this required that the posterior pdfs of different tips to be sampled jointly. A limiting factor in this work was that its high-dimensional state space added complexity to modeling and tracking computation. Kong et al. [8] employed a PF-based method similar to [7] to track MT tips. In this work, MT tip locations were estimated recursively using PF, and then MT bodies were segmented using active contours based on the estimations.

Although in [4] filament bodies were tracked accurately, we reported errors on tip location estimation because of the low SNR of filament tips. In this paper, we present a novel actin filament tracking algorithm which combines particle filters (PF) [9] with the stretching open active contours (SOAC) to address this problem. An example of our tracking results is shown in Fig. 1. By construction, SOACs stretch along bright ridges in an image. At each time step t, SOACs stretch along filament bodies and are forced to grow over distances that exceed the tip locations. Subsequently, particles are spread along each SOAC according to transition models, which predict the tip "length" (location) at time $t+1$, given the states and likelihoods of the particles at time t. Using the image information at time $t+1$, each particle is associated with a likelihood that the particle represents the correct tip. The particles' states and likelihoods are then used to estimate the posterior pdf describing the probability distribution of tip length at time $t+1$. Before tracking, this PF-based method requires the transition and likelihood models to be properly defined by providing an initial estimate of the value of the filament elongation rate, to within $\sim 20\%$ of the actual value.

The main contribution of this paper is that we reduce the state space of PF to a one dimensional space by implicitly modeling tip "length" as the state vector of our PF. By construction, tip locations are distributed at SOACs that grow along filament bodies; thus we only need track the "length" of tips. This novel framework naturally integrates filament body constraints to tip estimation. Experimental evaluation and comparison showed accurate and robust tracking performance of our algorithm.

2   Stretching Open Active Contour Models

In [4], open active contour models were presented to segment actin filaments. Let $\mathbf{r}(s) = (x(s), y(s)), s \in [0,1]$ parametrically represent an open curve. Treating this curve as an active contour, we seek to minimize its overall energy E, which consists of internal energy E_{int} and external energy E_{ext}, i.e., $E = E_{int} + k \cdot E_{ext}$, where k controls the relative contributions of the internal and external energy. The internal energy, $E_{int} = \int_0^1 (\alpha(s)|\mathbf{r}_s(s)|^2 + \beta(s)|\mathbf{r}_{ss}(s)|^2)ds$, controls the smoothness of the curve. The external energy, E_{ext}, represents external image constraints and consists of an image term E_{img} and an intensity-adaptive stretching term E_{str}, i.e., $E_{ext} = E_{img} + k_{str} \cdot E_{str}$, where k_{str} balances the contributions of E_{img} and E_{str}. The image term E_{img} is defined by the Gaussian filtered image, i.e., $E_{img} = G_\sigma * I$, to make the active contour converge to filament locations, which correspond to bright ridges in the images. The stretching term stretches the open active contour along a filament and stops stretching when its ends meet filament tips. Tip locations are determined by using an intensity-based criterion.

The main problem of [4] is that, in some very noisy TIRFM image sequences, the intensity-adaptive stretching term E_{str} may lead to large errors on tip estimation. Low contrast near filament tips may result in active contours "overgrowing" (see Fig. 2(a)), while intensity gaps on filament bodies may lead to active contours "under-growing" (see Fig. 2(b)). It was difficult to define an external energy term that copes with both scenarios for all filaments.

Although tips were difficult to be identified by intensity or contrast alone in noisy images, we observed that the over-grown active contours followed filament bodies accurately and were able to cover tip locations even when they over grew (See Fig. 2(c)). This means that we can search for tips along an over-grown active contour. Therefore, we propose a new stretching open active contour (SOAC) model similar to the one proposed in [4] but with a non-intensity-adaptive stretching term E'_{str}, which always makes a SOAC grow over distances that exceed the tip locations:

$$\nabla E'_{str}(\mathbf{r}(s)) = \begin{cases} \frac{\mathbf{r}_s(s)}{|\mathbf{r}_s(s)|} & s = 0, \\ -\frac{\mathbf{r}_s(s)}{|\mathbf{r}_s(s)|} & s = 1, \\ 0 & otherwise. \end{cases} \quad (1)$$

Therefore, the overall energy of a SOAC model is defined by

$$E = E_{int} + k \cdot \int_0^1 E_{img}(\mathbf{r}(s)) + k'_{str} \cdot E'_{str}(\mathbf{r}(s)) ds, \quad (2)$$

where k'_{str} is a constant that controls the stretching force that makes the active contour always grow over tips. The above SOAC model enables us to reduce the search space of filament tips to a one-dimensional space (along the SOAC's curve length) and naturally adds a continuous body constraint: a tip must be connected to a filament body.

3 Actin Filament Tracking Using Particle Filters

A SOAC model provides an estimation of filament body and therefore simplifies the problem of tip tracking to searching for and tracking tip patterns in a one-dimensional space along the SOAC curve's length. This is one of the major advantages when compared with approaches that work in a 4-dimensional space in [8] and the even higher dimensional space in [7]. To systematically search along an over-grown SOAC for the optimal tip location, we employ the widely used Sequential Importance Resampling (SIR) PF [10] to estimate the locations of both B-end and P-end of a filament.

3.1 Bayesian Tracking Based on Particle Filters

In the PF framework, the state vector of a target at time t, $X_t \in \mathbb{R}^n$, is given by $X_t = f_t(X_{t-1}, \mathbf{v}_{t-1})$, where $\mathbf{v}_{t-1} \in \mathbb{R}^n$ is an i.i.d. process noise vector, and $f_t : \mathbb{R}^n \times \mathbb{R}^n \to \mathbb{R}^n$ is a possibly nonlinear function that is modeled by a known transition model $P_t(X_t|X_{t-1})$. The measurements at time t, Z_t, relate to the state vector by $Z_t = h_t(X_t, n_t)$, where n_t is an i.i.d. measurement noise vector, and $h_t : \mathbb{R}^n \times \mathbb{R}^n \to \mathbb{R}^n$ is a possibly nonlinear function that is modeled by a known likelihood model $P_l(Z_t|X_t)$. It is assumed that the initial posteriori pdf $P(X_0|Z_0) \equiv P(X_0)$ is available as *a priori*.

The objective of tracking is then to recursively estimate X_t from measurements. Suppose that $P(X_{t-1}|Z_{1:t-1})$ at time $t-1$ is available. In principle, the pdf $P(X_t|Z_{1:t})$ can be obtained, recursively, in two stages: prediction and update.

Prediction: $\quad P(X_t|Z_{1:t-1}) = \int P_t(X_t|X_{t-1}) P(X_{t-1}|Z_{1:t-1}) dX_{t-1}, \quad (3)$

Update: $\quad P(X_t|Z_{1:t}) \propto P_l(Z_t|X_t) P(X_t|Z_{1:t-1}). \quad (4)$

In the SIR PF algorithm, at each time t, a group of N particles $\{X_{t-1}^{(i)}, w_{t-1}^{(i)}\}_{i=1}^{N}$ is propagated from $t-1$ to characterize $P(X_t|Z_{1:t})$ using the Monte Carlo principle:

$P(X_t|Z_{1:t}) \approx \sum_{i=1}^{N} w_t^{(i)} \delta(X_t - X_t^{(i)})$. It is usually assumed that $P(X_t|Z_t) = P(X_t|Z_{1:t})$.

Clearly, three aspects of the PF framework need to be specified:

- **The state vector** X_t, which models the system in a n-dimensional space;
- **The transition model** $P_t(X_t|X_{t-1})$, which models f_t;
- **The likelihood model** $P_l(Z_t|X_t)$, which models h_t.

For **the state vector** in our filament tip tracking problem, as we have simplified tip location estimation to a 1D space using SOAC, we propose to use the "length" of the tip at time t, S_t, as the state of our PF, *i.e.*, $X_t = S_t$. The "length" of a tip is defined as the filament length from the tip point to a reference point along the SOAC representing the filament. Reference points can be randomly chosen on SOACs during initialization. Tracking the length of a tip is equivalent to tracking its location on a SOAC.

For **the transition model**, because we choose tip length as the state vector, the transition model should describe the change of one tip's length over time. Therefore, it can also be interpreted as the tip elongation model. The two ends of an actin filament, the "barbed" (B-end) and "pointed" (P-end) end, respectively, grow at distinctively different rates. We model the transition probabilities of B-end and P-end tips separately. For the transition model of B-ends, we used a normal density, $P_{Bt}(X_t|X_{t-1}) \sim \mathcal{N}(X_{t-1} + \mu_b, \sigma_b^2)$, where μ_b is the average elongation rate of B-ends. Obviously, the more accurate the estimation of μ_b is, the more robust the tracking results are. For P-ends, because they grow much slower than B-ends, we set $P_{Pt}(X_t|X_{t-1}) \sim \mathcal{N}(X_{t-1}, \sigma_p^2)$.

When a SOAC has just been initialized, the B-end and the P-end of the filament it represents cannot be distinguished. Therefore in the first few frames, we dispatch half of the particles following the B-end transition model and the other half following the P-end model. After several tracking steps that take into account image measurement information, the B-end and P-end of the filament can be distinguished by comparing the posterior pdfs estimated using B-end and P-end particles respectively.

For **the likelihood model**, we use an appearance template based approach. In particular, we use a 10×4 pixel rectangle template containing a mean appearance image μ_T and a standard deviation image σ_T, both computed from manually selected tip image patches. When a filament A is intersecting another filament B, the tip of A would be occluded by B's body. This naturally implies that any pixel covered by filament B should have low confidence or certainty when being used to compute the likelihood of the tip of A. Therefore, at each time t, a confidence map M_t for each filament is created, in which pixels covered by other filaments are given the value 0.5, and all other pixels are given the value 1. The likelihood model is then defined by

$$P_l(Z_t|X_t) \propto \exp\left\{-\frac{1}{n}\sum_{i=1}^{n} \frac{M_t(\mathbf{s}_i)}{2\sigma_T(\mathbf{s}_i)} \cdot |F(X_t)(\mathbf{s}_i) - \mu_T(\mathbf{s}_i)|\right\}, \quad (5)$$

where n is the total number of pixels in the template tip patch, $\mathbf{s}_i$ is its ith pixel's coordinates, and $F(X_t)$ and M_t are the image patch and the confidence map patch of a tip with state X_t, respectively, after being translated and rotated to the template tip's coordinate.

3.2 SOAC Registration and Length Measurement

To perform measurements on the length and elongation rate of a tip, a reference point on the corresponding filament needs to be specified. However, a TIRFM image sequence show drift such as translation between contiguous frames [3]. To recover the same reference point on a filament over time, the converged SOACs in consecutive frames representing the filament are registered simultaneously using the Iterative Closest Points (ICP) algorithm [11].

4 The Algorithm

We summarize the proposed filament tracking algorithm as follows. Let $\mathbf{r}_{t-1}$ represent the SOAC active contour tracking the filament at time $t-1$. From the particle sample set $\{X_{t-1}^{(i)}, w_{t-1}^{(i)}\}_{i=1}^{N}$ at time step $t-1$ characterizing the pdf $P(X_{t-1}|Z_{t-1})$, we can construct a "new" sample-set $\{X_t^{(i)}, w_t^{(i)}\}_{i=1}^{N}$ approximating $P(X_t|Z_t)$ at time t:

- **Initialize** $\bar{\mathbf{r}}_t$ using $\mathbf{r}_{t-1}$ (Fig. 3(a)). Deform it by minimizing (2) and make sure both ends of $\bar{\mathbf{r}}_t$ grow over the tips of its corresponding filament (Fig. 3(b)).
- **Register** $\bar{\mathbf{r}}_t$ to $\mathbf{r}_{t-1}$ using the ICP method and recover the reference point on $\bar{\mathbf{r}}_t$ (Fig. 3(c-d)).
- **Select** a sample $\overline{X}_t^{(i)} = X_{t-1}^{(j)}$ with probability $w_{t-1}^{(j)}$.
- **Predict** $X_t^{(i)}$ to approximate $P(X_t|Z_{t-1})$ according to (3) by sampling from

$$P_{Bt}(X_t|X_{t-1} = \overline{X}_t^{(i)}) \quad \text{or} \quad P_{Pt}(X_t|X_{t-1} = \overline{X}_t^{(i)}), \quad (6)$$

depending on the tip type (B-end or P-end) the particle $\overline{X}_t^{(i)}$ represents (Fig. 3(e)).
- **Measure** and weight the new particle using the measurement Z_t according to (4) and (5). Then normalize all N particles to estimate $P(X_t|Z_t)$:

$$w_t^{(i)} = P_l(Z_t|X_t = X_t^{(i)}), \quad \text{then} \quad w_t^{(i)} = \frac{w_t^{(i)}}{\sum_{j=1}^{N} w_t^{(j)}}. \quad (7)$$

- **Estimate** the mean of $P(X_t|Z_t)$ at time t by

$$\mathcal{E}(X_t) \approx \sum_{i=1}^{N} w_t^{(i)} X_t^{(i)}. \quad (8)$$

- **Cut** $\bar{\mathbf{r}}_t$ according to $\mathcal{E}(X_t)$ to generate $\mathbf{r}_t$ (Fig. 3(f)).
- Go back to the initialization step for $t+1$.

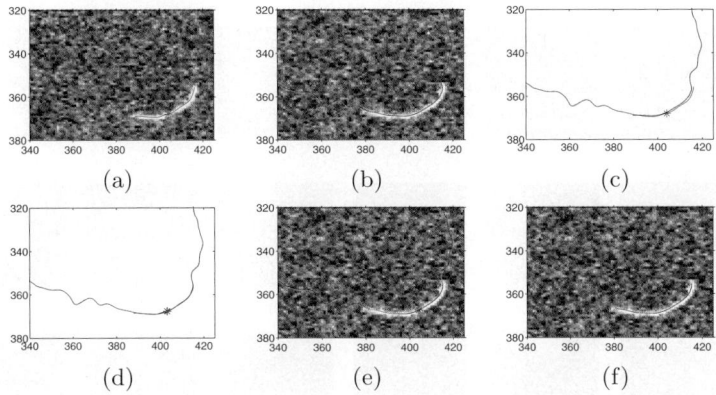

Fig. 3. Illustration of the algorithm. (a) A SOAC $\mathbf{r}_{t-1}$ (red) at time $t-1$, (b) initialize $\bar{\mathbf{r}}_t$ (blue) using $\mathbf{r}_{t-1}$ and deform it by minimizing (2), (c) before registration of $\mathbf{r}_{t-1}$ and $\bar{\mathbf{r}}_t$ (Red '*' denotes the reference point on $\mathbf{r}_{t-1}$), (d) after registration of $\mathbf{r}_{t-1}$ and $\bar{\mathbf{r}}_t$ (Blue '*' denotes the recovered reference point on $\bar{\mathbf{r}}_t$), (e) generate new particles (green) along $\bar{\mathbf{r}}_t$ according to $P(X_t|X_{t-1} = \overline{X}_t^{(i)})$, and measure each particle's likelihood probability $w_t^{(i)} = P(Z_t|X_t = X_t^{(i)})$, and (f) cut $\bar{\mathbf{r}}_t$ according to $\mathcal{E}(X_t)$ to generate $\mathbf{r}_t$.

5 Application to Experimental Data

5.1 Experimental Image Data

We used two TIRFM image sequences from [2]. In these experiments, polymerization of muscle Mg-ADP-actin was monitored in the presence of varying concentrations of inorganic phosphate (Pi) and actin monomers. The pixel size was 0.17 μm. There were 20 images in sequence I and and 34 images in sequence II. The time interval between frames was 30 sec in sequence I and 10 sec in sequence II.

5.2 Evaluation and Comparison with the Previous Method [4]

For both sequences, we set $\alpha = 0.05$, $\beta = 0.1$, $k = 0.6$, and $k'_{str} = 0.55$. μ_b for sequences I and II were set according to average elongation rates of B-ends measured by a manual method [3]. We set large values to σ_p and σ_b to avoid imposing any strong prior on tip length estimation. For sequence I, $\mu_b = 11.2524$ mon/sec, $\sigma_b = 4.5$ mon/sec, and $\sigma_p = 1$ mon/sec. For II, $\mu_b = 11.5760$ mon/sec, $\sigma_b = 5$ mon/sec, and $\sigma_p = 2.5$ mon/sec. We used 50 particles for each tip and initialized each SOAC using the segmentation method in [4] to obtain $P(X_0)$.

Fig. 4 illustrates 3 examples of our tracking algorithm. Taking advantage of temporal coherence and filament body constraints, our algorithm tracked filaments accurately and showed robust performance against filament intersection.

We observed that filament bodies were always tracked accurately by our algorithm. Therefore, we evaluated the algorithm by measuring errors on tip location estimation. We selected 10 and 5 actin filaments from image sequence I and II respectively to measure tracking errors. For all selected filaments, we manually

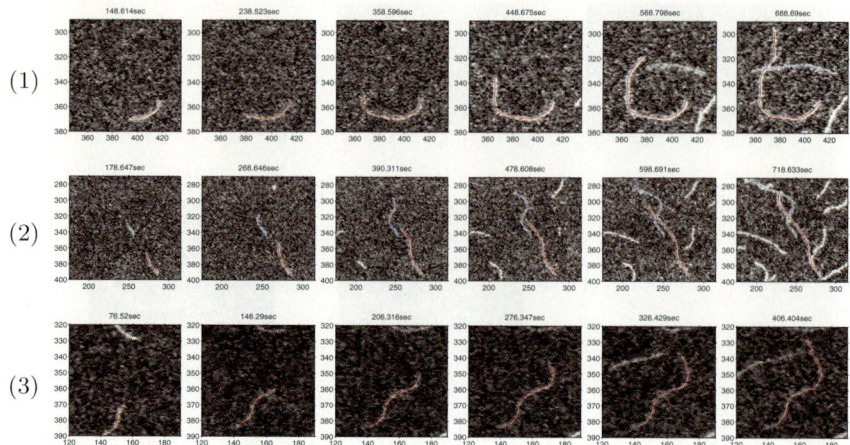

Fig. 4. Three examples of tracking filaments. (1-2) Tracking filaments in sequence I, and (3) tracking a filament in sequence II.

Table 1. Tip tracking error statistics of selected filaments in both image sequences I (Fig. 4(1-2)) and II (Fig. 4(3)). (Unit: pixel)

	Sequnce	Mean	Maximum	Standard Deviation	Number of Failures
Proposed Method	I	0.8789	3.5132	0.7211	0 out of 149
	II	1.7334	5.8342	1.4946	4 out of 170
Previous Method [4]	I	1.6732	10.2387	1.8776	4 out of 149
	II	2.9018	13.8472	2.3870	6 out of 170

labeled their two tips in each frame as ground truth and calculated L_2 distances between the ground truth and our algorithm's results. We also compared with tip location errors obtained by a previous method [4], which did not utilize temporal coherence and used an intensity criterion to determine tip locations. During the tracking process, when we observed a failure, which means a SOAC stretched onto a different filament, we reinitialized the SOAC in the next frame by hand and resumed tracking. Table 1 shows tip tracking error statistics of our algorithm and of the previous method; our new one-dimensional PF-based algorithm clearly outperforms the previous method.

6 Conclusion

In this paper, we introduce a novel actin filament tracking algorithm based on Stretching Open Active Contour (SOAC) models and one-dimensional Particle Filters (PF). Taking advantage of filament body estimated by the SOAC models, our method is able to find the tip using PF with a one-dimensional state vector. Such simplification naturally integrates filament body constraints to guarantee continuity between the estimated tip and body. A template based likelihood model and the stochastic nature of the PF framework also make our algorithm robust to noise and filament intersections. Experimental evaluation on TIRFM image sequences with low SNRs and comparison with a previous method demonstrate the accuracy and robustness of the proposed approach.

Acknowledgments. We would like to thank Ikuko Fujiwara (NHLBI/NIH) and Thomas Pollard (Yale) for providing the data, and Matthew Smith (Lehigh) for his suggestions. This work was supported by NIH grant R21GM083928.

References

1. Fujiwara, I., Takahashi, S., Tadakuma, H., Funatsu, T., Ishiwata, S.: Microscopic analysis of polymerization dynamics with individual actin filaments. Nat. Cell Biol. 4, 666–673 (2002)
2. Fujiwara, I., Vavylonis, D., Pollard, T.D.: Polymerization kinetics of ADP- and ADP-Pi-actin determined by fluorescence microscopy. Proc. Natl. Acad. Sci. USA 104, 8827–8832 (2007)
3. Kuhn, J.R., Pollard, T.D.: Real-time measurements of actin filament polymerization by total internal reflection fluorescence microscopy. Biophys. J. 88, 1387–1402 (2005)
4. Li, H., Shen, T., Smith, M., Fujiwara, I., Vavylonis, D., Huang, X.: Automated actin filament segmentation, tracking and tip elongation measurements based on open active contour models. ISBI (2009)
5. Hadjidemetriou, S., Toomre, D., Duncan, J.: Motion tracking of the outer tips of microtubules. Medical Image Analysis 12, 689–702 (2008)
6. Saban, M., Altinok, A., Peck, A., Kenney, C., Feinstein, S., Wilson, L., Rose, K., Manjunath, B.: Automated tracking and modeling of microtubule dynamics. ISBI 1, 1032–1035 (2006)
7. Smal, I., Draegestein, K., Galjart, N., Niessen, W., Meijering, E.: Particle filtering for multiple object tracking in dynamic fluorescence microscopy images: Application to microtubule growth analysis. IEEE Trans. on Medical Imaging 27, 789–804 (2008)
8. Kong, K., Marcus, A., Giannakakou, P., Wang, M.: Using particle filter to track and model microtubule dynamics. ICIP 5, 517–520 (2007)
9. Gordon, N., Salmond, D., Smith, A.: Novel approach to nonlinear/nongaussian Bayesian state estimation. IEE Proceedings-F (Radar and Signal Processing) 140, 107–113 (1993)
10. Isard, M., Blake, A.: Condensation–conditional density propagation for visual tracking. IJCV 29, 5–28 (1998)
11. Besl, P., McKay, H.: A method for registration of 3-D shapes. TPAMI 14, 239–256 (1992)

Toward Early Diagnosis of Lung Cancer

Ayman El-Baz[1], Georgy Gimel'farb[2], Robert Falk[3], Mohamed Abou El-Ghar[4], Sabrina Rainey[1], David Heredia[1], and Teresa Shaffer[1]

[1] Bioimaging Laboratory, Bioengineering Department, University of Louisville, Louisville, KY, USA
[2] Department of Computer Science, University of Auckland, Auckland, New Zealand
[3] Director, Medical Imaging Division, Jewish Hospital, Louisville, KY, USA
[4] Urology and Nephrology Department, University of Mansoura, Mansoura, Egypt

Abstract. Our long term research goal is to develop a fully automated, image-based diagnostic system for early diagnosis of pulmonary nodules that may lead to lung cancer. In this paper, we focus on generating new probabilistic models for the estimated growth rate of the detected lung nodules from Low Dose Computed Tomography (LDCT). We propose a new methodology for 3D LDCT data registration which is non-rigid and involves two steps: (i) global target-to-prototype alignment of one scan to another using the learned prior appearance model followed by (ii) local alignment in order to correct for intricate relative deformations. Visual appearance of these chest images is described using a Markov-Gibbs random field (MGRF) model with multiple pairwise interaction. An affine transformation that globally registers a target to a prototype is estimated by the gradient ascent-based maximization of a special Gibbs energy function. To handle local deformations, we displace each voxel of the target over evolving closed equi-spaced surfaces (iso-surfaces) to closely match the prototype. The evolution of the iso-surfaces is guided by a speed function in the directions that minimize distances between the corresponding voxel pairs on the iso-surfaces in both the data sets. Preliminary results show that the proposed accurate registration could lead to precise diagnosis and identification of the development of the detected pulmonary nodules.

1 Introduction

Because lung cancer is the most common cause of cancer deaths, fast and accurate analysis of pulmonary nodules is of major importance for medical computer-aided diagnostic systems (CAD).

Previous work. Tracking the temporal nodule behavior is a challenging task because of changes in the patient's position at each data acquisition, as well as effects of heart beats and respiration. In order to accurately measure how the nodules are developing in time, all these motions should be compensated by registering LDCT data sets taken at different time. Many methods have been proposed for solving medical image registration problems (see e.g. [1]) and to exclude the lung motions (see [2]). Moreover, it has been reported that the computer-assisted volume measurement is more reliable for small pulmonary nodules than the measurement by human experts [3]. Therefore, the remaining principal difficulty in monitoring and evaluating the nodule growth rate is automatic identification (or registration) of corresponding nodules in the follow-up scans. Registration of the two successive CT scans determines transformation of one image with respect to the other [4]. Some examples of previous works on registration of CT lung images are overviewed below.

Most of them exploit corresponding local structural elements (features) in the images. For the follow-up of small nodules, Brown et al. [5] developed a patient-specific model with 81% success for 27 nodules. Ko et al. [6] used centroids of local structures to apply rigid and affine image registration with 96% success for 58 nodules of 10 patients. To account for non-rigid motions and deformations of the lung, Woods et al. [7] developed an objective function using an anisotropic smoothness constraint and a continuous mechanical model. Feature points required by this algorithm are detected and registered as explained in [8], and then the continuous mechanical model is used to interpolate the image displacement.

2 Lung Motion Correction Models

2.1 Global Alignment

Basic Notation. Let $\mathcal{Q} = \{0, \ldots, Q-1\}$; $\mathbf{R} = [(x, y, z) : x = 0, \ldots, X-1; y = 0, \ldots, Y-1; z = 0, \ldots, Z-1]$, and $\mathbf{R_p} \subset \mathbf{R}$ be a finite set of scalar image signals (e.g. gray levels), a 3D arithmetic lattice supporting digital LDCT image data $g : \mathbf{R} \to \mathcal{Q}$, and an arbitrary-shaped part of the lattice occupied by the prototype, respectively. Let a finite set $\mathcal{N} = \{(\xi_1, \eta_1, \zeta_1), \ldots, (\xi_n, \eta_n, \zeta_n)\}$ of the (x, y, z)-coordinate offsets define neighboring voxels, or neighbors $\{((x + \xi, y + \eta, z + \zeta), (x - \xi, y - \eta, z - \zeta)) : (\xi, \eta, \zeta) \in \mathcal{N}\} \wedge \mathbf{R_p}$ interacting with each voxel $(x, y, z) \in \mathbf{R_p}$. The set $\mathcal{N}$ yields a 3D neighborhood graph on $\mathbf{R_p}$ that specifies translation invariant pairwise interactions between the voxels with n families $\mathcal{C}_{\xi,\eta,\zeta}$ of second-order cliques $c_{\xi,\eta,\zeta}(x, y, z) = ((x, y, z), (x + \xi, y + \eta, z + \zeta))$. Interaction strengths are given by a vector $\mathbf{V}^\mathsf{T} = \left[\mathbf{V}_{\xi,\eta,\zeta}^\mathsf{T} : (\xi, \eta, \zeta) \in \mathcal{N}\right]$ of potentials $\mathbf{V}_{\xi,\eta,\zeta}^\mathsf{T} = \left[V_{\xi,\eta,\zeta}(q, q') : (q, q') \in \mathcal{Q}^2\right]$ depending on signal co-occurrences; here T indicates transposition.

Data normalization. To account for possible monotone (order -preserving) changes of signals (e.g. due to different sensor characteristics), every LDCT data set is equalized using the cumulative empirical probability distribution of its signals.

Markov–Gibbs random field (MGRF) based appearance model. In a generic MGRF with multiple pairwise interaction, the Gibbs probability $P(g) \propto \exp(E(g))$ of an object g aligned with the prototype g° on $\mathbf{R_p}$ is specified with the Gibbs energy $E(g) = |\mathbf{R_p}|\mathbf{V}^\mathsf{T}\mathbf{F}(g)$ where $\mathbf{F}^\mathsf{T}(g)$ is the vector of scaled empirical probability distributions of signal co-occurrences over each clique family: $\mathbf{F}^\mathsf{T}(g) = [\rho_{\xi,\eta,\zeta}\mathbf{F}_{\xi,\eta,\zeta}^\mathsf{T}(g) : (\xi, \eta, \zeta) \in \mathcal{N}]$ where $\rho_{\xi,\eta,\zeta} = \frac{|\mathcal{C}_{\xi,\eta,\zeta}|}{|\mathbf{R_p}|}$ is the relative size of the family and $\mathbf{F}_{\xi,\eta,\zeta}(g) = [f_{\xi,\eta,\zeta}(q, q'|g) : (q, q') \in \mathcal{Q}^2]^\mathsf{T}$; here,

$f_{\xi,\eta,\zeta}(q,q'|g) = \frac{|\mathcal{C}_{\xi,\eta,\zeta;q,q'}(g)|}{|\mathcal{C}_{\xi,\eta,\zeta}|}$ are empirical probabilities of signal co-occurrences, and $\mathcal{C}_{\xi,\eta,\zeta;q,q'}(g) \subseteq \mathcal{C}_{\xi,\eta,\zeta}$ is a subfamily of the cliques $c_{\xi,\eta,\zeta}(x,y,z)$ supporting the co-occurrence $(g_{x,y,z} = q, g_{x+\xi,y+\eta,z+\zeta} = q')$ in g. The co-occurrence distributions and the Gibbs energy for the object are determined over $\mathbf{R}_p$, i.e. within the prototype boundary after an object is affinely aligned with the prototype. To account for the affine transformation, the initial image is resampled to the back-projected $\mathbf{R}_p$ by interpolation.

Learning the potentials. The MLE of $\mathbf{V}$ is proportional in the first approximation to the scaled centered empirical co-occurrence distributions for the prototype:

$$\mathbf{V}_{\xi,\eta,\zeta} = \lambda \rho_{\xi,\eta,\zeta} \left(\mathbf{F}_{\xi,\eta,\zeta}(g^\circ) - \frac{1}{Q^2}\mathbf{U} \right); \ (\xi,\eta,\zeta) \in \mathcal{N} \qquad (1)$$

where $\mathbf{U}$ is the vector with unit components. The common scaling factor λ is also computed analytically; it is approximately equal to Q^2 if $Q \gg 1$ and $\rho_{\xi,\eta,\zeta} \approx 1$ for all $(\xi,\eta,\zeta) \in \mathcal{N}$. In our case it can be set to $\lambda = 1$ because the registration uses only relative potential values and energies.

Learning the characteristic neighbors. To find the characteristic neighborhood set $\mathcal{N}$, the relative Gibbs energies $E_{\xi,\eta,\zeta}(g^\circ) = \rho_{\xi,\eta,\zeta} \mathbf{V}_{\xi,\eta,\zeta}^\mathsf{T} \mathbf{F}_{\xi,\eta,\zeta}(g^\circ)$ for the clique families, i.e. the scaled variances of the corresponding empirical co-occurrence distributions, are compared for a large number of possible candidates.

To automatically select the characteristic neighbors, we consider an empirical probability distribution of the energies as a mixture of a large "non-characteristic" low-energy component and a considerably smaller characteristic high-energy component: $P(E) = \pi P_{\text{lo}}(E) + (1-\pi) P_{\text{hi}}(E)$. Both the components $P_{\text{lo}}(E), P_{\text{hi}}(E)$ are of arbitrary shape and thus are approximated with linear combinations of positive and negative discrete Gaussians (EM-based algorithms introduced in [9] are used for both the approximation and the estimation of π). Example of the estimated characteristic neighbors is shown in Fig. 1.

Appearance-based registration. The desired affine transformation of an object g corresponds to a local maximum of its relative energy $E(g_\mathbf{a}) = \mathbf{V}^\mathsf{T} \mathbf{F}(g_\mathbf{a})$

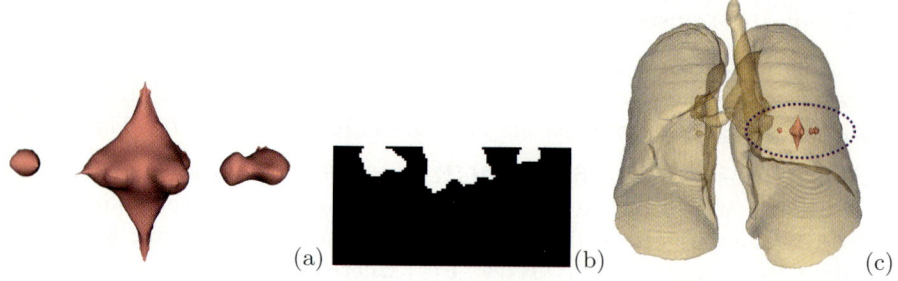

Fig. 1. The 3D neighborhood system (a) estimated for the lung tissues; its 2D cross section in the plane $\zeta = 0$ (b; in white) and its superposition onto the lungs reconstructed from the LDCT images (c)

under the learned appearance model $[\mathcal{N}, \mathbf{V}]$. Here, $g_\mathbf{a}$ is the part of the object image reduced to $\mathbf{R}_\mathbf{p}$ by the 3D affine transformation $\mathbf{a} = [a_{11}, \ldots, a_{34}]$: $x' = a_{11}x + a_{12}y + a_{13}z + a_{14}$; $y' = a_{21}x + a_{22}y + a_{23}z + a_{24}$; $z' = a_{31}x + a_{32}y + a_{33}z + a_{34}$. The initial transformation step is a pure translation with $a_{11} = a_{22} = a_{33} = 1$; $a_{12} = a_{13} = a_{21} = a_{23} = a_{31} = a_{32} = 0$, ensuring the most "energetic" overlap between the object and prototype. In other words, the chosen initial position $(a_{14}^*, a_{24}^*, a_{34}^*)$ maximizes the Gibbs energy. Then the gradient search for the local energy maximum closest to the initialization selects all the 12 parameters.

Figures 2(c,d) show the results of the global alignment of two segmented lungs. It is clear from Fig. 2(d) that the global alignment is not perfect due to local deformation.

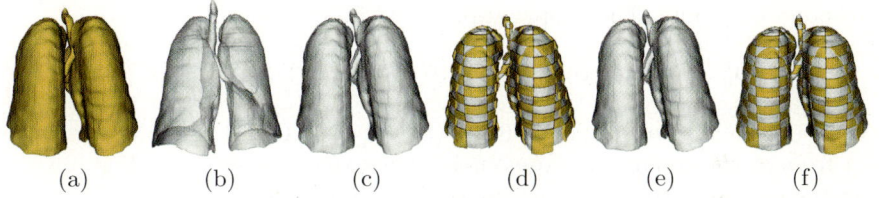

(a) (b) (c) (d) (e) (f)

Fig. 2. 3D global and local registration: (a) reference data, (b) target data, (c) target data after 3D affine transformation, (d) checkerboard visualization to show the motion of lung tissues, (e) results of our non-rigid registration, and (f) checkerboard visualization to show the quality of the proposed local deformation model.

2.2 Local Motion Model

To handle local deformations, we propose to deform the object over evolving closed equi-spaced surfaces (distance iso-surfaces) so that it closely matches the prototype. The evolution is guided by an exponential speed function and intends to minimize distances between corresponding voxel pairs on the iso-surfaces in both the images. The normalized cross correlation of the Gibbs energy is used to find correspondences between the iso-surfaces.

Our approach involves the following steps. First, a distance map inside the object is generated using fast marching level sets [10]. Secondly, the distance map is used to generate iso-surfaces (Fig. 3(b)). Note that the number of iso-surfaces is not necessarily the same for both the images and depends on the accuracy and the speed required by the user. The third step consists in finding correspondences between the iso-surfaces using the normalized cross correlation of the Gibbs energy. Finally, the evolution process deforms the iso-surfaces in the first data set (the target image) to match the iso-surfaces in the second data set (the prototype).

The following notation is used below for defining the evolution equation:

- $\mathbf{b}_{\mathbf{g}_1}^h = [\mathbf{p}_k^h : k = 1, \ldots, K] - K$ control points on a surface h on the reference data such that $\mathbf{p}_k = (x_k, y_k, z_k)$ form a circularly connected chain of line segments $(\mathbf{p}_1, \mathbf{p}_2), \ldots, (\mathbf{p}_{K-1}, \mathbf{p}_K), (\mathbf{p}_K, \mathbf{p}_1)$;

- $\mathbf{b}_{\mathbf{g}_2}^\gamma = [\mathbf{p}_n^\gamma : n = 1, \ldots, N]$ – N control points on a surface γ on the target data such that $\mathbf{p}_n = (x_n, y_n, z_n)$ form a circularly connected chain of line segments $(\mathbf{p}_1, \mathbf{p}_2), \ldots, (\mathbf{p}_{N-1}, \mathbf{p}_N), (\mathbf{p}_N, \mathbf{p}_1)$;
- $S(\mathbf{p}_k^h, \mathbf{p}_n^\gamma)$ – the Euclidean distance between a point on the surface h in the image $\mathbf{g}_1$ and the corresponding point on the surface γ in the image $\mathbf{g}_2$;
- $S(\mathbf{p}_n^\gamma, \mathbf{p}_n^{\gamma-1})$ – the Euclidean distance between a point on the surface γ in the image $\mathbf{g}_1$ and the nearest point on the surface $\gamma - 1$ in $\mathbf{g}_1$, and
- $\nu(.)$ – the propagation speed function.

The evolution $\mathbf{b}_\tau \to \mathbf{b}_{\tau+1}$ of a deformable boundary $\mathbf{b}$ in discrete time, $\tau = 0, 1, \ldots$, is specified by the system $\mathbf{p}_{n,\tau+1}^\gamma = \mathbf{p}_{n,\tau}^\gamma + \nu(\mathbf{p}_{n,\tau}^\gamma)\mathbf{u}_{n,\tau}$; $n = 1, \ldots, N$ of difference equations where $\nu(\mathbf{p}_{n,\tau}^\gamma)$ is a propagation speed function for the control point $\mathbf{p}_{n,\tau}^\gamma$ and $\mathbf{u}_{n,\tau}$ is the unit vector along the ray between the two corresponding points. The propagation speed function

$$\nu(\mathbf{p}_{n,\tau}^\gamma) = \min\left\{S(\mathbf{p}_k^h, \mathbf{p}_{n,\tau}^\gamma), S(\mathbf{p}_{n,\tau}^\gamma, \mathbf{p}_{n,\tau}^{\gamma-1}), S(\mathbf{p}_{n,\tau}^\gamma, \mathbf{p}_{n,\tau}^{\gamma+1})\right\}$$

satisfies the condition $\nu(\mathbf{p}_{n,\tau}^\gamma) = 0$ if $S(\mathbf{p}_k^h, \mathbf{p}_{n,\tau}^\gamma) = 0$ and prevents the current point from cross-passing the closest neighbor surfaces as shown in Fig. 3(a). The latter restriction is known as the smoothness constraint.

Again, the checkerboard visualization (Fig. 2(d)) of the data set in Fig. 2(a) and the aligned data set in Fig. 2(c) highlights the effect of the motion of lung tissues.

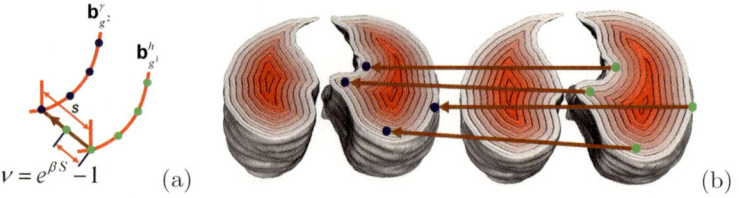

Fig. 3. (a) The proposed evolution scenario and (b) equi-spaced surfaces

3 Experimental Results and Conclusions

The proposed registration models were tested on the clinical datasets collected from 27 patients. Each patient has five LDCT scans, with the three months period between each two successive scans. This preliminary clinical database was collected by the LDCT scan protocol using a multidetector GE Light Speed Plus scanner with the following scanning parameters: slice thickness of 2.5 mm reconstructed every 1.5 mm, scanning pitch 1.5, pitch 1 mm, 140 KV, 100 MA, and F.O.V 36 cm.

After the two volumes at different time instants are registered, the task is to find out if the nodules are growing or not. For this purpose, the lung nodules were segmented after registration using our previous approach [11]. Once the nodules are segmented in the original and the registered image sequences, the

Table 1. Growth rate statistics for 14 patients with malignant nodules and 13 patients with benign nodules (p – statistical significance; μ – average rate, %; σ – standard deviation, %)

Scanning period	With the proposed registration					Without the registration				
	Malignant		Benign			Malignant		Benign		
	μ_M	σ_M	μ_B	σ_B	p	μ_M	σ_M	μ_B	σ_B	p
3 months	22	16	0.9	0.7	10^{-4}	5.6	4.8	2.8	1.9	0.1
6 months	49	20	2.9	2.3	10^{-4}	11	6.6	8.4	5.1	0.3
9 months	91	29	4.5	3.8	10^{-4}	24	9.3	17	11	0.1
12 months	140	32	5.4	4.3	10^{-4}	30	11	20	16	0.1

Table 2. Statistical analysis for the growth rate of the detected lung nodules for fourteen patients who have malignant nodules and thirteen patients who have benign nodules using ImageChecker commercial CT CAD system

Scanning period	Diameter-based follow up					Volume-based follow up				
	Malignant		Benign			Malignant		Benign		
	μ_M	σ_M	μ_B	σ_B	p	μ_M	σ_M	μ_B	σ_B	p
3 months	1.1	0.97	0.71	0.59	0.2229	6.15	3.91	3.67	2.73	0.0631
6 months	1.4	1.13	1.1	1.29	0.5254	11.7	4.37	9.27	4.17	0.1525
9 months	1.8	2.77	1.6	2.51	0.8461	21.9	9.93	16.17	9.97	0.0753
12 months	1.9	2.57	1.71	2.77	0.8548	31.3	12.3	22.21	12.7	0.0705

Table 3. Statistical analysis for the growth rate of the detected lung nodules for fourteen patients who have malignant nodules and thirteen patients who have benign nodules using the proposed approach in [12]

Scanning period	Malignant		Benign		
	μ_M	σ_M	μ_B	σ_B	p
3 months	9.25	7.5	4.91	2.93	0.0624
6 months	16.1	11.97	9.95	6.91	0.1183
9 months	23.7	16.43	13.87	9.85	0.0737
12 months	45.57	34.87	25.57	15.77	0.0699

volumes of the nodules are calculated using the Δx, Δy, and Δz values from the scanner (in our case, 0.7, 0.7, and 2.5 mm, respectively).

Our statistical analysis using the unpaired t-test shows that the difference between the average growth rate of malignant nodules and the average growth rate of benign nodules found with the proposed approach is statistically significant (as shown in Table 1). Also, Table 1 shows that no significant difference is found if the growth rate is measured without the data alignment step.

The advantages of using the proposed CAD system to estimate the growth rate of the detected lung nodules are highlighted by estimating the growth rate of the same detected lung nodules with ImageChecker commercial CT CAD system. This software provides two methods to monitor the detected lung nodules:

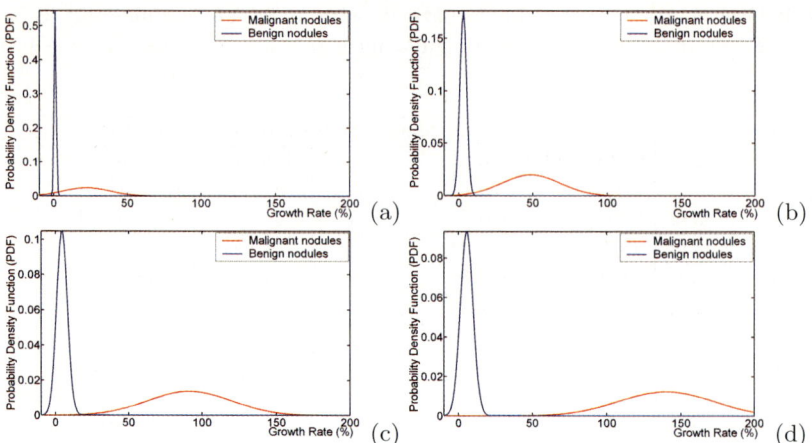

Fig. 4. Estimated probability density functions (probabilistic models) of the relative growth rates for 14 malignant and 13 benign nodules using our Linear Combination of Discrete Gaussian (LCDG) model [9]: (a) three months, (b) six months, (c) nine months, and (d) twelve months.

1) estimating the growth rate based on measuring the changes of the diameter of the largest cross section in the detected nodules and 2) estimating the growth rate based on measuring the volumetric changes of the detected nodules. The estimated growth rate using this CAD system is shown in Table 2. The main limitation of the ImageChecker CT CAD system is not considering the local deformation of the lung tissues from breathing and the heart beating. For this reason, the statistical analysis shown in Table 2 does not demonstrate a significant difference between the estimated growth rate of malignant lung nodules and the estimated growth rate of benign lung nodules, a difference which is detected by our proposed CAD system. The same limited ability to estimate the growth rate of the detected lung nodules exists in the most recent published work by Reeves et al. [12]. The statistical analysis of the estimated growth rates of the same detected nodules using the proposed approach in [12] is shown in Table 3. A traditional Bayes classifier based on the analysis of the growth rate of both benign and malignant nodules for 27 patients diagnosed 14 and 13 patients as malignant and benign, respectively. For simplicity, this classifier used a multivariate Gaussian model of the growth rate with the rates at 3, 6, 9, and 12 months as four discriminant features. The same patients were diagnosed by biopsy (the ground truth) showing that the classification was 100% correct. Therefore, the proposed image analysis techniques could be a promising supplement to the current technologies for diagnosing lung cancer.

We introduced a new approach for registering 3D spiral LDCT images that combines an initial affine global alignment of one scan (the target) to another scan (the reference) using the learned prior appearance model and subsequent local alignments that account for more intricate deformations.

References

1. Maintz, J., Viergever, M.: A Survey of Medical Image Registration. Journal of Medical Image Analysis 2, 1–36 (1998)
2. Ko, J., Naidich, D.: Computer-Aided Diagnosis and the Evaluation of Lung Disease. Journal of Thoracic Imaging 19(3), 136–155 (2004)
3. Kostis, W., Yankelevitz, D., Reeves, A., Fluture, S., Henschke, C.: Small Pulmonary Nodules: Reproducibility of Three-Dimensional Volumetric Measurement and Estimation of Time to Follow-Up CT. Radiology 231(2), 446–452 (2004)
4. Horn, B.: Closed-Form Solution of Absolute Orientation using Unit Quaternions. Journal of the Optical Society of America B 4(4), 629–642 (1987)
5. Brown, M., McNitt-Gray, M., Mankovich, N., Goldin, J., Hiller, J., Wilson, L., Aberle, D.: Method for Segmenting Chest CT Image Data using an Anatomical Model: Preliminary Results. IEEE TMI 16(6), 828–839 (1997)
6. Ko, J., Betke, M.: Chest CT: Automated Nodule Detection and Assessment of Change over Time-Preliminary Experience. Radiology 218, 267–273 (2001)
7. Woods, K., Fan, L., Chen, C., Wang, Y.: Model Supported Image Registration and Warping for Change Detection in Computer-Aided Diagnosis. In: Applied Imagery Pattern Recognition (AIPR) Annual Workshops, Washington DC (2000)
8. Fan, L., Chen, C.: An Integrated Approach to 3D Warping and Registration from Lung Images. In: Proceedings of SPIE Conf. Developments in X-Ray Tomography II (July 1999)
9. El-Baz, A., Gimel'farb, G.: EM Based Approximation of Empirical Distributions with Linear Combinations of Discrete Gaussians. In: Proc. of IEEE International Conference on Image Processing (ICIP 2007), San Antonio, Texas, USA, September 16–19, vol. IV, pp. 373–376 (2007)
10. Sethian, J.: Fast Marching Level Set Method for Monotonically Advancing Fronts. Proc. National Academy of Sciences, USA 93, 1591–1595 (1996)
11. El-Baz, A., Farag, A., Gimel'farb, G., Falk, R., Abou El-Ghar, M., Eldiasty, T.: A Framework for Automatic Segmentation of Lung Nodules from Low Dose Chest CT Scans. In: Proc. IAPR Int. Conf. on Pattern Recognition (ICPR 2006), Hong Kong, August 20–24, vol. 3, pp. 611–614 (2006)
12. Reeves, A., Chan, A., Yankelevitz, D., Henschke, C., Kressler, B., Kostis, W.: On Measuring the Change in Size of Pulmonary Nodules. IEEE TMI 25(4), 435–450 (2006)

Lung Extraction, Lobe Segmentation and Hierarchical Region Assessment for Quantitative Analysis on High Resolution Computed Tomography Images*

James C. Ross[1,2,3], Raúl San José Estépar[2,3], Alejandro Díaz[4,5],
Carl-Fredrik Westin[2,3], Ron Kikinis[3], Edwin K. Silverman[1,5], and George R. Washko[5]

[1] Channing Laboratory, Brigham and Women's Hospital, Boston, MA
[2] Laboratory of Mathematics in Imaging, Brigham and Women's Hospital,
Harvard Medical School, Boston, MA
[3] Surgical Planning Lab, Brigham and Women's Hospital, Boston, MA
[4] Pontificia Universidad Catolica de Chile, Chile
[5] Pulmonary and Critical Care Division, Brigham and Women's Hospital, Boston, MA

Abstract. Regional assessment of lung disease (such as chronic obstructive pulmonary disease) is a critical component to accurate patient diagnosis. Software tools than enable such analysis are also important for clinical research studies. In this work, we present an image segmentation and data representation framework that enables quantitative analysis specific to different lung regions on high resolution computed tomography (HRCT) datasets. We present an offline, fully automatic image processing chain that generates airway, vessel, and lung mask segmentations in which the left and right lung are delineated. We describe a novel lung lobe segmentation tool that produces reproducible results with minimal user interaction. A usability study performed across twenty datasets (inspiratory and expiratory exams including a range of disease states) demonstrates the tool's ability to generate results within five to seven minutes on average. We also describe a data representation scheme that involves compact encoding of label maps such that both "regions" (such as lung lobes) and "types" (such as emphysematous parenchyma) can be simultaneously represented at a given location in the HRCT.

1 Introduction

Regional assessment of lung disease is an important component of both diagnosis and therapy. Furthermore, localized quantitation of disease can provide insight into underlying disease mechanisms, and tools that offer such regional assessment are invaluable in large epidemiological studies. As an example, chronic obstructive pulmonary disease (COPD) is projected to be the 3rd leading cause of death worldwide by 2020 [1,2,3]. There are at least two distinct mechanisms of expiratory airflow obstruction in COPD subjects: emphysematous destruction of the lung parenchyma leading to airway collapse and intrinsic disease of the small airways [4,5]. The relative burden of airspace and airways disease can vary, however, within a cohort of subjects with similar lung function

---

* This work was supported by NIH grants U01-HL089897, U01-HL089856, K23HL089353-01A1, and the Parker B. Francis Foundation.

[6], and even regionally within the lungs of an individual [7]. Standard metrics, such as Forced Expiratory Volume in one second (FEV1), while reproducible and easy to measure are not necessarily indicative of the cause of airflow obstruction. Because of this, image based methods are useful for investigating subjects with COPD and helpful to define more homogeneous subsets of subjects within a cohort with comparable degrees of airflow obstruction.

Anatomically, the lungs consist of distinct lobes: the left lung is divided into upper and lower lobes, while the right lung is divied into upper, middle, and lower lobes. Each lobe has airway, vascular, and lymphatic supplies that are more or less independent of those supplies to other lobes. Hence, the lobes represent natural anatomic units over which to compute image-based disease metrics. Fissures (left oblique, right oblique, and right horizontal) define the boundaries between the lobes and present as 3D surfaces that have greater attenuation (i.e. are brighter) than the surrounding lung parenchyma in HRCT datasets. However, advanced disease states (emphysema), atelectasis, and certain imaging protocols (expiratory acquisitions) can make it extremely difficult to detect the fissures in certain regions, and the judgment of medical professionals is typically needed in order to define the location of these structures.

There have been a variety of lobe segmentation and fissure detection approaches developed to date. [8] uses fuzzy sets to define likely (oblique) fissure locations followed by a graph search to select the most probable fissure locations in 2D slices. Their method requires manual initialization, and results were reported on normal subjects. [9] first obtain a vessel segmentation from which they derive a distance map. The distance map, in conjunction with the original image and user interaction, drive watershed segmentation of the lobes. [10] perform lobe segmentation in a similar fashion but use a segmented airway tree to seed the watershed segmentation in an automatic framework. [11] generate ridge maps to enhance fissures and then use active open contours to delineate the fissures. Ten patients with pulmonary nodules were tested in their study. Algorithm run times were approximately five minutes and manual correction was needed in about 2.4% of the fissure regions. [12] use deformable mesh models to segment the lobes. They report accuracy results of 1 mm to 3 mm on a limited number of test sets.

In order to address segmentation failure modes that can be caused by extreme disease states, specific imaging protocols, or insufficiently segmented auxiliary structures (vessels or airways), manual interaction is needed. In this paper we present an interactive lung lobe segmentation scheme that enables fast, easy, and accurate segmentation in spite of such factors. The segmentation results are incorporated into an overall data representation framework that provides a compact way to simultaneously encode both lung regions (e.g. lobes) and types (e.g. parenchyma states). This representation provides a convenient way to interrogate the underlying CT data to assist with both diagnosis and exploratory research. In section 2 the lobe segmentation method and preprocessing steps are presented. The data representation framework is also explained. In section 3 image preprocessing and lobe segmentation examples are shown. We also conducted a study in which two pulmonologists used the lobe segmentation tool to produce segmentations across twenty HRCT datasets; results of this study are presented. Finally, conclusions are drawn in section 4.

2 Methods

In this section we begin by explaining the data representation scheme we use to encode segmentation results throughout the image processing pipeline. Next, we describe the image pre-processing steps required for the interactive lobe segmentation tool. Finally, we describe the lobe segmentation tool itself and discuss its usage and the underlying segmentation algorithm.

2.1 Label Map Representation

There are two abstract lung components of interest for the purposes of quantitative analysis: we refer to these as "regions" and "types". Currently, the regions we extract include the left upper and lower lobes; the right lower, middle and upper lobes; the left lung; the right lung; and the whole lung. These regions are naturally represented in a hierarchical framework, as depicted in the figure below. E.g., the left upper lobe is a part of the left lung, which is a part of the whole lung. The types currently represented include airway, vessel, normal parenchyma, and emphysematous parenchyma. The label maps produced by the segmentation routines (described below) are represented as 16-bit data; the least significant eight bits are used to encode the lung region while the most significant eight bits encode the lung type. This enables up to 256 regions and 256 types to be encoded within a single dataset. Extensions to the list of regions given above could include each lobe's set of sub-lobes, e.g., while extensions to the list of types could include a range of disease states (ground glass parenchyma, reticular parenchyma, etc.) as well as other basic anatomical types (airway lumen, airway wall, etc). The table below provides an example numbering scheme. As an example the 16-bit value corresponding to 00000110 00000100 (a base ten value of 1540) corresponds to reticular tissue in the right upper lobe while the 16 bit value 00000000 00000010 (a base ten value of 2) corresponds simply to right lung.

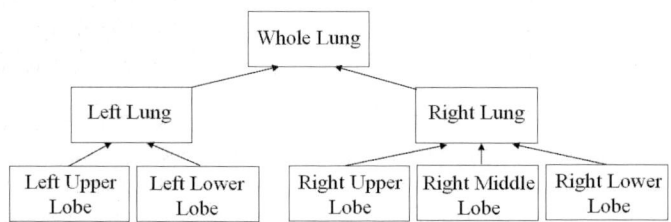

Fig. 1. Lung Region Hierarchy Diagram

2.2 Offline Image Processing

We employ a completely automatic image processing pipeline to generate initial segmentations of regions and types of interest. Prior to segmentation, the HRCT dataset is pre-processed with a median filter using a 3x3x3 kernel. The lung mask is then segmented using an approach very similar to that outlined in [13]. Briefly, this involves initial gray level thresholding using Otsu's method followed by morphological closing to fill in high

Table 1. Regions and Types Numbering Scheme

Region	8-Bit Value	Type	8-Bit Value
Undefined	0	Undefined	0
Whole Lung	1	Normal Parenchyma	1
Right Lung	2	Airway	2
Left Lung	3	Vessel	3
Right Upper Lobe	4	Emphysematous	4
Right Middle Lobe	5	Ground Glass	5
Right Lower Love	6	Reticular	6
Left Upper Lobe	7	Nodular	7
Left Lower Lobe	8		

attenuating areas within the lung field. These high attenuating areas tend mostly to be pulmonary vessels, so we assign these voxels a type value of "vessel" with the understanding that in some cases diseased lung parenchyma (due to edema or fibrosis) may be labeled vessel as well. We label the data as such in the eventuality that voxels labeled as "vessel" may be able to initialize more sophisticated vessel segmentation routines, but it should be emphasized that vessel segmentation is not the current objective.

In order to properly label airways outside the lung field (trachea and main bronchi), we apply connected component region growing to segment the airways. The patient orientation is obtained from the input DICOM dataset; this allows a search for the trachea from the correct end of the dataset: axial slices are iteratively considered until a small foreground structure in the center of the image is detected. Spatial consistency over several slices ensures that the object in question is indeed the trachea and not a spurious foreground object. Once this region of the trachea is determined, an initial threshold and seed location are selected to initialize the region growing algorithm. Region growing is repeated iteratively, and at each iteration the volume of the extracted airway tree is computed. Provided that the change in volume from one iteration to the next is within a certain tolerance, iteration continues with progressively higher threshold values. The final threshold is the one that lies at the boundary between acceptable airway segmentation and segmentation "explosion" due to leakage into parenchyma. To differentiate between airways that lie

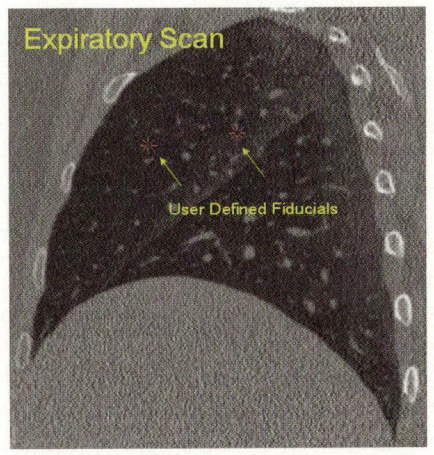

Fig. 2. User-defined points along right horizontal fissure

within the parenchyma and those that lie outside the lung field, each axial slice is considered in turn. Connected components is performed to identify regions labeled as lung and those segmented as airways. If the perimeter of an airway component is surrounded by at least 75% lung region, that entire component is assigned the region "whole lung", otherwise the assigned region is "undefined". Following the approach outlined in [13], minimum cost paths are determined using Dijkstra's algorithm in order to separate the left and right lungs. Given the known patient orientation in the image field, the lung regions are further labeled as "left" and "right".

2.3 Interactive Lobe Segmentation

We have developed a novel interactive lung lobe segmentation tool that enables a user to quickly, easily, and accurately generate segmentations of the left upper and lower lobes and right upper, middle, and lower lobes. This tool has been incorporated as a plugin for the Slicer3 software application. From the user's perspective, use of the tool involves loading the HRCT dataset and corresponding lung label map produced by the offline image processing pipeline. Next, the user simply scrolls through the HRCT data and clicks on points along three major fissures: left oblique, right oblique, and right horizontal. Figure 2 gives an example of two user-defined points along the right horizontal fissure. The dataset shown is an expiratory acquisition, and it is easy to appreciate from this example how faint fissures can be in such scans. Only a handful of points is necessary in most cases. Once these points have been selected, the segmentation algorithm is invoked, and the results are displayed for user verification. Additional points may then be added in areas of misalignment.

The underlying algorithm driving the lobe segmentation method employs thin plate splines (TPS) [14] to define height surfaces corresponding to the three fissures. The equation of the height surface is given by

$$f(x,y) = a_1 + a_2 x + a_3 y + \sum_{i=1}^{n} w_i U(|P_i + (x,y)|) \tag{1}$$

where $U(r) = r^2 \log r$ is the radial basis function. The coefficient vector, $\mathbf{a} = (a_1, a_2, a_3)$, and the weight vector, $\mathbf{w} = (w_1, \ldots, w_n)$ are determined from the n user-defined points, P, such that the height function's bending energy, E, is minimized.

$$E = \iint_{R^2} \left(\frac{\partial^2 f}{\partial x^2}\right)^2 + \left(\frac{\partial^2 f}{\partial x \partial y}\right)^2 + \left(\frac{\partial^2 f}{\partial y^2}\right)^2 dx dy \tag{2}$$

Intuitively, TPS provide an interpolation scheme whereby a minimally curved surface is defined such that it passes through all the user-selected points. A separate 3D surface is defined for each of the three fissures. The region of support for the left oblique fissure is the projection of the left lung region onto the axial plane and similarly for the fissures in the right lung. Using the height surface equation given above, voxels in the lung field falling on the surface (within the tolerance of a voxel width) are assigned a type value of "oblique fissure" or "horizontal fissure" depending on which user defined point set is being considered. We impose the anatomically-based constraint that the right horizontal fissure is only defined as such in regions where its height function value is above that of the right oblique fissure. Connected component region labeling is then used to label the upper and lower lobes in the left lung from the lung regions that lie above and below the left oblique fissure, respectively. Similar logic is applied to label the regions in the right lung. Note that during this region relabeling operation, the types assigned from the offline processing (airway and vessel) remain unchanged.

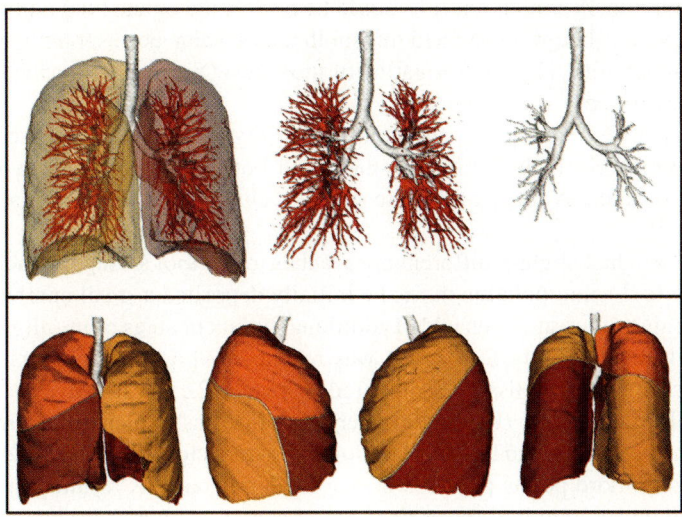

Fig. 4. Region and Type Segmentation. Top row shows example results from the automatic processing stage. Bottom row shows lobe segmentation results produced with the interactive lobe segmentation tool.

3 Results

Figure 4 shows results produced from the automatic processing stage (top row) and the interactive lobe segmentation tool (bottom row). The image in the upper left depicts all regions (left and right lung) and types (airways and vessels) extracted during this stage. Vessel and airway types are isolated and displayed in the upper middle image, and airway type is depicted in the upper right. It should be emphasized that the lobe segmentation results (bottom row) are merged with the output of the offline, automatic image processing stage, so the final label map includes regions left upper lobe, left lower lobe, right upper lobe, right middle lobe, right lower lobe; and types airway, vessel, oblique fissure, and horizontal fissure.

The utility of the region-type framework can be illustrated by figure 3 in which the following region-type pairs are isolated: (undefined, airway), (left upper lobe, airway), (left lower lobe, airway), etc. Alternatively, the user could have isolated all airways in the left lung, or simply the entire segmented airway tree, all with a single label

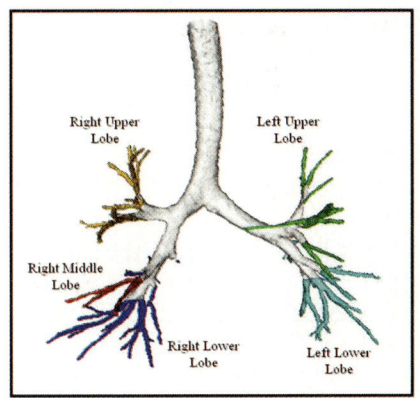

Fig. 3. Airways and Lobe Regions

map representation. A similar analysis could be performed on the lung parenchyma: by assigning all voxels below a specified threshold a type value corresponding to "emphysematous parenchyma" [15], interrogation of the dataset for disease localization can be efficiently performed.

The results of the lobe segmentation tool's usability study are summarized in table 2. Twenty datasets were included in the study, and both inspiratory and expiratory exams were considered. A range of disease states (including severe emphysema) are also represented.

The two users had slightly different approaches to the tool's usage. Reader 1 tended to rely on the tool's interpolation more: he initially deposited a small number of points, executed the algorithm, and then added additional points in areas of misalignment. This was repeated until a satisfactory result was reached. While this approach ultimately required fewer points per fissure (compared to reader 2), the iterative nature caused longer overall usage times. (Usage time here is defined as the length of time between the first clicked point and the final declaration of a satisfactory result). Reader 2 initially deposited many more points per fissure than reader 1, but this resulted in a better fit surface at the outset, required fewer fixes, and resulted in shorter usage times overall. Note that algorithm run time is mainly a function of the HRCT dataset size, and the dependence on the number of user-defined points is negligible.

Table 2. Lobe Segmentation Results. Cases are numbered and indicated as either inspiratory (i) or expiratory (e). The first three columns for each reader represent the number of points selected for the left oblique fissure (LO), the right oblique fissure (RO), and the right horizontal fissure (RH). Euclidean distances reflect the agreement between the two readers for each of the three fissures.

	Reader 1				Reader 2				Euclidean Distance (mm)			
	LO	RO	RH	Usage Time (minutes)	LO	RO	RH	Usage Time (minutes)	LO	RO	RH	Algorithm Time (seconds)
Case 1 (e)	12	8	8	6	10	16	8	7	1.75 ± 2.72	2.58 ± 2.36	4.08 ± 3.69	45
Case 2 (i)	10	13	14	7	10	21	11	7	0.98 ± 0.98	3.60 ± 3.41	2.96 ± 3.75	53
Case 3 (e)	8	24	9	9	26	41	13	10	4.17 ± 5.15	4.35 ± 4.81	2.97 ± 3.39	48
Case 4 (i)	6	18	7	9	20	26	14	5	2.83 ± 2.69	2.68 ± 2.72	2.39 ± 2.15	46
Case 5 (e)	8	13	6	6	13	18	5	3	2.75 ± 2.59	1.10 ± 1.32	0.80 ± 0.70	26
Case 6 (i)	11	15	9	5	14	17	7	5	1.86 ± 1.73	0.85 ± 0.98	4.51 ± 3.93	41
Case 7 (e)	9	16	15	6	13	19	10	4	1.45 ± 1.54	0.81 ± 0.81	6.44 ± 8.15	26
Case 8 (i)	10	15	9	6	18	15	7	5	1.61 ± 1.76	2.19 ± 2.15	1.21 ± 1.14	33
Case 9 (e)	16	22	15	10	8	23	14	4	1.25 ± 1.27	3.74 ± 4.60	2.27 ± 1.90	32
Case 10 (i)	9	13	14	9	16	15	12	4	0.99 ± 1.07	4.01 ± 3.75	4.32 ± 7.73	46
Case 11 (e)	12	20	11	7	17	23	19	4	1.32 ± 1.23	1.29 ± 1.24	0.66 ± 0.81	51
Case 12 (e)	9	12	20	10	17	18	13	4	3.32 ± 3.25	1.69 ± 2.60	3.02 ± 2.73	35
Case 13 (e)	12	31	10	11	19	22	17	3	1.82 ± 1.75	2.21 ± 2.95	7.19 ± 6.41	45
Case 14 (i)	11	16	11	6	13	17	15	7	1.59 ± 1.51	1.23 ± 1.40	4.02 ± 4.91	50
Case 15 (e)	20	12	6	6	13	20	11	4	5.18 ± 7.17	2.43 ± 2.63	2.43 ± 2.22	40
Case 16 (e)	6	17	6	5	11	30	14	8	1.59 ± 1.55	1.88 ± 2.10	13.7 ± 13.8	43
Case 17 (i)	9	20	8	8	10	41	13	8	2.08 ± 2.03	4.21 ± 4.82	2.02 ± 2.00	53
Case 18 (e)	13	15	6	5	13	23	11	5	1.85 ± 1.78	1.24 ± 1.18	4.45 ± 3.68	50
Case 19 (i)	17	17	6	7	29	24	16	6	1.34 ± 1.36	1.72 ± 1.85	1.65 ± 1.41	54
Case 20 (e)	11	24	7	8	22	43	14	12	1.84 ± 1.97	1.37 ± 1.34	19.4 ± 18.67	46
Average	10.95	17.05	9.85	7.3	15.6	23.6	12.2	5.75	2.08 ± 2.26	2.26 ± 2.45	4.52 ± 4.66	43.15

Despite the two approaches used by readers 1 and 2, the overall segmentation results are in very good agreement across the set of exams. This is reflected by the Euclidean distances between fissures presented in table 2. Disagreement is most noticeable for the right horizontal fissure. This is not surprising given that minor (horizontal) fissures are incomplete more often than major (oblique) fissures [16]. In such cases readers have to make boundary decisions in the near absence of image features.

4 Conclusion

We have presented a novel lung lobe segmentation tool that requires minimal user input and enables users to quickly and accurately produce lobe segmentations in spite of severe disease states and imaging protocols that can obscure fissure image signatures. The tool enables satisfactory results to be produced on HRCT datasets (which can consist of several hundred slices) in a matter of minutes. We also described a data representation scheme that provides a flexible framework for regional image quantitation.

References

1. Gulsvik, A.: The global burden and impact of chronic obstructive pulmonary disease worldwide. Monaldi. Arch. Chest. Dis. 56(3), 261–264 (2001)
2. Pauwels, R.A., Buist, A.S., Ma, P., Jenkins, C.R., Hurd, S.S.: Global strategy for the diagnosis, management, and prevention of chronic obstructive pulmonary disease: National heart, lung, and blood institute and world health organization global initiative for chronic obstructive lung disease (GOLD): executive summary. Respir Care 46(8), 798–825 (2001)
3. Mannino, D.M.: COPD: epidemiology, prevalence, morbidity and mortality, and disease heterogeneity. Chest 121(5 Suppl.), 121S–126S (2002)
4. Hogg, J.C., Macklem, P.T., Thurlbeck, W.M.: Site and nature of airway obstruction in chronic obstructive lung disease. N. Engl. J. Med. 278(25), 1355–1360 (1968)
5. Cosio, M.G., Hale, K.A., Niewoehner, D.E.: Morphologic and morphometric effects of prolonged cigarette smoking on the small airways. Am. Rev. Respir. Dis. 122(2), 265–321 (1980)
6. Washko, G., Criner, G., Mohsenifar, Z., Sciurba, F., Sharafkhaneh, A., Make, B., Hoffman, E., Reilly, J.: Assessing pulmonary function with CT scanning in patients with emphysema. Proc. Am. Thorac. Soc. 2(A259) (2005)
7. Hasegawa, M., Nasuhara, Y., Onodera, Y., Makita, H., Nagai, K., Fuke, S., Ito, Y., Betsuyaku, T., Nishimura, M.: Airflow limitation and airway dimensions in chronic obstructive pulmonary disease. Am. J. Respir. Crit. Care Med. 173(12), 1309–1315 (2006)
8. Zhang, L., Reinhardt, J.M.: Detection of lung lobe fissures using fuzzy logic. In: Chen, C.T., Clough, A.V. (eds.) Medical Imaging 1999: Physiology and Function from Multidimensional Images. Proc. of SPIE, vol. 3660, pp. 188–199 (1999)
9. Kuhnigk, J.M., Hahn, H., Hindennach, M., Dicken, V., Krass, S., Peitgen, H.O.: Lung lobe segmentation by anatomy-guided 3D watershed transform. In: Sonka, M., Fitzpatrick, M. (eds.) Medical Imaging 2003: Image Processing. Proc. of SPIE, vol. 5032, pp. 1482–1490 (2003)
10. Ukil, S., Hoffman, E.A., Reinhardt, J.M.: Automatic lung lobe segmentation in x-ray CT images by 3D watershed transform using anatomic information from the segmented airway tree. In: Fitzpatrick, M., Reinhardt, J.M. (eds.) Medical Imaging 2005: Image Processing. Proc. of SPIE, vol. 5747, pp. 556–567 (2005)
11. Wang, J., Betke, M., Ko, J.P.: Pulmonary fissure segmentation on CT. Med. Image Anal. 10(4), 530–547 (2006)
12. Blaffert, T., Barschdorf, H., Von Berg, J., Dries, S., Franz, A., Klinder, T., Lorenz, C., Renisch, A., Wiemker, R.: Lung lobe modeling and segmentation with individualized surface meshes. In: Reinhardt, J.M., Pluim, J. (eds.) Medical Imaging 2008: Image Processing. Proc. of SPIE, vol. 6914 (2008)

13. Hu, S., Hoffman, E., Reinhardt, J.: Automatic lung segmentation for accurate quantitation of volumetric x-ray CT images. IEEE Transactions on Medical Imaging 20(6), 490–498 (2001)
14. Bookstein, F.: Principal warps: thin-plate splines and the decomposition of deformations. IEEE Transactions on Pattern Analysis and Machine Intelligence 11(6) (June 1989)
15. Muller, N., Staples, C., Miller, R.: "Density mask": an objective method to quantitate emphysema using computed tomography. Chest 94, 782–787 (1988)
16. Aziz, M., Ashizawa, K., Nagaoki, K., Hayashi, K.: High resolution CT anatomy of the pulmonary fissures. Journal Thoracic Imaging 19(3), 186–191 (2004)

Learning COPD Sensitive Filters in Pulmonary CT

Lauge Sørensen[1], Pechin Lo[1], Haseem Ashraf[2], Jon Sporring[1], Mads Nielsen[1], and Marleen de Bruijne[1,3]

[1] Department of Computer Science, University of Copenhagen, Denmark
{lauges,pechin,madsn,sporring,marleen}@diku.dk
[2] Department of Respiratory Medicine, Gentofte University Hospital, Denmark
[3] Biomedical Imaging Group Rotterdam, Erasmus MC, The Netherlands

Abstract. The standard approaches to analyzing emphysema in computed tomography (CT) images are visual inspection and the relative area of voxels below a threshold (RA). The former approach is subjective and impractical in a large data set and the latter relies on a single threshold and independent voxel information, ignoring any spatial correlation in intensities. In recent years, supervised learning on texture features has been investigated as an alternative to these approaches, showing good results. However, supervised learning requires labeled samples, and these samples are often obtained via subjective and time consuming visual scoring done by human experts.

In this work, we investigate the possibility of applying supervised learning using texture measures on random CT samples where the labels are based on external, non-CT measures. We are not targeting emphysema directly, instead we focus on learning textural differences that discriminate subjects with chronic obstructive pulmonary disease (COPD) from healthy smokers, and it is expected that emphysema plays a major part in this. The proposed texture based approach achieves an 69% classification accuracy which is significantly better than RA's 55% accuracy.

1 Introduction

The traditional tools for diagnosis of chronic obstructive pulmonary disease (COPD) are pulmonary function tests (PFT)s. These are cheap and fast to acquire but suffer from several limitations, including insensitivity to early stages of COPD and lack of reproducibility [1]. More recently, computed tomography (CT) imaging has been used for direct measurement of one the components of the disease, namely emphysema, which is characterized by gradual loss of lung tissue and appears as low attenuation areas within the lung tissue. There are two common approaches for assessing emphysema in CT images: visual assessment, including sub-typing of emphysema based on radiological experience [2], and measures derived from the CT attenuation histogram, with the most widely used measure being relative area of voxels below a certain threshold (RA) [2].

RA disregards potentially valuable information in the CT image, such as spatial relations between voxels. Various alternatives have been suggested for analyzing emphysema in CT images. One such approach is analysis of bullae size distribution [3]. Another approach is supervised texture classification where a classifier is trained on manually annotated regions of interest (ROI)s [4,5,6,7]. The output of a trained classifier can be used for COPD quantification by fusion of individual ROI posterior probabilities [7].

Supervised learning requires a training set with labeled data which is usually acquired by manual annotation. However, having human observers manually annotating ROIs can be problematic. First of all, it is a subjective process suffering from inter-observer variability. This problem can partly be addressed by consensus readings of several experts. Another drawback is the time needed for doing the annotations, and when the data set is large, manual annotation is infeasible. Further, analysis will be limited to current knowledge and experience of experts, and there can be a bias towards typical cases in the annotated data set. In the emphysema case, this means restricting ourselves to the three known radiographic subtypes of emphysema [2].

In this work, we explore the possibility of diagnosing COPD in volumetric CT images of the lung based on texture classification without manual labeling. PFTs are used to define two subject groups, a healthy and a COPD group, and ROIs are randomly sampled from these two groups and labeled according to group membership. A supervised learning framework is applied for learning filters that are able to separate the two groups. This approach is less committed, objective, and can potentially uncover new textural patterns, or emphysema subtypes, as being part of COPD.

Classification is based on the k nearest neighbor (kNN) classifier using dissimilarity between sets of feature histograms as distance, and the features are based on a rotation invariant, multi-scale Gaussian filter bank [8]. The classification framework used here is similar to the one used in [6], but with a larger set of filters and in 3D instead of 2D. The obtained results are compared to RA in the experiments.

2 Selection of Training Samples

The classification framework relies on a grouping of the CT images into different subject groups, according to non-CT measures, and a lung segmentation S obtained from each CT image I. ROIs are sampled at random within the lung fields in the images and assigned labels, ω_i, according to subject group membership. The lung segmentation S is used for two purposes. First of all, it is used for limiting the random sampling to the lung fields. Secondly, it is used for allowing only lung parenchyma voxels to contribute to the obtained feature histograms as described in Section 3. In this work, we use PFTs to group the CT images, and S is extracted from I using thresholding and morphological smoothing, similar to [9].

3 Texture Measures

Each ROI is represented by a set of feature histograms representing distributions of filter responses computed in the ROI. The filtering is done by normalized convolution [10] with a binary mask to exclude contribution from larger non-parenchyma structures, such as the trachea, the main bronchi, and the exterior of the lung. A rotation invariant, multi-scale Gaussian filter bank [8] comprising eight basis filters is used.

3.1 Filters

Eight different measures of local image structure are used as base filters: the Gaussian function G_σ; the three eigenvalues of the Hessian $\lambda_{i,\sigma}, i = 1, 2, 3$, ordered such that $|\lambda_{1,\sigma}| \geq |\lambda_{2,\sigma}| \geq |\lambda_{3,\sigma}|$; gradient magnitude $||\nabla G_\sigma||_2 = \sqrt{I_{x,\sigma}^2 + I_{y,\sigma}^2 + I_{z,\sigma}^2}$, where $I_{x,\sigma}$ denotes the partial first order derivative of image I w.r.t. x at scale σ; Laplacian of the Gaussian $\nabla^2 G_\sigma = \lambda_{1,\sigma} + \lambda_{2,\sigma} + \lambda_{3,\sigma}$; Gaussian curvature $K_\sigma = \lambda_{1,\sigma} \lambda_{2,\sigma} \lambda_{3,\sigma}$; and the Frobenius norm of the Hessian $||H_\sigma||_F = \sqrt{\lambda_{1,\sigma}^2 + \lambda_{2,\sigma}^2 + \lambda_{3,\sigma}^2}$.

The filtering is performed by normalized convolution [10] with a Gaussian function

$$I_\sigma = \frac{(S(\mathbf{x})I(\mathbf{x})) * G_\sigma(\mathbf{x})}{S(\mathbf{x}) * G_\sigma(\mathbf{x})},$$

where $*$ denotes convolution and segmentation S computed from image I is used as an indicator function, indication whether voxel $\mathbf{x} = [x, y, z]^T$ is a lung parenchyma voxel or not. Derivatives are computed on the filtered images using finite differences.

3.2 Histogram Estimation

The filter responses are quantized into feature histograms. The bins edges are derived using adaptive binning [11]. This technique locally adapts the histogram bin widths to the data set at hand such that each bin contains the same mass when computing the histogram of all data while disregarding class labels. Only voxels within a lung segmentation S are used, and the resulting histogram is normalized to sum to one.

4 Classification

Classification is performed using the kNN classifier with summed histogram dissimilarity as distance

$$D(\mathbf{x}, \mathbf{y}) = \sum_{i=1}^{N_f} L(f_i(\mathbf{x}), f_i(\mathbf{y})), \tag{1}$$

where N_f is the number of feature histograms, $L(\cdot, \cdot)$ is a histogram dissimilarity measure, and $f_i(\mathbf{x}) \in \mathbb{R}^{N_b}$ is the i'th feature histogram with N_b bins estimated from an ROI centered on $\mathbf{x}$. Two histogram dissimilarity measures L are considered: L1-norm and L2-norm. The L1-norm and L2-norm are instances of the p-norm

$$L_p(H, K) = ||H - K||_p = \left(\sum_{i=1}^{N_b} |H_i - K_i|^p \right)^{1/p},$$

with $p = 1$ or $p = 2$ and where $H \in \mathbb{R}^{N_b}$ and $K \in \mathbb{R}^{N_b}$ are histograms each with N_b bins.

The posterior probability of belonging to class ω_i given that the current ROI is centered on voxel $\mathbf{x}$ is estimated in the kNN classifier by $P(\omega_i|\mathbf{x}) = k_{\omega_i}(\mathbf{x})/k$, where $k_{\omega_i}(\mathbf{x})$ is the number of nearest neighbors according to (1) belonging to class ω_i obtained from a total of k nearest neighbors.

5 Experiments

5.1 Data

Experiments are conducted using 296 low-dose volumetric CT images (tube voltage 140 kV, exposure 40 mAs, slice thickness 1 mm, and in-plane resolution ranging from 0.72 to 0.78 mm) from 296 different (ex-)smokers enrolled in the Danish Lung Cancer Screening Trial [12].

Two subjects groups, $\omega_i = \{\text{healthy}, \text{COPD}\}$, are defined based on the GOLD criteria [13]. These criteria use two PFTs based measures: expiratory volume in one second over forced vital capacity (FEV$_1$/FVC), and forced expiratory volume in one second corrected for age, sex, and height (FEV$_1$%pred). The healthy group is defined by FEV$_1$%pred ≥ 80 and FEV$_1$/FVC ≥ 0.7. The COPD group is defined by FEV$_1$%pred $< 80\%$ and FEV$_1$/FVC < 0.7, which corresponds to GOLD stage II or higher [13]. The healthy group contains 144 CT images and the COPD group contains 152 CT images. For each CT image, 50 cubic $r \times r \times r$ ROIs are sampled at random, thus a total of 14800 ROIs are used in the experiments. A separate set of 10 ROIs per subject is sampled to compute the adaptive binning described in Section 3.2.

Since PFTs are not very reproducible [1], the grouping is enhanced by ensuring that the criteria are fulfilled at two time instances; both when the CT images were acquired and one year after.

5.2 Training and Parameter Selection

There are several parameters to set in the classification system: ROI size r, number of histogram bins N_b, k in the kNN classifier, histogram dissimilarity measure L, and which filters, out of the ones described in Section 3.1, to use at which scales σ. In this work, we use $N_b = \sqrt[3]{\text{number of voxels in the ROI}} = r$ bins. This ensures that the standard deviation across bins is proportional to the standard deviation within bins. The best combination of $r = \{21, 31, 41\}$,

$L = \{L_1, L_2\}$, and $k = \{25, 35, 45\}$ is learned using cross-validation, and sequential forward feature selection (SFS) is used for determining the optimal filter subset for each combination. The scales of the filters are sampled exponentially according to $\sigma_i = 0.6(\sqrt{2})^i$ mm, $i = 0, \ldots, 6$. Together with the original intensity, this amounts a total of 57 feature histograms considered in the feature selection.

The CT images in the training set are divided into two sets by randomly placing half the images of each group in each set. The classification system is trained, and parameters are tuned by using one set as prototypes in the kNN classifier and by choosing the features and parameter settings that minimize the classification error on the other set.

5.3 Evaluation

The performance is estimated using 3-fold cross-validation, training the classifier as described above and applying the best performing kNN classifier, in terms of validation error, with the training set as prototypes to the test set. The results are evaluated in three ways. First, by maximum a posteriori classification accuracy on the ROIs. For the remaining cases, each subject is measured by posterior fusion: the mean healthy posterior probability is computed across all sampled ROIs in the subject. The second evaluation is maximum a posteriori classification accuracy on subject level, and the third is the ability to separate the healthy group of subjects from the COPD group according to a rank sum test on the mean healthy posterior.

Since the texture based CT measurements are proposed as an alternative to RA, we compare the obtained results to RA, computed both on the sampled ROIs and on whole lungs. The best RA for ROI classification, RA_i, is determined using cross-validation on the same data sets as used when training the kNN classifier on the range $i = [-960, -950, \ldots, -890]$ HU. Thresholds in this range are commonly used when measuring emphysema in CT [2]. The best percentage threshold used for classification based on RA is also determined during this procedure.

5.4 Results

The filters selected by SFS using the best parameter setting are shown in Table 1. Three of the filters are selected in two out of three folds. The selected optimal kNN parameters are $r = 41$ in all three folds and ordered by fold $L = L_2, L_1, L_2$ and $k = 35, 45, 35$. The selected optimal RA parameters are, ordered by fold, HU threshold $= -890, -960, -890$ and percentage threshold $= 32, 15, 47$. ROI classification accuracies, subject classification accuracies, areas under the receiver operating characteristic curve (AUC), and p-values for difference between groups according to a rank sum test are shown in Table 2. RA using -950 HU is also included for the sake of completeness. kNN achieves significantly higher ROI and subject classification accuracy than RA, $p < 10^{-4}$ according to McNemar's test. RA is able the pick up an overall group effect but has poor discrimination ability on a subject level. Figure 1(a) shows receiver operating characteristic (ROC) curves for the kNN classifier on the ROIs as well as for RA on the whole

Table 1. Selected filters in kNN in the cross-validation procedure

Fold	Selected filters
1	$\nabla^2 G_{0.6}, \lambda_{2,0.6}, \lambda_{3,0.6}, \lambda_{2,0.85}, \|\nabla G_{2.4}\|_2, \lambda_{1,2.4}, \nabla^2 G_{3.4}, K_{3.4}, \|\nabla G_{4.8}\|_2$
2	$K_{0.6}, G_{1.2}, \|\nabla G_{1.2}\|_2, \|\nabla G_{4.8}\|_2, K_{4.8}$
3	$\nabla^2 G_{0.6}, \|H_{0.6}\|_F, \|\nabla G_{1.7}\|_2, \lambda_{1,1.7}, G_{2.4}, K_{4.8}$

Table 2. Classification accuracies, AUCs, and p-values from a rank sum test

Measure	ROI accuracy	Subject accuracy	AUC	p-value
kNN	0.58	0.69	0.75	$< 10^{-4}$
RA$_{\text{learned}}$ (ROIs)	0.53	0.55	-	-
RA$_{890}$ (whole lung)	-	-	0.58	0.012
RA$_{950}$ (whole lung)	-	-	0.59	0.012

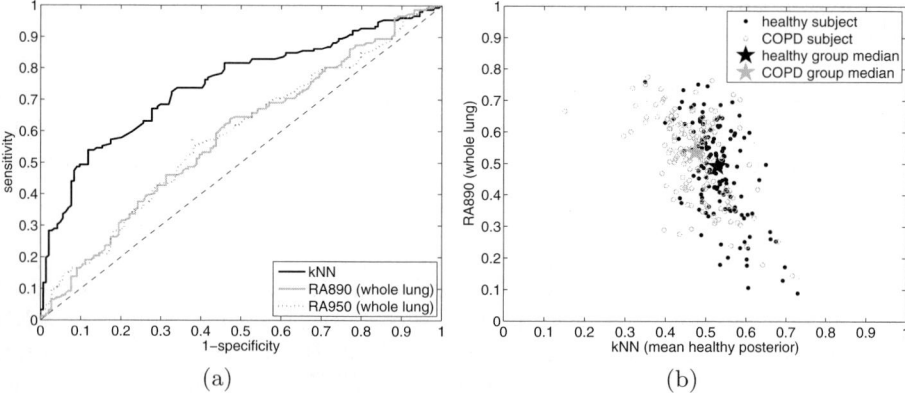

Fig. 1. (a) ROC curves at subject level. The curve for kNN is based on mean healthy posterior computed for each subject. (b) Scatter plot of mean kNN healthy posterior versus RA$_{890}$.

lung field. In the case of kNN, the parameter being varied is the healthy posterior threshold, and in the case of RA, the parameter is the threshold on the percentage of low attenuation voxels. AUC is clearly larger for the kNN classifier compared to RA. Figure 1(b) shows the COPD measures obtained by mean kNN healthy posterior and RA$_{890}$. The separation between the groups is much better for kNN as indicated by the classification accuracies and p-values in Table 2.

6 Discussion

The proposed texture based method outperforms RA in all comparisons. The classification accuracies in Table 2 are significantly higher, both at ROI and at subject level. When computing RA on the full lung, which is the common way of applying RA [2], more information is used than is available to the kNN classifier, and even in these cases RA performs worse.

The ROI classification accuracies in Table 2 are relatively low when compared to accuracies reported in the literature [4,5,6,7]. However, it is important to note that in the cited cases, the ROIs and labels are obtained by manual labeling of "interesting" areas in CT images. In this work, no manual labeling has been done, instead the labels were obtained by taking random samples of lung tissue within the lung fields. We expect the COPD group to also contain samples with no apparent lung disease pattern in a random sampling setup, hence, the classes are likely to overlap more when using this approach.

Intensity can be directly related to emphysema since emphysematous regions have lower intensities due to loss of lung tissue, and therefore original and smoothed intensities are considered important features. Nevertheless, intensity is not selected in the first cross-validation fold, but the Laplacian of the Gaussian which approximates the zero-order information at a larger scale is selected and may compensate for this. Three filters are selected in two out of three cross-validation folds: Laplacian of the Gaussian, $\nabla^2 G_{0.6}$, gradient magnitude, $||G_{4.8}||_2$, and Gaussian curvature $K_{4.8}$. $\nabla^2 G_{0.6}$ can be seen as a blob detector at low scale, and it may be small low attenuation areas within the lung tissue that are picked up by this filter. $||G_{4.8}||_2$ measures large scales edges and $K_{4.8}$ measures large scale blobs.

Emphysema is not uniformly distributed within the lungs. Paraseptal emphysema is located in the periphery of the lung, and centrilobular emphysema is predominantly in the upper lobes [2]. It would therefore be interesting to see whether the COPD related textural differences found in this work are localized in specific regions of the lungs.

Subjects were grouped using PFTs, and thus the classification system is trained to imitate diagnosis of COPD based on PFT. As can be seen from Figure 1(b) and the reported numbers, the learned filters achieve this to some degree. The result is a quantitative measure of COPD which may be more sensitive and reproducible than PFT. This facilitates study of disease development and progression in large cohorts such as current lung cancer screening trials, which may help improve the understanding of pathogenesis of COPD and eventually lead to improved diagnosis, prognosis, and treatment of individuals.

In summary, we conclude that it is possible to learn COPD sensitive filters in CT in a less committed, data-driven manner without, the often tedious, manual annotation of data. A kNN classifier using texture measures based on these filters is capable of separating healthy subjects from subjects with COPD, when these are diagnosed based solely on PFTs.

Acknowledgments. This work is partly funded by the Danish Council for Strategic Research (NABIIT), the Netherlands Organisation for Scientific Research (NWO), and AstraZeneca, Lund, Sweden.

References

1. Dirksen, A., Holstein-Rathlou, N.H., Madsen, F., Skovgaard, L.T., Ulrik, C.S., Heckscher, T., Kok-Jensen, A.: Long-range correlations of serial FEV1 measurements in emphysematous patients and normal subjects. J. Appl. Physiol. 85(1), 259–265 (1998)
2. Webb, W.R., Müller, N., Naidich, D.: High-Resolution CT of the Lung, 3rd edn. Lippincott Williams & Wilkins (2001)
3. Blechschmidt, R.A., Werthschützky, R., Lörcher, U.: Automated CT image evaluation of the lung: a morphology-based concept. IEEE Trans. Med. Imaging 20(5), 434–442 (2001)
4. Mendonça, P.R.S., Padfield, D.R., Ross, J.C., Miller, J.V., Dutta, S., Gautham, S.M.: Quantification of emphysema severity by histogram analysis of CT scans. In: Duncan, J.S., Gerig, G. (eds.) MICCAI 2005. LNCS, vol. 3749, pp. 738–744. Springer, Heidelberg (2005)
5. Xu, Y., Sonka, M., McLennan, G., Guo, J., Hoffman, E.A.: MDCT-based 3-D texture classification of emphysema and early smoking related lung pathologies. IEEE Trans. Med. Imaging 25(4), 464–475 (2006)
6. Sørensen, L., Shaker, S.B., de Bruijne, M.: Texture classification in lung CT using local binary patterns. In: Metaxas, D., Axel, L., Fichtinger, G., Székely, G. (eds.) MICCAI 2008, Part I. LNCS, vol. 5241, pp. 934–941. Springer, Heidelberg (2008)
7. Park, Y.S., Seo, J.B., Kim, N., Chae, E.J., Oh, Y.M., Lee, S.D., Lee, Y., Kang, S.H.: Texture-based quantification of pulmonary emphysema on high-resolution computed tomography: Comparison with density-based quantification and correlation with pulmonary function test. Investigative Radiology 43(6), 395–402 (2008)
8. ter Haar Romeny, B.M.: Applications of scale-space theory. In: Gaussian Scale-Space Theory, pp. 3–19. Kluwer Academic Publishers, Dordrecht (1997)
9. Hu, S., Hoffman, E., Reinhardt, J.: Automatic lung segmentation for accurate quantitation of volumetric X-ray CT images. IEEE Trans. Med. Imaging 20(6), 490–498 (2001)
10. Knutsson, H., Westin, C.F.: Normalized and differential convolution: Methods for interpolation and filtering of incomplete and uncertain data. In: CVPR, June 1993, pp. 515–523 (1993)
11. Ojala, T., Pietikäinen, M., Harwood, D.: A comparative study of texture measures with classification based on featured distributions. Pattern Recognition 29(1), 51–59 (1996)
12. Pedersen, J.H., Ashraf, H., Dirksen, A., Bach, K., Hansen, H., Toennesen, P., Thorsen, H., Brodersen, J., Skov, B.G., Døssing, M., Mortensen, J., Richter, K., Clementsen, P., Seersholm, N.: The Danish randomized lung cancer CT screening trial–overall design and results of the prevalence round. J. Thorac. Oncol. 4(5), 608–614 (2009)
13. Rabe, K.F., Hurd, S., Anzueto, A., Barnes, P.J., Buist, S.A., Calverley, P., Fukuchi, Y., Jenkins, C., Rodriguez-Roisin, R., van Weel, C., Zielinski, J.: Global strategy for the diagnosis, management, and prevention of chronic obstructive pulmonary disease: GOLD executive summary. Am. J. Respir. Crit. Care Med. 176(6), 532–555 (2007)

Automated Anatomical Labeling of Bronchial Branches Extracted from CT Datasets Based on Machine Learning and Combination Optimization and Its Application to Bronchoscope Guidance

Kensaku Mori[1,2], Shunsuke Ota[1], Daisuke Deguchi[1], Takayuki Kitasaka[2,3], Yasuhito Suenaga[1,2], Shingo Iwano[4], Yosihnori Hasegawa[2,4], Hirotsugu Takabatake[5], Masaki Mori[6], and Hiroshi Natori[7]

[1] Graduate School of Information Science, Nagoya University,
kensaku@is.nagoya-u.ac.jp
[2] Innovative Research Center for Preventive Medical Engineering, Nagoya University
[3] Faculty of Management and Information Science, Aichi Institute of Technology
[4] Graduate School of Medicine, Nagoya University
[5] Sapporo Minami-Sanjyo Hospital
[6] Sapporo Kosei Hospital
[7] Nishioka Hospital

Abstract. This paper presents a method for the automated anatomical labeling of bronchial branches extracted from 3D CT images based on machine learning and combination optimization. We also show applications of anatomical labeling on a bronchoscopy guidance system. This paper performs automated labeling by using machine learning and combination optimization. The actual procedure consists of four steps: (a) extraction of tree structures of the bronchus regions extracted from CT images, (b) construction of AdaBoost classifiers, (c) computation of candidate names for all branches by using the classifiers, (d) selection of best combination of anatomical names. We applied the proposed method to 90 cases of 3D CT datasets. The experimental results showed that the proposed method can assign correct anatomical names to 86.9% of the bronchial branches up to the sub-segmental lobe branches. Also, we overlaid the anatomical names of bronchial branches on real bronchoscopic views to guide real bronchoscopy.

1 Introduction

A bronchoscope is a flexible endoscope for observing the inside of the bronchus. A chest physician inserts a bronchoscope into the airway through the mouth or the nose to perform a diagnosis, a biopsy, or for treatment. However, the bronchus has a complex tree structure, so physicians easily get disoriented. A system that can guide physicians is strongly expected to be developed. On the other hand, a high resolution CT has also become available after the release of a multi-detector CT scanner. Such CT and bronchoscopic images can be combined, it would be possible to assist bronchoscopic procedures. Several research groups have been working on the development of bronchoscopic navigation systems that utilize pre-operative CT images as maps. If we can overlay the anatomical names of branches currently being observed or paths to target locations [1] on real bronchoscope images, it would be helpful for physicians.

Several research groups have developed automated anatomical labeling procedures for bronchial tree structures [2,3,4]. Anatomical labeling is performed by comparing input bronchial tree structures with branching pattern models. Kitaoka et al. [2] developed a matching algorithm of branching models and input tree structures using a weighted maximum clique search approach. However, their algorithm does not work well when the tree structures of the input bronchial branches differ from those of model. To cope with this problem, Mori et al. [3] developed a method that can handle variations of branching patterns by introducing multiple branching pattern models. In their method, if we assign anatomical names to a large number of cases, we must also prepare a large number of models to obtain accurate results. Ota presented a method for anatomical labeling based on machine learning [5]. In this method, we considered branch names as categories of the machine learning. However if a mislabeling occurs at a branch, the consequent branches are also mislabeled in the previous method [5]. Such mislabeling often occurs in the right main lobe part of the left lobe part where many branches show similar features in the method [5].

To solve the above problems, we propose a novel approach for anatomical labeling by introducing combination optimization. Classifiers that output branch name candidates with likelihoods are constructed by learning the feature vectors of the bronchial branch names of the learning datasets. The best combination of branch names are obtained under anatomical constraint.

2 Method

2.1 Overview

Figure 1 shows the processing flow of our proposed method. We construct classifiers that output bronchial branch name candidates with likelihoods using learning datasets. A machine learning approach is utilized here. In the anatomical labeling process, we compute the feature values of bronchial branches extracted from CT images. Then we compute the bronchial branch name candidates with the likelihoods for each bronchial branch using the classifiers. Finally, we determine the anatomical names for each branch by a combination optimization technique. In both the learning and test (labeling) phases, we extract the bronchus regions and the bronchial tree structure from the 3D CT images by Kitasaka's method [6]. The starting point of the tree structure is the trachea. We represent the i-th bronchial branch as $\mathbf{b}_i$ ($i = 1, 2, \cdots, N$. N is the number of bronchial branches.)

For assisting real bronchoscopy, we overlay the following anatomical names of the bronchial branches: (a) where a bronchoscope currently exists; (b) child

Automated Anatomical Labeling of Bronchial Branches

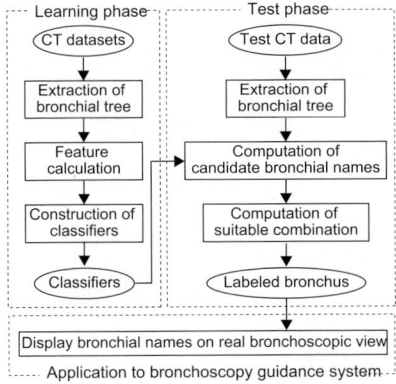

Fig. 1. Flowchart of proposed method

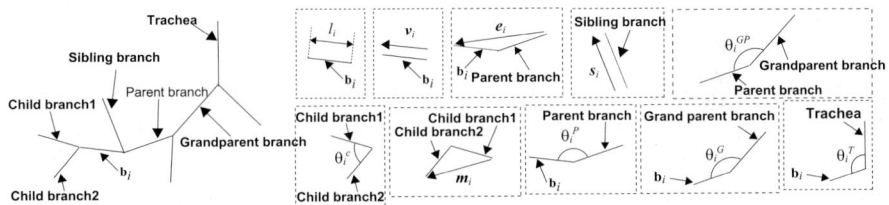

Fig. 2. Ten feature values used in the proposed method

branches of the current branch; and (c) the path to the target point (a set of anatomical names where an bronchoscope should be visited to reach the target point.)

2.2 Feature Values Computed at Each Bronchial Branch

We compute the following ten feature values for $\mathbf{b}_i$ shown in Fig. 2: (1) l_i: length of $\mathbf{b}_i$, (2) $\mathbf{v}_i$: running direction of $\mathbf{b}_i$, (3) $\mathbf{m}_i$: averaged direction of the running direction of the child branches of $\mathbf{b}_i$, (4) $\mathbf{e}_i$: relative coordinate of the end point of $\mathbf{b}_i$ against the parent branch of $\mathbf{b}_i$, (5) $\mathbf{s}_i$: running direction of sibling branches of $\mathbf{b}_i$, (6) θ_i^c : angle between child branches of $\mathbf{b}_i$, (7) θ_i^G: angle between $\mathbf{b}_i$ and its grandparent branch, (8) θ_i^P: angle between $\mathbf{b}_i$ and its parent branch, (9) θ_i^{GP}: angle between grandparent branch of $\mathbf{b}_i$ and parent branch of $\mathbf{b}_i$, and (10) θ_i^T : angle between trachea and $\mathbf{b}_i$.

2.3 Learning Phase (Training of Classifiers)

Preparation of Learning Datasets. We prepare learning datasets by computing the feature values of the bronchial branches extracted from the CT images. We also manually assign anatomical names to each bronchial branch.

710   K. Mori et al.

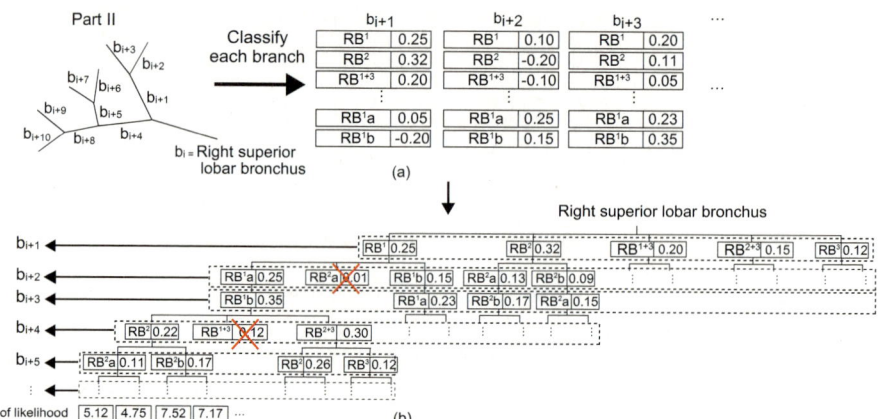

Fig. 3. Illustration of procedures for anatomical labeling of bronchial branches using a combinatorial optimization approach: (a) Example for classifying branches in region II; (b) Example for constructing a combination tree

Construction of Classifiers Using Multi-class AdaBoost. We construct classifiers that output bronchial branch name candidates with likelihoods. These classifiers are constructed using a multi-class AdaBoost technique [7]. Thresholding is used as a weak classifier of AdaBoost. We divide the airway tree into six parts: bronchi of: ((i) central area, (ii) right upper lobe part, (iii) right middle lobe part, (iv) right lower lobe part, (v) left upper lobe part, and (vi) left lower lobe part, For each part, classifiers $\mathbf{H}_\alpha$ ($\alpha = \text{I}, \cdots, \text{VI}$) are constructed and trained by learning datasets. Part division is performed to reduce the number of branch name combinations computed in the labeling procedure.

2.4   Test Phase (Anatomical Labeling)

Generation of List of Bronchial Branch Name Candidates. When we classify bronchial branch $\mathbf{b}_i$ existing in part α by classifier $\mathbf{H}_\alpha$, the classifier outputs set $(\mathcal{B}_i^\alpha)$ of pair $(\mathcal{L}_j)$ of category (L_j) and the likelihood of category (l_j) for branch $\mathbf{b}_i$. This process is formulated as

$$\mathcal{B}_i^\alpha = \left\{ \left(L_i^j, l_i^j\right) = \mathcal{L}_i^j : j = 1, 2, \cdots, N_\alpha \right\} = \mathbf{H}_\alpha(\mathbf{b}_i), \tag{1}$$

where N_α shows the number of categories existing in part α. The above process is illustrated in Fig. 3(a). In this example, the process generates sets of a pair of the bronchial branch name candidates (categories) and the likelihoods for all bronchial branches existing in part II using classifier $\mathbf{H}_\text{II}$.

Construction of Combination Tree. We generate combination tree $\mathcal{T}$ that enumerates the multiple pairs of a bronchial branch name candidate and its likelihood as nodes by

$$\mathcal{T} = \left\{ t_i^j = (L_i^j, l_i^j) : i = 1, 2, \cdots, W_j, j = 1, 2, \cdots, D \right\} \tag{2}$$

from the processing results of the previous step. The anatomical constraint of the bronchial tree is considered in the construction of $\mathcal{T}$. Here, we represent the branch name candidate as L_i^j and its likelihood as l_i^j. Also, we denote the number of nodes at the j-th depth of $\mathcal{T}$ and the depth of $\mathcal{T}$ as D.

The actual procedure for constructing combination tree $\mathcal{T}$ is explained by Fig. 3(b). First, we construct a combination tree whose root is the origin branch of each part. In the figure, the root branch is $\mathbf{b}_i$=right superior lobar bronchus. Then we traverse the bronchial tree from $\mathbf{b}_i$ by depth-first search and add a pair of bronchial branch name candidate and its likelihood at the same depth of $\mathcal{T}$ as the node. In this process, we eliminate nodes added to the combination tree using the rule of the branch names between a parent and a child or siblings. For example, in Fig. 3, $\mathbf{b}_{i+2}$ is a child branch of $\mathbf{b}_{i+1}$, If the branch name candidate of $\mathbf{b}_{i+1}$ is "RB^1 (= Rt. B^1)", $\mathbf{b}_{i+2}$ cannot be labeled "RB^2_a". Hence, we do not add this node. Similarly, $\mathbf{b}_{i+4}$ is a sibling branch of $\mathbf{b}_{i+1}$. If the branch name candidate of $\mathbf{b}_{i+1}$ is "RB^1", $\mathbf{b}_{i+2}$ cannot be labeled "RB^{1+3}". Therefore, we do not add this node. By considering anatomical constraint, computation time can be reduced related to the construction of $\mathcal{T}$.

Anatomical Labeling Using Combination Tree. Anatomical labeling is finally performed by finding path $\mathcal{L}^*$ showing the maximum of the sum of the likelihoods along with it in $\mathcal{T}$. This process is formulated as

$$\mathcal{L}^* = \arg\max_{\mathcal{L} \in \mathcal{T}} \left(l_i^1 + l_j^2 + \cdots + l_k^D \right), \tag{3}$$

where path $\mathcal{L} = \{t_i^1, t_j^2, \cdots, t_k^D\}$ is a set of nodes that exists on a path from the root node to the terminal node.

2.5 Application to Bronchoscope Guidance System

We utilize anatomical labeling results to overlay the anatomical names of a branch and its child branches currently being observed on the real bronchoscopic images in the bronchoscopy guidance system. Deguchi's method [8] was used to obtain the branch currently being observed. Furthermore, we compute the insertion path of a bronchoscope by a set of bronchial branch name [3] and overly it on a real bronchoscopic image. During a real bronchoscopy, the bronchoscope location is marked on the path overlaid on real bronchoscopic images. If the bronchoscope deviates off from the pre-planned path, the system shows a "WRONG WAY" message,

3 Experiments

We applied the proposed method to 90 cases of 3D CT images. The bronchial regions and branching structures were obtained by Kitasaka's method and manually corrected. To train the classifiers, anatomical names were manually assigned. The number of training data is not sufficient, because there are so many variation

Table 1. Accuracy of methods in [3], [5] and proposed ones (A) and (B) in each lobe (TR: trachea, LM: left main bronchus, RM: right main bronchus, RU: right upper, RL: tight middle and lower, LU: left upper and LL: left lower lobes)

	Accuracy of segmental (subsegmental) branch for each part [%]					
	TR, RB, LB	RU	RM	LU	LL	TOTAL
Previous [3]	100	73.6	83.5	90.5	76.7	83.5
Previous [5]	100 (100)	86.9 (85.2)	89.6 (81.7)	98.4 (91.6)	87.7 (79.0)	91.3 (84.3)
Proposed (a)	100 (100)	81.8 (78.2)	93.1 (86.2)	98.5 (92.6)	89.8 (81.1)	92.2 (86.9)
Proposed (b)	100 (100)	81.9 (78.9)	85.2 (73.0)	91.1 (77.2)	79.2 (75.1)	85.6 (78.6)

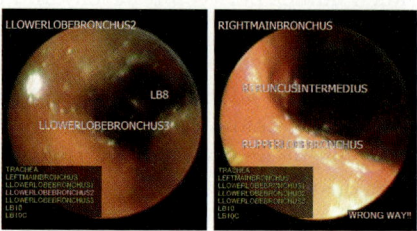

Fig. 4. Application of anatomical labeling in a bronchoscopy guidance system. Cases of inserting a bronchoscope to (right) correct path and (left) incorrect path.

in bronchial branch names. A branch called LB^7 rarely exists. Since the number of samples belonging to such categories is very small, this affects the learning of the classifiers, because the feature values obtained from such branches show sparse distribution in the feature space. Therefore, we organized two experiments: (a) adding 100 pairs of samples to all categories generated by normal random and (b) no addition of samples. We used the means and the variances of the feature values of each category as the means and the variances of the normal random. For both cases, we measured the accuracy of the anatomical labeling for branches up to the segmental branches and the sub-segmental branches under the leave-one-out method. For comparison, we also performed the anatomical labeling procedures described in [3,5]. Table 1 shows the labeling results. Here accuracy is computed by (the number of branched correctly labeled) / (the total number of branches)

We utilized the anatomical labeling results in the bronchoscopy guidance system. Figure 4 shows examples of such a bronchoscopy guidance system using an EM tracker. The system shows the bronchial branch names at appropriate positions on the real bronchoscopic images. Figure 4 (right) shows the case where a bronchoscope was inserted into the planned branch and (left) is where the bronchoscope was inserted into the wrong branch.

4 Discussion and Conclusion

This paper presented a method for anatomical labeling using combination optimization to precisely assign anatomical names to branches of a large number

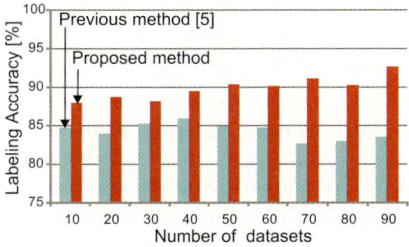
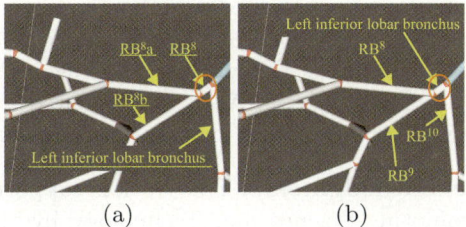

Fig. 5. Comparison of accuracy between previous[3] and proposed methods when number of datasets is increased

Fig. 6. Examples of results of anatomical labeling. White lines represent bronchial branches: (a) previous method [9], and (b) proposed one. Underlines show mislabeled branches.

of cases. To confirm the efficacy of the introduction of the machine learning approach in anatomical labeling, we measured the labeling accuracy by changing the number of cases. We randomly selected 10 to 90 cases and calculated the labeling accuracy by the previous method [3] (model-based approach) and the proposed method (machine learning approach.) The results are shown in Fig. 5. In the previous method, labeling accuracy became maximum when the number of cases was 40 and dud not change much for larger cases. In contrast, when we increase the number of cases in the proposed method, the labeling accuracy also increased. As stated in Section 1, we expected to improve the labeling accuracy by such a large number of cases.

Figure 6 shows the labeling results of the method described in [5] and the proposed methods. In this figure, the underlined branch names show incorrectly labeled branches. The branch name having the maximum likelihood of a target branch, which is surrounded by a circle and whose correct name is 'left inferior lobar bronchus' is RB^8. Hence, the previous method assigned RB^8 to the target branch, and the branches beyond it are mislabeled. On the other hand, the sum of the likelihood for labeling the target branch as 'left inferior lobar bronchus' is higher than that of RB^8, so the proposed method was able to correctly label it. As shown in Table 1, the proposed method improved labeling accuracy in most lung part except for RU. Labeling accuracy is significantly improved in RM and LL regions. If a mislabeling occurs at a branch in the previous method [5], the consequent branches were also mislabeled. Such mislabeling often occurred in RM and LL regions where many branches show similar features, On the other hand, the proposed method prevented such mislabeling by combination optimization.

We can see that the labeling accuracy is improved by adding samples artificially generated by normal random because some branches (categories), especially the branches of the right lower and the left lower lobes have a very small amount of samples. In such case, samples are sparsely distributed in the feature space. Consequently the learning process is affected. Further investigation for such cases is needed.

This paper presented a method for automated anatomical labeling of bronchial branches extracted from 3D CT images. We applied the proposed method to 90 cases of 3D chest CT images. Labeling accuracy was 86.9% for branches up to the sub-segmental level. Also, we presented a method to display anatomical names on real bronchoscopic images. Future work includes evaluation using more cases.

Acknowledgments. This work is supported by Special Coordination Funds for Promoting Science and Technology by the MEXT, Grant-in-aid for Scientific Research by JSPS and Grant-in-aid for Cancer Research by MHLW, Japan.

References

1. Kiraly, A.P., Helferty, J.P., Hoffman, E.A., McLennan, G., Higgins, W.E.: Three-Dimensional Path Planning for Virtual Bronchoscopy. IEEE Trans. Med. Imaging 23, 1365–1379 (2004)
2. Kitaoka, H., Park, Y., Tschirren, J., Reinhardt, J.M., Sonka, M., McLennan, G., Hoffman, E.A.: Automated nomenclature labeling of the bronchial tree in 3D-CT lung images. In: Dohi, T., Kikinis, R. (eds.) MICCAI 2002. LNCS, vol. 2489, pp. 1–11. Springer, Heidelberg (2002)
3. Mori, K., Ema, S., Kitasaka, T., Mekada, Y., Ide, I., Murase, H., Suenaga, Y., Takabatake, H., Mori, M., Natori, H.: Automated nomenclature of bronchial branches extracted from CT images and its application to biopsy path planning in virtual bronchoscopy. In: Duncan, J.S., Gerig, G. (eds.) MICCAI 2005. LNCS, vol. 3750, pp. 854–861. Springer, Heidelberg (2005)
4. Tschirren, J., McLennan, G., Palagyi, K., Hoffman, E.A., Sonka, M.: Matching and Anatomical Labeling of Human Airway Tree. IEEE Trans. Med. Imaging 24, 1540–1547 (2005)
5. Ota, S., Deguchi, D., Kitasaka, T., Mori, K., Suenaga, Y., Hasegawa, Y., Imaizumi, K., Takabatake, H., Mori, M., Natori, H.: Augmented display of anatomical names of bronchial branches for bronchoscopy assistance. In: Dohi, T., Sakuma, I., Liao, H. (eds.) MIAR 2008. LNCS, vol. 5128, pp. 377–384. Springer, Heidelberg (2008)
6. Kitasaka, T., Mori, K., Hasegawa, J., Toriwaki, J.: A Method for Extraction of Bronchus Regions from 3D Chest X-ray CT Images by Analyzing Structural Features of the Bronchus. FORMA 17, 321–338 (2002)
7. Li, L.: Multiclass Boosting with Repartitioning. In: Proc. of the 23rd Int'l Conf. on Machine Learning, pp. 569–576 (2006)
8. Deguchi, D., Ishitani, K., Kitasaka, T., Mori, K., Suenaga, Y., Takabatake, H., Mori, M., Natori, H.: A method for bronchoscope tracking using position sensor without fiducial markers. In: Proc. of SPIE, vol. 6511, p. 65110N-1-12 (2007)

Multi-level Ground Glass Nodule Detection and Segmentation in CT Lung Images

Yimo Tao[1,2], Le Lu[1], Maneesh Dewan[1], Albert Y. Chen[1,3], Jason Corso[3], Jianhua Xuan[2], Marcos Salganicoff[1], and Arun Krishnan[1]

[1] CAD R&D, Siemens Healthcare, Malvern, PA USA
[2] Dept. of Electrical and Computer Engineering, Virginia Tech, Arlington, VA USA
[3] Dept. of CSE, University at Buffalo SUNY, Buffalo, NY USA

Abstract. Early detection of Ground Glass Nodule (GGN) in lung Computed Tomography (CT) images is important for lung cancer prognosis. Due to its indistinct boundaries, manual detection and segmentation of GGN is labor-intensive and problematic. In this paper, we propose a novel multi-level learning-based framework for automatic detection and segmentation of GGN in lung CT images. Our main contributions are: firstly, a multi-level statistical learning-based approach that seamlessly integrates segmentation and detection to improve the overall accuracy for GGN detection (in a subvolume). The classification is done at two levels, both voxel-level and object-level. The algorithm starts with a three-phase voxel-level classification step, using volumetric features computed per voxel to generate a GGN class-conditional probability map. GGN candidates are then extracted from this probability map by integrating prior knowledge of shape and location, and the GGN object-level classifier is used to determine the occurrence of the GGN. Secondly, an extensive set of volumetric features are used to capture the GGN appearance. Finally, to our best knowledge, the GGN dataset used for experiments is an order of magnitude larger than previous work. The effectiveness of our method is demonstrated on a dataset of 1100 subvolumes (100 containing GGNs) extracted from about 200 subjects.

1 Introduction

Ground Glass Nodule(GGN) is a hazy area of increased attenuation in CT lung images, often indicative of bronchioloalveolar carcinoma (BAC) [1], that does not obscure underlying bronchial structures or pulmonary vessels. These faint pulmonary nodules are reported to have a higher probability of becoming malignant than solid nodules [1]. Hence early detection [2] and treatment of GGN are important for improving the prognosis of lung cancer. Furthermore, recent studies have shown that tracking the growth pattern of GGNs is informative and useful for quantifying and studying the progress of diseases over time [3]. Therefore, it is highly desirable to have algorithms that not only detect the GGN but are also capable of segmenting the GGN with good accuracy. However, due to their indistinct boundaries and similarity to its surrounding structures, consistent labeling of GGN at voxel-level is difficult for both computers and radiologists, with high inter- and intra-person errors [4]. On the other hand, the appearances of GGN on CT images, such as its shape, pattern and boundary, are very different from solid nodules. Thus, algorithms developed exclusively for solid nodule segmentation are likely to produce inaccurate results when directly applied to GGN. [5] addresses a GGN segmentation method using Markov random field representation and shape analysis based vessel removal method, but no GGN detection was exploited in this approach. [4] adopts the probability density functions (PDF) for modeling and segmenting GGN and PDFs are shown to be valid of distinguishing GGN and other lung parenchyma. An interactive 2D semi-automatic segmentation scheme is proposed in [6], which allows measuring the pixel opacity value of the GGN quantitatively, by constructing a graph Laplacian matrix and solving a linear equation system. This may be quite labor-intensive for radiologists to go through slices in order to obtain the final GGN nodule boundaries and opacity values.

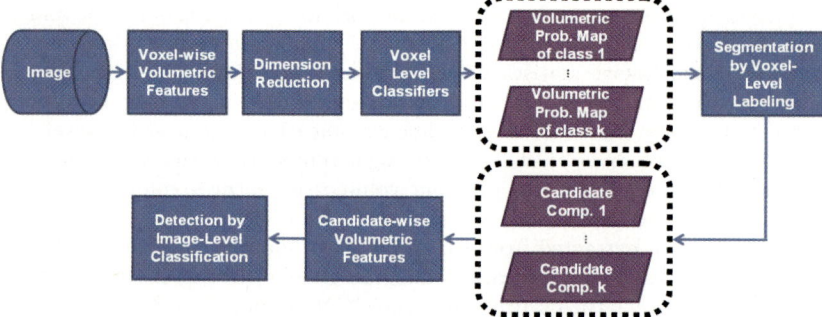

Fig. 1. Flow chart of the proposed approach

In this work, we propose a novel multi-level learning based approach for automatic segmentation and detection for GGN. Our method is composed of two parts as shown in Fig. 1: (1) voxel-wise soft labeling/segmentation, and (2) object-scale image classification/detection. The voxel-level GGN and non-GGN class labeling and segmentation works as follows: given a candidate sub-volume, our system will label each voxel with the probability likelihood of whether it comes from a "healthy" (non-GGN) or "diseased" (GGN) tissue by examining a 3D sliding window centered at that voxel; this labeled or probability weighted image can be viewed as a segmentation map of the GGN region in the original image. After this, the object-level image classification/detection module takes the label map along with other raw information and then classifies the whole sub-volume as positive (containing GGN) or negative. Thus only if the whole sub-volume is classified as positive or "diseased", we will conclude that detection has occurred. Although the method is designed for combined segmentation and detection of GGNs, it can be generalized to other medical imaging problems as well. The presented multi-level probabilistic aggregation process is partially motivated by earlier work in natural scene recognition and object detection [7,8].

The other key aspects of our work is that we use an comprehensive set of features to capture GGN appearance, and the experimental evaluation is done on a much larger dataset compared to previous studies. Note that our algorithm works at a sub-volume level, and it assumes that a candidate generation or interest point detection algorithm is run on a CT volume to obtain locations (typically hundreds) around which isotropic sub-volumes of fixed size ($60\times60\times60$ voxels) are extracted. This is typical in a computer-aided detection (CAD) system. In this paper, we focus on detection and segmentation at this sub-volume (SV) level, which is an integral and important part of the CAD system.

2 Methods

2.1 Voxel-Wise Volumetric Features

Our system computes a comprehensive collection of gray-level and texture features from a cubic sub-volume of interest (sVOIs) of size $7\times7\times7$ voxels across the larger sub-volume (SV). These features are briefly described below:

Gray Level Co-occurrence Matrix (GLCM) [9] is widely used for analyzing texture of 2D image. The co-occurrence matrix stores the co-occurrence frequencies of the pairs of gray levels, which are configured by a distance d and orientation o. Its extension to 3D cases is also practicable, as shown in [10]. The 3D method directly searches for gray level pairs in 26 directions on multiple planes to construct the co-occurrence matrix, whereas the 2D method exploits 8 directions in a single 2D plane. We then extract eight features from the constructed GLCM, including energy, entropy, correlation, inverse difference moment, inertia, cluster shade, cluster prominence, and Haralick correlation [9].

Local Binary Pattern (LBP) is an intensity- and rotation-invariant generalization of the GLCM method. We employ the volumetric LBP-Top [11] technique, an extension of the two-dimensional LBP operator, for parenchymal texture analysis in CT images.

Wavelets are another important and commonly used feature descriptor for texture analysis, due to their effectiveness in capturing localized spatial and frequency information and multi-resolution characteristics. Here, we extract mean intensities in the decomposed eight bands using 3D Harr wavelet. **Vesselness** and **Blobness**, computed based on the eigen-analysis of hessian matrix, have also been employed for vascular or blob-like structure detection or enhancement. We implement a 3D multi-scale version of Blobness and Vesselness feature extraction module for handling both bright and dark objects. Note that the Wavelets, Vesselness and Blobness depend on their own scales of spatial supporting settings, and the actual neighborhood may be larger or smaller than the size of $7\times7\times7$.

We also extract two groups of first order **gray-level features**, composed of **(i) gray level statistics features**, including minimum, maximum, mean, standard deviation, skewness and kurtosis, and **(ii) pixel index ratios**, including the ratios of low density pixels within (-1024, -950] Hounsfield unit(HU), medium density values within (-950, -765] HU, and medium-high density values within (-765, -450] HU.

Since the intensity values in the CT scans usually have a large range from -1024 to 1024 HU, texture feature calculation directly on HU values is computationally intensive and sensitive to noise. Therefore, we preprocess images using the multi-level thresholding *Otsu* method [12] to adaptively merge together image regions with similar gray levels. The resulting image is represented by individual texture primitives coded by a smaller gray-level domain. All texture-based features are extracted from this preprocessed image.

2.2 Segmentation by Voxel-Level Labeling

We treat the segmentation of GGN as a probabilistic voxel-level labeling problem. For each input sub-volume (SV), a total 39 volumetric intensity-texture features are calculated for each scanned sVOI of size $7\times7\times7$ voxels. Based on our 3D annotation maps of GGN and Non-GGN, feature vectors are split into positives and negatives and fed into an off-line learning process to train a probabilistic Gaussian mixture density model, in the lower-dimensional feature space after supervised dimension reduction. Finally the classifier takes each SV and produces its corresponding volumetric GGN-class probability map.

For the voxel-level labeling/classification problem, the size of training samples (as scanned volume of size $7\times7\times7$ voxels) can be really large (greater than 100,000). This requires choosing classifiers with good scalability. We choose linear discriminant analysis (LDA) along with Gaussian Mixture Models (GMM) as our classifier, i.e., GMM is used to learn the distribution of the classes in the LDA projected subspace. For each of the binary GGN and Non-GGN class, LDA is first exploited to further project the extracted features into a lower dimension, and GMM consisting of k-Gaussian distributions of different means and variances are then fit according to the training data, using Expectation-Minimization with multiple random initialization trials. Note that, the positive GGN class probability maps (PDM) are sufficient to extract and detect GGNs. The negative probability map is redundant and discarded. Note that, we perform model selection to choose the number k of Gaussian functions using the Bayesian Information criterion (BIC) and value of k is 3 and 5 for positive and negative class respectively. Other functions, e.g., t-distribution can also be explored, but we plan to investigate that in future work.

As there are many different types of tissues inside the CT lung image, such as vessel, airways, and normal parenchymal, the single-layer LDA classifier may have many false positives originating from this multi-tissue background. To reduce these GGN false positives, a multi-phase classification approach is adopted. It starts with the positive class output probability map from single phase, and treat it as a new image. This output image contains for each voxel a probability that it belongs to the structure to be enhanced (GGN). Next, another round of voxel-level feature extraction/selection and LDA-GMM training process is conducted using both the original image and the output image from the previous phase(s). All these intensity-texture features, in the joint image and PDM domain, are used to train a new classifier. This process can be iterated many times, as a simplified "Auto-Context" [13]. The rationale behind this approach is that the structure to be enhanced will be more distinctive in the (intermediate) enhanced image than in the original image. Therefore adding features from these weighed images will result in potentially more discriminative features between the positive regions and the spurious responses from the previous phase(s).

The multi-phase "Auto-Context" like process not only improves the overall performance but can also be used to speed up supervised enhancement by rejecting well classified training samples from the next phase. A simple classifier (e.g., using very few features) can be used in the first phase(s) to quickly throw away "easy" voxels and only the more difficult voxels are considered in the next phase(s). The classification thresholds on normalized probability values are automatically estimated by setting an operating point on receiver operating characteristic curve (ROC) for high recall and moderate false positive deduction.

2.3 Object-Level Labeling and Detection

At this stage, the goal is to locate and extract GGN candidates on the computed 3D probability map from the previous voxel-labeling step. The multiscale blobness filtering, with a larger smoothing kernel (than the voxel-level step) is used to capture the GGN shape. It is applied on each voxel to obtain a volumetric blobness likelihood map. Then, we multiply the voxel-level probability map with this blobness shape likelihood map to obtain another probability map which we refer to as shape-prior refined probability map (SPM). The SPM helps suppress spurious responses (false positives). The Otsu thresholding method[12] is applied again for discrete quantitization of SPM. We use connected component labeling to obtain disjointed objects as GGN candidates. Simple volume size based rules is used to reduce the number of candidate so that multiple candidates per volume are kept as the inputs to our object level classifier. We also incorporate the position prior information into candidate selection procedure.

For training, the manually annotated GGN segmentation is used to assign labels to the connected component candidates as true or false GGNs. The above-mentioned candidate generation procedure is also applied on negative volumes (without GGN) to obtain more negative samples for training. Given that each GGN candidate is associated with its discrete binary 3D mask, 39 intensity-texture features (mentioned in Section 2.1), are recomputed within this binary supporting region. Note that, these features are not computed on the 7×7×7 window as done earlier for the voxel-level classification stage. Many features are aggregations of local statistics over a spatial neighborhood so that they are size-scalable. In addition, we also calculate the volume size, the sphericity, and the mean on the PDM per candidate to form the final feature vector. For simplicity, we use the same LDA+GMM classifier as in section 2.2 to train GGN/non-GGN connected component candidate detector.

3 Results

Data. We collected total 1100 lung CT subvolumes, including 100 positive samples with GGN and 1000 negative samples without GGN. These subvolumes were randomly sampled from the outputs of a GGN candidate generator algorithm (discussed earlier in Section 1), on 153 healthy and 51 diseased patients. All subvolumes were sampled to produce approximately 0.6mm isotropic voxel resolution. GGN masks on randomly selected 60 positive samples were annotated. The remaining 40 positive subvolumes (with no ground truth of GGN masks) along with 300 randomly selected negative subvolumes were used only for the hold-out performance testing of GGN detection at the final classification stage.

Voxel-scale Classification & Labeling. We further splited these 60 positive subvolumes (with annotated GGN masks) and other 700 negative volumes into two parts for training and testing the voxel scale classification. Voxel scale data samples (as 7×7×7 boxes) were extracted on a 7×7×7 sampling grid, augmented with manually labeled GGN annotation masks. The training dataset had 40 positive and 500 negative subvolumes for the three-phase classifier training in section 2.2 (with likelihood ratio testing threshold settings as 0.05, 0.1 and 0.2 respectively for high recall and moderate false positive reduction). And the remaining subvolumes were used for testing. Table. 1 showed the voxel-level accuracies for the first phase classifier, first two phase classifiers, and all three phase classifiers. It was clearly evident that the further reduction of false positive samples, with increasing classification phases, substantially improved the overall classification performance. The ROC curve for the first phase classifier was shown in Fig. 2, with Area Under Curve (AUC) as 0.9412. We empirically found that the performance is stable with the sVOI size in a range of 5 to 15 voxels (note that the default value is 7).

To measure the level of agreement between human annotations and the segmented GGN (with Otsu thresholding and connected component), the *Jaccard* similarity coefficient (JC) and the volume similarity (VS) were exploited. The JC was defined as:

$$JC = \frac{X \cap Y}{X \cup Y} \qquad (1)$$

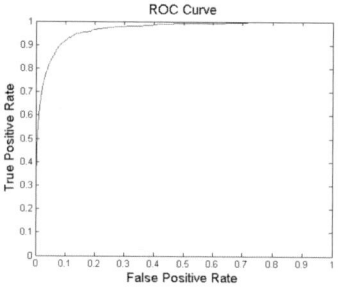

Fig. 2. The top level voxel-level GGN classification ROC curve

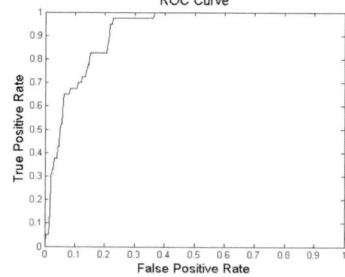

Fig. 3. The object-level classification ROC curve for GGN detection

Table 1. The multi-level voxel scale classification accuracy performance

	First Phase	First Two Phases	All Three Phases
GGN Samples	99.82%	96.62%	89.87%
Negative Samples	56.53%	80.86%	92.93%
Overall	65.37%	84.22%	92.28%

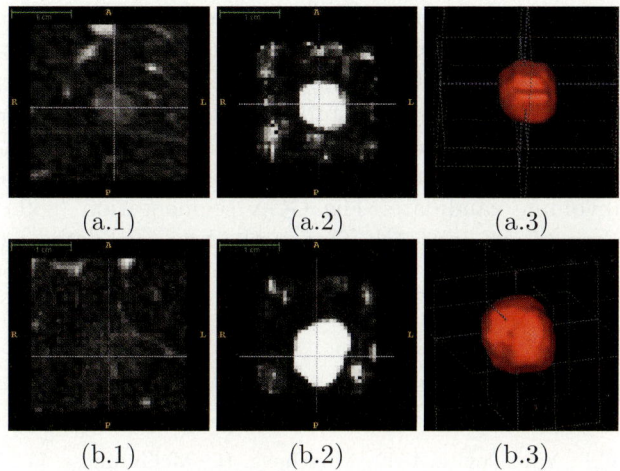

(a.1) (a.2) (a.3)

(b.1) (b.2) (b.3)

Fig. 4. Results the voxel-level classification: (a.1) and (b.1) The original CT images, (a.2) and (b.2) The volumetric probability map produced by voxel-scale classifiers, (a.3) and (b.3) the rendered segmentation of GGN

where JC measured the degree of overlap between two sets: X and Y and JC=1 when the two sets were totally overlapped. The VS was defined as:

$$VS = 1 - \frac{|\ ||X|| - ||Y||\ |}{||X|| + ||Y||} \qquad (2)$$

where VS measured the degree of similarity in the volume size of two sets X and Y, and the operator $||.||$ denoted the volume size of a set. It was equal to one, when the two sets had equal volumes. We reserved 20 positive GGN subvolumes for testing these two metrics, and used the remaining 40 positive subvolumes with all the negative volumes to train the voxel-level classifier. The average JC coefficient was 0.68, and the average VS was 0.865.

Object-scale Classification & GGN Detection. Fig. 3 showed the object level GGN classification performance with AUC as 0.914. For the hold-out testing set, 33 out of 40 GGN subvolumes were correctly detected, with a false negative rate is about 20%. We believed this result is promising and we planed to explore more descriptive features and other types of classifiers (e.g., SVM, boosting) to further investigate this problem. As compared with [4], the most relevant previous work in which only 10 GGN nodules were used for both training and testing, our studied GGN dataset is 10 times larger (i.e., 60 for training and 40 for testing). [6] uses 40 2-D CT image slices from 11 patients. Finally, illustrative examples of GGN labeling and segmentation were shown in Fig. 4.

4 Conclusion

In this paper, we presented a novel multi-level learning-based approach for automatic GGN detection that fuses segmentation and detection to improve the overall accuracy. We exploited a comprehensive set of features to encapsulate the GGN appearance. Our approach proposed a two-level classification by first generating a GGN class PDM at a voxel scale, then extracting object scale descriptors from this PDM, and then finally classifying the existence of GGN within CT subvolume candidate. The GGN segmentation (soft) mask was a desired byproduct of our approach. Our method was validated using extensive evaluations on a much larger GGN dataset than previously reported, of 1100 lung CT subvolumes from about 200 patients.

References

1. Henschke, C.I., Yankelevitz, D.F., Mirtcheva, R., McGuinness, G., McCauley, D., Miettinen, O.S.: CT Screening for Lung Cancer Frequency and Significance of Part-Solid and Nonsolid Nodules. Amer. Jour. Roentgenology 178(5) (2002)
2. Godoy, M., Ko, J., Kim, T., Naidich, D., Bogoni, L., Florin, C., Groot, P., White, C., Vlahos, I., Park, S., Salganicoff, M.: Effect of computer-aided diagnosis on radiologists detection performance of subsolid pulmonary nodules on ct: Initial results. In: American Roentgen Ray Society, ARRS (2009)
3. Park, C., Goo, J., Lee, H., Lee, C., Chun, E., Im, J.: Nodular ground-glass opacity at thin-section ct: Histologic correlation and evaluation of change at follow-up. RadioGraphics 27(2), 391–408 (2007)
4. Zhou, J., Chang, S., Metaxas, D., Zhao, B., Ginsberg, M., Schwartz, L.: Automatic detection and segmentation of ground glass opacity nodules. In: Larsen, R., Nielsen, M., Sporring, J. (eds.) MICCAI 2006. LNCS, vol. 4190, pp. 784–791. Springer, Heidelberg (2006)
5. Zhang, L., Fang, M., Naidich, D., Novak, C.: Consistent interactive segmentation of pulmonary ground glass nodules identified in ct studies. In: SPIE Medical Imaging (2004)
6. Zheng, Y., Kambhamettu, C., Bauer, T., Steiner, K.: Estimation of ground-glass opacity measurement in CT lung images. In: Metaxas, D., Axel, L., Fichtinger, G., Székely, G. (eds.) MICCAI 2008, Part II. LNCS, vol. 5242, pp. 238–245. Springer, Heidelberg (2008)
7. Lu, L., Toyama, K., Hager, G.: A two level approach for scene recognition. In: IEEE Conf. CVPR, pp. 688–695 (2005)
8. Leibe, B., Leonardis, A., Schiele, B.: Robust object detection with interleaved categorization and segmentation. Int. J. of Computer Vision 77, 259–289 (2008)
9. Haralick, R.: Statistical and structural approaches to texture. Proceedings of the IEEE 67, 786–804 (1979)

10. Xu, Y., Sonka, M., MnLenan, G., Guo, J., Hoffman, E.: MDCT-based 3-d texture classification of emphysema and early smoking related lung pathologies. IEEE Transactions on Medical Imaging 25(4) (2006)
11. Zhao, G., Pietiküinen, M.: Dynamic texture recognition using local binary patterns with an application to facial expressions. IEEE Transactions on Pattern Analysis and Machine Intelligence 29(6) (2007)
12. Otsu, N.: A threshold selection method from gray-level histograms. IEEE Transactions on Systems, Man, and Cybernetics 9, 62–66 (1979)
13. Tu, Z.: Auto-context and its application to high-level vision tasks. In: IEEE Conf. CVPR, pp. 1–8 (2008)

Global and Local Multi-valued Dissimilarity-Based Classification: Application to Computer-Aided Detection of Tuberculosis

Yulia Arzhaeva[1,2], Laurens Hogeweg[1], Pim A. de Jong[1], Max A. Viergever[1], and Bram van Ginneken[1]

[1] Image Sciences Institute, University Medical Center Utrecht, The Netherlands
[2] CSIRO Mathematical and Information Sciences, Australia
yulia.arzhaeva@csiro.au

Abstract. In many applications of computer-aided detection (CAD) it is not possible to precisely localize lesions or affected areas in images that are known to be abnormal. In this paper a novel approach to computer-aided detection is presented that can deal effectively with such weakly labeled data. Our approach is based on multi-valued dissimilarity measures that retain more information about underlying local image features than single-valued dissimilarities. We show how this approach can be extended by applying it locally as well as globally, and by merging the local and global classification results into an overall opinion about the image to be classified. The framework is applied to the detection of tuberculosis (TB) in chest radiographs. This is the first study to apply a CAD system to a large database of digital chest radiographs obtained from a TB screening program, including normal cases, suspect cases and cases with proven TB. The global dissimilarity approach achieved an area under the ROC curve of 0.81. The combination of local and global classifications increased this value to 0.83.

1 Introduction

Pulmonary tuberculosis (TB) is a major cause of death and illness worldwide, with 9.2 million new cases and 1.7 million deaths reported in 2006 [1]. Chest radiography is increasingly important in the fight against TB, especially because the rates of sputum-negative TB are rapidly increasing in populations with a high incidence of HIV/AIDS. On chest radiographs, TB often presents itself through subtle diffuse textural abnormalities. With the advent of digital radiography, computer-aided detection (CAD) systems can be developed that could facilitate mass population TB screening.

However, little research has been done in this area. In [2] texture analysis within the lung fields was used but this required experts to manually delineate abnormal areas, in order to train the system to discern normal regions from abnormal. Although such an approach may lead to a powerful CAD system, obtaining manual delineations of ill-defined diffuse lesions is laborious and likely to produce an unreliable ground truth. Our work focuses on classification of weakly labeled images, i.e. when the exact locations of abnormalities in training data are unknown and, therefore, local feature-based classifiers cannot be trained. Our approach circumvents the problem of the absence of local ground truth by using the distances, or dissimilarities, between estimated distributions of local features in the global classification of images. We estimate these differences per feature and therefore build a multi-valued dissimilarity-based (MVDB) classification system.

The underlying assumption of the MVDB method is that local feature distributions are sufficiently different for normal and abnormal images. However, this assumption is not likely to hold for cases with subtle small abnormalities only. We hypothesize that subdividing the lung fields into smaller parts and applying the MVDB classification to these parts separately, and subsequently combining these local opinions, may improve the sensitivity of the method to such abnormalities and increase overall classification performance. It should be noted that obtaining ground truth labels for fixed large lung subdivisions is easier than obtaining manual delineations of lesions. In this work, we apply the method to a large database of digital radiographs from a TB screening program. The proposed modification of the MVDB classification is general and applicable to other image classification tasks that involve local analysis.

2 Methods

2.1 Multi-valued Dissimilarity-Based Classification

Dissimilarity-based classification uses dissimilarity representations of objects instead of traditional feature vectors, that is, objects are represented by their pairwise comparisons. This is a natural way to describe a class of similar objects. A pairwise comparison is done by computing a measure of dissimilarity, or distance, between two objects. In the standard dissimilarity-based classification [3], each training object is represented as a vector of distances to a set of prototype objects. Then, any traditional classifier can be trained on dissimilarity representations of training objects and applied to the dissimilarity representation of a new object. This may not be an efficient strategy for classifying objects characterized by a large set of descriptors, such as numerous local texture features, because it reduces the abundance of local information in two objects to just one dissimilarity value between them.

MVDB classification is built on similar principles but reduces the loss of information compared to standard dissimilarity-based classification. While the standard dissimilarity-based method accumulates the distance over all the object descriptors, the MVBD method is based on computing a distance for every descriptor individually.

Let x and y be two objects characterized by n one- or multi-dimensional descriptors f_i, and $d_i = d(f_i^x, f_i^y)$ be the value of dissimilarity between corresponding descriptors of x and y, where d is a dissimilarity measure. Then, a vector $D(x, y) = (d_1, \ldots, d_n)$ is called the dissimilarity representation of object x with respect to object y. To construct a classifier on such representations, let us consider a training set T, and a set of prototype objects R of size r, $R = \{p_1, \ldots, p_r\}$, where $R \subseteq T$. For each $x \in T$, r different representations $D(x, p_k)$, $1 \leq k \leq r$, can be obtained, and consequently r classifiers can be trained on T using $D(x, p_k)$ as input. A test object, subsequently, can be classified r times using its prototype-bound representations. To obtain a final classification solution for a test object, the outputs of r classifiers must be combined. Combining classifiers benefits from complementary information provided by different dissimilarity representations. In this study we combine the posterior probabilities resulting from different classifiers with the sum rule:

$$P(c|x) = \frac{1}{r} \sum_{k=1}^{r} P_k(c|x), \qquad (1)$$

where $P(c|x)$ is a posterior probability that the object x belongs to a class c, and $P_k(c|x)$ is a posterior probability yielded by the classifier k.

Figure 1 schematically depicts the steps of the MVDB classification. To apply this method to an image classification task that involve local texture analysis, we describe each image by the distributions of its local texture features. These features are extracted at numerous locations inside the image, and their individual distributions are estimated by histograms. From the set of training images, r prototype images are selected, either randomly, or by following a systematic approach. Since the sum rule, used to combine the results of individual classifiers, is known to be less sensitive than other combiners to the errors of individual classifiers [4], we believe, the random selection of prototypes is a reasonable starting approach. Dissimilarities, computed between corresponding feature histograms of the image and a prototype, constitute a dissimilarity representation of the image.

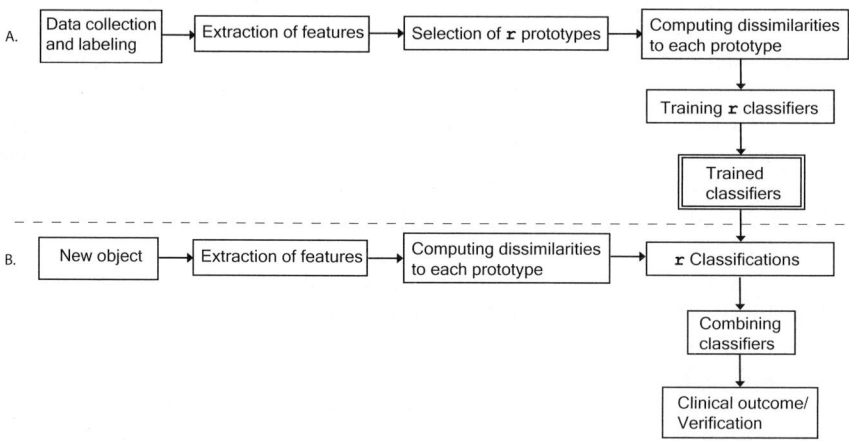

Fig. 1. Flow chart of the MVDB classification. (A) Training phase. (B) Testing phase.

2.2 Local Classification to Improve Global Results

Sometimes image descriptors, such as the local feature histograms, are too generalizing. This is true when an object whose presence we want to detect is too small with respect to the whole image. With the detection of TB, the texture feature histograms computed over the whole lung fields might not be sensitive enough to reflect the presence of subtle localized lesions in the lungs. We assume that the discriminating ability of descriptors will increase if they are computed over smaller image parts. When it is practical to obtain the ground truth for training images on a finer scale, e.g. class labels for a fixed image partition, we propose the following modification of the MVDB classification scheme.

1. Images are partitioned, and the ground truth is obtained for each part.
2. The MVDB scheme is applied to each image part separately, and, optionally, to the whole images too.
3. The classification results are combined to obtain an overall image solution.

Here, the combination rule might be different from the one in step 5 of the testing phase of the original scheme. In this paper we use the vote rule for the abnormal class ($c = 1$), and compute the posterior probability of the normal class($c = 0$) such as $P(c = 0|x) = 1 - P(c = 1|x)$, where x is the test object. The vote rule for computing $P(c = 1|x)$ is

$$P(c|x) = \max(P_0(c|x), \max_{l=1}^{L} P_l(c|x_l)), \ c = 1, \qquad (2)$$

where x_l, $1 \leq l \leq L$, are L image subdivisions, P_l is the result of applying the MVDB classification to x_l, and P_0 is the result of applying the MVDB classification to the whole image. The choice for the vote rule for the detection of abnormal images is intuitive because if any part of the image is abnormal then the whole image is abnormal. The use of P_0 in Eq. 2 is optional and is not needed if the performances of all regional classifiers are considerably better than that of the global classifier. It should also be noted that, for a certain region, only a fraction of abnormal images will have abnormalities in that particular region. Therefore, a high classification performance on one of the regions is not enough to obtain an equally high performance after combining. In addition to improving the image classification performance, the application of the MVDB to the regions allows one to obtain a prediction on which regions are likely to contain abnormalities.

3 Experiments

3.1 Materials

All images used in this work were posterior-anterior chest radiographs collected from a TB screening program among a high risk population. Radiographs were acquired with mobile digital thorax units (Delft Imaging Systems, the Netherlands) developed for cost-effective thorax examination and TB preventive screening. Images have a resolution of 2048×2048 and 12 bits data depth. Each image was read by two radiologists, and a person whose radiograph was considered TB suspect by one of them or both was contacted to undergo further tests. For a subset of the cases, positive microbiological culture tests were available and a definite diagnosis of TB could be established.

We collected all TB suspect and TB proven cases between 2002 and 2005, and a similar amount of randomly selected normal radiographs, excluding radiographs of children. Before collection, radiographs were anonymized. Normal and TB suspect images were re-read by a third radiologist, who classified a part of the cases differently. Re-classified images were excluded from the study. Finally, our database contained 256 normal radiographs (223 males, 33 females, ages 18–70 yrs, median age 41), 178 TB suspect radiographs (155 males, 23 females, ages 16–101 yrs, median age 35), and 37 radiographs with microbiologically proven TB (30 males, 7 females, ages 16–43 yrs, median age 29).

3.2 Local Feature Extraction

For practical considerations, images were downsized to 1024×1024. Prior to feature extraction, lung fields were automatically segmented from the radiographs using multi-resolution pixel classification, with settings as given in [5]. In order to train this segmentation procedure, lung fields were segmented manually from 20 radiographs not used otherwise in this study.

Next, local texture features were extracted from a large number of regions of interest (ROIs). At first, images were filtered with a multiscale filter bank of Gaussian derivatives, and subsequently central moments of histograms were calculated from each ROI in the original and the filtered images. The following parameters were chosen: Gaussian derivatives of orders $0, 1$ and 2 at five scales, $\sigma = 1, 2, 4, 8, 16$ pixels; overlapping circular ROIs with a radius of 32 pixels placed on a grid with 8×8 pixel spacing inside the lung fields; and four central moments, namely, the mean, standard deviation, skewness and kurtosis. Before filtering, pixel values in the lung fields were mirrored outside the lungs symmetrically with respect to the lung borders in order to prevent contamination of extracted features due to strong filter responses at the lung border. Two position features were added that defined x and y coordinates of the ROI centers relative to the center of the mass of a lung field. In total, 126 features were extracted from each ROI, and the number of ROIs per image ranged from 1920 to 8680.

3.3 Lung Partitioning

In order to perform the MVDB classification on lung subdivisions, each lung field was automatically divided into 4 equal-sized regions (see Figure 2). The regions around hilum (regions 4 and 8) included lung pixels overlapping with a circle placed at the lungs' center of mass. The radius of the circle was separately chosen for the left and right lung, such that the overlap covered one quarter of the pixels of that lung. The rest of each lung field was horizontally divided into three equal-sized parts. The third radiologist assessed regions in all the TB suspect and TB proven images, and assigned a region to class 1 if a TB-related abnormality was present in the region, or to class 0 otherwise.

3.4 Classification

Training and test images were randomly selected from the available normal and TB suspect data, so that the training and test sets each contained 128 normal and 89 abnormal images. The second test set was formed from the same normal images as in the first test set and all 37 radiographs with proven TB. We randomly selected 10 normal and 10 abnormal radiographs to serve as prototype images. For region classification, the same division into training and test sets was used, but the random selection of prototypes was performed separately for each region, so that 10 normal and 10 abnormal regions were selected each time. Prototypes were always selected from the training images. Normal prototype regions were selected from normal training images only. Normal regions from abnormal images were excluded from the training set during region classifications.

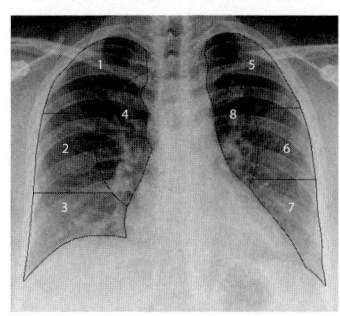

Fig. 2. Division of the lung fields into eight regions

The histograms of each local feature were obtained by a suitable binning of the range of feature values, either across the lung fields, or across a particular region. The range of possible values of each feature was estimated on prototypes and split into equal intervals - 128 for the lung fields, 64 for regions. A dissimilarity between two histograms was computed using χ^2 statistics as a dissimilarity measure:

$$d_{\chi^2}(h,k) = \sum_i \frac{\left(h(i) - m(i)\right)^2}{m(i)}, \quad (3)$$

where $h = \{h(i)\}$ and $k = \{k(i)\}$ are two corresponding histograms, i is a bin index, and $m(i) = \frac{h(i)+k(i)}{2}$. Dissimilarity representations were classified by the linear discriminant classifier. Classification was preceded by a principal component analysis (PCA) retaining 99% of variance to the dissimilarity representation, for the purpose of dimensionality reduction.

The MVDB method was compared with a straightforward approach where an image classification was composed of classification of each ROI and subsequent fusion of ROIs' posterior probabilities. In this approach, local feature vectors extracted from ROIs as described in Section 3.2 were used as input of the linear discriminant classifier preceded by the PCA. The division into training and test images was the same as for the MVDB experiments. ROIs from training images got the class labels of lung subdivisions they belonged to. An overall image decision was obtained by integrating all ROIs' posterior probabilities using the 95% percentile rule.

4 Results

The classification performance was estimated by means of the area under the receiver operating characteristic (ROC) curve, A_z [6]. A_z values for two test sets

Table 1. The performances of the MVDB classification and fusion, in terms of A_z

Test set	Lungs	Regions								Vote rule
		1	2	3	4	5	6	7	8	
Normal vs. suspect TB	**0.81**	0.79	0.71	0.85	0.66	0.82	0.81	0.72	0.77	**0.83**
Normal vs. proven TB	**0.70**	0.85	0.71	0.95	0.64	0.66	0.43	0.49	0.65	**0.74**

are presented in Table 1. The first column contains the results of the application of the MVDB classification to the whole lung fields. In the columns titled "1" to "8", A_z values for corresponding lung regions (see Figure 2) are listed. The final classification performance computed after combining global and local posterior probabilities by voting is given in the last column.

Combining global and local classification decisions slightly improves the overall classification performance compared to the results after applying the MVDB method to the whole lung fields only. To illustrate the gain of using the combination of local and global classifications, an example of a region with a slight diffuse abnormality is shown in Figure 3. This region was correctly classified as abnormal by the MVDB method applied locally (posterior probability $p_{c=1} = 0.89$), while an image containing this region was initially misclassified as normal by a global MVDB classifier ($p_{c=1} = 0.24$). After combing global and local results, the image received a probability of 0.89 of being abnormal.

The straightforward classification approach achieved $A_z = 0.77$ on the first test set and $A_z = 0.64$ on the second test set. This demonstrates the advantage of the MVDB method for classification of weakly labeled images.

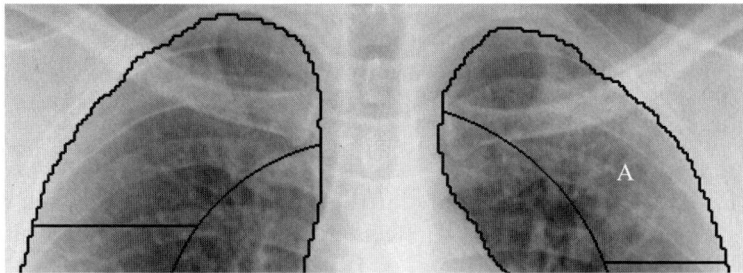

Fig. 3. An example of a correctly classified abnormal region (white "A" marks a proven TB lesion). An opposite region in the other lung is normal.

5 Discussion and Conclusions

The results presented in Table 1 demonstrate that the classification performance on the whole lung fields, as well as the performance of the combining scheme is considerably better on the first test set than on the second one. This observation can be explained in two ways. Firstly, the training set did not contain proven TB cases and so the test set with proven TB cases is expected to perform worse. Adding proven TB cases to the training set is expected to improve the performance of the CAD system. Secondly, there were TB proven images with extremely subtle abnormalities in our collection. Such images are difficult for humans and CAD systems to classify.

The other observation is that the local performances vary greatly for both test sets, from 0.66 to 0.85 on the first set, and from 0.42 to 0.95 on the second set. Such a variation can happen due to low numbers of abnormal samples for some regions in a test set (e.g. the second test set contained only 3 abnormal regions "7" and only 3 abnormal regions "3"). Each misclassification then drastically influences an A_z value for such regions. For some regions, the number of abnormal samples in the training set was also limited, which in general negatively affected the MVDB classification performance on such regions. Future work will include the collection of a much larger data set which we expect to be beneficial for our combination scheme. In future, we should also investigate whether performing the selection of prototypes systematically can improve the results of our method, and how its performance is influenced by the number of prototypes.

In conclusion, we have shown that the multi-valued dissimilarity-based classification is a practical tool that enables a CAD system to deal with weakly labeled images. Combining global and local classification decisions has a potential to improve the overall classification performance. We have been the first to apply such a scheme to the automated detection of tuberculosis in a large database of digital chest radiographs.

References

1. World Health Organization: WHO Report 2008: Global Tuberculosis Control, Surveillance, Planning, Financing (2008)
2. van Ginneken, B., Katsuragawa, S., ter Haar Romeny, B.M., Doi, K., Viergever, M.A.: Automatic detection of abnormalities in chest radiographs using local texture analysis. IEEE Transactions on Medical Imaging 21(2), 139–149 (2002)
3. Pekalska, E.: Dissimilarity representations in pattern recognition. PhD thesis, Delft University, the Netherlands (2005)
4. Kittler, J., Hatef, M., Duin, R.P.W., Matas, J.: On combining classifiers. IEEE Transactions on Pattern Analysis and Machine Intelligence 20(3), 226–239 (1998)
5. van Ginneken, B., Stegmann, M., Loog, M.: Segmentation of anatomical structures in chest radiographs using supervised methods: a comparative study on a public database. Medical Image Analysis 10(1), 19–40 (2006)
6. Metz, C.: ROC methodology in radiologic imaging. Investigative Radiology 21(9), 720–733 (1986)

Noninvasive Imaging of Electrophysiological Substrates in Post Myocardial Infarction

Linwei Wang[1], Heye Zhang[2], Ken C.L. Wong[1], Huafeng Liu[3], and Pengcheng Shi[1]

[1] Computational Biomedicine Laboratory
Rochester Institute of Technology, Rochester, New York, USA
[2] Bioengineering Institute, University of Auckland, Auckland, New Zealand
[3] State Key Laboratory of Modern Optical Instrumentation
Zhejiang University, China

Abstract. The presence of injured tissues after myocardial infarction (MI) creates substrates responsible for fatal arrhythmia; understanding of its arrhythmogenic mechanism requires investigation of the correlation of local abnormality between phenomenal electrical functions and inherent electrophysiological properties during normal sinus rhythm. This paper presents a physiological-model-constrained framework for imaging post-MI electrophysiological substrates from noninvasive body surface potential measurements. Using *a priori* knowledge of general cardiac electrical activity as constraints, it simultaneously reconstruct transmembrane potential dynamics and tissue excitability inside the 3D myocardium, with the central goal to localize and investigate the abnormality in these two different electrophysiological quantities. It is applied to four post-MI patients with quantitative validations by gold standards and notable improvements over existent results.

1 Introduction

The presence of injured tissues after myocardial infarction (MI) creates substrates responsible for fatal cardiac arrhythmia, such as ventricular tachycardia (VT) and fibrillation. Personalized imaging of post-MI electrophysiological substrates, particularly the correlation of local abnormality between phenomenal electrical function and inherent electrophysiological properties [1], is critical for assessing arrhythmia susceptibility of each individual.

Endocardial catheter mapping of purposely-induced VT measures electrical conduction on patient's endocardium; it guides catheter ablation with low success rate and risk of sudden death [2]. Substrate voltage mapping is free from inducing VT because the electroanatomical delineation of arrhythmogenic substrate is based on the characteristics of electrograms recorded on epi- or endocardium during sinus rhythm [2]. Electrical impedance mapping reflects bulk electrical properties of heart surfaces that vary with the evolution of MI [3]. These techniques define the extent of substrate on heart surfaces, but do not depict 3D substrate structure or reveal substrate undetectable by surface recordings. Besides, their spatial resolution is limited by the number of electrodes.

High-resolution contrast-enhanced MRI noninvasively reveals infarcted tissues with spatially complicated structures and tissue heterogeneity [1]. However, anatomical scar identified by MRI is not necessarily identical with critical electrophysiological substrates. Besides, contrast-enhanced MRI involves relatively expensive practice, use of harmful contrast agent such as gadolinium (Gd), and high false-positive identification because MI is not the only condition leading to contrast delayed Gd-enhancement [4].

Body surface potential mapping (BSPM) provides standard noninvasive observations of cardiac electrical activity with relatively simple procedure and economical equipments. Existing efforts in BSPM-driven cardiac electrophysiological reconstruction, when applied to post-MI substrate imaging, only focus on cardiac electrical functions. Electrophysiological reconstruction on heart surfaces assumes the substrate to be homogeneous and defines its extent only on heart surfaces [5]. Using a spherical infarct model, [6] estimated its location and size from BSP by deterministic optimization. The predefined infarct shape, however, does not allow flexible data-driven descriptions of intricate 3D infarct structures. We have developed a physiological-model-constrained framework that statistically combines general knowledge and patient's data for personalized imaging of volumetric TMP dynamics. It evaluates infarct solely based on abnormality of estimated TMP dynamics [7].

In this paper, we further develop our framework for noninvasive imaging of not only the phenomenal electrical function but also the inherent tissue property of the 3D myocardium for individual subjects. To obtain preliminary knowledge about local TMP abnormality, volumetric TMP dynamics is firstly estimated from BSPM data under the constraints of normally-parametrized physiological models. This initial TMP estimates is used to initialize simultaneous estimation of TMP and tissue excitability using BSPM data; abnormality in the two estimates is localized for investigation of their correlation and identification of electrophysiological substrates. Experiments are performed on four post-MI patients, where infarct location and extent are validated with the gold standard and compared to existent results on the same data sets.

2 Methodology

2.1 State Space System of Cardiac Electrophysiology

A priori physiological knowledge is used to constrain the reconstruction of subject-specific volumetric cardiac electrophysiological details. It is modeled on personalized heart-torso structures, where the volumetric myocardial TMP activity model for general spatiotemporal TMP dynamics is developed from [8]:

$$\begin{cases} \frac{\partial \mathbf{U}}{\partial t} = -\mathbf{M}^{-1}\mathbf{K}\mathbf{U} + k\mathbf{U}(\mathbf{U}-a)(1-\mathbf{U}) - \mathbf{U}\mathbf{V} \\ \frac{\partial \mathbf{V}}{\partial t} = -e(\mathbf{V} + k\mathbf{U}(\mathbf{U}-a-1)) \end{cases} \quad (1)$$

and TMP-to-BSP model for the mapping of BSP from volumetric TMP by [7]:

$$\mathbf{\Phi} = \mathbf{H}\mathbf{U} \quad (2)$$

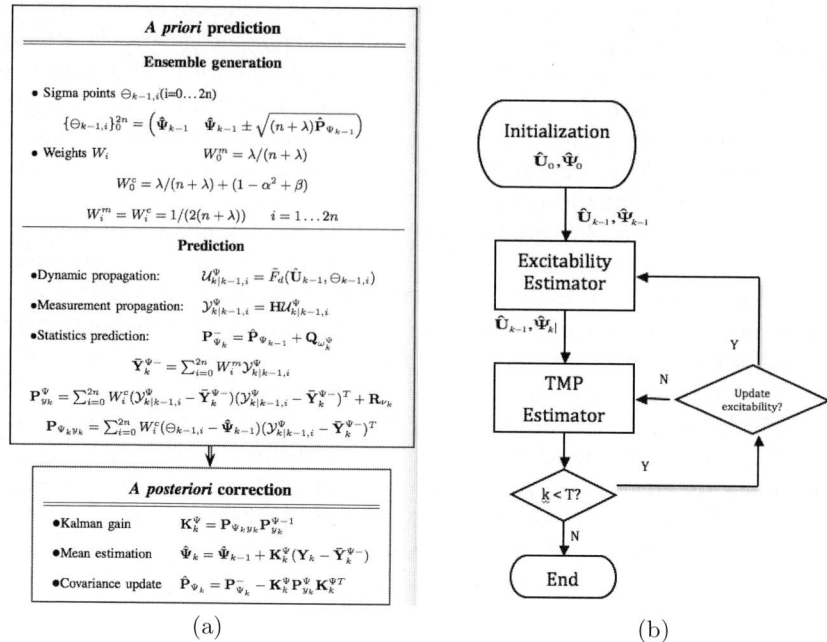

Fig. 1. (a) Flow of excitability estimation algorithm at the kth iteration. $\mathbf{Q}_{\omega_k^\psi}$ and $\mathbf{R}_{\nu_k}$: pre-specified covariance matrices for ω_k^ψ and ν. (b) Dual estimator of TMP dynamics and tissue excitability. T: total number of estimation steps.

where vectors **U** and **V** consist of TMP and recovery current on all meshfree points, and $\mathbf{\Phi}$ includes BSP from all vertices on the body surface. Matrices **M** and **K** account for intercellular electrical propagation; they encode 3D myocardial structure and its conductive anisotropy. **H** contains geometrical and conductivity information in personalized heart-torso structures. Parameters e, k and a determine TMP shapes, particularly, a represents myocardial tissue excitability and its increased value corresponds to reduced excitability.

To take into account modeling and data uncertainties (ω_k and ν_k), the physiological system is discretized into stochastic state space representation :

$$\mathbf{X}_k = F_d(\mathbf{X}_{k-1}, \mathbf{\Psi}_{k-1}) + \omega_k \quad (3)$$
$$\mathbf{Y}_k = \tilde{\mathbf{H}}\mathbf{X}_k + \nu_k \quad (4)$$

where $\mathbf{X}_k = \left(\mathbf{U}_k^T \ \mathbf{V}_k^T\right)^T$ and $\mathbf{Y}_k = \mathbf{\Phi}_k$. $\mathbf{\Psi}$ consists of unknown parameter a from all meshfree points, assumed to be spatially inhomogeneous but temporally invariant with random disturbance ω_{Ψ_k}:

$$\mathbf{\Psi}_k = \mathbf{\Psi}_{k-1} + \omega_{\Psi_k} \quad (5)$$

With increasing severity of injury after MI, temporal TMP shape is characterized by changes such as progressively reduced potential duration (PD) and delayed

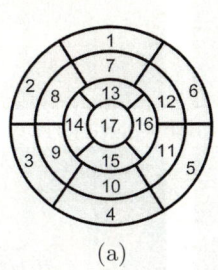 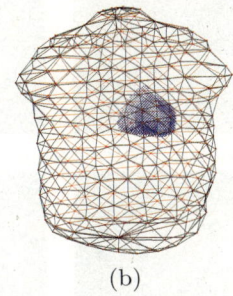

Fig. 2. (a) Standard 17-segement division of LV wall (polor map). Segments 1−6 lie in the basal layer, 7−12 the middle layer, 13−16 the apical layer and 17 the apex. At each layer, the segment labeling moves from anterior, septal, inferior to lateral part of the LV. (b) Personalized heart-torso model in case 2, where the ventricles are represented with 1373 meshfree points and the torso by triangulated body surface with 370 vertices.

activation time (AT) until the absence of activation in necrotic tissues. This loss of myocardial viability is also reflected as decreased tissue excitability.

2.2 Dual Estimation of TMP Dynamics and Tissue Excitability

To obtain preliminary approximation of local TMP abnormality without personalized prior knowledge, TMP dynamics is firstly estimated from BSP under constraints of normally-parameterized models (1,2) as described in [7]. AT and PD are calculated from TMP shapes, the order of which are then indexed by normalized iAT and iPD (points with earliest activation and longest TMP duration are indexed at $iAT = 0$ and $iPD = 0$, respectively). Differences of iAT and iPD between TMP estimates and simulated normal TMPs, dAT and dPD, measure the abnormality of local TMP dynamics as $dComb = (dAT + dPD)/2$. Parameter a on points with distinctly high value of $dComb$ are assigned with large value 0.3 for impaired excitability, while the others are valued from $0.14 - 0.17$ according to TMP heterogeneity across the heart wall. This vector of $\boldsymbol{\Psi}_0$, with $\mathbf{U}_0$ determined by locations of *normal* earliest ventricular activation, is used to initialize dual $\mathbf{U}$ and $\boldsymbol{\Psi}$ estimation.

Excitability estimator is developed similarly to TMP estimator in [7]. As described in Fig 1 (a), at each iteration k with previous estimates $\hat{\boldsymbol{\Psi}}_{k-1}$ and $\hat{\mathbf{P}}_{\Psi_{k-1}}$, an ensemble set $\{\ominus_{k-1,i}\}_{i=0}^{2n}$ is generated from $\hat{\boldsymbol{\Psi}}_{k-1}$ and $\hat{\mathbf{P}}_{\Psi_{k-1}}$ with n as the dimension of $\hat{\boldsymbol{\Psi}}$. It is passed through the system models (1, 2) with previous TMP estimates $\hat{\mathbf{U}}_{k-1}$ to generate new ensemble sets $\{\mathcal{U}_{k|k-1,i}^{\Psi}\}_{i=0}^{2n}$ and $\{\mathcal{Y}_{k,i}^{\Psi}\}_{i=0}^{2n}$. They are used to predict statistics of the unknowns, which are then corrected to final estimates of $\hat{\boldsymbol{\Psi}}_k$ and $\hat{\mathbf{P}}_{\Psi_k}$ using KF update rules. Dual $\mathbf{U}$-$\boldsymbol{\Psi}$ estimator loosely couples TMP estimator and excitability estimator sequentially in time (Fig 1 (b)): at iteration k with TMP estimates $\hat{\mathbf{U}}_{k-1}$ and excitability estimates $\hat{\boldsymbol{\Psi}}_{k-1}$, excitability estimator utilizes $\hat{\mathbf{U}}_{k-1}$ to update $\hat{\boldsymbol{\Psi}}_{k-1}$ as described above; TMP estimator then utilizes the updated $\hat{\boldsymbol{\Psi}}_k$ for estimating $\hat{\mathbf{U}}_k$ and $\hat{\mathbf{P}}_{u_k}$ [7].

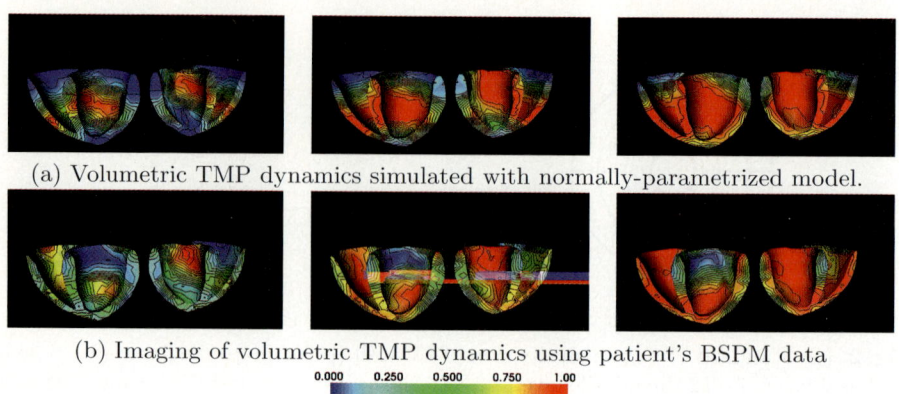

(a) Volumetric TMP dynamics simulated with normally-parametrized model.

(b) Imaging of volumetric TMP dynamics using patient's BSPM data

Fig. 3. Comparison of volumetric TMP imaging results (b) with simulated normal TMP dynamics (a) in case 2. The color bar encodes normalized TMP values and black contours represent TMP isochrones. From left to right: $8.0ms$, $12.3ms$ and $16.7ms$ after the onset of ventricular activation.

2.3 Substrate Imaging and Quantitative Evaluation

To investigate the correlation of abnormality between TMP dynamics and tissue excitability, we measure TMP abnormality by iAT and iPD of the TMP estimates as $iComb = (iAT + iPD)/2$, and similar thresholding method in initialization is used for distinguishing points with abnormally late AT and short PD. Abnormal value in tissue excitability directly reflect myocardial inviability, where increasing severity of injury is represented by $a > 0.25$ until the total loss of viability in necrotic tissues with $a > 0.5$ [8].

For comparisons with gold standard and the existing works, we evaluate the center and extent of infarcted tissues with abnormal excitability. Using the standard 17-segment division of LV (Fig 2 (a)) [9], we identify segments containing infarct substrate and calculate its extent (EP) by dividing the number of infarcted meshfree points by the total number of meshfree points. Substrate centroid (CE) is localized as the segment containing the center of infarcted meshfree points weighted by excitability estimates. Segment overlap (SO) with gold standard measures the percentage of correct identification.

3 Experiments

3.1 Experimental Data and Data Processing

MRI and BSP data are collected from 4 post-MI patients (case $1-4$) [10]. Cardiac MRI of each patient contains 10 slices rom apex to base of the heart, with 8mm inter-slice spacing and 1.33mm/pixel in-plane resolution. After hand-tracing epi-/endo-cardial contours and building a smoothed mesh for the heart surfaces, we drop a could of $1000-2000$ meshfree points inside the surface mesh to represent the 3D heart wall. Myocardial conductive anisotropy is considered

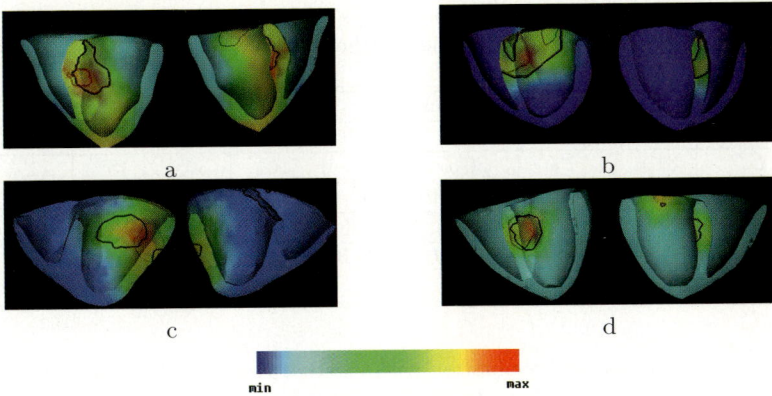

Fig. 4. Superimposed imaging of local abnormality in TMP dynamics and tissue excitability of the 3D myocardium ((a)-(d): case 1-4). Black contour encircles region of abnormal TMP functions. Color encodes tissue excitability; higher value represents lower excitability. Half-transparent visualization is used for better observationl.

by mapping volumetric fiber structures from the mathematical fibrous model in [11]. The torso is assumed to be an isotropic and homogeneous volume conductor, described by triangulated body surface with 370 apexes and obtained by deforming a reference torso model to match patient's MRI data [12]. Fig 2 (b) illustrates the personalized heart-torso model in case 2.

BSP is recorded by 123 electrodes with known anatomical locations and interpolated to 370 apexes on the body surface. Complete BSP sequences consist of a single averaged PQRST complex sampled at 2k Hz, out of which QRST interval for *ventricular* electrical activity is selected as framework inputs. It is interpolated in time and scaled in magnitude to adapt to the discretization step and normalized TMP value of the TMP activity model (1). There are no available gold standards of volumetric TMP activity or tissue excitability. Instead, after examining Gd-enhanced cardiac MRI, cardiologists provid us infarct center (CE), extent (EP) and affected segments for 4 cases (Table 1) [10].

3.2 Results

In volumetric TMP imaging results of case 2 (Fig 3 (b)), septal-inferior part of basal-middle LV exhibits distinct conduction delay compared to normal TMP dynamics simulated in the patient's heart (Fig 3 (a)). Fig 4 (b) illustrates the superimposed TMP and excitability abnormality, where the region of abnormal TMP functions is encircled with black contours and the color encodes tissue excitability. Fig 4 (a), (c) and (d) list results for case 1, 3 and 4, respectively: infarct collects in septal-anterior part of basal LV and septal part of middle LV in case 1, the inferior part of basal-middle LV and lateral part of middle-apical LV in case 3, and in anterior-basal, septal-middle LV in case 4. These results are in accordance with gold standards. Similar to the observations in [1], while

Table 1. Comparison of MI evaluation results with gold standards (Ref). Definition of the evaluation parameters is explained in the text.

	case 1		case 2		case 3		case 4	
	Ref	Results	Ref	Results	Ref	Results	Ref	Results
EP	31%	17%	30%	20%	52%	30%	15%	11%
CE	8	9	3/4/9/10	9	10/11	11	15	9
SO	N/A	97%	N/A	100%	N/A	100%	N/A	100%
segments	1-3,8-9 13-15	1-3,8-9 13-15,17	3,4,9,10	3,4,9,10	3-5,9-12 15-16	5,10-12 16	1,9-11 15,17	1,9

Table 2. Comparison of MI evaluation with existent results. EPD and CED are the difference between those as estimated and as determined from gold standards.

	Current results		Previous results	Mneimneh		Dawoud		Farina	
	case 3	case 4	case 3	case 3	case 4	case 3	case 4	case 3	case 4
EPD	22%	4%	24%	25%	2%	17%	26%	43%	14%
CED	0	1	0	0	1	1	2	1	1
SO	100%	100%	90%	90%	25%	56%	30%	40%	17%

abnormal electrical functions occurs within infarct zone, border zone exhibits normal electrical functions. The extent of injured tissues, therefore, is not the only measure for myocardial arrhythmia susceptibility. It is the distribution of tissue *heterogeneity* and the direction of electrical activation that work in concert to provoke arrhythmia.

Table 1 compares gold standards with our quantitative evaluation of infarct based on tissue excitability. In case 1, we correctly identify all infarcted segments but *overestimate* the infarct extent down to the apex (false positive at segment 17) and localize CE 1 segment away from gold standards. In case 2, we precisely identify the 4 infarcted segments and correctly localize CE. In case 3, we correctly localizes CE and highlights 5 out of 9 infarcted segments, *underestimating* the infarct extent in inferior LV. Among the two separate infarct mass in case 4, our results only identify the anterior-basal part and a small portion in inferior-middle LV. In summary, the presented framework provides close localization of CE and identifies substrate with high precision SO (low false positive identifications). Because calculation of EP may differ between gold standards and our approach, the reason for its discrepancies remains unclear.

Table 2 compares the current results with our previous MI evaluation which solely depends on volumetric TMP estimates [7], as well as existent results of case 3 and 4 obtained using case 1 and 2 for training. In brief, Dawoud *et al* solved the problem by epicardial potential imaging from BSP [5], Farina *et al* estimated the site and size of spherical infarct models [6], and Mneimneh *et al* produced the best results using simple ECG signal analysis [13]. In both cases, our results are comparable to the best results and substantially improved over the other two reconstruction results. Note that our framework has not required any training. In the future, proper training is a possible strategy for improving its performance. Compared to our previous work [7], simultaneous estimation of volumetric TMP dynamics and tissue excitability improves the accuracy of infarct identification (improved EP and SO).

4 Conclusions

Our framework enables investigation of the correlation between electrical functions and tissue property inside specific subject's heart; it helps assessing the arrhythmia susceptibility of individual subjects. Future works will analyze the pathophysiological implications of the current substrate imaging results and the extension to a wider category of pathologies. Since cardiac electrical conduction depends on both the active membrane properties of cardiac cells (*e.g.*, excitability) and passive properties determined by myocardial architectural features (*e.g.*, conductivity), future studies will investigate whether it is possible, and if so, how to separately estimate post-MI excitability and conductivity using BSPM data.

References

1. Ashikaga, H., Sasano, T., Dong, J., et al.: Magnetic resonance-based anatomical analysis of scar-related ventricular tachycardia. implications for catheter ablation. Circ. 101, 939–947 (2007)
2. Volkmer, M., Ouyang, F., Deger, F., et al.: Substrate mapping vs. tachycardia mapping using carto in patients with coronary artery disease and ventricular tachycardia: impact on outcome of catheter ablation. Europace 8, 968–976 (2006)
3. Fallert, M.A., Mirotznik, M.S., Downing, S.W., et al.: Myocardial electrical impedance mapping of ischemic sheep hearts and healing aneurysms. Circ. 87, 199–207 (1993)
4. Arai, A.E.: False positive or true positive troponin in patients presenting with chest pan but normal coronary arteries: Lessons from cardiac MRI. European Heart Journal 28, 1175–1177 (2007)
5. Dawoud, F.D.: Using inverse electrocardiography to image myocardial infarction. In: Proc. Comput. Cardiol. (2007)
6. Farina, D.: Model-based approach to the localization of infarction. In: Proc. Comput. Cardiol. (2007)
7. Wang, L., Wong, K.C.L., Zhang, H., Shi, P.: Noninvasive functional imaging of volumetric cardiac electrical activity: A human study on myocardial infarction. In: Metaxas, D., Axel, L., Fichtinger, G., Székely, G. (eds.) MICCAI 2008, Part I. LNCS, vol. 5241, pp. 1042–1050. Springer, Heidelberg (2008)
8. Aliev, R.R., Panfilov, A.V.: A simple two-variable model of cardiac excitation. Chaos, Solitions & Fractals 7(3), 293–301 (1996)
9. Cerqueira, M.D., Weissman, N.J., Dilsizian, V., et al.: Standardized myocardial segmentation and nomenclature for tomographic imaging of the heart. Circ. 105, 539–542 (2002)

10. Goldberger, A.L., Amaral, L.A.N., Glass, L., et al.: Physiobank, physiotoolkit, and physionet components of a new research resource for complex physiological signals. Cric. 101, e215–e220 (2000)
11. Nash, M.: Mechanics and Material Properties of the Heart using an Anatomically Accurate Mathematical Model. PhD thesis, Univ. of Auckland, New Zealand
12. Cheng, L.: Non-invasive Electrical Imaging of the Heartl. PhD thesis, Univ. of Auckland, New Zealand (2001)
13. Mneimneh, M.A., Povinelli, R.J.: Rps/gmm approach toward the localization of myocardial infarction. In: Proc. Comput. Cardiol. (2007)

Unsupervised Inline Analysis of Cardiac Perfusion MRI

Hui Xue[1,*], Sven Zuehlsdorff[2], Peter Kellman[3], Andrew Arai[3],
Sonia Nielles-Vallespin[4], Christophe Chefdhotel[1], Christine H. Lorenz[1],
and Jens Guehring[1]

[1] Imaging and Visualization, Siemens Corporate Research, Princeton, NJ, USA
[2] CMR R&D, Siemens Medical Solutions USA, Inc., Chicago, IL, USA
[3] Laboratory of Cardiac Energetics, National Institutes of Health, Bethesda, MD, USA
[4] MED MR PLM AW Cardiology, Siemens AG Healthcare Sector, Erlangen, Germany
`hui-xue@siemens.com`

Abstract. In this paper we first discuss the technical challenges preventing an automated analysis of cardiac perfusion MR images and subsequently present a fully unsupervised workflow to address the problems. The proposed solution consists of key-frame detection, consecutive motion compensation, surface coil inhomogeneity correction using proton density images and robust generation of pixel-wise perfusion parameter maps. The entire processing chain has been implemented on clinical MR systems to achieve unsupervised inline analysis of perfusion MRI. Validation results are reported for 260 perfusion time series, demonstrating feasibility of the approach.

1 Introduction

Myocardial first pass perfusion magnetic resonance imaging (MRI) has proven its clinical significance in the diagnosis of known and suspected ischemic heart disease, particularly in combination with cardiac delayed enhancement imaging [1]. However, the clinical routine to evaluate myocardial perfusion still relies on radionuclide imaging, such as Single Photon-Emission Computed Tomography (SPECT).

Despite many advantages over radionuclide techniques, MR perfusion imaging is still not widely used in clinical routine. Certain technical challenges prevent this technique to be added to the clinical workflow. Among them is complex cardiac motion caused by respiration, irregular heart rates, and imperfect cardiac gating. Due to these factors, a motion compensation procedure has to be applied prior to computing the myocardial signal intensity (SI) curves (Fig. 1) on a pixel-by-pixel basis. Another imperfection is B1-field inhomogeneity caused by non-uniform characteristics of the receiver coils. While qualitative visual reading is often not compromised by this effect [2], inhomogeneity can result in errors of quantitative or semi-quantitative analysis [1], which aims to estimate perfusion parameters, such as up-slope (SLOPE), area-under-curve (AUC) or myocardial blood flow.

The long and labor-intensive analysis process is also an important barrier to clinical utilization of MR stress perfusion imaging. Typically, clinical assessment requires sufficient coverage of the left ventricle (LV), while, due to the limited imaging efficiency of

---

[*] Corresponding author.

current MR scanners, a typical MR perfusion sequence acquires several two-dimensional (2D) images to approximate the coverage of LV. A minimum of three short-axis slices covering the basal, mid-ventricular, and apical portions of the LV is recommended [3]. To maintain sufficient temporal resolution during the first-pass of the contrast bolus, each slice should be imaged every one to two heart beats for a total duration of approximately 60s. As a result, a typical perfusion study can produce ~250 images. To generate signal time-intensity curves in order to estimate perfusion parameters, manual delineation of the endo- and epicardium is required due to cardiac motion. This process is time-consuming, and can be even worse in patients who are unable to hold their breath and require the data acquisition to be performed in a free breathing fashion.

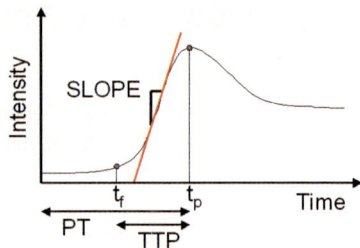

Fig. 1. Signal intensity curve and perfusion parameters. For each pixel the signal-time curve is analyzed and parameters like upslope (SLOPE), time-to-peak (TTP), peak time (PT) and area-under-curve (AUC, area under the curve between foot and peak) can be calculated. t_f and t_p are foot time and peak time.

To overcome these challenges, various image processing approaches are being investigated, mainly focusing on motion compensation of myocardium, including rigid-body image registration [4], ICA (independent component analysis) based correction [5], active contour [6] and active shape models [7]. However, few of these studies have yet obtained widespread usage and even fewer efforts were made so far to automate more comprehensive perfusion analysis workflows. Therefore, we propose an unsupervised perfusion analysis system, consisting of key-frame detection, consecutive motion compensation (MOCO), surface coil inhomogeneity correction (SCC) using proton density images, an Expectation-maximization (EM) algorithm, and robust parameter map generation. To maximize the clinical applicability, the proposed solution does not rely on assumptions about myocardial anatomy; therefore it can cope with different slice positions (basal, mid-ventricular and apical). Also, the processing pipeline can handle three widely used MR perfusion sequences including TurboFLASH (Turbo Fast Low Angle Shot), TrueFISP (True Fast Imaging with Steady state Precession), and GRE-EPI (Gradient Echo type Echo Planar Imaging). Finally, to provide clinicians with access to the proposed techniques, the algorithms are implemented within the Image Calculation Environment (ICE) as an inline processing chain on Siemens MR system.

2 Methods

2.1 Sequence Design

A flexible MR perfusion pulse sequence was implemented and tested on two clinical 1.5T scanners (Siemens MAGNETOM Espree and Avanto). The sequence supports different acquisition techniques, such as TurboFLASH, TrueFISP, and GRE-EPI hybrid. In order to enable a fully integrated inhomogeneity correction, the pulse sequence was modified to first acquire a small number (e.g. 2) of proton density (PD) weighted images before the start of the conventional first pass perfusion acquisition (Fig. 2). The slice prescription for the PD and perfusion images is identical. With the ap-

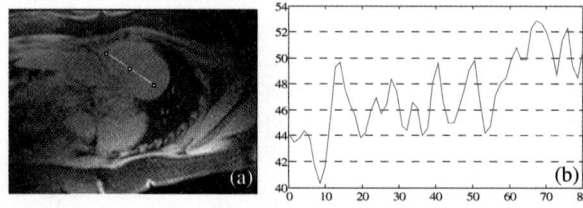

Fig. 2. (a) Example proton density image acquired before the normal perfusion acquisition. (b) Intensity profile across the heart region (yellow line). The intensity bias can be clearly observed.

proximation that the proton density across the myocardial anatomy is constant [1], the intensity changes of PD images can be positively related to local surface coil sensitivity.

2.2 Key-Frame Detection

The first step of the proposed workflow aims at detecting a *key-frame* for a perfusion series. This key-frame will be defined as the reference image, and relative motion between other phases and this reference image will be corrected. To improve the motion compensation, this key-frame should be a frame in which the myocardium has good contrast compared to the blood pool and surrounding tissues. We propose a key-frame selection approach which is based on the observation that during the contrast uptake the image intensity in regions where the contrast bolus enters will have higher standard deviation (SD) along the time dimension. As the first step, the standard deviation image for the perfusion series is computed. Although inconsistent myocardial motion can degrade the sharpness of myocardium, the contrast between myocardium and surrounding tissues in the SD image is found to be consistently noticeable. This observation holds true for the described perfusion MR pulse sequences. The next step is to select a frame having similar contrast as the SD image. For this purpose, the cross correlation ratios (CC) between every phase in the perfusion series and the SD image are computed. During the passing of contrast bolus, the CC ratio continues to increase and reaches its peak around the time point where the myocardium blood perfusion is maximized. We therefore pick the phase corresponding to the maximal CC ratio as the key-frame.

2.3 Consecutive Motion Compensation

We have found that the registration is more robust if two slices to be aligned have similar contrast. Therefore, a consecutive motion compensation strategy is developed to improve the performance of registration. As shown in Fig. 3, motion compensation starts from the key-frame and its direct neighbors (previous and next). After the first registration is finished, the next image is registered to its warped neighbor that has been transformed into the key-frame coordinate system. The complete series is corrected by consecutively performing multiple 2D-2D registrations between temporally adjacent slices. Considering the temporal resolution of perfusion studies is usually one to two heart beats, adjacent frames consistently show similar contrast, even during the first pass of contrast agents.

A fast variational non-rigid registration algorithm [8] is applied as the working-engine of perfusion motion compensation. This approach can be considered as an extension of the classic optical flow method. In this framework, a dense deformation field is estimated as the solution to a calculus of variation problem, which is solved by performing a compositional update step corresponding to a transport equation. The regularization is added by low-pass filtering the gradient images which are in turn used as velocity field to drive the transport equation. To speedup the convergence and avoid local minima, a multi-scale image pyramid is created. We selected the local cross correlation as the image similarity measure, as its explicit derivative can be more efficiently calculated than mutual information and still general enough to cope with intensity fluctuation and imaging noise between two adjacent perfusion frames.

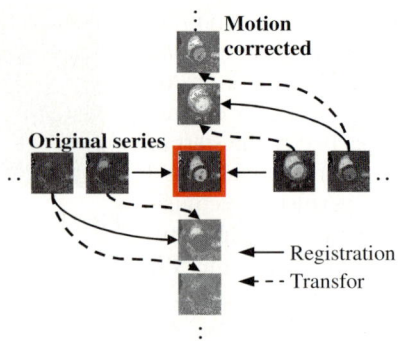

Fig. 3. An illustration of consecutive motion compensation. Motion compensation starts from the key-frame and its direct neighbors. Every image is aligned to its transformed previous neighbor. In this scheme, registration is performed between two perfusion phases with similar contrast.

2.4 Surface Coil Inhomogeneity Correction

To correct the variation in intensity due to the surface coil sensitivities, the proton density (PD) images are first registered to the key-frame. All motion compensated PD images are then averaged to improve the signal-to-noise ratio (SNR). To estimate the inhomogeneity field from the averaged PD images, we propose an algorithm to interleave tissue classification and bias estimation using Expectation-Maximization (EM) algorithm and B-Spline Free Form Deformation (BFFD).

The EM algorithm [9] consists of an expectation step (E-step) which performs the classification and a maximization step (M-step) which updates the parameter estimation. Assuming a Gaussian distribution and given initial parameters, the algorithm iteratively maximizes the data likelihood and updates the tissue classification. In the context of PD image based bias correction, we decided based on experimental evidence to classify PD images into three classes: background (BG), tissue with low intensity (TL) and tissue with high intensity (TH) because the contrast level in PD images is not sufficient to delineate specific tissue classes and the purpose here is not to get a detailed segmentation. We found this three-class assumption is robust for separating the regions of background and lung from organ tissues. To improve the accuracy of inhomogeneity estimation, all background pixels are then excluded from further computations.

We assume a multiplicative bias field. For a pixel i, its measured intensity is x_i. Defining the bias field at location i as b_i, the unbiased signal r_i can be estimated by $x_i = r_i \cdot b_i$. Using the notation $\tilde{x}_i = \log(x_i)$, the image formation model can become additive $\tilde{x}_i = \tilde{r}_i + \tilde{b}_i$. Then corresponding mean and sigma become $\tilde{\mu}_k$ and $\tilde{\sigma}_k$.

A B-Spline Free-Form Deformation is applied to approximate the bias field. In this representation, a dense 2D bias field is parameterized at a sparse control point lattice. Define the field-of-view (FOV) of the PD image as follows: $\Omega_s = \{(x,y)|0 \leq x \leq X, 0 \leq y \leq Y\}$ and ϕ_s denotes a grid of control points $\varphi_{p,q}$ with the grid spacing being $\Delta_x \times \Delta_y$. This spacing between adjacent control points is uniform for each coordinate direction. The 2D tensor of uniform 1D cubic B-splines is used to represent the spatial-variant bias ratio $\tilde{b}_i$:

$$T_{local}(\tilde{b}_i) = \sum_{m=0}^{3}\sum_{n=0}^{3} B_m(u) B_n(v) \varphi_{p+m,q+n} \quad (1)$$

Where (x, y) is the coordinate of pixel i, and $p = \lfloor x/\Delta_x \rfloor - 1$, $q = \lfloor y/\Delta_y \rfloor - 1$, $u = x/\Delta_x - \lfloor x/\Delta_x \rfloor$, and $v = y/\Delta_y - \lfloor y/\Delta_y \rfloor$. B_m represents the m-th basis function of the B-spline. The basis functions of cubic B-splines have limited support. Therefore changing a control point in the grid affects only a 4×4 region around that control point.

Unlike the formula in [11] where a polynomial with infinite support is used to approximate the bias field, we choose not to explicitly optimize the control point value during M-step, because it leads to solving a linear system for every pixel in the image due to the local support of B-Spline. To find the optimal control point value, we estimate a 'bias-free' image, similar to [11]:

$$\tilde{r}_i^{(m)} = \frac{\sum_{i=1}^{3} p^{(m)}(k|x_i) \cdot \tilde{\mu}_k^{(m)}}{\sum_{i=1}^{3} p^{(m)}(k|x_i)} \quad (2)$$

where $\tilde{r}_i^{(m)}$ denotes the estimated real signal at pixel location i for iteration m. Then the bias for this iteration can be estimated as $\tilde{b}_i^{(m)} = approx(\tilde{x}_i^{(m)} - \tilde{r}_i^{(m)})$. $approx(\cdot)$ is the FFD approximation step, which calculates the optimal control point value $\tilde{\varphi}_{i,j}^{(m)}$ (a detailed formula can be found in [10]). Given the estimated bias field, the corrected signal can be updated as $\tilde{x}_i^{(m+1)} = \tilde{x}_i^{(m)} - \tilde{b}_i^{(m)}$. Once the iteration converges or a maximum number of iterations is reached, the final bias field and corrected PD image are calculated by an exponential operator. As an illustration, Fig. 4 shows the estimated multiplicative bias field and corrected intensity profile for the PD image in Fig. 2.

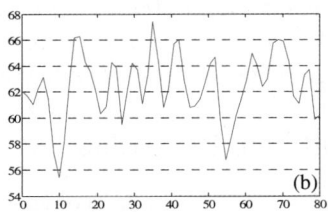

Fig. 4. Estimated (a) bias field and (b) corrected intensity profile (b) for Fig. 2. This bias field is used to correct the entire perfusion time series.

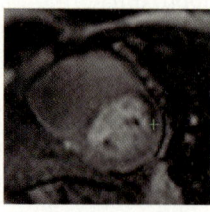 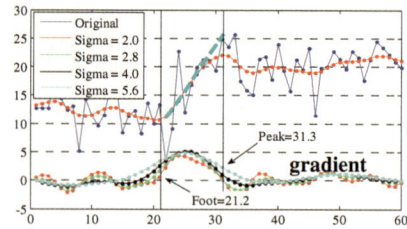

Fig. 5. An illustration of multi-scale perfusion parameter estimation. Although the pixel-wise time-intensity curve shows drastic fluctuation due to imaging noise, the multi-scale strategy is able to detect the first uptake of contrast bolus. Left: a perfusion time series with clear perfusion deficit; Right: the SI curve for a selected point (marked by the green cross) and detected contrast uptake.

2.5 Perfusion Parametric Map Generation

The final step of the proposed workflow is to calculate perfusion parameter maps. Instead of computing perfusion parameters for every myocardial segment, we developed a robust map generation algorithm based on the scale-space theory, which estimates perfusion parameters for each pixel in the image. Given a SI curve $s(t)$, a series of smoothed curves $s_i(t)$ are generated by convolution with Gaussian kernels $s_i(t) = s(t) * g_i(t)$, where $g_i(t)$ is a Gaussian function with the variance being $\sigma_i, i = 1,\ldots N$ and $\sigma_i < \sigma_j, 0 < i < j <= N$. Similarly the first-order derivative $s'_i(t)$ can be computed by convolution with the derivative of the Gaussian kernel. As no segment averaging is performed, the pixel-wise intensity curve $s(t)$ can be quite noisy (Fig. 5). To obtain a robust detection of first pass contrast bolus uptake, only the stable features that consistently appear across the whole scale space are kept. As the first step, all local maxima and zero-crossings of gradient $s'_1(t)$ are found as curve feature points. For each feature point, its appearance across all scales is checked using the concept of non-maximum suppression. The stable maximum with largest gradient is picked as the time-point corresponding to maximal up-slope. The foot time t_f is defined by the 20% of the maximal gradient, while the peak time t_p is determined by the first stable zero crossing point after the maximal up-slope, corresponding to the maximal intensity of first bolus uptake. Once the bolus uptake region is found, a weighted least-square fit is applied to this part of time-intensity curve and the optimal up-slope is estimated. The weight for intensity point t is defined as its gradient magnitude computed from $s'_i(t)$. A scatter interpolation strategy is finally applied to fill the 'holes' which often appear on the noisy background where the algorithm can not find enough stable features across the scale space.

3 Results and Discussion

Validation was performed on anonymized data from 40 subjects (3 institutions), with a total of 260 perfusion series. Three different MR perfusion imaging sequences (74 TurboFLASH, 12 TrueFISP, and 174 GRE-EPI) were used in these scans. All scans were performed with a minimum of three slice positions (basal, mid-ventricular and apical) and 2 PD images were acquired before the perfusion acquisition. We visually reviewed all datasets and classified them into two categories (no significant motion and with significant motion) according to the maximal motion magnitude presented in the series. Significant motion was not found in 92 series (35%) while the other 168 series (65%) clearly require motion compensation.

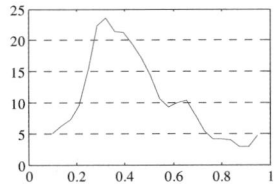

Fig. 6. Distribution of detected key-frames for the whole data cohort

The proposed analysis workflow was applied to all series and outputs of every processing step were inspected. For the key-frame detection, we found that the detected frames consistently showed good contrast between blood pool and myocardium. Fig. 6 shows the distribution of the key-frames, which is defined as the ratio between the index of key-frame and the length of the corresponding perfusion series. The mean of the key-frame ratio is 0.44 ± 0.19.

As demonstrated in Fig. 7 where an example of MR perfusion motion compensation is givxen, the jitter motion of myocardium was largely eliminated for those cases with significant motion. For cases where hearts remain stationary, we found no discernible errors were introduced by the algorithm. To quantitatively verify the motion compensation, we selected 30 series with significant motion (In-plane resolution: $1.4 \sim 2.4$ mm^2), covering all pulse sequences and slice positions. The quantitative evaluation was performed by manually delineating the left ventricle and myocardium. For every selected series, two single 2D frames

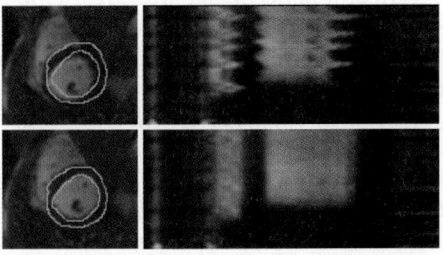

Fig 7. Motion compensation of a free-breathing series. First row: TrueFISP 2D slice overlaid with myocardium contour of key-frame and the intensity-time profile. Second row: the same slice after motion compensation and the corrected intensity-time profile.

were picked. One is the detected key-frame and the other frame was chosen when the myocardium motion was clearly discernible. Four statistical measures are computed to give a comprehensive quantification: a) T_{A-I} (the relative motion of the left ventricle center point along the Anterior-Inferior direction); b) T_{S-L} (the same motion along the Septal-Lateral direction); c) *Dice ratio* (the myocardium overlap ratio); d) *MBE* (the myocardium boundary errors, defined as the minimal distances between myocardium contours (endo and epi) extracted from the template and the registered slice). Table 1 summarizes the results, showing noticeable improvement after motion compensation.

Table 1. The quantitative measures of motion compensation

	T_{A-I} [mm]		T_{S-L} [mm]		Dice ratio		MBE [mm]	
	original	moco	original	moco	original	moco	original	moco
Mean	3.97	1.39	6.68	1.12	0.56	0.87	3.84	1.29
STD	3.26	1.03	4.69	0.83	0.20	0.04	3.19	1.24

moco: motion compensation.

The inhomogeneity correction fields estimated from the PD images were applied to the entire perfusion series to correct for the bias introduced by the surface coils. Visual inspection showed the reduction of intensity inhomogeneity that was consistently discernible throughout the datasets. To quantitatively verify the effects of bias correction, we selected the first frame of the perfusion acquisition and measured the intensity profile across the heart. We then fit a straight line to the data and estimated the absolute slope (AS) with and without bias correction. Because saturation recovery or inversion recovery pulses are normally applied to null the pre-contrast blood and tissue in the perfusion imaging, the intensity profile of the first phase often shows bias through the heart. For a group of 20 randomly selected series from the whole data cohort, the mean AS was originally 0.17 ± 0.13 and reduced to 0.06 ± 0.07 after the bias correction (Paired t-test, P<0.005, 95% CI: 0.05-0.18), which is consistent with our visual impression.

As the final step, four parameter maps (SLOPE, TTP, PT and AUC) were calculated for every test case. We found that the detection of bolus uptake was highly robust, which was verified by manually sampling the SI curves from blood pool and myocardium and comparing to the automated results. As an example, for patients without clear perfusion deficits, the maps show uniform myocardium, while real perfusion deficits can be clearly visualized (Fig. 8).

To make the proposed techniques accessible to clinicians, all processing steps were implemented within the Image Calculation Environment (ICE) of Siemens MRI systems. The inline perfusion analysis starts immediately after the reconstruction of MR signals. Original time series, corrected time series, and derived parameter maps are stored in the image database after processing. The entire processing chain was implemented to support concurrent calculation via simultaneous multi-threading. The processing time for a perfusion study with three series is typically less than 1min. The proposed system is under the clinical evaluation currently taken at four institutes (Langone Medical Centre, University of New York; Laboratory of Cardiac Energetics, National Institute of Health; University Medical Centre of Ohio State, Department of Cardiology, HELIOS-Klinikum Berlin-Buch). Among the overall positive feedback, clinicians strongly favor the robustness of proposed motion compensation, as many patients were scanned in the free/shallow breathing fashion.

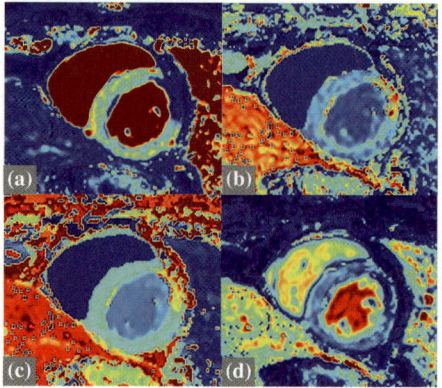

Fig. 8. Perfusion parameter maps (a-d: SLOPE, TTP, PT and AUC) for the series in Fig. 5. The deficit is clearly visualized.

References

1. Kellman, P., Arai, A.E.: Imaging Sequences for First Pass Perfusion-A Review. J. Cardio. MR 10, 525–537 (2007)
2. Guillemaud, R., Brady, M.: Estimating bias field of MR images. IEEE Trans. Med. Imaging 16, 238–251 (1997)

3. Puvaneswary, M.: Cardiac MR Imaging. Anshan Ltd. (2005)
4. Bracoud, L., Vincen, F., Pachai, C., Canet, E., Croisille, P., Revel, D.: Automatic Registration of MR First-Pass Myocardial Perfusion Images. In: Magnin, I.E., Montagnat, J., Clarysse, P., Nenonen, J., Katila, T. (eds.) FIMH 2003. LNCS, vol. 2674, pp. 215–223. Springer, Heidelberg (2003)
5. Milles, J., van der Geest, R.J., Jerosch-Herold, M., Reiber, J.H., Lelieveldt, B.P.: Fully automated registration of first-pass myocardial perfusion MRI using independent component analysis. Inf. Process Med. Imaging 20, 544–555 (2007)
6. Yang, G.Z., Burger, P., Panting, J., Gatehouse, P.D., Rueckert, D., Pennell, D.J., Firmin, D.N.: Motion and deformation tracking for short-axis echo-planar myocardial perfusion imaging. Med. Image Anal. 2(3), 285–302 (1998)
7. Stegmann, M.B., Olafsdottir, H., Larsson, H.B.: Unsupervised motion-compensation of multi-slice cardiac perfusion MRI. Med. Image Anal. 9(4), 394–410 (2005)
8. Chefd'hotel, C., Hermosillo, G., Faugeras, O.: Flows of diffeomorphisms for multimodal image registration. In: Proceedings of the IEEE ISBI (2002)
9. Dempster, A.P., Laird, N.M., Rubin, D.B.: Maximum likelihood from incomplete data via the EM algorithm. Journal of the Royal Statistical Society 39, 1–38 (1977)
10. XLee, S.Y., Wolberg, G., Shin, S.Y.: Scattered data interpolation with Multilevel B-Splines. IEEE Trans. Visualization and Computer Graphics 3(3), 228–244 (1997)
11. Van Leemput, K., Maes, F., Vandermeulen, D., Suetens, P.: Automated model-based bias field correction of MR images of the brain. IEEE Trans. Med. Imaging 18, 885–896 (1999)

Pattern Recognition of Abnormal Left Ventricle Wall Motion in Cardiac MR

Yingli Lu[1], Perry Radau[1], Kim Connelly[1,2], Alexander Dick[3], and Graham Wright[1]

[1] Imaging Research, Sunnybrook Health Sciences Centre, Toronto, ON, Canada
[2] Cardiology, St Michael's Hospital, Toronto, ON, Canada
[3] Cardiology, Sunnybrook Health Sciences Centre, Toronto, ON, Canada
yinglilu@gmail.com, perry.radau@gmail.com, connellyka@yahoo.ca,
Alexander.Dick@sunnybrook.ca,
gawright@sten.sunnybrook.utoronto.ca

Abstract. There are four main problems that limit application of pattern recognition techniques for recognition of abnormal cardiac left ventricle (LV) wall motion: 1) Normalization of the LV's size, shape, intensity level and position; 2) defining a spatial correspondence between phases and subjects; 3) extracting features; 4) and discriminating abnormal from normal wall motion. Solving these four problems is required for application of pattern recognition techniques to classify the normal and abnormal LV wall motion. In this work, we introduce a normalization scheme to solve the first and second problems. With this scheme, LVs are normalized to the same position, size, and intensity level. Using the normalized images, we proposed an intra-segment classification criterion based on a correlation measure to solve the third and fourth problems. Application of the method to recognition of abnormal cardiac MR LV wall motion showed promising results.

1 Introduction

Currently, diagnosis of abnormal left ventricle (LV) wall motion is generally based on visual inspection of the 4D (3D× temporal) dynamic cardiac magnetic resonance cine images. Studies have shown that this method may be inaccurate, time consuming and suffer from high inter-observer variability [1]. Therefore, methods of computer aided recognition of abnormal LV wall motion will clinically significant. Earlier literature [1,2,3,4] on recognition of abnormal LV wall motion are generally based on end-diastolic (ED) and end-systolic (ES) phases' wall thickening and motion information. Goals of this work are to introduce a novel application of pattern recognition techniques for computer aided recognition of abnormal LV wall motion. Unlike previous approaches, it utilizes the wall thickness and motion information from all cardiac phases.

There are four main problems that limit application of pattern recognition techniques to the problem of detecting abnormal LV wall motion. First, the LV's size, shape, intensity level and position require normalization. A subject's LV changes size, shape, intensity level and position throughout the cardiac cycle. And there is additional inter-subject variation. Second, it is important to determine a spatial correspondence between phases and subjects. The LV wall motion features can be extracted only after defining this correspondence. The third problem is feature extraction that is sensitive to wall motion but not sensitive to the following factors: thickness variation of the myocardium across subjects, as well as the size and position variation of the papillary muscles and endocardial trabeculations across phases and subjects. The final problem is discrimination of normal and abnormal wall motion and selection of a classification criterion. Without solving these four problems, it is difficult to use pattern recognition techniques to detect and classify LV wall motion.

In this work, we introduce a normalization scheme so that the LV from each slice is normalized to polar coordinates with a fixed size, intensity level and position. Because cardiac motion is a complex combination of wall thickening, circumferential shortening and longitudinal ventricular shortening, determining pixel-based spatial registration phases and subjects is difficult and complicated by the requirement of retaining information about abnormal wall motion. This problem is simplified by establishing segment correspondence instead, and this appropriately matches clinical wall motion scoring practice[5,6]. In the feature extraction stage, we propose an intra-segment correlation to measure each segment's wall motion relative to normal values. Training data is used to determine the correlation measure criterion for discrimination of abnormal wall motion.

2 Left Ventricle Normalization

There are four steps in the normalization scheme: reference points localization, spatial normalization, intensity normalization, and labeling of segments. It is assumed that epicardial contours are available, for example after application of the automated segmentation algorithm described in the previous works [9-13].

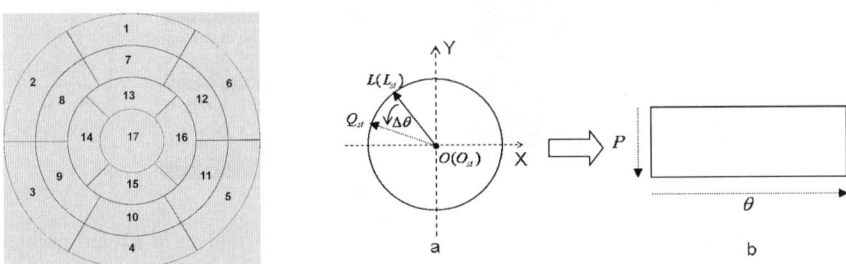

Fig. 1. AHA 17 myocardial segments   **Fig. 2.** Diagram of spatial normalization

Reference Points Localization. Because of the diversity of patients' body positions in the scanner and different heart positions in the thorax, we have to normalize different heart positions to the same. In this work, we used the AHA 17 segment reference [5, 6] (Refer to Fig.1). In which, the heart is divided into four parts cutting across the long axis of the LV: basal, mid-cavity, apical and apex. The basal and mid-cavity short axis slices are each divided radially into 6 segments, whereas the apical slice has 4 segments, and the 17th segment is the apex. According to the AHA 17 segment model, either junction between the right ventricular wall and the interventricular septum of the basal (and mid-cavity) slice on the ED phase can be used as reference point to identify different segments. In this work, the anterior end of the interventricular septum is used as the reference point. (Point L in Fig. 3a and 3e). For each subject, there are two sub-steps to locate the reference points of each phase:

Step1. Mark reference point L at the selected basal (or midcavity) slice's ED phase.

Step2. Calculate reference point of each phase (excluding ED). Given L and centroid O of the epicardium contour, we have the angle to the reference point L on the epicardium, $\angle XOL$ (Fig. 2a). For a given slice $slice_{st}$ and $\angle XOL$ and O_{st}, we can get the reference point L_{st} of $slice_{st}$ with the assumption that $\angle XO_{st}L_{st} = \angle XOL$ (Note: The slice at level s and phase t is defined as $slice_{st}$ $s = 1,2..., S$, $t = 1,2,...,T$, where S and T are the maximum slice and phase numbers respectively. O_{st} is the centroid of the plotted epicardial contour of $slice_{st}$).

Given reference points L_{st} of each subject, and combined with the 'spatial normalization' step, heart positions of different subjects can be localized.

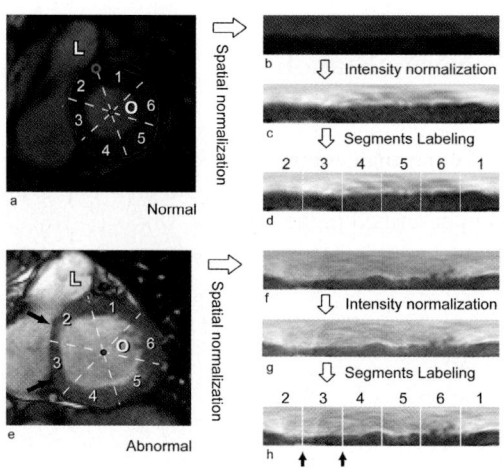

Fig. 3. Examples of the normalization procedure for a normal subject (**a-d**) and an abnormal wall motion patient (**e-h**). In **a** and **e**, the darker circular band is the myocardium, and the whiter pool is blood. In **a** and **e**, L is the reference point and O is the centroid of the LV. In **e** and **h**, the two black arrows point to the abnormal segment.

Spatial Normalization. An essential feature of the LV is the approximately radial wall motion and circular epicardial boundary, therefore the analysis is simplified by mapping the pixel intensities from Cartesian (x, y) to polar coordinates. In addition, the proposed mapping described below normalizes the size and shape of the myocardium by normalizing the length of each radial line from the LV centre to the epicardium.

This normalizes the images spatially for both intra- and inter-subject comparisons. For $slice_{st}$ of each subject, there are five steps:

Step 0. Set $col = 1, \theta = \angle XO_{st}L_{st}, Q_{st} = L_{st}$. col is defined as the output image column index.

Step 1. Plot line segment $O_{st}Q_{st}$ from O_{st} to Q_{st}.

Step 2. Interpolate the pixel intensity values along line segment $O_{st}Q_{st}$ to P points. Put the result in the col^{th} column of output image with P rows.

Step 3. Set $\theta = \theta + \Delta\theta$ along the counterclockwise direction. Update Q_{st} (on the LV epicardium boundary) by constraint $\angle XO_{st}Q_{st} = \theta$. Set $col = col + 1$.

Step 4. Repeat step1 and step3, until Q_{st} equals L_{st} (initial point).

After these steps, $slice_{st}$ has been normalized to a $P \times col$ rectangular image. See Fig. 3b and 3f for examples, with $\Delta\theta = 1°$, and $P = 60$. The result is a 60×360 image. By means of this spatial normalization, LVs of different subjects were normalized to the same position, since for all of the resultant images the left edge represents the line from the LV centre to the reference point L, the row represents the radial distance (normalized by the distance to the epicardium for that radial line) and the column is the counterclockwise polar angle.

Intensity Normalization. In order to normalize the intensity differences across slices, phases, subjects and scanners, each pixel has its intensity set to $(x - \mu)/\sigma$, where, x is the original intensity value, μ and σ are respectively the mean and the standard deviation of the rectangular image. (See Fig.3c and 3g.)

Segments Labeling. According to the AHA segment model (Fig.1), the basal segments 1 to 6 correspond to the blocks found by dividing evenly the rectangular image along the vertical direction, as labeled in Fig. 3d and 3h. The mid-cavity segments 7 to 12 have the same partitions as segments 1 to 6. The apical segments 13 to 16 correspond to the $1^{st} - 4^{th}$ rectangular block by dividing evenly the rectangular image along the vertical direction (Refer to [5]).

3 Intra-segment Correlation Based Classification

In the cardiac cycle, there are different phases alternating in a natural order, for instance, from systole to diastole. Motion patterns of the normal segment should be deviate away from motion patterns of the abnormal segment. For a specific segment, if we concatenate the normalized segment images of all the phases in column manner, we get a spatial-temporal segment image (e.g. Fig.4a, c). Comparing the motion pattern of the segment for normal (Fig. 4a) and abnormal cases (Fig. 4c), we found that from phase 4 to phase 18, the normal segment contracts more than the abnormal segment. For the normalized segment image of each phase $t(t = 1, 2, \cdots, T)$, a column vector U_t is calculated by averaging the vertical line intensity profile across θ angles of the segment (refer to Fig.2b). Subsequently the correlation coefficients CC_t between U_{ED} and

$U_t(t=1,2,\cdots,T)$ can be calculated to measure the motion pattern along all the t phases. (ED refers to the end diastolic phase, with $ED=1$ in Fig.4.) Fig. 4d shows the correlation coefficients of both normal and abnormal segments. This demonstrates that the contraction is greater (correlation is lower) in a normal segment than an abnormal segment from phase 4 to 18. Therefore, the CC_t of the abnormal segment has a motion pattern that deviates from the normal segment's $CC_t(t=1,2,\cdots,T)$. Accordingly, the CC_t measure can be use to discriminate the normal and abnormal segments, with a classification criterion derived from the training data. When a new patient is encountered, for each segment, the following steps summarized the recognition process: 1. LV normalization; 2. Calculate $U_t(t=1,2,\cdots,T)$; 3. Calculate $CC_t(t=1,2,\cdots,T)$; 4. Classify to normal or abnormal based on a predefined classification criterion.

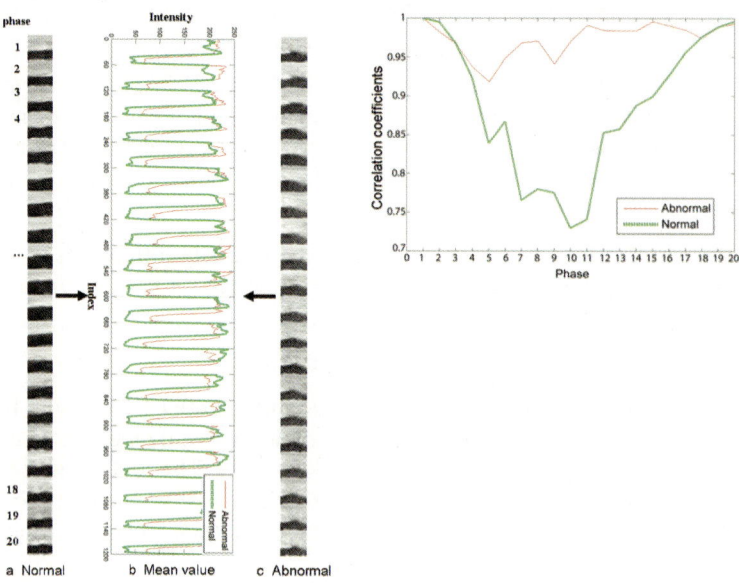

Fig. 4. Segment images from different phases concatenated in column from normal a) and abnormal c) subjects. b) U, intensity profiles of column image averaged across segment θ of the normal (green) and abnormal (red) segment. d) Intra-segment correlation coefficients of the normal and abnormal segment.

4 Experiments and Results

4.1 Data

For this study, the MRI of 17 patients were analyzed (2 female, 15 male, age: 64.8 ± 9.5). Cine Fiesta MR short axis (SAX) images were obtained with a 1.5T GE Signa MRI. All the images were obtained during 10-15 s breath-holds with a temporal resolution of 20 cardiac phases. Six to 12 SAX images were obtained from the atrioventricular ring to the apex (thickness=8mm, gap=8mm, FOV=320mm× 320mm, matrix=256×256). For all subjects, a single basal slice was selected for this preliminary study, and 12/17 patients had regional abnormal wall motion for the basal slice by expert visual assessment. Before normalization, contour points were placed manually with spline interpolation to plot the epicardial boundary. From the epicardial boundary the centroid of the LV is calculated. For each subject, in the LV segmentation step, the first input landmark point at the ED phase is recorded as reference point L. In this work, the anterior end of the interventricular septum was used as the reference point. In the spatial normalization step $\Delta\theta$ was set to $1°$ and P was set to 60, resulting in a 60×360 rectangular image in polar coordinates.

4.2 Experiments and Results

In order to determine a classification criterion for each segment, we calculated the $CC_t(t=1,2,\cdots,20)$ averaged across all subjects with the same assessment (normal or abnormal wall motion). Fig 5 shows plots of the averaged $CC_t(t=1,2,\cdots,20)$ for individual segments, demonstrating that the minimum value of the averaged normal CC_t falls between phase 6 and 10 and is always smaller than the minimum of the averaged abnormal CC_t. Accordingly, for segment 1-6, the classification criterion is defined as: If $\min(CC_t)(t=6,7,\cdots,10) < T_{segment}$ $(segment=1,2,\cdots,6)$, segment is classified as normal. Otherwise, the segment is classified as abnormal.

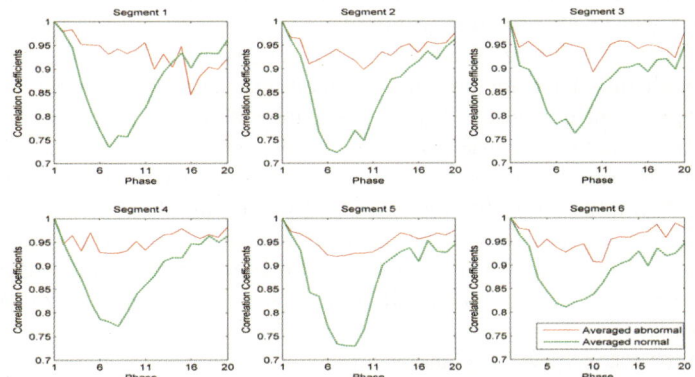

Fig. 5. Correlation coefficients. Each graph illustrates the wall motion of a segment as measured by the correlation CC_t between the phase t and end diastolic phase.

Table 1. Sensitivity, specificity and accuracy of segments 1-6

	Segment					
	1	2	3	4	5	6
Sensitivity	80%	85.7%	100%	75.0%	85.7%	100%
Specificity	91.7%	100%	90.9%	84.6%	90%	66.7%
Accuracy	88.2%	94.1%	94.1%	82.4%	88.2%	70.6%
Recognition time (10^{-4} s)	1.4	1.7	1.7	1.1	1.1	1.8

Table 2. Comparison with manual and other computer aided method

	Manual method in [1]	computer aided Method in [1]	Proposed method
Mean Sensitivity	80%	84%	87.1%(27/31)
Mean Specificity	76%	77%	85.9%(61/71)
Mean Accuracy	77%	79%	86.3%(88/102)

The performance of the proposed classification method was calculated on a per segment basis, where the expert reader's visual assessment served as ground truth. Segment classification results were used to calculate the sensitivity, specificity and accuracy, with a total of 17x6=102 segments (Table 1). Table 1 also shows that the computational time for recognition (normalization and discrimination) is approximately 10^{-4} second per segment on consumer hardware (2×2.8GHz Quad-core Intel Xeon Mac Pro, Apple) with non-optimized Matlab code (Mathworks). In Table 2, the performance of the proposed method was also evaluated by comparisons with previous work in [1]. These preliminary results are better than the manual and computer aided methods described in [1] as measured by sensitivity, specificity and accuracy.

5 Discussions and Conclusions

With the normalization scheme, LV images of different positions, sizes, shapes and intensity levels are normalized to myocardium coordinates with the same position, size, and intensity level, providing a foundation for pattern recognition of wall motion. Spatial correspondence is established for segments rather than pixels in this work. Although this does not provide for pixel-wise analysis of cardiac motion of non-rigid registration techniques [7], it is suitable for automated recognition of regional LV wall motion because the wall motion assessment required clinically is based on the AHA segment model [5,6]. This partially solves the second problem proposed in the introduction. In order to solve the third and fourth problems, for each segment, an intra-subject correlation measure was proposed. Since the correlation coefficients are calculated with an intra-segment manner, the variability of myocardial thickness between subjects and the papillary muscles, trabeculations' size and position will not be an issue.

Although the mean specificity and accuracy were relatively low for clinical use, as a preliminary attempt to use the pattern recognition method for assessment of regional LV wall motion, the results are still promising. Further improvements are desirable, including: 1) combining with automated or semi-automated methods to segment the LV; 2) training with mid-cavity and apical slices where papillary muscles are present; 3) a larger set of subjects, with separate training and validation sets; 4) more efficient methods of classification (e.g. support vector machine [8]). While a simple classification criterion was used in this work, the results are still promising due to the effectiveness of the normalization and feature extraction scheme.

Compared with the previous work on regional LV wall motion analysis methods [1, 2, 3, 4], main characteristics of the proposed method can be summarized as: 1) Segmentation of the endocardium is not required. Analyzing the radial profile in LV coordinates has been shown to be sufficient for detecting wall motion abnormalities in this patient study data set. 2) This method finds an appropriate balance between complexity and simplicity. A pixel-wise estimate of wall motion adds complexity of analysis and the detailed motion is not required for clinical assessment. An accurate location of the reference point to demarcate segments of each phase is difficult. Therefore, the proposed reference point location scheme was utilized, although it will lead to slight segment location errors due to the LV twisting and ventricular torsion. 3) The complete information from all phases and segments is utilized to determine a wall motion estimate comparable to the standard manual wall motion scores. 4) This method is a novel application of pattern recognition techniques to LV motion analysis.

In summary, a scheme has been proposed for abnormal LV wall motion detection by the techniques of pattern recognition. By the proposed LV normalization method, the LVs with different shapes, positions, sizes and intensity levels are normalized to rectangular images with same position, size and intensity level. This normalization scheme is a crucial bridge for the further applications of pattern recognition method to LV motion analysis. Following the normalization, an intra-segment correlation based classifier was used for recognition of segments with abnormal regional LV wall motion. The results demonstrate a promising method for recognition of abnormal LV wall motion that deserves more extensive validation.

References

1. Caiani, E.G., Toledo, E., MacEneaney, P., et al.: Automated interpretation of regional left ventricular wall motion from cardiac magnetic resonance images. Journal of Cardiovascular Magnetic Resonance 8(3), 427–433 (2006)
2. Saring, D., Ehrhardt, J., Stork, A., et al.: Computer-assisted analysis of 4D cardiac MR image sequences after myocardial infarction. Methods Inf. Med. 45(4), 377–383 (2006)
3. Suinesiaputra, A., Uzumcu, M., Frangi, A.F.: Detecting regional abnormal cardiac contraction in short-axis MR images using independent component analysis. In: Barillot, C., Haynor, D.R., Hellier, P. (eds.) MICCAI 2004. LNCS, vol. 3216, pp. 737–744. Springer, Heidelberg (2004)
4. Suinesiaputra, A., Frangi, A.F., Uzumcu, M.: Extraction of myocardial contractility patterns from short-axes MR images using independent component analysis. In: Sonka, M., Kakadiaris, I.A., Kybic, J. (eds.) CVAMIA/MMBIA 2004. LNCS, vol. 3117, pp. 75–86. Springer, Heidelberg (2004)
5. Cerqueira, M.D., Weissman, N.J., Dilsizian, V.: Standardized myocardial segmentation and nomenclature for tomographic imaging of the heart. J. Nucl. Cardiol. 9, 240–245 (2002)
6. Bogaert, J., Dymarkowski, S., Taylor, A.M.: Clinical Cardiac MRI, pp. 95–97. Springer, Heidelberg (2005)
7. Li, B., Young, A.A., Cowan, B.R.: GPU accelerated non-rigid registration for the evaluation of cardiac function. Med. Image Comp. Comp. Assist. Interv. 11(Pt 2), 880–887 (2008)
8. Burges, C.J.C.: A Tutorial on Support Vector Machines for Pattern Recognition. Data Mining and Knowledge Discovery 2, 121–167 (1998)
9. Fradkin, M., Ciofolo, C., Mory, B., Hautvast, G., Breeuwer, M.: Comprehensive segmentation of cine cardiac MR images. Med. Image Comp. Comp. Assist. Interv. 11(Pt 1), 178–185 (2008)
10. Ben Ayed, I., Lu, Y., Li, S., Ross, I.: Left ventricle tracking using overlap priors. Med. Image Comp. Comp. Assist. Interv. 11(Pt 1), 1025–1033 (2008)

11. Cocosco, C.A., Niessen, W.J., Netsch, T., Vonken, E.J., Lund, G., Stork, A., Viergever, M.A.: Automatic image-driven segmentation of the ventricles in cardiac cine MRI. J. Magn. Reson. Imaging 28(2), 366–374 (2008)
12. Lynch, M., Ghita, O., Whelan, P.F.: Segmentation of the Left Ventricle of the Heart in 3-D+t MRI Data Using an Optimized Nonrigid Temporal Model. IEEE Trans. Med. Imaging 27(2), 195–203 (2008)
13. Lu, Y., Radau, P., Connelly, K., Dick, A., Wright, G.M.: Segmentation of Left Ventricle in Cardiac Cine MRI: An Automatic Image-Driven Method. LNCS, vol. 5528, pp. 339–347. Springer, Heidelberg (2009)

Septal Flash Assessment on CRT Candidates Based on Statistical Atlases of Motion

Nicolas Duchateau[1,2], Mathieu De Craene[1,2], Etel Silva[3], Marta Sitges[3], Bart H. Bijnens[1,2,4], and Alejandro F. Frangi[1,2,4]

[1] CISTIB - Universitat Pompeu Fabra, Barcelona, Spain
[2] CIBER-BBN, Spain
[3] Hospital Clinic - IDIBAPS - University of Barcelona, Spain
[4] ICREA, Barcelona, Spain

Abstract. In this paper, we propose a complete framework for the automatic detection and quantification of abnormal heart motion patterns using Statistical Atlases of Motion built from healthy populations. The method is illustrated on CRT patients with identified cardiac dyssynchrony and abnormal septal motion on 2D ultrasound (US) sequences. The use of the 2D US modality guarantees that the temporal resolution of the image sequences is high enough to work under a small displacements hypothesis. Under this assumption, the computed displacement fields can be directly considered as cardiac velocities. Comparison of subjects acquired with different spatiotemporal resolutions implies the reorientation and temporal normalization of velocity fields in a common space of coordinates. Statistics are then performed on the reoriented vector fields. Results show the ability of the method to correctly detect abnormal motion patterns and quantify their distance to normality. The use of local p-values for quantifying abnormal motion patterns is believed to be a promising strategy for computing new markers of cardiac dyssynchrony for better characterizing CRT candidates.

1 Introduction

Cardiac Resynchronization Therapy (CRT) has been shown to efficiently restore the coordination and relaxation among cardiac chambers, leading to better survival in patients with advanced heart failure and evidence of ventricular conduction delays [1]. The main clinical challenge for CRT is currently the understanding of physiological mechanisms involved behind positive or negative response. Recently, a promising way of finding non-responders for CRT was presented in [2], who proposed a classification of patients into classes of dyssynchrony patterns, and evaluated the response of each of these groups. This analysis attempts to relate the patient to a population with a known electrical or mechanical dyssynchrony defect that is expected to be effectively corrected by CRT. In this perspective, the computation of distances from a new subject to well identified groups of patients is a novel strategy for improving CRT response rate.

Recent research in computational anatomy has lead to the design and evaluation of statistical tools that synthesize the average anatomy within a population as well as the statistical deviation from this average. Recent works used non-rigid registration techniques to build Statistical Atlases of Motion of the heart from magnetic resonance image sequences [3], in which the displacement fields reflect the movement of anatomical structures. The use of 4D transformation models was presented in [4] for motion tracking over sequences of images. Registration is performed between frames at time points t_i and t_0 ($i \neq 0$). Such a strategy can provide large displacements, which in an atlas perspective would require to perform statistics on the tangent space of diffeomorphisms, using the methods described in [5]. In addition, representing the motion in reference to the first frame does not take advantage of the strong correlation between consecutive frames, and introduces a lot of redundancy between time steps for statistical computations.

A diffeomorphic registration scheme using paths between pairs of consecutive frames was recently presented in [6] for the synchronization of 4D time-series of cardiac images, and allows spatially consistent comparison of the supposedly temporally aligned sequences. One drawback of this technique is the fact that the computed transformations are only available at the discrete timepoints where the frames of the sequences are defined. Combining pairwise matching terms with the computation of diffeomorphic paths [7] allows to follow the evolution of a shape over a 2D+t sequence, and therefore to track the anatomy over the continuous timescale. However, this method still needs spatio-temporal synchronization steps to apply it for atlas construction from various sequences, and needs to prove its feasability when applied to real ultrasound (US) data.

In this paper we propose a complete and flexible pipeline for the construction of atlases of motion from sequences of US images, and illustrate its use for clinically-oriented quantitative comparison. We take advantage of registration between pairs of consecutive frames to work under a small displacements hypothesis. Our strategy is motivated by the fact that low correlation exists between time-distant frames for the US modality, and by the good temporal resolution of the 2D US modality. While existing atlases of motion are based on displacement fields, we prefer velocities, directly related to cardiac function. Working with small displacements allows easier definition of velocities over the whole continuous timescale, and direct computation of classical statistics on these velocities, once they have been brought to the same spatio-temporal system of coordinates. The structure provided by the atlas is then used for chosen pathology comparison to a healthy population, in the context of looking for CRT responders. We apply the method to the characterization of one mechanism related to Left Ventricle (LV) dyssynchrony, namely Septal Flash (SF), a quick inward/outward movement of the septum with respect to the LV, which occurs during the electrical activation of the heart chambers. We chose to work with 2D+t US modality as it is the only one used in clinical practice with sufficient temporal resolution to accurately identify fast septal motion patterns. However, the concepts developed in this paper could readily be applied to 3D+t once the required temporal resolution is accessible in standard clinical acquisition protocols.

2 Computation of Cardiac Velocities

2.1 Intra-sequence Registration

In the following we will denote $S = \{S(t_1), ..., S(t_i), ..., S(t_N)\}$ the temporal series of 2D images for one given patient, which contains N images taken at time-points t_i. To track the anatomy along cardiac cycles, pairwise registration between consecutive frames provides an optimal sequence of transformations $\varphi_{t_i,t_{i+1}} : \boldsymbol{x} \mapsto \boldsymbol{x}'$ for each series, which map any point of image $S(t_i, \boldsymbol{x})$ to its corresponding point in the following frame $S(t_{i+1}, \boldsymbol{x}')$. Our non-rigid registration uses the Free-Form Deformation (FFD) method [8], which is made multi-resolution to improve its robustness to the position and spacing of control points. We used spacings of successively 26, 13 and 6.5 mm, and mutual information as matching term.

2.2 Small Displacements Hypothesis and Definition of Velocities

If the displacements are small, the logarithm [5] of a transformation $\log\left(\varphi_{t_i,t_{i+1}}\right)$ can be approximated at the first order by its corresponding displacement field $\varphi_{t_i,t_{i+1}} - \boldsymbol{Id}$. Velocities are directly obtained at the discrete time-points where the data is defined using

$$\forall i \quad (t_{i+1} - t_i) \cdot \boldsymbol{v}(t_i, .) = \log\left(\varphi_{t_i,t_{i+1}}\right) \approx \left(\varphi_{t_i,t_{i+1}} - \boldsymbol{Id}\right) \qquad (1)$$

and assumed to be stationary between consecutive time-points t_i and t_{i+1}, which means that:

$$\boldsymbol{v}(t, \widehat{\varphi}_{t_i,t}(\boldsymbol{x})) = \boldsymbol{v}(t_i, \boldsymbol{x}) \qquad (2)$$

where t_i is the closest time-point that precedes t at which the series S is defined. Equation 2 means that trajectories are linearly interpolated to provide $\widehat{\varphi}_{t_i,t}(\boldsymbol{x})$, the position at time t of the anatomical point that was at $\boldsymbol{x}$ at time t_i. Orientation and invertibility are preserved at any point $(t, \boldsymbol{x})$, as the log-exponential does with large displacements.

In our $t_i \to t_{i+1}$ registration approach, we can reasonably assume that the displacements are small. Such a choice is encouraged by the good temporal resolution of the 2D US modality. We validated this assumption by comparing the computed displacement fields and the logarithm of their relative transformations, using $D(\varphi_1, \varphi_2) = \frac{1}{card(\Omega)} \cdot \sum_{\boldsymbol{x}_j \in \Omega} \frac{|\varphi_2 \circ \varphi_1^{-1} - \boldsymbol{Id}|}{|\varphi_1 - \boldsymbol{Id}|}(\boldsymbol{x}_j)$ as normalized dissimilarity measure between two transformations φ_1 and φ_2, where Ω is the image domain. We previouly ensured these transformations are diffeomorphic, that-is-to-say they are invertible, smooth and with smooth inverse so that the logarithm can be computed. The results of this experiment are summarized in Fig.1, which presents the comparison of φ and $\log \varphi + \boldsymbol{Id}$ for all the frames of one series containing three cycles. To get a range of comparison, this experiment is also done for a $0 \to t_i$ registration strategy, which works with larger displacements, and for a SF patient.

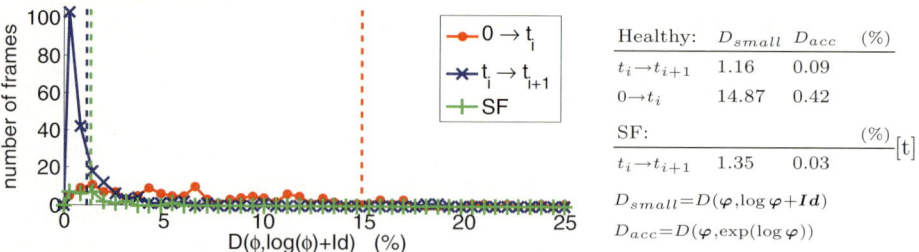

Fig. 1. Left: distribution of the dissimilarity measure D_{small} over the set of frames (*red* and *blue*: healthy volunteer, all the frames, $t_i \rightarrow t_{i+1}$ and $0 \rightarrow t_i$ approaches, *green*: SF patient, frames where SF occurs). Average over all the frames is in dashed line, and summed up in the table on the right. Table also contains D_{acc} for the assessment of logarithm computations accuracy.

2.3 Drift Correction

Drift artifacts from registration between pairs of consecutive frames are solved by applying for each cycle a correction involving a linear-in-time scaling of the transformation between frames which begin consecutive cycles, $\varphi_{T_j,T_{j+1}}$, where T_j is the time-point starting cycle j. This transformation aims at correcting probe motion during the acquisition, and adds robustness towards out-of-plane motion, as the assumption $\varphi_{T_j,T_{j+1}} = Id$ generally made in other works [4] is not verified in our database of 2D US sequences.

3 Statistics on Cardiac Velocities

3.1 Pre-processing Steps

For each patient, the registration steps provide velocities on which statistics can be computed directly. They should first be brought into the same system of spatio-temporal coordinates. In the following we use k index to refer to sample patient k, and we index variable names accordingly.

Temporal Normalization. On each sequence, two control points related to the cardiac cycle phases are identified on the corresponding Electrocardiogram (ECG) and then mapped to a normalized timescale: the onset of QRS complex, using ECG tools from GE EchoPac software, and aortic valve closure, observed in left-parasternal long-axis images and located on ECG for the apical 4-chamber view we use by ECG correspondence. This step will be automated in further work. Between the control points temporal data is then adjusted linearly to match the new timescale. Similar synchronization methods [9] also identified a set of control points over each sequence of MR images, but used image similarity. We preferred to rely on ECG information, as for US images the identification of these points using image data can be biased by respiratory or probe motion. In addition, the use of physiological events as temporal landmarks is believed to be more extendable to handle pathological subjects.

Spatial Reorientation. Velocities $v^k(t, x)$ are initially defined in the system of coordinates of patient k, but should be reoriented to be embedded in a reference system of coordinates before computing any statistics. We chose arbitrarily one series with good image quality as the reference. We first compute the transformation $\phi^{k \to ref}(t, x)$ which maps estimated images of patient k and reference ref at time t, using FFD. We ensured that the computed transformation is invertible by checking that its jacobian has a positive determinant. Using notations of Section 2.2, an image S is simply estimated at time t from the image at the closest preceding time-point t_i, with $\widehat{S}(t,.) = \widehat{\varphi}_{t_i,t}(S(t_i,.))$. Reorientation of velocity fields v^k is then achieved at every point (t, x) using a push-forward action on vector fields [10]:

$$\mathcal{P}_\phi(v) = \mathbf{D}\phi \cdot (v \circ \phi^{-1}) \qquad (3)$$

where $v = v^k$, $\phi = \phi^{k \to ref}$ and $\mathbf{D}$ the jacobian operator. We use the same computations for the inverse as in [5].

3.2 Statistical Computations

Once these pre-processing steps have been achieved, statistics can be directly computed on velocities. We first compute their average and variance to characterize the atlas population. Considering K different sample series $\{S^k | \ k = 1...K\}$, we obtain at any desired point (t, x) the average $\overline{v} = \frac{1}{K} \sum_{k=1}^{K} v^k$ and the covariance matrix $\Sigma_v = \frac{1}{K-1} \mathbf{V}^t \cdot \mathbf{V}$ from the set of velocities v^k. Here $\mathbf{V}^t = [(v^1 - \overline{v})|...|(v^K - \overline{v})]$ is the $2 \times K$ matrix whose columns are the centered velocity samples at (t, x), and ^{t} is the matrix transposition operator.

The atlas is then used for the comparison of the velocities of a given patient to the population used for its construction, through the computation at every desired point (t, x) of statistical indexes assessing abnormality. We chose as index the p-value obtained from Hotelling's t-square statistic [11]:

$$t^2 = \alpha \ (v - \overline{v})^t \cdot \Sigma_v^{-1} \cdot (v - \overline{v})$$

where $\alpha = K/(K+1)$, v is the velocity to compare to the atlas, and $\overline{v}$ and Σ_v are the average and the covariance matrix computed for the population atlas.

(pixels)	Healthy			SF		
	δ_{inter}	δ_{intra}	Δ_{track}	δ_{inter}	δ_{intra}	Δ_{track}
1. Basal inferoseptal	2.21	1.90	1.57	1.29	2.43	1.73
2. Mid inferoseptal	2.51	3.58	3.84	0.41	1.84	1.26
3. Apical septal	1.66	3.97	5.11	0.70	2.03	2.67
4. Apical	0.97	2.17	2.76	0.77	2.72	1.67
Average	1.84	2.91	3.32	0.79	2.26	1.83

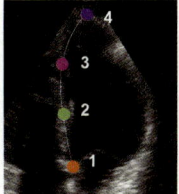

Fig. 2. Comparison between automatic and manual tracking: inter- and intra-operator standard deviation (δ_{inter} and δ_{intra}), and distance between automatically and manually tracked points (Δ_{track}).

4 Experiments on 2D US Sequences

We acquired 2D+t echocardiographic sequences in an apical 4-chamber view for two populations of patients, using a GE Vivid 7 machine. The atlas population was made up of 21 healthy volunteers. The second population included 4 CRT patients with visually assessed SF. The choice of the apical 4-chamber view is lead by the fact that it is the one used in clinical routine for the assessment of the inward/outward movement of the septum related to SF. Physiological differences between patients constrain the acquisition parameters, that will differ in terms of temporal resolution and image quality. For the atlas population, we acquired images with optimized resolution, that corresponds in average to a frame rate of 60 frames/s and a pixel size of 0.15×0.15 mm^2. For constraints related to the therapy, such settings were not reproducible for SF patients, acquired at a similar spatial resolution but at a lower frame rate (30 frames/s).

4.1 Atlas Construction

We first evaluated the quality of our intra-sequence registration by comparing it to manual landmarking. Three observers tracked 4 points along the septum that correspond to basal-inferoseptal, mid-inferoseptal, apical-septal and apical levels. Measurements were repeated 10 times for each point, and selection was done over one cycle of one healthy volunteer and one SF patient. Then each landmark was automatically tracked, starting from its average position in the first frame. Fig.2 presents the average in time of inter- and intra- observer variability, and compares it to the distance between automatically and manually tracked points. Automatic and manual tracking show comparable precision over all the selected points.

In order to check the efficiency of the synchronization scheme described in Section 3.1, we acquired 4 sequences for the same patient and checked that the

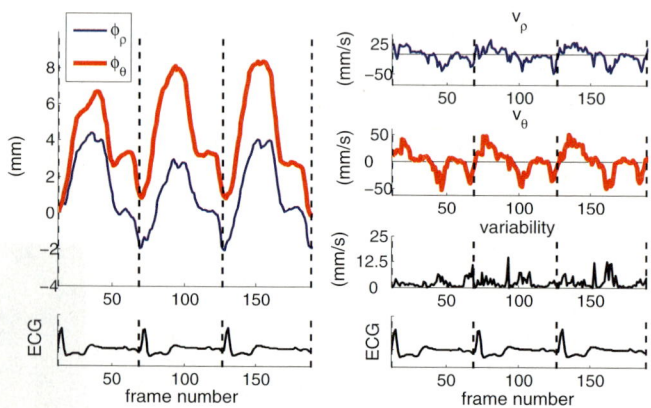

Fig. 3. Repeatability measurement for the spatio-temporal synchronization scheme. Left: radial (*thin blue*) and longitudinal (*thick red*) position of a tracked point at mid-inferoseptal level. Right: corresponding velocities. $\sqrt{Tr(\boldsymbol{\Sigma}_v)}$ is used as variability measure.

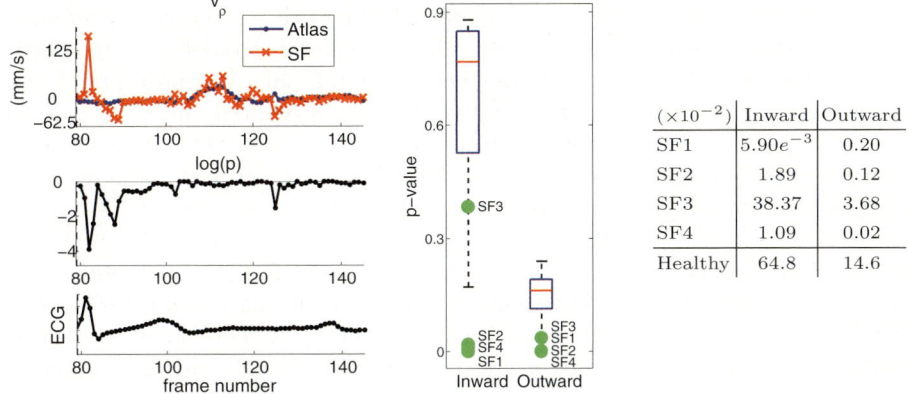

Fig. 4. Comparison of SF patients to the atlas, at mid-inferoseptal level. Left: radial velocity (*blue*: atlas average, *red*: SF1), and p-value plot along 1 cycle for SF1. Middle: p-value for the atlas population (*box plots*), and the 4 SF patients (*green dots*) at timepoints corresponding to maximum inward (left) and outward (right) patterns. Right: table summarizing these p-values for the atlas (average of the leave-one-out values) and the 4 SF patients.

estimated velocities overlap after the synchronization. These sequences contain 3 whole cycles, and are made of 204, 189, 209 and 218 frames, respectively, with varying orientation of the probe. Good repeatability is observed between the curves, using $\sqrt{Tr(\Sigma_v)}$ as variability measure (Fig.3).

4.2 Septal Flash Assessment

We built the atlas of motion using the whole set of synchronized healthy volunteers, and then compared velocity fields for the atlas and the 4 SF patients as described in Section 3.2. The comparison is shown at mid-inferoseptal level, where the fast inward/outward motion of the septum takes place (Fig.4). Velocity and p-value profiles are plotted for one SF patient to see when SF occurs relatively to the ECG. Low p-value means high degree of abnormality. From both plots we can notice a very large abnormal inward velocity when the septum is activated, which is almost immediately followed by a fast outward motion at the time when the infero-lateral wall contracts. Box plots in the middle and the recapitulative table on the right compare p-values for the 4 SF patients and p-values for the atlas population, which were obtained using leave-one-out cross-validation. On SF patient 3 abnormality is hard to assess, due to the poor image quality of the sequence and the limited magnitude of the SF. On all the other three SF patients, p-value enables efficient assessment of abnormality for the SF pattern.

5 Conclusion

In this paper, we proposed to apply atlas quantification techniques to characterize the septal flash mechanism, which proved its interest for understanding response to CRT. We proposed a complete framework for the construction of an atlas that represents motion in a standard spatio-temporal system of coordinates and compared cardiac velocities between CRT patients and a population of healthy subjects. Our experimental results demonstrated the ability of the atlas to assess local motion abnormalities in time and space. Our pipeline could easily be extended to strain measurements for a more advanced characterization of the mechanisms conditioning response to CRT.

Acknowledgments. This research has been partially funded by the Industrial and Technological Development Center (CDTI) under the CENIT Programme (CDTEAM Project) and the European Community's Seventh Framework Programme (FP7/2007-2013) under grant agreement n. 224495 (euHeart project).

References

1. Mullens, W., Grimm, R.A., Verga, T., Dresing, T., Starling, R.C., Wilkoff, B.L., Wilson Tang, W.H.: Insights From a Cardiac Resynchronization Optimization Clinic as Part of a Heart Failure Disease Management Program. J. Am. Coll. of Cardiology 53(9), 765–773 (2009)
2. Parsai, C., Bijnens, B.H., Sutherland, G.R., Baltabaeva, A., Claus, P., Marciniak, M., Paul, V., Scheffer, M., Donal, E., Derumeaux, G., Anderson, L.: Toward understanding response to cardiac resynchronization therapy: left ventricular dyssynchrony is only one of multiple mechanisms. Eur. Heart J. 30(8), 940–949 (2009)
3. Petitjean, C., Rougon, N., Cluzel, P., Prêteux, F., Grenier, P.: Quantification of myocardial function using tagged-MR and cine-MR images. Int. J. of Card. Im. 20(6), 497–508 (2004)
4. Ledesma-Carbayo, M.J., Kybic, J., Desco, M., Santos, A., Sühling, M., Hunziker, P.R., Unser, M.: Spatio-temporal nonrigid registration for ultrasound cardiac motion estimation. IEEE Trans. Med. Im. 24(9), 1113–1126 (2005)
5. Arsigny, V., Commowick, O., Pennec, X., Ayache, N.: A log-euclidean framework for statistics on diffeomorphisms. In: Larsen, R., Nielsen, M., Sporring, J. (eds.) MICCAI 2006. LNCS, vol. 4190, pp. 924–931. Springer, Heidelberg (2006)
6. Peyrat, J.-M., Delingette, H., Sermesant, M., Pennec, X., Xu, C., Ayache, N.: Registration of 4D time-series of cardiac images with multichannel diffeomorphic demons. In: Metaxas, D., Axel, L., Fichtinger, G., Székely, G. (eds.) MICCAI 2008, Part II. LNCS, vol. 5242, pp. 972–979. Springer, Heidelberg (2008)
7. Khan, A.R., Beg, M.F.: Representation of time-varying shapes in the large deformation diffeomorphic framework. In: ISBI, pp. 1521–1524 (2008)
8. Rueckert, D., Sonoda, L.I., Hayes, C., Hill, D.L., Leach, M.O., Hawkes, D.J.: Non-rigid registration using free-form deformations: application to breast MR images. IEEE Trans. Med. Im. 18(8), 712–721 (1999)
9. Perperidis, D., Mohiaddin, R.H., Rueckert, D.: Spatio-temporal free-form registration of cardiac MR image sequences. Med. Im. An. 9(5), 441–456 (2005)
10. Tu, L.W.: An Introduction to Manifolds, 1st edn., ch. 14. Springer, Heidelberg (2007)
11. Hotelling, H.: The Generalization of Student's Ratio. The Annals of Mathematical Statistics 2(3), 360–378 (1931)

Personalized Modeling and Assessment of the Aortic-Mitral Coupling from 4D TEE and CT

Razvan Ioan Ionasec[1,4,*], Ingmar Voigt[2,5], Bogdan Georgescu[1], Yang Wang[1], Helene Houle[3], Joachim Hornegger[5], Nassir Navab[4], and Dorin Comaniciu[1]

[1] Integrated Data Systems, Siemens Corporate Research, Princeton, USA
razvan.ionasec@siemens.com
[2] Software and Engineering, Siemens Corporate Technology, Erlangen, Germany
[3] Ultrasound, Siemens Medical Solutions, Mountain View, CA, USA
[4] Computer Aided Medical Procedures, Technical University Munich, Germany
[5] Chair of Pattern Recognition, Friedrich-Alexander-University, Erlangen, Germany

Abstract. The anatomy, function and hemodynamics of the aortic and mitral valves are known to be strongly interconnected. An integrated quantitative and visual assessment of the aortic-mitral coupling may have an impact on patient evaluation, planning and guidance of minimal invasive procedures. In this paper, we propose a novel model-driven method for functional and morphological characterization of the entire aortic-mitral apparatus. A holistic physiological model is hierarchically defined to represent the anatomy and motion of the two left heart valves. Robust learning-based algorithms are applied to estimate the patient-specific spatial-temporal parameters from four-dimensional TEE and CT data. The piecewise affine location of the valves is initially determined over the whole cardiac cycle using an incremental search performed in marginal spaces. Consequently, efficient spectrum detection in the trajectory space is applied to estimate the cyclic motion of the articulated model. Finally, the full personalized surface model of the aortic-mitral coupling is constructed using statistical shape models and local spatial-temporal refinement. Experiments performed on 65 4D TEE and 69 4D CT sequences demonstrated an average accuracy of 1.45mm and speed of 60 seconds for the proposed approach. Initial clinical validation on model-based and expert measurement showed the precision to be in the range of the inter-user variability. To the best of our knowledge this is the first time a complete model of the aortic-mitral coupling estimated from TEE and CT data is proposed.

1 Introduction

Aortic and mitral valves are the most commonly diseased valves, cumulating in 64 percent and 14 percent, respectively of the valvular heart disease case. The coupling of the aortic and mitral valvular annuli through fibrous tissue is evident and leads to strong functional and hemodynamical interdependency. Recent

---

[*] Corresponding author.

studies and findings demand that the dynamics and morphologies of the aortic and mitral valve must be considered simultaneously [1,2]. Reciprocal changes of the aortic and mitral annular areas have been reported and it was concluded, that the fibrous aortic-mitral continuity acts as an anchor for the valves. Together with the muscular portions of either annuli and their contraction during their reciprocal motion, it facilitates the opening and closing of the other valve during systole and diastole respectively [3]. Various findings and facts related to interventions on both valves emphasize the notion of their coupling. In transapical aortic valve replacement, the prosthese's stent must not be placed too far downwards into the directions of the left ventricle, as it would impair the mitral anterior leaflet's mobility [4]. Moreover another recent study pointed out, that mitral regurgitation can be positively affected by aortic valve replacement [5]. Understanding the dynamics and morphology of the aortic-mitral valvular apparatus is important as a base for diagnosis and treatment decisions, optimal design of prostheses and intervention outcome improvement.

Recently, personalized valve models have attracted great attention and are expected to significantly advance the management of patients with valve heart disease. To date, separate approaches were reported for modeling of both valves [6,7]. Veronesi et al.[3] reported a method, where both annuli were segmented with manual initialization and quantified. Up to now the full joint morphology and dynamics of both valves at the same time have not been studied due to the lack of suitable methods and tools.

In this paper we propose a new model driven approach for quantitative and visual assessment of the aortic-mitral complex, which models all relevant anatomical structures of both valves. For the first time a complete personalized model of the aortic-mitral coupling, non-invasively derived from 4D Computed Tomography (CT) and 4D Transoesophageal Echocardiography (TEE) acquisitions, accurately represents the valves' morphology and function. The personalized parameter estimation from input image sequences is performed efficiently using a robust and hierarchical learning-based algorithm. Our approach enables for integrated quantification, and has the potential to fuel research on mixed valve disease, cardiac pathophysiology and interventional procedures.

2 Physiological Modeling of the Aortic-Mitral Coupling

We propose a physiological model of the complete aortic-mitral apparatus capable to capture complex morphological, dynamic and pathological variations. The valves are coupled by a fibrous tissue [1] and work in synchrony [3,2] to regulate the blood flow in the left heart. The central anatomical structures are: aortic root and leaflets along with mitral anterior and posterior leaflets. To efficiently handle the anatomical complexity, the model representation and corresponding parameterization is constructed hierarchically and includes: a global piecewise affine model, a non-rigid articulated model and a full surface model.

The time dependent global position (c_x, c_y, c_z, t), orientation $(\alpha_x, \alpha_y, \alpha_z, t)$ and scale (s_x, s_y, s_z, t), are defined for each valve individually and illustrated as

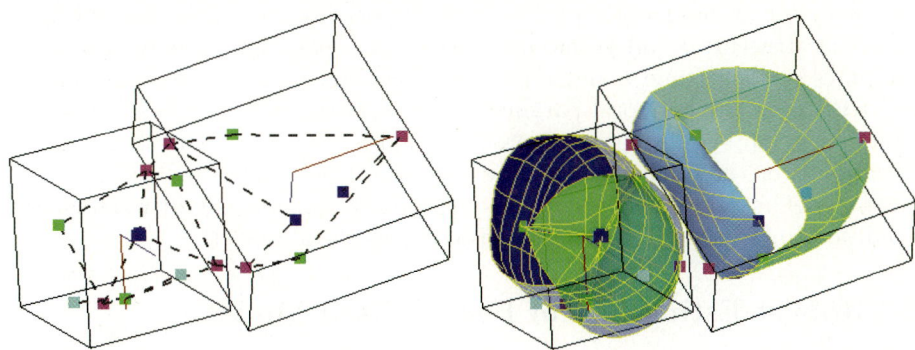

Fig. 1. Physiological model of the aortic-mitral coupling. **Left:** Non-rigid articulated model including the following landmarks: aortic and mitral commissures (green), aortic and mitral tips (blue), aortic hinges and mitral triagones (magenta) and coronary ostia (cyan). **Right:** Full surface model: aortic root (blue), aortic leaflets (green), anterior (light-blue) and posterior (light green) mitral leaflets.

bounding boxes in Fig. 1. Positions are given by the valve's barycenters, while scales are chosen to comprise the entire underlying anatomy. The long axes are defined by the normal vectors to the aortic-commissural plane and mitral-trigonal plane, while short axes point from the barycenters to the LR-commissure and mitral posteroannular midpoint, respectively.

The aortic and mitral valves execute a rapid opening-closing movement, which follows a complex and synchronized motion pattern. Normalized by the global parameters, the non-rigid motion is represented through an articulated model. It consists of 18 joints, which are relevant anatomical landmarks (see Fig. 1 Left). Each joint j is parameterized through the corresponding trajectory $\boldsymbol{a}_j$, given by the concatenation of the spatial coordinates, $\boldsymbol{a}^j(t) \in \mathbb{R}^3$, over time $t = 0, \cdots, n-1$:

$$\boldsymbol{a}^j = [\boldsymbol{a}^j(0), \boldsymbol{a}^j(1), \cdots, \boldsymbol{a}^j(t), \cdots, \boldsymbol{a}^j(n-1)] \quad (1)$$

The highest abstraction layer models the 3D surfaces of the anatomical structures: aortic root, left/right/none coronary leaflets for the aortic valve, and anterior/posterior leaflets for the mitral valve (see Fig. 1 **Right**). The aortic root connects the ascending aorta to the left ventricle outflow tract and is modeled as a cylindrical surface constrained by the hinges, coronary ostia and aortic commissures. Attached to the root are the three aortic leaflets, delineated by the corresponding tip, hinge and commissures, and modeled as paraboloids. The anterior and posterior leaflets of the mitral valve separate hemodynamically the left ventricle from the left atrium. The aortic mitral curtain, which anatomically links the two valves, ends into the left and right fibrous trigones. These, together with the mitral-commissures and corresponding tip are fixing the anterior leaflet. The posterior leaflet, divided into three scallops, is located between the mitral commissures, middle triagone and its corresponding tip. The saddled shaped mitral annulus is modeled implicitly by the upper margins of the mitral leaflets. For each structure k, all surfaces $C^k(u,v,t)$ are parameterized by spatial coordinates u,v and time t and represented by Non uniform rational B-splines (NURBS) [8]. The temporal parameter t extends the standard NURBS surface equation by applying the tensor product, and is used to capture the temporal variation over the cardiac cycle. The surface model is anchored to the articulated model introduced above and is constraint by anatomically-driven boundary condition to form a full 4D physiological aortic-mitral model.

3 Robust Estimation of Personalized Model

The model parameters introduced in section 2 are estimated from 4D patient specific data to obtain a personalized representation of the aortic-mitral apparatus. To maximize efficiency and comply with the hierarchical model definition, the estimation algorithm is based on robust learning methods and is divided in three stages: Global Localization and Motion Estimation, Trajectory Spectrum Learning and Dynamic Surface Model Fitting.

Global Localization and Motion Estimation. The global location and motion is represented by the 3D+t affine parameters $(c_x, c_y, c_z, \alpha_x, \alpha_y, \alpha_z, s_x, s_y, s_z, t)$, for each valve. These are estimated by combining anatomy detectors trained using the Marginal Space Learning (MSL) framework [9] with a variant of the Random Sample Consensus (RANSAC) [10]. MSL provides an efficient way of learning high dimensional models and fast online search by operating in subspaces of increasing dimensionality. Anatomical classifiers are sequentially learned on the subspaces: position, position + orientation and position + orientation + scale. The probabilistic boosting tree (PBT) [11], in combination with Haar and Steerable Features [9], is applied for training. The RANSAC estimator is employed to obtain a robust and time consistent global motion. Several high-probable hypotheses are obtained for each frame by scanning the trained MSL-based affine estimator over the input image sequence. Assuming a constant global motion, the candidate hypotheses are sequentially sampled as the current motion model parameters and the best fit from each frame is considered when computing the robust quality measure. The final inlier selection is given by the model with the maximum number of hypotheses within the pre-specified tolerance $\sigma = 7mm$, measured usign the L1 norm.

Trajectory Spectrum Learning. We propose a novel algorithm to estimate the non-rigid motion of the articulated model by performing learning and optimization in trajectory spectrum spaces [12]. The trajectory of each joint $\boldsymbol{a^j}$ in (1) can be represented by its corresponding discrete Fourier transform (DFT) coefficients:

$$\boldsymbol{s^j}(f) = \sum_{t=0}^{n-1} \boldsymbol{a^j}(t) e^{\frac{-j2\pi t f}{n}} \qquad (2)$$

where $\boldsymbol{s^j}(f)$ is the frequency spectrum of the x, y, or z components of the trajectory $\boldsymbol{a^j}(t)$, and $f = 0, 1, \cdots, n-1$. Consequently, the objective to find the trajectory $\boldsymbol{a}^j$, with the maximum posterior probability for a series of volumes I can be express as:

$$\arg\max_{\boldsymbol{a}^j} p(\boldsymbol{a}^j|I) = \arg\max_{\boldsymbol{s}^j} p(\boldsymbol{s}^j|I) = \arg\max_{\boldsymbol{s}^j} \\ p(\boldsymbol{s}^j(0),\cdots,\boldsymbol{s}^j(n-1)|I(0),\cdots,I(n-1)) \tag{3}$$

As the original search space is high dimensional, the learning and optimization is performed efficiently in orthogonal subspace with increased dimensionality spanned by the DFT bases functions. This incremental approach initially captures coarse level motion and gradually refines high-frequent deformations as the search space dimension increases. Starting with the initial space of the DC ($\boldsymbol{s}^j(0)$), we iteratively add frequency components $\boldsymbol{s}^j(f)$ and learn the posterior probability in each subsequent subspace until reaching the dimensionality of the original space, $n-1$. At a certain stage i, the subspace includes the spectrum component $\boldsymbol{s}^j(0),\ldots,\boldsymbol{s}^j(i)$ and the conditional probability is modeled by a trained detector D_i:

$$p(\boldsymbol{s}^j(i)|\boldsymbol{s}^j(0),\ldots,\boldsymbol{s}^j(i-1)) = D_i(\boldsymbol{s}^j(0),\ldots,\boldsymbol{s}^j(i)) \tag{4}$$

For each subspace, the detectors D_i are trained on positive and negative trajectories extracted from the training set, using the probabilistic boosting tree (PBT) algorithm in conjunction with steerable features [9].

The detection starts with a zero-spectrum and estimates incrementally the amplitude and phase of each DFT component $\boldsymbol{s}^j(f)$. At a certain stage i, high probability hypothesis are determined and preserved by D_i. Subsequently, the dimensionality of the search subspace is extended to $i+1$ with the spectrum component $\boldsymbol{s}^j(i+1)$ and the detection is repeated using D_{i+1}. The algorithm stops when the original space is reached and outputs the optimal trajectory spectrum ($\boldsymbol{s}^j(0),\cdots,\boldsymbol{s}^j(n-1)$). The location and motion of the model is obtained by reconstructed the trajectory $\boldsymbol{a}^j$ of each joint j applying the inverse DFT transformation [1]. The spectrum representation and corresponding decomposition enable efficient motion learning and optimization as the number of tested hypotheses during detection is significantly reduced by at least on magnitude.

Dynamic Surface Model Fitting. The full surface model is initialized by fitting the mean shape, learned from the training set, to the estimated articulated model from the previous section. Boundary detectors, trained using PBT and steerable features, deform locally the surfaces to obtain proper object delineation [9]. The resulting surfaces are projected on the corresponding shape space to impose the geometric smoothness constraint. The PCA-based shape model, which contains 80 modes, is computed from point correspondences maintained by model re-sampling within anatomical local coordinates (Sec. 2). To enhance temporal smoothness, a learned motion prior, combined with optical

---

[1] The non-rigid motion trajectories are reconstructed from the real coefficients of the DFT, while optimization runs in the complex space, considering both amplitude (real) and phase (imaginary)

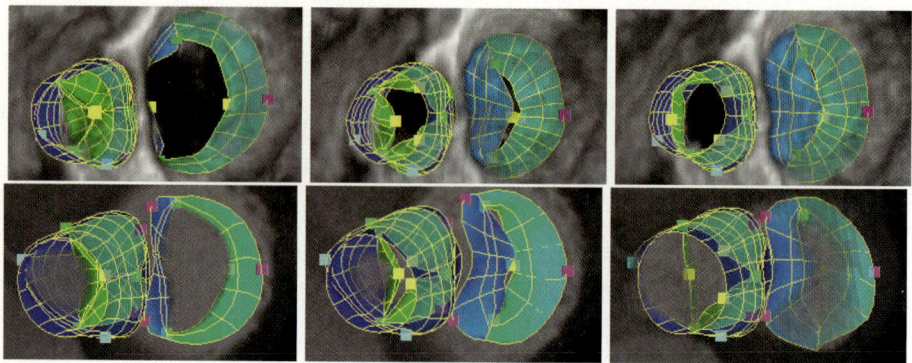

Fig. 2. Examples of the personalized model in TEE (**Top**) and CT (**Bottom**)

flow estimation, is applied to predict the propagated surfaces based on the previous frames [13]. The above procedure is repeated for each volume in the image sequences, in both forward and backward directions, to obtain a personalized dynamic surface model of the entire aortic-mitral apparatus.

4 Results

The proposed method for personalized aortic-mitral modeling was evaluated on 69 4D CT (690 volumes) and 65 4D TEE (1516 volumes) studies. The data set contains healthy as well as valves affected by various diseases, such as stenosis, regurgitation, prolapse and annular dilation. Both CT and TEE scans were acquired using heterogeneous protocols with various sizes and resolutions. Each study is associated with a manual performed annotation, which represents the ground-truth. This was obtained and refined together with clinical experts while gradually improving the semi-automated annotation system. Performance is reported on three-fold cross validation experiments.

The accuracy of the algorithm for the three estimation stages is presented in Table 1. Global location and motion parameters were estimated on low-resolution (3mm) images, with errors measured from the Euclidean distance of the bounding boxes' corner points between ground-truth and detected results. The accuracy of the non-rigid articulated model estimator is computed from the average Euclidean distance over all aortic and mitral joints. Performance for the full surface estimator is measured by the point-to-mesh distance. We obtain an average accuracy of 1.45 mm with a total computation time of 60 seconds for the personalized aortic-mitral coupling model (see Fig.2). The obtained system-error is compared to the inter-user variability in an experiment involving a randomly selected subset of 10 TEE sequences and models placed manually by 3 expert users. The barycentric distance and angle between the aortic and mitral valve were measured from the model in end-diastole and end-systole. Fig. 3 demonstrates that the system-error relative to the mean measurements of all experts lies for 90% of the cases within the 80% user-variability confidence interval.

Table 1. Errors for each detection stage in TEE (Left) and CT (Right)

	(mm)	Mean	Std.	Median	80%	Mean	Std.	Median	80%
Global Affine Parameters		6.95	4.12	5.96	8.72	8.09	3.32	7.57	10.4
Non-Rigid Articulated Model		3.78	1.55	3.43	4.85	2.93	1.36	2.59	3.38
Full Surface Model		1.54	1.17	1.16	1.78	1.36	0.93	1.30	1.53

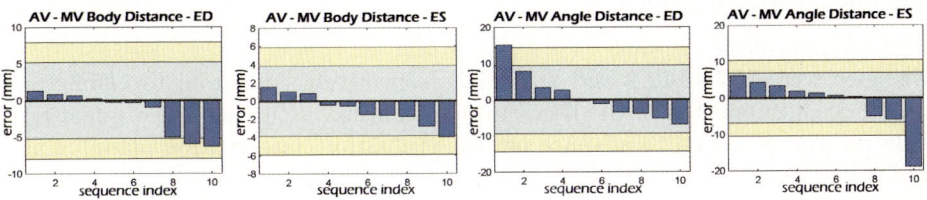

Fig. 3. System error compared to the inter-user variability. The sorted system error (blue bars) and the 80% (light blue area) and 90% (yellow) confidence intervals of the user variability determined from the standard deviation.

Table 2. Left: System-precision for various dimensions of the aortic-mitral coupling. **Right:** Bland-Altman plots for the aortic and mitral valves area.

	Mean	STD
VAJ (cm)	0.137	0.017
SV (cm)	0.166	0.043
STJ (cm)	0.098	0.029
AC (cm)	0.846	0.3
APD (cm)	0.325	0.219
AL-PM-D (cm)	0.509	0.37

The inter-modality consistency of the model-based quantification was demonstrated on studies of patients which underwent both imaging investigations, TEE and cardiac CT. A strong correlation, r=0.98, p<0.0001 and 0.97-0.99 confidence intervals, was obtained on standard measurements (aortic valve area, inter-commissural distances and root diameters at the sinotubular, ventricular-arterial junction and ventricular-arterial junction), derived from the personalized model in four different CT/TEE exams.

We demonstrated the quantitative capabilities of our approach by comparing model driven to expert measurements. Table 2 presents the system-precision for various dimensions of the aortic-mitral coupling: Diameters of the ventricular-arterial junction (VAJ), sinus of valsalva (SV) and sinotubular junction (SJ), aortic valve area (AV area), mitral valve area (MV area), mitral annular circumference (AC), anteroposterior diameter (APD), anterolateral-posteromedial diameter (AL-PM-D). The mean interannular angle and interannular centroid

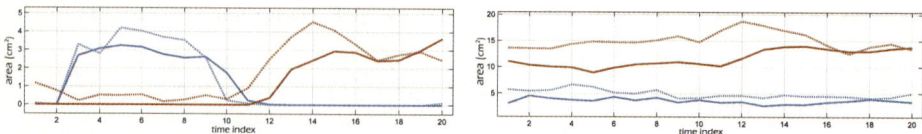

Fig. 4. Measurements obtained before (dotted lines) and after (solid lines) mitral annuloplasty. **Left:** Aortic (blue) and Mitral (red) valvular area. **Right:** Aortic (blue) and Mitral (red) annular area.

distance were 137.0±12.2 and 26.5±4.2, respectively compared to 136.2±12.6 and 25.0±3.2 reported in the literature [3]. Automatic, model-based quantification has the potential to advance patient evaluation, intervention planning and guidance.

Pre- and post-operative modeling for a patient who underwent mitral annuloplasty revealed the substantial effect on the aortic valve (not targeted during the procedure), confirming observations from [1,2,3]. The aortic and mitral valvular areas over the cardiac cycle are illustrated in Fig. 4 **Left**, which clearly shows the mitral-regurgitation cured after the intervention. The synchronous annuli deformation and indirect operation effects on the aortic morphology and dynamics are illustrated in Fig. 4 **Right**.

5 Discussion

Latest clinical research confirmed that the morphology, function and hemodynamic-activity of the aortic and mitral valves are strongly interconnected. In this paper, we introduced the first personalized model of the entire aortic-mitral apparatus derived from 4D TEE and 4D CT data. The full anatomy and dynamics are represented through a physiological-driven hierarchical model. From input volume sequences, we estimate the personalized parameters of the non-rigid motion and surface model by applying a robust an efficient machine learning algorithm. The presented approach enables for efficient and integrated quantification of the aortic-mitral complex. Extensive experiments performed on a large heterogeneous data set demonstrated the precision of 1.45mm and speed of 60 seconds for the proposed approach. Furthermore, clinical validation showed a strong inter-modality and inter-subject correlation for a comprehensive set of model-based measurements. The proposed method has the potential to significantly advance the joint examination, procedure planning and prosthetic valve design for both, aortic and mitral valves.

References

1. Lansac, E., Lim, K., Shomura, Y., Goetz, W., Lim, H., Rice, N., Saber, H., Duran, C.: Dynamic balance of the aortomitral junction. J. Thorac. Cardiovasc. Surg. 123, 911–918 (2002)

2. Timek, T., Green, G., Tibayan, F., Lai, F., Rodriguez, F., Liang, D., Daughters, G., Ingels, N., Miller, D.: Aorto-mitral annular dynamics. Ann. Thorac. Surg. 76, 1944–1950 (2003)
3. Veronesi, F., Corsi, C., Sugeng, L., Mor-Avi, V., Caiani, E., Weinert, L., Lamberti, C., Land, R.M.: A study of functional anatomy of aortic-mitral valve coupling using 3D matrix transesophageal echocardiography. Circ. Cardiovasc. Imaging 2(1), 24–31 (2009)
4. Gessat, M., Merk, D., Falk, V., Walther, T., Noettling, A., Burgert, O.: A planning system for transapical aortic valve implantation. In: Proc. SPIE Medical Imaging (2009)
5. Vanden-Eynden, F., Bouchard, D., El-Hamamsy, I., Butnaru, A., Demers, P., Carrier, M., Perrault, L., Tardif, J., Pellerin, M.: Effect of aortic valve replacement for aortic stenosis on severity of mitral regurgitation. Ann. Thorac. Surg. 83, 1279–1284 (2007)
6. Ionasec, R.I., Georgescu, B., Gassner, E., Vogt, S., Kutter, O., Scheuering, M., Navab, N., Comaniciu, D.: Dynamic model-driven quantitative and visual evaluation of the aortic valve from 4D CT. In: Metaxas, D., Axel, L., Fichtinger, G., Székely, G. (eds.) MICCAI 2008, Part I. LNCS, vol. 5241, pp. 686–694. Springer, Heidelberg (2008)
7. Voigt, I., Ionasec, R., Georgescu, B., Houle, H., Huber, M., Hornegger, J., Comaniciu, D.: Model-driven physiological assessment of the mitral valve from 4d tee. In: Proc SPIE Medical Imaging (2009)
8. Piegl, L., Tiller, W.: The NURBS book. Springer, London (1995)
9. Zheng, Y., Barbu, A., et al.: Fast automatic heart chamber segmentation from 3d ct data using marginal space learning and steerable features. In: International Conference on Computer Vision (2007)
10. Fischler, M., Bolles, R.: Random sample consensus: A paradigm for model fitting with applications to image analysis and automated cartography. Comm. of the ACM 24(6), 381–395 (1981)
11. Tu, Z.: Probabilistic boosting-tree: Learning discriminative methods for classification, recognition, and clustering. In: International Conference on Computer Vision, pp. 1589–1596 (2005)
12. Ionasec, R., Wang, Y., Georgescu, B., Voigt, I., Navab, N., Comaniciu, D.: Robust motion estimation using trajectory spectrum learning: Application to aortic and mitral valve modeling. In: International Conference on Computer Vision (submitted, 2009)
13. Yang, L., Georgescu, B., Zheng, Y., Meer, P., Comaniciu, D.: 3d ultrasound tracking of the left ventricle using one-step forward prediction and data fusion of collaborative trackers. In: IEEE Conference on Computer Vision and Pattern Recognition (2008)

A New 3-D Automated Computational Method to Evaluate In-Stent Neointimal Hyperplasia in In-Vivo Intravascular Optical Coherence Tomography Pullbacks

Serhan Gurmeric[1], Gozde Gul Isguder[1], Stéphane Carlier[2], and Gozde Unal[1]

[1] Faculty of Engineering and Natural Sciences, Sabanci University, Istanbul, Turkey
gozdeunal@sabanciuniv.edu
[2] St Maria hospital, Halle and UZ Brussel, Belgium

Abstract. Detection of stent struts imaged in vivo by optical coherence tomography (OCT) after percutaneous coronary interventions (PCI) and quantification of in-stent neointimal hyperplasia (NIH) are important. In this paper, we present a new computational method to facilitate the physician in this endeavor to assess and compare new (drug-eluting) stents. We developed a new algorithm for stent strut detection and utilized splines to reconstruct the lumen and stent boundaries which provide automatic measurements of NIH thickness, lumen and stent area. Our original approach is based on the detection of stent struts unique characteristics: bright reflection and shadow behind. Furthermore, we present for the first time to our knowledge a rotation correction method applied across OCT cross-section images for 3D reconstruction and visualization of reconstructed lumen and stent boundaries for further analysis in the longitudinal dimension of the coronary artery. Our experiments over OCT cross-sections taken from 7 patients presenting varying degrees of NIH after PCI illustrate a good agreement between the computer method and expert evaluations: Bland-Altmann analysis revealed a mean difference for lumen cross-section area of $0.11 \pm 0.70 mm^2$ and for the stent cross-section area of $0.10 \pm 1.28 mm^2$.

1 Introduction

Optical Coherence Tomography (OCT) is a recent modality, which measures the intensity of back-reflected infrared light instead of acoustical waves using an interferometer since the speed of light is much faster than that of sound [1]. OCT was found useful as an intravascular imaging technique, and compared to IVUS in several works [2,3]. The biggest advantage of OCT is its high resolution, on the order of 15 microns spatially, but at the cost of a decreased penetration depth of 1mm to 2mm. Both in vitro and in vivo studies [2,4] have shown that the resolution of OCT can differentiate between typical constituents of atherosclerotic plaques, such as lipid, calcium, and fibrous tissue better than IVUS [5], and can also resolve the thin fibrous cap that is thought to be responsible for plaque vulnerability[6].

Although Drug Eluting Stents (DES) suppress NeoIntimal Hyperplasia (NIH) strongly, in-stent restenosis after DES implantation still occurs [7]. Studies have shown that nonuniform circumferential stent strut distribution affects local drug concentration [8]. Number and distribution of the stent struts might also affect the magnitude of NIH after stent implantation in human coronary arteries [9]. Therefore, tracking of stent position/malapposition and neointimal tissue growth after stent implantation is clinically important.

To our knowledge, besides studies of stents by IVUS, there are no studies of strut distribution analysis on intracoronary OCT pullbacks to assist in the assessment of the degree of restenosis. The objective of this study was three-fold: (i) to explore the usability and performance of automatic computer methods to help with stent strut analysis in varying degrees of NIH scenarios; (ii) to compare the computer analysis with expert analysis to correlate the results in OCT images; (iii) to carry the 2D OCT pullback analysis to longitudinal dimension in 3D.

2 Method

OCT Imaging Protocol. Automated pullbacks at 1 mm/s were conventionally performed using a M2 OCT Imaging System (LightLab Imaging, Inc., Westford, MA, USA) running at a frame rate of 15.6/sec and a dedicated fibre-optic imaging wire (ImageWire^{TM}, LightLab Imaging Inc., Westford, MA, USA). Temporary blood clearance was obtained with a proximal occlusion balloon inflated to between 0.5-0.7 atm, while simultaneously flushing physiological saline through the distal lumen of the balloon catheter at a rate of 0.5ml/s. Images have an axial resolution of about 15 microns. In vivo OCT pullbacks were recorded as rectangular images of 200x752 pixels (200 angles with 752 samples each on each ray). These rectangular images were processed by our method and displayed after scan-conversion in a standard viewing format.

Study Population. Seven pullbacks performed in previously stented coronary segments of seven patients presenting varying degrees of NIH were the test cases of our automated methods.

2.1 OCT Pullback Image Analysis

Our approach consists of four different main parts: (i) preprocessing OCT cross-section images; (ii) initializing and propagating a spline inside the lumen region; (iii) detection of struts and reconstruction of the stent boundary; (iv) registration between consecutive OCT images for 3D reconstruction, and measurements for assessment of in-stent restenosis.

Preprocessing. It can be observed in a typical OCT image that brighter pixel groups represent vessel wall, plaque, and stent struts (Fig. 1). To enhance the desired information in the image, a 50 percentile of the histogram is selected as a threshold, and the image is thresholded followed by a median and a Gaussian filter to enhance and smooth the regions with struts and their shadows around the lumen (Fig 1-b and c).

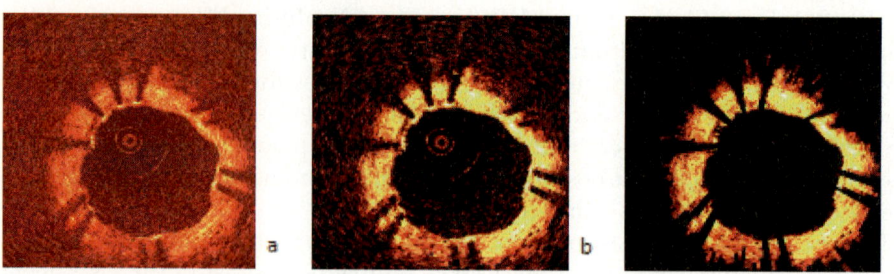

Fig. 1. (a) OCT display image; (b) Thresholded image; (c) Denoised image

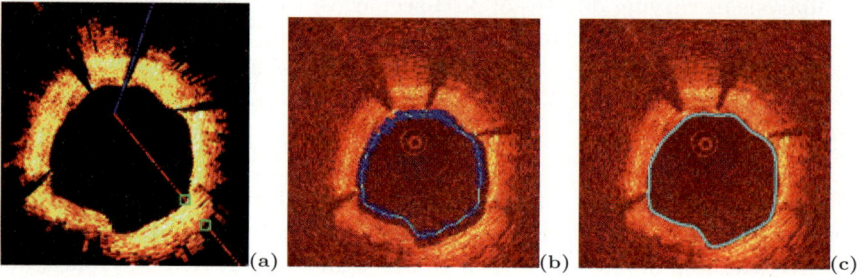

Fig. 2. (a) Ray shooting in prefiltered image; (b) Initial spline on ray intersection points; (c) Spline evolution and segmented lumen region

Lumen Segmentation. We developed a new and problem specific method for segmentation of the lumen region on an OCT cross-section image and creation of a band or a region of interest (ROI) in the arterial wall behind the lumen boundary, which facilitates stent strut detection. Particularly, strut shadows in this ROI are essential clues utilized in our algorithm. To segment the lumen region, we utilized a Catmull-Rom spline, which has four polynomial blending functions and whose control points are exactly on the spline contour. The interaction and initialization of this cubic hermite spline are practically well-suited to our problem for correction of the lumen contour and stent splines, if necessary.

Spline Initialization and Propagation. For detection of the ROI, i.e. the inner and outer boundaries of the observable bright band in the OCT image, we utilize two splines, and initialize the spline control points by shooting rays on the rectangular domain "denoised image" from the center coordinates of the display image to every angle, and analyzing the thickness of the ROI region in the arterial wall (Fig. 2-a). Two Catmull-Rom splines are constructed to separate strut and shadow zone of image. The control points are initialized at the inner side of the ROI (Fig. 2-b), and the spline propagates towards the lumen border and stops on the desired boundaries via an edge-based active contour framework as exemplified in Fig. 2-c.

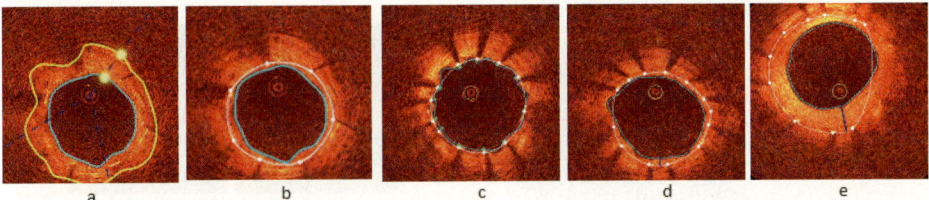

Fig. 3. (a) The ROI with start and end points for energy calculations; (b) Detected struts; Examples of strut detection, lumen and stent boundary reconstruction in 3 different scenarios: (c) NIH absent; (d) minimum amount of NIH; (e) moderate amount of NIH

Shadow and Strut Detection. One important observation is that the OCT cross-section images which contain stent struts, generally include shadows behind the struts. Analyzing the angular intensity energy distribution in the ROI provides clues to these shadows. To build such an energy map, rays from the image center are extended and the intersection points of these rays and the splines are computed. Interpolation of these two intersection coordinates (Fig. 3-a) and summation of corresponding image intensity values define the energy on a ray. Energy distribution over all the rays are analyzed: falling and rising of energy on these rays indicates the presence and absence of strut shadows. A second analysis over the detected shadow rays is carried out between the two splines to detect the exact strut positions over the original image. A strut on a shadow ray is the maximum bright intensity pixel group and mostly negative deep gradient vectors follow such a group (Fig. 3-b). The stent boundary is reconstructed by fitting another Catmull-Rom spline to the detected struts.

For different NIH scenarios, we designed two modes of our system: (i) the new stent implants and minimum NIH cases; (ii) mild to severe NIH cases. The shadow and strut detection then differs w.r.t. the interpolation of the angular energy calculation: either starts from first spline to the middle range of the ROI, or from the middle of the ROI towards the outer field, respectively. Thus the search range varies and the strut detection threshold parameters are heuristically determined and fixed for both modes (mode 1: 30% energy fall, 45% energy rise; mode 2: 45% energy fall, 35% energy rise) for all the experiments. A simple mode picking operation changes these parameters in the application. Examples are shown in Fig. 3 for strut detection, lumen and stent boundary reconstruction in three different scenarios: (c) virtually no NIH; (d) minimum amount of NIH; (e) moderate amount of NIH.

Calibration. Calibration of the OCT images was based on the known physical dimension of the imaging sheath (0.0019") inside which the fibre-optic rotates and that is visualized as a small circle in the middle of the display image and as a line on the rectangular image.

2.2 3D Reconstruction in the Longitudinal Dimension

During a pullback, as the catheter moves inside the arteries in-vivo, it inevitably translates and rotates and causes a misalignment between the two recorded

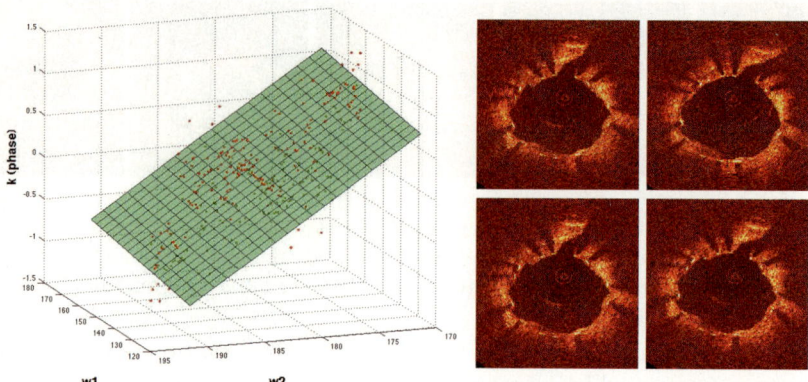

Fig. 4. Rotation estimation: Middle column: source image; Right top: reference image; Right bottom: rotated source image with the estimated rotation=-5.21 degrees; Left: fitted plane to phase ρ

consecutive cross-section images. Moreover, the catheter may go back and forth as the heart dilates and compresses. The result is a pulsatile and jagged longitudinal geometry of the vessel wall (see Fig 6-a). For an accurate 3D vessel geometry and longitudinal analysis, these catheter effects should be corrected. We address two of the cross-sectional catheter motion. The first is the translation of the catheter in the lumen due to varying vessel curvature. We account for this by aligning the OCT cross-section images w.r.t. their lumen border center of mass.

To address the rotation of the catheter during pullback, we estimated rotation between subsequent frames via a spectral correlation analysis method inspired by [10], where the translation on a rectangular image, which corresponds to a rotation on the display image, is calculated as follows: Let I be the rectangular image and I_t is the translated version of I with a 2D translation $\boldsymbol{t} = (t_1, t_2)$. The ratio between the Fourier transforms of the image I and I_t: $k(w_1, w_2) = F(I_t)/F(I) \cdot e^{-j<\boldsymbol{w},\boldsymbol{t}>}$, can be used to extract the phase: $\rho(\boldsymbol{w}) = \langle \boldsymbol{w}, \boldsymbol{t} \rangle = w_1 * t_1 + w_2 * t_2$, where $\boldsymbol{w} = (w_1, w_2)$ denotes the 2D frequency vector. The idea then is to estimate the amount of shift using the phase defined over the 2D frequency space by fitting a plane to the ρ function: $Aw_1 + Bw_2 + C\rho = D$. Here a translation between the two images in either the horizontal or the vertical direction can be detected over the plane aligned with one of the frequency axis w_1 or w_2. Practically, a least-squares estimator is used via a singular value decomposition. In the OCT rectangular images, the calculated slope B of the plane represents the estimated rotation value in radians (whereas D=0). In Fig. 4 an example is shown for rotation estimation between two subsequent OCT frames.

After the 2D registration, we reconstruct the 3D geometry of the stent and lumen borders by building triangular meshes over the stack of 2D rotated splines. On top of these, we render the stent struts approximated by a thin ellipsoid geometry. Our future goal here is to obtain 3D models of stent meshes, however, for the current work, we accounted for the lack of a mesh model by a filtering to eliminate struts that violate certain distance conditions away from the neighbor strut on adjacent frames. A transparent stent tube model is deformed to fit detected struts as will be depicted in the Results.

3 Results and Discussions

3.1 Assessment of Strut Distribution

39 OCT cross-sections from 7 pullbacks of 7 patients presenting varying degrees of NIH are selected. Manual strut detection is carried out by the expert in two ways: (i) via manual tracing using the reviewing software provided by the OCT manufacturer (LightLab Imaging, MA, USA), called as LL software here and taken as the gold standard; (ii) using our system with correction over the automatic results (the extracted splines can be corrected, stent struts can be added, removed or marked), abbreviated as the SF (Stent Follow-up) system. The two manual analysis (LL and SF) are compared with the automatic detection (ASF: Automatic Stent Follow-up) over this image set.

Figure 5 depicts a diagram for the measurements carried out in our experiments for the strut assessment. First, we count the total number of detected struts in each cross-section image. The percentage of correctly detected struts is set to 1 − normalized error, where the normalized error = |#struts marked by the physician − #struts detected by our algorithm| / |#struts marked by the physician|. Another parameter measured is the maximum angle between adjacent stent struts. As reported by Takebayashi et al. [9], this measurement correlates with the NIH thickness in IVUS-based studies. NIH thickness was also evaluated looking at the lumen cross-sectional area (L-CSA), the stent cross-sectional area (S-CSA), minimum, maximum, and average distance between the lumen boundary and the stent. Finally, stent eccentricity was calculated as the minimum divided by the maximum stent diameter.

Table 1 presents measurements of the lumen and the stent CSAs, and the number of stent struts with a comparison between the automatic detection (ASF), the expert's adjustment of the automatic results (SF), and the expert's manual measurements using the LightLab software (LL). Table 2 presents the rest of the measurements: the maximum inter-strut angle, the minimum, average, and maximum distances between the stent and the lumen borders, and the stent eccentricity, which were not available from the LL software.

Very good agreements were found between the computer methods and the expert evaluations for lumen CSA (mean difference following Bland-Altmann $=0.11 \pm 0.70 mm^2$; $r^2 = 0.98, p < 0.0001$) and the stent CSA (mean difference= $0.10 \pm 1.28 mm^2$; $r^2 = 0.85, p < 0.0001$). The average number of detected struts was 10.4 ± 2.9 per cross-section when the expert identified 10.5 ± 2.8 ($r^2 = 0.78, p < 0.0001$), with an overall accuracy in strut detection of $91 \pm 11\%$. For the given patient dataset: lumen CSA was on the average $6.05 \pm 1.87 mm^2$, stent CSA was $6.26 \pm 1.63 mm^2$, maximum angle between struts was on the average 85.96 ± 54.23^o, maximum, average, and minimum distance between the stent and

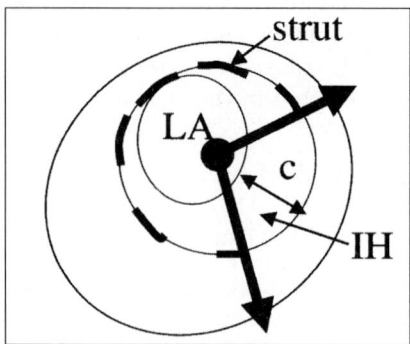

Fig. 5. Schematic of struts and related measurements calculated for stent follow-up analysis, adapted from [9]. Maximum interstrut angle, LA (lumen cross-sectional area: L-CSA), IH (=Stent CSA - L-CSA), distances between the lumen and the stent contours (here c is depicted: the maximum distance=thickness of the NIH).

Table 1. Strut assessment measurements compared among the expert manual detection with two different systems and the automatic detection. Values are mean ± std. ASF: Autodetection, SF: Expert manual adjustment, LL: Expert manual measurement.

	ASF	SF	LL
Lumen CSA, mm^2	5.78±1.76	6.09±1.85	6.05±1.87
Stent CSA, mm^2	6.59±1.91	6.33±1.66	6.26±1.63
Stent struts, n normalized to (0,1)	0.91±0.11	1.00±0.00	1.00±0.00

Table 2. Other strut assessment measurements compared between the expert manual detection and the automatic detection with our system. Values are mean ± std.

	ASF	SF
Max angle btw stent struts, °	75.09±26.63	85.96±54.23
Max distance btw stent and lumen border, mm	0.31±0.15	0.18±0.13
Avg distance btw stent and lumen border, mm	0.14±0.07	0.08±0.06
Min distance btw stent and lumen border, mm	0.02±0.04	0.01±0.02
Stent eccentricity	0.75±0.11	0.80±0.08

the lumen were $0.18 \pm 0.13 mm$, $0.08 \pm 0.06 mm$, and $0.01 \pm 0.02 mm$, respectively, and stent eccentricity was 0.80 ± 0.08.

Due to possible hindering of shadows by severe NIH, strut detection and stent boundary reconstruction becomes more challenging and more prone to errors than that of the lumen. This difficulty caused a lower match between the automatic and manual computations based on the stent boundary such as

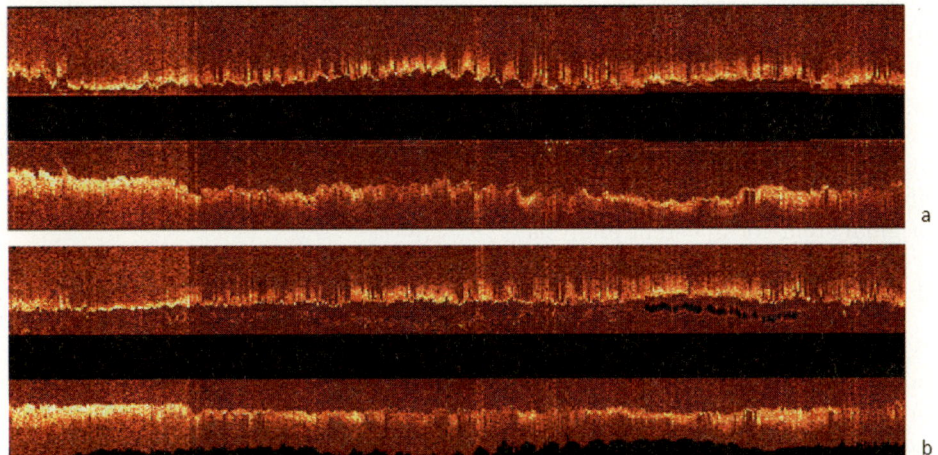

Fig. 6. Longitudinal cut view: (a) original; (b) center and rotation aligned pullback

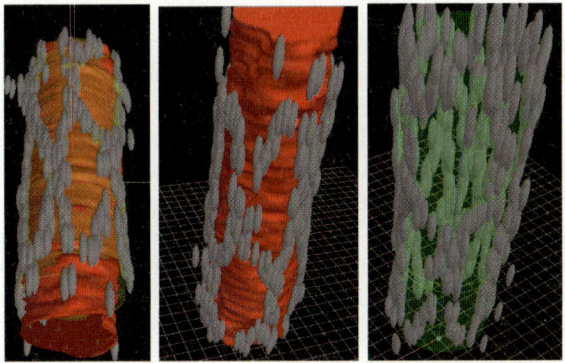

Fig. 7. Examples of 3D Reconstruction of the lumen boundary (red surface), the stent boundary (yellow surface depicted on the left) and the stent struts represented as gray ellipsoids. Green transparent mesh on the right represents the vessel wall.

the maximum distance calculation between the stent and the lumen border as observed in Table 2. Our work is ongoing for further improvements on such struts, which were missed with the shadow detection.

3.2 3D Reconstruction

The performance of the 2D OCT registration method (Sec 2.2) is validated on synthetic images: a binary ellipse image is generated and rotated with a known value to generate a second ellipse image, then the spectral correlation method is used to estimate the amount of rotation. The results were $\approx 98.5\%$ accurate for up to rotations of 0.8 radians. The proposed method has been applied to OCT pullbacks to account for catheter cross-sectional motion. Fig. 6 depicts a longitudinal view from the original pullback (a), the center and rotation aligned pullback (b), where the reduced jaggedness in the lumen boundaries can be observed.

Next, a 3D visualization is shown in Fig. 7 for the reconstructed lumen surface, and stent struts as a surface rendering. The mesh pattern of the stent is visible and presents a possibility of examining the 3D position of the stent w.r.t. the lumen boundary. We are currently working on including a 3D mesh model of the original stent for 3D stent analysis.

4 Conclusions

We presented a new spline-based segmentation for both the lumen and the stent boundaries, and an energy map based automatic stent strut detection algorithm in OCT pullbacks, to assist in the problem of strut distribution assessment. Our experimental results demonstrated that our algorithm works reasonably well on the segmentation of target boundaries in OCT images, and detected stent struts and their trailing shadows. A strut distribution analysis was carried out and a number of measures important for stent implant follow-up and monitoring of the neointimal tissue growth over struts were calculated. An extension to a 3D/longitudinal analysis is also illustrated. Part of our ongoing and future studies include extension of the spline segmentation to 3D, and using previously constructed models of stent meshes.

The conclusion from our study is that our new methods appear to offer a robust and reliable automated analysis of OCT pullbacks of coronary stented segments that might assist physicians in evaluating in-stent restenosis after PCI and study the vascular response of new stents and eluted drugs. A large-scale evaluation of OCT pullback stent analysis will be necessary to further correlate the degree of NIH and circumferential stent strut distribution, as suggested previously by IVUS [9].

References

1. Barlis, P., Schmitt, J.: Current and future developments in intracoronary optical coherence tomography imaging. EuroIntervention 4, 529–534 (2008)
2. Jang, I.: et al: Visualization of coronary atherosclerotic plaques in patients using optical coherence tomography: Comparison with intravascular ultrasound. American Journal of Cardiology 39, 604–609 (2002)
3. Patwari, P.: et al: Assessment of coronary plaque with optical coherence tomography and high-frequency ultrasound. American Journal of Cardiology 85, 641–644 (2000)
4. Yabushita, H.: et al: Characterization of human atherosclerosis by optical coherence tomography. Circulation 106, 1640–1645 (2002)
5. Rieber, J., Meissner, O., Babaryka, G., Oswald, S.R.M., Koenig, A., Schiele, T., Shapiro, M., Theisen, K., Reiser, M., Klauss, V., Hoffmann, U.: Diagnostic accuracy of optical coherence tomography and intravascular ultrasound for the detection and characterization of atherosclerotic plaque composition in ex-vivo coronary specimens: a comparison with histology. Coronary Artery Disease 17(5), 425–430 (2006)

6. Xu, C., Schmitt, J., Carlier, S., Virmani, R.: Characterization of atherosclerosis plaques by measuring both backscattering and attenuation coefficients in optical coherence tomography. Journal of Biomedical Optics 13(3) (2008)
7. Lemos, P., Saia, F., Ligthart, J., Arampatzis, C., Sianos, G., Tanabe, K., Hoye, A., Degertekin, M., Daemen, J., McFadden, E., Hofma, S., Smits, P., de Feyter, P., van der Giessen, W., van Domburg, R., Serruys, P.: Coronary restenosis after sirolimus-eluting stent implantation: morphological description and mechanistic analysis from a consecutive series of cases. Circulation 108, 257–260 (2003)
8. Hwang, C.W., Wu, D., Edelman, E.R.: Physiological transport forces govern drug distribution for stent-based delivery. Circulation 104, 600–605 (2001)
9. Takebayashi, H., Mintz, G., Carlier, S., Kobayashi, Y., Fujii, K., Yasuda, T., Costa, R., Moussa, I., Dangas, G., Mehran, R., Lansky, A., Kreps, E., Collins, M., Colombo, A., Stone, G., Leon, M., Moses, J.: Nonuniform strut distribution correlates with more neointimal hyperplasia after sirolimus-eluting stent implantation. Circulation 110, 3430–3434 (2004)
10. Hernandez, A., Radeva, P., Tovar, A., Gil, D.: Vessel structures alignment by spectral analysis of IVUS sequences. In: Proceedings of Computer Vision for Intravascular and Intracardiac Imaging, CVII (2006)

MKL for Robust Multi-modality AD Classification

Chris Hinrichs[1,2], Vikas Singh[1,2], Guofan Xu[3], and Sterling Johnson[3]

[1]Dept. of Computer Sciences   [2]Dept. of Biostatistics & Med. Informatics   [3]Dept. of Medicine
University of Wisconsin–Madison
{hinrichs,vsingh}@cs.wisc.edu, {gxu,scj}@medicine.wisc.edu

Abstract. We study the problem of classifying mild Alzheimer's disease (AD) subjects from healthy individuals (controls) using *multi-modal* image data, to facilitate early identification of AD related pathologies. Several recent papers have demonstrated that such classification is possible with MR or PET images, using machine learning methods such as SVM and boosting. These algorithms learn the classifier using one *type* of image data. However, AD is not well characterized by one imaging modality alone, and analysis is typically performed using several image types – each measuring a different type of structural/functional characteristic. This paper explores the AD classification problem using multiple modalities *simultaneously*. The difficulty here is to assess the relevance of each modality (which cannot be assumed a priori), as well as to optimize the classifier. To tackle this problem, we utilize and adapt a recently developed idea called Multi-Kernel learning (MKL). Briefly, each imaging modality spawns one (or more kernels) and we simultaneously solve for the kernel weights and a maximum margin classifier. To make the model robust, we propose strategies to suppress the influence of a small subset of outliers on the classifier – this yields an alternative minimization based algorithm for robust MKL. We present promising *multi-modal* classification experiments on a large dataset of images from the ADNI project.

1 Introduction

Alzheimer's Disease (AD) is a neurodegenerative disorder affecting over 5 million people in the United States, and is a leading cause of dementia worldwide. An emphasis in recent AD research, especially in the context of early diagnosis, has been placed on identifying markers of the disease (such as structural/functional changes in brain regions) using imaging data (*e.g.*, MR, FDG-PET). Large scale studies such as the ADNI project [1] are collecting imaging data and associated clinical biomarkers in an effort to facilitate the development and evaluation of new approaches, and the identification of new imaging biomarkers. These advances are expected to yield important insights into the progression patterns of AD. One aspect of the ADNI project in particular is the acquisition and analysis of *multi-modal* imaging data: this includes Magnetic Resonance (MR), 18fluorodeoxyglucose-Positron Emission Tomography (FDG-PET), and Pittsburgh Compound B (PIB) PET image scans of the participants. The rationale is that because different modalities reveal different aspects of the underlying neuropathology, information from one modality adds to the diagnosis based on the other. For example, a patient may show only slight hippocampal atrophy in the MR images, but the FDG-PET image may reveal increased hypometabolism in medial-temporal and parietal regions (which is more suggestive of AD). Our objective here is to design machine learning algorithms which are (by design) *cognizant of such multimodal imaging data*, and "learn" the patterns differentiating controls from AD or MCI subjects using multiple modalities *simultaneously*: for predicting cognitive decline, or for identifying early symptoms of AD pathology.

The analysis of imaging data, in AD and aging research, has traditionally been approached by manual indication of brain regions suspected to be related to AD neurodegeneration, and performing statistical analysis to determine if group means (in those regions) are different [2]. Another approach is to automatically identify the discriminative regions using Voxel-based Morphometry (VBM) [3]. However, the *diagnostic* potential of group analysis is somewhat limited, usually by the degree of overlap in the group distributions. Therefore, a significant emphasis is being placed on determining and exploiting the *predictive value* of imaging-based biomarkers for diagnosis at the level of individual subjects. In this direction, a number of groups are exploring the applicability of machine learning ideas to this important problem. For instance, in [4], Support Vector Machines (SVM) were used to perform classification of structural MR scans after nominal feature selection. This procedure gave good classification accuracy on the Baltimore Longitudinal data set (BLSA). Recently [5] also used linear SVMs to classify AD cases from other types of dementia using whole brain MR images. High accuracy was obtained on confirmed AD patients and slightly less where post-mortem diagnosis was unavailable. Vemuri *et al.* showed promising evaluations on another data set, obtaining 88-90% accuracy [6], (also using linear SVMs). The authors of [7] proposed an augmented form of Linear Program Boosting (LP Boosting) which takes into account spatial characteristics of medical images, also reporting good accuracy on the ADNI data set. Observe that all of these methods have specifically focused on using a *single imaging modality* (e.g., MR or PET) for classification. One way to adapt such algorithms to make use of multiple imaging modalities (or additional clinical/cognitive data) is to "concatenate" the set of images for each subject into *one* feature vector. Not only does this increase the dimensionality of the distribution significantly, but it also requires finding a suitable "normalization" of each modality (to preserve its information content). Otherwise, features derived from one image type may easily overwhelm features from the other.

Contributions. The key contributions of this paper are (A) We propose an efficient multi-modal learning framework for AD classification based on multi-kernel learning (MKL). We cast the data from each imaging modality as one (or more) kernels, and solve for the support vectors (to maximize the margin) and the relative weights (importance) of each kernel; (B) To account for outliers (possibly misdiagnosed cases), the algorithm also incorporates a robustness parameter to identify such examples, and discount their effect on the classifier. This is tackled via alternative minimization; (C) We report the first set of multi-modal experimental results using robust-MKL learning on the ADNI dataset.

2 Preliminaries

We briefly review the underlying model for Support Vector Machines, before discussing the MKL setting and our construction. The SVM framework relies on the assumption that the concept (or classifier) we seek to learn (between two classes of examples) is well separated by a gap or *margin* in a certain feature space, and the algorithm can minimize the test error of a decision boundary by *maximizing* the width of the margin in the set of training examples provided. The decision boundary or *separating hyper-plane*, is parameterized by a weight vector **w** and offset (or bias) b. The classifier decides the possible class label for an unlabeled example **x** by calculating the inner product $\langle \mathbf{w}, \mathbf{x} \rangle$, and evaluating whether it is greater or less than b. SVMs operate on the principle that we must not only place examples on the correct side of the decision hyper-plane, but each example must also be far from the hyper-plane. In this case, the width of the margin is proportional to $\frac{1}{||\mathbf{w}||_2}$, see [8]. When choosing among two (or more) such decision boundaries (where both correctly classify all training data), the one with a smaller ℓ_2-norm maximizes the margin and yields better accuracy. The SVM primal problem and corresponding dual problem are given as:

(primal)

$$\min_{\mathbf{w},\xi} \frac{||\mathbf{w}||}{2} + C\sum_i \xi_i \quad (1)$$

s.t. $y_i \mathbf{w}^T x_i + \xi_i \geq 1 \ \forall i$

$\xi_i \geq 0 \ \forall i$

(dual)

$$\max_{\alpha} \sum_i \alpha_i - \sum_{i,j} \alpha_i \alpha_j y_i y_j \underbrace{x_i^T x_j}_{\text{kernel}} \quad (2)$$

s.t. $0 \leq \alpha_i \leq C \ \forall i$

$\sum_i y_i \alpha_i = 0 \ \forall i$

2.1 Multi-kernel Learning

We first introduce Multi-kernel learning (MKL) [9], and then explain why it serves as a good basic formalization for our problem. In the next section, we will outline the main extensions. To motivate MKL, notice that in the dual of the SVM model (2), the dot product is replaced with a kernel function which expresses similarity among the the different data examples. This substitution offers a number of advantages, see [8]. Nonetheless, choosing the right kernel matrix for a given problem may not be straightforward, and typically requires adjustments. An attractive alternative is to represent each subset of features (e.g., each imaging modality) using its own kernel matrix and then seek an *optimal combination* of these kernels to form a *single* kernel matrix – one with the desirable properties of a good kernel (e.g., separable, maximizes the margin) for the complete data (i.e., all modalities). The process of choosing a set of coefficients, or sub-kernel weights, which are used to combine the candidate kernels into a single one, $\hat{K}$ while simultaneously optimizing the expected test error is called Multi-Kernel Learning (MKL). The problem is formulated as follows.

$$\min_{\mathbf{w_k},\xi,\beta,b} \left(\sum_k \beta_k ||\mathbf{w_k}||_2 \right)^2 + C \sum_i^N \xi_i \quad (3)$$

subject to $y_i \left(\sum_k \beta_k \mathbf{w_k}^T \phi_k(x_i) + b \right) + \xi_1 \geq 1 \ \forall i$

$\sum_k \beta_k = 1$

Here, the coefficients β_k are the sub-kernel weights. Notice that the squared ℓ_1-norm penalty on the individual sub-kernel weights combined with the ℓ_2-norm penalty on the weights in each individual view leads to sparsity among different kernels, but not among weights in each individual view [9]. In our AD classification problem, we use the set of images from each imaging modality to spawn a set of kernels. In other words, the distribution of the MR images of the set of subjects may give one (or a set of kernels). The same process is repeated for other types of images as well as any other form of demographic, clinical, or cognitive data available. The optimization problem then reduces to finding their weights (importance) while simultaneously maximizing the margin for the training data. The $\hat{K}$ hence calculated is the *combination* of *all* available kernels.

3 Algorithm

3.1 Outlier Ablation

In addition to finding the optimal combination of kernels, we must also identify and suppress the influence of one or more mislabeled subjects (examples) on the classifier. This is important in the AD classification problem because of: (1) Co-morbidity: In some cases, AD is coincident with other neurodegenerative diseases such as Lewy bodies; (2) While the image data may suggest signs of pathology characteristic of AD, these usually *precede* cognitive decline. As a result, the subject may be cognitively normal (and labeled as control). To ensure that the algorithm is robust for this problem and other applications, we would like to identify such outliers within the model. In order to do this, one option within the SVM setting is to replace the regular loss function with the "robust" hinge loss function which differs only in that the "penalty" is capped at 1.

$$\text{robust-hinge}(w, x, y) = \min(1, (1 - yw^T x)_+), \text{ where } y_i \in \{+1, -1\} \text{ are the class labels.} \quad (4)$$

This means that once an example falls on the wrong side of the classifier there is no additional increase in penalty. To address the non-convexity of (4) the authors in [10] replaced the usual hinge loss function with the $\eta-$hinge loss function, which uses a discount variable η_i for each example. That is,

$$\eta\text{-hinge}(w, x, y) = \eta(1 - yw^T x)_+ + (1 - \eta), \quad 0 \leq \eta \leq 1 \quad (5)$$

The result in [10] shows that η-hinge loss has the same optimum and value as robust-hinge loss. Our proposed model makes use of such a parameter to serve as both an outlier indicator and also to adjust the influence of this example on the classifier in the MKL setting. We present our optimization model next.

$$\min_{\eta} \min_{\mathbf{w}, \xi_i, \eta_{i,k}} \sum_k \|\mathbf{w_k}\|^2 + C \sum_i \xi_i - D \sum_{i,k} \eta_{i,k} \quad (6)$$

$$\text{s.t. } y_i(\sum_k \eta_{i,k} \mathbf{w_k}^T \phi_k(x)) + \xi_i \geq 1 \ \forall i$$

$$0 \leq \eta_{i,k} \leq 1 \ \forall i, k, \quad \xi_i \geq 0 \ \forall i,$$

Here, $\mathbf{w_k}$ is the set of weights for the kernel k, ξ_i is the slack for example i (similar to SVMs), and $\eta_{i,k}$ is the discount on example i's influence on training classification in view k (described in detail below).

Justification. Notice that η introduces a discount for every example's influence on the classifier *in each kernel*. This is balanced by the *positive reward* for making η as large as possible. Therefore, an example which is badly characterized in some kernels can *still be used* effectively in other kernels where it is more accurately characterized. In this way, the proposed model performs *automated* outlier suppression in the MKL setting.

3.2 Alternative Minimization

We note that while (6) accurately expresses our problem, efficiently optimizing the objective function is rather difficult. To address this problem, we "relax" this formulation by treating the discount coefficients η fixed at each iteration. The value is iteratively updated according to the following expression.

$$\eta_{i,k} = \frac{\left(y_i \sum_j \alpha_j y_j K_k(x_i, x_j)\right)_-}{\left|\sum_{i',j'} (y_{i'} \alpha_{j'} y_{j'} K_k(x_{i'}, x_{j'}))_-\right|} + 1 \qquad (7)$$

Here, the denominator represents a normalization over all examples within a single kernel. This is necessary because different kernels have different variances, which must be accounted for (since we are combining kernels). Subsequent to setting the η variables, (6) can be solved to optimality, and η is again updated in the next iteration.

4 Experimental Results

In this section, we evaluate our multi-modal learning framework on image scans from the ADNI dataset. The Alzheimer's disease neuroimaging initiative (ADNI) [1] is a landmark research study sponsored by the National Institutes of Health, to determine whether brain imaging can help predict onset and monitor progression of Alzheimer's disease. The study is ongoing and will cover a total of 800 patients (200 healthy controls, 400 MCI individuals, and 200 mild AD patients). For our evaluations, we used MR and PET scans of 159 patients (77 AD, 82 controls) from this dataset. The data also provides a diagnosis for each subject based on clinical evaluations, this was used for training the classifier, and for calculating the accuracy of the system.

To evaluate our algorithm, we adopted a two fold approach. First, we measured the goodness of this approach w.r.t. to outlier detection, especially with respect to its effect on unseen test examples. In order to do this, we analyzed the variation in the kernel matrices as a response to outlier identification and suppression. Second, we evaluated the efficacy of the multi-kernel framework (with outlier detection) as a classification system, w.r.t. its accuracy using ROC curves. We discuss our experiments next.

4.1 Evaluation of Outlier Detection

Here, we evaluate the usefulness of outlier detection in the classification model. Recall that an ideal input to any maximum margin classifier is a dataset where each class is separated from the other by a large margin. Since the MKL setup optimizes a collection of kernels, it is important to understand how a large margin in a data set translates to values in a kernel. To demonstrate this effect, we show two toy examples in Fig. 1. The first distribution is a setting where the classes are well separated (Fig. 1(a)): we see that

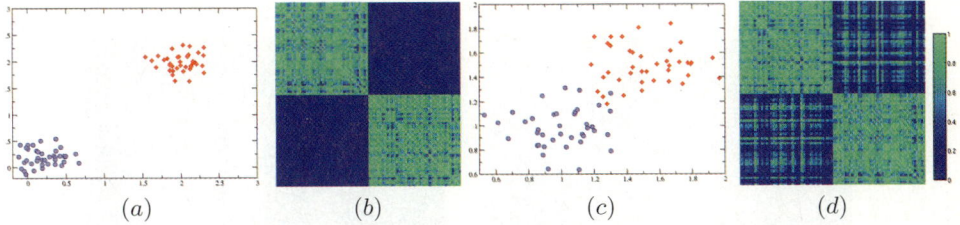

Fig. 1. Toy Example: (a) Well separated classes, (b) Kernel for well separated classes, (c) Overlapping Classes (d) Kernel for overlapping classes

the corresponding kernel matrix in Fig. 1(b) shows two distinct regions with high values (in green) for the two classes, where as the region pertaining to *inter-class* similarities shows no signal (in blue). In the second case (Fig. 1(c)), the classes are overlapping, which is also reflected in the kernel matrix being noisier as shown in Fig. 1(d).

A similar effect can be observed in the kernels of our dataset as a response to outlier detection. Fig. 2 shows how outlier detection improves the signal quality in the kernel matrices. Fig. 2 (a) and (c) display the uncorrected train and test kernel matrices created simply by summing-up the set of individual kernel matrices. Fig. 2 (b) and (d) show the corresponding outlier-ablated train and test kernels. For visualization, the dataset is re-ordered with respect to groups before kernel creation, so that the kernel shows contiguous blocks (similar to Fig. 1). In 2 (a), we see vertical and horizontal lines of lighter color in the interclass region of the kernel, corresponding to outlier subjects who have a *stronger resemblance to the opposite class*. This effect is mitigated to a significant extent with outlier detection in Fig. 2 (b). Next, we analyze the effect of outlier ablation on unseen test items. For this, the test kernel is constructed with the training examples as rows and test examples as columns. In the kernel for the uncorrected case in Fig. 2 (c), the vertical lines correspond to unseen outlier subjects, whereas the horizontal lines are attenuated, indicating that in presence of training data, the non-outlier subjects have sharper contrast (causing an improved confidence in classification). Finally, the test kernel (after outlier detection) shown in Fig. 2 (d) shows a stronger within-class signal, and does not attempt to correctly classify the outliers, thereby discounting their effect on the decision boundary as desired (recall hinge loss from (4)).

4.2 Efficacy of Multi-kernel Framework

ROC curves and accuracy results. First, we evaluate the classification accuracy of our robust multi-kernel learning framework for single modality classification, using MR and FDG scans individually as well as both these modalities in a combined setting. We used a set of eight kernels each (linear and Gaussian with varying values of σ) for MR and FDG PET: 16 in all. Feature selection was performed using a simple voxel-wise t-test, and thresholding based on the p-values. We performed 10-fold cross-validation, and report the average of various error measures such as accuracy, sensitivity, and sensitivity (average over 25 runs). Our results are summarized in Table 3. As expected, we can

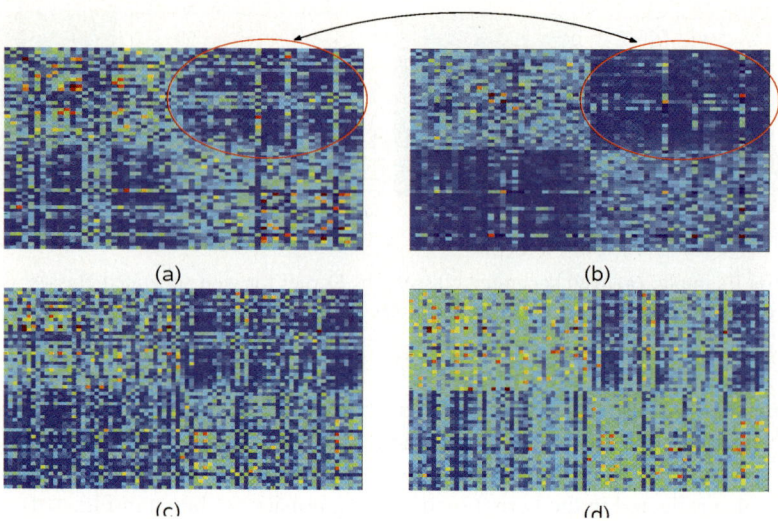

Fig. 2. (a) Sum of base kernel matrices on training examples. (b) Robust-MKL kernel matrix between training examples. Note that the two classes are clearly visible, and the vertical and horizontal lines corresponding to outliers are attenuated. (c) Sum of base kernel matrices on test examples. (d) Robust-MKL kernel matrix between test examples. Notice that while there are vertical lines corresponding to outlier test examples, the horizontal lines remain largely attenuated.

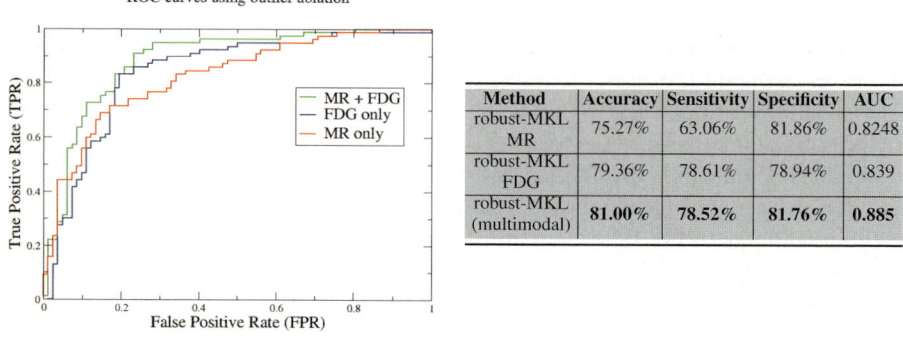

Method	Accuracy	Sensitivity	Specificity	AUC
robust-MKL MR	75.27%	63.06%	81.86%	0.8248
robust-MKL FDG	79.36%	78.61%	78.94%	0.839
robust-MKL (multimodal)	**81.00%**	**78.52%**	**81.76%**	**0.885**

Fig. 3. ROC curves and Accuracy results for the single modal and multimodal classification using robust MKL

clearly see that the robust multi-modal framework with MR and FDG PET data outperforms the accuracy obtained using only one imaging modality (even when we use multiple kernels with each image type). The area under the curve (AUC) for the proposed algorithm is 0.885 suggesting that it is an effective method for AD classification.

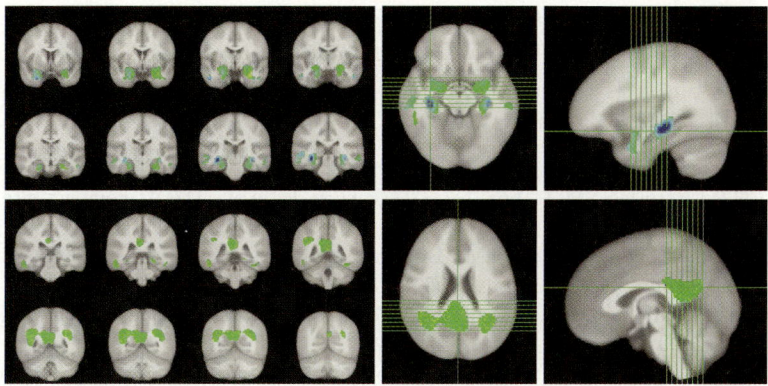

Fig. 4. (Top) Classifier weights for gray-matter probability images shown overlaid on a template. (Bottom) Classifier weights for FDG-PET images shown overlaid on a template. The images (left) show the discriminative regions as a mosaic. The images (right) are provided for 3-D localization.

Interpretation of discriminative brain regions. We evaluated the relative importance of various brain regions selected by the algorithm, and whether these regions are consistent with clinically accepted distributions of AD pathology. The classifier weights chosen by our algorithm are weights on different voxels, and therefore can be interpreted as distributions of weights on the brain regions. Fig. 4 shows the calculated weights for Gray Matter Probability (GMP) and FDG-PET images. For GMP, we see the hippocampus and hippocampal gyri are featured prominently, along with middle temporal regions. For FDG-PET, we see the posterior cingulate cortex and parietal lobules bilaterally are featured prominently. We find these results encouraging because the selected regions are all known to be affected in AD patients [11,12].

5 Conclusions

We have proposed a robust MKL framework for multi-modal AD classification. By framing each unique modality as one (or more) kernels, the scheme learns the kernel weights as well as a maximum margin classifier. Our framework also offers robustness to outliers, with the capability of automatically detecting them and partly discounting their influence on the decision boundary. Various sophisticated feature selection algorithms can be also be used as in [6] (discriminative image voxels) to further improve the accuracy of the model. Finally, rather than ad-hoc feature concatenation to make use of additional clinical and demographic data (if available), our algorithm allows an easy and intuitive incorporation – simply by constructing another kernel for such features.

Acknowledgments. This research was supported in part by the UW-Madison ICTR through an NIH Award (CTSA) 1UL1RR025011, a Merit Review Grant from the Department of Veterans Affairs, the Wisconsin Comprehensive Memory Program, and NIH grant AG021155. The authors also acknowledge the facilities and resources at the William S. Middleton Memorial Veterans Hospital. Data collection and sharing for this project was funded by the Alzheimer's Disease Neuroimaging Initiative (ADNI); CH was also supported by a UW-CIBM fellowship.

References

1. Jack, C.R., Bernstein, M.A., Fox, N.C., Thompson, P., et al.: The Alzheimer's disease neuroimaging initiative (ADNI): MRI methods. Journal of Magnetic Resonance Imaging (2008)
2. Apostolova, L.G., Thompson, P.M.: Brain mapping as a tool to study neurodegeneration. Neurotherapeutics 4(3), 387–400 (2007)
3. Ashburner, J., Friston, K.J.: Voxel-Based Morphometry - the methods. Neuroimage 11(6), 805–821 (2000)
4. Fan, Y., Resnick, S.M., Wu, X., Davatzikos, C.: Structural and functional biomarkers of prodromal Alzheimer's disease: a high-dimensional pattern classification study. Neuroimage 41(2), 277–285 (2008)
5. Klöppel, S., Stonnington, C.M., Chu, C., Draganski, B., et al.: Automatic classification of MR scans in Alzheimer's disease. Brain 131(3), 681–689 (2008)
6. Vemuri, P., Gunter, J.L., Senjem, M.L., Whitwell, J.L., et al.: Alzheimer's disease diagnosis in individual subjects using structural MR images: validation studies. Neuroimage 39(3), 1186–1197 (2008)
7. Hinrichs, C., Singh, V., Mukherjee, L., Chung, M.K., Xu, G., Johnson, S.C.: Spatially Augmented LPBoosting with evaluations on the ADNI dataset. Neuroimage (in press, 2009)
8. Schölkopf, B., Smola, A.: Learning with kernels: Support Vector Machines, Regularization, Optimization, and Beyond. MIT Press, Cambridge (2002)
9. Sonnenburg, S., Rätsch, G., Schäfer, C., Schölkopf, B.: Large scale multiple kernel learning. Journ. of Machine Learning Research 7, 1531–1565 (2006)
10. Xu, L., Crammer, K., Schuurmans, D.: Robust support vector machine training via convex outlier ablation. In: Proc. of AAAI (2006)
11. Jack, C., Petersen, R., Xu, Y., O'Brien, P., et al.: Rates of hippocampal atrophy correlate with change in clinical status in aging and AD. Neurology 55(4), 484–490 (2000)
12. Minoshima, S., Giordani, B., Berent, S., Frey, K.A.: et al.: Metabolic reduction in the posterior cingulate cortex in very early alzheimer's disease. Ann. Neurol., 85–94 (1997)

A New Approach for Creating Customizable Cytoarchitectonic Probabilistic Maps without a Template

Amir M. Tahmasebi[1], Purang Abolmaesumi[1], Xiujuan Geng[2],
Patricia Morosan[3], Katrin Amunts[4], Gary E. Christensen[5],
and Ingrid S. Johnsrude[6]

[1] School of Computing, Queen's University, Kingston, ON, Canada
tahmaseb@cs.queensu.ca
[2] Neuroimaging Research Branch, National Institute on Drug Abuse, NIH, USA
[3] Institute of Medicine, Research Center Juelich, Juelich, Germany
[4] Brain Imaging Center West, Germany
[5] Electrical and Computer Engineering, University of Iowa, USA
[6] Department of Psychology, Queen's University, Kingston, Canada

Abstract. We present a novel technique for creating template-free probabilistic maps of the cytoarchitectonic areas using a groupwise registration. We use the technique to transform 10 human post-mortem structural MR data sets, together with their corresponding cytoarchitectonic information, to a common space. We have targeted the cytoarchitectonically defined subregions of the primary auditory cortex. Thanks to the template-free groupwise registration, the created maps are not macroanatomically biased towards a specific geometry/topology. The advantage of the groupwise versus pairwise registration in avoiding such anatomical bias is better revealed in studies with small number of subjects and a high degree of variability among the individuals such as the post-mortem data. A leave-one-out cross-validation method was used to compare the sensitivity, specificity and positive predictive value of the proposed and published maps. We observe a significant improvement in localization of cytoarchitectonically defined subregions in primary auditory cortex using the proposed maps. The proposed maps can be tailored to any subject space by registering the subject image to the average of the groupwise-registered post-mortem images.

1 Introduction

Functional neuroimaging group studies usually involve a "normalization" step, in which brain image data from every subject are transformed to a common standard space. Such normalization compensates, at least in part, for the macroanatomical differences (sulci and gyri patterns) among individual brains within the group, with the expected consequence that the overlap of functional activation among subjects will be increased. However, function is determined more by the cyto-, myelo-, and connectional architecture of the brain [1,2], than by the configuration of gyri and sulci, and these microanatomical characteristics do not necessarily align with macroanatomy [3]. Recent progress in human brain mapping has

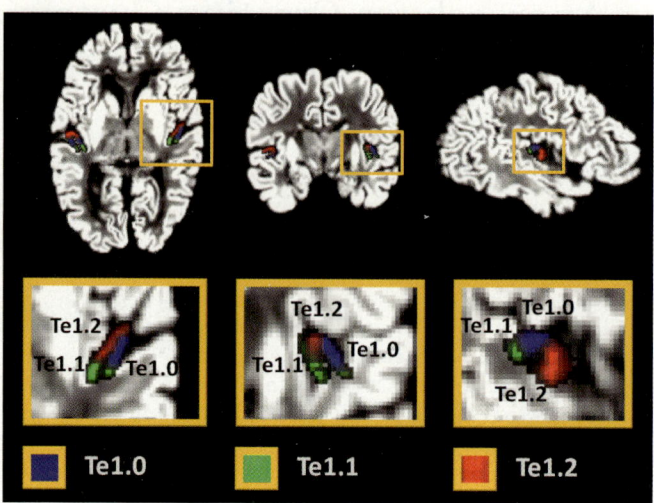

Fig. 1. Highlighted regions depicts Te1.0 (blue), Te1.1 (green), and Te1.2 (red) cytoarchitectonic subregions of the primary auditory cortex in a post-mortem brain

enabled observer-independent analysis of the cytoarchitecture of the cortex [4]. Integration of this detailed knowledge of microanatomy with functional observations seems a promising way forward for understanding the principles underlying functional organization in the brain [5]. A lack of information about intersubject microanatomical variability has been a major challenge in this endeavor. A common solution, given that microanatomical details are not easily obtainable from MR images, is the use of probabilistic maps of cytoarchitectonic data, derived from a number of post-mortem data sets registered to a standard stereotaxic space. To create a probability map, the structure of interest is first labeled in a group of individuals. Then, all the labeled volumes are transformed to a common space and overlapped to find the union of the labeled regions. Probability maps allow statistical assessment of the location of a particular region in any image that is being transformed to the spatial frame of the map. Moreover, they provide a way to predict the position of a functional activation focus and provide a method for analyzing data in an anatomically informed way (*i.e.*, region-of-interest-based analysis).

Maps of the motor and somatosensory cortices, auditory cortex, visual cortex, Broca's region and others have already been published [1,6] based on extensive and painstaking analysis of 10 post-mortem human brains (Juelich/Dusseldorf data sets). A list of available maps is given in [7]. In primary auditory cortex, Morosan and colleagues [8] developed maps of three subregions: Te1.0, Te1.1, and Te1.2, which all overlap with the anteriormost gyrus of Heschl (HG). Figure 1 shows the cross-sectional views for a post-mortem brain with the corresponding cytoarchitectonic labels of the three subregions. Morosan utilized an affine registration to transform the cytoarchitectonic labels to MNI space; however, due to intersubject anatomical variability of HG among the brains, the generated probability maps are diffuse, with large overlaps between maps of adjacent regions. Recently, Bailey et al. [9] proposed deformable registration of these three cytoarchitectonic data sets in order to create maps tailored to particular individuals. In that method, the cytoarchitectonic subregions are locally warped to the gyrus of Heschl in the subject brain. However, this technique requires manual segmentation of HG in the subject image which is time consuming, subjective, and requires anatomical expertise. Furthermore, entirely new probability maps must be generated for each new brain image. The method proposed here is completely automatic, and the probability map created can then be warped to the space of any other brain image.

In this work, we present a new approach for creating cytoarchitectonic probabilistic maps for microanatomical subregions that can also be customized for a specific subject space. The proposed technique utilizes a groupwise deformable registration [10] to warp the 10 post-mortem brains as well as the corresponding cytoarchitectonic information to a common space (i.e., group space). The groupwise registration has the advantage of avoiding the anatomical bias introduced by choosing a specific template in typical pairwise registration frameworks. The effect of the template bias in the resulting probability maps becomes even more dramatic when using a small group of subjects (such as the post-mortem brains) as the resulting maps necessarily give high probabilities where the anatomy is similar to the template and low probabilities elsewhere. On the other hand, in a groupwise registration, every brain in the study is given equal probability of presence in the final map. The constructed probability maps using the proposed method can be further tailored to the anatomy of an individual subject by using a deformable registration between the average of the warped post-mortem data and the subject image.

We evaluate and compare the *quality* of the proposed probability maps using a leave-one-out (LOO) method [11]. Maps were created based on nine data sets, and used to 'diagnose' the auditory subregion in the excluded data set. True positive, false positive, false negative, and true negative voxels were measured, and the sensitivity, specificity and positive predictive value (PPV) of the maps were calculated. The same measures were calculated between the published maps and the labeled regions in the post-mortem brains, with the necessary difference that the published maps (created from all 10 data sets) also comprise the data that was used to evaluate them. Note that this biases our results away from our prediction (that the new maps are better). Repeated-measures ANOVAs were conducted on each of the diagnostic measures. The proposed maps yielded significantly higher PPV and specificity compared to the published maps, whereas the two map types did not differ in sensitivity. Furthermore, the overlap between probability maps for adjacent subareas was analyzed and compared between the proposed and published maps. There was significantly less overlap between every pair of maps created by the proposed method compared to the published maps.

2 Materials and Methods

Figure 2 demonstrates an overview of the proposed approach. As shown in the figure, the procedure consists of two major parts: (a) creating probabilistic maps

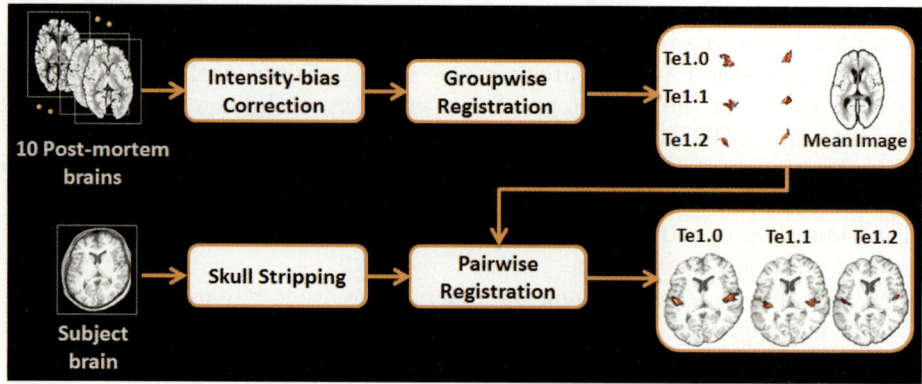

Fig. 2. Overview of the proposed approach for creating customized cytoarchitectonic probability maps for primary auditory cortex subregions: Te1.0, Te1.1, and Te1.2

in the group space; and (b) customizing the constructed maps for a specific subject brain. Both input data and the created outputs are in MNI space.

The 10 post-mortem human brains used in this study are from previously published work [6]: serial coronal brain sections stained for cell bodies were quantitatively analyzed. An observer-independent method was used to determine the areal border for each subregion. Results were digitized and mapped onto high-resolution structural MR images of the same post-mortem brains, creating three-dimensional labeled volumes of cytoarchitectonic regions. These areas are called Te1.0, Te1.1, and Te1.2, and all overlap somewhat with Heschl's gyrus. The post-mortem data was intensity-bias corrected using BrainSuite2 software[1] to achieve intensity matching among the regions with similar tissue type.

2.1 Cytoarchitectonic Probabilistic Map in Group Space

The post-mortem MR images were concurrently registered to a common space using implicit reference-based group (IRG) registration [10]. IRG is a recently developed groupwise registration technique that jointly estimates transformation from each image in the group to a "hidden" reference by optimizing the intensity difference of each pair of the deformed images. The intensity-bias correction step applied to the post-mortem data guarantees intensity matching between corresponding voxels of all images within the group. The cost function includes a similarity cost and a regularization constraint, defined as:

$$C = C_{similarity} + C_{reg} \qquad (1)$$

where

$$C_{similarity} = \sum_{i,j} \int \|(I_i(h_{iR}(x)) - I_j(h_{jR}(x)))\|^2 dx \qquad (2)$$

---

[1] BrainSuite2: http://brainsuite.usc.edu/

I_i represents the ith image in the group and $h_{iR}(x)$ is the transformation from image I_i to the implicit reference. C_{reg} is a small deformation linear-elastic constraint [12] to penalize transformations with large and unsmooth distortion. The transformed images converge to the implicit reference during the IRG registration eliminating the bias associated with selecting a specific reference image. The algorithm assumes a small deformation linear elastic model and uses the Fourier series to parameterize the deformation field. A spatial and frequency multi-resolution procedure is used to estimate the full resolution transformations to avoid local minima. Next, the resulting deformation fields are used to transform the corresponding cytoarchitectural labels to the same group space. A probability map was constructed by averaging the 10 warped subregions.

In order to customize the generated probability maps for a specific subject, one can use a deformable registration such as the normalization tool provided in SPM[2] to transform the subject to the space of the average post-mortem brain or vice versa. When conducting a group study, it is recommended that the group average image be registered to the groupwise averaged post-mortem image.

2.2 Evaluation Framework

Leave-One-Out Cross-Validation. The constructed probability maps as well as the post-mortem data were transformed to MNI space using the SPM software for validation. The quality of the proposed probability maps was evaluated using a leave-one-out method at two different thresholds: 20%, and 60% (for the published maps) and 22.2% and 66.67% (for the proposed maps). All combinations of nine out of 10 (10 cases) were used to create probability maps for three subregions of Te1.0, Te1.1, and Te1.2 using the proposed method. The created maps were then used to 'diagnose' each subregion in the excluded brain, and true positive (TP), false positive (FP), true negative (TN) and false negative (FN) voxels were calculated. Labeled voxels from the excluded brain that were correctly identified by the probability map are TP voxels. Labeled voxels that were not identified in the excluded brain are FN, and unlabeled voxels that were incorrectly classified as the target subregion by the probability map are FP. Finally, unlabeled voxels that are correctly identified by the probability map are TN. We measure the quality of the maps based on sensitivity (Sn), specificity (Sp) and positive predictive value (PPV):

$$Sn = \frac{TP}{TP+FN}, \quad Sp = \frac{TN}{TN+FP}, \quad PPV = \frac{TP}{TP+FP} \qquad (3)$$

The published maps were also used to evaluate the same post-mortem data; however, the published maps were evaluated on the same data that was used to constitute the maps. MANOVAs were used to identify significant differences on these measures between the two types of maps.

Between-Map Overlap. Any single voxel can only belong to one subregion. To the extent that voxels are shared between two adjacent Te1 maps and are

---
[2] Statistical Parametric Mapping: Wellcome Department of Cognitive Neurology, UK.

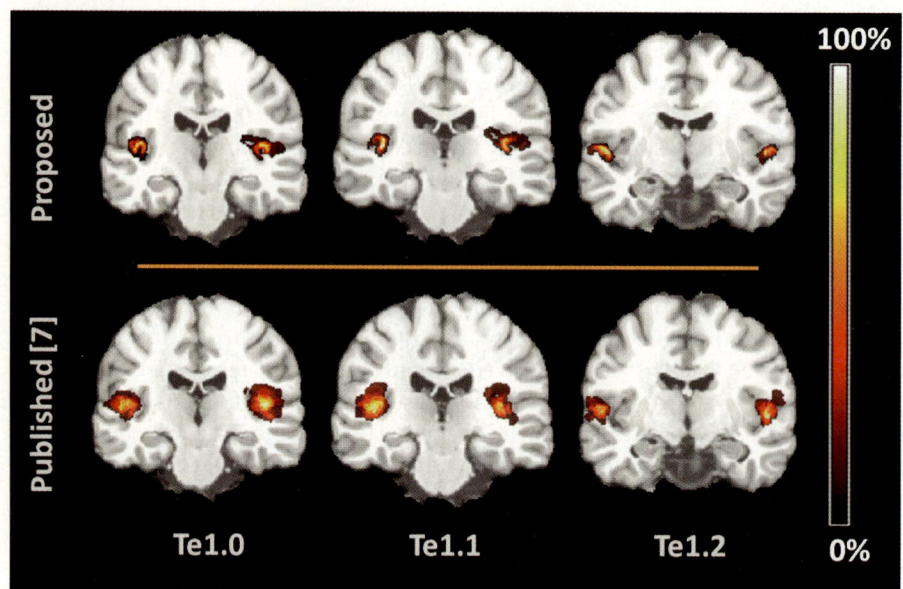

Fig. 3. Comparing cytoarchitectonic probability maps generated using the proposed method and the previously published maps [8], superimposed on Colin27 brain

assigned high probabilities by both maps, the maps do not segregate the regions well. We evaluate the two methods for such between-map overlap (*i.e.*, Te1.0/Te1.1, Te1.0/Te1.2, and Te1.1/Te1.2).

3 Results and Discussion

Figure 3 gives cross-sectional views of both the proposed and previously published probability maps for Te1.0, Te1.1, and Te1.2 subregions overlaid on Colin27 [13] brain image. White and black colors correspond to the highest and the lowest probabilities, respectively. As can be seen, the proposed probability maps are significantly denser in terms of the spatial expansion and more focused on Heschl's gyrus. Both proposed and published probability maps are more diffuse in the right hemisphere than left.

Sensitivity, specificity, and positive predictive values were calculated for both proposed and published maps. We consider left and right hemispheres separately. Four-factor MANOVAs (method: proposed vs. published; subregions of Te1: Te1.0, Te1.1, and Te1.2; hemisphere: left or right; threshold value: 2 levels) were conducted on each of the three diagnostic measures followed by post-hoc pairwise comparisons to identify significant differences. PPV (F(1,9)=113.442, $p < 0.05$) and specificity (F(1,9)=298.542, $p < 0.05$) were significantly higher for the proposed than the published maps; however, sensitivity did not differ; see Table 1. Significant difference in PPV despite no significant difference in sensitivity implies that the proposed maps are more conservative in labeling the cytoarchitecture in brain compared to published maps.

Table 1. Mean±std of the sensitivity, specificity and PPV values of the 10 test cases for both types of maps

Method	Sensitivity (mean±std)	Specificity (mean±std)	PPV (mean±std)
proposed	23.8 ± 1.1%	96.8 ± 0.3%	73.4 ± 2.1%
published	24.2 ± 1.4%	84.8 ± 0.6%	30.4 ± 3.6%

Table 2. Total percentage of the overlapping voxels and the critical voxels in every pair of the overlapping maps given for both methods

Overlapping Maps	Method	Overlap Percentage	Critical Voxels
Te1.0/Te1.1	Proposed	0.1%	0.0%
	Published	1.4%	21.0%
Te1.0/Te1.2	Proposed	0.6%	3.0%
	Published	1.0%	20.0%

Next, the percentage of the overlap between maps of adjacent subareas was calculated and compared between the proposed and published maps. All maps were thresholded at 40%, assuming overlap at lesser probabilities could arise for voxels on the edges of the maps. We define an overlapping voxel as "critical" if the probability value for both maps exceeds 50%. As can be observed from Table 2, there is a higher probability of overlapping voxels in the published maps exceeding this critical value compared to our proposed maps. Nonadjacent regions (Te1.1 and Te1.2) did not overlap in either map type.

4 Conclusions

The presented work demonstrates a novel approach for creating template-free customizable cytoarchitectonic probabilistic maps for Te1 subregions of the human primary auditory cortex. In anatomical/functional studies of the brain with a small number of subjects (such as the post-mortem data set), pairwise matching introduces a large bias factor in the registration results due to the high degree of intersubject morphological variability among the individuals. The template-free strategy of registration avoids such bias by simultaneous registration of all brains towards a virtual reference image that is iteratively updated. The proposed method of cytoarchitectonic probability map construction takes advantage of a novel groupwise registration to transform the labeled post-mortem data into a common space in a template-free fashion. The presented approach can be applied to any other area of the brain for which the corresponding cytoarchitectonic data is available from post-mortem subjects. For the Juelich data set, this includes motor cortex, somatomotor cortex, visual cortex, Broca's area and others. The proposed approach enables accurate and reliable testing of the hypothesis of architectonic-functional relationships in cognitive neuroscience.

These probability maps, after the data from a functional neuroimaging (*e.g.*, fMRI) subject has been registered to them, can be used to conduct a ROI-based statistical analysis by using them as weighted filters on the functional data. Such method of ROI-based functional analysis would allow for more precise and focused functional differentiation of small, adjacent subregions in the brain.

Acknowledgments. This work was partially supported by the Natural Sciences and Engineering Research Council (NSERC), Ontario Ministry of Research and Innovation, the Canadian Institutes of Health Research (CIHR), and NIH grant EB004126.

References

1. Amunts, K., Weiss, P., Mohlberg, H., et al.: Analysis of verbal fluency in microstructurally defined stereotactic space: The role of Brodmann's areas 44 and 45. J. Comp. Neurol. 16(2), 176 (2002)
2. Eickhoff, S., Amunts, K., Mohlberg, H., Zilles, K.: The human parietal operculum. II. stereotaxic maps and correlation with functional imaging results. Cereb. Cortex 16(2), 268–279 (2006)
3. Amunts, K., Zilles, K.: Advances in cytoarchitectonic mapping of the human cerebral cortex. Neuroimaging Clin. N. Am. 11, 151–169 (2001)
4. Amunts, K., Schleicher, A., Bürgel, U., Mohlberg, H., Uylings, H., Zilles, K.: Broca's region revisited: Cytoarchitecture and intersubject variability. J. Comp. Neurol. 412(2), 319–341 (1999)
5. Felleman, D., Essen, D.V.: Distributed hierarchical processing in the primate cerebral cortex. Cereb. Cortex 1, 1–47 (1991)
6. Zilles, K., Schleicher, A., Palomero-Gallagher, N., Amunts, K.: Quantitative analysis of cyto- and receptorarchitecture of the human brain. Brain Mapping: The Methods, 2nd edn., pp. 573–602 (2002)
7. Eickhoff, S., Paus, T., Caspers, S., Grosbras, M., Evans, A., Zilles, K., Amunts, K.: Assignment of functional activations to probabilistic cytoarchitectonic areas revisited. NeuroImage 36(3), 511–521 (2007)
8. Morosan, P., Rademacher, J., Schleicher, A., Amunts, K., Schormann, T., Zilles, K.: Human primary auditory cortex: Cytoarchitectonic subdivisions and mapping into a spatial reference system. NeuroImage 13(4), 684–701 (2001)
9. Bailey, L., Abolmaesumi, P., Tam, J., Morosan, P., Cusack, R., Amunts, K., Johnsrude, I.: Customised cytoarchitectonic probability maps using deformable registration: Primary auditory cortex. In: Ayache, N., Ourselin, S., Maeder, A. (eds.) MICCAI 2007, Part II. LNCS, vol. 4792, pp. 760–768. Springer, Heidelberg (2007)
10. Geng, X., Christensen, G., Gu, H., Ross, T., Yang, Y.: Implicit reference-based group-wise image registration and its application to structural and functional MRI. NeuroImage (in press, 2009)
11. Tahmasebi, A., Abolmaesumi, P., Wild, C., Johnsrude, I.: Quantification of intersubject variability in human brain: a validation framework for probabilistic maps. In: Proc. SPIE, vol. 7262, p. 726218 (2009)
12. Christensen, G., Johnson, H.: Consistent image registration. IEEE Trans. Med. Imag. 20, 568–582 (2001)
13. Holmes, C., Hoge, R., Collins, L., Woods, R., Toga, A., Evans, A.: Enhancement of MR images using registration for signal averaging. J. Comput. Assist. Tomogr. 22(2), 324–333 (1998)

A Computer-Aided Diagnosis System of Nuclear Cataract via Ranking

Wei Huang[1], Huiqi Li[2], Kap Luk Chan[1], Joo Hwee Lim[2], Jiang Liu[2], and Tien Yin Wong[3]

[1] School of Electrical and Electronic Engineering,
Nanyang Technological University, Singapore
[2] Institute for Infocomm Research, Agency for Science,
Technology and Research, Singapore
[3] National University of Singapore, Singapore National Eye Center and Singapore Eye Research Institute

Abstract. A novel computer-aided diagnosis system of nuclear cataract via ranking is firstly proposed in this paper. The grade of nuclear cataract in a slit-lamp image is predicted based on its neighboring labeled images in a ranked images list, which is achieved using an optimal ranking function. A new ranking evaluation measure is proposed for learning the optimal ranking function via direct optimization. Our system has been tested by a large dataset composed of 1000 slit-lamp images from 1000 different cases. Both experimental results and comparison with several state-of-the-art methods indicate the superiority of our system.

1 Introduction

Cataract, the clouding or opacity of normally clear human lens, is the leading cause of blindness globally. Based on locations of opacity, age-related cataracts can be categorized into three types: *posterior sub-capsular cataract, cortical cataract* and *nuclear cataract*, among which nuclear cataract (cataract formed in the nucleus) is the most common type [1]. In clinical diagnosis, a reasonable grade of nuclear cataract is often assigned by trained ophthalmologists to each *slit-lamp image* by comparing its opacity severity with a set of standard photos [2]. This grading scheme is often subjective (inter-observer agreement is only around 65% [2]) and time-consuming. Recently, there are research efforts towards automatic diagnosis of nuclear cataract to improve its grading objectivity and save workload [3], [4]. In [3], intensities on visual axis were used as features and *linear regression* was applied to grade nuclear cataract. In [4], more diverse features and advanced technique (*support vector machine* (svm) regression) were adopted. Both systems aim to output a final grade, but they offer little help to train junior ophthalmologists. One of the most important means to gain skills in clinics is practice and learning from similar cases.

In this paper, we, computer scientists and clinicians working closely together, propose a novel computer-aided diagnosis (CAD) system, which firstly regards nuclear cataract grading as a *ranking* task. The flowchart of our system is shown

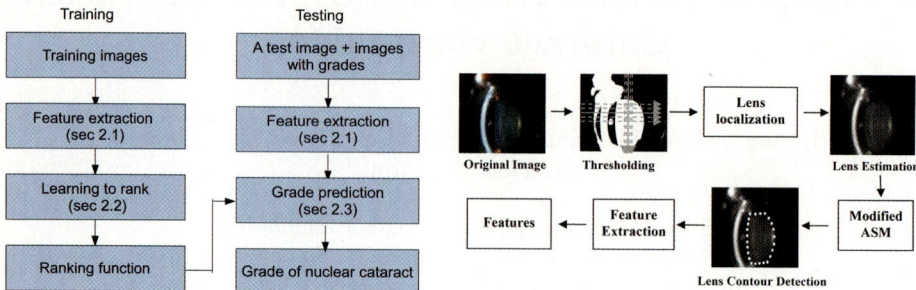

Fig. 1. Flowchart of our system

Fig. 2. Diagram of feature extraction scheme

in Fig. 1. Given a slit-lamp image to grade, ranking aims to sort the slit-lamp image together with other slit-lamp images, whose grades are known, to form a ranked images list according to their nuclear cataract severity measured by a *ranking function*. Grade of the slit-lamp image is then predicted using its neighboring images in the ranked list. In order to achieve an optimal ranking function for ranking these images, we incorporate the "*learning to rank*" technique [5], in which we propose a new ranking evaluation measure that can be directly optimized for learning ranking functions. This is different from many other traditional "learning to rank" methods, which adopt various complicated approaches, such as *adaptive boosting* [6], [7] or svm [8], to learn ranking functions, based on traditional ranking evaluation measures [9]. Our contribution lies in three aspects: (1) We firstly propose a novel CAD system that grades nuclear cataract in slit-lamp images via ranking using local features; (2) We propose a new ranking evaluation measure, and incorporate "learning to rank" technique to learn an optimal ranking function via direct optimization based on the new measure; (3) Our system has been tested by a large dataset composed of 1000 slit-lamp images from 1000 different cases. Experimental results have been compared with ones achieved from several state-of-the-art methods and evaluated with clinical ground truth.

2 Methodology

2.1 Local Feature Extraction from Slit-Lamp Images

Robust feature extraction is essential for any medical imaging application. Here we apply a model-based method to detect the anatomical contour of lens, and then, we extract local discriminative feature from detected regions following previously published clinical works [2], [10]. The whole process is illustrated in Fig. 2. The foreground of lens image is segmented by thresholding 20% - 30% brightest pixels in the grey image. Horizontal profile clustering and vertical profile clustering are employed to estimate lens structure as an ellipse, which is based on the largest cluster and used as the initialization of detected lens

Table 1. Description of feature extracted from each slit-lamp image

Feature Number	Description
1	mean intensity inside the lens contour
2 - 4	color information on posterior reflex in HSI color space
5	mean intensity within the central part of lens
6	intensity ratio between anterior lentil and posterior lentil

contour. After that, a modified *active shape model* (ASM) [11] is employed to further evolve the contour to better match the lens. Based on the lens structure detected by ASM, a 6-dimensional local feature vector is selected and extracted from each slit-lamp image. The specification of feature vector is described in Table 1.

2.2 Surrogate-NDCG and Ranking Function Learning

In this section, we aim to sort slit-lamp images to form a ranked images list according to their nuclear cataract severity. We incorporate the "learning to rank" technique here, to learn an optimal ranking function, which is used to rank images. In order to learn the function, we propose a new ranking evaluation measure, named *surrogate-NDCG* (*Normalized Discounted Cumulative Gain*), which can be directly optimized for learning ranking functions.

NDCG is a traditional position-based ranking evaluation measure, which can handle multiple-level relevance judgements [9]. It was chosen here because nuclear cataract grades annotated by ophthalmologists in our application are also multiple ordinal values. The definition of NDCG is as follows [9]:

$$NDCG = N_n^{-1} \times DCG = N_n^{-1} \sum_{x \in \chi} \frac{2^{r(x)} - 1}{log_2(1 + \pi(x))} \qquad (1)$$

where, x is a slit-lamp image and χ is the set of images to be ranked; $r(x)$ and $\pi(x)$ are the grade and position of image x in the ranked images list sorted by decreasing nuclear cataract severity, respectively; N_n is a normalization term denoting the maximum of DCG, which can be achieved when all images are sorted in a perfect order of decreasing severity. Unfortunately, optimization cannot be directly applied on NDCG for learning ranking functions, since the measure itself is neither continuous nor differentiable in terms of discrete position $\pi(x)$. Hence, many traditional state-of-the-art "learning to rank" methods [6], [7], [8] incorporate complicated techniques for learning ranking functions with indirect optimization based on NDCG.

To solve the problem, we first approximate position $\pi(x)$ as follows:

$$\pi(x) = 1 + \sum_{y \neq x, y \in \chi} \mathbf{1}\{s_{xy} < 0\}, \qquad s_{xy} = s_x - s_y = f(\theta, \hat{x}) - f(\theta, \hat{y}) \qquad (2)$$

where, s_x is the *score* of slit-lamp image x computed from ranking function $f(\theta, \hat{x})$, which is of a linear form ($f(\theta, \hat{x}) = \theta \hat{x}$) in this work; θ and $\hat{x}$ are parameters of $f(\theta, \hat{x})$ to learn and extracted feature of image x, respectively. $\mathbf{1}\{s_{xy} < 0\}$

is an *indictor function*, whose value is positive when $s_{xy} < 0$ and negative otherwise. Hence, when the score of image x is smaller than y's ($s_{xy} = s_x - s_y < 0$), $\mathbf{1}\{s_{xy} < 0\}$ becomes positive and $\pi(x)$ becomes larger, which matches the fact that images with lighter symptom (represented by smaller score s_x) should be ranked in the rear of a ranked images list (larger position $\pi(x)$) in a descending order of nuclear cataract severity.

Furthermore, we overcome the *step characteristics* of indictor function $\mathbf{1}\{s_{xy} < 0\}$ by approximating it via a continuous *hyperbolic tangent function*. In this way, we can achieve a new continuous approximated position $\hat{\pi}(x)$:

$$\hat{\pi}(x) = 1 + \sum_{y \neq x, y \in \chi} \mathbf{1}\{s_{xy} < 0\} \simeq 1 + \sum_{y \neq x, y \in \chi} \frac{exp(-2\alpha s_{xy}) - 1}{exp(-2\alpha s_{xy}) + 1} \quad (3)$$

where, $\alpha > 0$ is a scaling constant. Hence, our new continuous and differentiable ranking evaluation measure *surrogate-NDCG* ($\widehat{NDCG}$) can be achieved:

$$\widehat{NDCG} = N_n^{-1} \sum_{x \in \chi} \frac{2^{r(x)} - 1}{log_2(1 + \hat{\pi}(x))} \quad (4)$$

Our method to directly optimize $\widehat{NDCG}$ for learning ranking functions is listed in Table 2. The key step is to compute gradient of $\widehat{NDCG}$ with respect to θ ($\nabla \widehat{NDCG}(\theta)$) in step 6. After applying the *chain rule*, the gradient is as follows:

$$\nabla \widehat{NDCG}(\theta) = \frac{\partial \widehat{NDCG}}{\partial \theta} = N_n^{-1} \sum_{x \in \chi} \frac{\partial \frac{2^{r(x)}-1}{log_2(1+\hat{\pi}(x))}}{\partial \hat{\pi}(x)} \cdot \frac{\partial \hat{\pi}(x)}{\partial \theta}$$

$$= N_n^{-1} \sum_{x \in \chi} \left(-\frac{2^{r(x)} - 1}{(log_2(1 + \hat{\pi}(x)))^2} \cdot \frac{1}{(1 + \hat{\pi}(x))ln2} \right) \cdot$$

$$\left(\sum_{y \neq x, y \in \chi} \frac{-4\alpha \cdot exp\left(-2\alpha(f(\theta,\hat{x}) - f(\theta,\hat{y}))\right)}{\left[exp\left(-2\alpha(f(\theta,\hat{x}) - f(\theta,\hat{y}))\right) + 1\right]^2} \cdot \left(\frac{\partial f(\theta,\hat{x})}{\partial \theta} - \frac{\partial f(\theta,\hat{y})}{\partial \theta} \right) \right) \quad (5)$$

Detailed derivation is omitted here. The formula of step 7 in Table 2 shows the actual implementation of maximizing NDCG by minimizing the negative of it. For inputs in Table 2, we also apply a series of n positive scaling constants $\{\alpha_1, \ldots, \alpha_n\}$ as candidates of α in Equation 3. Therefore, $(n \times T)$ ranking functions $f(\theta, \hat{x})$ can be learned as outputs from Table 2. In a following validation step, NDCG value (Equation 1) of each outputted ranking function is calculated from its ranked images list, which is achieved by applying the specified ranking function to rank validation images. The one with the highest NDCG value will be chosen as the optimal ranking function $f_{opt}(\theta, \hat{x})$.

2.3 Automatic Diagnosis of Nuclear Cataract

Using the optimal ranking function $f_{opt}(\theta, \hat{x})$ achieved from section 2.2, a slit-lamp image x to grade can be sorted together with other slit-lamp images with

Table 2. Learning ranking functions via direct optimization on $\widehat{NDCG}$

Inputs	1.	m training sets of slit-lamp images x and their grades r(x)
	2.	Iteration times: T
	3.	Learning rate: η
	4.	n scaling constants candidates $\{\alpha_1, \ldots, \alpha_n\}$
Algorithm		
	1.	For $\alpha \in \{\alpha_1, \ldots, \alpha_n\}$
	2.	Initialize parameters θ of ranking function $f(\theta, \hat{x})$ as θ_0
	3.	For t = 1 to T
	4.	Set $\theta = \theta_{t-1}$
	5.	For i = 1 to m, apply *gradient descent* approach:
	6.	Feed (x, r(x)) to Equation 5 for computing $\nabla \widehat{NDCG}(\theta)$
	7.	Update parameter $\theta = \theta - \eta \cdot \nabla \widehat{NDCG}(\theta)$
	8.	End for 5
	9.	Set $\theta_t = \theta$
	10.	End for 3
	11.	End for 1
Outputs		$(n \times T)$ learned ranking functions $f(\theta, \hat{x})$ with $(n \times T)$ learned θ

known grades, to form a ranked images list in the order of nuclear cataract severity. After that, grade g_{x_i} of the slit-lamp image x located at position i in the ranked images list can be predicted by using both scores computed from ranking function $f_{opt}(\theta, \hat{x})$ and grades $g_{x_{i-1}}$ and $g_{x_{i+1}}$ of its neighboring images in the ranked images list as follows:

$$g_{x_i} = \begin{cases} g_{x_{i+1}} & \text{if } g_{x_{i+1}} = g_{x_{i-1}} \\ g_{x_{i+1}} + \frac{s_{x_i} - s_{x_{i+1}}}{s_{x_{i-1}} - s_{x_{i+1}}} \times (g_{x_{i-1}} - g_{x_{i+1}}) & \text{if } g_{x_{i-1}} > g_{x_{i+1}} \\ g_{x_{i-1}} + \frac{s_{x_{i-1}} - s_{x_i}}{s_{x_{i-1}} - s_{x_{i+1}}} \times (g_{x_{i+1}} - g_{x_{i-1}}) & \text{if } g_{x_{i-1}} < g_{x_{i+1}} \end{cases} \quad (6)$$

3 Experiments and Discussion

3.1 Data Description

Our CAD system has been tested by a large dataset composed of 1000 slit-lamp images from 1000 different cases including both normal and pathological conditions achieved from a population-based study, the *Singapore Malay Eye Study* (SiMES) [12]. All images were captured using a Topcon DC-1 digital slit-lamp camera with FD-21 flash attachment. The slit-lamp images were saved as 24-bit color images with the size of 2048 × 1536 pixels. Clinical ground truth were provided by ophthalmologists using *Wisconsin cataract grading system* [2].

3.2 Ranking Experiments and Statistical Analysis

After feature extraction, the 1000 images are divided into 5 subsets for *five-fold cross validation*; there are 3 training sets, 1 validation set and 1 testing set respectively. We empirically set $m = 30$, $T = 200$, $\eta = 0.01$ and

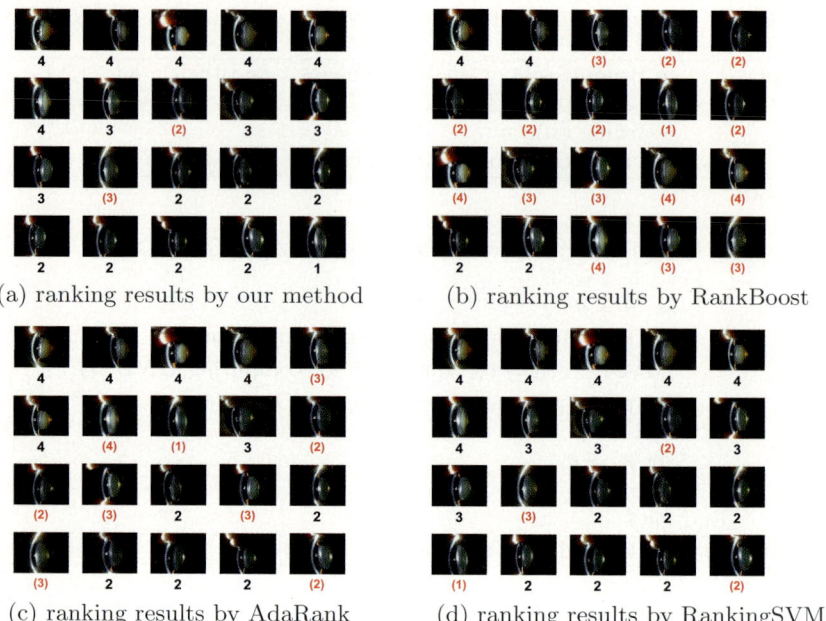

Fig. 3. An example of ranking the same 20 slit-lamp images (ranking errors are highlighted in red within brackets; the clinical ground truth is 4: 1st-6th images; 3: 7th-11th images; 2: 12th-19th images; 1: 20th image)

$\alpha \in \{0.1, 0.2, 0.5, 1, 1.5, 2, 2.5, 5, 7, 10\}$ as inputs in Table 2. There are three state-of-the-art "learning to rank" methods for ranking comparison, including *RankBoost* [6], *AdaRank* [7] and *RankingSVM* [8]. Related parameters setting are equivalent to ours. For these three methods, 4 subsets beside the testing set were used for training as there were no validations included. An example of ranking the same 20 testing images is shown in Fig. 3. The number below each image is its clinical ground truth. In this testing set, 4 represents the severest symptom of nuclear cataract, while 1 is the lightest. It can be seen that our method achieved the best ranking performance (only 2 ranking errors) among all methods (RankBoost: 16 errors; AdaRank: 9 errors; RankingSVM: 4 errors).

To evaluate our method quantitatively, we utilized ranking evaluation measure NDCG (Equation 1), and results are listed in Table 3.2. We can easily see that RankingSVM and our method achieve better performance than RankBoost and AdaRank, although comparison between RankingSVM and our method is not clear. Thus, a statistical test is conducted to further discern which method is superior from statistical point of view. After performing one-way *analysis of variance* (ANOVA), the *p-value* is nearly 0, which casts serious doubts on the null hypothesis that RankingSVM and our method share the same NDCG means. Hence, a series of post-hoc *multiple comparison tests* are applied and partial results are listed in Table 3.2. The estimated NDCG mean of our method is

Table 3. NDCG of all methods on five-fold cross validation test (mean±variance)

Fold	Our Method	RankBoost	AdaRank	RankingSVM
1	**0.9770±0.0013**	0.8068±0.0046	0.9078±0.0028	0.9769±0.0013
2	**0.9693±0.0018**	0.8077±0.0033	0.9105±0.0026	0.9597±0.0022
3	0.9169±0.0028	0.7421±0.0110	0.8779±0.0081	**0.9206±0.0038**
4	**0.9729±0.0009**	0.8075±0.0051	0.9523±0.0011	0.9714±0.0014
5	0.9396±0.0025	0.7536±0.0064	0.9064±0.0049	**0.9410±0.0019**

Table 4. Multiple comparison test results of our method against other methods

Method I	Method II	Estimated Mean Diff. (I-II)	95% Confidence Int.
Our Method	RankBoost	0.1708	[0.1401, 0.2016]
Our Method	AdaRank	0.0454	[0.0147, 0.0762]
Our Method	RankingSVM	**0.0017**	**[-0.0291, 0.0325]**

0.0017 higher, and a 95% confidence interval is [-0.0291, 0.0325], which shows that for less than 50% cases (about 44.8% if the confidence interval is uniformly distributed), RankingSVM performs better. For the majority, ours is superior.

3.3 Nuclear Cataract Grading from Ranking

To evaluate automatic diagnosis performance of our CAD system, we used the same 1000 slit-lamp images dataset for grading test. Grades in our system are computed from Equation 6 based on ranking results achieved from section 3.2. The mean error between predicted grades of our system and ophthalmologists' clinical ground truth is only 0.541. The grading accuracy measuring grading errors within one integer grade (clinically important) is 91.4%. Experimental results show that our CAD system is promising in grading nuclear cataract of slit-lamp images from a large dataset.

4 Conclusion

A novel computer-aided diagnosis (CAD) system of nuclear cataract via ranking is firstly proposed in this paper. Grade of a slit-lamp image is predicted using its neighboring images in a ranked images list, which is achieved using a learned ranking function via direct optimization based on a new proposed ranking evaluation measure. Our system has been tested by a large images dataset composed of 1000 slit-lamp images from 1000 different cases. Results show that our system performs better than several state-of-the-art methods. Our system can also be utilized as a training tool for junior clinicians to learn diagnostic decision from similar images (neighboring images in the ranked images list), which have already been diagnosed by senior clinicians. It can be used in research to analyze difference diagnosis with similar symptoms as well.

Acknowledgments. We would like to acknowledge Singapore A*STAR SBIC SiRIAN grant for providing the clinical images and ophthalmologists from Singapore Eye Research Institute for valuable clinical inputs. We want to express our gratitude to Prof. Paul Mitchell, Prof. Jie Jin Wang and Ms Ava Tan from the University of Sydney, Australia for providing technical inputs and providing the ground truth of cataract grading.

References

1. World Health Organization (WHO): Magnitude and Causes of Visual Impairments (2002), http://www.who.int/mediacentre/factsheets/fs282/en/index.html
2. Klein, B., Klein, R., Linton, K., Magli, Y., Neider, M.: Assessment of Cataracts from Photographs in the Beaver Dam Eye Study. Ophthalmology 97(11), 1428–1433 (1990)
3. Fan, S., Dyer, C.R., Hubbard, L., Klein, B.: An automatic system for classification of nuclear sclerosis from slit-lamp photographs. In: Ellis, R.E., Peters, T.M. (eds.) MICCAI 2003. LNCS, vol. 2878, pp. 592–601. Springer, Heidelberg (2003)
4. Li, H., Lim, J., Liu, J., Wong, T.-Y., Tan, A., Wang, J., Paul, M.: Image Based Grading of Nuclear Cataract by SVM Regression. In: SPIE Proceeding of Medical Imaging, vol. 6915, 691536–691536(8) (2008)
5. Agarwal, S., Cortes, C., Herbrich, R.: Proceeding of NIPS Workshop on Learning to Rank (2005)
6. Freund, Y., Iyer, R., Schapire, R., Singer, Y.: An Efficient Boosting Algorithm for Combining Preference. Journal of Machine Learning Research 4, 933–969 (2003)
7. Xu, J., Li, H.: AdaRank: A Boosting Algorithm for Information Retrieval. In: ACM SIGIR, pp. 391–398 (2007)
8. Joachims, T.: Optimizing Search Engines using Clickthrough Data. In: ACM SIGKDD, pp. 133–142 (2002)
9. Jarvelin, K., Kekalainen, J.: IR evaluation methods for retrieving highly relevant documents. In: ACM SIGIR, pp. 41–48 (2000)
10. Chylack, L., Wolfe, J., Singer, D., Leske, M.: The Lens Opacities Classification System III. Archives of Ophthalmology 111, 831–836 (1993)
11. Li, H., Chutatape, O.: Boundary detection of optic disk by a modified ASM method. Pattern Recognition 36(9), 2093–2104 (2003)
12. Foong, A., Saw, S., Loo, J., et al.: Rationale and Methodology for a Population-based Study of Eye Diseases in Malay People: The Singapore Malay Eye Study (SiMES). Ophthalmic Epidemiology 14(1), 25–35 (2007)

Automated Segmentation of the Femur and Pelvis from 3D CT Data of Diseased Hip Using Hierarchical Statistical Shape Model of Joint Structure

Futoshi Yokota[1], Toshiyuki Okada[2], Masaki Takao[3], Nobuhiko Sugano[3], Yukio Tada[1], and Yoshinobu Sato[3]

[1] Graduate School of Engineering, Kobe University, Japan
[2] Medical Center for Translational Research, Osaka University Hospital, Japan
[3] Graduate School of Medicine, Osaka University, Japan

Abstract. Segmentation of the femur and pelvis from 3D data is prerequisite of patient specific planning and simulation for hip surgery. Separation of the femoral head and acetabulum is one of main difficulties in the diseased hip joint due to deformed shapes and extreme narrowness of the joint space. In this paper, we develop a hierarchical multi-object statistical shape model representing joint structure for automated segmentation of the diseased hip from 3D CT images. In order to represent shape variations as well as pose variations of the femur against the pelvis, both shape and pose variations are embedded in a combined pelvis and femur statistical shape model (SSM). Further, the whole combined SSM is divided into individual pelvis and femur SSMs and a partial combined SSM only including the acetabulum and proximal femur. The partial combined SSM maintains the consistency of the two bones by imposing the constraint that the shapes of the overlapped portions of the individual and partial combined SSMs are identical. The experimental results show that segmentation and separation accuracy of the femur and pelvis was improved using the proposed method compared with independent use of the pelvis and femur SSMs.

1 Introduction

Segmentation of the femur and pelvis from 3D images is an important preprocessing of patient specific planning and simulation for hip surgery. Although healthy hips are relatively easy to be segmented, osteoarthrosis of the hip mainly caused by congenital hip dysplasia needs to be dealt with for clinical application such as preoperative planning for total hip arthroplasty (THA). In the 3D images of patients with the above described disease, bone deformation and joint space narrowing are highly severe, and the boundaries of the femur and pelvis around the joint space are quite difficult to be identified. While 2D X-ray images are typically used for preoperative planning of THA, 3D analysis is quite useful to deal with such highly deformed hips. In the current segmentation methods, manual interactions are involved to determine the boundaries around the joint space. Our aim is to automate segmentation of 3D images of deformed hips due to the disease described above.

Automated segmentation of the pelvic bone from 3D images using a statistical shape model (SSM) was reported [1]. For the diseased hip, however, segmentation accuracy is insufficient around the joint space due to lack of boundary information. Some previous works embed spatial relationships between multiple adjacent objects such as the femur and pelvis into SSMs [2][3]. Frangi et al. constructed a SSM of multiple objects by regarding combined multiple objects as one single shape [2]. Yang et al. explicitly modeled the relations between adjacent objects [3]. These methods deal with the relations among whole objects and suitable for stable segmentation of multiple objects due to high specificity of shape representation. In case of the hip joint, the pelvis and femur have close relations locally around the joint space, and thus modeling whole-object relations is inefficient with respect to accuracy of shape representation. To overcome this issue, Okada et al. addressed the problem of embedding local spatial relations into SSMs [4]. However, these methods do not deal with intra-patient variability of the spatial relations such as pose variations in joint motion.

In this paper, we propose a method for embedding pose variations of joint motion of the diseased hip into multi-object SSMs and its application to automated segmentation from 3D images. We construct a hierarchical SSM of the hip, in which Frangi's method is firstly applied to construct a combined pelvis-femur SSM of the whole hip, and then Okada's method is utilized to enforce the constraint of local spatial relations around the joint space on individual femur and pelvis SSMs. We aim at stable and accurate segmentation especially around the joint space by applying a coarse-fine strategy using the hierarchical hip SSM.

2 Methods

Figure 1 shows coronal views and 3D renderings of CT images of normal and diseased hips. In the normal hip, which is the non-diseased side of a patient data, it is observable in the image that the femoral head and acetabulum are separated by the joint space. In the diseased hip, however, the femoral head is highly deformed and it is difficult to identify the joint space only using local image features. In addition, the shape deformation due to osteoarthrosis of the hip shows a characteristic tendency as the disease progresses. Therefore, anatomical prior information is essential in order to determine the boundaries appropriately.

Anatomical prior information is typically embedded in a SSM. However, the pelvis and femur are interrelated in the hip joint and their spatial relations are changeable under the constraints of the range of motion. Since the pose of the femur against the pelvis is unknown in CT image, not only their shape variations but also the pose variations between them need to be incorporated into statistical modeling. In the following, the detailed methods of the statistical modeling and its use for segmentation are described.

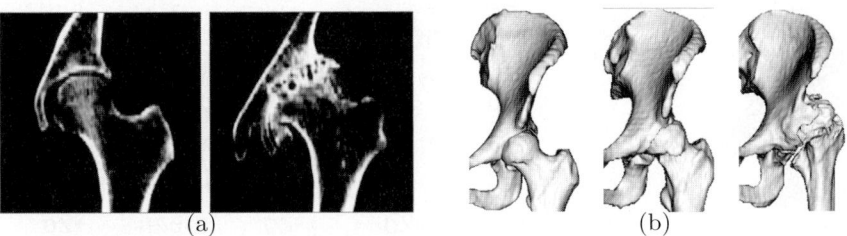

Fig. 1. Coronal views and 3D renderings of CT images of normal and diseased hips. (a) Coronal views. Left: normal hip. Right: diseased hip. (b) 3D renderings. Left: normal hip. Middle: mildly diseased hip. Right: severely diseased hip.

2.1 Statistical Modeling of Pose and Shape Variations

We assume that a sufficient number of the surface models of the pelvis and femur of different patients are available, which are constructed from manually segmented regions in the training CT datasets and represented in the pelvis and femur coordinate systems, respectively, defined based on anatomical landmarks. Further, we assume that inter-patient non-rigid registration is performed among the surface models [5].

In order to embed the pose variations into SSMs, possible pose variations are simulationally generated for each patient dataset. Although the hip joint is well-approximated by a spherical joint if it is healthy, sphere approximation is often inappropriate for the diseased hip joint as shown in Fig. 1(b). We assume that the joint space region, which is defined as a region between the acetabular and femoral boundaries manually traced from CT images, consists of the acetabular and femoral cartilages. Further, we assume that the thickness distribution of the femoral cartilage is uniform while the acetabular cartilage is not. The latter assumption is based on Zoroofi's observation that the acetabular cartilage is mainly damaged in the diseased hip, which was obtained through quantitative MR image analysis [6]. In order to generate possible poses for the diseased case based on the assumptions, we define the distance map of the joint space on the acetabular surface as the distribution of the distance from each point on acetabular surface to the nearest point of the femoral head surface. We regard the distance map in the pose at the CT image acquisition as the template. To generate possible poses of the femur against the pelvis, translation $\mathbf{t}_j$ is estimated for each of systematically generated arbitrary rotations, R_j, so that the calculated distance map is as close as possible to that of the template using the following equation:

$$\mathbf{t}_j = \operatorname{argmin}_{\mathbf{t}} C(\mathbf{t}; R_j) = \operatorname{argmin}_{\mathbf{t}} \sum_{k=1}^{N} \{d(\mathbf{p}_k, F) - d(\mathbf{p}_k, R_j F + \mathbf{t})\}^2 \quad (1)$$

where $d(\mathbf{x}, Y)$ denotes the distance from point $\mathbf{x}$ to surface Y, $\mathbf{p}_k$ is each point on the acetabular surface, F is the femoral head surface, and R_j is each generated

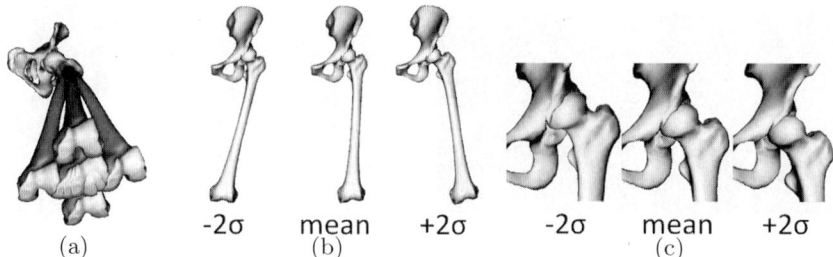

Fig. 2. Training dataset and two characteristic modes of the constructed combined pelvis and femur SSM. (a) Generated poses of the femur against the pelvis. (b) First mode of SSM. (c) Forth mode of SSM.

rotation matrix. The center of gravity of the femoral head is used for the center of rotation. The femur is rotated along the three axes based on the anatomical coordinate system (e.g., flexion and extension). $C(\mathbf{t}; \mathrm{R}_j)$ is minimized using Levenberg-Marquardt method.

For each patient data, n poses $(\mathbf{t}_j, \mathrm{R}_j)$ $(j = 1, \cdots, n)$ of the femur against the pelvis are generated. Figure 2(a) shows examples of poses generated from one patient data. Given m patient data, principal component analysis is applied for $n \times m$ training datasets to construct the combined pelvis and femur SSM where both the shape and pose variations are embedded. Figure 2(b) shows the first mode that represents main variations of both femur pose and pelvis shape. Figure 2(c) shows the fourth mode that mainly represents typical deformation of osteoarthrosis of the hip caused by hip dysplasia.

2.2 Hierarchical Multi-organ SSM of the Hip Joint

Specificity and generality are often regarded as criteria of shape representation. The former is related to the ability of representing only a specific category of shapes while the latter is the ability of representing any shapes in the category. The combined SSM is considered to be advantageous on specificity compared with independent pelvis and femur SSMs because it represents only consistent spatial relations of the acetabular and femoral head shapes while inconsistent relations can be accepted especially around the joint space by using the independent SSMs. On the other hand, the independent SSMs are advantageous on generality because more shape variations can be represented by independent use of them.

In order to take the both advantages, a hierarchical multi-organ SSM is constructed, which has the combined SSM at the upper level of hierarchy and the independent SSMs are at the lower level (Fig. 3). In order to embed constraints for maintaining the consistency into the independent SSMs, a partial combined SSM of the acetabulum and proximal femur is constructed using the method described in subsection 2.1 so that pose variations of the acetabulum and proximal femur are embedded. The partial combined SSM is utilized so as to enforce

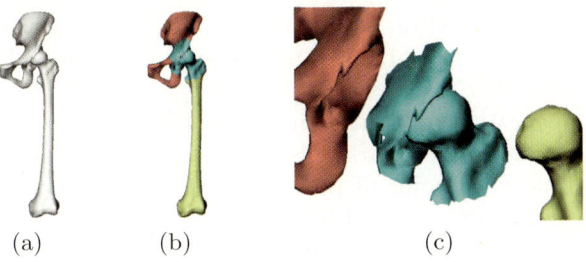

Fig. 3. Hierarchical division of the hip joint shape for hierarchical statistical shape model. (a) Upper level. (b) Lower level. (c) Partial combined SSM of the acetabulum and proximal femur.

the consistency constraint that the shape variations of independent pelvis and femur SSMs are consistent with those of the partial combined SSM. By enforcing the consistency constraint, it is expected that specificity only around the joint space is improved while generality of the independent SSMs for other parts is still maintained.

Let $\mathbf{s}_p$ and $\mathbf{s}_f$ be shape parameter vectors in SSMs of the pelvis and femur, respectively. Let $S_p(\mathbf{s}_p)$ and $S_f(\mathbf{s}_f)$ be polygon surfaces of the pelvis and femur SSMs generated by $\mathbf{s}_p$ and $\mathbf{s}_f$, respectively. Let $\mathbf{s}_{js}$ and $S'_{js}(\mathbf{s}_{js})$ be the shape parameter vector and the generated surface of the combined partial SSM, and let $S'_a(\mathbf{s}_{js})$ and $S'_{pf}(\mathbf{s}_{js})$ be the surfaces, which are included in $S'_{js}(\mathbf{s}_{js})$, corresponding to the acetabulum and proximal femur, respectively. Let $S_a(\mathbf{s}_p)$ and $S_{pf}(\mathbf{s}_f)$ be the surfaces, included in $S_p(\mathbf{s}_p)$ and $S_f(\mathbf{s}_f)$, corresponding to $S'_a(\mathbf{s}_{js})$ and $S'_{pf}(\mathbf{s}_{js})$, respectively. The consistency constraints are realized by adding the term $C_c(\mathbf{s}_p, \mathbf{s}_f, \mathbf{s}_{js})$ given by

$$C_c(\mathbf{s}_p, \mathbf{s}_f, \mathbf{s}_{js}) = d\left(S_a(\mathbf{s}_p), S'_a(\mathbf{s}_{js})\right)^2 + d\left(S_{pf}(\mathbf{s}_f), S'_{pf}(\mathbf{s}_{js})\right)^2 \qquad (2)$$

to the cost function for segmentation, shape recovery, and so on, where $d(S_1, S_2)$ denotes average distance between corresponding nodes in polygon surfaces S_1 and S_2. Using this term, the femur and pelvis surfaces generated from the independent pelvis and femur SSMs are constrained by consistent joint space surfaces generated using the combined partial acetabulum and proximal femur SSM.

2.3 Coarse-Fine Segmentation Procedure

Using the hierarchical SSM, coarse-fine segmentation is performed. Four anatomical landmark points are manually specified in CT images to determine the pelvis coordinate system. After this manual specification, fully-automated segmentation is performed as described below.

Firstly, initialization is performed. The combined SSM is fitted to the boundary edge points of roughly segmented bone regions extracted using simple thresholding of CT images in order to obtain initial parameter setting for subsequent segmentation processes. Let $\mathbf{s}$ be the shape parameter vector of SSM, E be a set of edge points to be fitted to SSM surface defined by $\mathbf{s}$, and $C_D(\mathbf{s}, E)$ be a cost function defined based on the average distance between the SSM surface generated with **s** and edge points E. SSM fitting is performed by obtaining **s** which minimizes $C_D(\mathbf{s}, E)$.

Secondly, segmentation by SSM fitting is performed at the upper level. Edge detection is performed based on intensity profile analysis along perpendicular direction at each surface point of previously estimated SSM, and SSM fitting to the detected edges are repeated for a fixed number of times. And then, the final result of the upper hierarchical level, that is, fitting result to the combined pelvis and femur SSM, is inherited to the lower level as its initial conditions.

Finally, segmentation by SSM fitting is performed at the lower level. Simultaneous fitting of pelvis and femur SSMs is performed under the consistency constraint, which is realized by adding the term described in subsection 2.2 (Equation (2)) to the cost function, which is given by

$$C(\mathbf{s}_p, \mathbf{s}_f, \mathbf{s}_{js}) = C_D(\mathbf{s}_p, E_p) + C_D(\mathbf{s}_f, E_f) + \lambda C_c(\mathbf{s}_p, \mathbf{s}_f, \mathbf{s}_{js}) \qquad (3)$$

where λ is a weight parameter for the consistency constraint. Similarly to the previous step, this fitting process is repeated for a fixed number of times.

3 Results

We used 22 CT datasets of female patients of osteoarthrosis of the hip caused by hip dysplasia. Any CT datasets did not include hip implants. By utilizing the mirror-transformed contralateral side, 44 hemi-hips were used for construction of SSMs of the hemi-pelvis and femur. Typically, one side was non-diseased, that is, normal, or mildly diseased compared with the other side. Therefore, the datasets included normal hips to some extent.

In addition to the standard pose in CT imaging, six additional poses of the femur were generated. That is, seven poses were used for one hemi-hip dataset. ±10 degrees rotations around each of the three axes were generated and appropriate translations were estimated for each rotation using Equation (1). $308(=7\times 44)$ datasets, which involve both shape and pose variations, were used for SSM construction.

In order to construct the combined partial SSM, the acetabulum and proximal femur regions were defined as regions within 50 mm from the approximated femoral head center in the reference data used for inter-patient nonrigid registration. Using 44 hemi-hips, leave-two-out cross validations were performed to evaluate segmentation accuracy. The reason of using leave-gtwoh-out method was because two hemi-hips of the same patient used for accuracy evaluation should not be used for SSM construction. We tested several parameter values for the weight of the consistency constraint, and $\lambda = 0.01$ was selected.

Table 1 shows accuracy evaluation results of one conventional method, that is, the independent pelvis and femur SSMs, and two proposed methods, that is, the combined pelvis and femur SSM, and the hierarchical hip joint SSM. Manually traced boundaries were used for the gold standard, and the average distance between estimated and gold standard boundaries was used for an error measure.

Table 1. Evaluation results of segmentation accuracy. Averages of 44 datasets of average distance [mm] are shown in each SSM. The result of the proposed method around the joint space is shown as bold fonts.

Region of evaluation	Whole hip shape	Around joint space
Independent pelvis and femur SSMs	1.26 mm	2.26 mm
Combined pelvis and femur SSM	1.51 mm	2.00 mm
Hierarchical SSM	1.20 mm	**1.78 mm**

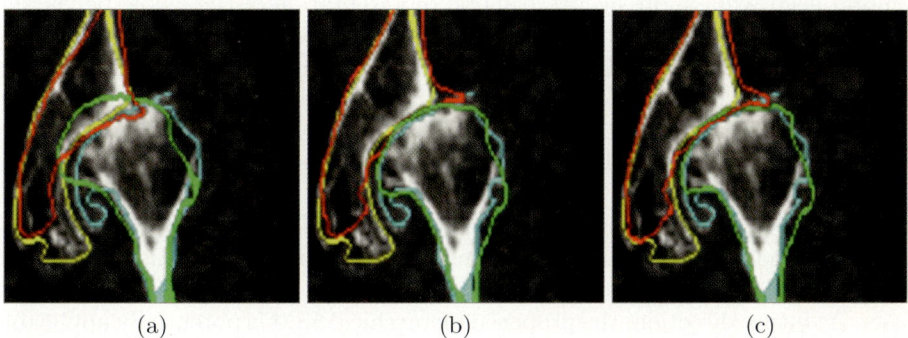

(a)   (b)   (c)

Fig. 4. Results of an illustrative case. (a) Conventional independent pelvis and femur SSMs. (b) Combined pelvis and femur SSM. (c) Hierarchical SSM. Red and green contours are estimated regions of pelvis and femur, respectively. Yellow and cyan contours are gold standards.

To evaluate the effectiveness of proposed method, we measured the accuracy around the joint space in addition to the whole pelvis and femur shapes. When we used the conventional method, additional manual specification in the CT images was necessary to determine the femur coordinate system. Around the joint space, the error was significantly reduced using the hierarchical SSM (1.78 mm) and slightly reduced using the combined SSM (2.00 mm) compared with the conventional method (2.26 mm). The accuracy was improved (more than 0.3 mm) in 23 cases, worse (more than 0.3 mm) in 2 cases, and not changed largely (within 0.3 mm difference) in 19 cases out of 44 cases by using the hierarchical SSM in spite that additional manual specifications for the femur coordinate system setting was necessary in the conventional method.

Figure 4 shows coronal views of a typical case. Similar to this figure, it was confirmed that the consistency constraint effectively worked to maintain the consistency between the acetabulum and femoral head boundaries in most cases.

4 Discussion and Conclusions

We have described a method for modeling statistical prior information of the diseased hip joint structure and its use for automated segmentation from 3D CT images. In order to deal with unknown pose between the pelvis and femur, not only shape variations but also pose variations of the two bones are embedded into a SSM to construct the combined pelvis and femur SSM, which is further hierarchically decomposed into the individual pelvis and femur SSMs and a combined acetabulum and proximal femur SSM. The amount of error reduction for the proposed SSMs (21% reduction) was compareble to that of previously published related method [4] in a similar situation (24% reduction). We validated that the consistency constraint enforced by the combined acetabular and proximal femur SSM is effective to maintain specific relationships between the acetabulum and femoral head while more accurate shape representation of the whole pelvis and femur becomes possible. The performance of the proposed method depends on the training datasets. Only two cases in which the conventional method significantly outperformed the proposed one in the error measure were those with highly severe deformation (although it is more precise to say that the both methods failed). It is considered that the training datasets did not cover these cases. Excepting few highly severe cases for which training datasets were supposed to be insufficient, however, accuracy improvement was larger for cases with moderate deformation (0.64-mm improvement) than non-diseased cases (0.49-mm improvement). Therefore, the proposed method was more effective for diseased cases. As future direction, the proposed hierarchical SSM is potentially applicable to other joint structures if the range of motion of the joint can be appropriately modeled.

References

1. Heiko, S., Dagmar, K., Markus, H., Hans, L., Stefan, Z., Hans, C.H.: Automatic Segmentation of the Pelvic Bones from CT Data Based on a Statistical Shape Model. In: Eurographics Workshop on Visual Computing for Biomedicine, Delft, pp. 93–100 (2008)
2. Frangi, A.F., Rueckert, D., Schnabel, J.A., Niessen, W.J.: Automatic Construction of Multiple-Object Three-Dimensional Statistical Shape Models: Application to Cardiac Modeling. IEEE T. Med. Imaging 21(9), 1151–1166 (2002)
3. Jing, Y., Staib, L.H., Duncan, J.S.: Neighbor-constrained Segmentation with Level Set based 3-D Deformable Models. IEEE T. Med. Imaging 23(8), 940–998 (2004)
4. Okada, T., Yokota, K., Hori, M., Nakamoto, M., Nakamura, H., Sato, Y.: Construction of hierarchical multi-organ statistical atlases and their application to multi-organ segmentation from CT images. In: Metaxas, D., Axel, L., Fichtinger, G., Székely, G. (eds.) MICCAI 2008, Part I. LNCS, vol. 5241, pp. 502–509. Springer, Heidelberg (2008)
5. Haili, C., Anand, R.: A new point matching algorithm for non-rigid registration. Comput. Vis. Image Und. 89, 114–141 (2003)
6. Zoroofi, R.A., Sato, Y., Nishii, T., Nakanishi, K., Tanaka, H., Sugano, N., Yoshikawa, H., Nakamura, H., Tamura, S.: Automated Segmentation of Acetabular Cartilage in MR images of the Hip. Technical Report, Institute of Electronics, Information and Communication Engineers. pp. 63–68 (2005)

Computer-Aided Assessment of Anomalies in the Scoliotic Spine in 3-D MRI Images

Florian Jäger[1], Joachim Hornegger[1], Siegfried Schwab[2,*], and Rolf Janka[2,*]

[1] Department of Computer Science, Chair of Pattern Recognition and Erlangen Graduate School in Advanced Optical Technologies (SAOT), University of Erlangen, Germany
jaeger@informatik.uni-erlangen.de
[2] Radiologic Institute, University of Erlangen, Germany

Abstract. The assessment of anomalies in the scoliotic spine using Magnetic Resonance Imaging (MRI) is an essential task during the planning phase of a patient's treatment and operations. Due to the pathologic bending of the spine, this is an extremely time consuming process as an orthogonal view onto every vertebra is required. In this article we present a system for computer-aided assessment (CAA) of anomalies in 3-D MRI images of the spine relying on curved planar reformations (CPR). We introduce all necessary steps, from the pre-processing of the data to the visualization component. As the core part of the framework is based on a segmentation of the spinal cord we focus on this. The proposed segmentation method is an iterative process. In every iteration the segmentation is updated by an energy based scheme derived from Markov random field (MRF) theory. We evaluate the segmentation results on public available clinical relevant 3-D MRI data sets of scoliosis patients. In order to assess the quality of the segmentation we use the angle between automatically computed planes through the vertebra and planes estimated by medical experts. This results in a mean angle difference of less than six degrees.

1 Introduction

MRI is being used increasingly to investigate children with scoliosis. Although there may be a hereditary component to true idiopathic scoliosis, the condition has no known cause and is not associated with dysraphism. However, in the infantile and juvenile age group the incidence of spinal cord anomalies like tethered cord, syringomyelia, Chiari malformations, diastematomyelia and meningocele / myelomeningocele ranges from 17.6 to 26% [1,2]. Furthermore there can be structural changes of the vertebral bodies like wedge vertebra or hemivertebra. As MRI can visualize all these abnormalities it can be extremely important in the pre-operative planning of scoliosis. Failure to detect abnormalities of the

---

[*] The authors gratefully acknowledge funding of the Erlangen Graduate School in Advanced Optical Technologies (SAOT) by the German National Science Foundation (DFG) in the framework of the excellence initiative.

neuraxis prior to treatment of scoliosis, particularly with instrumentation that lengthens the spine, can have serious neurological consequences.

With the introduction of 3-D spin echo sequences (SPACE, Siemens, Erlangen, Germany) MRI of the scoliotic spine can be acquired with only two sequences (upper spine and lower spine). However, due to the extreme bending of the vertebral column in all three axes the manual assessment of the spine is a very time consuming process. In some cases it is even impossible for the radiologist to analyze pathological changes within the spine manually. Furthermore, it can be very difficult to specify the anatomic localization of the viewed vertebra.

In this article we introduce a framework for CAA of the spine. We show that it is possible to statistically model the spinal channel and cord. Using this model we perform a segmentation of the spinal channel and cord. Upon this we build an application that enables the physician to assess the scoliotic spine nearly as fast and precise than a non-scoliotic spine which should improve the pre-operative work-up of this young patient group.

Most state-of-the-art methods for the localization of the spine in tomographic images do a segmentation of the vertebra (e.g. [3]). In general, these approaches use assumptions about the spinal appearance that are not fulfilled in data sets of scoliosis patients. Particulary the shape of the scoliotic spine is altered considerably. Thus, all assumptions concerning the typical "s" shape and with that the orientation of the vertebra are no longer valid. Additionally, the shape of the vertebra can vary in a wider range than in the non-scoliotic case. Two typical examples of spinal images of scoliosis patients are shown in Figure 1. Additionally, there are a few methods for segmentation of the spinal cord [4,5]. The computation of the centerline presented in this article does not depend on any prior information about the shape of the spine nor on the shape of the vertebra. Further on, it is not restricted to the used MRI protocol but can be adapted to other modalities in a straight forward manner. The only requirement is that the spinal channel or the spinal cord are visible within the images.

2 Method

The system for the CAA of spine anomalies can be separated into four parts pre-processing of the data sets, the segmentation of the spinal channel/cord, the labeling of the vertebra and finally the visualization of the data.

2.1 Pre-processing

Our experiments show that it is enough to use the following standard state-of-the-art pre-processing methods. In order to be able to directly use signal intensities additional to structural components within the images, we apply Homomorphic Unsharp Masking (HUM). This compensates the influence of coil inhomogeneities during the acquisition of the 3-D MRI images. The kernel size used was about 30 mm [6]. Sequentially, we use a signal intensity standardization approach to correct inter-scan intensity variations within the data sets. The

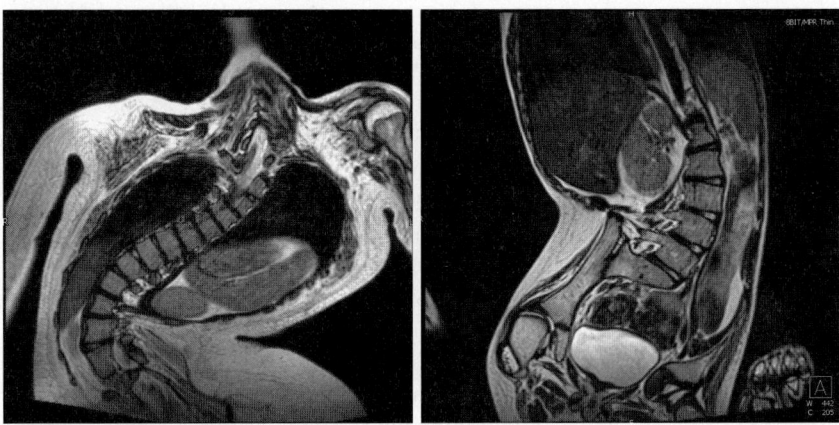

Fig. 1. Coronar slices from two 3-D MRI spine images showing typical scoliotic spines

method used is based on the non-rigid alignment of image histograms [7]. Finally, a median filter is applied to the data sets to reduce noise present in the images. All these methods can be applied during the segmentation step on a per voxel basis. Thus, only voxels that are required for the segmentation of the spinal channel/cord are processed. This yields a reduced computational cost.

2.2 Segmentation Method

The proposed method for the segmentation of the spinal channel and cord is an iterative process. The basic idea is that in each iteration step the segmentation is propagated with respect to the minimization of an energy function. This function is based on local signal intensities as well as local structural information like image gradients and the distance to the current approximation of the spinal centerline. The spatial coherence is statistically modeled by posteriori probabilities that can easily be formulated as Gibbs distributions.

Initialization Step. For the initialization of the presented method the radiologist has to set a seed point within the spinal channel. From this seed point an adaptive region growing is started. The upper and lower intensity boundary of the segmentation is increased/decreased by one in each growing step until a defined number of voxels N_0 is contained within the segmented region. Afterwards we apply morphologic closing to the initial segmentation S_0 to fill potential holes due to signal intensity variations within the images. Heuristics show that $N_0 = 300$ is enough. All segmentation S_i are binary images with a value of one for voxels within the segmented region and zero as background value.

Iteration Step. First, in every iteration i the centerline c_i is approximated using the segmented region S_{i-1} from the previous iteration. The estimation of c_i is done by thinning the segmentation S_{i-1} using the method presented by Lee in [8] and a sequential polynomial least-squares approximation of the $x-$, $y-$ and $z-$ component of the skeleton voxels. In general a polynomial degree of four to six is sufficient.

The second phase in every iteration i is the minimization of the energy function U given the previous segmentation S_{i-1} and the parametric centerline c_i. The objective function is derived from MRF theory [9]. The optimal solution is defined by the maximum of the probability function $P(S_i) = Z^{-1} \exp(-U(S_i))$ with Z being a normalization constant, $U(S_i) = \sum_{\boldsymbol{x}} V(s_{\boldsymbol{x}}|S_i)$ being the objective energy function and $s_{\boldsymbol{x}}$ being the state of the voxel $\boldsymbol{x}$. There are two different states: occupied ($s_{\boldsymbol{x}} = 1$) if the voxel is part of the spinal channel/cord and free ($s_{\boldsymbol{x}} = 0$) otherwise. Using S_{i-1} as initialization we assume that we are within the area of attraction of the correct minimum [10]. For this reason a local gradient descent strategy can be used for optimization. S_i is set to S_{i-1} initially. Then for all voxels $\boldsymbol{x}$ neighboring S_i the energy for the occupied state e_1 and the energy for the free state e_0 is computed. If $e_1 < e_0$ the voxel $\boldsymbol{x}$ is added to the segmented area in S_i. This is repeated until no more voxels change from state free to occupied. First this is done for the segmentation of the spinal channel. This segmentation is then used as initialization for the segmentation of the spinal cord.

The potential $V(s_{\boldsymbol{x}}|S_i)$ is composed by the following four parts. The first part of the potential is called smoothness prior as it controls the homogeneity of the segmentation result. It can be formulated as

$$V_s(s_{\boldsymbol{x}}|S_i) = 1.0 - \frac{1}{|\mathcal{N}_{\boldsymbol{x}}|} \sum_{\{\boldsymbol{x}' \in \mathcal{N}_{\boldsymbol{x}} | s_{\boldsymbol{x}'} = s_{\boldsymbol{x}}\}} 1 \quad (1)$$

with $\mathcal{N}_{\boldsymbol{x}}$ being the neighborhood of $\boldsymbol{x}$ and $|\cdot|$ the cardinality. This means that $V_s(s_{\boldsymbol{x}}|S_i)$ is zero if all voxels in the neighborhood of $\boldsymbol{x}$ have the state $s_{\boldsymbol{x}}$. If all neighboring voxels have a different state than $s_{\boldsymbol{x}}$ the potential is one.

The second one uses knowledge about the intensity range of the spinal channel and cord. The intensities are modeled by normal distributions $N(\mu_c, \sigma_c^2)$ and $N(\mu_o, \sigma_o^2)$ with μ_c and σ_c being the parameters of the spinal channel and μ_o, σ_o of the cord respectively. Thus, the resulting intensity potential V_v of a voxel $\boldsymbol{x}$ can be formulated as

$$V_v(s_{\boldsymbol{x}}|S_i) = (-1)^{s_{\boldsymbol{x}}+1} \left(|\mathcal{I}(\boldsymbol{x}) - \mu_{\{c,o\}}| - 2\sigma_{\{c,o\}} \right) / (2\sigma_{\{c,o\}}) \quad (2)$$

where $\mathcal{I}$ is the MRI volume of the spine. For $s_{\boldsymbol{x}} = 1$ the potential has the minimum -1 if $\mathcal{I}(\boldsymbol{x}) = \mu_{\{c,o\}}$, it is zero if $\mathcal{I}(\boldsymbol{x}) = \mu_{\{c,o\}} \pm 2\sigma_{\{c,o\}}$ and positive if the signal intensity differs more than $2\sigma_{\{c,o\}}$ from $\mu_{\{c,o\}}$. If the voxel's state is $s_{\boldsymbol{x}} = 0$, the maximum is 1 and falls down linearly to $-\infty$. Consequently, voxels having an intensity between $\mu_{\{c,o\}} \pm \sigma_{\{c,o\}}$ are preferred to be within the segmentation; voxels with intensities that differ more than $\sigma_{\{c,o\}}$ from the mean $\mu_{\{c,o\}}$ tend to belong to the background.

The third part of the potential utilizes the relative position of the voxel to the current centerline estimation c_i. With $d_c(\boldsymbol{x})$ being the Euclidean distance from the voxel $\boldsymbol{x}$ to the centerline c_i the potential V_c can be written as

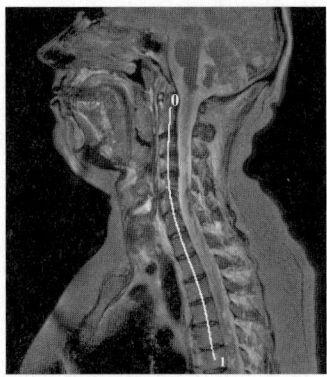 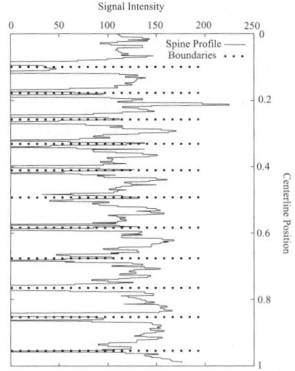

Fig. 2. The left image shows a 12 mm thick MIP in the spinal region including the computed centerline through the vertebra (white line). The data set shown is preprocessed. This centerline is used to compute the boundary positions of the vertebra. In the righthand plot the signal intensities along the centerline are shown. Additionally the estimated boundaries of the vertebra are illustrated (dotted lines). The computed threshold was $\theta = 70.3$.

$$V_c(s_{\boldsymbol{x}}|S_i) = (-1)^{s_{\boldsymbol{x}}+1}(d_c(\boldsymbol{x}) - r)/r \qquad (3)$$

where $r/2$ is the average radius of the spinal channel/cord. As a result $V_c(s_{\boldsymbol{x}} = 1|S_i) < V_c(s_{\boldsymbol{x}} = 0|S_i)$ for voxels that are closer than $r/2$ to the approximated center line c_i and $V_c(s_{\boldsymbol{x}} = 1|S_i) > V_c(s_{\boldsymbol{x}} = 0|S_i)$ if the distance is larger. The minimal value of V_c for the occupied state is -1; the maximal value of the potential for $s_{\boldsymbol{x}} = 0$ is 1.

Finally, the last part of the potential uses the scalar product between the propagation direction of the segmentation and the gradient of the image intensities. As propagation direction we use the gradient of the segmentation image S_i at the voxel $\boldsymbol{x}$. Thus, the potential can be defined as

$$V_g(s_{\boldsymbol{x}}|S_i) = (-1)^{s_{\boldsymbol{x}}}(1 - |(\nabla \mathcal{I}(\boldsymbol{x}))^T \nabla S_i(\boldsymbol{x})|/m) \qquad (4)$$

where m is the maximal tolerable magnitude of the gradient. If the gradients are aligned parallel or anti-parallel or if the image gradient is zero, the potential for $s_{\boldsymbol{x}} = 1$ has its minimal value -1 and its maximal value 1 for $s_{\boldsymbol{x}} = 0$.

2.3 Labeling of the Vertebra and Visualization

In order to label the vertebra within the images, we compute an intensity profile p on the ventral side of the estimated centerline. Then we apply a threshold θ to the computed profile p. From this an initial guess about the positions of the vertebra is computed. Finally, this guess is refined using the average distances between the vertebra. The profile as well as the estimated boundaries of the vertebra are illustrated in Figure 2. As there is no slice where the whole centerline through the vertebra can be seen we use a 12 mm thick Maximum Intensity Projection

(MIP) to be able to cover the whole spine in the illustration. The original slice thickness was 1 mm.

For the visualization, the computed centerline is approximated by splines. Using the parametric approximation we can compute MPRs that are orthogonal to the backbone for every position of the spinal channel/cord. An illustration of the presentation of the MPRs is shown in Figure 3.

3 Results

Data Sets. All data sets were acquired during clinical routine. In total we used 20 3-D MRI SPACE data sets from the spine including ten volumes showing the upper spine and ten data sets covering the lower spine. All images were acquired with a repetition time of TR = 1000ms and an echo time of TE = 130ms. The volumes had a isotropic in-plane resolution between 0.8 mm× 0.8 mm and 1.3 mm× 1.3 mm and a slice thickness of 1 mm. The image matrix had a size of 384 × 384. Every scan consists of 60 up to 160 slices. All used data sets are publicly available at our homepage[1].

Evaluation Method. The whole processing chain was implemented in C++ and integrated into the ITK Framework (http://www.itk.org). For a better presentation of the results and to increase the usability for radiologists everything was integrated into the medical visualization platform InSpace3D. The experiments were performed on a 2.00 GHz Intel Core2 CPU with 2 GB RAM. The whole processing chain took about 5-20s depending on the size and the bending of the backbone.

The focus of this work is an easy-to-use framework for CAA of anomalies in the scoliotic spine. For this reason it is important that radiologists have an orthogonal view onto every vertebra. Thus, we use the following quality measure for evaluation. First, for every vertebra v within the images, a medical expert defines a ground truth plane with normal $\boldsymbol{n_g}^v$. Then, the corresponding planes with normal $\boldsymbol{n_a}^v$ are computed using the proposed segmentation method. In order to measure the distance between the corresponding planes we use the angle

$$d_v = \arccos |(\boldsymbol{n_g}^v)^T \cdot \boldsymbol{n_a}^v| \qquad (5)$$

between the normal vectors. The range of d_v is $[0°, \ldots, 90°]$. If both planes are aligned perfectly parallel or anti-parallel the angle between the normal vectors is $d_v = 0$ degree. If, on the other hand, the corresponding planes are orthogonal, $d_v = 90$. The quality q of the proposed segmentation method is computed by

$$q = \frac{1}{V} \sum_{i=1}^{V} d_i \qquad (6)$$

with V being the number of ground truth planes. It reflects the mean angular deviation of the ground truth to the automatically computed planes.

---
[1] http://www5.informatik.uni-erlangen.de/~spine/

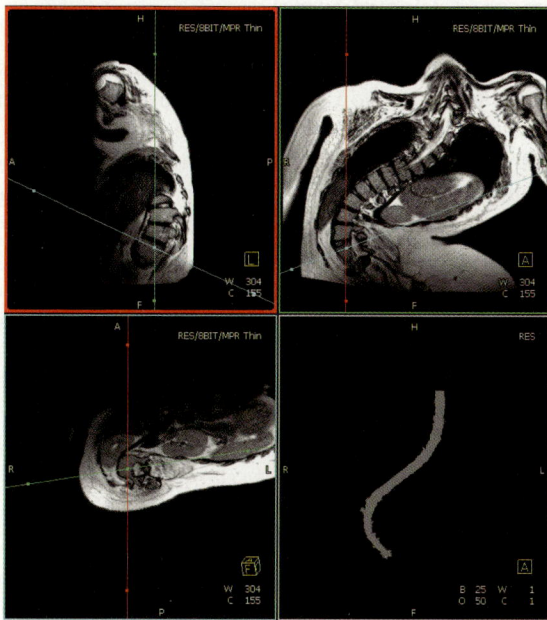

Fig. 3. The figure shows the presentation of the computed MPRs. The upper two images show the sagittal plane and the coronal plane respectively. The second row shows the plane orthogonal to the spinal cord. Finally, the result of the segmentation of the spinal cord is presented in a 3-D view (lower right).

Evaluation Results. In total planes through $V = 181$ different vertebra were defined by the radiologist. Using the proposed quality measure for our segmentation method yielded a mean distance of $q = 5.74°$ with a standard deviation of $\sigma_q = 6.13°$. The minimal deviation was 0.42° and the maximal deviation was 20.15 degrees (lower spine: $\mu_l = 6.98°$, $\sigma_l = 7.69$, $\min_l = 0.83°$, $\max_l = 20.15°$, upper spine: $\mu_u = 5.14°$, $\sigma_u = 5.22$, $\min_u = 0.42°$, $\max_u = 17.19°$). If it is assumed that an average vertebra has a size of about $30 \times 30 \times 20 mm^3$ this means that there is a distance between the two planes of less than 2mm at the border of an average vertebra.

Additionally, a second radiologist defined $V = 61$ planes through vertebra that were also labeled by the first radiologist. These planes were used to compute the inter-observer variability of both radiologists. This resulted in a mean angular deviation of $q_o = 2.94°$ ($\sigma_{q_o} = 1.99°$, $\min = 0.48°$, $\max = 9.38°$).

The results show that the proposed algorithm works very reliable for the upper spine. Especially in the lower lumbar area and the pelvic region the results get slightly worse. The reason for this is that the medulla ends in this region and separate nerve cords are left. Thus, there is a higher probability that the segmentation follows these cords away from the backbone. In clinical routine this is not a big problem, as these regions are irrelevant for diagnostics in general.

4 Discussion and Conclusion

We presented a novel approach for the segmentation of the spinal cord based on MRF theory. The segmentation is used to compute planes orthogonal to the vertebra column for CAA of anomalies in the scoliotic spine. The advantage of our method is that we do not use any segmentation of the vertebra itself or information about their relative positioning. Thus, even an extreme bending of the spine or pathologic changes of the vertebra structure can be compensated easily. Further on, the method presented works on 3-D volumes and is not restricted to a good visible coverage of the spine in a single slice. Additionally, no training step is required. Thus, the method can easily adapt if the acquisition protocol changes or other modalities like CT are used.

The proposed framework enables the radiologist to easily assess anomalies in the scoliotic spine. The errors in orientation observed are small enough for clinical usage. Furthermore, the majority of false centerline estimations occurs in the pelvic region of the spine that is only of little diagnostic interest. The observed errors can further be reduced by post-processing like a rough segmentation of the vertebra using the approximated centerline to improve their pose estimation.

References

1. Lewonowski, K., King, J.D., Nelson, M.D.: Routine use of magnetic resonance imaging in idiopathic scoliosis patients less than eleven years of age. Spine 17(Suppl. 6), 109–116 (1992)
2. Gupta, P., Lenke, L.G., Bridwell, K.H.: Incidence of neural axis abnormalities in infantile and juvenile patients with spinal deformity. is a magnetic resonance screening necessary? Spine 23, 206–210 (1998)
3. Peng, Z., Zhong, J., Wee, W., Lee, J.: Automated vertebra detection and segmentation from the whole spine MR images. In: IEEE-EMBS, New York City, USA, pp. 2527–2530. IEEE, Los Alamitos (2006)
4. McIntosh, C., Hamarneh, G.: Spinal crawlers: Deformable organisms for spinal cord segmentation and analysis. In: Larsen, R., Nielsen, M., Sporring, J. (eds.) MICCAI 2006. LNCS, vol. 4190, pp. 808–815. Springer, Heidelberg (2006)
5. Coulon, O., Hickman, S.J., Barker, G.J., Miller, D.H., Arridge, S.R.: Quantification of spinal cord atrophy from magnetic resonance images via a b-spline active surface model. Magn. Reson. Med. 47(6), 1176–1185 (2002)
6. Brinkmann, B.H., Manduca, A., Robb, R.A.: Optimized homomorphic unsharp masking for MR grayscale inhomogeneity correction. IEEE Trans. Med. Imag. 17(2), 161–171 (1998)
7. Jäger, F., Hornegger, J.: Nonrigid registration of joint histograms for intensity standardization in magnetic resonance imaging. IEEE Trans. Med. Imag. 28(1), 137–150 (2009)
8. Lee, T.C., Kashyap, R.L., Chu, C.N.: Building skeleton models via 3-d medial surface/axis thinning algorithms. CVGIP 56(6), 462–478 (1994)
9. Li, S.Z.: Markov Random Field Modeling in Image Analysis. Computer Science Workbench. Springer, Tokyo (2001)
10. Fetita, C.L., Prêteux, F.J.: Quantitative 3d ct bronchography. In: ISBI, Washington, DC, USA, pp. 221–224. IEEE, Los Alamitos (2002)

Optimal Graph Search Segmentation Using Arc-Weighted Graph for Simultaneous Surface Detection of Bladder and Prostate[*]

Qi Song[1], Xiaodong Wu[1,2], Yunlong Liu[1], Mark Smith[2], John Buatti[2], and Milan Sonka[1,2,3]

[1] Department of Electrical & Computer Engineering
[2] Department of Radiation Oncology
[3] Department of Ophthalmology & Visual Sciences,
University of Iowa, Iowa City, IA 52242, USA
{qi-song,xiaodong-wu,milan-sonka}@uiowa.edu

Abstract. We present a novel method for globally optimal surface segmentation of multiple mutually interacting objects, incorporating both edge and shape knowledge in a 3-D graph-theoretic approach. Hard surface interacting constraints are enforced in the interacting regions, preserving the geometric relationship of those partially interacting surfaces. The soft smoothness *a priori* shape compliance is introduced into the energy functional to provide shape guidance. The globally optimal surfaces can be simultaneously achieved by solving a maximum flow problem based on an arc-weighted graph representation. Representing the segmentation problem in an arc-weighted graph, one can incorporate a wider spectrum of constraints into the formulation, thus increasing segmentation accuracy and robustness in volumetric image data. To the best of our knowledge, our method is the first attempt to introduce the arc-weighted graph representation into the graph-searching approach for simultaneous segmentation of multiple partially interacting objects, which admits a globally optimal solution in a low-order polynomial time. Our new approach was applied to the simultaneous surface detection of bladder and prostate. The result was quite encouraging in spite of the low saliency of the bladder and prostate in CT images.

1 Introduction

In the United States, prostate cancer is one of the most common cancers in men, accounting for about 25% of all newly diagnosed cases [1]. Precise target delineation is critical for a successful 3-D radiotherapy treatment planning for prostate cancer treatment. Automatic segmentation techniques are urgently needed due to large amounts of 3-D image data that require increased time for manually contouring.

---

[*] This work was supported in part by NSF grants CCF-0830402 and CCF-0844765, and NIH grants R01-EB004640 and K25-CA123112. We would like to thank Dr. Honghai Zhang' help with pre-segmentation of prostate CT image data.

The segmentation of pelvic structure is of particularly difficulty. It involves soft tissues that present a large variability in shape and size. Those soft tissues also have similar intensity and have seriously mutual influence in position and shape. Many attempts have been tried in this area, such as registration approach (e.g. [2]), implicit and explicit models (e.g. [3,4,5]), and bayesian formulation (e.g. [6]). None of these methods can produce a globally optimal solution with respect to a task-specific objective function. Freedman et al. [7] developed an interactive approach based on graph cut method [8]. Their method incorporating soft shape prior allows for a global optimum. However, it focuses on only single object (bladder) segmentation and is at least non-trivial to incorporate mutually interacting surface constraints to simultaneously segment multiple object surfaces. We are thus motivated to propose a novel method incorporating both edge and shape information for globally optimal segmentation of bladder and prostate.

Our work is a non-trivial extension of the framework proposed by Wu et al. [9] and Li et al. [10]. Instead of only employing node weights in the graph to represent the desired segmentation properties, we propose in this paper an arc-weighted graph representation, which utilizes the weights of both graph nodes and arcs to incorporate a wider spectrum of constraints, e.g., the soft smoothness *a priori* shape compliance presented in this paper and other prior shape knowledge. Hard surface interacting constraints are enforced in interacting regions to preserve geometric relationships between partially interacting boundary surfaces of prostate and bladder. Soft smoothness shape compliance is further employed to incorporate shape information. Two mutually interacting optimal surfaces are then computed by solving a maximum flow problem.

Yin et al. [11] have developed a framework based on the graph-searching approach for knee-joint segmentation of bones and cartilages. Their work yet was still limited to using the *node-weighted* graph representation. Li et al. [12] adopted the arc-weighted graph representation to incorporate the elliptic shape model priors and smoothness penalty for simultaneous delineation multiple surfaces of a *single* object. Most recently, graph-cut based segmentation methods have attracted a lot of attention. One of the most influential work is Boykov and Funka-Lea's interactive segmentation algorithm for d-D images based on minimum s-t cuts [8], which is topologically flexible and shares some elegance with the level set methods. However, incorporating *a priori* shapes and simultaneous detection of mutually interacting surfaces into the Boykov framework and any other previous graph-based methods is at least non-trivial. Also, unlike the graph cut method, our proposed method requires less/no human interaction.

2 Optimal Segmentation of Multiple Mutually Interacting Objects Incorporating Both Edge and Shape Knowledge

To present our method in a comprehensible manner, in this section we consider the task of detecting a terrain-like surface representing the boundary of a

3-D object in a volumetric image. Note that the simpler principles used for this illustration are directly applicable to arbitrarily-irregularly meshed surfaces. We introduce a soft smoothness *a priori* shape compliance term into the energy function using an arc-weighted graph model to substantially extended the graph-searching framework [9,10]. The extension makes it possible to incorporate a wider spectrum of constraints.

2.1 Problem Formulation

Consider a volumetric image $\mathcal{I}(X, Y, Z)$ of size $X \times Y \times Z$. For each (x, y) pair, the voxel subset $\{\mathcal{I}(x, y, z) | 0 \leq z < Z\}$ forms a column parallel to the z-axis, denoted by $Col(x, y)$. Each column has a set of neighborhoods for a certain neighbor setting, e.g., four-neighbor relationship [10]. The surface of particularly interest in $\mathcal{I}$, denoted $S(x, y)$, is the terrain-like surface which intersects with exactly one voxel of each column of voxels parallel to the z-axis. A surface is considered feasible if it satisfies certain smoothness constraints. Specifically, if $\mathcal{I}(x_1, y_1, z_1)$ and $\mathcal{I}(x_2, y_2, z_2)$ are two voxels on the surface from neighboring columns in the x-direction, then $|z_1 - z_2| \leq \Delta_x$, where Δ_x is a specified smoothness parameter. Similar constraints exist for neighboring columns in the y-direction.

Let $\Gamma = [0..X-1] \times [0..Y-1]$ denote the grid domain of image $\mathcal{I}$. We enforce a surface interacting constraints for each pair of the sought surfaces S_i and S_j in mutually interacting region $R_{ij} \subseteq \Gamma$, on which both S_i and S_j are interacting each other. For any $(x, y) \in R_{ij}$, if $\mathcal{I}(x, y, z) \in S_i$ and $\mathcal{I}(x, y, z') \in S_j$, then we have $\delta_{ij}^l \leq z' - z \leq \delta_{ij}^u$, where $\delta_{ij}^l \geq 0$ and $\delta_{ij}^u \geq 0$ are two specified surface interacting constraints. An edge-based cost $c_i(x, y, z)$ is assigned to each voxel $\mathcal{I}(x, y, z)$ for each target surface S_i, which is inversely related to the likelihood that the desired surface contains the voxel. Yet utilizing only image edge information may not be sufficient. To make full use of priori information and incorporate a wider spectrum of constraints, we introduce into the objective function a soft smoothness *a priori* shape compliance energy term $\mathcal{E}_{smooth}(S)$ for surface S, with $\mathcal{E}_{smooth}(S) = \int_\Gamma \phi(\nabla S)$, where ϕ is a smoothness penalty function. Assume that $\mathcal{N}$ is a given neighborhood system on Γ. For any $p(x, y) \in \Gamma$, let $S(p)$ denote the z-coordinate of the voxel $\mathcal{I}(x, y, z)$ on S. Then, the discrete form of *a priori* shape compliance smoothness energy $\mathcal{E}_{smooth}(S)$ can be expressed as $\Sigma_{(p,q) \in \mathcal{N}} f_{p,q}(|S(p) - S(q)|)$, where $f_{p,q}$ is a non-decreasing function associated with two neighboring columns of p and q that penalizes the shape changes of S on p and q. Then our **enhanced optimal surface detection (EOSD)** problem seeks an optimal set S of λ surfaces in $\mathcal{I}$ such that (1) each individual surface satisfies hard smoothness constraints; (2) each pair of surfaces satisfies surface interacting constraints; and (3) the cost $\alpha(S)$ induced by S, with the form

$$\alpha(S) = \sum_{i=1}^{\lambda} \sum_{\mathcal{I}_i(x,y,z) \in S_i} c_i(x, y, z) + \sum_{i=1}^{\lambda} \sum_{(p,q) \in \mathcal{N}} f_{p,q}^{(i)}(|S_i(p) - S_i(q)|) \quad (1)$$

is minimized. In this paper, we focus on the linear smoothness penalty functions, i.e., $f_{p,q}(h) = a \cdot h + b$ (a and b are a constant, $h = 0, 1, 2, ...$) between two neighboring columns $Col(p)$ and $Col(q)$.

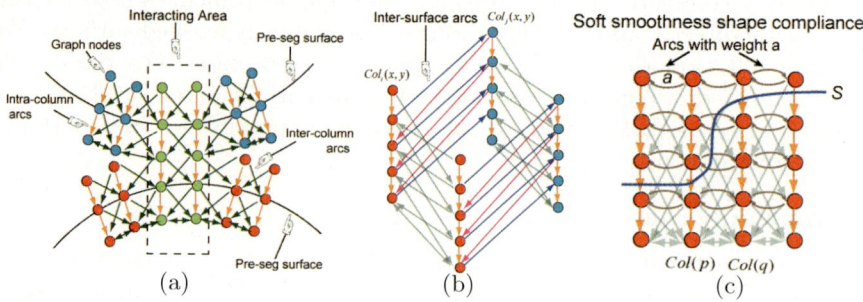

Fig. 1. Graph construction for mutually interacting objects. An example 2-D slice from a 3-D image is presented. (a) Intra-column arcs (yellow arrows) and inter-column arcs(green arrows). The hard smoothness parameter is set 1. (b) Inter-surface arcs (blue and red arrows) on the interacting region. For visualization, the slice on the interacting region is duplicated and visualized in two separated slices. The distance between two surfaces ranges from $\delta_{ij}^l = 1$ to $\delta_{ij}^u = 2$. (c) Incorporating a linear smoothness penalty. The feasible surface S cuts the arcs with a total weight of $2a$ on the neighboring columns $Col(p)$ and $Col(q)$, which measures the smoothness shape compliance term of $\alpha(S)$ for the two neighboring columns. Green arrow shows the hard smoothness constraints (inter-column arcs) with parameter 2.

2.2 The Arc-Weighted Graph Representation for Incorporating *A Priori* Shape Knowledge

In the original graph-searching model [9,10], only the node weights in a graph was used to represent the desired segmentation properties, e.g., edge-based image costs. To incorporate *a prior* shape knowledge, we utilize the weights of both graph nodes and arcs (directed graph edges) to represent the desired segmentation properties. The basic idea is to reduce the EOSD problem to the minimum s-excess problem [9]. A directed graph G containing λ node-disjoint subgraphs $\{G_i = (V_i, E_i) : i = 1, 2, ..., \lambda\}$ is defined, in which every node $V_i(x, y, z) \in V_i$ represents exactly one voxel $\mathcal{I}(x, y, z)$. Both intra-column arcs and inter-column arcs are added to ensure the monotonicity of the target surfaces and the hard smoothness constraints (Fig.1(a)), as described in [10]. To enforce the surface interacting constraints between any two sought surfaces S_i and S_j on the given mutually interacting region R_{ij}, the inter-surface arcs with $+\infty$ weights are added (Fig.1(b)). Suppose for the two sought surfaces S_i and S_j, the prior knowledge puts S_i below S_j and the distance between S_i and S_j ranges from δ_{ij}^l to δ_{ij}^u. A directed arc is put from each node $V_j(x, y, z)$ with $(x, y) \in R_{ij}$ and $z < Z - \delta_{ij}^l$ to node $V_i(x, y, z + \delta_{ij}^l)$ in G_i. This ensures that if voxel $\mathcal{I}(x, y, z)$ lies on surface S_j, then the voxel $\mathcal{I}(x, y, z')$ on S_i must be no "lower" than voxel $\mathcal{I}(x, y, z + \delta_{ij}^l)$ (i.e., $z' \geq z + \delta_{ij}^l$). On the other hand, each node $V_i(x, y, z)$ with $(x, y) \in R_{ij}$ and $z \geq \delta_{ij}^l$ has an arc to $V_j(x, y, z')$ with $z' = \max\{0, z - \delta_{ij}^u\}$, making sure that if $\mathcal{I}(x, y, z)$ is on S_i, then the voxel of $Col(x, y)$ on S_j must be no "lower" than voxel $\mathcal{I}(x, y, z')$. To incorporate the linear smoothness penalty, for any two neighboring columns $Col(p)$ and $Col(q)$ with $p = (x,y)$ and $q = (x',y')$, node $V_i(x,y,z)$ has one arc to node $V_i(x',y',z)$ as well as one arc from $V_i(x',y',z)$ to $V_i(x,y,z)$, each with an arc-weight of a for all $z = 1, ..., Z-1$. If a feasible surface S_i intersects columns $Col(p)$ and $Col(q)$ at $S_i(p)$ and $S_i(q)$, respectively, a total weight of $a \cdot (|S_i(p) - S_i(q)|)$ contributes to the corresponding cut in G, which is equivalent to the soft smoothness penalty $f_{p,q}^{(i)}(|S_i(p) - S_i(q)|)$ for the minimization problem while considering that b is a constant for any feasible surface S_i (Fig.1(c)). Thus, the linear smoothness penalty is incorporated.

The weight of each node in the graph is set as described in [10]. With this constructed graph G, an optimal cut $\mathcal{C}^* = (A^*, \bar{A}^*)$ $(A^* \cup \bar{A}^* = V)$ in G minimizing the total weight of nodes in A^* plus the total arc weight of $\mathcal{C}^*$ defines an optimal set $\mathcal{S}^*$ of λ surfaces in $\mathcal{I}$ minimizing the objective function $\alpha(\mathcal{S}^*)$. Note that $\mathcal{C}^*$ can be computed efficiently using the maximum flow algorithm in a low-order polynomial time [9]. The optimal λ surfaces can then be recovered by computing the upper envelope of the optimal cut $\mathcal{C}^*$.

3 Simultaneous Surface Detection of Bladder and Prostate

In this section, we apply our optimal graph searching method developed in Section 2 for simultaneous segmentation of bladder and prostate in 3-D CT images. Our approach mainly consists of two stages: (a) Pre-segmentation of the objects of interest. An approximation of target surfaces can be obtained, which gives useful information about the topological structures of the target objects. (b) Accurate delineation using graph optimization based on the pre-segmented surface mesh. The use of surface mesh allows our method to readily incorporate shape priors and the known topology.

3.1 Pre-segmentation of Bladder and Prostate

A 3-D geodesic active contour method [13] was conducted for pre-segmentation of the bladder. Three user-defined points were required as an initial input. The prostate shows a much better coherency in shape than bladder. Hence we computed the mean shape of the prostate from the training set of eight 3-D manual segmentation. Then an approximate bounding box of interest for prostate is interactively defined and the obtained mean shape was roughly fitted into the never-before seen CT images using rigid transformations as the pre-segmentation result. Note that the pre-segmentation results only serve to provide a basic topological structure information, thus we do not require accurate segmentation at this stage. The statement was proved in the following experiments. Overlapping between pre-segmented prostate and bladder is also allowed, which can be resolved in the graph optimization step.

3.2 Graph Construction and Optimization

From pre-segmentation results, two triangulated meshes were generated using isosurfacing algorithm (e.g., marching cubes) to specify neighboring relations among voxels on sought surfaces. As described in Section 2.2, to utilize our arc-weighted graph representation for mutually interacting surface detection, a one-to-one correspondence between two surface meshes needed to be computed on "interacting regions", which were defined according to the distance between two pre-segmented surfaces. Note that prostate and bladder are always almost attached to each other or with a very small distance away. Thus we simply projected the pre-segmented prostate surface mesh on the interacting region to the mesh of the pre-segmented bladder boundary surface. Then we use the projected mesh patch to replace the original bladder surface mesh on the interacting region. Thus, a one-to-one mesh correspondence on interacting region was established since two new meshes on that area have exactly the same topological structure.

For each vertex of the two triangulated meshes, a vector of voxels (columns) was created. The number of nodes on each column depends on the required resolution. For columns outside the interacting region, the normal at each mesh vertex was used as the column (sampling) direction. For each mesh vertex on the interacting region, a column of voxels that captures both prostate and bladder boundaries, was computed along the average normal of the pre-segmented prostate mesh for enforcing the surface interacting constrains between the bladder and prostate boundaries.

A weighted directed graph G was then constructed as in Section 2.2. To incorporate the shape priori knowledge, we employed a linear soft smoothness penalty $f_{p,q}(h) = a \cdot h + b$ ($h = 0, 1, 2, ...$) between two neighboring columns $Col(p)$ and $Col(q)$, where a and b are constant parameters. In our experiments, we set $a = 5$ and $b = 0$ according to the experimental results on the training set.

Cost function design plays an important role for successful surface detection. In our segmentation, the gradient-based cost function was employed for edge-based costs. The negative magnitude of the gradient of the image $\mathcal{I}$ was computed at each voxel as $c_{edge} = |\nabla \mathcal{I}|$.

Observe that intensities of bladder and prostate are generally higher than surrounding tissues. A Sobel kernel was used to favor a bright-to-dark transition.

4 Experiments and Results

21 3-D CT images from different patients with prostate cancer were employed for validation. No contrast agent was filled. 8 datasets were randomly selected as the training set to build a shape model of prostate. Segmentation experiments were carried out on the remaining 13 datasets. The resolution of image ranges from $0.98 \times 0.98 \times 3.00 \ mm^3$ to $1.60 \times 1.60 \times 3.00 \ mm^3$.

The computed results were compared with the expert tracing outlines. We employed the methods similiar to those used in [3] for the quantitative measures, which include the following: (1) The *probability of detection* v_d, calculated as the fraction of the expert-defined target object that was contained by our computed result; (2) The *probability of false alarm* v_{fa}, calculated as the fraction of our computed target object that lies outside the expert-defined result; and (3) The *unsigned surface distance error* s_d, computed as the distance between the expert-defined surface and our computed surface, which was expressed

Table 1. Overall quantitative results for the bladder-prostate segmentation

	With soft smoothness			Without soft smoothness		
	v_d	v_{fa}	$s_d(mm)$	v_d	v_{fa}	$s_d(mm)$
Bladder	0.958	0.115	1.04±1.00	0.958	0.120	1.09±1.02
Prostate	0.852	0.136	1.38±1.08	0.800	0.122	1.48±1.17

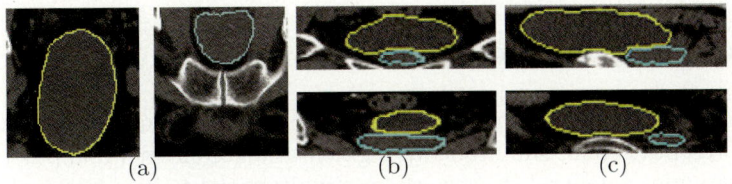

(a) (b) (c)

Fig. 2. The bladder (yellow) and prostate (blue) segmentation results. (a) Transverse view. (b) Coronal view. (c) Sagittal view.

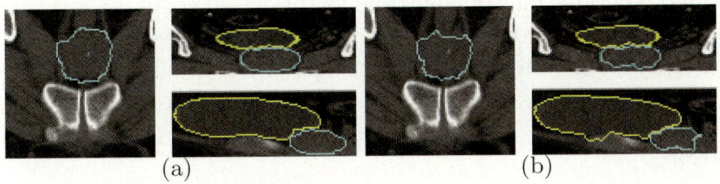

(a) (b)

Fig. 3. Comparison of simultaneous bladder-prostate segmentation. (a) Linear smoothness penalty used. (b) No soft smoothness penalty. Identical hard smoothness constraints and cost functions were used.

as mean±standard deviation. To test the effectiveness of using soft smoothness *a priori* shape compliance energy, experiments were conducted for all image datasets with and without using the soft-smoothness term.

The result is shown in Table. 1. Our approach generally produced a high-quality segmentation (i.e., v_d near 0.9, v_{fa} near 0.1), which is similar to the inter-expert variability as reported in [5,14]. By using the soft smoothness term, segmentation results for prostate were obviously improved in 9 out of 13 datasets. The improvement for bladder was relatively small.

Illustrative results of our experiments are shown in Fig. 2(a)-(c) for three views. From all views, our surface interacting constraints work quite well with no overlapping of prostate and bladder on the interacting region. Fig. 3 shows the comparison of simultaneous bladder-prostate segmentation segmentation results with and without soft smoothness term, exhibiting expected improvement.

A nature question is that how sensitive the final segmentation is to pre-segmentation result. To answer this question, two different experiments were conducted. First, pre-segmentation results of bladder and prostate were perturbed by 2 voxels separately in each of the in-plane directions, resulting in 12 pre-segmented results for each dataset. Second, pre-segmentation results were scaled up by a factor of 1.1 and scaled down by 0.9 for the bladder and the prostate separately, resulting in 4 more pre-segmentions for each dataset. The experiments were done on one randomly chosen dataset. For all 16 perturbed and scaled pre-segmentations, the final segmentations remain successful, and the mean unsigned surface distance error was 1.10 mm for bladder and 1.13 mm for prostate, which are comparable to the original results: 1.09 mm for bladder and 1.07 mm for prostate.

5 Discussion and Conclusion

In this paper, we introduce a novel graph-searching method using an arc-weighted graph representation for simultaneous segmentation of bladder and prostate. Our method provides a general framework for simultaneous segmentation of multiple partially interacting surfaces belonging to multiple objects in an optimal fashion with respect to a task-specific objective function. The arc-weighted graph representation allows an easy incorporation of a wider spectrum of constraints while utilizing weighted combinations of edge- and shape-based costs. 13 3-D CT datasets were employed for validation. The result is quite impressive considering the difficulty of the segmentation for pelvic structures.

References

1. Jemal, A., Siegel, R., Ward, E., Hao, Y., Murray, T., Thun, M.J.: Cancer statistics. Lancet 353, 267–272 (2008)
2. Malsch, U., Thieke, C., Bendl, R.: Fast elastic registration for adaptive radiotherapy. In: Larsen, R., Nielsen, M., Sporring, J. (eds.) MICCAI 2006. LNCS, vol. 4191, pp. 612–619. Springer, Heidelberg (2006)
3. Freedman, D., Radke, R.J., Zhang, T., Jeong, Y., Lovelock, D.M., Chen, G.T.Y.: Model-based segmentation of medical imagery by matching distributions. IEEE Trans. Medical Imaging 24(3) (2005)
4. Dam, E., Fletcher, P.T., Pizer, S.M., Tracton, G., Rosenman, J.: Prostate shape modeling based on principal geodesic analysis bootstrapping. In: Barillot, C., Haynor, D.R., Hellier, P. (eds.) MICCAI 2004. LNCS, vol. 3217, pp. 1008–1016. Springer, Heidelberg (2004)
5. Costa, M.J., Delingette, H., Novellas, S., Ayache, N.: Automatic segmentation of bladder and prostate using coupled 3D deformable models. In: Ayache, N., Ourselin, S., Maeder, A. (eds.) MICCAI 2007, Part I. LNCS, vol. 4791, pp. 252–260. Springer, Heidelberg (2007)
6. Rousson, M., Khamene, A., Diallo, M.H., Celi, J.C., Sauer, F.: Constrained surface evolutions for prostate and bladder segmentation in CT images. In: Liu, Y., Jiang, T.-Z., Zhang, C. (eds.) CVBIA 2005. LNCS, vol. 3765, pp. 251–260. Springer, Heidelberg (2005)
7. Freedman, D., Zhang, T.: Interactive graph cut based segmentation with shape priors. In: CVPR 2005, vol. 1, pp. 755–762 (2005)
8. Boykov, Y., Funka-Lea, G.: Graph cuts and efficient N-D image segmentation. Int. Journal of Computer Vision 70(2), 109–131 (2006)

9. Wu, X., Chen, D.Z.: Optimal net surface problems with applications. In: Widmayer, P., Triguero, F., Morales, R., Hennessy, M., Eidenbenz, S., Conejo, R. (eds.) ICALP 2002. LNCS, vol. 2380, p. 1029. Springer, Heidelberg (2002)
10. Li, K., Wu, X., Chen, D.Z., Sonka, M.: Optimal surface segmentation in volumetric images - a graph-theoretic approach. IEEE Trans. Pattern Anal. Machine Intell. 28(1), 119–134 (2006)
11. Yin, Y., Zhang, X., Sonka, M.: Optimal multi-object multi-surface graph search segmentation: full-joint cartilage delineation in 3D. In: MIUA 2008, pp. 104–108 (2008)
12. Li, K., Jolly, M.P.: Simultaneous detection of multiple elastic surfaces with application to tumor segmentation in CT images. In: SPIE 2008, vol. 6914 (2008)
13. Caselles, V., Kimmel, R., Sapiro, G.: Geodesic active contours. International journal on computer vision 22, 61–97 (1997)
14. Fiorino, C., Reni, M., Bolognesi, A., Cattaneo, G.M., Calandrino, R.: Intra- and inter- observer variability in contouring prostate and seminal vesicles: Implications for conformal treatment planning. Radiotherapy Oncol. 47(3), 285–292 (1998)

Automated Calibration for Computerized Analysis of Prostate Lesions Using Pharmacokinetic Magnetic Resonance Images[*]

Pieter C. Vos, Thomas Hambrock, Jelle O. Barenstz, and Henkjan J. Huisman

Department of Radiology, University Medical Centre Nijmegen, Netherlands
p.vos@rad.umcn.nl

Abstract. The feasibility of an automated calibration method for estimating the arterial input function when calculating pharmacokinetic parameters from Dynamic Contrast Enhanced MRI is shown. In a previous study [1], it was demonstrated that the computer aided diagnoses (CADx) system performs optimal when per patient calibration was used, but required manual annotation of reference tissue. In this study we propose a fully automated segmentation method that tackles this limitation and tested the method with our CADx system when discriminating prostate cancer from benign areas in the peripheral zone.

A method was developed to automatically segment normal peripheral zone tissue (PZ). Context based segmentation using the Otsu histogram based threshold selection method and by Hessian based blob detection, was developed to automatically select PZ as reference tissue for the per patient calibration.

In 38 consecutive patients carcinoma, benign and normal tissue were annotated on MR images by a radiologist and a researcher using whole mount step-section histopathology as standard of reference. A feature set comprising pharmacokinetic parameters was computed for each ROI and used to train a support vector machine (SVM) as classifier.

In total 42 malignant, 29 benign and 37 normal regions were annotated. The diagnostic accuracy obtained for differentiating malignant from benign lesions using a conventional general patient plasma profile showed an accuracy of 0.65 (0.54-0.76). Using the automated segmentation per patient calibration method the diagnostic value improved to 0.80 (0.71-0.88), whereas the manual segmentation per patient calibration showed a diagnostic performance of 0.80 (0.70-0.90).

These results show that an automated per-patient calibration is feasible, a significant better discriminating performance compared to the conventional fixed calibration was obtained and the diagnostic accuracy is similar to using manual per-patient calibration.

1 Introduction

Several studies have indicated that multimodal MRI increases the prostate cancer (PCa) localization accuracy of the radiologist. The accuracy is, however,

---

[*] This work was funded by grant **KUN 2004-3141** of the Dutch Cancer Society.

dependent on the experience of the radiologist [2,3,4]. To help improve the diagnostic accuracy of the (unexperienced) radiologist, we are investigating the possible additional value of CADx. Previously [1], the feasibility was demonstrated of an in-house developed CADx system that calculates the malignancy likelihood of a given suspicious area in the peripheral zone of the prostate using T1-w DCE-MRI at 1.5T. Discrimination of malignant and benign regions was performed using a SVM as classifier that was trained with features extracted from quantitative pharmacokinetic (PK) maps as well as T1 estimates. The study showed that a diagnostic accuracy of 0.83 (0.75-0.92) was obtained by a standalone CADx, which is comparable to an expert radiologist performance.

Pharmacokinetic (PK) DCE-MRI could further improve PCa differentiation by reducing inter patient and inter MR scanner fluctuations compared to conventional DCE-MRI. PK tissue parameters are estimated by fitting a tracer physiologic compartment model to the observed DCE-MRI data that is driven by a plasma profile. Various techniques for estimating plasma profiles exist. Quite some PK estimators do not include per patient calibration, but use a general patient plasma profile (fixed calibration) [5,6]. Huisman et al. [7] demonstrated that the plasma profile varies per patient and thus, fixed calibration can cause fluctuation among patient when estimating the PK parameters. In [8], it was shown that the CADx system performs significantly better using per patient calibration instead of fixed calibration. The presented method was, however, dependent on manual annotation of healthy tissue before a malignancy likelihood could be calculated. This study addresses that limitation by presenting a more objective and automated calibration method and investigates its effect on the diagnostic accuracy of the CADx system.

The purpose of this study was to investigate the feasibility of a CADx system capable of objectively discriminating PCa from non-malignant disorders located in the peripheral zone of the prostate using an automated per patient calibration method.

2 Method

2.1 Pharmacokinetic Modeling

Analysis of DCE-MRI data requires knowledge of the concentration of the contrast agent in the blood plasma. Without calibration (or fixed calibration), inter-patient plasma profile variability causes fluctuations in PK estimates, which are not related to the tissue condition. When using a power injector the most likely cause of differences in plasma curves are differences in body weight (total distributional volume), heart rate, vascular condition. Removing the plasma shape can be regarded as a form of patient calibration whereas fixed calibration uses a fixed plasma function over all patients.

The parametric model for analyzing contrast agent concentration time curves in DCE-MRI is the two compartment model of Tofts et al. [9]. The observed concentration-time curve can be expressed as:

$$C_v(t) = h(t; t_0, V_e, K^{trans}, Washout) \otimes C_p(t), \tag{1}$$

where $C_v(.)$ denotes the observed tracer concentration, $h(.)$ the tissue impulse response, $C_p(t)$ the plasma input function and $t_0, V_e, K^{trans}, Washout$ are parameters from the model. The reference tissue method estimates the plasma input function by:
$$\hat{C}_p(t) = C_{ref,v}(t)/h_{ref,v}(t), \qquad (2)$$
where $C_{ref,v}(.)$ represents the observed plasma profile for tissue v and $h_{ref,v}(.)$ a reference plasma profile for tissue v based on literature. The reference tissue method is considered to be a robust technique [10].

2.2 Automated Per Patient Calibration

In a previous study [8], it was demonstrated that using PZ as reference tissue gave good results for estimating PK parameters. In this study a method was developed to auto segment PZ. The method is divided into two stages. First, the location of the prostate is detected using a blob detection method. In the second stage, this location is further refined to segment a PZ region.

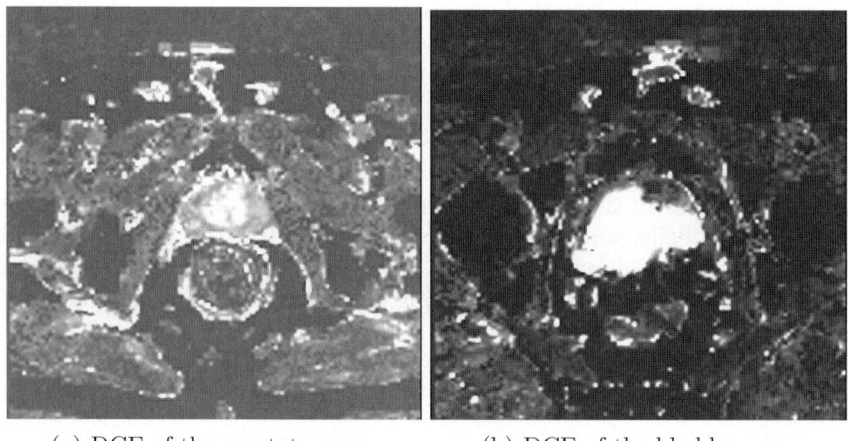

(a) DCE of the prostate area.   (b) DCE of the bladder area.

Fig. 1. Rational for modeling an early and large enhancing blob in the pelvic area

Automated Localization of the Prostate. The prostate can be modelled as a large enhancing area (or blob) in the pelvis. Figure 1(a) demonstrates this model where the prostate can easily be detected by a human observer. Large and strong enhancements can be observed in the transition zone of the prostate making it suitable for detection. First experimental results showed however, that this assumption is not only true for the prostate. Because the acquisition time for the DCE-MRI can be rather long (3 min), contrast agent also arrives in the bladder, resulting in a comparably large enhancing blob, as demonstrated in figure 1(b). The prostate model is therefore extended by including the arrival time of the contrast agent (t_0 of $C_v(t)$). Otsu's automatic threshold selection method from gray-level histograms ([11]) is used to segment early enhancing structures in the relative enhancement image $V(x)$:

$$V_O(\mathbf{x}) = \begin{cases} V(\mathbf{x}), & t_0(x) < th_{Otsu} \\ 0 \end{cases} \quad (3)$$

A common approach to detect blobs is to consider the Taylor expansion of V_O at multiscale for a given neighborhood of pixel x [12],

$$V_O(\mathbf{x} + \delta\mathbf{x}, \sigma) \approx V_O(\mathbf{x}, \sigma) + \delta\mathbf{x}^T \nabla_\sigma + \delta\mathbf{x}^T H_\sigma \delta\mathbf{x}, \quad (4)$$

where ∇_σ and H_σ are the gradient vector and Hessian vector of an image at scale σ. Here, V_O is convolved using derivatives of Gaussians:

$$\frac{\delta}{\delta \mathbf{x}} V_O(\mathbf{x}, \sigma) = \sigma V_O(\mathbf{x}) \frac{\delta}{\delta \mathbf{x}} G(\mathbf{x}, \sigma). \quad (5)$$

Next, from H_σ eigenvalues $\lambda_{\sigma,k}$ are computed, corresponding the the k-th normalized vector $\hat{u}_{\sigma,k}$ and analyzed to determine the likelihood of a pixel $\mathbf{x}$ belonging to a blob. This analysis is based on the following likelihood function (for bright blob, dark background):

$$P(\mathbf{x}, \sigma) = |\lambda_1(x)||\lambda_2(x)||\lambda_3(x)|, \quad (6)$$

that is, all three eigen values should be large to represent a blob. A multiscale approach is adopted after which the maximum response is selected:

$$P(\mathbf{x}) = \max_{\sigma_{min} \leq \sigma \leq \sigma_{max}} P(\mathbf{x}, \sigma). \quad (7)$$

The center location of the prostate x_{pc} containing the highest probability is then selected by $x_{pc} = arg\max_x P(\mathbf{x})$. In figure 2(a) a probability map is shown that is used for the prostate detection.

Automated Segmentation of Normal Peripheral Zone Tissue. In the second stage of the method, a context based segmentation is performed to extract normal peripheral zone tissue. The method is based on the model that the PZ is mainly dorsal located of x_{pc}. Thus, we define a box-mask below x_{pc} with height, width and depth set to σ to mask V_O. Here, σ corresponds with the size of the prostate and is the scale at which $P(x_{pc})$ was found by the blob detector:

$$S(x_{pc}) = arg\max_\sigma (P(x_{pc}, \sigma)) \quad (8)$$

Figure 2(b) demonstrates this model. Simple thresholding of extrema and removal of sharp edges using a gradient magnitude filter can now be applied to the box-mask which results in the segmentation of normal peripheral zone tissue, as demonstrated in figures 2(c) and 2(d).

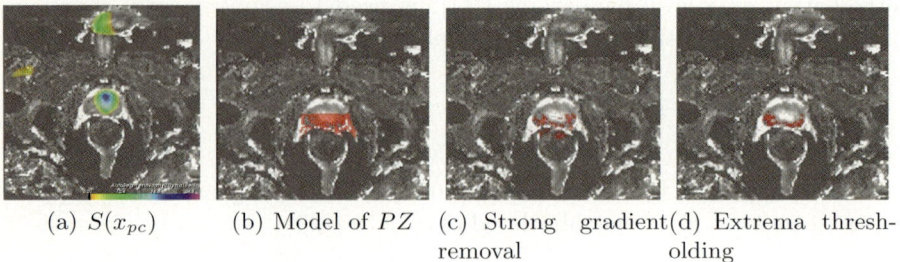

(a) $S(x_{pc})$ (b) Model of PZ (c) Strong gradient removal (d) Extrema thresholding

Fig. 2. Example case of context based segmentation of normal peripheral zone tissue

2.3 CADx Performance Evaluation

The features K^{trans}, V_e and $Washout$ were computed and used to train a SVM as classifier [9]. The features were combined into a single malignancy likelihood estimate using the SVM. The output of the classifier was used as a measure of likelihood of malignancy. The discriminating performance of the CADx system was estimated by means of the area under the receiver operator characteristics (ROC) curve (AUC). The prospective performance of the lesion analysis with per patient and fixed calibration were estimated by means of leave-one-patient-out (LOPO) cross validation. LOPO avoids training and testing on the same data and to emphasize the prospective value, one whole patient case was drawn from the set. The LOPO involves training on all but one case, estimating the likelihood of that left-out case, and repeating the procedure until each case has been tested individually. The bootstrap technique was used to compute 95% confidence intervals for the AUC and significance level for the paired difference [13].

2.4 Experiment

The study set consisted of 38 consecutive patients that were selected between January 2007 and October 2008. These patients had biopsy-proven PCa and underwent dynamic contrast-enhanced MR imaging at 3.0T, complementary to the routine staging MR imaging examination of the prostate. Patients were included in the study only if they were candidates for radical retropubic prostatectomy within 6 weeks after MR imaging. The study was approved by the institutional review board, and informed consent was obtained from all patients prior to MR imaging. Exclusion criteria were: previous hormonal therapy, lymph nodes positive for metastases at frozen section analysis, contraindications to MR imaging (e.g., cardiac pacemakers, intracranial clips), contraindications to endorectal coil insertion (e.g., anorectal surgery, inflammatory bowel disease).

Images were acquired with a 3.0T whole body MR scanner (TrioTim, Siemens Medical Solutions, Erlangen, Germany). A pelvic phased-array as well as a balloon-mounted disposable endorectal surface coil (MedRad®, Pittsburgh, PA, USA) inserted and inflated with approximately 80 cm³ of Perfluorocarbon (FOMBLIN LC08), were used for receiving. The machine body coil was used for

RF transmitting. An amount of 1 mg of glucagon (Glucagon®, Novo Nordisk, Bagsvaerd, Denmark)) was administered directly before the MRI scan, to all patients to reduce peristaltic bowel movement during the examination.

High-spatial-resolution T2-weighted fast spin-echo imaging in the axial, sagittal and coronal planes, covering the prostate and seminal vesicles, was performed. 3D T1-weighted spoiled gradient echo images were acquired before and during an intravenous bolus injection of paramagnetic gadolinium chelate (0.1 mmol/kg, gadopentetate, Magnevist®; Schering, Berlin, Germany) using a power injector (Spectris, Medrad®, Pittsburgh, PA, US) with an injection rate of 2.5 ml/second followed by a 15 ml saline flush for 300 sec every 3 seconds. Fitting the DCE-MRI is decribed elsewhere [14].

Whole-mount step-section histology tumor maps were used as ground truth for annotating PCa (with a relevant diameter of at least 5mm), non-malignant suspicious enhancing (NS) and normal (N) regions on T2-w images for all patients in consensus by two readers.

3 Results

One patient case was excluded because the DCE examination had failed. In total 42 malignant regions were annotated in the peripheral zone. The number of NS regions annotated in the peripheral zone was 29. The number of normal peripheral zone regions was 38.

The effect of the per patient calibration on the diagnostic performance was first evaluated by pairwise scatterplots of PK parameters of the lesions. It is noticeable in figure 3(a) that without calibration the clusters overlap more than the clusters in figure 3(c) where manual calibration is included. Figure 3(b) shows similar results for automatic patient calibration. Furthermore, the N and NS

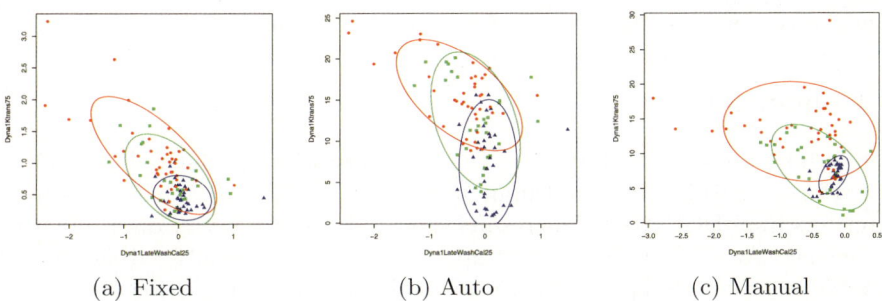

(a) Fixed   (b) Auto   (c) Manual

Fig. 3. Pairwise scatterplots of 2 kinetic parameters, $Washout$ versus K^{trans}, for the whole database with squares representing NS regions, spheres as malignant regions and triangles as N regions for the different calibration methods used. The ellipsoids summarize the three clusters by fitting a bivariate normal distribution and displaying the outline at 2 times standard deviation radius. It is noticeable that the clusters overlap one another when fixed calibration is used, whereas manual and automated per patient calibration demonstrate a noticeable clustering of features.

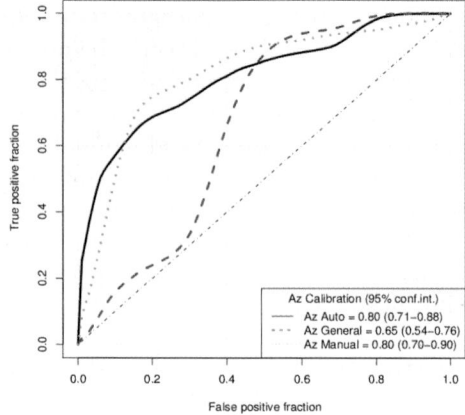

Fig. 4. ROC curves showing the discriminating performance of the CADx system using the different calibration methods fixed, automated per patient and manual per patient calibration

clusters have a smaller covariance when patient calibration is used. An effect on the diagnostic performance can therefore be expected. The different distributions demonstrate the strong effect of the chosen calibration method.

The performance of discriminating malignant lesions from NS areas with fixed, manual and automatic calibration is demonstrated in the ROC curves shown in figure 3. Here, the focus is on the characterization of NS and malignant regions, because it is more challenging and clinically relevant. The diagnostic accuracy was 0.65 (95% confidence intervals = 0.54-0.76)) when fixed calibration was used. The diagnostic accuracy improved significantly for both manual per patient calibration, Az=0.80 (0.70-0.90), as for automated per patient calibration, Az=0.80 (0.71-0.88). The marginal difference between the automated and manual calibration means that they perform similar, which was the intended goal.

4 Conclusion

In this study, we have demonstrated the feasibility of an automated calibration method for estimating the arterial input function when calculating pharmacokinetic parameters from DCE-MRI. The results show a significant better discriminating performance (Az=0.80 (0.71-0.88)) compared to the conventional fixed calibration. The performance is similar to using the manual per patient calibration.

References

1. Vos, P., Hambrock, T., Hulsbergen-van de Kaa, C., Fütterer, J., Barentsz, J., Huisman, H.: Computerized analysis of prostate lesions in the peripheral zone using dynamic contrast enhanced MRI. Med. Phys. 35(3), 888–899 (2008)
2. Hricak, H., Choyke, P., Eberhardt, S., Leibel, S., Scardino, P.: Imaging prostate cancer: a multidisciplinary perspective. Radiology 243(1), 28–53 (2007)

3. Fütterer, J., Heijmink, S., Scheenen, T., Veltman, J., Huisman, H., Vos, P., de Kaa, C., Witjes, J., Krabbe, P., Heerschap, A., Barentsz, J.: Prostate Cancer Localization with Dynamic Contrast-enhanced MR Imaging and Proton MR Spectroscopic Imaging. Radiology 241(2), 449–458 (2006)
4. Chan, I., Wells, W., Mulkern, R., Haker, S., Zhang, J., Zou, K., Maier, S., Tempany, C.: Detection of prostate cancer by integration of line-scan diffusion, T2-mapping and T2-weighted magnetic resonance imaging; a multichannel statistical classifier. Med. Phys. 30(9), 2390–2398 (2003)
5. Weinmann, H.J., Laniado, M., Mutzel, W.: Pharmacokinetics of GdDTPA/ dimeglumine after intravenous injection into healthy volunteers. Physiol. Chem. Phys. Med. NMR 16(2), 167–172 (1984)
6. Brix, G., Semmler, W., Port, R., Schad, L.R., Layer, G., Lorenz, W.J.: Pharmacokinetic parameters in CNS Gd-DTPA enhanced MR imaging. J. Comput. Assist. Tomogr. 15(4), 621–628 (1991)
7. Huisman, H., Veltman, J., Boetes, C., Karssemeijer, N., Blickman, H., Barentsz, J.: Computer-aided diagnosis of breast MRI using pharmacokinetic modeling. RSNA, SSC17–09 (2006)
8. Vos, P.C., Hambrock, T., Fütterer, J.J., van de Kaa, C.A.H., Barentsz, J., Huisman, H.H.: Effect of calibration on computerized analysis of prostate lesions using quantitative dynamic contrast-enhanced magnetic resonance imaging. In: SPIE, vol. 6514, 65140U (2007)
9. Tofts, P., Brix, G., Buckley, D., Evelhoch, J., Henderson, E., Knopp, M., Larsson, H., Lee, T., Mayr, N., Parker, G., Port, R., Taylor, J., Weisskoff, R.: Estimating kinetic parameters from dynamic contrast-enhanced T(1)-weighted MRI of a diffusable tracer: standardized quantities and symbols. J. Magn. Reson. Imaging 10(3), 223–232 (1999)
10. Kovar, D., Lewis, M., Karczmar, G.: A new method for imaging perfusion and contrast extraction fraction: input functions derived from reference tissues. J. Magn. Reson. Imaging 8(5), 1126–1134 (1998)
11. Otsu, N.: A threshold selection method from gray-level histograms. EEE Trans. Sys., Man., Cyber. 9(1), 62–66 (1979)
12. Frangi, A.F., Niessen, W.J., Vincken, K.L., Viergever, M.A.: Multiscale vessel enhancement filtering. In: Wells, W.M., Colchester, A.C.F., Delp, S.L. (eds.) MICCAI 1998. LNCS, vol. 1496, p. 130. Springer, Heidelberg (1998)
13. Rutter, C.: Bootstrap estimation of diagnostic accuracy with patient-clustered data. Acad. Radiol. 7(6), 413–419 (2000)
14. Hittmair, K., Gomiscek, G., Langenberger, K., Recht, M., Imhof, H., Kramer, J.: Method for the quantitative assessment of contrast agent uptake in dynamic contrast-enhanced MRI. Magn. Reson. Med. 31(5), 567–571 (1994)

Spectral Embedding Based Probabilistic Boosting Tree (ScEPTre): Classifying High Dimensional Heterogeneous Biomedical Data*

Pallavi Tiwari[1], Mark Rosen[2], Galen Reed[3], John Kurhanewicz[3], and Anant Madabhushi[1]

[1] Department of Biomedical Engineering, Rutgers University, USA
pallavit@eden.rutgers.edu, anantm@rci.rutgers.edu
[2] Department of Radiology, University of Pennsylvania, USA
[3] Department of Radiology, University of California, San Francisco, USA

Abstract. The major challenge with classifying high dimensional biomedical data is in identifying the appropriate feature representation to (a) overcome the curse of dimensionality, and (b) facilitate separation between the data classes. Another challenge is to integrate information from two disparate modalities, possibly existing in different dimensional spaces, for improved classification. In this paper, we present a novel data representation, integration and classification scheme, Spectral Embedding based Probabilistic boosting Tree (ScEPTre), which incorporates Spectral Embedding (SE) for data representation and integration and a Probabilistic Boosting Tree classifier for data classification. SE provides an alternate representation of the data by non-linearly transforming high dimensional data into a low dimensional embedding space such that the relative adjacencies between objects are preserved. We demonstrate the utility of ScEPTre to classify and integrate Magnetic Resonance (MR) Spectroscopy (MRS) and Imaging (MRI) data for prostate cancer detection. Area under the receiver operating Curve (AUC) obtained via randomized cross validation on 15 prostate MRI-MRS studies suggests that (a) ScEPTre on MRS significantly outperforms a Haar wavelets based classifier, (b) integration of MRI-MRS via ScEPTre performs significantly better compared to using MRI and MRS alone, and (c) data integration via ScEPTre yields superior classification results compared to combining decisions from individual classifiers (or modalities).

1 Introduction

Biomedical data such as gene expression, dynamic contrast enhanced Magnetic resonance Imaging (MRI) and Spectroscopy (MRS) suffer from the curse of dimensionality owing to the presence of large redundant, non-discriminative features within a relatively small sample space. A major challenge is to identify

---
* Work made possible via grants from Coulter Foundation (WHCF 4-29368), New Jersey Commission on Cancer Research, National Cancer Institute (R21CA127186-01, R03CA128081-01), and the Society for Imaging Informatics in Medicine (SIIM).

appropriate feature representation methods and thus facilitate accurate classification. The default data representation choice for spectral and signal classification has been wavelets [1] or Principal Component Analysis (PCA) which is a linear dimensionality reduction method.

It has been shown previously that PCA fails to capture the inherent non-linear structure of high dimensional biomedical data [2]. For such cases, non linear DR methods such as Spectral Embedding (SE) [3] are more appropriate, since they reduce data dimensionality by assuming a non-linear relationship between high dimensional data samples. The objective behind SE is to non-linearly map objects $c, d \in C$ that are adjacent in the M dimensional ambient space ($\boldsymbol{F}(c), \boldsymbol{F}(d)$) to adjacent locations in the low dimensional embedding ($\boldsymbol{S}(c), \boldsymbol{S}(d)$), where $\boldsymbol{S}(c), \boldsymbol{S}(d)$ represent the β-dimensional dominant Eigen vectors corresponding to c, d ($\beta << M$). Such non-linear mapping captures the inherent structure of the high dimensional data manifold such that object proximity and local geometries are preserved in the reduced Eigen space. These methods can also employ a wide range of similarity kernels and hence can be applied to representing diverse data including imaging, spectral, and omics.

With the wide array of multi-scale, multi-functional, multi-modal data now available for disease characterization, one of the challenges in integrated disease diagnostics is to homogeneously represent the different data streams (eg. imaging, spectroscopy, omics) to enable data fusion and classification. For example, consider the difficulties in fusing T2-weighted (w) MRI data (structural information) with MRS data (metabolic information) which involves combining scalar MR image intensity information with a high dimensional metabolic vector from the same spatial location. Data-fusion algorithms are classified broadly as data level integration and decision level integration [4]. At data level integration, original features ($\boldsymbol{F}_A(c)$) and ($\boldsymbol{F}_B(c)$) from two disparate modalities A and B are combined either via vector concatenation $\boldsymbol{F}_{AB}(c) = [\boldsymbol{F}_A(c), \boldsymbol{F}_B(c)]$ or some sort of averaging. In decision level integration, individual classifications ($\mathbf{h}_A$) and ($\mathbf{h}_B$) from each modality A, B are combined. Decision level integration strategies however tend to implicitly treat the data channels as independent and may result in sub optimal fusion and classification.

2 Novel Contributions of This Work

In this paper, we present an integrated data representation, fusion and classification scheme, **S**pectral **E**mbedding based **P**robabilisitic Boosting **T**ree (ScEPTre), that enables (a) homogeneous representation of multiple, disparate, high dimensional biomedical data modalities in a reduced dimensional space, and (b) fusion of disparate features from heterogeneous modalities of differing dimensionalities to obtain improved classification. Data representation and fusion in ScEPTre is performed using Spectral Embedding (SE), while the Probabilistic Boosting Tree (PBT) algorithm is used for classification. The PBT classifier generates a tree structure by recursively training each node of the tree using AdaBoost such that each node is a strong classifier [5]. PBT has the advantage of computing discriminative probabilities where hard decisions cannot be made.

In this work, we demonstrate the applicability of ScEPTre to first automatically represent and classify prostate MRS and MRI individually, followed by the data fusion of the two modalities for prostate cancer (CaP) detection. We also demonstrate that ScEPTre on MRS for CaP detection significantly outperforms classification via wavelets, the traditional method of data representation for spectral data. The contributions of this work are:

- A novel data representation scheme (ScEPTre) which enables data fusion and classification by first homogeneously representing heterogeneous data with different dimensionality within the spectrally embedded space.
- ScEPTre is shown to perform better in terms of representing high dimensional spectral data compared to the wavelet representation and yields better classification compared to decision level integration.

3 Methodological Description of ScEPTre

3.1 Spectral Embedding of High Dimensional Biomedical Data

The aim of Spectral Embedding [3] is to find an embedding vector $\boldsymbol{S}^{SE}(c_i)$, $\forall c_i \in C$, $i \in \{1,\ldots,|C|\}$, such that the relative ordering of the distances between objects in high dimensional space is maximally preserved in the lower dimensional space. Thus, if locations $c_i, c_j \in C, i, j \in \{1,\ldots,|C|\}$, are adjacent in the high dimensional feature space $\boldsymbol{F}(c_i), \boldsymbol{F}(c_j)$ respectively, then $||\boldsymbol{S}^{SE}(c_i) - \boldsymbol{S}^{SE}(c_j)||_2$ should be small, where $||.||_2$ represents the Euclidean norm. This will only be true if the distances between all $c_i, c_j \in C$ are preserved in the low dimensional mapping of the data. To compute the optimal embedding, we first define adjacency matrix $W_{SE} \in \Re^{|C|\times|C|}$ as

$$W_{SE}(i,j) = e^{-||\boldsymbol{F}(c_i)-\boldsymbol{F}(c_j)||_2}, \forall c_i, c_j \in C, i,j \in \{1,\ldots,|C|\}. \tag{1}$$

$\boldsymbol{S}^{SE}(c_i)$ is then obtained from the maximization of the function:

$$E(\mathcal{X}_{SE}) = 2\gamma \times trace\left[\frac{\mathcal{X}_{SE}(D-W_{SE})\mathcal{X}_{SE}^{\mathsf{T}}}{\mathcal{X}_{SE}D\mathcal{X}_{SE}^{\mathsf{T}}}\right], \tag{2}$$

where $\mathcal{X}_{SE} = \left[\boldsymbol{S}^{SE}(c_1); \boldsymbol{S}^{SE}(c_2); \ldots; \boldsymbol{S}^{SE}(c_n)\right], n = |C|$ and $\gamma = |C| - 1$. Additionally, D is a diagonal matrix where $\forall c \in C$, the diagonal element is defined as $D(i,i) = \sum_j W_{SE}(i,j)$. The embedding space is defined by the Eigenvectors corresponding to the smallest m Eigenvalues of $(D - W_{SE})\mathcal{X}_{SE} = \lambda D \mathcal{X}_{SE}$. The matrix $\mathcal{X}_{SE} \in \Re^{|C|\times\beta}$ of the first β Eigenvectors is constructed, and $\forall c_i \in C, \boldsymbol{S}^{SE}(c_i)$ is defined as row i of $\mathcal{X}_{SE}$.

3.2 Multi-modal Data Fusion in the Embedding Space

In [4], it has been suggested that data level integration can be achieved by aggregating features from two disparate sources ($\boldsymbol{F}_1(c)$ and $\boldsymbol{F}_2(c)$) into a single feature vector $\boldsymbol{E}(c)$ before classification. While this may be a reasonable strategy when $|\boldsymbol{F}_1(c)|=|\boldsymbol{F}_2(c)|$, it may not be optimal when the feature vectors are of very different dimensionalities. ScEPTre enables data fusion between different dimensional feature vectors $\boldsymbol{F}_1(c)$, $\boldsymbol{F}_2(c)$ by first independently spectrally embedding them ($|\boldsymbol{S}_1^{SE}(c)| = |\boldsymbol{S}_2^{SE}(c)|$) so that the combined feature vector $[\boldsymbol{S}_1(c), \boldsymbol{S}_2(c)]$ can then be used for classification.

3.3 PBT Classifier

The PBT algorithm [5] is a combination of the Adaboost and decision trees classifiers. It iteratively generates a tree structure of length L in the training stage where each node of the tree is boosted with T weak classifiers. The hierarchical tree is obtained by dividing new samples in two subsets of $\tilde{\boldsymbol{F}}_{Right}$ and $\tilde{\boldsymbol{F}}_{Left}$ and recursively training the left and right sub-trees using Adaboost. To solve for overfitting, error parameter ϵ is introduced such that samples falling in the range $[\frac{1}{2} - \epsilon, \frac{1}{2} + \epsilon]$ are assigned to both subtrees with probabilities $(\boldsymbol{F}(c), p(1|c)) \rightarrow \tilde{\boldsymbol{F}}_{Right}(c)$ and $(\boldsymbol{F}(c), p(0|c)) \rightarrow \tilde{\boldsymbol{F}}_{Left}(c)$, where the function $p(Y|c)$ represents the posterior class conditional probability of c belonging to class $Y \in \{0, 1\}$. The algorithm stops when misclassification error hits a pre-defined threshold θ.

During testing, the conditional probability of the sample is calculated at each node based on the learned hierarchical tree. The discriminative model is obtained at the top of the tree by combining the probabilities associated with probability propagation of the sample at various nodes yielding a posterior conditional probability value $p(1|c)$, $p(0|c) \in [0, 1]$, for each sample c as belonging to one of the two classes.

4 ScEPTre for Prostate Cancer Detection Using Integrated MR Imaging and Spectroscopy

4.1 Notation and Data Description

A total of 15 1.5 Tesla (T) T2-w MRI and corresponding MRS studies were obtained prior to radical prostatectomy from University of California, San Francisco. We represent the 3D prostate T2-w scene by $\hat{\mathcal{C}} = (\hat{C}, \hat{f})$, where $\hat{C}$ is a 3D grid of voxels $\hat{c} \in \hat{C}$ and $\hat{f}(\hat{c})$ is a function that assigns an intensity value to every $\hat{c} \in \hat{C}$. We also define a spectral scene $\mathcal{C} = (C, \boldsymbol{F})$ where C is a 3D grid of MRS metavoxels, $c \in C$ and $\boldsymbol{F}$ is a spectral vector associated with each $c \in C$. Note that multiple voxels are present within the region R_{cd} between any two adjacent metavoxels $c, d \in C$. For the sake of convenience we represent R_{cd} as $R(c)$, where $\hat{c} \in R(c)$. Figure 1(a) shows a MRS spectral grid superposed on a T2-w MRI slice with expert annotated class labels $Y(c) \in \{1, 2, 3, 4, 5\}$ based on a clinical standardized 5-point scale [6] which classifies each spectra as definitely benign (1), probably benign (2), equivocal (3), probably cancer (4) and definitely cancer (5). In this work, all spectra labeled (4, 5) were assumed to be CaP and all spectra labeled as (1, 2) were assumed as benign. The 15 studies comprised 1331 class 1, 2 and 407 class 4, 5 spectra.

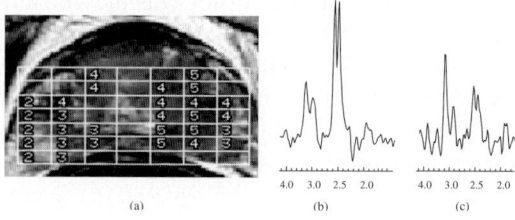

Fig. 1. (a) MRS metavoxels $c \in C$ superposed on the corresponding T2-w MRI section. Representative spectra from (b) class 2 (probably benign) and (c) class 4 (probably CaP) are shown. Note that classifying such similar looking spectra manually is a challenging, error prone, and laborious task for radiologists.

4.2 Feature Extraction of MRI and MRS

(a) Feature Extraction from MRS. Instead of extracting features derived from MRS spectral peaks, we consider the spectra in its totality. Thus, each $c \in C$, $\boldsymbol{F}(c) = [f_\alpha(c) | \alpha \in \{1, ...U\}]$ represents the MR spectral vector, reflecting the frequency component of each of the U metabolites.

(b) Feature Extraction from MRI. 38 texture features scenes were extracted motivated by previous demonstration of their utility in discriminating between the CaP and non-CaP classes [7]. We calculated the feature scenes $\hat{\mathcal{G}}_u = (\hat{C}, \hat{f}_u)$ for each $\hat{C}$ by applying the feature operators Φ_u, $u \in \{1, \ldots, 38\}$ within a local neighborhood associated with every $\hat{c} \in \hat{C}$. Hence $\hat{f}_u(\hat{c})$ is the feature value associated with feature operator Φ_u at voxel $\hat{c}$. 13 gradient, 12 first order statistical and 13 Haralick features were extracted at each $\hat{c} \in \hat{C}$. We define a T2-w MRI texture feature vector for each metavoxel $c \in C$ by taking the average of the feature values within the corresponding metavoxel as $g_u(c) = \frac{1}{|R(c)|} \sum_{\hat{c} \in R(c)} \left[\hat{f}_u(\hat{c})\right]$ where $|R(c)|$ represents the cardinality of the set of voxels contained in the space between any 2 adjacent meta-voxels. The corresponding feature vector is then given as $\boldsymbol{G}(c) = [g_u(c) | u \in \{1, \ldots, 38\}], \forall c \in C$.

4.3 Data Representation, Fusion, and Classification via ScEPTre

(a) Data Representation. For each $c \in C$, $\boldsymbol{G}(c)$, $\boldsymbol{F}(c)$ is reduced to β dimensional feature vectors $\boldsymbol{S}^{T2}$ and $\boldsymbol{S}^{MRS}$, corresponding to the spectrally embedded T2-w and MRS vectors [8].

(b) Data Fusion. Owing to the physical and dimensional differences in the MRS and T2-w MRI features, the MRS-MRI meta-classifier is created in the joint T2-w MRI and MRS embedding space where the physicality of the object features has been removed. A direct concatenation of the T2-w MRI and MRS embedding coordinates can be obtained as $\boldsymbol{S}^{T2MRS} = [\boldsymbol{S}^{T2}(c), \boldsymbol{S}^{MRS}(c)]$. The concatenated feature vector $\boldsymbol{S}^{T2MRS}(c)$ is then used for classification.

(c) Classification. PBT generates a posterior conditional probability for CaP, $p(w_T|\ \boldsymbol{S}^\phi)$, $\phi \in \{T2, MRS, T2MRS\}$ for each spectral location $c \in C$, based on the embedding vector $\boldsymbol{S}^\phi(c)$, where w_T represents CaP class (4, 5 spectra). We define $\mathbf{h}^{\phi,\rho}(c)$ as the binary prediction result at each threshold $\rho \in [0,1]$ such that $\mathbf{h}^{\phi,\rho}(c) = 1$ when $p(w_T|\boldsymbol{S}^\phi) \geq \rho$, 0 otherwise.

PBT was trained using $\theta = 0.45$ and $\epsilon = 0.4$ as suggested in [5]. Five weak classifiers were used to train each node of PBT using AdaBoost for length $L = 5$. Since samples for each class (1, 2 and 4, 5) were not equally distributed within the dataset, the number of training samples ($\Pi \in \{100, 200, 300\}$) from each class was varied to evaluate the classifier with respect to training and the remaining were used for testing. A randomized cross validation strategy comprising 25 runs was used to evaluate PBT performance for each set of training data ($\Pi \in \{100, 200, 300\}$). For each training set, Receiver Operating Characteristic (ROC) curves were computed and mean μ^{AUC} and standard deviation σ^{AUC} of area under curve (AUC) were computed over 25 runs. The experiments were repeated for different numbers of embedding dimensions ($\beta \in \{5, 10, 15\}$).

5 Results and Discussion

Figure 2(a) shows average ROC curves obtained for $\mathbf{h}^{T2}$, $\mathbf{h}^{MRS}$, and $\mathbf{h}^{T2MRS}$ across 25 runs of randomized cross validation for $\beta = 10$ using 300 training samples from each class (1, 2 and 4, 5). The highest AUC value corresponds to the classifier $\mathbf{h}^{T2MRS}$ (shown in black), while the lowest is for $\mathbf{h}^{T2}$ (shown in red). Figure 2(b) shows average ROC curves obtained from $\mathbf{h}^{T2MRS}$ and $\hat{\mathbf{h}}^{T2MRS}$ for $\beta = 10$ using 300 training samples from each class across 25 cross validation runs. AUC and accuracy values for $\mathbf{h}^{T2}$, $\mathbf{h}^{MRS}$, and $\mathbf{h}^{T2MRS}$ averaged over 25 cross validation runs are summarized in Table 1 with corresponding standard deviations for $\beta = \{5, 10, 15\}$. Our quantitative evaluation demonstrate that CaP classification obtained via ScEPTre employing multi-modal integration of MRI-MRS outperforms classification obtained via, (a) wavelets, (b) MRI, MRS alone, and (c) decision level integration of MRI-MRS.

5.1 MRS via ScEPTre and Wavelet Based PBT Classification

Discrete wavelet transform (DWT) based representation of MRS was compared against the spectral embedding representation. DWT transforms a M dimensional spectral signal $\boldsymbol{F}(c)$ into a feature vector $\boldsymbol{S}^{WT}(c)$ containing M wavelet coefficients using a set of basis functions. Each wavelet coefficient is calculated by taking the dot product of spectral vector $\boldsymbol{F}(c)$ with one of the N basis functions, derived from the mother wavelet by a series of translations and dilations. The top m of M largest wavelet coefficients were used for classification with the PBT to distinguish between cancer (4, 5) and benign spectra (1, 2). Different values of $N \in \{3, 4, 5, 6, 7, 8, 9\}$ were employed in the spectral representation. Quantitative results indicate that ScEPTre on MRS performs better compared to a wavelet-based PBT classifier, both in terms of accuracy and AUC. ScEPTre using $\mathbf{h}^{MRS}$ results in μ^{AUC}=0.8743 ($\beta = 10$, $\Pi = 300$) compared to $\mathbf{h}^{WT}$ ($N = 7$, $\Pi = 300$) which yields $\mu^{AUC} = 0.7725$.

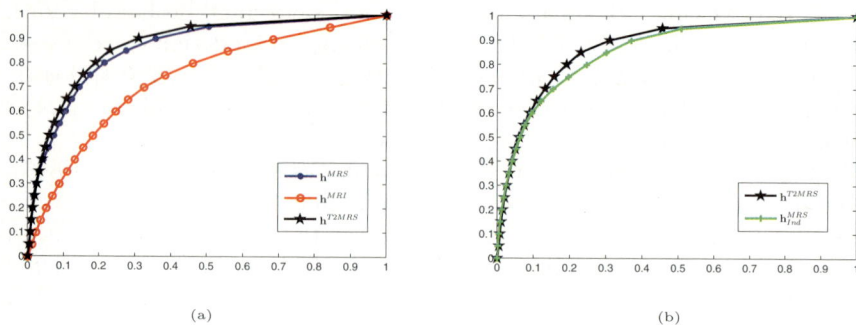

Fig. 2. Average ROC curves across 300 training samples over 25 cross validation runs for classifiers (a) $\mathbf{h}^{T2}$, $\mathbf{h}^{MRS}$, $\mathbf{h}^{T2MRS}$, and (b) $\mathbf{h}^{T2MRS}$, $\hat{\mathbf{h}}^{T2MRS}$. The best performance in both (a) and (b) corresponds to the classifier (shown in black) based on data level integration of structural and metabolic data ($\mathbf{h}^{T2MRS}$).

Table 1. Table shows the μ^{AUC}, σ^{AUC} and accuracy results for 300 training samples from each class using ScEPTre on $\mathbf{h}^{T2}$, $\mathbf{h}^{MRS}$, $\mathbf{h}^{T2MRS}$ respectively, for $\beta \in \{5, 10, 15\}$

β	Accuracy			AUC		
	$\mathbf{h}^{T2}$	$\mathbf{h}^{MRS}$	$\mathbf{h}^{T2MRS}$	$\mathbf{h}^{T2}$	$\mathbf{h}^{MRS}$	$\mathbf{h}^{T2MRS}$
5	56.53 ± 5.53	65.35 ± 4.5	67.62 ± 3.5	65.13 ± 3.13	76.32 ± 1.87	75.82 ± 2.09
10	67.72±3.42	79.44±3.33	**79.51±2.54**	73.27±2.36	86.17±1.91	**87.43±1.41**
15	71.12± 4.47	81.52 ± 2.53	**83.64 ± 2.61**	73.89 ± 1.73	87.49 ± 1.49	**90.27 ± 1.52**

5.2 ScEPTre Based MRI-MRS Meta-classification Compared to MRI/MRS Alone

As is apparent from Figure 2 and Table 1, MRI-MRS data fusion ($\mathbf{h}^{T2MRS}$) using ScEPTre significantly outperformed classification obtained by both T2-w MRI ($\mathbf{h}^{T2}$) and MRS ($\mathbf{h}^{MRS}$) individually.

5.3 Data Level Integration vs. Decision Level Integration

The higher AUC values for $\mathbf{h}^{T2MRS}$ compared to $\hat{\mathbf{h}}^{T2MRS}$ suggests that data level integration is superior to decision level classification. Paired student t-tests were also conducted for AUC at the operating point of the average ROC curves, with the null hypothesis being no improvement in performance of $\mathbf{h}^{T2MRS}$ when compared to the other 3 classifiers ($\mathbf{h}^{T2}$, $\mathbf{h}^{MRS}$, $\hat{\mathbf{h}}^{T2MRS}$). Significantly superior performance ($p < 0.05$) was observed for $\mathbf{h}^{T2MRS}$ suggesting that integrating structural textural features and metabolic information at the data-level offers the most optimal results for CaP detection.

6 Concluding Remarks and Future Directions

In this paper, we presented ScEPTre, an integrated data representation, integration and classification scheme which is capable of (a) accurately representing high dimensional biomedical data, (b) integrating two heterogeneous multimodal datasets embedded in different dimensionalities, and (c) yielding superior data-level integration compared to decision level combination. Data representation was employed using spectral embedding, a non-linear dimensionality reduction scheme which extracts meaningful class relationships embedded in the data. Data integration in ScEPTre is then performed by concatenating Eigen feature vectors obtained from the different modalities, subsequently classified via a Probabilistic Boosting Tree. In this work we presented the application of ScEPTre for representation, integration and classification of MRS and MRI for prostate cancer detection. Results show that ScEPTre on MRS significantly outperforms a classifier that uses wavelets to represent the MRS data. We also demonstrated that integration of MRI-MRS using ScEPTre performs better than both MRI and MRS alone, and ScEPTre based data fusion is superior to decision level integration from a classification perspective.

References

1. Unser, M., Aldroubi, A.: A review of wavelets in biomedical applications. Proceedings of the IEEE 84, 626–638 (1996)
2. Lee, G., Madabhushi, A., Rodriguez, C.: Investigating the efficacy of nonlinear dimensionality reduction schemes in classifying gene and protein expression studies. IEEE Trans. on Comp. Biol. and Bioinf. 5, 368–384 (2008)
3. Shi, J., Malik, J.: Normalized cuts and image segmentation. IEEE PAMI 22(8), 888–905 (2000)
4. Rohlfing, T., Pfefferbaum, A., Sullivan, E.V., Maurer Jr., C.R.: Information fusion in biomedical image analysis: Combination of data vs. Combination of interpretations. In: Christensen, G.E., Sonka, M. (eds.) IPMI 2005. LNCS, vol. 3565, pp. 150–161. Springer, Heidelberg (2005)
5. Tu, Z.: Probabilistic boosting-tree: Learning discriminative models for classification, recognition, and clustering. ICCV 2, 1589–1596 (2005)
6. Jung, J., Coakley, F., Vigneron, D., Swanson, M., Qayyum, A., Kurhanewicz, J., et al.: Prostate depiction at endorectal MR Spectroscopic Imaging: investigation of a standardized evaluation system. Radiology 233, 701–708 (2004)
7. Madabhushi, A., Feldman, M., Metexas, D., Tomaszeweski, J., Chute, D.: Automated Detection of Prostatic Adenocarcinoma from High-Resolution Ex Vivo MRI. IEEE TMI 2412, 1611–1625 (2005)
8. Tiwari, P., Madabhushi, A., Rosen, M.A.: A hierarchical unsupervised spectral clustering scheme for detection of prostate cancer from magnetic resonance spectroscopy (MRS). In: Ayache, N., Ourselin, S., Maeder, A. (eds.) MICCAI 2007, Part II. LNCS, vol. 4792, pp. 278–286. Springer, Heidelberg (2007)

Automatic Correction of Intensity Nonuniformity from Sparseness of Gradient Distribution in Medical Images

Yuanjie Zheng[1], Murray Grossman[2], Suyash P. Awate[1], and James C. Gee[1]

[1] Penn Image Computing and Science Laboratory (PICSL),
Department of Radiology, University of Pennsylvania School of Medicine,
Philadelphia, PA, USA
[2] Department of Neurology, University of Pennsylvania School of Medicine,
Philadelphia, PA, USA

Abstract. We propose to use the sparseness property of the gradient probability distribution to estimate the intensity nonuniformity in medical images, resulting in two novel automatic methods: a non-parametric method and a parametric method. Our methods are easy to implement because they both solve an iteratively re-weighted least squares problem. They are remarkably accurate as shown by our experiments on images of different imaged objects and from different imaging modalities.

1 Introduction

Intensity nonuniformity is an artifact in medical images, perceived as a smooth variation of intensities across the image. It is also referred to as intensity inhomogeneity, shading or bias field. This artifact can be produced by different imaging modalities, such as magnetic resonance (MR) imaging, computer tomography (CT), X-ray, ultrasound, and transmission electron microscopy (TEM), etc. Although intensity inhomogeneity may not be noticeable to human observer, it can degrade many medical image analysis methods like segmentation, registration, and feature extraction, etc.

There exist different kinds of methods to correct the intensity nonuniformity in medical images. In the recent detailed review [1], they are classified into filtering based methods to remove image contents unrelated to the nonuniformity, surface fitting based methods based on the intensities of major tissues or the image gradients [2], segmentation based methods performed by iterating on the two processes of image segmentation and bias field's fitting [3,4], and image intensity histogram based methods through maximizing the high frequency of the image intensity distribution or minimizing the image entropy [5,6], etc.

In this paper, we propose to apply the sparseness property of the gradient probability distribution in medical images to the automatic estimation of the bias field. The sparse distribution is typically characterized by a high kurtosis and two heavy tails. From this prior knowledge, we obtain a non-parametric method and a parametric method. The two methods are simple to implement. They both work by solving an iteratively re-weighted least squares (IRLS) problem. In each iteration, only a linear equations system needs to be solved. The two novel methods are also remarkably accurate, as shown by our results on simulated and real MR brain images, real CT lung images, and real TEM rabbit retina images.

2 Sparseness of Image Gradient Distribution

Recent research has shown that images of real-world scenes obey a sparse probability distribution in their gradients [7,8]. This sparseness property is extremely robust and characterized with a high kurtosis and two heavy tails in the gradient distribution. It stems from the assumption on the image that adjacent pixels have similar intensities unless separated by edges, i.e. the widely known piecewise constancy property of image.

This sparse distribution can be modeled with different ways, e.g. the exponential function [8], as expressed below

$$p(x) = e^{-|x|^\alpha} \qquad (1)$$

where the parameter $\alpha < 1$ and can be fit from the gradient histogram.

We compute the image gradient histogram with the optimal bin size computed by the method in [9], and then use it to fit α in Eq. (1) with the maximum likelihood [10].

3 Methods

We use this sparseness property of gradient distribution in medical images to estimate the bias field in order to correct the intensity nonuniformity. To be concise, we provide the explanations of the 2D image case. However, the modifications to the 3D volume are straightforward.

3.1 Problem Definition

Considering the noise free case, a given 2D medical image Z is the product of the intensity nonuniformity free image I and a bias field B, as expressed below

$$Z(i,j) = I(i,j)B(i,j), \qquad (2)$$

where (i,j) index pixel in the image, and if M and N represent the total numbers of rows and columns, respectively, we have $1 \leq i \leq M$ and $1 \leq j \leq N$.

In the process of correcting the intensity nonuniformity, our goal is to estimate B in Eq. (2) for each pixel. This is a classic ill-posed problem because the number of unknowns (I and B) is twice the number of equations. To make it solvable, we need to add constraints on both I and B.

Instead of computing B directly, we solve for its logarithm as in [8]. Let $\mathcal{Z} = \ln Z$, $\mathcal{I} = \ln I$, and $\mathcal{B} = \ln B$. Then, we have

$$\mathcal{Z}(i,j) = \mathcal{I}(i,j) + \mathcal{B}(i,j). \qquad (3)$$

We denote the gradients of $\mathcal{Z}$, $\mathcal{I}$, and $\mathcal{B}$ for each pixel (i,j) by $\psi^{\mathcal{Z}}(i,j)$, $\psi^{\mathcal{I}}(i,j)$, and $\psi^{\mathcal{B}}(i,j)$, respectively. Then,

$$\psi^{\mathcal{Z}}(i,j) = \psi^{\mathcal{I}}(i,j) + \psi^{\mathcal{B}}(i,j). \tag{4}$$

Given an image $\mathcal{Z}$ with the intensity nonuniformity, we find a maximum a posteriori (MAP) solution to $\mathcal{B}$. Using Bayes' rule, this amounts to solving the optimization problem

$$\mathcal{B} = \arg\max_{\mathcal{B}} P(\mathcal{B}|\mathcal{Z}) \propto \arg\max_{\mathcal{B}} P(\mathcal{Z}|\mathcal{B})P(\mathcal{B}). \tag{5}$$

Different specifications of $P(\mathcal{Z}|\mathcal{B})$ and $P(\mathcal{B})$ in Eq. (5) may lead to different algorithms to solve the bias field $\mathcal{B}$. The conditional probability $P(\mathcal{Z}|\mathcal{B})$ can be determined by some prior knowledge on the nonuniformity free image $\mathcal{I} = \mathcal{Z} - \mathcal{B}$, while $P(\mathcal{B})$ can be set from some prior information on the field $\mathcal{B}$.

To compute $P(\mathcal{Z}|\mathcal{B})$, we impose the sparseness prior of the image gradient distribution explained in Eq. (1) on $\mathcal{I}$ as below

$$P(\mathcal{Z}|\mathcal{B}) = P\left(\psi^{\mathcal{I}}\right) = e^{-|\psi^{\mathcal{I}}|^{\alpha}}, \quad \alpha < 1. \tag{6}$$

From Eq. (4), we have

$$\psi^{\mathcal{I}}(i,j) = \psi^{\mathcal{Z}}(i,j) - \psi^{\mathcal{B}}(i,j). \tag{7}$$

Substituting Eq. (7) into Eq. (6), yields

$$P(\mathcal{Z}|\mathcal{B}) = e^{-\sum_{(i,j)} |\psi^{\mathcal{Z}}(i,j) - \psi^{\mathcal{B}}(i,j)|^{\alpha}}. \tag{8}$$

To determine $P(\mathcal{B})$, there are basically two ways: non-parametric method and parametric method. Non-parametric method does not assume any model on $\mathcal{B}$ and estimate for each pixel while enforcing spatially local smoothness. $P(\mathcal{B})$ can be expressed explicitly by $\mathcal{B}$ values based on the smoothness constraints. Parametric method represents $\mathcal{B}$ with some model functions and estimate the parameters of the model. $P(\mathcal{B})$ is represented by the parameters of the model through enforcing some prior constraints on the model, or is eliminated when no prior constraint is necessary in the model.

3.2 Non-parametric Method

We impose a smoothness prior over $\mathcal{B}$:

$$P(\mathcal{B}) = e^{-\lambda_s \sum_{(i,j)} \left(\mathcal{B}_{xx}(i,j)^2 + \mathcal{B}_{yy}(i,j)^2\right)}, \tag{9}$$

where λ_s is a parameter (e.g. 0.8) determining how smooth the resulting $\mathcal{B}$ will be, and $\mathcal{B}_{xx}(i,j)$ and $\mathcal{B}_{yy}(i,j)$ are the second order derivatives at pixel (i,j) along the horizontal direction and vertical direction, respectively.

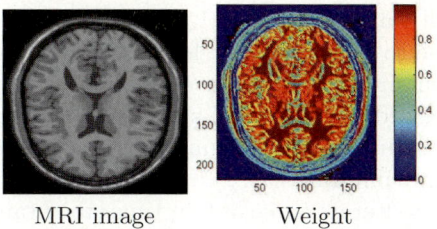

MRI image   Weight

Fig. 1. Computed weights (Eq. (13)) in the non-parametric method after the 3rd iteration of the IRLS algorithm, shown by color coding with the spectrum in the color bar (right).

The maximization of Eq. (5) becomes the the minimization of the below object function

$$\mathcal{O} = \sum_{(i,j)} |\psi^{\mathcal{Z}}(i,j) - \psi^{\mathcal{B}}(i,j)|^{\alpha} + \lambda_s \left(\sum_{(i,j)} \mathcal{B}_{xx}(i,j)^2 + \sum_{(i,j)} \mathcal{B}_{yy}(i,j)^2 \right). \quad (10)$$

The minimization of Eq. (10) does not have a closed-form solution because the exponent α in the first term is less than one as mentioned in Eq. (1). To solve it, most nonlinear optimization techniques [11] can be directly applied, however, they would be very time-consuming and easy to be trapped into a local minimum considering the large number of unknowns in Eq. (10) (it equals to the number of pixels). In order to get a good solution in less time to this minimization problem, we employ the iteratively re-weighted least squares (IRLS) technique [12,8]. IRLS poses the optimization as a sequence of standard least squares problems, each using a weight factor based on the solution of the previous iteration. Specifically, at the kth iteration, the energy function using the new weight can be written as

$$\mathcal{O} = \sum_{(i,j)} w_k(i,j) \left(\psi^{\mathcal{Z}}(i,j) - \psi^{\mathcal{B}}(i,j) \right)^2 + \lambda_s \left(\sum_{(i,j)} \mathcal{B}_{xx}(i,j)^2 + \sum_{(i,j)} \mathcal{B}_{yy}(i,j)^2 \right), \quad (11)$$

where weight $w_k(i,j)$ is computed in terms of the optimal $\mathcal{B}_{k-1}$ from the last iteration as

$$w_k(i,j) = e^{-S_1}(1 - e^{-S_2}),$$
$$S_1 = |\psi^{\mathcal{Z}}(i,j) - \psi^{\mathcal{B}_{k-1}}(i,j)|, \quad S_2 = \alpha (S_1)^{\alpha-1} \quad (12)$$

It is easy to see that minimizing $\mathcal{O}$ in Eq. (11) is to make the gradient of $\mathcal{B}$ equal to the gradient of $\mathcal{Z}$ at each pixel while enforcing spatially local smoothness on $\mathcal{B}$. However, it is well known that this kind of problem has no unique solution because adding a constant value on $\mathcal{B}$ will not influence $\mathcal{O}$ value. To tackle it, we add another constraint as shown in the new object function below

$$\mathcal{O} = \sum_{(i,j)} w_k(i,j) \left(\psi^{\mathcal{Z}}(i,j) - \psi^{\mathcal{B}}(i,j) \right)^2$$
$$+ \lambda_s \left(\sum_{(i,j)} \mathcal{B}_{xx}(i,j)^2 + \sum_{(i,j)} \mathcal{B}_{yy}(i,j)^2 \right) + \epsilon \sum_{(i,j)} \mathcal{B}(i,j)^2, \quad (13)$$

where ϵ is a very small value, e.g. 0.00001. This constraint makes $\mathcal{B}$ as small as possible (i.e. $\mathcal{B}$ as close to 1 as possible), leading $\mathcal{B}$ to a unique solution.

The object function in Eq. (13) is a standard least-squares problem. We can always obtain a closed-form optimal solution by solving a linear equations system. Details of the solution can be found in the supplementary file.

In our experiments, we initialize $\mathcal{B}(i,j) = 0$ (i.e. $B(i,j) = 1$) for all pixels (i,j), and find that it suffices to iterate three or four times to obtain satisfactory results. We also observed that the re-computed weights at each iteration k are higher at pixels whose gradients in $\mathcal{Z}$ are more similar to the ones in the estimated $\mathcal{B}_{k-1}$. Thus, the solution is biased towards smoother regions whose gradients are relatively smaller. Fig. 1 shows the weights recovered at the final iteration for an MR image.

3.3 Parametric Method

Different models are suitable to represent the nonuniformity field $\mathcal{B}$, considering its smoothly changing property, like the cubic B-splines [5], thin-plate splines, and the the bivariate polynomial, etc. We choose the bivariate polynomial for its efficiency shown by [2], for which the model in degree D (e.g. 4) is

$$\mathcal{B}(i,j) = \sum_{t=0}^{D} \sum_{l=0}^{t} a_{t-l,l} x_{(i,j)}^{t-l} y_{(i,j)}^{l} \qquad (14)$$

where $\{a_{t-l,l}\}$ are parameters determining the polynomial, and $x_{(i,j)}$ and $y_{(i,j)}$ are the values of pixel (i,j) on the x-axis and y-axis, respectively. Note that the number of elements in $\{a_{t-l,l}\}$ is $(D+1)(D+2)/2$.

We apply the IRLS scheme used in the non-parametric method to estimating model parameters in the parametric method. Considering the fact that the model in Eq. (14) already incorporates the spatial smoothness on $\mathcal{B}$, the smoothness constraints on $\mathcal{B}$ values can be eliminated. The object function in each iteration of the IRLS is then written as

$$\mathcal{O} = \sum_{(i,j)} w_k(i,j) \left(\psi^{\mathcal{Z}}(i,j) - \psi^{\mathcal{B}}(i,j) \right)^2 + \epsilon \sum_{t=0}^{D} \sum_{l=0}^{t} a_{t-l,l}^2 \qquad (15)$$

where we add the regularization on $\{a_{t-l,l}\}$ in order to get a unique solution as explained in Eq. (13), and the weights $w_k(i,j)$ are computed with Eq. (12).

The object function in Eq. (15) is also a standard least-squares problem relative to $\{a_{t-l,l}\}$, and its minimization also has a closed-form solution by solving a linear equations system. It can be seen from the fact that gradient on $\mathcal{B}$ is linear to $\{a_{t-l,l}\}$. More details of the solution can be found in the supplementary file. In our experiments, we initialize $\{a_{t-l,l}\}$ to zero, and it suffices for three or four times to obtain satisfactory results.

The proposed non-parametric and parametric methods are both easy to implement and run fast. The two methods iterate only three or four times on solving a weighted least square problem with the IRLS technique. The weighted least square problem is solved by resolving a linear equations system for which the solution can be represented by some operations of matrices. We note that the operations of sparse matrices are needed for solving Eq. (13).

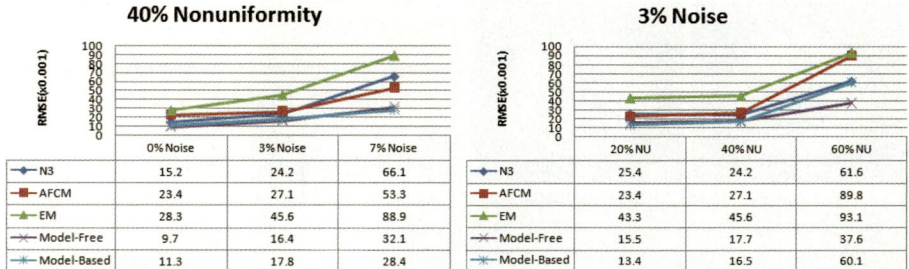

Fig. 2. The statistics of Root Mean Squared Error (RMSE) in estimation of the bias field in the simulated MR brain data sets at different levels of noise and nonuniformity

4 Results

To implement our algorithms, the matrix operations in Eq. (13) were performed with the TAUCS [1], a library of sparse linear solvers.

We provide both quantitative evaluations with simulated data sets and visual evaluations with real data sets on our algorithms. For all experiments, we use $\alpha = 0.71$ in the sparse distribution model (Eq. (1)), that was estimated from 84 MR human brain images and 45 CT human lung images. These images were chosen to be free of the intensity nonuniformity guaranteed by visual inspections. In addition, we run our algorithms on a lower resolution image down-sampled from the given image and then reconstruct the resulting bias field to the original size by interpolation, as in [5]. In the experiments, the gradients along the two axis for 2D image and the three axes for 3D volume are all used.

4.1 Quantitative Evaluation

We test our algorithms on the 3D MR volumes obtained from the BrainWeb Simulated Brain Database[2], for which the ground truth of the bias field is known. The Root Mean Squared Error (RMSE) between the estimation and the ground truth is computed. The results of our algorithms are compared with the widely used N3 [5], AFCM [3], and EM based method [4].

The simulated data sets are obtained with the following settings: T1, T2 and PD modalities, slice thickness of 1 mm, 0%, 3% and 7% noise levels, and 20% and 40% intensity nonuniformity levels. As a preprocessing, the extra-cranial tissues were removed from all 3D volumes according to the ground-truth memberships of the tissues provided on the BrainWeb website. In order to get data sets with more severer intensity nonuniformity effects, we constructed the 60% intensity nonuniformity level by linearly scaling the range values of the ground truth to 0.70 ... 1.30 as explained on the website, and then enforcing it on the volumes download with the different noise levels and with 0% intensity nonuniformity.

---

[1] http://www.tau.ac.il/ stoledo/taucs/
[2] http://www.bic.mni.mcgill.ca/brainweb/

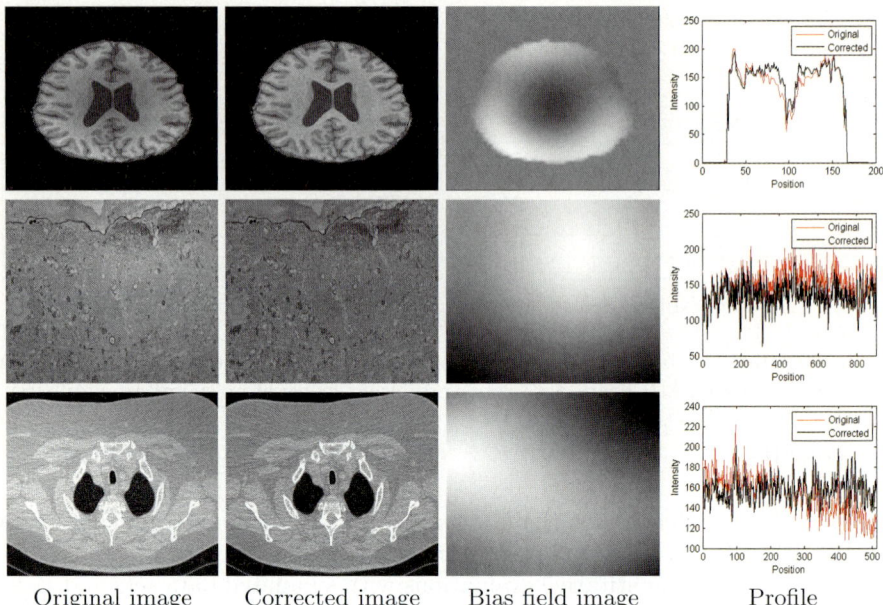

Original image   Corrected image   Bias field image   Profile

Fig. 3. Corrections of the bias field by our non-parametric method on one MR brain image (up), one TEM image (middle) from rabbit retina, and one CT lung image (down). The profiles are drawn on a horizontal line of the image.

Before computing the RMSE statistics, the multiplicative factor [5] is removed from the resulting bias field by minimizing the mean square distance between the result and the ground truth. Therefore, only the shape differences account for the errors.

We found that the chosen methods all perform very similarly on different imaging modalities. Therefore, we averaged the RMSE statistics over the three modalities. From the results shown in Fig. 2, we can see that our methods can improve the estimation accuracies relative to the standard methods. Moreover, our methods seem more robust to noise. Compared between the two new methods, the parametric method resists noise better but may produce larger errors when the nonuniformity is very severer. It is because a severer bias field may go beyond the representation ability of the model in Eq. (14).

4.2 Visual Evaluation

We also run our algorithms on real data: 9 MR brain volumes, 2 TEM images from the rabbit retina, and 5 CT lung volumes, for which the intensity nonuniformity artifacts can be visually perceived. Due to the lacking of the ground truth of the bias fields, we evaluate the results by visual inspections through observing the intensity profile on selected lines.

We found that both of our two new methods can efficiently correct the bias field in images from different modalities and of different imaged objects, resulting in flatter profiles. We put some results by the non-parametric method in Fig. 3.

5 Conclusion and Future Work

Based on the sparseness of the gradient distribution in medical images, we proposed a non-parametric approach and a parametric approach for the automatic correction of the intensity nonuniformity. They are easy to implement and remarkably accurate. Similar strategy has already been used successfully vignetting correction in [8].

Considering the fact that the sparseness property can be treated as a robust prior knowledge of an ideal image or even an ideal deformation field, our paper may also inspire several more works following the line of using this property in medical image inpainting, image segmentation, and image registration.

Acknowledgments. The authors gratefully acknowledge NIH support of this work via grants EB006266, DA022807 and NS045839.

References

1. Vovk, U., Pernus, F., Lika, B.: A review of methods for correction of intensity inhomogeneity in MRI. IEEE Transactions on Medical Imaging 26(3), 405–421 (2007)
2. Tasdizen, T., Jurrus, E., Whitaker, R.T.: Non-uniform illumination correction in transmission electron microscopy. In: MICCAI Workshop on Microscopic Image Analysis with Applications in Biology (2008)
3. Pham, D.L., Prince, J.L.: Adaptive fuzzy segmentation of magnetic resonance images. IEEE Transactions on Medical Imaging 18(9), 737–752 (1999)
4. Zhang, Y., Smith, S., Brady, M.: Hidden markov random field model and segmentation of brain MR images. IEEE Transactions on Medical Imaging 20, 45–57 (2001)
5. Sled, J.G., Zijdenbos, A.P., Evans, A.C.: A nonparametric method for automatic correction of intensity nonuniformity in MRI data. IEEE Transactions on Medical Imaging 17(1), 87–97 (1998)
6. Styner, M., Brechbuhler, C., Szekely, G., Gerig, G.: Parametric estimate of intensity inhomogeneities applied to MRI. IEEE Transactions on Medical Imaging 19, 153–165 (2000)
7. Olshausen, B.A., Field, D.J.: Emergence of simple-cell receptive field properties by learning a sparse code for natural images. Nature 381, 607–609 (1996)
8. Zheng, Y., Yu, J., Kang, S.B., Lin, S., Kambhamettu, C.: Single-image vignetting correction using radial gradient symmetry. In: CVPR (2008)
9. Shimazaki, H., Shinomoto, S.: A method for selecting the bin size of a time histogram. Neural Computation 19(6), 1503–1527 (2007)
10. Aldrich, J.: R.a. fisher and the making of maximum likelihood 1912-1922. Statistical Science 12(3), 162–176 (1997)
11. Nocedal, J., Wright, S.J.: Numerical Optimization. Springer, Heidelberg (2006)
12. Meer, P.: Robust techniques for computer vision, pp. 107–190. Prentice-Hall, Englewood Cliffs (2005)

Weakly Supervised Group-Wise Model Learning Based on Discrete Optimization*

René Donner[1,2], Horst Wildenauer[3], Horst Bischof[2], and Georg Langs[1]

[1] Computational Image Analysis and Radiology Lab, Department of Radiology,
Medical University of Vienna, Austria
rene.donner@meduniwien.ac.at
[2] Institute for Computer Graphics and Vision,
Graz University of Technology, Austria
[3] Pattern Recognition and Image Processing Group,
Vienna University of Technology, Austria

Abstract. In this paper we propose a method for the weakly supervised learning of *sparse appearance models* from medical image data based on *Markov random fields (MRF)*. The models are learnt from a single annotated example and additional training samples without annotations. The approach formulates the model learning as solving a set of MRFs. Both the model training and the resulting model are able to cope with complex and repetitive structures. The weakly supervised model learning yields sparse MRF appearance models that perform equally well as those trained with manual annotations, thereby eliminating the need for tedious manual training supervision. Evaluation results are reported for hand radiographs and cardiac MRI slices.

1 Introduction

The reliable, fast segmentation of anatomical structures is a central issue in medical image analysis. It has been tackled by a number of powerful approaches. Among them are Active Shape Models / Active Appearance Models [1], Active Feature Models [2], Graph-Cuts [3], Active Contours [4], or Level-Set approaches [5]. There are two main open issues with the current approaches in model based localization and segmentation: **1.** The usually limited capture range of model search, that requires some sort of initialization, making application specific heuristics necessary, and **2.** the learning of the model, which is only possible with a substantial amount of user supervision. This is of particular importance for medical data, which exhibits ambiguous appearance and complex structure. In this paper we propose an approach that tackles both of these points by formulating the learning of a model in a discrete optimization framework.

The approach proposed in this paper is related to two lines of previous work **1)** Group-wise registration approaches: in [6] the authors establish a mapping on a

---

* This work has been supported by the Austrian National Bank Fond project Computer Based Quantification of Osteoporosis and Bone Alignment, MU Vienna, TU Graz.

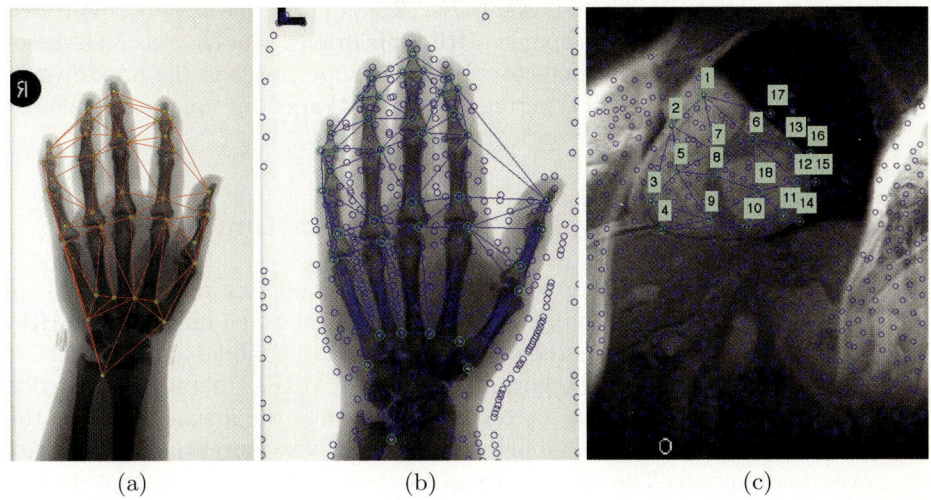

Fig. 1. (a) Example of an annotation consisting of M manually selected interest points used for model building. (b) Examples of the SAM hand model match on the hand data sets. (c) Match of a SAM model trained on heart MRs on a test image. Each model node has been assigned to an interest point in the target image such that the overall MRF confidence for the match is maximized.

spherical reference manifold, [7] which employs piece-wise affine deformations to map the entire data, [8] which uses congealing to obtain a model of appearance variation from a set of images, or [9] where correspondences between sets of interest points in a population of examples are obtained. **2)** Work that integrates discrete optimization for the analysis of image populations: in [10] MRFs are used as an efficient way of encoding deformations for the registration of pairs of images, in [11] Sparse MRF Appearance Models (SAMs) localize objects and structures in images with shape and appearance models based on MRFs. They use a sparse representation of the object category consisting of a statistical model of local appearance descriptors and localize geometry. The information encoded in the model and the results of the search image analysis are used to construct an MRF whose solution represents the optimal mapping of the model to the image, i.e. the best localization.

The contribution of this paper is a method that learns a sparse model of shape and appearance based on Markov random fields in a weakly supervised fashion. Instead of relying on the tedious, and potentially in-accurate annotation of the entire training data, only a single instance is annotated, to define the structure of interest. Based on this initial annotation the algorithm extends the model to the remaining training examples by iteratively including high confidence matches in the emerging model which is encoded as an MRF. The method results in a model quality equivalent to manually constructed sparse MRF appearance models, as is shown in Sec. 4. We report results for two medical data sets employing combined GVFpoints [11] and Harris corners as well interest points based on superpixels [12].

The paper is structured as follows: In Sec. 2 we outline the weakly supervised learning approach building on Sparse MRF Appearance Models. Sec. 3 discusses how to employ interest point detectors based on superpixels in the SAM framework. In Sec. 4 we present the experimental evaluation of our approach, followed by conclusion and outlook in Sec. 5.

2 Model Learning by Discrete Optimization

The learning method is based on modeling the shape and appearance variation of an object population and encoding the model's relation to an image in an MRF. The MRF's solution represents the optimal mapping of a model to an image, i.e. the best localization. During the learning phase such MRFs are solved repeatedly, optimizing the set of landmark correspondences across the images, while at the same time converging to a final model which optimally captures the properties of the entire training set. The appearance of the training examples is captured by local descriptors. The model consists of a set of landmarks, each associated with a model point descriptor $\overline{\mathbf{D}}_m$, and a set of edges connecting these landmarks. The edges hold the geometry information in the form of Gaussian distributions of model edge lengths $(\overline{l}_a, l_a^\sigma)$ and model angles $(\overline{\beta}_{a1}, \overline{\beta}_{a2}, \beta_{a1}^\sigma, \beta_{a2}^\sigma)$ as well as appearance descriptors $\overline{\mathbf{E}}_a$.

Shape and Appearance Model Matching by MRFs. The costs of matching of a model to an example image are encoded in the confidence function

$$C(\mathbf{S}) = \sum_{m=1\ldots M} \mathbf{C}(m, \mathbf{S}(m)) + \sum_{a=1\ldots A} \mathbf{E}(a, \mathbf{S}(a)), \qquad (1)$$

which consists of *unary* terms $\mathbf{C}$ describing the M model landmarks similarities, *binary* terms $\mathbf{E}$ capturing the similarities of the A model edges to the target edges. To estimate $\mathbf{C}$ and $\mathbf{V}$ a set of interest points $\{\mathbf{p}_1, \ldots, \mathbf{p}_N\}$ is extracted from the image with the corresponding local appearance descriptor. The MRF's solution, the so called *labeling* $\mathbf{S}$ maximising C, assigns each model node m to an interest point t in the target image.

The quality of a (model point m, target point t)-match $c_{m,t}$ equals the negative distance between the local target descriptor $\mathbf{D}_t$ and the model point descriptor $\overline{\mathbf{D}}_m$: $c_{m,t} = -\|\mathbf{D}_t - \overline{\mathbf{D}}_m\|$. All mutual distances between model and potential target correspondences are computed, resulting in $\mathbf{C} \in \mathbb{R}^{M \times N}$ encoding the label qualities for each of the nodes. The qualities of the AN^2 edges in the model constitute $\mathbf{E} \in \mathbb{R}^{A \times N^2}$. The quality of an edge e between two labels n_i, n_j in $\mathbf{E}(a, e) = e_{conf}^a$ is computed by comparing its length l_e and relative angles β_{e1}, β_{e2} with the corresponding (circular) Gaussian distributions of the model edge length $(\overline{l}_a, l_a^\sigma)$ and model angles $(\overline{\beta}_{a1}, \overline{\beta}_{a2}, \beta_{a1}^\sigma, \beta_{a2}^\sigma)$. The confidence for the edge's appearance equals the negative distance between the edge descriptor and the model edge descriptor $\overline{\mathbf{E}}_a$. Each of the confidences is then normalized by operator n(.) to a maximum of 0 and a median of -1 (Eqs. 2,5,6). The overall confidence of edge e representing the model edge a is finally set to the minimum of the confidences for length, angles and descriptor, thus removing unlikely candidates:

$$e^a_{lengthConf} = \text{n}\left(e^{-(l_e - \bar{l}_a)^2/(2 * l_a^{\sigma 2})} - 1\right) \tag{2}$$

$$e^a_{angleConf1} = e^{-(\beta_{e1} - \bar{\beta}_{a1})^2/(2 * \beta_{a1}^{\sigma\,2})} \tag{3}$$

$$e^a_{angleConf2} = e^{-(\beta_{e2} - \bar{\beta}_{a2})^2/(2 * \beta_{a2}^{\sigma\,2})} \tag{4}$$

$$e^a_{angleConf} = \text{n}\left(min(e^a_{angleConf1}, e^a_{angleConf2}) - 1\right) \tag{5}$$

$$e^a_{descriptorConf} = \text{n}\left(-\|E_e - \overline{\mathbf{E}}_a\|\right) \tag{6}$$

$$e^a_{conf} = min(e^a_{lengthConf}, e^a_{angleConf}, e^a_{descriptorConf}) \tag{7}$$

Weakly Supervised Learning of the Model

Given the sparse appearance model estimate $\mathcal{E}_{J^k}$ defined by the landmarks from labeling $\langle \mathbf{S}_i | i \in J^k \rangle$, initially derived from the manually annotated image $J^1 = \{j^*\}$, we can assign a confidence $C_i(\mathcal{E}_{J^k})$ for the matching of the model estimate to the training images $i \notin J^k$ and thus to the corresponding target interest point (labelings $\mathbf{S}_i$). For the initial variances of the model's distributions lower bounds are used.

Based on the configuration of the landmarks we can check for the validity of the resulting labeling, allowing for the exclusion of outliers, i.e. the labelings have to conform to the model topology and the selected labels have to be unique.

Given a set of valid model confidences $C_i(\mathcal{E}_{J^k})$ and corresponding labelings $\mathbf{S}_i$ the labeling

$$\mathbf{S}_i^* = \underset{\mathbf{S}_i}{\operatorname{argmin}}\, C_i(\mathcal{E}_{J^k}) \tag{8}$$

is added to the model set J^k to compute a new model estimate $\mathcal{E}_{J^{k+1}}$ with $J^{k+1} = J^k \cup i$. This new model estimate is again used to compute labelings for the remaining training images until J comprises all training images for which valid matches can be computed, resulting in the final model estimate $\mathcal{E}^*$. This model is then evaluated by leave-one-out cross-validation on the whole data set (Sec. 4).

3 Capturing Local Appearance

In this work we employ local descriptors to capture the appearance of the examples during learning. For this various approaches exist, of which we investigate two: In [11] *gradient vector flow* was utilized to detect interest points (GVF-points), and describe their local appearance. The second method is based on super-pixels and can be employed for data where GVFpoints are not well suited and an even distribution of interest points is crucial.

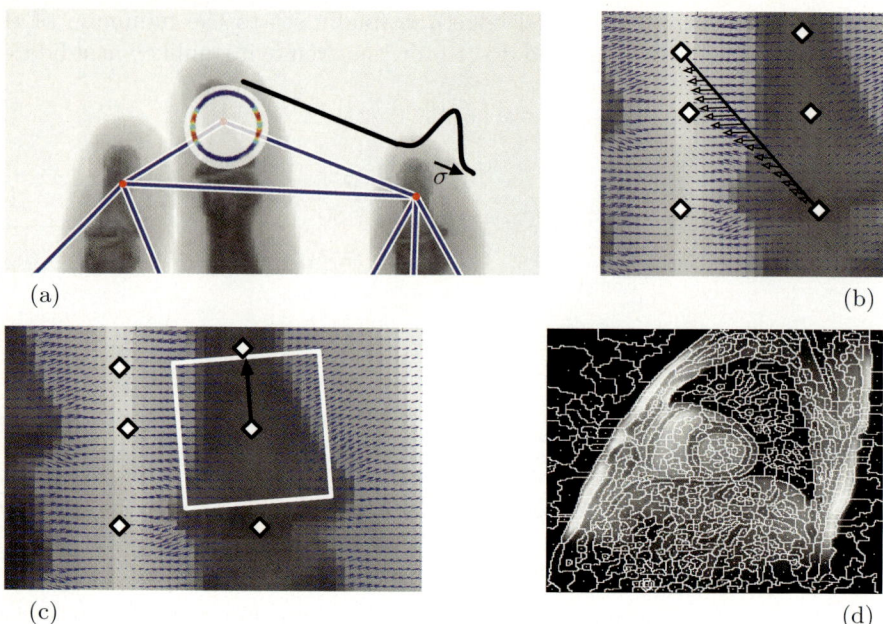

Fig. 2. (a) Illustration of the angle and length statistics learnt for a sparse appearance model node in relation to its neighbors. GVFpoints (b) point and (c) edge descriptors extracted from the GVF field. (d) Example of the watershed superpixels and the resulting interest points (centroids) for the cardiac MR data set.

1. Local Descriptors from GVF and descriptors are located at the approximate centers of homogeneous regions, thus representing rotationally oder mirror symmetric structures like the cross-sections of human organs and skeletal structures. Around each interest point patches are extracted from the vector field according to their orientation as depicted in Fig. 2. To enhance the specificity of local cliques of interest points, GVFpoints can be combined with complementary information like the one derived from a Harris corner detector (Fig.1).

2. Local Descriptors from Superpixels Locally operating interest point detectors face considerable problems when confronted with medical imaging data obtained by MR or X-rays. Besides low contrast and strong noise, these images can be often characterized by a dominance of irregular, semi-local image structures. In such a setting, local intensities no longer provide stable cues for identifying discriminative features.

Recently [12] proposed Laplacian of Gaussians-based (LoG, i.e., mean curvature) watershed regions in the context of multi-scale image over-segmentation. The application of this technique leads to a complete segmentation into regularly shaped, spatially evenly distributed semi-local interest regions as shown in Fig.2 (d). Note that the watersheds approximate true region boundaries very well. Also, the method is able to pick out important image structures of different sizes. Given an image $\mathbf{I}$, the LoG at position $\mathbf{x}$ is defined as $\nabla^2 \mathbf{I}(\mathbf{x}, t) =$

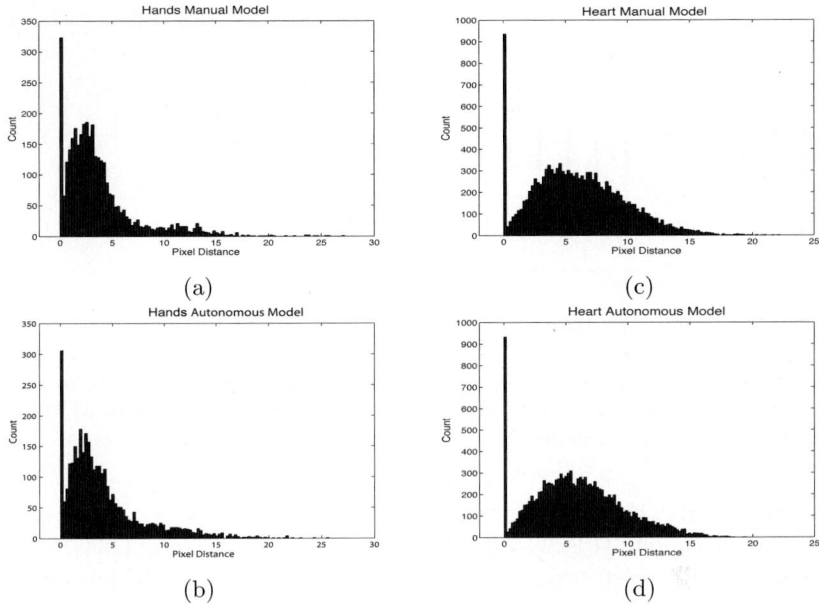

Fig. 3. Result histograms for the pixel distances of result landmarks to ground truth landmarks for the two datasets

$\mathbf{I}_{xx}(\mathbf{x}, t) + \mathbf{I}_{yy}(\mathbf{x}, t)$, where $\mathbf{I}_{xx}$ and $\mathbf{I}_{xx}$ denote the second-order partial derivatives at Gaussian blurring scale t. The LoG produces strong negative/positive responses for bright/dark blob and ridge-like structures. Using this, interest points are extracted as follows: **1)** Detection of spatial extrema (seed points) in the LoG response. Discard low contrast extrema with small minimum absolute difference to adjacent pixels. **2)** Segment the image into regions assigned to positive or negative mean curvature. This is achieved by applying the watershed to the negative absolute Laplacian $-|\nabla^2 \mathbf{I}(\mathbf{x}, t)|$ using the seeds from 1. **3)** Interest points are obtained as centroids of all pixels within a region. This is insensitive to small shape variations of the regions. In practice we found a dense representation of the image to give the best registration results. Due to the very moderate scale variations in our data, scale adaption was not necessary. We simply extract interest points at several predefined scales retaining the one with ≈ 800 interest points.

4 Experiments

The proposed approach was evaluated on 2 medical data sets[1]: **1)** For a set of 12 hand radiographs (300×450 pixels) 39 landmarks were used consisting of both GVFpoints and interest points derived from a Harris corner detector. **2)** 14 Slices

---

[1] The implementation is available from the author's website:
http://www.cir.meduniwien.ac.at/donner-software/

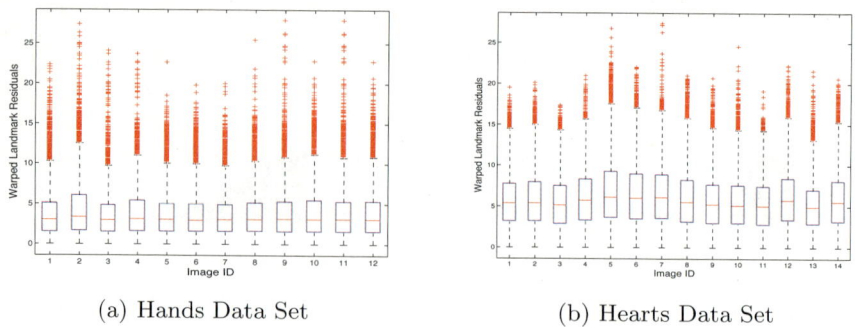

(a) Hands Data Set (b) Hearts Data Set

Fig. 4. Boxplot depicting the results of the leave-one-out cross-validation for different models. For each model, a different image from the training set was used as annotated start image. Note how the model's performance does not depend on the start image.

from cardiac MRs [13] with a resolution of 256x256 pixels were used together with superpixel points (Fig. 1) with 18 interest points selected. This data set is very challenging to conventional interest point detectors due to low contrasts, very weak gradients and large variations throughout the set, impeding a single parameter set to yield reasonable interest points. In contrast, the super pixel based interest points proved to give reliable and descriptive locations, performing equally well on all images in the data set. The number of superpixels was ≈ 800 for the heart data set while the total number of interest points for the hand data amounted to ≈ 1000.

For each data set, the SAMs were run with in a leave-one-out cross validation framework **a)** using the manual annotations of all T training images to construct the sparse appearance model and **b)** by employing the weakly supervised model learning approach starting from a single, manual annotation of a randomly selected image and constructing the final model as outlined in Sec. 2. **c)** Additionally, the influence of which image was annotated was investigated.

To measure the accuracy of the method, ground truth annotations (centers of the fingers joints, inner and outer boundary of the left ventricle) were warped between all possible $n(n-1)$ image pairs according to the diffeomorphic fields imposed by the SAM matching results on the two images. The residual pixel distances between the warped landmarks to the fixed ground truth were recorded. This measure illustrates the ability of the models to capture the intrinsic structure of the data and the success of the SAMs to yield an accurate match.

Results. The results for the experiments **a)** and **b)** are displayed in Fig. 3(a-d). Subfigures (a) and (b) allow to compare the performance of the manual model vs. the semi-automatic approach on the hand data set, while (c,d) show the results for the cardiac MR data set. The mean / median / max values for the hand models (a) 3.77 / 2.80 / 27.22 and (b) 4.15 / 3.03 / 25.70 demonstrate the equivalent model matching capacity of both approaches. For heart MRs, (c) 6.01 / 5.71 / 22.2 and (d) 5.98 / 5.70 / 19.54 consistently show an equal or better performance of the semi-automatic approach, resulting in less outliers. Fig. 4 shows that the proposed model learning approach is insensitive to the choice of the single annotated bootstrap image. This provides a high degree of robustness for practical applications. The results clearly indicate the power of the proposed weakly supervised model learning approach for SAMs to overcome the need for the manual annotation of the whole training set. The runtimes for the proposed approach are about 1 hour / 3 hrs for the heart / hand data sets for the model learning phase, and around 10-20sec for a single localization.

5 Conclusion and Outlook

We present an approach for the weakly supervised learning of sparse appearance models based on MRFs. The method requires only a single annotation, and learns a model that represents appearance and geometric behavior from an training population. The method is closely related to SAMs, but yields models without the need for supervised training. It has the potential to solve the localization requirements present in many state-of-the-art image analysis approaches, being especially well suited for medical applications exhibiting complex and ambiguous structures that make manual annotation, and standard local optimization approaches, unfeasible. Together with super pixel based local descriptors this forms the prerequisite for building 3D SAMs for widespread application, as the shape annotation of 3D data is far more demanding and currently prohibits the wide adoption of model based approaches in this domain.

References

1. Cootes, T.F., Edwards, G.J., Taylor, C.J.: Active appearance models. IEEE Trans. PAMI 23(6), 681–685 (2001)
2. Langs, G., Peloschek, P., Donner, R., Reiter, M., Bischof, H.: Active Feature Models. In: Proc. ICPR, pp. 417–420 (2006)
3. Boykov, Y., Jolly, M.P.: Interactive graph cuts for optimal boundary & region segmentation of objects in N-D images. In: Proc. ICCV, pp. 105–112 (2001)
4. Kass, M., Witkin, A., Terzopoulos, D.: Snakes: Active contour models. International Journal on Computer Vision 1, 321–331 (1988)
5. Paragios, N., Deriche, R.: Geodesic Active Contours and Level Sets for the Detection and Tracking of Moving Objects. IEEE PAMI 22(3) (2000)
6. Davies, R.H., Twining, C.J., Cootes, T.F., Waterton, J.C., Taylor, C.J.: 3D statistical shape models using direct optimisation of description length. In: Heyden, A., Sparr, G., Nielsen, M., Johansen, P. (eds.) ECCV 2002. LNCS, vol. 2352, pp. 3–20. Springer, Heidelberg (2002)
7. Cootes, T., Twining, C., Petrović, V., Taylor, C.: Groupwise construction of appearance models using piece-wise affine deformations. In: BMVC 2005 (2005)
8. Zöllei, L., Learned-Miller, E.G., Grimson, W.E.L., Wells, W.M.: Efficient population registration of 3D data. In: Liu, Y., Jiang, T.-Z., Zhang, C. (eds.) CVBIA 2005. LNCS, vol. 3765, pp. 291–301. Springer, Heidelberg (2005)

9. Langs, G., Donner, R., Peloschek, P., Bischof, H.: Robust autonomous model learning from 2D and 3D data sets. In: Ayache, N., Ourselin, S., Maeder, A. (eds.) MICCAI 2007, Part I. LNCS, vol. 4791, pp. 968–976. Springer, Heidelberg (2007)
10. Glocker, B., Komodakis, N., Tziritas, G., Navab, N., Paragios, N.: Dense image registration through MRFs and efficient linear programming. Medical Image Analysis 12(6), 731–741 (2008)
11. Donner, R., Mičušík, B., Langs, G., Bischof, H.: Sparse MRF Appearance Models for Fast Anatomical Structure Localisation. In: Proc. BMVC (2007)
12. Wildenauer, H., Micusik, B., Vincze, M.: Efficient texture representation using multi-scale regions. In: ACCV, pp. 65–74 (2007)
13. Stegmann, M.B.: An annotated dataset of 14 cardiac MR images. Technical report, Technical University of Denmark, DTU (2002)

ECOC Random Fields for Lumen Segmentation in Radial Artery IVUS Sequences

Francesco Ciompi[1,2], Oriol Pujol[1,2], Eduard Fernández-Nofrerías[3], Josepa Mauri[3], and Petia Radeva[1,2]

[1] Dep. of Applied Mathematics and Analysis, University of Barcelona, Spain
[2] Computer Vision Center, Campus UAB, Bellaterra, Barcelona, Spain
[3] University Hospital "Germans Trias i Pujol", Badalona, Spain
f.ciompi@cvc.uab.es

Abstract. The measure of lumen volume on radial arteries can be used to evaluate the vessel response to different vasodilators. In this paper, we present a framework for automatic lumen segmentation in longitudinal cut images of radial artery from Intravascular ultrasound sequences. The segmentation is tackled as a classification problem where the contextual information is exploited by means of *Conditional Random Fields* (CRFs). A multi-class classification framework is proposed, and inference is achieved by combining binary CRFs according to the *Error-Correcting-Output-Code* technique. The results are validated against manually segmented sequences. Finally, the method is compared with other state-of-the-art classifiers.

1 Introduction

In order to evaluate the effects of drugs and vasodilators administration, the morphological alteration of the artery must be analyzed after the drug treatment. The most indicative parameter that can be used to evaluate the drug effectiveness is the change of lumen volume. Intravascular Ultrasound (IVUS) is an imaging technique that allows to explore both arterial vessel morphology and composition; as such, it is suitable to perform the required measurement.

Most of the proposed approaches for automatic lumen segmentation devolve upon active contour models the organization and interpolation of image features belonging to the vessel border. Ad-hoc solutions, statistical and probabilistic models including a-priori knowledge of the vessel geometry are also considered. In [1,2] the gray level probability density function of the vessel structures, following Rayleigh distribution, is used. In [3] a cost function over the edge image of the vessel is defined, to perform a graph search based approach in which each pixel is a node, determining the border as the minimum cost path. In [4] a shape space is constructed from statistical analysis of morphology on training data and borders are constrained to a smooth closed geometry. In [5] the lumen detection is achieved by classifying blood areas using Adaboost.

The appearance of the lumen morphology in IVUS images is often corrupted, mainly due to the effect of the guide of the catheter and calcifications in the

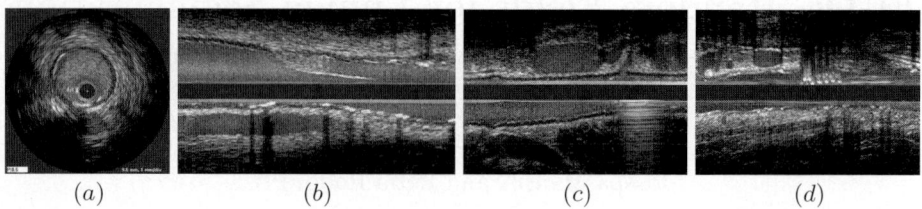

Fig. 1. Short-axis IVUS image (a). Examples of corrupted areas in IVUS longitudinal cuts: presence of outer arteries or veins (b), bifurcations and texture distortions (c), calcifications and lack of continuity in vessel structure (d).

vessel wall. Furthermore, the presence of bifurcations or outer vessels, apparently identical to the lumen area, can lead to an erroneous segmentation, especially when the border appearance is subtle (see Fig. 1). Some of the existing automatic lumen detectors cope with these problems by including *a-priori* knowledge or spatial constrains related to the geometrical morphology of the vessel; other methods perform a pre-emptive detection of calcifications, bifurcations or guide effects, in order to predict where a correction on vessel geometry has to be applied.

The method proposed in this paper is intended to overcome the need of ad-hoc corrections or case-specific knowledge by formulating the segmentation process as a classification problem, exploiting the contextual information over the vessel geometry. The contextual information helps the inference in ambiguous cases by exploiting the relationships among connected image points. To exploit this, we propose to apply *Conditional Random Fields* (CRFs) [6], a discriminative graphical model that estimates an a-posteriori probability function by considering the observation of each node in the graph and both predictions and observations of nodes in its neighborhood. The use of a CRF model as basic classifier allows to design a framework in which different classes, together with their spatial relationship, can be learnt from a set of labeled examples. In order to differentiate the lumen area from the rest of the vessel structure, usually corrupted by the phenomena discussed above, we design a multi-class model where lumen, vessel interfaces and outer tissue are represented as separate classes in a supervised learning framework. The multi-class definition of the problem is here solved by means of the Error-Correcting-Output-Code (ECOC) [7] technique. Finally, the whole lumen structure detected by the ECOC Random Field (ECOC-RF) is delineated by an active contour model.

Summarizing, the novelty of the proposed methodology consists in defining the lumen detection and segmentation as a multi-class classification problem using an ECOC-based supervised framework. Moreover, in order to cope with the ambiguity of local image configuration, we take profit of the image context by using CRF as a classifier able to make inference basing on local image features and neighborhood relationships. Finally, the vessel region is regularized by a deformable model.

2 Methodology

2.1 Classes Definition

Looking at the longitudinal cut, different structures can be observed: *blood region*, *interfaces* and the *outer part* of the vessel. The class defined as *interfaces* actually consists in the *intima*, typically identified by a transition from the darker blood texture to a brighter area, and *media-adventitia* interfaces, characterized by a dark band separating the internal vessel membrane from the outer tissue. Given the different appearance of these interfaces as well as the fact that they can be visible only in some regions of the image, we split the *interface* class into two sub-classes. Since even the manual segmentation of interfaces is difficult, the sub-classes definition (*border*$_1$ and *border*$_2$) is based on a *k-means* unsupervised classifier [8]. The unsupervised clustering is solely used to define the two sub-classes before the training process. Therefore, a 4 classes classification problem is defined.

2.2 Features Extraction for Conditional Random Fields

CRFs as binary classifier requires a graphical representation $\mathcal{G} = (\mathcal{S}, \mathcal{E})$ (*lattice*) of the input data, where $\mathcal{S}$ is the set of nodes, corresponding to each block of the lattice and $\mathcal{E}$ indicates edges, corresponding to the interconnections among nodes. In this case, the lattice is constructed by dividing the longitudinal cut into squared blocks of fixed size W. Features are first extracted from the whole image, then a feature vector $\mathbf{x}_i$ is assigned to each node $\mathcal{S}_i \subset \mathcal{S}$ by considering the *median* value of each feature in the block. The feature selection process proposed in [5] has been used to select, among a wide set of texture descriptors, the most discriminant features for the proposed problem, resulting in *Gabor* filters [9], *Local Binary Patterns* [10], *Sobel* filter in the $\hat{x}$ direction, *mean value*, *standard deviation* and the *ratio* among these two values on the grey-levels of the image, computed by a sliding windows of size H. Finally, the *First Order Absolute Moment* (FOAM) of the grey levels [11] is also used. FOAM is an operator that computes a vector always pointing towards the strongest gray-level discontinuity and assuming magnitude close to zero when applied to the discontinuity itself. Features extraction process results in a 10-dimensional *observation* vector.

2.3 Conditional Random Fields

Once the graph has been constructed, the observation vector $\mathbf{x}_i \in X$ and the label $y_i \in Y = \{-1, +1\}$ can be assigned to each node $\mathcal{S}_i$. The probability function modeled by CRFs for a given binary classification problem can be estimated as:

$$P(y|\mathbf{x}, \theta) = \frac{1}{Z(\mathbf{x})} \exp(\sum_{i \in \mathcal{S}} A(y_i, \mathbf{x}, \theta_S) + \sum_{i \in \mathcal{S}} \sum_{j \in \mathcal{N}_i} I(y_i, y_j, \mathbf{x}, \theta_E)),$$

where A is the *association potential*, modeling the relationship among the observation $\mathbf{x}$ from an image region (node) with the label y for the region, while I is the *interaction potential*, modeling the relationship among different nodes. $\mathcal{N}_i$ is the neighborhood of the node $\mathcal{S}_i$ and $\theta = \{\theta_S \cup \theta_E\}$ is a parameters vector that has to be estimated; $Z(\mathbf{x})$ is an observation-dependent normalization function. A typical estimation of the parameter vector is given by $\theta^* = argmax_\theta P(y|\mathbf{x}, \theta)$.

2.4 Error Correcting Output Code

The presented CRF is able to model a conditional probability for a binary classification problem, while 4 classes are foreseen in our approach. Error Correcting Output Code [7] is a technique that combines N binary classifiers to solve a K-classes classification problem. For each class a particular *codeword* $c_k = \{1, 0, -1\}^{1 \times N}$ is obtained ($k = 1, ..., K$). Based on a chosen coding strategy, a matrix $\mathbf{M}$ is designed, in which each column represents a binary classifier (*dichotomy*) and each row represents a class. A value 1 in position $\mathbf{M}(k, j)$ means that the jth dichotomy classifies an unknown example as belonging to the class k, a value -1 means that the it belongs to the class $q \neq k$ and a 0 value means that we do not care about classification result, regarding class k. Therefore, to classify an unknown example, the distance between the obtained codeword and each row m_k of the matrix $\mathbf{M}$ is computed: the inferred class will be the value k reporting the minimum distance. The number of classifier, using the *one-versus-one* coding technique is $K(K-1)/2$. In a 4 classes problem, 6 binary classifiers must be trained (see Fig. 2).

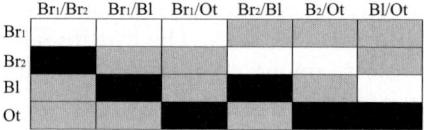

Fig. 2. Error-Correcting-Output-Codes matrix used in a 4 classes (rows) classification problem using 6 binary classifiers (columns) with *one-vs-one* coding technique. A white box represents a 1 value, a grey box represents a 0 value and a black box a -1 value. $Br_{1,2} = border_{1,2}$, Bl = *blood*, Ot = *outer tissue*.

2.5 ECOC Random Fields for Automatic Lumen Detection

Given the graphical representation of the input images, following [12] we define the *node* features vector $\mathbf{h}_i = [1, \mathbf{x}_i]$ and the *edge* feature vector $\mathbf{h}_{ij} = [1, |\mathbf{x}_i - \mathbf{x}_j|]$, where $\mathbf{x}_i$ and $\mathbf{x}_j$ are the observations for the nodes $\mathcal{S}_i$ and $\mathcal{S}_j$, respectively. Since the classes $border_1$ and $border_2$ result from an unsupervised clustering process, no spatial relationships is expected. For this reason, the discrimination among these two classes is devolved upon an AdaBoost classifier [13] trained with examples defined by the k-*means* unsupervised classifier. Conditional Random Fields are instead trained to learn spatial dependencies on the other binary problems. Following [12,14], potential functions are defined as $A(y_i, \mathbf{x}) = \exp(y_i \theta_N^T \mathbf{h}_i)$ and $I(y_i, y_j, \mathbf{x}) = \exp(y_i y_j \theta_E^T \mathbf{h}_{ij})$.

The training process basically consists in estimating $\theta^* = argmax_\theta P(y|\mathbf{x}, \theta)$ or, equivalently $\theta^* = argmin_\theta \mathcal{L}(\theta)$, where $\mathcal{L}(\theta)$ is the *negative Log-posterior* of the parameters given the data and the labels (see [12] for details); θ_N is initialized by logistic regression, while θ_E is empirically initialized to a constant value 0.1.

The *inference* on the whole graph is performed by *Loopy Belief Propagation* [15] for each binary CRF model, thus generating, together with the result provided by AdaBoost, a 6 elements codeword. The definition of different areas of the image is achieved by decoding the codeword using *Attenuated Euclidean Distance* [16]. Lumen regions are thus defined and inference for each node is implicitly related to the contextual information of the neighborhood.

In order to achieve the final lumen segmentation, an active contour model is applied on the vessel structure provided by the ECOC-RF classification, using a gravity map as external energy function [17]. This step is necessary in order to regularize the prediction by filtering some spurious points and, most importantly, by including long term interactions among classified regions. In this way, the local estimation, assumed to be robust due to the exploited contextual information, is constrained by nodes in the neighborhood and by farther nodes as well. It is worth to note that, differently from classical proposed approach, the active contour model is here applied on a higher information level, i.e. the segmentation obtained by the classification rather than the grey level information provided by the image. In our case the role of the active model consists in interpreting the results proposed by the multi-class classification rather than to infer a solution.

3 Validation and Results

A wide set of IVUS images sequences from radial arteries have been acquired at the University Hospital "German Trias i Pujol" (Badalona, Spain); 5 study cases, presenting the more challenging segmentation have been selected, consisting in 10 sequences. Since the amount of data and the vessel structures variety in a single sequence is large, the used data set is highly representative. Longitudinal cuts have been extracted from each sequence and lumen area has been segmented by two experts; areas in which both segmentations agreed have been considered as *ground truth*. Textural features described in section 2.2 are extracted using the following parameters: $(W, H) = (5, 100)$ px, $(\sigma_{gabor}, \phi_{gabor}, F_{gabor}) = \{(12.7205, 0.0442, 0); (6.3602, 0.0442, 0); (3.1801, 0.3536, 3\pi/4); (1.5901, 0.3536, 3\pi/4)\}$, $(R_{LBP}, P_{LBP}) = (4,32)$ and $(\sigma_{1_{FOAM}} = \sigma_{3_{FOAM}}) = 15$ px. We follow the *Leave-One-Patient-Out* cross-validation technique. At each fold, manual and automatic segmentation are compared and the error in lumen area detection is computed. For each point x of the border delimiting the lumen area, the error $\Delta_B(x) = m_B(x) - a_B(x)$ is computed; $m_B(x)$ and $a_B(x)$ are the manual and automatic border detection, respectively. Evaluated parameters are: $max|\Delta_B(x)|$, *mean value* and the *standard deviation* of $\Delta_B(x)$. Furthermore, contiguous patches corresponding to 1.5 *sec* of observations ($\simeq 0.8\ mm$) have been considered in each sequence and lumen area in both manual and automatic

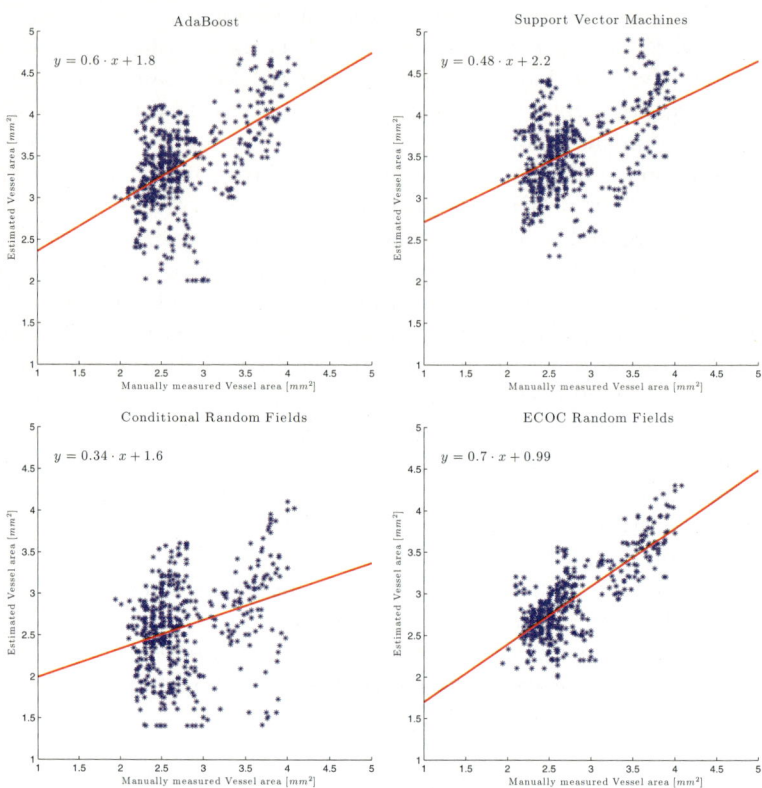

Fig. 3. Manual vs Automatic lumen area measurement, in mm^2, for the classifiers considered in the comparison. The straight line fitting points is also indicated.

segmentation have been computed (Fig. 3). The correlation coefficient ρ between the automatically predicted area and the ground truth area is also computed (see Table 1).

Given the classification-based nature of the proposed method, a comparison with other *state-of-the-art* classifiers is straightforward. For this reason, we also classified the lumen region by using AdaBoost [13] and Support Vector Machine (SVM) [18] binary classifiers in the *blood-vs-outer tissue* problem. Furthermore, a single binary CRF model for the same binary problem has been considered in the comparison. AdaBoost classifier has been trained with up to 50 Decision Stumps while the SVMlight[1] implementation with RBF kernel has been used for SVM (γ and C have been tuned according to [19]). CRF has been trained by Stochastic Gradient Descent [12] (batch size = 6, $\eta = 10^{-6}$). Table 1 reports the performance parameters for the considered methods. Figure 4 shows some examples of lumen detection in the critical cases achieved by the ECOC-RF proposed method.

---

[1] http://svmlight.joachims.org/

Table 1. Results of compared methods

	Δ_B ($|mean| \pm std$)	$max(|\Delta_B|)$	ρ
AdaBoost	0.32 ± 0.32 mm	1.3 mm	0.54
SVM	0.40 ± 0.33 mm	1.3 mm	0.49
CRF	0.08 ± 0.41 mm	0.8 mm	0.31
ECOC-RF	0.08 ± 0.24 mm	1.0 mm	0.77

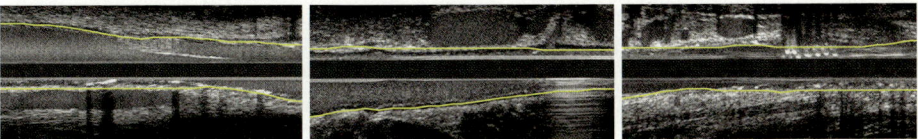

Fig. 4. ECOC-RF lumen segmentation results on the challenging examples of Fig. 1

4 Discussions and Conclusions

The proposed ECOC-RF method outperforms the other considered approaches (see Table 1). We can observe that a single CRF achieves a mean segmentation error lower than AdaBoost and SVM, although attaining a higher standard deviation. ECOC-RF solves this problem, thanks to the strength given by the multi-class definition. Moreover, a high correlation among computed lumen areas and ground truth is exhibited. It is worth to note that the clouds of point in the ECOC-RF case (see Fig. 3) is more compact and close to fitting straight line, thus showing much higher correlation between manual and automatic measurements in the proposed method respect to other strategies. The comparison with AdaBoost and SVM shows the benefits of exploiting contextual information in discriminative approaches while the comparison with a binary CRF justifies the use of a multi-class framework.

A novel method for automatic lumen detection based on multi-class classification on IVUS images has been presented integrating in the same framework CRF, ECOCs and deformable models. The contextual information on longitudinal cut images has been used, together with a long term regularization, in order to solve problems due to the corruption in the vessel appearance. The comparison with other state-of-the-art methods clearly shows the superiority of a discriminant multi-class contextual model, resulting in the most accurate segmentation.

Radial artery volume computation can be easily performed by means of the proposed method, allowing to study the effect of different drugs administration. The promising results on the contextual-based classification of arterial vessel suggest to deeply investigate its applicability to IVUS image analysis. The proposed methodology could also be applied to coronary artery lumen segmentation and can represent the basis for accurate assessment of vessel border properties.

References

1. Cardinal, M.H.R., Meunier, J., Soulez, G., Maurice, R.L., Therasse, E., Cloutier, G.: Intravascular ultrasound image segmentation: a three-dimensional fast-marching method based on gray level distributions. TMI 25(5), 590–601 (2006)
2. Brusseau, E., de Korte, C.L., Mastik, F., Schaar, J., van der Steen, A.F.W.: Fully automatic luminal contour segmentation in intracoronary ultrasound imaging–a statistical approach. TMI 23(5), 554–566 (2004)
3. Sonka, M., Zhang, X., Siebes, M., Bissing, M.S., Dejong, S.C., Collins, S.M., McKay, C.R.: Segmentation of intravascular ultrasound images: a knowledge-based approach. TMI 14(4), 719–732 (1995)
4. Unal, G., Bucher, S., Carlier, S., Slabaugh, G., Fang, T., Tanaka, K.: Shape-driven segmentation of the arterial wall in intravascular ultrasound images. TITB 12(3), 335–347 (2008)
5. Rotger, D., Radeva, P., Fernández-Nofrerías, E., Mauri, J.: Blood detection in ivus images for 3d volume of lumen changes measurement due to different drugs administration. In: CAIP, pp. 285–292 (2007)
6. Lafferty, J., Mccallum, A., Pereira, F.: Conditional random fields: Probabilistic models for segmenting and labeling sequence data. In: Proc. 18th ICML, pp. 282–289. Morgan Kaufmann, San Francisco (2001)
7. Dietterich, T.G., Bakiri, G.: Solving multiclass learning problems via error-correcting output codes. JAIR 2, 263–286 (1995)
8. Macqueen, J.B.: Some methods of classification and analysis of multivariate observations. In: Proceedings of the Fifth Berkeley Symposium on Mathematical Statistics and Probability, pp. 281–297 (1967)
9. Bovik, A.C., Clark, M., Geisler, W.S.: Multichannel texture analysis using localized spatial filters. TPAMI 12(1), 55–73 (1990)
10. Ojala, T., Pietikäien, M., Mäenpää, T.: Multiresolution gray-scale and rotation invariant texture classification with local binary patterns. TPAMI 24(7), 971–987 (2002)
11. Demi, M., Bianchini, E., Faita, F., Gemignani, V.: Contour tracking on ultrasound sequences of vascular images. PRIA 18(4), 606–612 (2008)
12. Vishwanathan, S.V.N., Schraudolph, N.N., Schmidt, M.W., Murphy, K.P.: Accelerated training of conditional random fields with stochastic gradient methods. In: ICML 2006, pp. 969–976. ACM, New York (2006)
13. Schapire, R.E.: The boosting approach to machine learning: An overview (2002)
14. Kumar, S., Hebert, M.: Discriminative fields for modeling spatial dependencies in natural images. In: Advances in Neural Information Processing Systems (2003)
15. Yedidia, J.S., Freeman, W.T., Weiss, Y.: Understanding belief propagation and its generalizations, 239–269 (January 2002)
16. Escalera, S., Pujol, O., Radeva, P.: On the decoding process in ternary error-correcting output codes. TPAMI 99(1) (2009)
17. Pujol, O.: A semi-Supervised Statistical Framework and Generative Snakes for IVUS Analysis. PhD thesis, Autonomous University of Barcelona (2004)
18. Boser, B.E., Guyon, I.M., Vapnik, V.N.: A training algorithm for optimal margin classifiers. In: COLT, pp. 144–152 (1992)
19. Rifkin, R., Klautau, A.: In defense of one-vs-all classification. JMLR 5, 101–141 (2004)

Dynamic Layer Separation for Coronary DSA and Enhancement in Fluoroscopic Sequences

Ying Zhu[1,*], Simone Prummer[2], Peng Wang[1], Terrence Chen[1], Dorin Comaniciu[1], and Martin Ostermeier[2]

[1] Siemens Corporate Research Inc., Princeton, NJ, USA
[2] Siemens AG, Health Care, MED AX PLM-I, Forchheim, Germany
yingzhu@siemens.com

Abstract. This paper presents a new technique of coronary digital subtraction angiography which separates layers of moving background structures from dynamic fluoroscopic sequences of the heart and obtains moving layers of coronary arteries. A Bayeisan framework combines dense motion estimation, uncertainty propagation and statistical fusion to achieve reliable background layer estimation and motion compensation for coronary sequences. Encouraging results have been achieved on clinically acquired coronary sequences, where the proposed method considerably improves the visibility and perceptibility of coronary arteries undergoing breathing and cardiac movements. Perceptibility improvement is significant especially for very thin vessels. Clinical benefit is expected in the context of obese patients and deep angulation, as well as in the reduction of contrast dose in normal size patients.

1 Introduction

Digital subtraction angiography (DSA) is a fluoroscopy technique to clearly visualize blood vessels by subtracting a pre-contrast image called *mask* from later images once the contrast medium has been introduced. In this work, we introduce a new technique called coronary DSA (cDSA) to better visualize coronary vessels in 2D dynamic fluoroscopic sequences of the heart. Using a small number of pre-contrast masks, cDSA produces sequences of dynamic coronary arteries by separating and subtracting sequences of moving background layers. cDSA is an important technique with broad applications in image guided cardiovascular intervention. Fig. 1 shows two applications of cDSA. First, the separation of background and coronary layers enables the function of fade-in and fade-out of the dynamic background structures, thus giving clinicians more options in displaying the coronary arteries in motion during cardiac interventions or for diagnosis purpose. Second, with the coronary layer extracted from fluoroscopic sequences, we are able to virtually enhance the contrast medium for improved visibility and perceptibility of coronary arteries, which brings clinical benefits in the context of obese patients and deep angulation.

---
[*] Corresponding author.

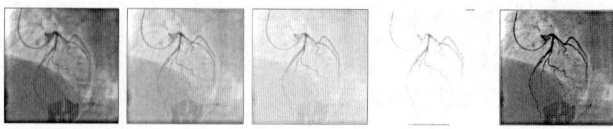

Fig. 1. cDSA applications. From left to right: original image, two images with fading background layer, coronary layer, coronary enhanced image.

A main challenge for cDSA is to deal with complex motion caused by cardiac, breathing and patient table movements. In cardiac fluoroscopic sequences, both static bone tissues and tissues undergoing a mixture of cardiac and respiratory movements can be seen in transparency. Existing techniques of motion correction [4] remain largely insufficient in dealing with such complex motion. Related work has been reported in dealing with transparent motion [1,2,5,6]. In [7], a technique based on non-parametric motion estimation has been proposed, where a dense motion field is used for motion correction between a mask and a contrast image, and learning-based method is used to facilitate motion estimation.

We present a Bayesian framework for tracking the moving layer of dynamic background structures to achieve coronary subtraction in cardiac fluoroscopic sequences. Dense motion estimation between mask images and a contrast image are used to predict the background layer of the contrast image, and predictions from multiple masks are statistically fused to obtain the final estimation of the background layer. Compared to the method in [7] which selects one mask image for motion compensation, the Bayesian framework improves the accuracy of background layer estimation through uncertainty propagation and statistical fusion of motion compensation from multiple masks.

2 Method

In X-ray imaging, the intensity of the energy flux undergoes exponential attenuation through layers of tissues, resulting in multiplicative transparency [4]. With logarithmic postprocessing, fluoroscopic images are represented by an additive model consisting of multiple layers. In cDSA, only two layers are considered to simplify the problem, a coronary layer defined as the transparent layer containing coronary arteries filled with contrast medium, and a background layer defined as the transparent layer containing background structures. Denote $I_t(\mathbf{x})$, $I_{C,t}(\mathbf{x})$ and $I_{B,t}(\mathbf{x})$ as the contrast-filled frame, its coronary layer and background layer at time t respectively, where $\mathbf{x}$ is the pixel location. The additive layer composition model is expressed as $I_t(\mathbf{x}) = I_{C,t}(\mathbf{x}) + I_{B,t}(\mathbf{x})$. The goal is to remove the background layer to obtain the layer of coronary arteries while both layers are undergoing cardiac, respiratory and other types of movements. The proposed Bayesian framework is illustrated in Fig. 2. First, prior to contrast injection, a small number of images are acquired at different cardiac and breathing phases to serve as static masks for background estimation. Second, once the contrast medium has been introduced, motion estimation is performed between each mask

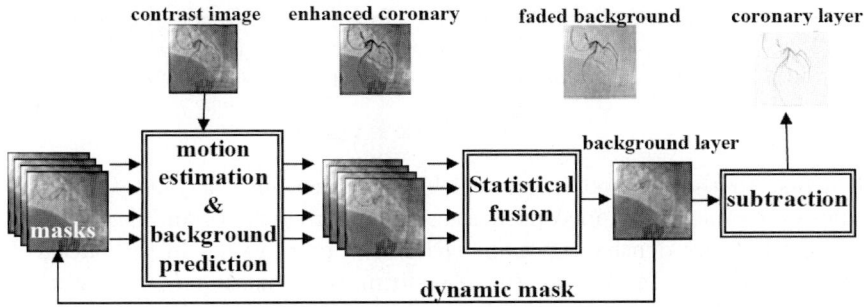

Fig. 2. Bayesian framework of dynamic layer separation

and a contrast image, and the resulting motion field is used to predict the background layer of the contrast image. Predictions from multiple masks are fused statistically to obtain a final estimate of the background layer. At last, the coronary layer is estimated by subtracting the background estimate from the contrast image. In processing a fluoroscopic sequence, layer estimates obtained from previous frames are also used as dynamic masks to predict the background layer of a current frame. In this framework, we assume that the C-arm remains still. New masks have to be reacquired for cDSA when change of angulation occurs.

2.1 Background Motion Estimation

We use the non-parametric approach introduced in [7] to estimate the motion between a mask image I_m and a contrast image $I_t(\mathbf{x})$. First, a technique of learning-based vessel segment detection is applied to the contrast image to roughly separate the image areas of vessels from the region of background structures and to exclude most of the vessel areas from motion estimation. Second, the Lucas-Kanade-Fusion algorithm is applied to estimate a dense motion field $\mathbf{v}(\mathbf{x})$ between the mask image and the background region of the contrast image. The algorithm combines the Lucas-Kanade algorithm which iteratively estimates incremental motion and the covariance-based filtering technique to retain spatial smoothness and consistency of the motion field. For every pixel $\mathbf{x}$, the algorithm computes an estimate of the displacement vector $\widehat{\mathbf{v}}(\mathbf{x})$ locally. In addition, the algorithm also estimates its covariance $C(\widehat{\mathbf{v}}(\mathbf{x}))$ to characterize the uncertainty in the motion estimation. In homogeneous image areas with lack of textures or areas with vessel pixels excluded from motion calculation, the motion estimates tend to be unreliable and their covariance matrices have large eigenvalues.

2.2 Background Layer Prediction with Uncertainty Propagation

Given the motion estimation $\widehat{\mathbf{v}}(\mathbf{x})$ and its covariance $C(\widehat{\mathbf{v}}(\mathbf{x}))$, the probability distribution of the motion vector $\mathbf{v}(\mathbf{x})$ can be approximated as a Gaussian distribution with mean $\widehat{\mathbf{v}}(\mathbf{x})$ and covariance $C(\widehat{\mathbf{v}}(\mathbf{x}))$.

$$\mathbf{v}(\mathbf{x}) \sim N(\widehat{\mathbf{v}}(\mathbf{x}), C(\widehat{\mathbf{v}}(\mathbf{x}))); \quad E[\mathbf{v}(\mathbf{x})] = \widehat{\mathbf{v}}(\mathbf{x}), \quad Cov[\mathbf{v}(\mathbf{x})] = C(\widehat{\mathbf{v}}(\mathbf{x})) \tag{1}$$

Pixel values in the background layer $I_{B,t}(\mathbf{x})$ are predicted from the mask image.

$$I_{B,t}(\mathbf{x}) = I_m(\mathbf{x} + \mathbf{v}(\mathbf{x})) \tag{2}$$

In contrast to the method in [7] which only takes into account the mean of the motion estimates, we incorporate second order statistics and derive the prediction probability density functions (PDFs) of pixel values in the background layer $p(I_{B,t}(\mathbf{x})|I_m)$. In general, the transformation function $I_m(\mathbf{x} + \mathbf{v}(\mathbf{x}))$ is a nonlinear function of $\mathbf{v}(\mathbf{x})$ and techniques such as linearization and unscented transformation [3] are required to parameterize the means and covariances of the probability distribution. Due to the computational complexity of the unscented transformation, we choose to linearize the transformation function as follows.

$$\begin{aligned} I_m(\mathbf{x} + \mathbf{v}(\mathbf{x})) &\approx I_m(\mathbf{x} + \widehat{\mathbf{v}}(\mathbf{x})) + \nabla^T I_m(\mathbf{x} + \widehat{\mathbf{v}}(\mathbf{x}))[\mathbf{v}(\mathbf{x}) - \widehat{\mathbf{v}}(\mathbf{x})] \\ \nabla I_m(\mathbf{x} + \widehat{\mathbf{v}}(\mathbf{x})) &= [\partial_x I_m(\mathbf{x} + \widehat{\mathbf{v}}(\mathbf{x})), \partial_y I_m(\mathbf{x} + \widehat{\mathbf{v}}(\mathbf{x}))]^T \end{aligned} \tag{3}$$

where $\nabla I_m(\mathbf{x} + \widehat{\mathbf{v}}(\mathbf{x}))$ denotes the gradient vector of the transformed image $I_m(\mathbf{x} + \widehat{\mathbf{v}}(\mathbf{x}))$. The mean and variance of $I_{B,t}(\mathbf{x})$ (2) are approximated as

$$\begin{aligned} E[I_{B,t}(\mathbf{x})|I_m] &= I_m(\mathbf{x} + \widehat{\mathbf{v}}) \\ Var[I_{B,t}(\mathbf{x})|I_m] &= \nabla^T I_m(\mathbf{x} + \widehat{\mathbf{v}}(\mathbf{x})) \cdot C(\widehat{\mathbf{v}}(\mathbf{x})) \cdot \nabla I_m(\mathbf{x} + \widehat{\mathbf{v}}(\mathbf{x})) \end{aligned} \tag{4}$$

Through linearization of the transformation function, the uncertainties in motion estimation are propagated to the prediction of background pixel values. The prediction PDF is approximated by a Gaussian distribution.

$$p(I_{B,t}(\mathbf{x})|I_m) = N(I_{B,t}(\mathbf{x}); E[I_{B,t}(\mathbf{x})|I_m], Var[I_{B,t}(\mathbf{x})|I_m]) \tag{5}$$

2.3 Statistical Fusion with Multiple Mask Images

In cardiac interventional procedures, sequences of fluoroscopic images showing cardiovascular structures in motion are acquired to provide real-time image guidance. Multiple image frames are often captured before a contrast medium flows into coronary arteries. These pre-contrast frames capture the background layer from different cardiac and respiratory phases and are used as static mask images. To deal with large image motion caused by deep breathing, we also include the estimated background layers from previous contrast frames as dynamic mask images.

Denote $\{I_{m,i}(\mathbf{x}) : i = 1, \cdots, n_s\}$ as the static mask images acquired at time $t_1, \cdots, t_{n_s}$, and $\{I_{D,k}(\mathbf{x}) = I_{B,t-k}(\mathbf{x}) : k = 1, \cdots, n_d\}$ as the dynamic mask images coming from the estimated background layers of frames $t-1, \cdots, t-n_d$. Through motion estimation and uncertainty propagation, we obtain multiple prediction PDFs of the background layer.

$$\begin{aligned} p(I_{B,t}(\mathbf{x})|I_{m,t_i}) &= N(I_{B,t}(\mathbf{x}); m_{t,t_i}(\mathbf{x}), \sigma^2_{t,t_i}(\mathbf{x})) \quad (i = 0, \cdots, n_s) \\ p(I_{B,t}(\mathbf{x})|I_{D,k}) &= N(I_{B,t}(\mathbf{x}); m_{t,t-k}(\mathbf{x}), \sigma^2_{t,t-k}(\mathbf{x})) \quad (k = 1, \cdots, n_d) \end{aligned} \tag{6}$$

where $m_{t,t_i}(\mathbf{x}) = E[I_{B,t}(\mathbf{x})|I_{m,i}]$, $\sigma^2_{t,t_i}(\mathbf{x}) = Cov[I_{B,t}(\mathbf{x})|I_{m,i}]$, $m_{t,t-k}(\mathbf{x}) = E[I_{B,t}(\mathbf{x})|I_{D,k}]$, $\sigma^2_{t,t-k}(\mathbf{x}) = Cov[I_{B,t}(\mathbf{x})|I_{D,k}]$ are the estimated mean and covariance of background pixel values. Fusing multiple estimates of the background layer, we obtain the linear minimum-mean-square-error (MMSE) estimate as

$$\widehat{I}_{B,t}(\mathbf{x}) = \frac{\sum_{i=0}^{n_s} \sigma^{-2}_{t,t_i}(\mathbf{x}) m_{t,t_i}(\mathbf{x}) + \sum_{k=1}^{n_d} \sigma^{-2}_{t,t-k}(\mathbf{x}) m_{t,t-k}(\mathbf{x})}{\sum_{i=0}^{n_s} \sigma^{-2}_{t,t_i}(\mathbf{x}) + \sum_{k=1}^{n_d} \sigma^{-2}_{t,t-k}(\mathbf{x})} \quad (7)$$

and the estimation of coronary layer is obtained through subtraction

$$\widehat{I}_{C,t}(\mathbf{x}) = I_t(\mathbf{x}) - \widehat{I}_{B,t}(\mathbf{x}) \quad (8)$$

With the background layer separated from the coronary layer, it is straightforward to fade out the background layer or to enhance the coronary layer by layer composition.

$$\alpha_C \widehat{I}_{C,t} + \alpha_B \widehat{I}_{B,t} \quad (\alpha_C \geq 1, 0 \leq \alpha_B \leq 1) \quad (9)$$

To fade out the background layer, we set $\alpha_C = 1$ and decrease α_B. To virtually enhance the contrast, we set $\alpha_B = 1$ and increase α_C.

3 Experimental Results

Fluoroscopic sequences of 30 patients acquired during cardiovascular intervention have been used to evaluate the proposed cDSA method. The sequences were acquired on Angiographic C-arm systems (AXIOM Artis, Siemens Medical Solution) from different rotational angles and included cases of patients holding breath, deep breathing as well as table movements. Since the proposed cDSA technique was planned at the end of the imaging chain for general use cases, the test sequences were not selected particularly by disease phenotypes. Nevertheless, they contain cases of stenosis, lesions and stent placement. Each image frame has either 512×512 pixels or 1024×1024 pixels, and the pixel size is either $0.17mm$ or $0.28mm$. Frames at the beginning of each sequence and before the contrast medium starts to flush into the coronaries are sampled to define static mask images used in processing the following frames. The number of mask images ranges from 3 to 9 frames in each sequence, and they are uniformly sampled from half to one cardiac cycle. There are between 18 to 150 frames per sequence showing intra-coronary flow of the contrast medium, and in total there are 1829 such frames used to compute performance metrics. All testing frames are scaled to 8-bit images with gray values between 0 and 255.

To evaluate the performance of the background layer estimation, we computed the mean squared error (MSE) of the background estimation in each frame, i.e. the mean squared difference between estimated background pixels and the actual background pixels of a testing frame I_t in the background region Ω_t of the frame, $MSE = \frac{1}{|\Omega_t|} \sum_{\mathbf{x} \in \Omega_t} ||\widehat{I}_{B,t}(\mathbf{x}) - I_t(\mathbf{x})||^2$. The histogram of the MSE over 1829

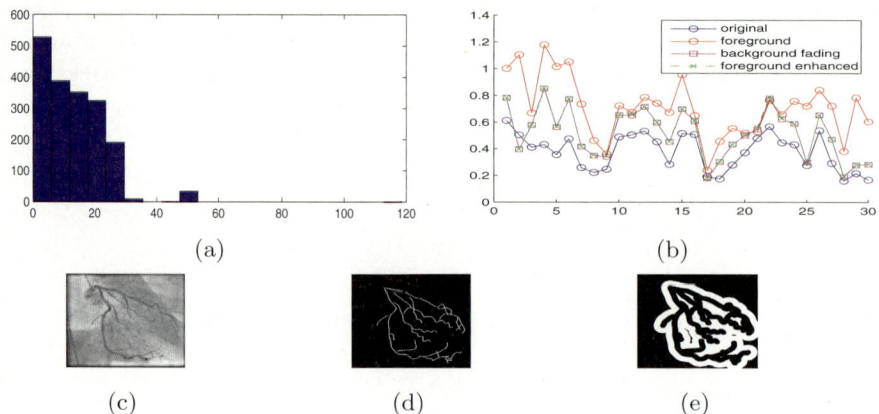

Fig. 3. Performance metrics. (a) Histogram of MSEs over 1829 testing frames. (b) JM distances measured in the original images, images with faded background layers and images with enhanced coronary layers. (c) A test frame. (d) Annotated vessel pixels (in white) and (e) Background pixels (in white) used to compute JM distance.

testing frames is shown in Fig. 3-1. MSEs of the $50th$, $60th$, $70th$, $80th$ and $90th$ percentiles are 11.77, 16.02, 18.07, 21.34 and 24.40 respectively, which corresponds to 3.43, 4.00, 4.25, 4.62 and 4.94 of gray value difference. The mean MSE is 13.06 and the standard deviation is 10.00. To evaluate how cDSA improves the visibility conditions around coronary arteries, we use Jeffries-Matusita (JM) distance to measure the difference in the gray values between coronary arteries and surrounding background areas. In each testing sequence, we manually annotated coronary arteries in a contrast-filled frame. The distribution of pixel values in the areas occupied by coronary vessels (Fig. 3-(d)) was computed as p_C. The distribution of the gray values of background pixels in the areas surrounding coronary vessels (Fig. 3-(e)) was computed as p_B. The JM distance is defined as $JM(p_C, p_B) = [\int_{\mathbf{z}} (\sqrt{p_C(\mathbf{z})} - \sqrt{p_B(\mathbf{z})})^2]^{1/2}$. The JM distance measures how well the two gray value distributions are separated from each other. It is bounded between 0 and $\sqrt{2}$. Higher values of the JM distance is related to better visibility conditions around coronary arteries. The JM distances measured on the original images, the coronary layers, the images with faded background layers

Table 1. Mean, median and standard deviation (std) of JM distances over original images, coronary layers, images with faded background layers, images with enhanced coronary layers

cDSA	mean	median	std
original ($\alpha_C = \alpha_B = 1$)	0.3845	0.4262	0.1366
coronary layer ($\alpha_C = 1, \alpha_B = 0$)	0.7170	0.7289	0.2244
faded background ($\alpha_C = 1, \alpha_B = 0.5$)	0.5239	0.5604	0.1865
enhanced coronary ($\alpha_C = 2, \alpha_B = 1$)	0.5271	0.5706	0.1869

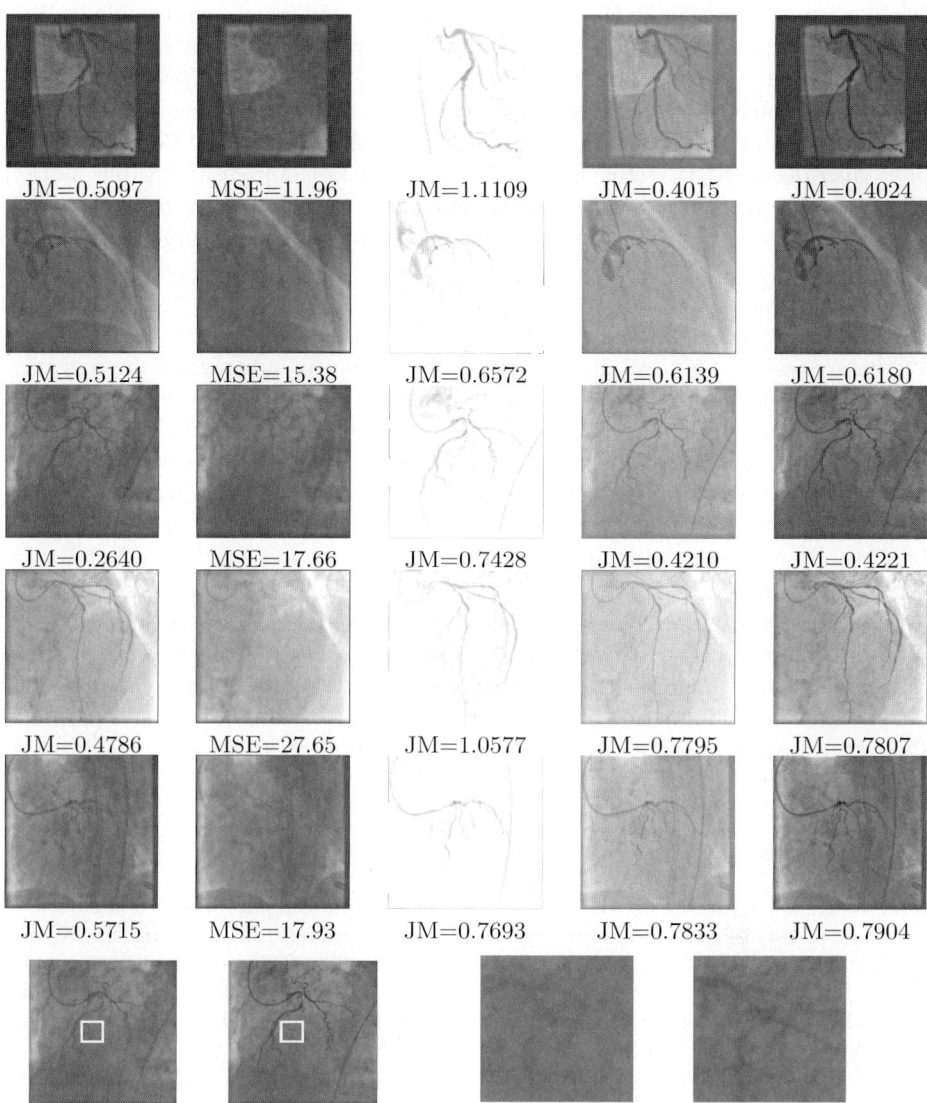

Fig. 4. cDSA results. Column 1: original images; column 2: background layer estimation; column3: coronary layer estimation; column 4: images with faded background; column5: images with enhanced coronary layers. Last row from left to right: original image and coronary enhanced image with white boxes enclosing thin vessels, zoom in on patches of thin vessels from original image and coronary enhanced image.

and the images with enhanced coronary layers are plotted in Fig. 3-(b). Their mean, median and standard deviation are further compared in Table 1.The JM distances measured on the coronary layers are consistently higher compared to the JM distances measured on the original images. In 90% of the cases, the JM distances are improved by both fading out the background layers and enhancing the coronary layers, suggesting improved visibility conditions achieved by cDSA. Fig. 4 shows several image results of layer separation, fade-out of background layers and enhancement of coronary layers. The visibility and perceptibility of the coronary arteries is considerably improved through enhancing coronary layers. In particular, thin vessels are made more visible by the cDSA method. We have also observed that the use of dynamic masks compensates table motion considerably due to the fact that image motion between adjacent frames is small even though over time the accumulated image motion can be large.

4 Discussion

We have presented a novel method for coronary digital subtraction angiography in $2D$ dynamic fluoroscopic sequences. Through dense motion estimation and statistical fusion, a Bayesian framework is proposed to estimate the moving layers of background structures in cardiac fluoroscopic sequences and to obtain the layer of coronary arteries through subtraction. Using this method to separate coronary layers from background structures, we are able to fade out the background layer or virtually enhance the contrast by enhancing the coronary layers to improve the image quality. Encouraging results have been obtained in terms of visibility and perceptibility improvement of coronary vessels and thin vessels in particular. The clinical benefits are expected for cardiac intervention in the context of obese patients and deep angulation. In addition, the ability of coronary enhancement also allows for the reduction of the contrast medium used in normal size patients. Our future study includes the evaluation of cDSA on cases involving diluted contrast medium.

References

1. Auvray, V., Liénard, J., Bouthemy, P.: Multiresolution parametric estimation of transparent motions and denoising of fluoroscopic images. In: Duncan, J.S., Gerig, G. (eds.) MICCAI 2005. LNCS, vol. 3750, pp. 352–360. Springer, Heidelberg (2005)
2. Ju, S.X., Black, M.J., Jepson, A.D.: Skin and Bones: Multi-layer, Locally Affine, Optical Flow and Regularization with Transparency. In: Proc. IEEE Conf. Computer Vision and Pattern Recognition, pp. 307–314 (1996)
3. Julier, S.J., Uhlmann, J.K.: A New Extension of the Kalman Filter to Nonlinear Systems, pp. 182–193 (1997)
4. Meijering, E.H.W., Niessen, W.J., Viergever, M.A.: Retrospective Motion Correction in Digital Subtraction Angiography: A Review. IEEE Trans. Medical Imaging 18(1), 2–21 (1999)
5. Sarel, B., Irani, M.: Separating Transparent Layers Through Layer Information Exchange. In: Proc. European Conf. on Computer Vision, pp. 328–341 (2004)
6. Szeliski, R., Avidan, S., Anandan, P.: Layer Extraction from Multiple Images Containing Reflections and Transparency. In: Proc. IEEE Conf. Computer Vision and Pattern Recognition, pp. 246–253 (2000)
7. Zhu, Y., Prummer, S., Chen, T., Ostermeier, M., Comaniciu, D.: Coronary DSA: Enhancing Coronary Tree Visibility through Discriminative Learning and Robust Motion Estimation. In: SPIE Medical Imaging (2009)

An Inverse Scattering Algorithm for the Segmentation of the Luminal Border on Intravascular Ultrasound Data

E. Gerardo Mendizabal-Ruiz[1], George Biros[2], and Ioannis A. Kakadiaris[1]

[1] Computational Biomedicine Lab, Departments of Computer Science, Electrical and Computer Engineering, and Biomedical Engineering, University of Houston, Houston, TX
[2] Department of Biomedical Engineering and School of Computational Science and Engineering, Georgia Institute of Technology, Atlanta, GA

Abstract. Intravascular ultrasound (IVUS) is a catheter-based medical imaging technique that produces cross-sectional images of blood vessels and is particularly useful for studying atherosclerosis. In this paper, we present a novel method for segmentation of the luminal border on IVUS images using the radio frequency (RF) raw signal based on a scattering model and an inversion scheme. The scattering model is based on a random distribution of point scatterers in the vessel. The per-scatterer signal uses a differential backscatter cross-section coefficient (DBC) that depends on the tissue type. Segmentation requires two inversions: a calibration inversion and a reconstruction inversion. In the calibration step, we use a *single* manually segmented frame and then solve an inverse problem to recover the DBC for the lumen and vessel wall (κ^l and κ^w, respectively) and the width of the impulse signal σ. In the reconstruction step, we use the parameters from the calibration step to solve a new inverse problem: for each angle Θ_i of the IVUS data, we reconstruct the lumen-vessel wall interface. We evaluated our method using three 40MHz IVUS sequences by comparing with manual segmentations. Our preliminary results indicate that it is possible to segment the luminal border by solving an inverse problem using the IVUS RF raw signal with the scatterer model.

1 Introduction

Intravascular ultrasound (IVUS) is an invasive catheter imaging technique capable of providing high-resolution, cross-sectional images of the interior of human blood vessels. The IVUS catheter consists of a solid-state or mechanically-rotated transducer that emits ultrasound pulses and receives acoustic echoes (i.e., A-line) at a discrete set of angles (commonly 240 to 360). The envelopes of the received signals are computed, log-compressed, and then geometrically transformed to obtain the disc-shaped B-mode IVUS image.

Segmentation of IVUS images refers to the delineation of the lumen/intima and media/adventita borders. This process is necessary for assessing the vessel and plaque characteristics. Given that IVUS sequences may be hundreds to thousands of frames long, manual segmentation of a complete sequence is prohibitively time-consuming. Thus, methods for automatic segmentation of IVUS images are needed.

Contributions. In this paper, we present a novel method for segmentation of the luminal border on IVUS data. using the radio frequency (RF) raw signal based on a scattering model and an inversion scheme. The main contribution of this work is a method for the segmentation that relies on a physics-based modeling of the IVUS signal instead of the IVUS B-mode images as in previous approaches. We evaluated our method using three 40MHz IVUS sequences by comparing the automatic segmentation result with manual segmentation. Our preliminary results indicate that it is possible to segment the luminal border by solving an inverse problem using the IVUS RF raw signal with a scatterer model.

Limitations. The model we present is quite simplistic both in the scattering approximation and in the spatial distribution of the scatterers. This is especially true in the lumen border. Also, shadow artifacts and side branches can create problems in the reconstruction.

Related work. Previous approaches for IVUS data analysis can be divided into two classes: image processing-based analysis and physics-based analysis. For the first class, the majority of methods relate to segmentation of the different layers of the vessel. Most reported successful approaches are based on contour detection by the minimization of a cost function. Recent proposed methods include those by Unal *et al.* [1] based on active shape models, Mendizabal-Ruiz *et al.* [2] using a probabilistic approach, Downe *et al.* [3] based on a 3-D graph search, and Papadogiorgaki *et al.* [4] based on wavelets. The input to all of the previous IVUS segmentation methods is the gray scale B-mode image. The limitation of these methods is a consequence of the fact that the appearance of the B-mode image depends on the characteristic of the IVUS system and the parameters used for the B-mode transformation. Thus, no segmentation method is guaranteed to perform correctly on IVUS images from different systems.

The second class of method relates to tissue classification from IVUS data. Although there are methods that work with the B-mode image [5,6], the most successful approaches are those focused on the characterization of atherosclerotic plaque composition by analysis of the ultrasound RF signal. Nair *et al.* [7] proposed a method known as "virtual histology" (IVUS-VH). Kawasaki *et al.* [8] proposed another method of tissue classification using the integrated backscatter (IB) parameter. O'Malley *et al.* and Katouzian *et al.* [9,10] explored methods for blood characterization. Mendizabal-Ruiz *et al.* [11] presented a method for the identification of contrast agent. However, none of these methods is designed for segmentation of the lumen/intima or media/adventitia.

2 Methods

For modeling the reflected IVUS signal, we chose to use the model employed by Rosales *et al.* [12]. This model assumes that the IVUS signal can be obtained from a physical model based on the transmission and reflection of ultrasound waves that radially penetrate the arterial structure. Since the wavelength produced by IVUS transducers is very large in comparison to the dimension of the structures of the vessel, this model assumes that structures can be modeled as a finite set of point scatterers with an associated differential backscattering cross-section coefficient (DBC). Although the signal in the transducer comes from a three-dimensional distribution of scatterers, in this paper we process the A-line scans independently and we consider two-dimensional distributions of scatterers. Consider an ultrasound pulse P_0 emitted at time t_0 with speed c

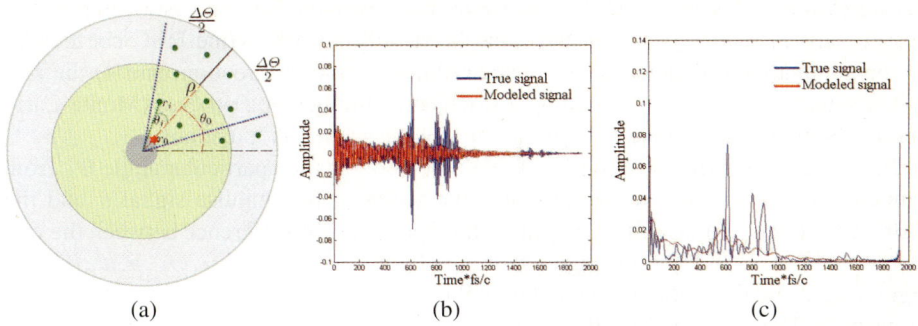

Fig. 1. (a) Scatterers interacting with the ultrasound beam on IVUS. (b) Raw real and modeled IVUS signals for a single angle. (c) Positive envelope of real and modeled IVUS signals for a single angle.

from the IVUS transducer with coordinates (r_0, θ_0), and that interacts at time t_i with a scatterer located at a position (r_i, θ_i) with a DBC of $\kappa(r_i, \theta_i)$ (Fig. 1(a)). The reflected pulse P_i is a replica of the transmitted sound pulse P_0 that will return to the transducer at time $(t_i - t_0)$ and will be out of phase with respect to P_0 by $\frac{2r_i}{c}$, where c is the speed of sound in the medium. The ultrasound beam will interact with scatterers along its radial direction along an angular window given by $\Delta\Theta = \sin^{-1}(1.22\frac{\lambda}{D})$ (Fig. 1(a)), where $\lambda = \frac{c}{f}$ is the wavelength, f is the transducer frequency and D is the transducer diameter. Assuming Born approximation scattering, we use the principle of superposition to represent the total scattered wave as a sum of reflections from individual point scatterers [13]. Then, using this model, the ultrasound reflected signal for each transducer's angular position Θ_k at time t for a finite set of N scatterers with coordinates (r_i, θ_i) where $\theta_i \in \{\Theta_k - \frac{\Delta\Theta}{2}, \Theta_k + \frac{\Delta\Theta}{2}\}$ and DBC $\kappa(r_i, \theta_i)$ is given by: $\hat{s}(t, \Theta_k) = C\sum_{i=1}^{N} \frac{\kappa(r_i,\theta_i)\exp(-\mu r_i)}{r_i} \exp\left(\frac{-(t-\frac{2r_i}{c})^2}{2\sigma^2}\right) \sin\left(\omega t - \frac{2r_i}{c}\right)$, where μ is the attenuation coefficient, C defines the transducer constant parameters, and $\omega = 2\pi f$ is the angular velocity of the impulse function with width σ.

Recovering of the impulse signal width and the DBCs: The width of the impulse signal σ is a parameter that depends on the characteristics of the particular IVUS transducer employed. However, since this parameter is not allays available, it is necessary to recover it from the IVUS data. Fontaine *et al.* [13,14] attempted to recover the scattering characteristics of blood, however, there is no consensus in the literature on the DBC values for blood. As we are mostly interested in reconstructing the lumen-wall interface, we use a two-step procedure that first calibrates scattering parameters and then inverts for the interface. We can therefore ignore the transducer-constant parameter C, since this is a constant and will only affect the scale of the resulting values. Additionally, we normalize the signal using the number of scatterers. Our modeled signal, then, is given by: $\hat{S}(t, \Theta_k) = \frac{1}{N}\sum_{i=1}^{N} \frac{\kappa(r_i,\theta_i)\exp(-\mu r_i)}{r_i} \exp\left(\frac{-(t-\frac{2r_i}{c})^2}{2\sigma^2}\right) \sin\left(\omega t - \frac{2r_i}{c}\right)$.

Specifically, our segmentation method requires two inversion steps: a calibration inversion (Algorithm 1) and a reconstruction inversion (Algorithm 2). Both steps employ the following assumptions: 1) there are only two layers within the vessel: lumen and vessel wall; 2) scatterers within the same layer will have the same DBC coefficient; 3) the attenuation coefficient μ is constant along the radial direction; and 4) the real IVUS signal can be approximated by a stochastic minimization process (Monte Carlo approach) on which we take random samples of the scatterers' positions.

If we know the radial position ρ_k of the lumen border for a particular angle Θ_k from a manual segmentation, we can compute the width of the impulse signal σ and the DBCs for lumen κ^l and wall κ^w by the minimization of the difference between the real IVUS signal $S(t, \Theta_k)$ and the signal computed with our model $\hat{S}(t, \Theta_k, \sigma, \kappa^l, \kappa^w)$. A significant difficulty is that we cannot treat the distribution of scatterers in a deterministic fashion. The scatterers' positions are the result of a spatial stochastic point process. Therefore, the minimization of the differences of the signals should be approached in a stochastic sense. There are many alternative methodologies for that purpose (e.g., stochastic optimization, Bayesian methods). In this paper, we consider the optimal parameter values as functions of the scatterer locations. Then, for each angle k we generate ξ samplings of scatterers' positions and minimize sum of the errors between the real IVUS signal and each of the ξ modeled signals. Specifically, we solve the problem:

$$\min_{\sigma_k, \kappa_k^l, \kappa_k^w} \frac{1}{2} \sum_t \sum_{i=1}^{\xi} (E(t, \Theta_k) - \hat{E}_i(t, \Theta_k, \sigma, \kappa^l, \kappa^w))^2 , \qquad (1)$$

where $E(t, \Theta_k)$ and $\hat{E}_i(t, \Theta_k, \sigma, \kappa^l, \kappa^w)$ are the positive envelopes for the real and the modeled signals, respectively. Finally, we compute the median for each of the resulting parameters.

Segmentation: The radial position ρ_k of the lumen border for each angle Θ_k can be recovered in a similar way. We use the parameters computed on the first inversion and we find ρ_k by the minimization of the sum of differences between the real IVUS signal $S(t, \Theta_k)$ and the signals computed with our model $\hat{S}_i(t, \Theta_k, \rho_k)$ for each sampling ξ. Specifically, we solve:

$$\min_{\rho_k} \frac{1}{2} \sum_t \sum_{i=1}^{\xi} (E(t, \Theta_k) - \hat{E}_i(t, \Theta_k, \rho_k))^2 . \qquad (2)$$

The sampling of the scatterers' positions is done by dividing the vessel into P partitions, and on each partition we place a number of scatterers N_P in random positions using a uniform distribution. The number of scatterers N_P for each partition is determined by the area occupied by the partition and the density β_α (number of scatterers by unit area) corresponding to the layer α on which the partition is present.

The resulting curve might not be smooth due to noise. Moreover, artifacts (guidewire and shadows) and side branches may generate invalid points (outliers with respect to the curve points). Since we expect the number of invalid points to be small (these artifacts are present in small sections of the curve), we remove these outliers by applying clustering on the resulting curve points and eliminating the points corresponding to the smallest cluster. Finally, in order to constrain the curve to be smooth, we use an L_1-minimization method combined with spectral smoothing [15] that also adds the property of periodicity to the curve.

Algorithm 1. Calibration step

Require: IVUS raw signal and manual segmentation of a *single* frame, initial point $x = \{\kappa_0^l, \kappa_0^w \sigma_0\}$, attenuation coefficient μ, scatterer densities for lumen and wall (β_l and β_w, respectively), angular window $\Delta\Theta$, number of partitions N_P, and number of scatterers sampling ξ_1.

1: Extract information about the IVUS data (i.e., frequency of the transducer f, sampling frequency fs, maximum radius R_m and number of angles N_θ).
2: Obtain the radius of the lumen ρ_i for all angles Θ_i from the manual segmentation.
3: **for** i=1 to N_θ **do**
4:    **for** j=1 to ξ_1 **do**
5:       Place random point scatterers within the P partitions of the lumen and wall area using the corresponding densities β_l and β_w.
6:    **end for**
7:    Compute the DBC for the lumen and wall scatterers (κ_i^l and κ_i^w) and the width of the impulse signal σ_i by solving Eq. (1).
8: **end for**
9: Compute the median of the values obtained from each angle $\hat{\kappa}^l$, $\hat{\kappa}^w$, and $\hat{\sigma}$.
10: **return** $\hat{\kappa}^l$, $\hat{\kappa}^w$, and $\hat{\sigma}$.

3 Results

We tested our method on 90 frames corresponding to three 40MHz IVUS sequences obtained from different rabbits' aortas. In order to be consistent with our first assumption, we ignored the section of the IVUS signal corresponding to the sheathing transducer (ringdown artifact). For the catheter used to acquired the data (Boston Scientific), the diameter of the transducer was approximately 0.9 *mm*, while the angular window that we used for generating results was $\Delta\Theta = 2.9°$. Since our goal was to recover the lumen boundary, we used the typical attenuation coefficient for blood (i.e., 0.02 *np/cm* at 1MHz) [16]. For our data frequency (40MHz), the attenuation coefficient μ corresponded to 0.8 *np/cm*. The minimization was done using a simplex method. We used the voxel approach to create random scatterers [17]. Since in our experiments we had a radial resolution of $\delta_r = c/f = 0.04$ *mm*, we set the voxel size to $V = 16 \cdot 10^{-4}$ *mm*^{2}. Experiments on syntectic data indicated that the exact value for the densities was not a determinant for the performance of our model provided $\beta_l \leq \beta_w$ (assuming a smaller density on lumen). Moreover, we chose the density values $\beta_l = 219$ and $\beta_w = 636$ according to the ratio of densities that we could expect on these tissues based on typical values for RBCs and epithelial cells [18]. The density used for the segmentation step was arbitrarily set constant to $\beta_s = 1000$ for all the partitions P. The numbers of scatterer position samplings ξ used for parameter recovering and lumen segmentation were $\xi_1 = 20$ and $\xi_2 = 10$, respectively.

The computed parameters ($\hat{\kappa}^l$, $\hat{\kappa}^w$, $\hat{\sigma}$) for the first sequence were ($1.19 \cdot 10^{-9}$, $3.54 \cdot 10^{-9}$, $6.33 \cdot 10^{-8}$), for the second sequence were ($1.28 \cdot 10^{-9}$, $2.77 \cdot 10^{-9}$, $6.94 \cdot 10^{-8}$) and for the third sequence were ($1.03 \cdot 10^{-9}$, $2.84 \cdot 10^{-9}$, $5.29 \cdot 10^{-8}$). Figures 1 (b,c) depict an example of a real IVUS signal and the adjusted signal using our model respectively. Figure 2 depicts examples of segmentation results. The segmentation results on the 90

Algorithm 2. Reconstruction step

Require: IVUS raw signal of the frame to be segmented, initial point $x = \{\rho_o\}$, attenuation coefficient μ, scatterer density β_s, angular window $\Delta\Theta$, DBC coefficients for lumen and wall (κ^l and κ^w, respectively), width of the impulse signal σ, number of partitions N_P, and number of sampling ξ_2.

1: Extract the information about IVUS data (i.e., frequency of the transducer f, sampling frequency fs, Number of angles N_θ, maximum radius R_m).
2: **for** i=1 to N_θ **do**
3:    **for** j=1 to ξ_2 **do**
4:       Place random point scatterers within the P partitions along the radius using the corresponding density β_P.
5:    **end for**
6:    Find the lumen border $\hat{\rho}_i$ by solving Eq. (2).
7: **end for**
8: **return** $\hat{\rho}$.

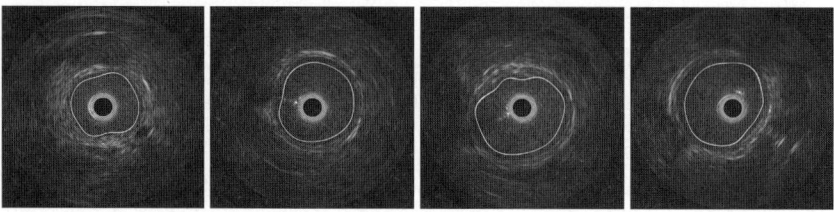

Fig. 2. Examples of segmentation results

frames were evaluated by comparing the agreement between areas corresponding to lumen on each frame by our method (A) with manual segmentations from two expert observers (O_1 and O_2). The mean Dice similarity coefficient was $s = 90.27$. In addition, we performed linear regression and Bland-Altman analysis, for which we report the inter-observer and automatic mean biases (mean area difference) and variabilities. The coefficient of determination (R^2, where R is the linear correlation) for area differences between O_1 and O_2 (O_1,O_2) was R^2=0.98, and R^2=0.93 and R^2=0.93 for (A,O_1) and (A,O_2), respectively. The bias of the area differences for (O_1,O_2) was $(1.80 \pm 0.93) \cdot 10^5\ mm^2$, for (A,$O_1$) the bias was $(-5.80 \pm 3.16) \cdot 10^5\ mm^2$, and for (A,$O_2$) was $(-3.99 \pm 2.71) \cdot 10^5\ mm^2$. Figure 3 depicts the results of this analysis.

4 Discussion

The IVUS RF signal may vary between different systems and even between different sequences, since a different IVUS catheter is used every time. However, due the fact that we calibrate our method for each sequence using a one-frame manual segmentation on the parameter's recovery step, our method can overcome this limitation. The model we use is quite simplistic both in the scattering approximation and in the spatial distribution of the scatterers. This is especially true in the lumen border resulting in a

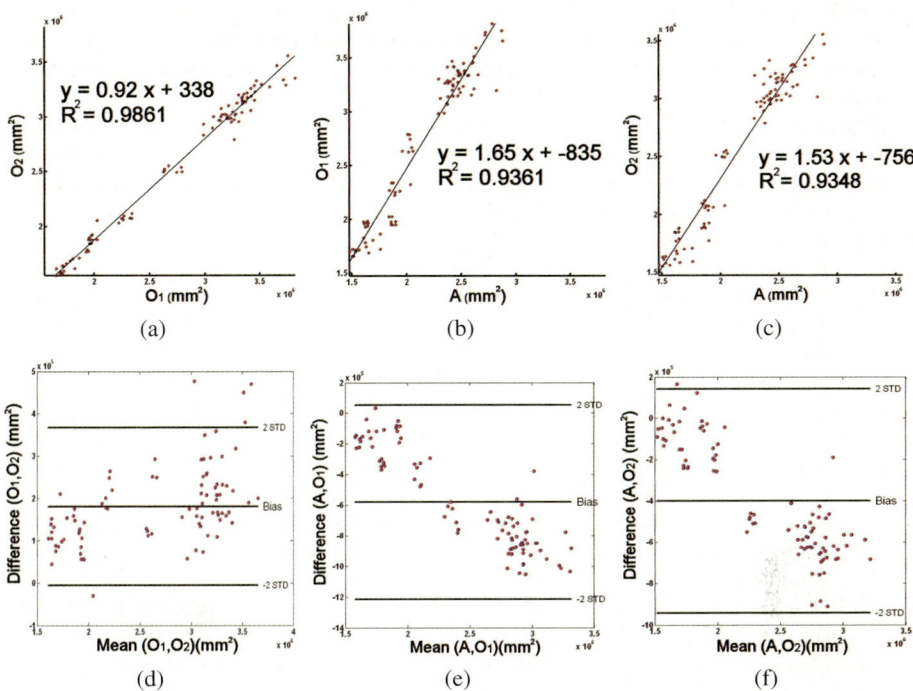

Fig. 3. Linear regression plot (a-c) and Bland-Altman plot (d-f) for O_1 vs O_2 (a,d), A vs. O_1 (b,e) and A vs. O_2 (c,f). Each point correspond to one of the 90 segmented frames.

under-segmentation by our method. Another limitation of our method relates to do with the time required to solve the inverse problems that limits the possibility of using the method on real time.

5 Conclusion

We have presented a novel method for segmentation of the luminal border on IVUS using a physics-based approach as opposed to an image-analysis based approach. To the best of our knowledge, this is the first method that segments IVUS images using the RF signal instead of B-mode images. Our preliminary results indicate that is possible to segment the luminal border by solving an inverse problem using the IVUS RF raw signal with a scatterer model. Future work includes the inclusion of additional layers, alternate methods for placing the scatterers, and comparison with image-based IVUS segmentation methods.

References

1. Unal, G., Bucher, S., Carlier, S., Slabaugh, G., Fang, T., Tanaka, K.: Shape-driven segmentation of the arterial wall in intravascular ultrasound images. IEEE Transactions on Information Technology in Biomedicine 12(3), 335–347 (2008)

2. Mendizabal-Ruiz, E.G., Rivera, M., Kakadiaris, I.A.: A probabilistic segmentation method for the identification of luminal borders in intravascular ultrasound images. In: Proc. IEEE Conference on Computer Vision and Pattern Recognition, Anchorage, AK, Jun. 2008, pp. 1–8 (2008)
3. Downe, R., Wahle, A., Kovarnik, T., Skalicka, H., Lopez, J., Horak, J., Sonka, M.: Segmentation of intravascular ultrasound images using graph search and a novel cost function. In: Proc. 2nd MICCAI Workshop on Computer Vision for Intravascular and Intracardiac Imaging, New York, September 10, 2008, pp. 71–79 (2008)
4. Papadogiorgaki, M., Mezaris, V., Chatzizisis, Y., Giannoglou, G., Kompatsiaris, I.: Image analysis techniques for automated IVUS contour detection. Ultrasound in Medicine and Biology 34(9), 1482–1498 (2008)
5. Roodaki, A., Taki, A., Setarehdan, S.K., Navab, N.: Modified wavelet transform features for characterizing different plaque types in IVUS images; a feasibility study. In: Proc. 9th International Conference on Signal Processing, Beijing, China, October 2008, pp. 789–792 (2008)
6. Katouzian, A., Baseri, B., Konofagou, E.E., Laine, A.F.: An alternative approach to spectrum-based atherosclerotic plaque characterization techniques using intravascular ultrasound (IVUS) backscattered signals. In: Proc. 2nd MICCAI Workshop on Computer Vision for Intravascular and Intracardiac Imaging, New York (2008)
7. Nair, A., Kuban, B., Tuzcu, E., Schoenhagen, P., Nissen, S., Vince, D.: Coronary plaque classification with intravascular ultrasound radiofrequency data analysis. Circulation 106(17), 2200–2206 (2002)
8. Kawasaki, M., Takatsu, H., Noda, T., Sano, K., Ito, Y., Hayakawa, K., Tsuchiya, K., Arai, M., Nishigaki, K., Takemura, G., Minatoguchi, S., Fujiwara, T., Fujiwara, H.: In vivo quantitative tissue characterization of human coronary arterial plaques by use of integrated backscatter intravascular ultrasound and comparison with angioscopic findings. Circulation 105, 2487–2492 (2002)
9. O'Malley, S.M., Naghavi, M., Kakadiaris, I.A.: One-class acoustic characterization applied to blood detection in IVUS. In: Proc. Medical Image Computing and Computer-Assisted Intervention, Brisbane, Australia, pp. 202–209 (2007)
10. Katouzian, A., Baseri, B., Konofagou, E., Laine, A.: Automatic detection of blood versus non-blood regions on intravascular ultrasound (IVUS) images using wavelet packet signatures. In: Proc. Medical Imaging 2008: Ultrasonic Imaging and Signal Processing, San Diego, CA (Feburary 2008)
11. Mendizabal-Ruiz, E.G., Kakadiaris, I.A.: One-class acoustic characterization applied to contrast agent detection in IVUS. In: Proc. Medical Image Computing and Computer-Assisted Intervention Workshop on Computer Vision for Intravascular and Intracardiac Imaging, New York, September 10 (2008)
12. Ramirez, M., Ivanova, P., Mauri, J., Pujol, O.: Simulation model of intravascular ultrasound images. In: Proc. Medical Image Computing and Computer-Assisted Intervention, Saint-Malo, France, pp. 200–207 (2004)
13. Fontaine, I., Bertrand, M., Cloutier, G.: A system-based approach to modeling the ultrasound signal backscattered by red blood cells. Biophysical Journal 77(5), 2387–2399 (1999)
14. Fontaine, I., Savery, D., Cloutier, G.: Simulation of ultrasound backscattering by red cell aggregates: Effect of shear rate and anisotropy. Biophysical Journal 82(4), 1696–1710 (2002)
15. Rice, J.R., White, J.S.: Norms for smoothing and estimation. Society for Industrial and Applied Mathematics Review, 243–256 (1964)
16. Shung, K.K., Smith, M.B., Tsui, B.: Principles of medical imaging. Academic Press, London (1992)
17. Lim, B., Bascom, P., Cobbold, R.: Particle and voxel approaches for simulating ultrasound backscattering from tissue. Ultrasound in Medicine and Biology 22(9), 1237–1247 (1996)
18. Shung, K., Thieme, G.: Ultrasonic scattering in biological tissues. CRC Press, Boca Raton (1993)

Image-Driven Cardiac Left Ventricle Segmentation for the Evaluation of Multiview Fused Real-Time 3-Dimensional Echocardiography Images

Kashif Rajpoot[1,*], J. Alison Noble[1], Vicente Grau[1],
Cezary Szmigielski[2], and Harald Becher[2]

[1] Institute of Biomedical Engineering, University of Oxford, Oxford, UK
[2] Department of Cardiovascular Medicine, University of Oxford, Oxford, UK
{kashif,noble}@robots.ox.ac.uk, vicente.grau@oerc.ox.ac.uk,
cezary.szmigielski@cardiov.ox.ac.uk, harald.becher@orh.nhs.uk

Abstract. Real-time 3-dimensional echocardiography (RT3DE) permits the acquisition and visualization of the beating heart in 3D. Despite a number of efforts to automate the left ventricle (LV) delineation from RT3DE images, this remains a challenging problem due to the poor nature of the acquired images usually containing missing anatomical information and high speckle noise. Recently, there have been efforts to improve image quality and anatomical definition by acquiring multiple single-view RT3DE images with small probe movements and fusing them together after alignment. In this work, we evaluate the quality of the multiview fused images using an image-driven semi-automatic LV segmentation method. The segmentation method is based on an edge-driven level set framework, where the edges are extracted using a local-phase inspired feature detector for low-contrast echocardiography boundaries. This totally image-driven segmentation method is applied for the evaluation of end-diastolic (ED) and end-systolic (ES) single-view and multiview fused images. Experiments were conducted on 17 cases and the results show that multiview fused images have better image segmentation quality, but large failures were observed on ED (88.2%) and ES (58.8%) single-view images.

1 Introduction and Literature

Echocardiography provides a simple, real-time, low-cost, and completely harmless way to assess the cardiac function. It is now possible to capture the 3D volume sequences of the heart by acquiring real-time 3-dimensional echocardiography (RT3DE) images using a matrix-array ultrasound transducer. Although it has been shown that RT3DE improves reproducibility in comparison to 2D echocardiography [1], it has still not been adopted for routine clinical use for cardiac function analysis. It is expected that reliable and robust automatic methods for left ventricle (LV) endocardial surface extraction will aid the uptake of RT3DE in the clinics.

---

[*] Kashif Rajpoot is funded by a PhD scholarship from Higher Education Commission, Pakistan.

Cardiac segmentation from RT3DE images is an active area of research and a variety of solutions have been proposed. The major LV segmentation methods for RT3DE images fall into 3 broad categories: edge-driven, region-driven and prior-model driven. In the edge-driven approaches [2,3], a snake-like deformable model [4] is attracted towards the boundary edges usually detected from intensity-gradient based edge detectors. In the region-driven approaches [5,6], image intensities for the LV blood-cavity and myocardium tissue are modeled using a statistical distribution. On the other hand, prior-model driven methods [7,8] construct a statistical model of shape and/or appearance from a training set of RT3DE volumes and use this model to guide LV segmentation. However, it is very difficult to capture the true shape variability of the heart due to its complex nature. Furthermore, it is very challenging to represent the different pathologies in the statistical model. In contrast, both the edge- and region-driven approaches are purely image-driven techniques and they are fully dependent upon the image quality and the anatomical information in the image. This may imply that the segmentation method will be unsuccessful on poor- or average-quality images, due to the problems caused by speckle, missing anatomical boundaries, limited field-of-view (FOV) and intensity dropout (see Fig. 1(b)-(e)). Moreover, quite often a close initialization of the surface is needed in the edge-driven approaches either via registration [2] or manual landmark selection [3].

There have been recent efforts to improve RT3DE image quality by image fusion [9] or compounding [10]. This involves acquiring multiple single-view RT3DE images from different probe positions over the chest cavity and following a 2-step approach to (i) register and (ii) combine them together. Recently, we have developed a wavelet-based multiview RT3DE image fusion method [11] that showed improvements in the signal-to-noise ratio, contrast, and anatomical information. It can also extend the FOV thus permitting a complete 3D coverage of large hearts.

In this work, we use the multiview RT3DE fused images for LV endocardial surface extraction. For this purpose, we introduce an edge-driven level set [4] based LV segmentation framework while the edges are derived from a local-phase inspired feature detector [12] designed for low-contrast echocardiography images. The key contribution of the paper is to objectively assess the quality of multiview fused images against single-view images for automated segmentation.

The paper begins with the details of RT3DE image fusion and the proposed segmentation approach in Section 2. Experimental results and their validation are presented in Section 3. The paper finishes with concluding remarks in Section 4.

2 Methods

2.1 Multiview RT3DE Image Fusion

We give a brief description of the multiview RT3DE image fusion process here; full details can be found in [11]. The standard single-view RT3DE images are acquired from different transducer positions from the apical view acoustic window (see Fig. 1(a)). The first full-volume image sequence (1) is acquired by placing the transducer probe near the LV apex. Two more full-volume sequences (2,3) are acquired by translating the probe from the apex towards the lateral wall of the LV by approximately 1cm and 2cm, respectively. Another full-volume sequence (4) is acquired by translating the probe from the apex towards the interventricular septum by approximately 1cm. Finally, two more volume sequences (5,6) are captured by moving the probe one intercostal space above and below the first probe position. In some cases, more than one volume was acquired from the same probe position by a slight angular tilt of the probe.

The acquired multiple single-view images are then aligned using a multiresolution rigid registration algorithm using normalized cross-correlation as a similarity measure and the Powell method as the optimization technique. The first full volume acquired near the apical position is used as the reference volume for registration. Once the image correspondence has been established, the aligned images are then combined together in a way that aims at preserving the salient structures [11]. A wavelet analysis technique is used to decompose each single-view image into its low- and high-frequency components. The fusion is then performed in the wavelet domain, treating the low- and high-frequency wavelet coefficients differently. It was shown in [11] that the fusion improves the anatomical information (measured as the number of relevant features detected in an image) by about 16%. Fig. 1(b)-(f) show example results of image fusion on 2D image slices.

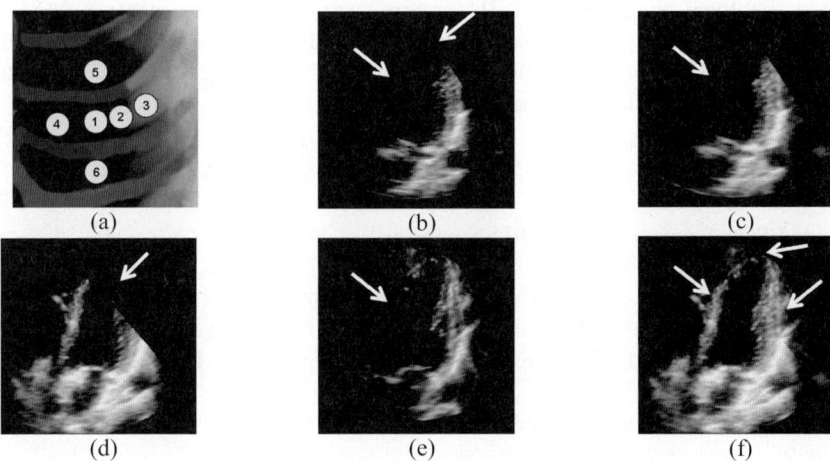

Fig. 1. Single-view image acquisition and example 2D image results of multiview RT3DE fusion. (a) Image acquisition protocol (probe locations indicated 1 to 6 over chest), (b)-(e) 2D slices from aligned single-view volumes – arrows indicate the missing anatomical information, (f) fused image – arrows depict the filled-in anatomical information due to fusion.

2.2 LV Segmentation

The LV segmentation problem is posed as a deformable surface evolution model [4]:

$$S_t(t, u) = F_{image} + F_{regularization} \quad (1)$$

where $S_t(t, u)$ is the surface at time t parameterized by u, F_{image} is the image based force and $F_{regularization}$ is the surface regularization force. Following the level set (LS) methods based derivation of Casselles et al. [4], a higher-dimensional implicit surface embedding function φ can be introduced and surface evolution (1) becomes the solution of a partial differential equation (PDE):

$$\frac{\partial \varphi}{\partial t} = \alpha g_I \|\nabla \varphi\| + \beta \kappa g_I \|\nabla \varphi\| + \gamma \nabla g_I . \nabla \varphi \qquad (2)$$

where the first term on the right is a balloon force (controlling the growth or shrinkage of the LS), the second term is a curvature-based smoothness term, and the last term is the advection term controlling the attachment of the deformable model to the image edges. In (2), α, β and γ are the weights for the balloon force, the curvature force κ and the advection force, respectively. Here, g_I is an edge-indicator function that decreases monotonically with the gradient magnitude of the image I [13]:

$$g_I = f_{map}\left(\frac{\|\nabla(G_\sigma * I)\|}{max\|\nabla(G_\sigma * I)\|}\right), \qquad f_{map}(x) = \left[1 + (x/v)^\lambda\right]^{-1} \qquad (3)$$

where $G_\sigma * I$ denotes convolution of image I with a Gaussian kernel of variance σ, v is the edge contrast parameter, and λ is the edge exponent parameter.

For echocardiography, the intensity-gradient based edge-indicator function g_I of (3) is not the best option due to the highly noisy nature of these images. Instead, we adapted the local-phase inspired 3D feature asymmetry (*FA*) measure [12]. This feature detector is designed for detecting step-like edges (i.e., asymmetric endocardial borders) from low-contrast and noisy echocardiography images. For the computation of the edge-indicator function, we substitute I with FA in (3):

$$g_{FA} = f_{map}\left(\frac{\|\nabla(G_\sigma * FA)\|}{max\|\nabla(G_\sigma * FA)\|}\right)$$

thus our LS surface evolution PDE becomes:

$$\frac{\partial \varphi}{\partial t} = \alpha g_{FA} \|\nabla \varphi\| + \beta \kappa g_{FA} \|\nabla \varphi\| + \gamma \nabla g_{FA} . \nabla \varphi \qquad (4)$$

To solve (4), we used the Yushkevich et al. implementation of LS methods [13].

2.3 Post-processing of LV Surface

The level set based LV endocardial surface extraction method described in the previous section is purely edge-driven. The process works by initializing a sphere inside the LV cavity and allowing it to expand under the influence of balloon force until stopped by the edges. However, there are many false features in the cavity: for example, the edges due to the papillary muscle or the apical region (see Fig. 2(a)). This is a cause of problems in the extraction of the true endocardial surface. We therefore perform a post-processing operation on the LS segmentation. The post-processing steps are described in the following.

1. *Apex point selection.* The apex region is a difficult region for an edge-driven endocardial segmentation method because of its very complex shape and lack of boundary definition. Post-segmentation, the middle slice apical 4-chamber plane is presented to the user for manual selection of a point near the apex using a single mouse click. A small sphere is generated at this location having a radius of 3-voxels (see Fig. 2(b)), which aids the operation of the next step.

2. *Surface fitting.* The LS segmented surface is not smooth because of the papillary muscles and the trabeculae near the endocardium. We perform a hypersurface fitting (tessellation-based linear interpolation) to the LS segmented surface, which now includes the sphere at the apex location from last step (see Fig. 2(c)).
3. *Surface smoothness.* Commonly, the clinicians expect the endocardial surface to be a smooth surface delineating the endocardium. For this purpose, we perform a Gaussian-smoothing step to smooth the endocardial surface (see Fig. 2(d)).

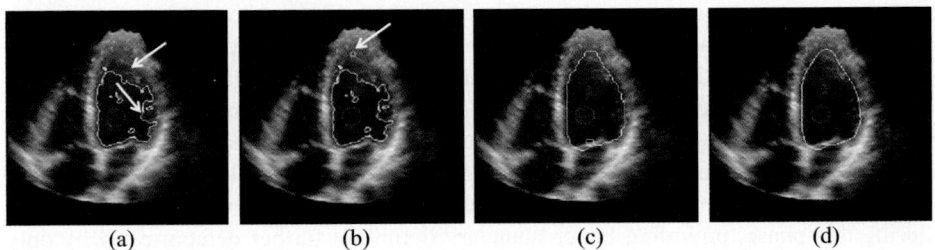

Fig. 2. Post-processing operations shown on a 2D end-diastolic slice. Red circle inside the LV cavity is the initial contour placed automatically. (a) LS segmentation (arrows indicate the problematic regions), (b) apex adjustment (arrow indicates the placement of sphere), (c) segmentation after surface fitting, and (d) smoothed final segmentation.

3 Experimental Results

3.1 Data and Experimental Setup

Volumetric images (17 cases) were obtained from healthy young subjects using the Philips iE33 scanner (Philips Medical Systems, Andover, USA) with a matrix-array transducer (3-5 MHz), acquiring a full-volume sequence by ECG-gating over 4 heartbeats. The usual spatial dimensions are 224x208x208 voxels. For each case, 3 to 8 single-view images were acquired and fused using the wavelet fusion (see 2.1). To assess the fused image for automatic quantification, the LV segmentation method (see 2.2) was applied to the fused image and one single-view image (the reference volume as in 2.1). For almost all of the subjects, the reference single-view image was of better quality (in terms of anatomical information) than the other single-view images.

End-diastolic (ED) and end-systolic (ES) frames for each dataset were identified by an expert cardiologist. The segmentation method was applied to the ED and ES phases of both fused and reference single-view images. The segmentation was initialized automatically as a sphere of 10-voxels radius at the centre of the image. The automatic initialization in this way was inside the LV cavity for all the cases except for two ED images, in which case manual initialization was needed. The successful convergence (the ability to reach near the LV endocardial border) of the segmentation method was quantified and the clear failures of the method were visually classified according to the possible causes: (i) LV cavity speckle noise, (ii) boundary leakage due to insufficient boundary information at the endocardial border, and (iii) both leakage and noise. To validate the successful segmentation cases, the fused images were also manually segmented by an expert cardiologist using commercial software (CardioView, TomTec, Germany) to obtain measurements for ED volume (EDV), ES volume (ESV), and ejection fraction (EF). LV trabeculations and papillary muscles were included within the LV cavity. In addition, magnetic resonance images (MRI) from all the cases were acquired for reference and the EDV, ESV, and EF measurements were calculated by an expert cardiologist.

3.2 Results

Fig. 3 shows example segmentation results on both single-view and fused images, demonstrating the lack of sufficient information in the single-view images for a successful segmentation. On the other hand, the same segmentation method works successfully on a fused image. Table 1 summarizes the segmentation failures for single-view images, while there were no failures on the fused images. For single-view images, the algorithm failed in most cases at both end-diastole (88.2%) and end-systole (58.8%). There were fewer failures at ES because the myocardium is thicker during this phase, providing better boundary definition further demonstrated by only 30% failures at ES due to leakage or leakage and noise compared to 60% failures at ED. The absolute difference in EDV, ESV, and EF measurements is given in Table 2. The RT3DE EDV and ESV are underestimated compared to MRI, which has been reported before [1]. The EDV differences with automatic RT3DE (55.9 ± 23.1) and manual RT3DE (64.5 ± 19.9) in comparison to MRI are considerably underestimated, probably due to large MRI EDVs (205.8 ± 19.7) because the scanned subjects were young athletes having large hearts. However, the clinically important EF measure is within the known reproducibility range [1] (see Table 2). Fig. 4 presents Bland-Altman analysis demonstrating that there is a good statistical agreement between the automatic and manual RT3DE and MRI measurements.

Table 1. Failure of segmentation on single-view images (17 datasets) and its quantification. There were no failures on multiview fused images.

	End-diastolic phase	End-systolic phase
Total Failure	88.2% (**15**)	58.8% (**10**)
Cavity noise	40% (6)	70% (7)
Boundary leakage	13% (2)	20% (2)
Leakage + noise	47% (7)	10% (1)

Table 2. Absolute differences in quantification of EDV, ESV, and EF (*17* datasets). AEcho – Automatic measurements. MEcho – Manual measurements. MRI – MRI measurements. The differences are given as average ± standard deviation.

	AEcho vs. MEcho	MEcho vs. MRI	AEcho vs. MRI
EDV (mL)	14.6 ± 6.9	64.5 ± 19.9	55.9 ± 23.1
ESV (mL)	9.1 ± 6.2	20.0 ± 9.7	18.0 ± 11.5
EF (%)	5.9 ± 4.9	5.0 ± 7.0	8.3 ± 4.9

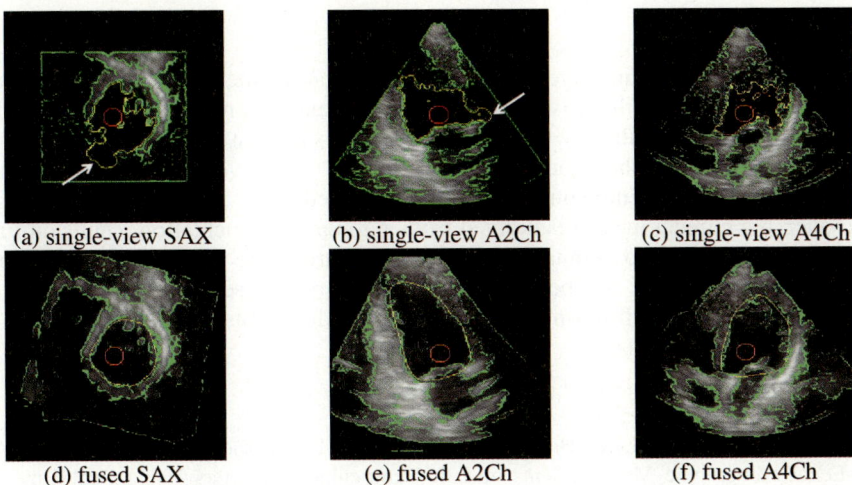

Fig. 3. Segmentation results on orthogonal planes. Red – automatic initialization. Green – edge-indicator features. Yellow – segmentation result. SAX – Short-axis plane. A 2Ch – Apical 2-chamber plane. A4Ch – Apical 4-chamber plane. Arrows indicate failure of the segmentation due to leakage. No post-processing was performed on the single-view image due to failure.

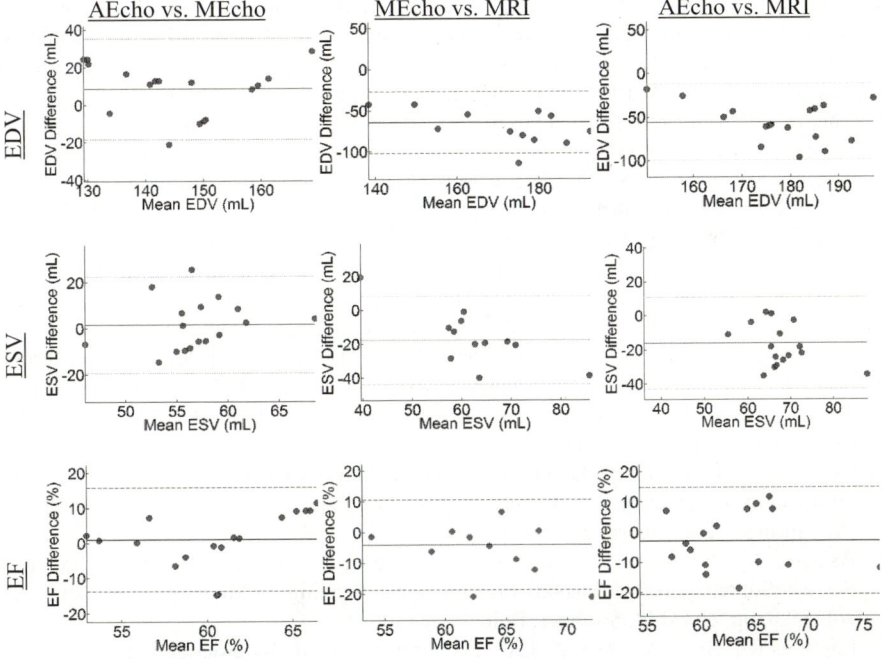

Fig. 4. Bland-Altman analysis of EDV (mL), ESV (mL), and EF (%). Average difference and 95% confidence interval are displayed as solid and dashed lines, respectively.

4 Conclusions

This work introduced an edge-driven LS segmentation method while using local-phase derived edges as the driving force. The segmentation method was then applied for the evaluation of multiview fused RT3DE images against the conventional single-view RT3DE images. The experiments indicate that a relatively simple segmentation method does much better on the multiview fused than in single-view images. Moreover, the clinical measures derived from automatic segmentation results on fused images are very close to manually computed measures. The results thus demonstrate that the fused images are better suited for automated segmentation because of improved anatomical definition and noise reduction due to fusion.

References

1. Jenkins, C., Bricknell, K., Hanekom, L., Marwick, T.: Reproducibility and Accuracy of Echocardiographic Measurements of Left Ventricular Parameters Using Real-Time 3-D Echocardiography. Journal of the American College of Cardiology 44 (2004)
2. Zagrodsky, V., Walimbe, V., Castro-Pareja, C., Qin, J.X., Song, J.-M., Shekhar, R.: Registration-Assisted Segmentation of Real-Time 3-D Echocardiographic Data Using Deformable Models. IEEE Transactions on Medical Imaging 24, 1089–1099 (2005)
3. Corsi, C., Saracino, G., Sarti, A., Lamberti, C.: Left Ventricular Volume Estimation for Real-Time Three-Dimensional Echocardiography. IEEE Trans. MI 21, 1202–1208 (2002)
4. Casselles, V., Kimmel, R., Sapiro, G.: Geodesic Active Contours. IJCV 22, 61–79 (1997)
5. Angelini, E.D., Homma, S., Pearson, G., Holmes, J.W., Laine, A.F.: Segmentation of RT3D Ultrasound for Quantification of Ventricular Function: A Clinical Study on Right and Left Ventricles. Ultrasound in Med. & Biol. 31, 1143–1158 (2005)
6. Zhu, Y., Papademetris, X., Sinusas, A.J., Duncan, J.S.: Segmentation of myocardial volumes from real-time 3D echocardiography using an incompressibility constraint. In: Ayache, N., Ourselin, S., Maeder, A. (eds.) MICCAI 2007, Part I. LNCS, vol. 4791, pp. 44–51. Springer, Heidelberg (2007)
7. Stralen, M.V., Leung, K.Y.E., Voormolen, M.M., et al.: Automatic Segmentation of the Left Ventricle in 3D Echcoardiography Using Active Appearance Models. In: IEEE Ultrasonics Symposium, pp. 1480–1483 (2007)
8. Hansegard, J., Orderud, F., Rabben, S.I.: Real-Time Active Shape Models for Segmentation of 3D Cardiac Ultrasound. Computer Analysis of Images & Patterns (2007)
9. Soler, P., Gerard, O., Allain, P., Saloux, E., Angelini, E., Bloch, I.: Comparison of Fusion Techniques for 3D+T Echocardiography Acquisitions from Different Acoustic Windows. Computers in Cardiology, 141–144 (2005)
10. Grau, V., Noble, J.A.: Adaptive multiscale ultrasound compounding using phase information. In: Duncan, J.S., Gerig, G. (eds.) MICCAI 2005. LNCS, vol. 3749, pp. 589–596. Springer, Heidelberg (2005)
11. Rajpoot, K., Noble, J.A., Grau, V., Szmigielski, C., Becher, H.: Multiview RT3D Echocardiography Image Fusion. In: Functional Imaging & Modeling of Heart. LNCS, vol. 5528, pp. 134–143. Springer, Heidelberg (2009)
12. Rajpoot, K., Grau, V., Noble, J.A.: Local-phase Based 3D Boundary Detection using Monogenic Signal and its Application to RT3D Echocardiography Images. In: ISBI (2009)
13. Yushkevich, P.A., Piven, J., Hazlett, H.C., Smith, R.G., Ho, S., Gee, J.C., Gerig, G.: Userguided 3D Active Contour Segmentation of Anatomical Structures: Significantly Improved Efficiency and Reliability. NeuroImage 31 (2006)

Left Ventricle Segmentation via Graph Cut Distribution Matching

Ismail Ben Ayed[1], Kumaradevan Punithakumar[1], Shuo Li[1], Ali Islam[2], and Jaron Chong[3]

[1] GE Healthcare, London, ON, Canada
[2] St. Joseph's Health Care, London, ON, Canada
[3] University of Western Ontario, London, ON, Canada

Abstract. We present a discrete kernel density matching energy for segmenting the left ventricle cavity in cardiac magnetic resonance sequences. The energy and its graph cut optimization based on an original first-order approximation of the Bhattacharyya measure have not been proposed previously, and yield competitive results in nearly real-time. The algorithm seeks a region within each frame by optimization of two priors, one geometric (distance-based) and the other photometric, each measuring a distribution similarity between the region and a model learned from the first frame. Based on global rather than pixelwise information, the proposed algorithm does not require complex training and optimization with respect to geometric transformations. Unlike related active contour methods, it does not compute iterative updates of computationally expensive kernel densities. Furthermore, the proposed first-order analysis can be used for other intractable energies and, therefore, can lead to segmentation algorithms which share the flexibility of active contours and computational advantages of graph cuts. Quantitative evaluations over 2280 images acquired from 20 subjects demonstrated that the results correlate well with independent manual segmentations by an expert.

1 Introduction

Accurate segmentation of the left ventricle (LV) cavity in magnetic resonance (MR) sequences is very important for complete diagnosis of cardiovascular diseases [1], [3]. Manual segmentation of all images is prohibitively time-consuming. Therefore, automatic or semi-automatic algorithms are highly desired. Albeit an impressive research effort has been devoted to the LV [1]–[15], current methods are still not sufficiently fast and flexible for routine clinical use, mainly because of the difficulties inherent to MR cardiac images [4]. Existing methods are based, among others, on active contours [1]–[3], [5]–[11], active appearance/shape models [12], [14], and registration [15]. Generally, the problem is stated as an energy optimization. In this connection, optimization of active contour functionals has been the most prevalent and flexible choice in the literature because it allows introducing a wide range of photometric and geometric[1] constraints on the solution [1]–[3], [5]–[11]. Generally, these constraints reference a sum over the target region or its boundary of *pixelwise* correspondences between the

---
[1] Geometric constraints reference object shape, position, and size.

image and geometric/photometric models learned from a training set. Pixelwise photometric information cannot distinguish connected cardiac regions having almost the same photometric profile [1]–[3], for instance the papillary muscles within the cavity and the myocardium (cf. the examples in Fig. 1). Therefore, most of existing methods bias the solution towards a finite set of shapes learned *a priori*. Although very effective in some cases, training-based algorithms may have difficulty in capturing the substantial subject variations in a clinical context [1], [3], [4]. The ensuing results are bounded to the characteristics, variability, and mathematical description of the training set. For instance, a pathological case outside the set of learned shapes may not be recovered, and photometric models have to be updated for new acquisition protocols and sequences.

To relax dependence on a statistical training, the studies in [1]–[3] investigated active contour optimization of *intensity matching* criteria, given a user-provided segmentation of one frame. In [3], the authors propose to maintain a constant photometric environment in the vicinity of the cavity boundary propagated over the sequence. Based on a global similarity measure between distributions, the method in [1], [2] maintains over a cardiac sequence a constant overlap between the intensity distributions of the cavity and myocardium, which led to promising results for mid-cavity images. Based only on the current data, these methods allow more flexibility in clinical use, although at the price of a user initialization. Furthermore, in the context of general-purpose methods, recent studies have shown that the use of *global* distribution-matching measures outperforms standard segmentation techniques based on pixelwise information, and is less sensitive to inaccuracies in estimating the models [16]–[18]. As such, it can relax the need of complex training. Unfortunately, optimization of a global measure with respect to segmentation is *NP-hard* [21], and the problem has been commonly addressed with active contours [1], [2], [16]–[18], which lead to computationally intensive algorithms. Along with an incremental contour evolution, the methods in [1], [2], [16]–[18] require a large number of updates of computationally onerous integrals, namely, the distributions of the regions defined by the contour at each iteration and the corresponding measures. Active contour methods rely on stepwise gradient descent. As a result, the algorithms are notoriously slow, converge to a local minimum, and depend on the choice of an approximating numerical scheme of contour evolution and the corresponding parameters.

This study investigates a *discrete* distribution-matching energy defined over a binary labeling, based on the Bhattacharyya kernel, and containing two priors, one geometric (distance-based) and the other photometric, each measuring a distribution similarity between the target region and a model. The ensuing problem is *NP-hard*, and the energy does not afford an analytical form amenable to graph cut optimization. To address efficiently the problem, we propose an original first-order approximation of the Bhattacharyya measure by introducing an auxiliary labeling, thereby computing a global graph cut optimum in nearly real-time. Unlike active contours, the algorithm does not compute iterative integral updates. It requires only a graph cut. The energy removes the need of a training, and prevents the papillary muscles from being included in the myocardium. Based on a distance distribution, the geometric prior handles intrinsically variations of the LV without biasing the solution towards a finite set of shapes, and relaxes optimization over geometric transformations. Furthermore, the proposed first-order analysis can be used for other intractable energies and, therefore, can lead to segmentation algorithms which share the flexibility of active contours and computational advantages of graph cuts. Evaluations and comparisons with [1] demonstrated that the proposed method brings improvements in accuracy and computational efficiency.

2 Formulation

Consider a MR cardiac sequence containing N image functions[2] $\mathbf{I}_p^n = \mathbf{I}^n(p) : \mathcal{P} \subset \mathbb{N} \to \mathcal{I}$, $n \in [1..N]$, with $\mathcal{P}$ the positional array and $\mathcal{I}$ the space of photometric variables. Our purpose is to automatically detect the cavity of the heart in each frame $n \in [2..N]$ (cf. Fig. 1). For $n \in [2..N]$, we state the problem as the minimization of a *discrete* cost function with respect to a binary variable (labeling), $\mathcal{L}^n(p) : \mathcal{P} \to \{0,1\}$, which defines a variable partition of $\mathcal{P}$: the *heart cavity* $\mathbf{C}^n$ corresponding to region $\{p \in \mathcal{P} / \mathcal{L}^n(p) = 1\}$ and its complement, the *background* $\mathbf{B}^n$ corresponding to region $\{p \in \mathcal{P} / \mathcal{L}^n(p) = 0\}$. The optimal labeling is sought by minimizing an original energy designed to address the problems related to cardiac MR images and containing two *kernel density matching* terms, an *intensity matching* term and a *distance matching* term. To introduce our energy, we first consider the following definitions for any labeling $\mathcal{L} : \mathcal{P} \to \{0,1\}$, any image $\mathbf{I} : \mathcal{P} \to \mathcal{I}$, and any space of variables $\mathcal{I}$.

- $\mathbf{P}^{\mathcal{I}}_{\mathcal{L},\mathbf{I}}$ is the kernel density estimate (KDE) of the distribution of image data $\mathbf{I}$ within region $\mathbf{R}_{\mathcal{L}} = \{p \in \mathcal{P} / \mathcal{L}(p) = 1\}$

$$\forall i \in \mathcal{I}, \quad \mathbf{P}^{\mathcal{I}}_{\mathcal{L},\mathbf{I}}(i) = \frac{\sum_{p \in \mathbf{R}_{\mathcal{L}}} K(i - \mathbf{I}_p)}{\mathbf{A}_{\mathcal{L}}}, \quad \text{with } K(y) = \frac{1}{\sqrt{2\pi\sigma^2}} exp^{-\frac{y^2}{2\sigma^2}}, \quad (1)$$

$\mathbf{A}_{\mathcal{L}}$ is the number of pixels within $\mathbf{R}_{\mathcal{L}}$: $\mathbf{A}_{\mathcal{L}} = \sum_{\mathbf{R}_{\mathcal{L}}} 1$, and σ is the width of the Gaussian kernel. Note that choosing K equal to the Dirac function yields the histogram.

- $\mathcal{B}(f,g)$ is the *Bhattacharyya coefficient*[3] measuring the amount of overlap (similarity) between two distributions f and g: $\mathcal{B}(f,g) = \sum_{i \in \mathcal{I}} \sqrt{f(i)g(i)}$.

We assume that a segmentation of frame $\mathbf{I}^1$, i.e., a labeling $\mathcal{L}^1$ defining a partition $\{\mathbf{C}^1, \mathbf{B}^1\}$, is given. Using this prior information from the first frame in the current data, the intensity/geometry model distributions of the cavity are learned, and embedded in the following distribution matching constraints to segment subsequent frames.

Intensity matching term. Given the learned model distribution of intensity, which we denote $\mathbf{M}^{\mathcal{I}} = \mathbf{P}^{\mathcal{I}}_{\mathcal{L}^1,\mathbf{I}^1}$, the purpose of this term is to find for each subsequent frame $\mathbf{I}^n$ a region $\mathbf{C}^n$ whose intensity distribution most closely matches $\mathbf{M}^{\mathcal{I}}$. To this end, we minimizes the following intensity matching function with respect to $\mathcal{L}$:

$$\mathcal{B}^{\mathcal{I}}(\mathcal{L}, \mathbf{I}^n) = -\mathcal{B}(\mathbf{P}^{\mathcal{I}}_{\mathcal{L},\mathbf{I}^n}, \mathbf{M}^{\mathcal{I}}) = -\sum_{i \in \mathcal{I}} \sqrt{\mathbf{P}^{\mathcal{I}}_{\mathcal{L},\mathbf{I}^n}(i) \mathbf{M}^{\mathcal{I}}(i)} \quad (2)$$

Distance matching term. The purpose of this term is to constrain the segmentation with prior geometric information (shape, scale, and position of the cavity) obtained

---
[2] The number of frames N is typically equal to 20 or 25.
[3] Note that the values of $\mathcal{B}$ are always in $[0, 1]$, where 0 indicates that there is no overlap, and 1 indicates a perfect match between the distributions.

from the learning frame. Let c be the centroid of cavity $\mathbf{C}^1$ in the learning frame and $\mathbf{D}(p) = \frac{\|p-c\|}{N_\mathbf{D}} : \mathcal{P} \to \mathcal{D}$ a *distance image* measuring at each point $p \in \mathcal{P}$ the normalized distance between p and c, with $\mathcal{D}$ the space of distance variables and $N_\mathbf{D}$ a normalization constant. Let $\mathbf{M}^\mathcal{D} = \mathbf{P}^\mathcal{D}_{\mathcal{L}^1,\mathbf{D}}$ the model distribution of distances within the cavity in the learning frame. We propose to find a region $\mathbf{C}^n$ whose distance distribution most closely matches $\mathbf{M}^\mathcal{D}$ by minimizing:

$$\mathcal{B}^\mathcal{D}(\mathcal{L}, \mathbf{D}) = -\mathcal{B}(\mathbf{P}^\mathcal{D}_{\mathcal{L},\mathbf{D}}, \mathbf{M}^\mathcal{D}) = -\sum_{d \in \mathcal{D}} \sqrt{\mathbf{P}^\mathcal{D}_{\mathcal{L},\mathbf{D}}(d) \mathbf{M}^\mathcal{D}(d)} \tag{3}$$

Note that this geometric prior is invariant to rotation, and embeds *implicitly* uncertainties with respect to scale via the kernel width σ in (1). The higher σ, the more scale variations allowed. In our experiments, $\sigma = 2$ was sufficient to handle effectively variations in the scale of the cavity (cf. the examples in Fig. 1). The proposed geometric prior relaxes (1) complex learning/modeling of geometric characteristics and the need of a training set and (2) *explicit* optimization with respect to geometric transformations.

The proposed energy function. We propose to minimize an energy containing the intensity/distance matching terms and a regularization term for smooth segmentation boundaries. For each $n \in [2..N]$, the algorithm computes the optimal labeling $\mathcal{L}^n_{opt}$ minimizing the following discrete cost function over all $\mathcal{L} : \mathcal{P} \to \{0,1\}$:

$$\mathcal{F}(\mathcal{L}, \mathbf{I}^n) = \underbrace{\mathcal{B}^\mathcal{I}(\mathcal{L}, \mathbf{I}^n)}_{Intensity\ Matching} + \underbrace{\mathcal{B}^\mathcal{D}(\mathcal{L}, \mathbf{D})}_{Geometry\ Matching} + \underbrace{\lambda \mathbf{S}(\mathcal{L})}_{Smoothness} \tag{4}$$

where $\mathbf{S}(\mathcal{L})$ is related to the length of the partition boundary given by [22]:

$$\mathbf{S}(\mathcal{L}) = \sum_{\{p,q\} \in \mathcal{N}} \frac{1}{\|p-q\|} \delta_{\mathcal{L}(p) \neq \mathcal{L}(q)}, \text{ with } \delta_{x \neq y} = \begin{cases} 1 & \text{if } x \neq y \\ 0 & \text{if } x = y \end{cases} \tag{5}$$

and $\mathcal{N}$ is a neighborhood system containing all unordered pairs $\{p,q\}$ of neighboring elements of $\mathcal{P}$. λ is a positive constant that balances the relative contribution of $\mathbf{S}$.

Global and efficient graph cut optimization. Optimization of the distribution matching functions in $\mathcal{F}(\mathcal{L}, \mathbf{I}^n)$ is not directly amenable to graph cut computation. It is an *NP-hard* problem. Furthermore, gradient-based optimization procedures are computationally very expensive and difficult to apply. To solve this problem efficiently, we propose a *first-order approximation* of the Bhattacharyya measures in $\mathcal{F}(\mathcal{L}, \mathbf{I}^n)$ by introducing an *auxiliary*[4] labeling which corresponds to an arbitrary, fixed partition. For any labeling $\mathcal{L}$, we rewrite the intensity matching term minus a constant as follows:

$$\mathcal{B}^\mathcal{I}(\mathcal{L}, \mathbf{I}^n) - \underbrace{\mathcal{B}^\mathcal{I}(\mathcal{L}_a, \mathbf{I}^n)}_{Constant} \approx \underbrace{\sum_{p \in \mathcal{P}} \delta \mathcal{B}^\mathcal{I}_{p,\mathcal{L}_a,\mathcal{L}}}_{Variations\ of\ \mathcal{B}^\mathcal{I}} \approx -\frac{1}{2} \sum_{p \in \mathcal{P}} \sum_{i \in \mathcal{I}} \sqrt{\frac{\mathbf{M}^\mathcal{I}(i)}{\mathbf{P}^\mathcal{I}_{\mathcal{L}_a,\mathbf{I}^n}(i)}} \delta \mathbf{P}^\mathcal{I}_{p,\mathcal{L}_a,\mathcal{L}}(i), \tag{6}$$

---

[4] Note that $\mathcal{L}_a$ is an arbitrary fixed labeling which can be obtained from a given segmentation of the first frame.

where $\delta\mathcal{B}^{\mathcal{I}}_{p,\mathcal{L}_a,\mathcal{L}}$ (respectively $\delta\mathbf{P}^{\mathcal{I}}_{p,\mathcal{L}_a,\mathcal{L}}(i)$) is the *elementary variation* of $\mathcal{B}^{\mathcal{I}}(\mathcal{L}_a, \mathbf{I}^n)$ (respectively $\mathbf{P}^{\mathcal{I}}_{\mathcal{L}_a,\mathbf{I}^n}(i)$) that corresponds to changing the label of pixel p from $\mathcal{L}_a(p)$ to $\mathcal{L}(p)$. Elementary variation $\delta\mathcal{B}^{\mathcal{I}}_{p,\mathcal{L}_a,\mathcal{L}}$ is computed in the rightmost approximation of (6) with the *first-order expansion* of the Bhattacharyya measure $\mathcal{B}^{\mathcal{I}}(\mathcal{L}, \mathbf{I}^n)$. Now we compute elementary variations $\delta\mathbf{P}^{\mathcal{I}}_{p,\mathcal{L}_a,\mathcal{L}}(i)$, $i \in \mathcal{I}$, using the expression of the kernel density estimate in (1), which yields after some algebraic manipulations:

$$\delta\mathbf{P}^{\mathcal{I}}_{p,\mathcal{L}_a,\mathcal{L}}(i) = \begin{cases} \delta_{\mathcal{L}_a(p)\neq 1} \frac{K(i-\mathbf{I}^n_p) - \mathbf{P}^{\mathcal{I}}_{\mathcal{L}_a,\mathbf{I}^n}(i)}{\mathbf{A}_{\mathcal{L}_a}+1} & \text{if } \mathcal{L}(p) = 1 \\ \delta_{\mathcal{L}_a(p)\neq 0} \frac{\mathbf{P}^{\mathcal{I}}_{\mathcal{L}_a,\mathbf{I}^n}(i) - K(i-\mathbf{I}^n_p)}{\mathbf{A}_{\mathcal{L}_a}-1} & \text{if } \mathcal{L}(p) = 0 \end{cases} \quad (7)$$

where $\delta_{x\neq y}$ given by (5). Finally, using (7) in (6) and after some manipulations, the intensity matching term reads as the sum of *unary penalties* plus a constant:

$$\mathcal{B}^{\mathcal{I}}(\mathcal{L}, \mathbf{I}^n) \approx constant + \sum_{p\in\mathcal{P}} \mathbf{b}^{\mathcal{I}}_{p,\mathbf{I}^n}(\mathcal{L}(p)), \quad (8)$$

with $\mathbf{b}^{\mathcal{I}}_{p,\mathbf{I}}$ given, for any image $\mathbf{I}: \mathcal{P} \to \mathcal{I}$ and any space of variables $\mathcal{I}$, by

$$\mathbf{b}^{\mathcal{I}}_{p,\mathbf{I}}(1) = \frac{\delta_{\mathcal{L}_a(p)\neq 1}}{2(\mathbf{A}_{\mathcal{L}_a}+1)} \left(\mathcal{B}^{\mathcal{I}}(\mathcal{L}_a, \mathbf{I}) - \sum_{i\in\mathcal{I}} K(i-\mathbf{I}_p) \sqrt{\frac{\mathbf{M}^{\mathcal{I}}(i)}{\mathbf{P}^{\mathcal{I}}_{\mathcal{L}_a,\mathbf{I}}(i)}} \right)$$

$$\mathbf{b}^{\mathcal{I}}_{p,\mathbf{I}}(0) = \frac{\delta_{\mathcal{L}_a(p)\neq 0}}{2(\mathbf{A}_{\mathcal{L}_a}-1)} \left(\sum_{i\in\mathcal{I}} K(i-\mathbf{I}_p) \sqrt{\frac{\mathbf{M}^{\mathcal{I}}(i)}{\mathbf{P}^{\mathcal{I}}_{\mathcal{L}_a,\mathbf{I}}(i)}} - \mathcal{B}^{\mathcal{I}}(\mathcal{L}_a, \mathbf{I}) \right) \quad (9)$$

Using a similar computation for the distance matching term, adopting the same notation in (9) for distance image $\mathbf{D}$, and ignoring the constants, our problem reduces to optimizing the following sum of unary and pairwise (submodular) penalties:

$$\mathcal{L}_{opt} = \arg\min_{\mathcal{L}:\mathcal{P}\to\{0,1\}} \sum_{p\in\mathcal{P}} \{\mathbf{b}^{\mathcal{I}}_{p,\mathbf{I}^n}(\mathcal{L}(p)) + \mathbf{b}^{\mathcal{D}}_{p,\mathbf{D}}(\mathcal{L}(p))\} + \lambda \mathbf{S}(\mathcal{L}) \quad (10)$$

In combinatorial optimization, a *global optimum* of the sum of unary and pairwise (submodular) penalties can be computed efficiently in *low-order polynomial time* by solving an equivalent max-flow problem [20]. In our case, it suffices to build a *weighted* graph $\mathcal{G} = \langle \mathbf{N}, \mathbf{E} \rangle$, where $\mathbf{N}$ is the set of nodes and $\mathbf{E}$ the set of edges connecting these nodes. $\mathbf{N}$ contains a node for each pixel $p \in \mathcal{P}$ and two additional terminal nodes, one representing the foreground region (i.e., the cavity), denoted $\mathbf{T_F}$, and the other representing the background, denoted $\mathbf{T_B}$. Let $\mathbf{w}_{p,q}$ be the weight of the edge connecting neighboring pixels $\{p,q\}$ in $\mathcal{N}$, and $\{\mathbf{w}_{p,\mathbf{T_F}}, \mathbf{w}_{p,\mathbf{T_B}}\}$ the weights of the edges connecting each pixel p to each of the terminals. By setting the edge weights as follows:

$$\mathbf{w}_{p,\mathbf{T_F}} = \mathbf{b}^{\mathcal{I}}_{p,\mathbf{I}^n}(0) + \mathbf{b}^{\mathcal{D}}_{p,\mathbf{D}}(0); \quad \mathbf{w}_{p,\mathbf{T_B}} = \mathbf{b}^{\mathcal{I}}_{p,\mathbf{I}^n}(1) + \mathbf{b}^{\mathcal{D}}_{p,\mathbf{D}}(1); \quad \mathbf{w}_{p,q} = \frac{\lambda}{\|p-q\|},$$

we compute, using the max-flow algorithm of Boykov and Kolmogorov [20], a minimum cut $\mathcal{C}^n_{opt}$ of $\mathcal{G}$, i.e., a subset of edges in $\mathbf{E}$ whose removal divides the graph into two disconnected subgraphs, each containing a terminal node, and whose sum of edge weights is minimal. This minimum cut, which assigns each node (pixel) p in $\mathcal{P}$ to one of the two terminals, induces an optimal labeling $\mathcal{L}_{opt}^n$ ($\mathcal{L}_{opt}^n(p) = 1$ if p is connected to $\mathbf{T_F}$ and $\mathcal{L}_{opt}^n(p) = 0$ if p is connected to $\mathbf{T_B}$), which minimizes globally the approximation in (10) and, therefore, the proposed energy function.

3 Experimental Evaluations and Comparisons

We applied the method to 120 short axis cardiac cine MR sequences acquired from 20 subjects: a total of 2280 images including apical, mid-cavity and basal slices were automatically segmented, and the results were compared to independent manual segmentations by an expert. Using the same datasets, we compared the accuracy and computational load/time of the proposed method with the recent LV segmentation in [1]. Similar to [1], the proposed method relaxes the need of a training, and model distributions were learned from a user-provided segmentation of the first frame in each sequence. The regularization and kernel width parameters were unchanged for all the datasets: λ is fixed equal to 0.15, and kernel width σ is set equal to 2 for distance distributions, and equal to 10 for intensity distributions. In Fig. 1, we give a representative sample of the results for 2 subjects. Although it uses information from only one frame in the current data, the method handles implicitly variations in the scale/shape of the

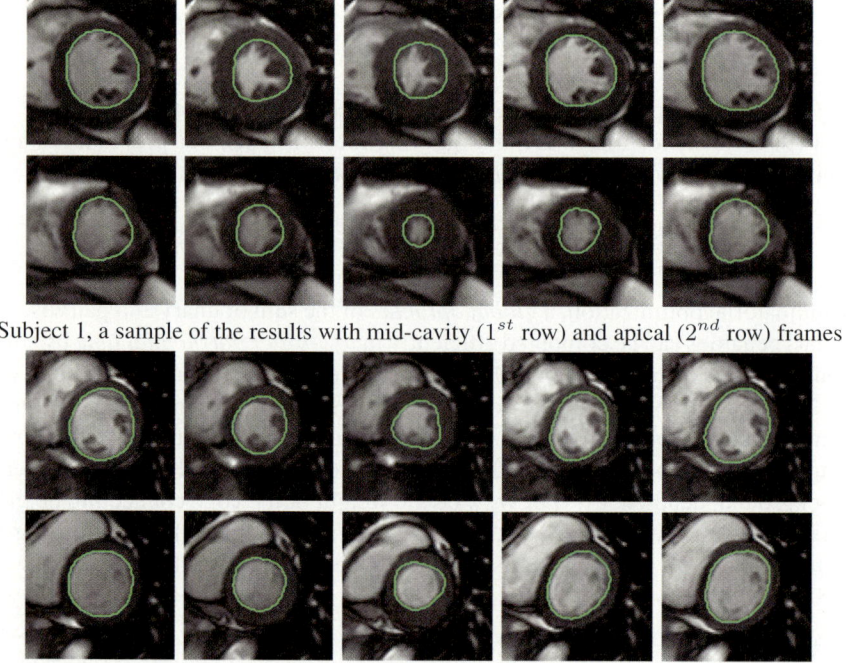

Subject 1, a sample of the results with mid-cavity (1st row) and apical (2nd row) frames

Subject 2, a sample of the results with mid-cavity (1st row) and basal (2nd row) frames

Fig. 1. A representative sample of the results for 2 subjects

Table 1. *Dice metrics (DM expressed as mean $\pm$ standard deviation) and Reliability function ($\mathcal{R}(d) = Pr(DM > d)$). The higher the DM and $\mathcal{R}$, the better the performance.*

Performance measure	DM	$\mathcal{R}(0.80)$	$\mathcal{R}(0.85)$	$\mathcal{R}(0.90)$
Proposed method	0.91 ± 0.04	0.97	0.93	0.80
Method in [1]	0.88 ± 0.09	0.89	0.85	0.72

Table 2. Computation time (CPU) and number of kernel density estimations (KDEs) for the proposed method and the curve evolution method in [1]

Computation time/load	Average CPU/frame	Average CPU/subject	Nb of KDEs/frame
Proposed method	$0.08\ sec$	$9.62\ secs$	1
Method in [1]	$4.33\ secs$	$494.45\ secs$	300

cavity and prevents the papillary muscles from being included erroneously in the myocardium. Therefore, its relaxes the need of complex training and optimization over geometric transformations.

Dice metric. We evaluated the *Dice Metric* (DM) commonly used to measure the similarity (overlap) between manual and automatic segmentations [1], [6], [7]. Let $\mathbf{V_a}$, $\mathbf{V_m}$ and $\mathbf{V_{am}}$ be the volumes[5] of, respectively, the automatically segmented cavity, the corresponding hand-labeled cavity, and the intersection between them. DM is given by[6]: $DM = \frac{2\mathbf{V_{am}}}{\mathbf{V_a}+\mathbf{V_m}}$. The proposed method yielded a DM equal to 0.91 ± 0.04 for all the data analyzed (DM is expressed as mean $\pm$ standard deviation). Table 1 reports DM statistics for the proposed method and [1]. Using the same data, the method in [1] yielded a DM equal to 0.88 ± 0.09. Fig. 2 (a) depicts the DM for a representative sample of the analyzed volumes. The proposed method led to a significant improvement in average accuracy. Note that an average DM higher than 0.80 indicates an excellent agreement with manual segmentations [7], and an average DM higher than 0.90 is, generally, difficult to obtain because the small structure of the cavity at the apex decreases significantly the DM [6]. For instance, the study in [6] reports a DM equal to 0.81 ± 0.16 whereas the authors in [7] report a DM equal to 0.88 ± 0.06.

Reliability. we examined quantitatively and comparatively the *reliability* of the algorithm by evaluating the *reliability function*–i.e., the complementary cumulative distribution function (ccdf)–of the obtained Dice metrics, defined for each $d \in [0, 1]$ as the probability of obtaining DM higher than d over all volumes: $\mathcal{R}(d) = Pr(DM > d)$ =(number of volumes segmented with DM higher than d)/(total number of volumes). $\mathcal{R}(d)$ measures how reliable the algorithm in yielding accuracy d. For the proposed method and [1], we report in Table 1 the reliability of different accuracy levels ($d = 0.80, d = 0.85, d = 0.90$), and plot $\mathcal{R}$ as a function of d in Fig. 2 (c). Our algorithm led to a higher reliability curve and 8% improvement in reliabilities. For instance, we obtained $\mathcal{R}(0.80) = 0.97$, i.e, an excellent agreement ($DM > 0.80$) in 97% of the cases, whereas the method in [1] achieved 89% of the cases with a similar accuracy.

---

[5] The volume is measured by the sum of areas of the cavity region in 6 segmented images.
[6] DM is always in $[0, 1]$. DM equal to 1 indicates a perfect match between segmentations.

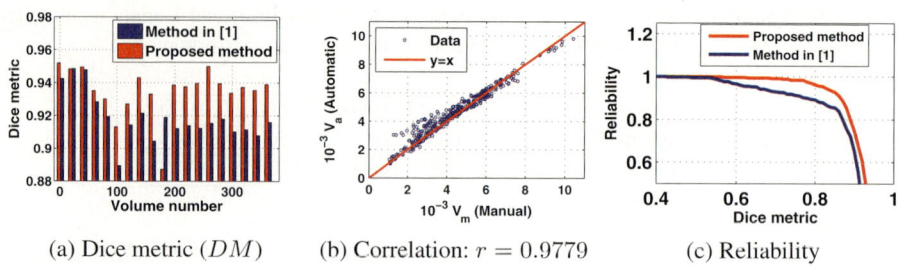

(a) Dice metric (DM)   (b) Correlation: $r = 0.9779$ (c) Reliability

Fig. 2. Comparisons of manual and automatic segmentations of 2280 images (380 volumes) acquired from 20 subjects. (a) Dice metric (DM) in a representative sample of the tested volumes for the proposed method and [1]. (b) Automatic volumes versus manual volumes for the proposed method: the obtained *correlation coefficient* is $r = 0.9779$. (c) Reliability ($\mathcal{R}(d) = Pr(DM > d)$) for the proposed method and [1]. The proposed method led to a *higher* reliability curve.

Correlation coefficient. The proposed method yielded a high correlation between manual and automatic segmentations: $r = 0.9779$. The linear regression plot, displayed in Fig. 2 (b) with the identity line, illustrates this correlation.

Computation time/load. Although based on distribution measures, the algorithm led to nearly *real-time* segmentation. Running on a 2 GHz machine, it needs $0.08\ sec$ to process a frame ($12.5\ images/sec$). Table 2 reports the computation time/load for the proposed method and [1]. The proposed approximation leads to a significant decrease in computation load because it requires only a joint kernel density estimation (KDE) and graph cut, whereas the curve evolution in [1] requires approximately 300 KDEs.

References

1. Ben Ayed, I., Li, S., Ross, I.: Embedding Overlap Priors in Variational Left Ventricle Tracking. IEEE Trans. on Medical Imaging (available online) (in press, 2009)
2. Ben Ayed, I., Lu, Y., Li, S., Ross, I.: Left ventricle tracking using overlap priors. In: Metaxas, D., Axel, L., Fichtinger, G., Székely, G. (eds.) MICCAI 2008, Part I. LNCS, vol. 5241, pp. 1025–1033. Springer, Heidelberg (2008)
3. Hautvast, G., Lobregt, S., Breeuwer, M., Gerritsen, F.: Automatic Contour Propagation in Cine Cardiac Magnetic Resonance Images. IEEE Trans. on Medical Imaging 25(11), 1472–1482 (2006)
4. Jolly, M.-P.: Automatic recovery of the left ventricular blood pool in cardiac cine MR images. In: Metaxas, D., Axel, L., Fichtinger, G., Székely, G. (eds.) MICCAI 2008, Part I. LNCS, vol. 5241, pp. 110–118. Springer, Heidelberg (2008)
5. Fradkin, M., Ciofolo, C., Mory, B., Hautvast, G., Breeuwer, M.: Comprehensive segmentation of cine cardiac MR images. In: Metaxas, D., Axel, L., Fichtinger, G., Székely, G. (eds.) MICCAI 2008, Part I. LNCS, vol. 5241, pp. 178–185. Springer, Heidelberg (2008)
6. Lynch, M., Ghita, O., Whelan, P.F.: Segmentation of the Left Ventricle of the Heart in 3-D+t MRI Data Using an Optimized Nonrigid Temporal Model. IEEE Trans. on Medical Imaging 27(2), 195–203 (2008)
7. Pluempitiwiriyawej, C., Moura, J.M.F., Lin Wu, Y.-J., Ho, C.: STACS: new active contour scheme for cardiac MR image segmentation. IEEE Trans. on Medical Imaging 24(5), 593–603 (2005)

8. Sun, W., Çetin, M., Chan, R., Reddy, V., Holmvang, G., Chandar, V., Willsky, A.S.: Segmenting and tracking the left ventricle by learning the dynamics in cardiac images. In: Christensen, G.E., Sonka, M. (eds.) IPMI 2005. LNCS, vol. 3565, pp. 553–565. Springer, Heidelberg (2005)
9. Kausa, M.R., von Berga, J., Weesea, J., Niessenb, W., Pekar, V.: Automated segmentation of the left ventricle in cardiac MRI. Medical Image Analysis 8(3), 245–254 (2004)
10. Paragios, N.: A level set approach for shape-driven segmentation and tracking of the left ventricle. IEEE Trans. on Medical Imaging 22(6), 773–776 (2003)
11. Fritscher, K.D., Pilgram, R., Schubert, R.: Automatic cardiac 4D segmentation using level sets. In: Frangi, A.F., Radeva, P.I., Santos, A., Hernandez, M. (eds.) FIMH 2005. LNCS, vol. 3504, pp. 113–122. Springer, Heidelberg (2005)
12. Andreopoulos, A., Tsotsos, J.K.: Efficient and Generalizable Statistical Models of Shape and Appearance for Analysis of Cardiac MRI. Medical Image Analysis 12(3), 335–357 (2008)
13. Jolly, M.-P.: Automatic Segmentation of the Left Ventricle in Cardiac MR and CT Images. International Journal of Computer Vision 70(2), 151–163 (2006)
14. Zambal, S., Hladůvka, J., Bühler, K.: Improving segmentation of the left ventricle using a two-component statistical model. In: Larsen, R., Nielsen, M., Sporring, J. (eds.) MICCAI 2006. LNCS, vol. 4190, pp. 151–158. Springer, Heidelberg (2006)
15. Zhuang, X., Rhode, K.S., Arridge, S.R., Razavi, R., Hill, D.L.G., Hawkes, D.J., Ourselin, S.: An atlas-based segmentation propagation framework using locally affine registration – application to automatic whole heart segmentation. In: Metaxas, D., Axel, L., Fichtinger, G., Székely, G. (eds.) MICCAI 2008, Part II. LNCS, vol. 5242, pp. 425–433. Springer, Heidelberg (2008)
16. Ben Ayed, I., Li, S., Ross, I.: A Statistical Overlap Prior for Variational Image Segmentation. International Journal of Computer Vision (available online) (in press, 2009)
17. Zhang, T., Freedman, D.: Improving performance of distribution tracking through background mismatch. IEEE Trans. on Pattern Anal. and Machine Intell. 27(2), 282–287 (2005)
18. Freedman, D., Zhang, T.: Active contours for tracking distributions. IEEE Transactions on Image Processing 13(4), 518–526 (2004)
19. Boykov, Y., Funka-Lea, G.: Graph Cuts and Efficient N-D Image Segmentation. Int. J. of Computer Vision 70(2), 109–131 (2006)
20. Boykov, Y., Kolmogorov, V.: An experimental comparison of min-cut/max-flow algorithms for energy minimization in vision. IEEE Trans. on Pattern Anal. and Machine Intell. 26(9), 1124–1137 (2004)
21. Rother, C., Kolmogorov, V., Minka, T., Blake, A.: Cosegmentation of Image Pairs by Histogram Matching–Incorporating a Global Constraint into MRFs. In: CVPR(1), pp. 993–1000 (2006)
22. Boykov, Y., Kolmogorov, V.: Computing geodesics and minimal surfaces via graph cuts. In: ICCV, pp. 26–33 (2003)

Combining Registration and Minimum Surfaces for the Segmentation of the Left Ventricle in Cardiac Cine MR Images

Marie-Pierre Jolly, Hui Xue, Leo Grady, and Jens Guehring

Siemens Corporate Research, Imaging and Visualization Department Princeton, NJ
marie-pierre.jolly@siemens.com

Abstract. This paper describes a system to automatically segment the left ventricle in all slices and all phases of cardiac cine magnetic resonance datasets. After localizing the left ventricle blood pool using motion, thresholding and clustering, slices are segmented sequentially. For each slice, deformable registration is used to align all the phases, candidates contours are recovered in the average image using shortest paths, and a minimal surface is built to generate the final contours. The advantage of our method is that the resulting contours follow the edges in each phase and are consistent over time. We demonstrate using 19 patient examples that the results are very good. The RMS distance between ground truth and our segmentation is only 1.6 pixels (2.7 mm) and the Dice coefficient is 0.89.

1 Introduction

Cardiovascular disease is now the largest cause of death in the modern world and is an important health concern. Physicians use non invasive technologies such as magnetic resonance (MR) imaging to observe the behavior of the heart and more specifically the left ventricle (LV). They want to quantify important measures such as blood pool volume over time, myocardial mass, ejection fraction, cardiac output, peak ejection rate, filling rate, myocardial thickening, which can all be computed with an outline of the LV. Manual outlining in all images is very cumbersome however and most physicians limit it to the end-diastolic (ED) and end-systolic (ES) phases, which is enough to calculate ejection fraction, but not enough to estimate some of the other quantities. This paper proposes a system to automatically segment the LV in all slices and all phases of a cardiac MR cine study.

MR cine consists of 4D (3D+T) data and the segmentation of all the images can be tackled in various ways. Some researchers have attempted 4D segmentation [1]. We believe however that this approach is not feasible, since it is very difficult to build a model that is general enough to cover all possible shapes and dynamics of the LV and a model-free approach would not be constrained enough. The opposite approach of segmenting each image individually [2] results in little cohesion between images and unsmooth contours over time. The intermediate approach used very often of segmenting the LV in one phase on all slices [3,4]

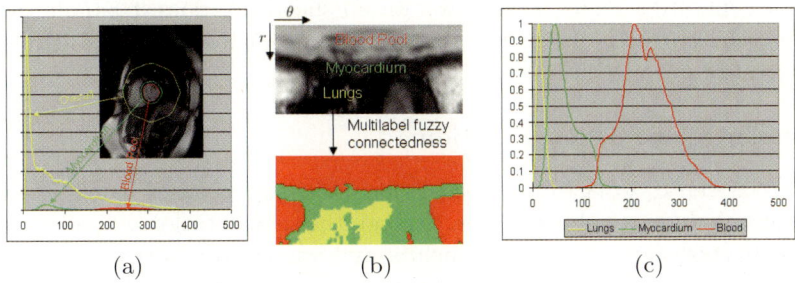

Fig. 1. Gray level analysis: (a) Original histograms; (b) Polar image and multiseeded fuzzy connectedness region labeling; (c) Final histograms

can be quite difficult. When a model is used, it needs to be carefully trained for all possible LV shapes and all possible MR acquisition protocols. Conversely, image-base techniques tend to be ad-hoc. We have chosen instead to segment all phases in one slice and propagate the segmentation between slices. This method can take advantage of the strong temporal correlation between phases to segment individual slices. For temporal propagation, researchers have proposed using a dynamic model of the LV [5,6] while other methods incorporate a tracking component into the recovery for process [7,8]. We use deformable registration to align all phases and generate an average image for segmentation. We use minimal surfaces to enforce consistency between phases so that contours follow image edges in each phase and are smooth over time.

We will describe the different steps of the algorithm and demonstrate on 19 patient datasets that the segmented contours are very close to manually defined ground truth contours.

2 Left Ventricle Segmentation

The proposed algorithm is divided into the following steps: 1) Heart and left ventricle blood pool detection; 2) Polar space transformation; 3) Gray scale analysis; 4) Segmentation of the first slice, which comprises of deformable registration to align all the phases, segmentation of the average temporal image and minimal surface segmentation of all phases; and 5) Segmentation of the other slices. We will describe each of these steps in more details in the next sections.

2.1 Heart and Left Ventricle Blood Pool Detection

For the detection of the heart and the LV blood pool, we use the method proposed by Jolly [9]. It uses the first harmonic of the Fourier transform in each slice to detect the beating heart. Then, blood-like connected components are extracted using Otsu thresholding and characterized by their shape, temporal behavior, position, etc. Finally, isoperimetric clustering is used to group connected components between slices and form the LV blood pool. This process does not generate a blood pool region on all slices, nor does it handle the papillary muscles correctly in the blood pool region, but it is a good starting point for the rest of our algorithm.

2.2 Polar Space Transformation

We have chosen to work in polar space for multiple reasons. First, the contours to be recovered are roughly circular. Second, the segmentation will be performed using a shortest path algorithm which is well known to be biased toward small contours in Cartesian space. In polar space however, all contours have the same size since they start on one side of the image and end on the other, so there is no bias on the length of the contour. Finally, the images in Cartesian space are around 256×256 while in polar space, they are around 50×90 making the processing much faster. The center and maximum radius of the polar space are calculated from the blood pool estimates.

2.3 Gray Level Analysis

Because no two MR acquisitions are the same, it is important to determine the gray level properties of the images in the current dataset. We use the multiseeded fuzzy connectedness approach proposed in [10] to build histograms for the lungs, myocardium and blood pool distributions. The process is illustrated in Fig. 1. Approximate histograms are built using the blood pool regions recovered in Section 2.1, the pixels in a small ring around those regions, and a larger region (largely consisting of lung pixels). The pixels in the center of the main peaks in those histograms are used as seeds for the multiseeded fuzzy connectedness algorithm which groups pixels into homogeneous regions (roughly corresponding to blood, myocardium and lungs). The final histograms are built from these regions.

3 Segmentation of the First Slice

The first slice in the dataset (the most basal slice) intersects with the valve plane. This makes it difficult to segment and often, the LV cannot be detected by the first step in Section 2.1. Consequently, we first segment the first slice on which an LV blood pool was detected. It is usually a clean slice, below the valve plane, without many papillary muscles inside the blood pool. It is a very good candidate to start the segmentation process.

3.1 Deformable Registration

To segment a slice, we first register all the phases in the slice and generate an average image. To calculate the deformation field between two phases, a variational non-rigid registration algorithm [11] is applied. This approach can be viewed as an extension of the classical optical flow method in which a dense deformation field is estimated as the solution to a calculus of variations problem

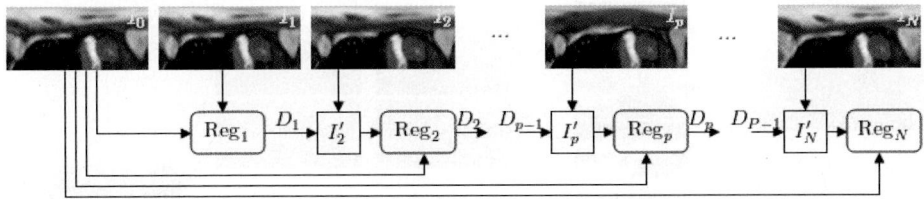

Fig. 2. Strategy to capture the large deformations between pairs of phases (especially ED and ES) during registration in polar space

where the cost function is defined as the sum of an image similarity measure (local cross correlation ratio) and regularization terms.

The registration algorithm is applied to the polar images because the contours will be recovered in polar space and the intrinsic motion of the myocardium is mostly radial [12]. To account for the fact that, in polar space, the pixels in the first column of the image are neighbors of the pixels in the last column of the image, we use the tiling boundary condition on the images to calculate derivatives.

Due to the large myocardial contraction during the R-R intervals and the finite capture range of non-rigid registration, a simple registration from the ED phase often fails to fully recover the myocardium deformation in other phases (especially the ES phase). We propose the strategy illustrated in Fig. 2 to overcome this limitation. After a phase is selected as the reference image, the next phase is first registered to this reference. Then, the second registration is initialized with the deformation field from the first registration, which is equivalent to first transforming the second phase to the reference coordinate system using a partially accurate deformation field and then running the registration between those to recover the remaining deformation.

3.2 Segmentation in the Average Temporal Image

The endocardium and epicardium contours are recovered independently in the average image using a shortest path algorithm for which the main difficulty is to define the cost function. In this case, the strong gradient between the papillary muscles and the blood should be avoided as the contour should stay behind the papillary muscles. Also, the gradient which might be stronger between the lungs and the fat than between the myocardium and the fat is not a good indicator of the epicardium.

Since it is impossible to design the best cost function that will work in all possible cases, we have chosen to use multiple cost functions to recover multiple contour candidates as illustrated in Fig. 3. First, the phases are aligned separately to the ED and ES phases and averaged to produce the ED and ES average images $I_{ED}(x)$ and $I_{ES}(x)$. Then, for each average image, we compute two different myocardium probabilities: a) the distribution probability $\mathcal{M}^H(x)$ is the response of the myocardium histogram to the pixels in the average image; b)

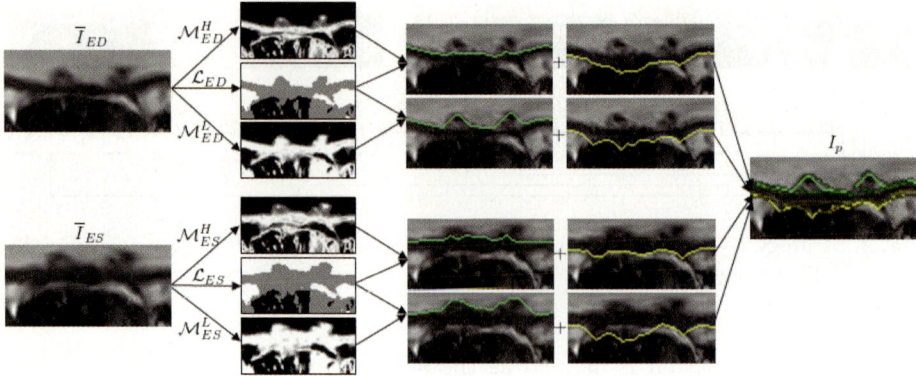

Fig. 3. Segmentation of the average images to generate multiple candidate contours

the label probability $\mathcal{M}^L(x)$ is the average of the label images $\mathcal{L}_p(x)$ produced by the multiseeded fuzzy connectedness algorithm. Finally, gradient images are computed in the following way. For the endocardium, $g^{\text{endo}}(x)$ is the gradient of $\mathcal{M}(x)$ where gradients in the wrong direction are eliminated because the probability is expected to be bright inside the myocardium. Also pixel transitions in $\mathcal{L}(x)$ from myocardium below to non myocardium above are highlighted. For the epicardium, $g^{\text{epi}}(x)$ is the sum of the gradient of $\mathcal{M}(x)$ and the gradient of $I(x)$. Again, gradients in the wrong direction are eliminated and pixel transitions in $\mathcal{L}(x)$ from blood (lung) below to non blood (non lung) above are highlighted.

The endocardium is recovered first using the gradient cost function defined as $G(x) = \frac{1}{|g(x)|^2 + \epsilon}$. Then, for the epicardium, three criteria are minimized, namely the gradient cost function, the number of pixels between the two contours not labeled as myocardium in $\mathcal{L}(x)$, and the variation in the thickness of the myocardium. We use Dijkstra's algorithm to recover the shortest path. All the pixels in the leftmost column in the image are initialized as starting points on the path and as soon as a path reaches a pixel in the rightmost column, the algorithm terminates. The contours generated by the shortest path algorithm using the two different probability images for the two average images are transfered back to all the phases using the corresponding deformation fields to obtain four different candidate contours per phase. These contours are then combined using a minimal surface algorithm.

3.3 Minimal Surface Segmentation of All Phases

The minimal surface algorithm was developed by Grady [13] to extend the shortest path algorithm to 3D. This extension of the shortest path algorithm accepts one or more closed 2D contours as input and produces the global minimal surface, with respect to the cost function, having these 2D contours as its boundary.

The cost function is defined as follows for each phase p. It is important to follow the edges of the current frame, so the directed gradient images $g_p^{\text{endo}}(x)$ and $g_p^{\text{epi}}(x)$ of the probability images $\mathcal{M}_p^H(x)$ and $\mathcal{M}_p^L(x)$ for the current phase and the gradient cost function $G_p(x) = \frac{1}{|g_p(x)|^2 + \epsilon}$ are computed as described earlier.

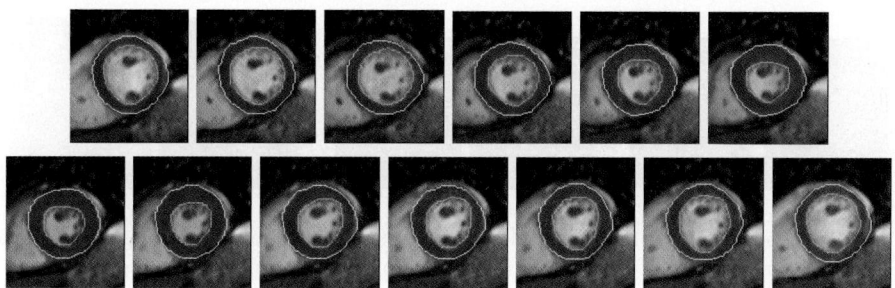

Fig. 4. Segmentation of the first slice (cropped for better viewing)

Then, pixels on the candidate contours are retained based on how likely there are of belonging to the final contour. For the endocardium, since we want the contour to stay behind the papillary muscles, the most promising pixels are farther from the center of the contour. In polar coordinates, these pixels have a larger row position. Let $i(x)$ be the row position of pixel x and let $i_1(x)$ (resp. $i_2(x)$) be the row position of the top most (resp. bottom most) contour in the same column as pixel x. The likelihood of a pixel on a candidate contour is defined as $F_p^{\text{endo}}(x) = \alpha(i(x) - i_1(x)) + \beta$. The situation is more complicated for the epicardium because there are many missing and spurious edges. Once the endocardium has been recovered, we determine the average thickness T of the myocardium using all epicardium candidates in that phase. The likelihood of a pixel on a candidate contour is defined as $F_p^{\text{epi}}(x) = \|i(x) - (i^{\text{endo}}(x) + T)\|$. In addition, if there are no good edges for the epicardium in a particular area, the pixels T away from the endocardium become good candidate by setting $F_p^{\text{epi}}(i^{\text{endo}}(x) + T, j) = 0$. The distance map from these candidate pixels is computed and multiplied to the gradient cost functions to generate the final cost function for the minimal surface algorithm.

To initialize the contours for the minimal surface algorithm, we apply Dijkstra's algorithm in the ED phase to generate a 2D contour. The 3D volume consists of all phases with the ED phase as the first phase and ED phase added again as the last phase. This way, the algorithm is initialized with two contours and the minimal surface is generated between them. In order to not bias the algorithm with the initial contour, we apply a second pass where the initial contour is the ES contour from the first pass and the 3D volume goes from the ES phase to the ES phase. Once the contours have been segmented, they are converted back to Cartesian space. Fig. 4 shows an example of the segmentation in the first slice.

4 Segmentation of the Other Slices

The segmentation of the other slices is very similar. The slices are propagated in both directions from the first slice to the apex and to the base. To begin, we apply the deformable registration to align the ED and ES phases of the current

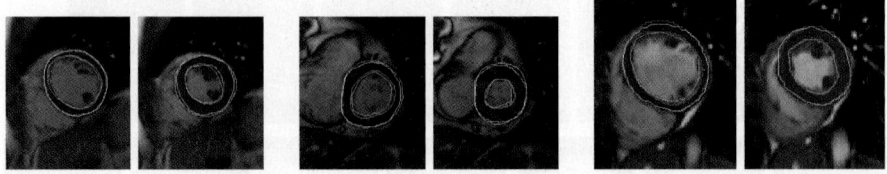

Fig. 5. Segmentation in mid-ventricle slices (cropped for better viewing): automatic contours are shown brighter and ground truth contours are shown dimmer

slice to the previous slice. The contours in the ED and ES phases from the previous slice are transferred to the current slice by applying the deformation field to define shape priors. When the candidate contours are recovered using the shortest path algorithms in the ED and ES average images, the distance maps around the prior contours are combined with the gradient cost functions as follows:

$$\hat{G}_k^{\text{endo}}(x) = G_k^{\text{endo}}(x)(D_k^{\text{endo}}(x) + 1)$$
$$\hat{G}_k^{\text{epi}}(x) = G_k^{\text{epi}}(x)(D_k^{\text{epi}}(x) + 1) \qquad k = ED, ES.$$

Finally, the candidate contours (including the prior contours) are combined using the minimal surface algorithm. Segmentation examples are shown in Fig. 5 where automatic contours are shown in bright while ground truths are dimmer.

5 Experiments

To evaluate the performance of the algorithm, we have collected 19 patient datasets from 4 different clinical sites. Two experts manually outlined the endocardium and epicardium in the ED and ES phases for all the datasets. They worked together to produce a single contour set that was agreed upon. We ran our fully automatic algorithm and generated the segmentation contours. The algorithm is quite fast, it takes 1 minute to segment an average dataset with 200 images (0.3 s per image) on a dual core laptop (2.33GHz and 2GB RAM).

The contours were compared in the following way. To compute the distance between two contours, we first sample the contours so that their vertices are one pixel apart. For each vertex on each contour, we compute the distance to the closest point (not necessarily a vertex) on the other contour. We then plot the cumulative histogram of these distances for all patients (all vertices on all contours) and compute the root mean square (RMS) of these distances. We also compute the average Dice coefficient. Fig. 7 shows the summary of results for all contours, the endocardium and epicardium contours, the most basal slices, the most apical slices, and the mid-ventricular slices. The cumulative histograms are to be read in the following way: a point (x, y) on the curve says that $x\%$ of all distances are below y pixels (pixel sizes for the 19 datasets varied between 1.32 and 2.47 mm).

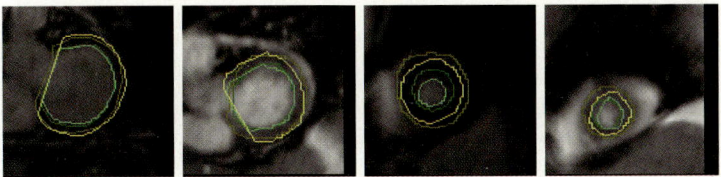

Fig. 6. Segmentation results in the most basal and most apical slices

	RMS (pixels)	RMS (mm)	Dice
overall	1.61	2.70	0.89
endocardium	1.48	2.48	0.88
epicardium	1.74	2.91	0.91
basal slices	1.65	2.76	0.92
apical slices	2.36	3.92	0.78
mid slices	1.34	2.24	0.93
Pixel sizes: 1.32 - 2.47 mm			

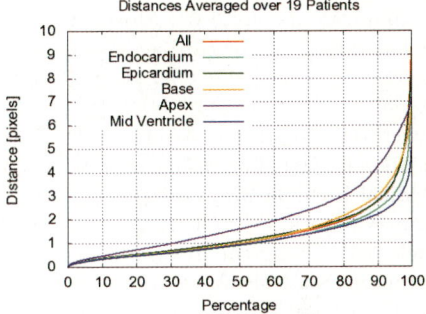

Fig. 7. Distance between ground truth and automatic contours (the RMS distance should be small, the Dice coefficient should be large), a point (x, y) in the graph indicates that $x\%$ of all distances are below y

The curves show that the error is around 1 pixel ($\approx$ 2 mm) half of the time and around 2 pixels ($\approx$ 4 mm) 80% of the time. There are very few large errors which means that they occur in a few places and can easily be manually edited. We observe that there is not much difference between endocardium and epicardium: the algorithm recovers both contours equally well. The algorithm performs well in the basal slices, but the error is much larger in the apical slices, and it can be seen in the graph in Fig. 7 that the largest 10% of the distances are significantly lower when those slices are ignored. Actually, very few people in the literature have considered such slices as the ones seen in Fig. 6 where the outflow tract can be seen in the base and the LV blood pool moves in and out of the slice between ED and ES (no ground truth was defined on the ES phases of those slices) and where the endocardium is very small in the apical slices.

6 Conclusions

We have proposed a fully automatic system to segment the left ventricle myocardium from cine MR images. The method combines deformable registration, shortest paths, and minimal surfaces. We demonstrated on 19 datasets that the results look very good and the errors are small enough that the system can be used in clinical settings. In the future, we would like to combine this short axis segmentation with a long axis segmentation (similar to [4]) as it will help in resolving the more difficult cases in the basal and apical slices.

References

1. Lorenzo-Valdés, M., Sanchez-Ortiz, G., Elkington, A., Mohiaddin, R., Rueckert, D.: Segmentation of 4D cardiac MR images using a probabilistic atlas and the EM algorithm. Medical Image Analysis 8 (2004)
2. Jolly, M.: Automatic segmentation of the left ventricle in cardiac MR and CT images. International Journal of Computer Vision 70(2) (2006)
3. Mitchell, S., Lelieveldt, B., van der Geest, R., Bosch, H., Reiber, J., Sonka, M.: Multistage hybrid active appearance model matching: Segmentation of the left and right ventricles in cardiac MR images. IEEE Trans. Medical Imaging 20(5) (2001)
4. Fradkin, M., Ciofolo, C., Mory, B., Hautvast, G., Breeuwer, M.: Comprehensive segmentation of cine cardiac MR images. In: Metaxas, D., Axel, L., Fichtinger, G., Székely, G. (eds.) MICCAI 2008, Part I. LNCS, vol. 5241, pp. 178–185. Springer, Heidelberg (2008)
5. Lynch, M., Ghita, O., Whelan, P.F.: Segmentation of the left ventricle of the heart in 3-D+t MRI data using an optimized nonrigid temporal model. IEEE Trans. Medical Imaging 27(2) (2008)
6. Sun, W., Çetin, M., Chan, R., Willsky, A.: Segmentation of the evolving left ventricle by learning the dynamics. In: ISBI (2008)
7. Paragios, N.: A level set approach for shape-driven segmentation and tracking of the left ventricle. IEEE Trans. Medical Imaging 22(6) (2003)
8. Lorenzo-Valdés, M., Sanchez-Ortiz, G.I., Mohiaddin, R.H., Rueckert, D.: Atlas-based segmentation and tracking of 3D cardiac MR images using non-rigid registration. In: Dohi, T., Kikinis, R. (eds.) MICCAI 2002. LNCS, vol. 2488, p. 642. Springer, Heidelberg (2002)
9. Jolly, M.-P.: Automatic recovery of the left ventricular blood pool in cardiac cine MR images. In: Metaxas, D., Axel, L., Fichtinger, G., Székely, G. (eds.) MICCAI 2008, Part I. LNCS, vol. 5241, pp. 110–118. Springer, Heidelberg (2008)
10. Jolly, M.P., Grady, L.: 3D general lesion segmentation in CT. In: ISBI (2008)
11. Hermosillo, G., Chefd'hotel, C., Faugeras, O.: Variational methods for multimodal image matching. International Journal of Computer Vision 50(3) (2002)
12. Noble, N., Hill, D., Breeuwer, M., Schnabel, J., Hawkes, D., Gerritsen, F., Razavi, R.: Myocardial delineation via registration in a polar coordinate system. In: Dohi, T., Kikinis, R. (eds.) MICCAI 2002. LNCS, vol. 2488, p. 651. Springer, Heidelberg (2002)
13. Grady, L.: Computing extact discrete minimal surfaces: Extending and solving the shortest path problem in 3D with application to segmentation. In: CVPR (2006)

Left Ventricle Segmentation Using Diffusion Wavelets and Boosting

Salma Essafi[1,2], Georg Langs[3], and Nikos Paragios[1,2]

[1] Laboratoire de Mathématiques Appliquées aux Systèmes,
Ecole Centrale de Paris, France
[2] GALEN Group, INRIA Saclay-Ile de France, Orsay, France
[3] Computational Image Analysis and Radiology Lab, Department of Radiology,
Medical University of Vienna, Austria
salma.essafi@ecp.fr, georg.langs@meduniwien.ac.at,
nikos.paragios@ecp.fr

Abstract. We propose a method for the segmentation of medical images based on a novel parameterization of prior shape knowledge and a search scheme based on classifying local appearance. The method uses diffusion wavelets to capture arbitrary and continuous interdependencies in the training data and uses them for an efficient shape model. The lack of classic visual consistency in complex medical imaging data, is tackled by a manifold learning approach handling optimal high-dimensional local features by Gentle Boosting. Appearance saliency is encoded in the model and segmentation is performed through the extraction and classification of the corresponding features in a new data set, as well as a diffusion wavelet based shape model constraint. Our framework supports hierarchies both in the model and the search space, can encode complex geometric and photometric dependencies of the structure of interest, and can deal with arbitrary topologies. Promising results are reported for heart CT data sets, proving the impact of the soft parameterization, and the efficiency of our approach.

1 Introduction

Data acquired by medical imaging modalities has a level of richness that needs computer based methods to extract relevant information in a consistent and efficient manner. The automatic and accurate delineation of the left ventricle (LV) is a prominent example for a critical component of computer-assisted cardiac diagnosis. Information with respect to the ejection fraction, the wall motion, and the valve behavior can be very useful toward predicting and avoiding myocardial infarction. Existing segmentation approaches include the use of a shortest path algorithm along with shape matching which was considered in [1],or an alternative shape representation using level set functions was proposed in [2].

These methods depend heavily on the accuracy of the inter-subject registration for group comparison and the parameterization of the shape. A promising line of research considering wavelets for the representation of shapes was initiated in [3] by build hierarchical active shape models of 2-D anatomical objects using 1-D wavelets, which are then used for shape based image segmentation. A further extension was proposed in [4] where spherical wavelets are used to characterize shape variation in a local fashion in the space and frequency domain.

Two crucial components of image model based methods are the parameterization of the shape manifold, and the capturing and representation of the appearance in the training and search data. The model based segmentation approach proposed in this paper accounts for the systematic behavior of shape variation and image support in anatomical structures, with a parameterization that goes beyond pre-defined reference manifolds. For the parameterization of complex structures it is worthwhile to not rely on a reference manifold with an a priori topology, but to learn the appropriate topology from the training data. For this we have to determine the intrinsic topology of a shape for which multiple examples are available, and have to encode this information in the shape model, to use it in the representation and during segmentation.

We propose a method that integrates local voxel classification and global search models. We model and parameterize shape variation of structures with arbitrary topology, by using diffusion wavelet shape models [5] to represent the shape variation with a learnt parameterization based on mutual distance. The approach deals with complex and soft connectivity properties of objects by encoding their interdependencies with a diffusion kernel [6]. The topology is learned from the training data instead of using a priori choices like e.g., a sphere and represents the shape variation by means of diffusion wavelets [7]. A detailed explanation of diffusion wavelet shape models, including variants of the parameterization can be found in [8].

During search this model is used together with a GentleBoost classifier [9] trained on the local appearance of the individual landmarks describing the anatomical structure. The method obtains an accurate delineation of partially visible surfaces and complex texture, that cannot be achieved with registration based methods. The shape representation is based on a finite set of landmarks, that can be repeatedly identified and exhibit significant differentiation to the background on different examples of the anatomical structure, and more particularly for CT cardiac volumes. During the search the hierarchical diffusion wavelet shape model [8] is fitted to new data based on local appearance captured by the classifier. Related approaches combining local features with standard shape models are [10], or [11]. The method computes a local feature vector for every voxel and maps it via a GentleBoost classifier [9] to a probability that the voxel belongs to a specific landmark in the object. The classifier is trained from the training data set segmentations. The probabilistic output is constrained by the shape model. The mapping onto the diffusion wavelet coefficient space ensures valid results with regard to the training data. The result of this procedure is a probability for each voxel regarding its match to the structure to be segmented, conditioned on both local and global information. We report results on CT left heart ventricle data sets, that illustrate the impact of the soft parameterization, as well as the global classifier based search.

2 Hierarchical Shape Model Building

We model the shape variation observed in the training data by means of diffusion wavelets. Wavelets represent a robust mathematical tool for hierarchically decomposing functions into different frequency components. We refer the reader to [12] for complete

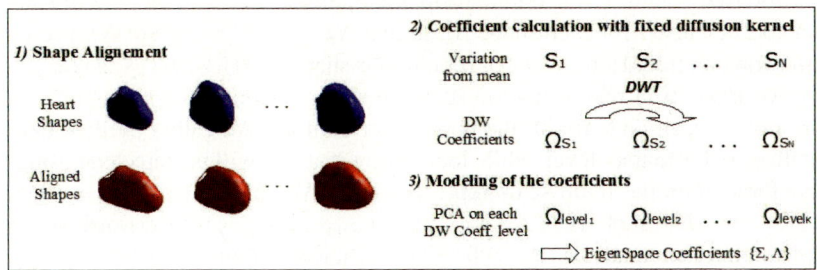

Fig. 1. Scheme of Diffusion Wavelet Coefficient Process

description of the theory. The major advantage of wavelets is the compact support of basis functions on one hand, and on the inherently hierarchical representation based on multi-resolution modeling of processes at different spatial and temporal scales. The diffusion wavelet technique introduced by [7] associates multi-scale representation of training data as well as the topological information captured by means of a diffusion kernel [6]. Diffusion wavelets enable local as well as global variation detection, which makes it useful and suitable for our application.

For the modeling of the variation, we consider the heart volumes as a finite set of landmarks. Starting from m landmark positions, $\mathbf{H}_i = \langle \mathbf{x}_1^i, \mathbf{x}_2^i, \ldots \mathbf{x}_m^i, \rangle$, are known in n training volume images $\mathbf{V}_1, \mathbf{V}_2, \ldots, \mathbf{V}_N$. Our data comprises $\mathcal{H} = \{\mathbf{H}_1, \mathbf{H}_2, ..., \mathbf{H}_N\}$, where $\mathbf{x}_j^i \in \mathbb{R}^d$, and we refer to $\mathbf{H}_i \in \mathbb{R}^{dm}$ a shape. Since we are only interested in the non-rigid deformation, all anatomical shapes are aligned by Procrustes analysis, which produces the series of examples H_i^p, from which we compute the mean shape $\bar{H}^p$ (Fig. 1). Once registered, the shapes are used through their deviation S_i from the mean shape, $S_i = H_i^p - \bar{H}^p$, where $\bar{H}^p$ represents the volumes mean shape.

We now specify a topology over the set of landmarks. For this we use a hierarchical geometric graph framework introduced in [6]. It applies the concept of diffusion to capture mutual relations between nodes in a Markov chain, and derives the global structure of a shape. In our case, this structure is the neighborhood relation between landmarks of the shape, that determines the domain upon which the wavelet representation is built. Diffusion maps grant a canonical representation of high-dimensional data. By this we are able to represent spatial relations as well as the data behavior. The structure is encoded in a diffusion operator $\Delta \in \mathbb{R}^{m \times m}$. Combining those two diffusion approaches leads us to a prior knowledge of global and local training population variation [8]. The diffusion operator Δ is built on the set of points embedded in a metric space utilizing their mutual distance in the mean shape, and reflects all pairwise relations between individual points in the shape set.

After defining the diffusion operator Δ, we build the according *diffusion wavelet tree*. For this we apply general multi resolution construction for efficiently computing, representing and compressing Δ^{2j}, for $j > 0$. The latter are dyadic powers of Δ, and we use them as dilation operators to move from one level to the next, which is a simple way of compressing high orders of the diffusion operator. The process of constructing the diffusion wavelet, the tree and the coefficients is described in detail in [7].

Once the tree is built based on the diffusion operator, we can compute the diffusion wavelet coefficients Ω for each shape S_i, so that $\Omega_{S_i} = \Psi^{-1} S_i$, where Ψ represents the diffusion wavelet tree. Hence we can rebuild our shape as $H_i^p = \bar{H}^p + \Psi \Omega_{S_i}$.

Now we move to a representation scale by scale, in order to construct a model of the variation at each level for all the population training. We gather the low frequency information in the coarser level, while localized variations will be detected through high level coefficients in the multi scale representation. We define $\Omega_{level\,j}$ at every scale j, with $(1 \leq j \leq K)$, such as $\Omega_{level\,j} = \{\Omega_{S_i/level=j}\}_{i=1...N}$. Afterward we perform principle component analysis (PCA) for the coefficients of all scales.

The eigenspace resulting from this PCA will be referred as $\{\Lambda, \Sigma\}$, where more precisely will have $\Sigma = \{\sigma_j\}_{j=1...K}$, and the corresponding eigenvalues $\Lambda = \{\lambda_j\}_{j=1...K}$ of the covariance matrix of the diffusion wavelets coefficients at each level j, and the according coefficients $\Omega_{level\,j}^*$ that represent each training shape in this coordinate system. Hence in each level the coefficients would be expressed such as:

$$\Omega_{level\,j} = \bar{\Omega}_{level\,j} + \sigma_j \left(\sigma'_j . \Omega_{level\,j}^*\right) \qquad (1)$$

Finally we can activate the shape reconstruction process: (1) we compute the diffusion wavelet coefficients $\Omega_{S_i\,Rec}$ in each level,(2) we remodel the shape based on the diffusion wavelet tree, and get the reconstructed shape: $\Upsilon_i^p = \bar{H}^p + \Psi \Omega_{S_i\,Rec}$.

3 Segmentation Based on Image Information and the Model Prior

The segmentation of the LV is challenging mostly due to the similar visual properties with the other chambers of the heart cavity, as well as the presence of papillary muscles. The use of edge-driven terms with regional statistics along either with deformable contours or active shape and appearance models. In the first case, computational complexity is an issue and the proper handling of papillary muscles is problematic. In the second case, one has to deal with either the linearity of the sub-space or the fact that building appearance modes requires appearance normalization and too many samples. We adopt recent developments in machine learning that explores the use of weak classifiers and arbitrary image features. In the context of the heart muscle, our feature space involves the (i) gradient phase and magnitude, (ii) structure tensor plus their (iii) curvature [13] and (v) the responses to Gabor filters with different phases and orientations.

3.1 Learning a Classifier for Appearance Modeling

Starting from this feature space, we apply Gentle Adaboost [9] to obtain a local appearance prior for the search in new data. The boosting process aims to build a strong classifier by combining a number of weak classifiers, which need only be better than chance. For this we call upon a sequential learning process: at each iteration, we add a weak classifier. It is the basic learning algorithm introduces by Viola, Jones in [14]. Our classification problem evolves as a two class training set that can be represented as: $S = \{(x_i, y_i)\}_{i=1}^{l} \subset \mathbb{R}^N \times \{-1, +1\}$.

Given these classifiers, we use them to locate landmarks during the segmentation process. The classifiers detect landmarks present on the ventricle muscle wall against

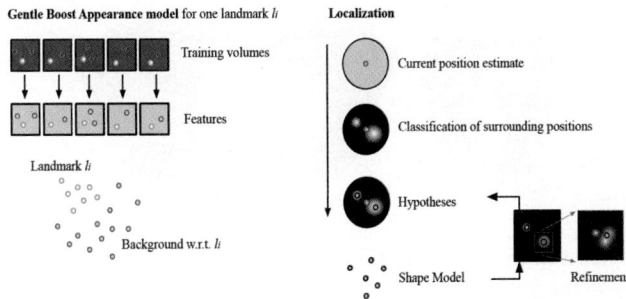

Fig. 2. Scheme of the appearance model: Based on local features, and a classifier we can assign each position in the volume an evidence value for landmarks presence. This results in a set of hypotheses for landmark positions, that are verified by the shape model constraint.

background. This is a very different strategy in comparison to standard search methods [15]. The main search strategy is: extract features from the volume, for each landmark obtain a few candidate positions with a very strong classifier response, fit the DW model to these candidates, and determine the candidate configuration with the highest plausibility with regard to the shape prior. After continue with the local search at the current landmark estimates constraint by the DW model. During the shape model fitting we check which candidates have the highest plausibility with the trained DW model.

In Fig. 2 the scheme of the model search is depicted. For each landmark the search volume $\mathbf{V}$ is projected into a hypothesis space $\mathbf{V}_i^H$ that reflects the evidence for the landmark presence for each point in the volume. This results in a position hypothesis $\hat{\mathbf{x}}_i$ for each landmark. The set of landmark hypotheses $\langle \hat{\mathbf{x}}_1, \ldots, \hat{\mathbf{x}}_n \rangle$ is tested with the diffusion wavelet shape model, resulting in a position prediction for each landmark. These predictions are used to generate new hypotheses based on the local image support $\mathbf{V}_i^{H'}$ and the shape model. The hypothesis space is the classifier response on each position in the volume. During the progressing search we just consider the neighborhood of the current landmark location estimate during the last iteration.

3.2 The Segmentation Algorithm

Let us summarize the learning and search concepts introduced in this paper. The method consists of a training phase and an execution step. First, the shape model and parameterization, and the local classifiers for the appearance representation are learnt. During search they are used to locate and segment structures in new image data.

Learning: During the training both geometry and appearance of the structure of interest are learned.
- Given n examples of the structure of interest location and the corresponding images, we represent the shape variability through diffusion wavelets.
- Using the same examples, we compute the selected feature images for each training example for different resolutions. For each landmark, at each resolution, we construct a set of training samples containing local features and

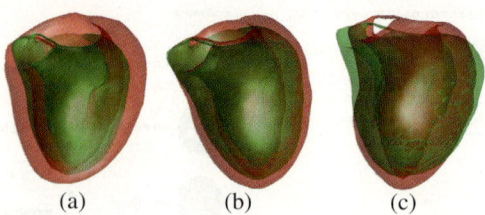

Fig. 3. Reconstructed surfaces for Heart CT data using projected wavelet coefficients on PCA eigenspace, representing 99% of the total variance at finest level. The surfaces are showing the $\pm 3 sqrt(\lambda_i)$ from left to right. Figure is dedicated to the sagital view.

corresponding labels which indicate if the position is the landmark location or the background, i.e., whether it is on the ventricle wall or on the background. Let's note here that background voxels are chosen randomly in the volume except the particular landmark positions for training.
- To train for the fine local differentiation we take into consideration only the neighborhood of every landmark candidate in each training image. We train a classifier for each landmark and retain only the ones with solid performance or wide-margins between the different classes.

Segmentation: Using both geometric and appearance priors and the corresponding feature space in the image we perform the structure delineation as follows: the process is initiated with the mean shape, and proceeds in an iterative manner,
- Perform a local search for the most probable landmark positions using the trained classifiers
- Constrain the solution using the diffusion wavelet coefficient constraints, and repeats the previous search steps until convergence.

This results in landmark location estimates in the search image, that are based on the appearance, and the shape constrained learned during the training phase.

4 Experimental Validation

To assess the performance of our approach, we consider a data set that includes 25 CT volumes of the heart, with an approximate voxel spacing of 1.5 mm, for which 90 anatomical standard of reference landmarks, and a set of 1451 control points for the left ventricle was available, in addition to the ground truth segmentation from experts concerning the diastole as well as the systole.

We have run our algorithm in a leave-one-out cross validation fashion. For the diffusion wavelet building part, we obtain 9 diffusion wavelet levels of decomposition for the shape prior. As for the initialization of our framework, we used the mean shape displaced by a random translation of 30 mm.

To evaluate the efficiency of our method, we computed two error measures: (i) the Hausdorff distance revealing the maximum error between the standard of reference and our model reconstruction, as well as (ii) mean distance error of the detected landmarks. In Fig.4.a, one can see that the Hausdorff distance error decreases with an increasing

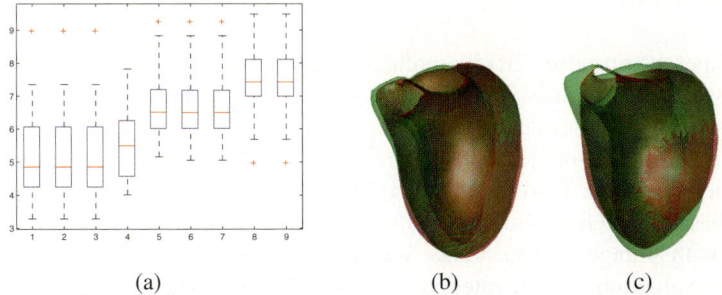

(a)   (b)   (c)

Fig. 4. Multiscale Diffusion Wavelets Reconstruction. (a) Hausdorff Error Distance (in voxel) of reconstructed heart at each diffusion scale for all data in the training set. (b) Data, green: ground truth segmentation, red: reconstruction result for finest scale and (c) coarsest wavelet scale.

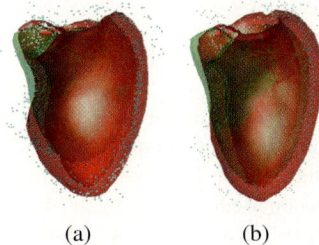

(a)   (b)

Fig. 5. Model search result for Heart muscle. Ground truth in green, in red: search results. (a) standard Gaussian search approach, and (b) method presented in this paper.

number of diffusion wavelet levels used for reconstruction. When we consider the mean reconstruction error over all data, we reach a distance of 2.2313 voxel in the image for the finest level, while as for the coarsest level we obtain 2.7073 voxel. The comparison of detection results for different numbers of levels used during reconstruction can be seen in Fig.4. Note that diffusion wavelets have been shown to outperform standard Gaussian models in terms of search error in [5] on muscle MRI data.

During the search validation experiments, we consider a multi-resolution approach for each landmark patch which goes from 5*5 pixels to 20*20 pixels in 4 steps. We obtain 200 landmarks candidates, for 15 training hearts and 10 testing examples. Experiments were carried out using Gentle Adaboost, which is adequate to deal with a large number of negative examples as well as the rather limited size of our training set.

In the quantitative assessment of the search/segmentation algorithm explained in Sec.3, we obtain a lowest error of 4.72 voxel between ground truth and relative segmented volume. In a typical segmentation scenario, the method takes approximately 68 seconds in average through non-optimized code implemented in Matlab 7.5, on a 2GHz DELL Duo Computer with 2Gb RAM. One should note here that we are working toward search in very large data sets, while searching for small complex structures, thus the efficiency of gradient descent of ASM is limited. In an ideal case one would combine the trade off between the reconstruction accuracy and the classification error to choose the best candidate for the search segmentation.

5 Conclusion

In this paper we propose a 3D hierarchical shape prior segmentation framework based on diffusion wavelets and local appearance classifiers. The diffusion wavelets are able to represent subtle inter-dependencies in the training data, by clustering coefficients, and representing the topology of the structure by a diffusion kernel, instead of a fixed pre-defined manifold. The conjunction of the diffusion wavelet constraint with a search method based on a GentleBoost classifier leads to an effective segmentation scheme. It can deal with ambiguous appearance and complex structures. Future work will focus on extensive evaluation, and the integration of efficient optimization techniques in addition to the studied priors to obtain a more flexible and powerful paradigm for representing shapes of arbitrary topologies, and the search in large data sets.

References

1. Jolly, M.: Automatic segmentation of the left ventricle in cardiac MR and CT images. IJCV 70(2), 151–163 (2006)
2. Paragios, N.: A Variational Approach for the Segmentation of the Left Ventricle in Cardiac Image Analysis. International Journal of Computer Vision 50(3), 345–362 (2002)
3. Davatzikos, C., Tao, X., Dinggang, S.: Hierarchical active shape models, using the wavelet transform. IEEE Transactions on Medical Imaging 22, 414–423 (2003)
4. Nain, D., Haker, S., Bobick, A., Tannenbaum, A.: Multiscale 3-d shape representation and segmentation using spherical wavelets. IEEE Trans. Med. Imaging 26(4), 598–618 (2007)
5. Essafi, S., Langs, G., Deux, J.F., Rahmouni, A., Bassez, G., Paragios, N.: Wavelet-driven knowledge-based MRI calf segmentation. In: Proceedings of ISBI (2009)
6. Coifman, R.R., Lafon, S.: Diffusion maps. Appl. Comput. Harmon. Anal. 21, 5–30 (2006)
7. Coifman, R.R., Maggioni, M.: Diffusion wavelets. Appl. Comput. Harmon. Anal. 21, 53–94 (2006)
8. Essafi, S., Langs, G., Paragios, N.: Hierarchical 3d diffusion wavelets shape priors. In: IEEE International Conference in Computer Vision, ICCV 2009 (2009)
9. Friedman, J., Hastie, T., Tibshirani, R.: Additive logistic regression: A statistical view of boosting. Annals of statistics, 337–374 (2000)
10. Scott, I.M., Cootes, T.F., Taylor, C.J.: Improving appearance model matching using local image structure. In: Taylor, C.J., Noble, J.A. (eds.) IPMI 2003. LNCS, vol. 2732, pp. 258–269. Springer, Heidelberg (2003)
11. Qian, Z., Metaxas, D.N., Axel, L.: A learning framework for the automatic and accurate segmentation of cardiac tagged MRI images. In: CVBIA, pp. 93–102 (2005)
12. Meyer, Y.: Wavelets - Algorithms and applications. Applied Mathematics (1993)
13. Rieger, B., Timmermans, F.J., van Vliet, L.J., Verbeek, P.W.: On curvature estimation of iso surfaces in 3d gray-value images and the computation of shape descriptors. IEEE Transactions on Pattern Analysis and Machine Intelligence 26(8), 1088–1094 (2004)
14. Viola, P., Jones, M.: Robust real-time object detection. International Journal of Computer Vision (2001)
15. Cootes, T.F., Taylor, C.J., Cooper, D.H., Graham, J.: Active shape models-their training and application. Computer Vision and Image Understanding 61, 38–59 (1995)

3D Cardiac Segmentation Using Temporal Correlation of Radio Frequency Ultrasound Data

Maartje M. Nillesen[1], Richard G.P. Lopata[1], Henkjan J. Huisman[2], Johan M. Thijssen[1], Livia Kapusta[3], and Chris L. de Korte[1]

[1] Clinical Physics Laboratory, Department of Pediatrics
m.m.nillesen@cukz.umcn.nl
[2] Department of Radiology
[3] Pediatric Cardiology, Department of Pediatrics
Radboud University Nijmegen Medical Centre

Abstract. Semi-automatic segmentation of the myocardium in 3D echographic images may substantially support clinical diagnosis of heart disease. Particularly in children with congenital heart disease, segmentation should be based on the echo features solely since *a priori* knowledge on the shape of the heart cannot be used. Segmentation of echocardiographic images is challenging because of the poor echogenicity contrast between blood and the myocardium in some regions and the inherent speckle noise from randomly backscattered echoes. Phase information present in the radio frequency (rf) ultrasound data might yield useful, additional features in these regions. A semi-3D technique was used to determine maximum temporal cross-correlation values locally from the rf data. To segment the endocardial surface, maximum cross-correlation values were used as additional external force in a deformable model approach and were tested against and combined with adaptive filtered, demodulated rf data. The method was tested on full volume images (Philips, iE33) of four healthy children and evaluated by comparison with contours obtained from manual segmentation.

1 Introduction

Three-dimensional (3D) segmentation of the endocardial surface could be a helpful tool for clinical assessment of 3D echocardiographic images. Segmentation may not only serve as an important tool for assessment of cardiac output and other functional parameters but also as a preprocessing step for tissue characterization, strain imaging and diagnosis of congenital deformities. Since manual segmentation of the left ventricle in 3D ultrasound image sequences is time-consuming and is subject to inter-expert variability, (semi-) automatic segmentation techniques are required (see [1] for an overview). The influence of speckle noise and the poor contrast in echogenicity between the blood and the heart wall in regions where the muscle fibers are mainly parallel to the propagation direction of the ultrasound beam, impose strong demands on the segmentation algorithm. Automatic segmentation purely based on differences in echogenicity will be problematic in these low echogenicity regions as the contrast between blood and myocardial tissue is absent. Therefore, a technique using temporal information might be beneficial.

Segmentation techniques using shape and appearance models of the left ventricle have been described [2] to overcome these segmentation problems. However, in children with congenital deformities of the heart, inclusion of *a priori* knowledge about the average shape of the left ventricle will lead to erroneous segmentation results. The addition of temporal information by using cross-correlation techniques might facilitate segmentation in these problematic low contrast regions. Few segmentation methods use the rich phase information available in the radio frequency (rf) signal [3], [4], [5]. Yan et al.[6] propose the use of maximum correlation coefficients obtained from a phase sensitive speckle tracking method for segmentation of the left ventricle.

This study builds on the work of Yan et al. [6] and Nillesen et al. [7] using a combination of maximum cross-correlation values and adaptive mean squares (AMS) filter values as external forces of a gradient-based deformable simplex mesh model. The cross-correlation values were obtained from a semi-3D coarse-to-fine displacement algorithm (developed for strain estimation). This combined method was compared with segmentation results using correlation or AMS values as an external force separately. All results were evaluated by comparing them with manual segmentation.

2 Materials and Methods

Echocardiographic image sequences of the left ventricle were obtained in four healthy children. Echographic imaging was approved by the local ethics committee and parents gave their informed consent for using the data. Transthoracic full volume image sequences (ECG-gated, volume rate ≈50 Hz) were obtained in long/short axis views. Rf-data were acquired directly after receive beam-forming using an iE33 ultrasound system (Philips Medical Systems, Bothell, WA, USA), equipped with an rf-interface and a pediatric X7-2 matrix array transducer (2-7 MHz). Rf-data were sampled at 16 MHz and transmitted to an external hard disk. The data were band pass filtered (FIR least squares filter [2-5 MHz]) to prevent disturbance by clutter and noise from frequencies outside the frequency band of the transducer. For constructing echograms, the data were amplitude demodulated using the Hilbert transform method.

2.1 Temporal Cross-Correlation of the Radio Frequency Signal

As velocity of the blood flow is expected to be higher than velocity of the surrounding myocardial tissue, rf-signals will correlate less for fast moving blood than for myocardial tissue. Temporal correlations might thus be used as a feature for distinguishing between blood and the heart muscle. For 3D strain imaging purposes, the cross-correlation function (CCF) of 2D windows of rf-data was calculated [8], [9] using two subsequent full volumes. The peak of the cross-correlation function reveals the displacement of a 2D segment of rf-data in the next time frame in 2D space. A 2D coarse-to-fine displacement estimation algorithm was expanded into an iterative semi-3D approach. 2D reference windows of 50 x 5 (axial x lateral) samples within the axial-azimuth plane were matched with a search area of 150 x 11 samples in the next frame. Both the CCF and the axial and lateral displacements were estimated. Next, the axial displacements were used as an offset to estimate axial and elevational displacements and the CCF in the axial-elevational plane. Hence, the displacements in three orthogonal directions in 3D space were assessed. This semi-3D approach was preferred over a full-3D approach since the iterative 2D cross-correlation calculation imposed a lower computational load and no significant difference in performance and precision was found between both methods [9]. The maximum cross-correlation (MCC) values were found for each window. Window overlap in the axial direction was 75%, resulting in a cross-correlation image of 147 x 62 x 56 samples. This corresponds to a pixel resolution of 600μm in the axial direction.

2.2 3D Adaptive Filtering

Besides the maximum cross-correlation values, adaptive filtering was used as a more conventional method to optimize the distinction between blood and myocardium. 3D Adaptive Mean Squares filtering of the amplitude demodulated data was applied in the spatial domain. The 3D filter kernel size was related to image speckle size and contained approximately 5 x 2 x 2 (axial x lateral x elevational) speckles. The AMS filter incorporates knowledge about speckle statistics of blood and myocardium in an adaptive manner: homogeneous regions are filtered strongly, i.e. speckle noise is reduced, whereas in inhomogeneous regions the degree of filtering is low, such that transitions between blood and myocardium are preserved. The AMS filter has been proven to be effective for segmentation of echocardiographic images when using gradient based deformable models [7].

2.3 Deformable Model

A deformable simplex mesh model [10] was used for segmentation of the left ventricle. In this model, each vertex of the mesh $p_i = (x_i, y_i, z_i)$ is displaced in an iterative manner according to the discrete approximation of the Newtonian law of motion:

$$p_{i+1} = p_i + \alpha F_{int} + F_{ext} \qquad (1)$$

F_{ext} is an external force derived from the image data that steers the simplex mesh onto boundary structures. In this study, F_{ext} consisted of an adaptive filtering based component and the newly defined maximum cross-correlation component:

$$F_{ext} = \beta F_{grad_{AMS}} + \delta F_{grad_{MCC}} + \kappa F_{speed_{AMS}} + \lambda F_{speed_{MCC}} \qquad (2)$$

Both AMS and MCC images were used to compute gradient and speed forces (see [11],[12] for a general description of gradient and speed forces). F_{int} is a regularization force and controls the smoothness of the surface [10]. Weighting factors

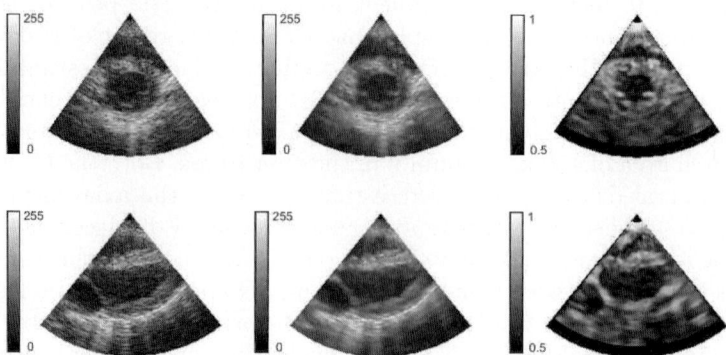

Fig. 1. Short *(upper panel)* and long *(lower panel)* axis views from a full volume dataset for the two external force types of the deformable model. *Left:* demodulated rf-data. *Middle:* data after adaptive filtering. *Right:* maximum cross correlation values.

$\alpha, \beta, \delta, \kappa$ and λ were used to balance the different forces. Whereas adaptive filtering and computation of the cross-correlation was performed by processing the data along the scan-lines, computation of the external and internal forces, as well as the deformation of the simplex mesh was performed on the data in scan-converted (i.e., sector) format. Initialization of the mesh was done by interactive placement of a small spherical mesh in the center of the left ventricle.

Fig. 1 shows long and short axis views from a full volume dataset for the two external force types of the model. In this figure, the original demodulated rf-data, the data after adaptive filtering and the cross-correlation image are shown. Image data were visualized in scan-converted format, in order to obtain realistic anatomical views.

2.4 Evaluation

The method was evaluated by comparing left ventricular cavity contours as obtained from the segmentation method with contours obtained from manual segmentation. Papillary muscles were excluded from the left ventricular cavity. Contours were extracted from the 3D volume segmented by the deformable model and compared to manual segmentation for long axis (LAX) view and three short axis (SAX) cross sections (at base, mid and apical level). Three different force types were compared: using AMS force only (original model, $\beta \neq 0, \kappa \neq 0, \delta = \lambda = 0$), using cross-correlation force only ($\beta = \kappa = 0, \delta \neq 0, \lambda \neq 0$), and the combined model ($\beta = \kappa = \delta = \lambda \neq 0$). The mismatch ratio based on the Dice coefficient was computed for all three force types to the express dissimilarity between manual (Ref) and automatic segmentation (Seg):

$$Mismatch_{Dice} = 1 - \frac{2(Ref \cap Seg)}{(Ref + Seg)} \qquad (3)$$

3 Results

3D segmentation of the left ventricle was performed in four full volume images obtained from four healthy children (6, 7, 8 and 9 years old) in the end systolic phase of the heart cycle. For each dataset, the three different force types (AMS, MCC and a combination of both AMS and MCC) were tested using the deformable model. For each dataset, the same initial position of the mesh in the center of the left ventricle was used for all three segmentation methods.

Fig. 1 illustrates that the contrast between blood and the myocardium is higher for the cross-correlation values than for the adaptive filtered data. Also endocardial regions with low echogenicity seem to have better contrast between blood and myocardium in the correlation image. Fig. 2 shows the effect of the maximum cross-correlation on the segmentation results. In this figure, segmentations of the endocardial surface in the long axis view (LAX) and three short axis views (SAX base, mid and apex) are given for an illustrative example. It can be clearly seen that for this dataset, segmentation exclusively based on the AMS data leads to overestimation of the dimension of the ventricular cavity at the apical side of the long axis view (compare mismatch ratios in Table 1, column 2, LAX). Segmentation solely based on maximum cross-correlation leads to incorrect segmentation and underestimation of the endocardial dimension, see middle panel. Combination of AMS and cross-correlation force (lower panel) improves

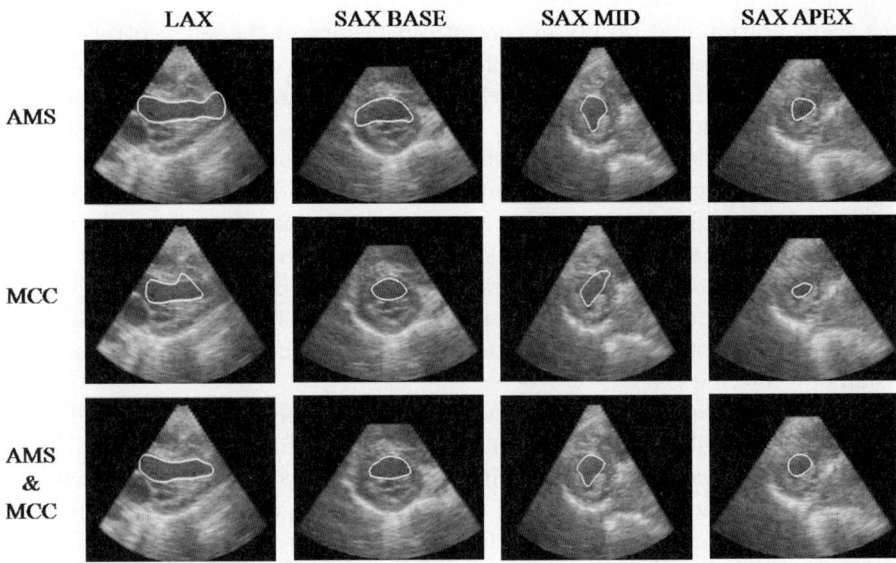

Fig. 2. Segmentation results for three settings of the deformable model for one dataset. Long and short axis views overlaid with contours of the segmented endocardial surface using AMS *(upper)*, maximum cross correlation (MCC) *(middle)* and an equally weighed combination of AMS and MCC force *(lower)*.

Table 1. Mismatch ratios for segmentation by adaptive mean squares (AMS), maximum cross-correlation (MCC) and AMS/MCC combined methods. Long axis (LAX) view and short axis (SAX) view images for the data set of Fig. 2.

Mismatch ratios	LAX	SAX Base	SAX Mid	SAX Apex
AMS	0.23	0.25	0.23	0.13
MCC	0.22	0.14	0.16	0.27
AMS & MCC	0.12	0.14	0.15	0.12

Table 2. Average mismatch ratios (n = 4) for segmentation by adaptive mean squares (AMS), maximum cross-correlation (MCC) and AMS/MCC combined methods for long axis (LAX) view and short axis (SAX) view images

Average mismatch ratios	LAX	SAX Base	SAX Mid	SAX Apex
AMS	0.18	0.16	0.22	0.15
MCC	0.17	0.14	0.17	0.26
AMS & MCC	0.11	0.12	0.14	0.13

the segmentation and results in correct dimensions of the left ventricle. Also in the short axis views, combination of AMS and cross-correlation results in better segmentation of the endocardial surface. Corresponding mismatch ratios for this dataset (see Table 1) revealed that the segmentation results improved (i.e., the mismatch ratio decreased) when the cross-correlation force was added to the AMS force. Using the cross-correlation force on its own resulted in underestimation of the endocardial surface, whereas a segmentation that only used the AMS filtered data resulted in crossing boundaries in the low contrast regions. Table 2 summarizes the mismatch ratios for the four different views (LAX, SAX base, mid and apex), averaged over all four datasets. According to this table, the combination of AMS and MCC force yielded the most accurate segmentation results for all views.

To demonstrate the effect of the MCC force, the gray levels of manually drawn myocardial and blood pool regions were compared for AMS and MCC values. Figure 3 compares AMS against MCC values for myocardial regions with high and low echogenicity (apical), and a blood pool region, respectively It can be seen from this figure that the AMS force is highly distinctive in the case of blood vs. myocardial tissue with high echogenicity. However, for low contrast regions of the heart muscle, for example near the apex, blood and myocardium can no longer be classified by using the AMS values, whereas in this case, MCC still can be used to distinguish blood form myocardial tissue.

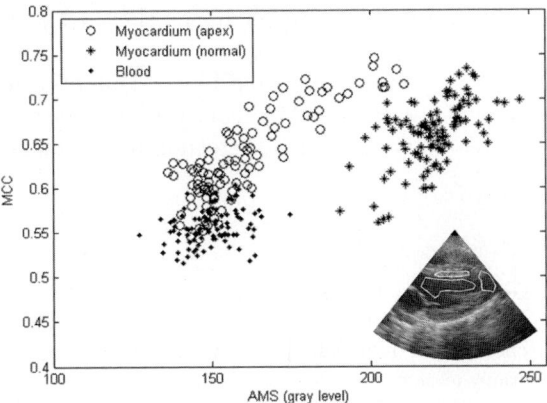

Fig. 3. Comparison between AMS *(horizontal axis)* and MCC *(vertical axis)* values for high and low contrast myocardial regions vs. blood pool region. Manually drawn regions are shown in the echogram *(bottom right)*.

4   Discussion and Conclusion

In this study, we developed a method that enables segmentation of anatomical structures in the heart of children by incorporating temporal information in the model. According to these preliminary results, maximum temporal cross-correlation values, based on the rf-signal, have additional value for the segmentation of cardiac tissue. Since correlation can still be high in areas with low echogenicity, inclusion of this parameter in the deformable simplex model as an extra feature facilitates segmentation in regions where contrast between blood pool and endocardial border is too low to perform gray-level based segmentation. This is illustrated by the proper segmentation of the apical region in Fig. 2. The complimentary character of the MCC and AMS is demonstrated in Fig. 3. In high quality images (without low contrast regions), the AMS force already yielded adequate segmentation results and the cross-correlation force did have no additional value as indicated by the mismatch ratios for AMS and the combination of MCC and AMS in the apical short axis view (Table 1).

A deformable model that only uses the cross-correlation force underestimated the blood pool region. This is most likely caused by the larger windows used in the computation of correlation values and because of the blood close to the heart wall 'adhering' to the moving heart muscle, leading to a higher correlation value, i.e., lower MCC contrast, in blood regions close to the endocardial border.

Presently, the method has been tested in the end-systolic phase where deformation of the heart is small, because with the current echo systems, the frame rate of full volume imaging is still limited in terms of the accuracy of cross-correlation values throughout the entire cardiac cycle. For example, the cross-correlation based model could be used in the end-systolic and end-diastolic phase as a more robust initialization for segmentation of the other frames in the cardiac cycle. In future, the method will be extended to more frames during the cardiac cycle.

Acknowledgments. This work is supported by the Dutch Technology Foundation (STW), project 06466 and Philips Medical Systems. The authors would like to thank Bob Rijk for his assistance with the echographic image acquisitions.

References

1. Noble, J.A., Boukerroui, D.: Ultrasound Image Segmentation: A Survey. IEEE Trans. Med. Imag. 25(8), 987–1010 (2006)
2. Bosch, J.G., Mitchell, S.C., Lelieveldt, B.P., Nijland, F., Kamp, O., Sonka, M., Reiber, J.H.: Automatic segmentation of echocardiographic sequences by active appearance motion models. IEEE Trans. Med. Imag. 21(11), 1374–1383 (2002)
3. Boukerroui, D., Basset, O., Baskurt, A., Giminez, G.: A multiparametric and multiresolution segmentation algorithm of 3-D ultrasonic data. IEEE Trans. Ultrason. Ferroelectr. Freq. Control 48(1), 64–77 (2001)
4. Davignon, F., Deprez, J.F., Basset, O.: A parametric imaging approach for the segmentation of ultrasound data. Ultrasonics 43(10), 789–801 (2005)
5. Dydenko, I., Friboulet, D., Gorce, J.M., D'Hooge, J., Bijnens, B., Magnin, I.E.: Towards ultrasound cardiac image segmentation based on the radiofrequency signal. Med. Image Anal. 7(3), 353–367 (2003)
6. Yan, P., Jia, C.X., Sinusas, A., Thiele, K., O'Donnell, M., Duncan, J.S.: LV segmentation through the analysis of radio frequency ultrasonic images. Inf. Process Med. Imaging 20, 233–244 (2007)
7. Nillesen, M.M., Lopata, R.G.P., Gerrits, I.H., Kapusta, L., Huisman, H.J., Thijssen, J.M., de Korte, C.L.: Segmentation of the heart muscle in 3D pediatric echocardiographic images. Ultrasound Med. Biol. 33(9), 1453–1462 (2007)
8. Chen, X., Xie, H., Erkamp, R., Kim, K., Jia, C., Rubin, J.M., O'Donnell, M.: 3-D correlation-based speckle tracking. Ultrason Imaging 27(1), 21–36 (2005)
9. Lopata, R.G.P., Nillesen, M.M., Gerrits, I.H., Thijssen, J.M., Kapusta, L., de Korte, C.L.: 4D cardiac strain imaging: methods and initial results. In: Proceedings of the IEEE International Ultrasonics Symposium, New York, U.S.A., pp. 872–875 (2007)
10. Delingette, H.: General object reconstruction based on simplex meshes. International Journal of Computer Vision 32(2), 111–146 (1999)
11. Böttger, T., Kunert, T., Meinzer, H.P., Wolf, I.: Application of a new segmentation tool based on interactive simplex meshes to cardiac images and pulmonary MRI data. Acad. Radiol. 14(3), 319–329 (2007)
12. Nillesen, M.M., Lopata, R.G.P., de Boode, W.P., Gerrits, I.H., Huisman, H.J., Thijssen, J.M., Kapusta, L., de Korte, C.L.: In vivo validation of cardiac output assessment in non-standard 3D echocardiographic images. Phys. Med. Biol. 54(7), 1951–1962 (2009)

Improved Modelling of Ultrasound Contrast Agent Diminution for Blood Perfusion Analysis

Christian Kier[1], Karsten Meyer-Wiethe[2], Günter Seidel[2], and Alfred Mertins[1]

[1] Institute for Signal Processing, University of Lübeck, Germany
kier@isip.uni-luebeck.de
[2] Department of Neurology, University Medical Center Schleswig-Holstein,
Lübeck, Germany

Abstract. Ultrasound contrast imaging is increasingly used to analyze blood perfusion in cases of ischemic or cancerous diseases. Among other imaging methods, the diminution harmonic imaging (DHI), which modells the diminution of contrast agent due to ultrasound pulses, is the most promising because of its speed. However, the current imaging quality of DHI is insufficient for reliable diagnoses.

In this paper, we extend the mathematical DHI model to include the part of the intensity signal which is due to tissue reflections and other effects not based on the contrast agent and its concentration in the blood. We show in a phantom experiment with available perfusion ground truth the vast improvements in accuracy of the new model. Our findings also strongly support the theory of a linear relationship between the perfusion speed and the determined perfusion coefficient, which is a large step towards quantitative perfusion measurements.

1 Introduction

Ultrasound (US) perfusion analysis with ultrasound contrast agents (UCA) is a growing field. Its applications cover all major areas in the body, e.g. heart, liver, or brain [1,2]. Due to the use of ultrasound it has several advantages over the use of CT/MRI–based methods, for instance reduced time and cost, and the applicability to critically ill patients as a bedside method. However, the imaging quality is not yet on the level accustomed by CT or MRI.

The most widely used imaging method is based on analyzing the kinetics of a UCA bolus. Studies have shown its diagnostic significance [3]. Its main drawback however is its long duration, which also makes it prone to movement artifacts [4]. Other methods are based on continuous UCA infusion, such as the diminution method. It uses high-power US pulses to destroy a substantial part of the contrast agent with each pulse. A steady state is reached after a couple of pulses, in which every pulse destroys as much UCA as is washed in during the interframe interval. Instead of covering a whole bolus, which takes up to 60 s, the DHI method acquires only 6–10 images at an interframe interval of 150–1000 ms. The first approach to model the DHI method and extract perfusion-related parameters appeared in [5], where the model was fitted to the data by

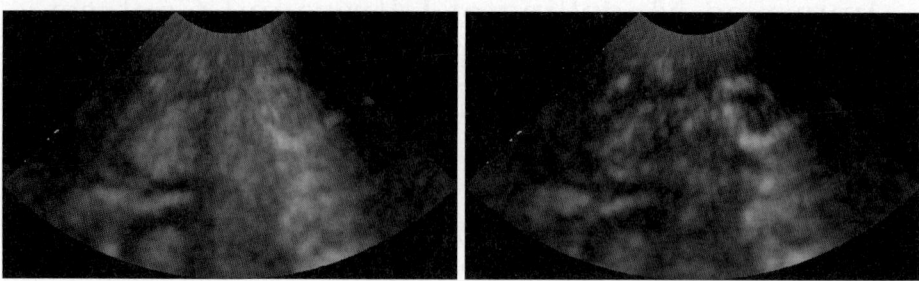

Fig. 1. First (left) and last (right) image of an exemplary transcranial DHI sequence

least squares methods. An improvement was made by [6] to be able to directly calculate the parameters and avoid the time-consuming fitting process. Other approaches tried to determine the perfusion in a general way, independent of the actual UCA concentration and insonation pattern used [7]. However, they do not seem to have found wide acceptance.

This paper is organized as follows: Section 2 explains the DHI method in detail and presents our model extensions and their implications. In Section 3, the results of a phantom study are shown to prove the higher accuracy of the new model. Finally, in Section 4 the results are discussed and conclusions are drawn.

2 Methods

2.1 Diminution Harmonic Imaging

To improve the SNR, ultrasound harmonic imaging makes use of the fact that the ultrasound attenuation varies over frequency. The use of UCA amplifies this effect. UCA consist mainly of gas-filled microbubbles that nonlinearly scatter ultrasound and hence improve harmonic imaging. Depending on the US pulse energy, the microbubbles are even destroyed, which also generates a nonlinear echo. While the US pulse is sent with a center frequency of 1.8MHz, the probe records also harmonic frequencies which are mainly due to contrast agent. Since contrast agent can only be found in the blood circulation, this procedure is well suited for perfusion imaging. Analyzing a varying contrast agent concentration in an US image sequence provides information about the actual perfusion in the imaging plane.

The DHI method is based on continuous contrast agent infusion leading to a constant UCA concentration in the blood. A series of US pulses reduces the UCA concentration, since microbubbles are destroyed due to the high sound pressure using this method. After approximately 5 pulses, the UCA concentration approaches an equilibrium, in which an US pulse destroys as much contrast agent as is flowing into the image plane during one interpulse interval. Fig. 1 shows the first and last image from an exemplary DHI sequence (in this case from the brain). The intensity decrease is clearly shown although in some high blood flow velocity regions, like the posterior cerebral artery, the intensity almost did not change.

2.2 Mathematical Model

Our model is specific to the DHI process, which we consider special even among ultrasound perfusion analysis models. As opposed to many other perfusion analysis approaches, the DHI process directly depends on the insonation pattern. Hence, the measurement itself drastically influences the measured process.

As shown in Fig. 1, in some regions the image intensity does not change very much or decreases only to a certain level. This is due to the fact that the US system receives not only UCA echos but also tissue signals. Although quite obvious, this baseline intensity I_b was to our knowledge not yet modelled explicitly. Instead, its incorporation with the model was considered unnecessary [5].

Furthermore, the UCA concentration is modelled while only the image intensity $I(n)$ is observable. Although considered the most critical precondition, past publications did not make an assumption on the relationship between UCA concentration and image intensity, but used the intensity values directly. Due to equally distributed UCA and unchanged acoustic power and insonation plane, the remaining fraction of UCA d is assumed to be constant. Hence, a linear relationship between the UCA concentration $C(n)$ and the UCA-dependent image intensity $I_c(n)$ can be assumed, which is supported by our experimental results:

$$I(n) := I_c(n) + I_b \qquad (1)$$
$$I_c(n) := k \cdot C(n) \qquad (2)$$

where n is the index for an insonation pulse, since the process can only be observed at discrete intervals. Three factors influence the UCA concentration $C(n)$ in the insonation plane: blood wash-in, wash-out, and UCA destruction by US pulses. Hence, it can be modelled as the following function in the sampled tissue/blood volume:

$$C(n+1) = C(1) \cdot \underbrace{\left(1 - e^{-p \cdot \Delta t}\right)}_{Inflow} + C(n) \cdot \underbrace{d}_{Destruction} \cdot \underbrace{e^{-p \cdot \Delta t}}_{Outflow}. \qquad (3)$$

Here, Δt denotes the time between two pulses, d gives the amount of contrast agent that is not destroyed by the pulse ($0 \leq d \leq 1$), and p is the perfusion coefficient so that e^{-p*dt} is the fraction of blood that is exchanged. Since the acquisition time is below 2 seconds, p is assumed to be constant. The process is illustrated in Fig. 2. To calculate the concentration in the nth step directly, the following closed form exists:

$$C(n) = C(1) \cdot \left(x^{n-1} + y \cdot \frac{x^{n-1} - 1}{x - 1}\right), \text{ with} \qquad (4)$$
$$x = d \cdot e^{-p \cdot \Delta t} \quad \text{and} \quad y = 1 - e^{-p \cdot \Delta t}.$$

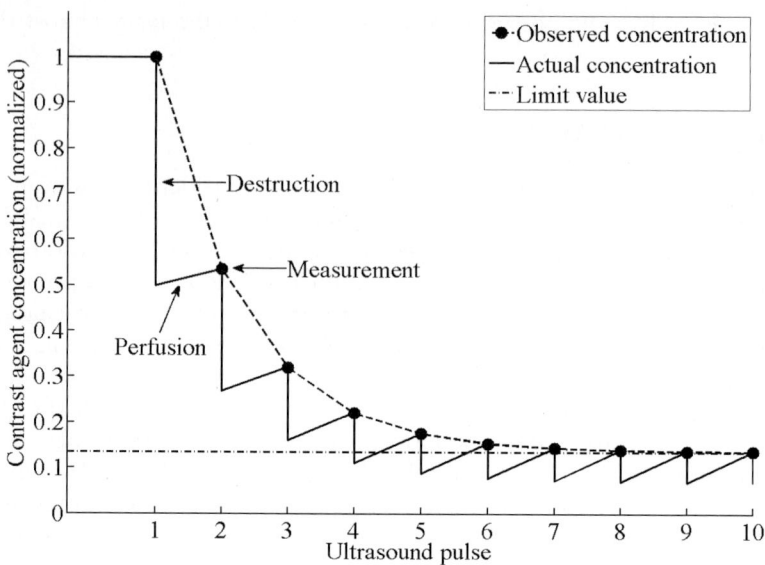

Fig. 2. Illustration of the DHI process with observed and actual concentration

The state of equilibrium between inflow, outflow and destruction that is eventually reached results in a constant intensity I_∞:

$$I_\infty := \lim_{n\to\infty} I(n) \stackrel{(1)}{=} \lim_{n\to\infty} I_c(n) + I_b \stackrel{(2)}{=} \lim_{n\to\infty} k \cdot C(n) + I_b$$

$$\stackrel{(4)}{=} k \cdot C(1) \left[\lim_{n\to\infty} x^{n-1} + \lim_{n\to\infty} y \cdot \frac{x^{n-1}-1}{x-1} \right] + I_b \qquad (5)$$

$$\stackrel{p \geq 0}{=} I_c(1) \cdot \frac{-y}{x-1} + I_b = I_c(1) \cdot \frac{e^{-p \cdot \Delta t} - 1}{d \cdot e^{-p \cdot \Delta t} - 1} + I_b.$$

Equation 5 shows that the relation between $I_c(n)$ and $C(n)$ does not have to be explicitly calculated. After solving equation 5 for p we have:

$$p = \frac{1}{\Delta t} \ln \frac{I_{c\infty} d - I_c(1)}{I_{c\infty} - I_c(1)} \qquad \text{with} \quad I_{c\infty} := \lim_{n\to\infty} I_c(n)$$

$$\stackrel{(1)}{=} \frac{1}{\Delta t} \ln \frac{I_\infty d - I(1) + I_b(1-d)}{I_\infty - I(1)} \qquad (6)$$

In this equation, $I(1)$ and I_∞ can be taken from the US image series. The baseline intensity I_b and the destruction coefficient d are still missing. For this, we develop the following limit:

$$L_n := \lim_{\Delta t \to 0} \frac{I(n+1) - I_b}{I(n) - I_b} \lim_{\Delta t \to 0} \frac{I_c(n+1)}{I_c(n)}$$

$$= \lim_{\Delta t \to 0} \frac{kC(1)\left[x^n + y\frac{x^n-1}{x-1}\right]}{kC(1)\left[x^{n-1} + y\frac{x^{n-1}-1}{x-1}\right]} = \frac{d^n}{d^{n-1}} = d \qquad (7)$$

Since equation 7 is valid for all n, we can equalize two arbitrary L_n to solve this equation for I_b. We select $n = 1$ and $n = 2$ since at these frames flow effects are relatively small while the absolute destruction value is largest:

$$L_1 = L_2$$
$$\frac{I(2) - I_b}{I(1) - I_b} = \frac{I(3) - I_b}{I(2) - I_b} \qquad (8)$$
$$I_b = \frac{I(2)^2 - I(3)I(1)}{2I(2) - I(3) - I(1)}$$

Finally, we can obtain all values from the US image series and calculate I_b. Using equation 7, we obtain d also. To correct for possible errors due to image noise, we set I_b to the highest value (255 with 8 bit grayscale images) when the denominator in equation 8 is zero and also constrain I_b to the minimum of the time-intensity-curve.

3 Results

To validate our new method, we performed experiments with a flow phantom as well as examinations on humans to determine the brain perfusion.

3.1 Phantom Experiments

We designed a simple open-circuit flow model with a dialysis cartridge as a capillary phantom. The cartridge consisted of 9000 capillaries with an internal diameter of 200 μm. The fluid (nondegassed water at 22 °C) was driven by a programmable pump, which was connected to a roller pump head, providing continuous nonpulsatile flow at defined flow volumes. To avoid flotation of the UCA in the capillary-free entry section of the cartridge, it was fixed in a vertical position. The UCA was applied using a perfusion pump.

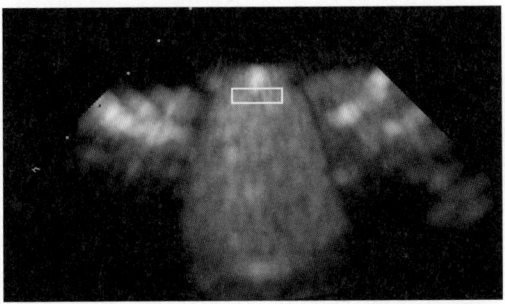
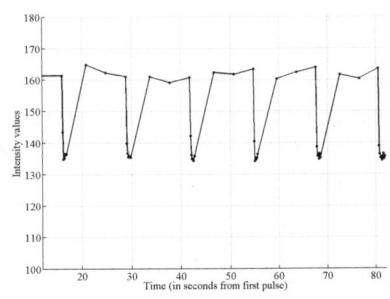

Fig. 3. Placement of the ROI (left) and exemplary time-intensity-curve (right) for the phantom experiment

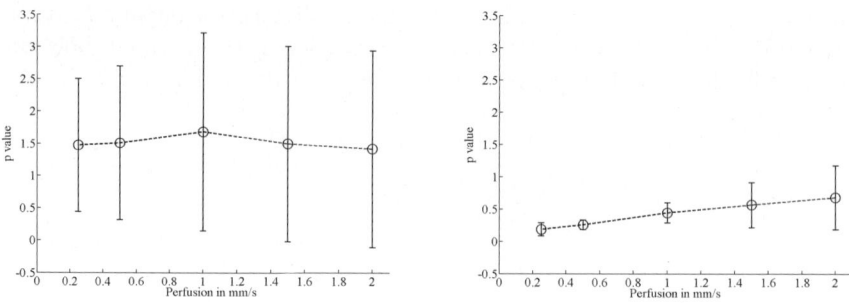

Fig. 4. Existing (left) and new (right) perfusion coefficient plotted over the known perfusion velocity

Using a custom-made probe holder, the US probe was held in place at an insonation angle of 90° to the phantom, providing a cross-sectional view. Harmonic imaging was performed with a SONOS 5500 US system (Philips Medical Systems, Best, The Netherlands) and a 1.8–3.6 MHz sector transducer (S4 probe, Philips) in the conventional harmonic imaging mode (T-INT, insonation at 1.8 MHz, receiver tuned to 3.6 MHz). The mechanical index (MI) was 1.6. Gain and transmit power settings were kept constant during the session. Standardized insonation conditions were provided by an acoustic stand-off.

Five flow velocities (0.25, 0.5, 1, 1.5, and 2 mm/s) were investigated at five frame rates (1, 1.33, 2, 4 and 6.67 Hz). The rapid, destructive US sequences were followed by three pulses at 0.25 Hz to allow replenishment of intact microbubbles into the insonation plane. To assess the repeatability of the measurements, each combination was repeated 6 times during one single session.

To exclude attenuation phenomena that occur in deeper regions of the flow model, we analyzed contrast data of a rectangular region of interest (ROI), which was placed at a distance of 30 mm from the probe. Fig. 3 shows the placement of the ROI as well as an exemplary time-intensity curve of one sequence.

The obtained images were used to calculate p in the ROI according to the model given in [6] and for our new method. Since in the phantom experiment we have the perfusion ground truth available, we put the calculated p values in relation to the known perfusion velocities. The most impressive results are shown in Fig. 4. It is clearly visible that the new perfusion coefficient correlates highly to the perfusion velocity which is not the case for the existing model.

The appearance of the new perfusion coefficient also strongly supports the theory of a linear relationship. Fitting a line onto the obtained values of p gives

$$P = 3.47 \cdot p + 0.44 \tag{9}$$

with P being the known perfusion velocity.

3.2 Brain Perfusion

Among applications of perfusion analysis, determining brain perfusion with transcranial sonography is considered most challenging, since US images suffer from

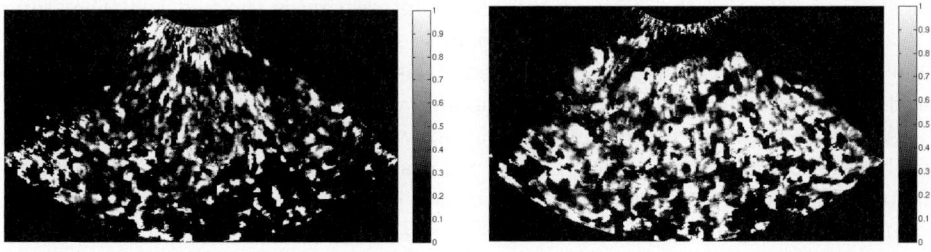

Fig. 5. Visualizations of the perfusion coefficient for a healthy subject (left) and a patient suffering from an ischemic stroke (right)

a low SNR due to the high impedance of the skull. When acquiring a DHI sequence, the penetration depth of the ultrasound beam is set to 10 cm. Thus, two sequences are necessary to cover the diencephalic imaging plane from both hemispheres of a patient.

Fig. 5 shows two visualizations of the perfusion coefficient for two different subjects. Both sequences have been acquired in an axial imaging plane with the US probe at the temporal acoustic bone window at a frame rate of 6.67 Hz. Values of p were calculated with the new method and visualized as gray-level images. The most interesting part of the brain regarding pathological brain perfusion is close to the skull, i.e. close to the top in the US frame, because (a) most perfusion deficits occur in this area and (b) the lower part of the US image area increasingly suffers from the UCA attenuation or shadowing effect and hence can be ignored in the further analysis.

The images may be difficult to grasp, but in comparison it becomes evident that a large region to the top of the right image, i.e. at the cortex of the ischemic stroke patient, has a perfusion coefficient value of zero. That means this region is not perfused at all which was also confirmed by an MRI examination of this patient.

This visualization is of course only semi-quantitative and does not incorporate the findings from Section 3.1. A fully quantitative mapping using the relationship given in equation 9 is not feasible, since many influencing factors hinder the comparison of the phantom experiment with the human examination.

4 Discussion and Conclusions

Compared to currently used diagnostic procedures the presented method features fast and inexpensive perfusion analysis by means of ultrasound image sequences. An examination can be performed directly at the patient's bedside under minimal strain for the patient. Especially noteworthy is the short examination time of the DHI method compared to other US imaging methods. Besides further stress reduction for the patient it helps in providing stable insonation conditions and thus makes it the most promising method among its competitors.

Our model extension greatly enhances prediction accuracy for the perfusion coefficient and supports the theory of a linear relation to the underlying perfusion as shown in the *in vitro* experiments. Most interesting is the fact that the standard deviation of the perfusion coefficient is smaller the lower the perfusion is. These regions of malperfused, i.e. ischemic, tissue are of high diagnostic interest and a high accuracy is especially important.

Although setup to mimic human microcirculation conditions, transfering the findings of the *in vitro* to the *in vivo* case is still a challenging task, since many factors influence the relationship determined in equation 9. Besides imaging parameters, such as mechanical index, UCA-related parameters have to be considered, i.e. the type of UCA, its concentration etc. Furthermore, patient-related paramters exist, like the accessibility of the acoustic bone window. However, our findings are a great step towards fully quantitative perfusion analysis of microcirculation with ultrasound. Still, comprehensive phantom studies are needed to provide a basis to cover all parameter combinations.

To summarize, our method is very promising. The ultrasound-based diminution harmonic imaging method provides a fast and inexpensive alternative among different modalities for microcirculation evaluation. Because of the general approach it is not restricted to cerebral microcirculation and can be applied to every organ that is reachable by ultrasound.

References

1. Hancock, J., Dittrich, H., Jewitt, D., Monagham, M.: Evaluation of myocardial, hepatic, and renal perfusion in a variety of clinical conditions using an intravenous ultrasoundcontrast agent (optison) and second harmonic imaging. Heart 81(6), 636–641 (1999)
2. Seidel, G., Meyer, K.: Impact of ultrasound contrast agents in cerebrovascular diagnostics. European Journal of Ultrasound 16(1-2), 81–90 (2002)
3. Krogias, C., Postert, T., Meves, S., Wilkening, W., Przuntek, H., Eyding, J.: Semiquantitative analysis of ultrasonic cerebral perfusion imaging. Ultrasound in Medicine & Biology 31(8), 1007–1012 (2005)
4. Maciak, A., Kier, C., Seidel, G., Meyer-Wiethe, K., Hofmann, U.G.: Detecting stripe artifacts in ultrasound images. Journal of Digital Imaging (2007)
5. Wilkening, W., Postert, T., Federlein, J., Kono, Y., Mattrey, R., Ermert, H.: Ultrasonic assessment of perfusion conditions in the brain and in the liver. In: Proc. IEEE Ultrasonics Symposium, San Juan, Puerto Rico, October 2000, vol. 2, pp. 1545–1548 (2000)
6. Kier, C., Meyer-Wiethe, K., Seidel, G., Aach, T.: Ultrasound cerebral perfusion analysis based on a mathematical model for diminution harmonic imaging. Methods of Information in Medicine 46(3), 308–313 (2007)
7. Williams, Q.R., Noble, J.A.: A spatio-temporal analysis of contrast ultrasound image sequences for assessment of tissue perfusion. In: Barillot, C., Haynor, D.R., Hellier, P. (eds.) MICCAI 2004. LNCS, vol. 3217, pp. 899–906. Springer, Heidelberg (2004)

A Novel 3D Joint Markov-Gibbs Model for Extracting Blood Vessels from PC–MRA Images

Ayman El-Baz[1], Georgy Gimel'farb[2], Robert Falk[3], Mohamed Abou El-Ghar[4], Vedant Kumar[1], and David Heredia[1]

[1] Bioimaging Laboratory, University of Louisville, Louisville, KY, USA
[2] Department of Computer Science, University of Auckland, Auckland, New Zealand
[3] Director, Medical Imaging Division, Jewish Hospital, Louisville, KY, USA
[4] Urology and Nephrology Department, University of Mansoura, Mansoura, Egypt

Abstract. New techniques for more accurate segmentation of a 3D cerebrovascular system from phase contrast (PC) magnetic resonance angiography (MRA) data are proposed. In this paper, we describe PC–MRA images and desired maps of regions by a joint Markov-Gibbs random field model (MGRF) of independent image signals and interdependent region labels but focus on most accurate model identification. To better specify region borders, each empirical distribution of signals is precisely approximated by a Linear Combination of Discrete Gaussians (LCDG) with positive and negative components. We modified the conventional Expectation-Maximization (EM) algorithm to deal with the LCDG. The initial segmentation based on the LCDG-models is then iteratively refined using a MGRF model with analytically estimated potentials. Experiments with both the phantoms and real data sets confirm high accuracy of the proposed approach.

1 Introduction

Accurate cerebrovascular segmentation using non-invasive MRA is a valuable tool for early diagnostics and timely treatment of intracranial vascular diseases. Among three common MRA techniques, such as time-of-flight MRA (TOF–MRA), phase contrast angiography (PCA), and contrast enhanced MRA (CE-MRA), only TOF–MRA and PCA use flowing blood as an inherent contrast medium, while for CE-MRA a contrasting substance has to be injected into the circulatory system. Our work is motivated by the wide use of PCA and TOF–MRA in clinical practice.

Today's most popular techniques for segmenting blood vessels from MRA data can be roughly classified in two categories: deformable models and statistical methods. The former iteratively adjust an initial boundary surface to blood vessels by optimizing an energy function that depends on image gradient and surface smoothness [1]. Topologically adaptable surfaces make classical deformable models more efficient in segmenting intracranial vasculature [2]. Geodesic active contours implemented with level set techniques offer flexible topological adaptability to segment MRA images [3] including more efficient adaptation to local geometric structures represented e.g. by tensor eigenvalues [4]. Fast segmentation of blood vessel surfaces is obtained by inflating a 3D balloon with fast marching methods [5]. In [6] they used a marked point-based segmentation algorithm to extract the coronary tree from 2D X-ray angiography.

The latter extract the vascular tree automatically, but their accuracy depends on underlying probability models. The MRA images are multi-modal in the sense that particular modes of the marginal probability distribution of signals are associated with regions-of-interest. To the best of our knowledge, the only adaptive statistical approaches for extracting blood vessels from the MRA data were proposed by Noble and her group [7,8]. The marginal distribution is modeled with a mixture of two Gaussian and one uniform or Rician components for the stationary CSF and bones, brain tissues, and arteries, respectively. The uniform component presumes the blood flow is strictly laminar. In [9] they presented a segmentation algorithm to extract the vascular system from TOF–MRA images. Their approach is based on using a mixture of Gaussian and Rayleigh distributions to approximate the normalized histogram of TOF-MRA images.

2 Joint Markov-Gibbs Model of PC–MRA Images

Let $\mathbf{R} = \{(i,j,z) : 1 \leq i \leq I, 1 \leq j \leq J, 1 \leq z \leq Z\}$ denote a finite arithmetic grid supporting grayscale PC–MRA images $\mathbf{g} : \mathbf{R} \to \mathbf{Q}$ and their region maps $\mathbf{m} : \mathbf{R} \to \mathbf{X}$. Here, $\mathbf{Q} = \{0, \ldots, Q-1\}$ and $\mathbf{X} = \{1, \ldots, X\}$ are the sets of gray levels and region labels, respectively, where Q is the number of gray levels and X is the number of image classes. The MGRF model of images to segment is given by a joint probability distribution of PC–MRA images and desired region maps $P(\mathbf{g}, \mathbf{m}) = P(\mathbf{m})P(\mathbf{g}|\mathbf{m})$. Here, $P(\mathbf{m})$ is an unconditional distribution of maps and $P(\mathbf{g}|\mathbf{m})$ is a conditional distribution of images, given a map. The Bayesian MAP estimate of the map, given the image $\mathbf{g}$, $\mathbf{m}^* = \arg\max_{\mathbf{m}} L(\mathbf{g}, \mathbf{m})$ maximizes the log-likelihood function:

$$L(\mathbf{g}, \mathbf{m}) = \log P(\mathbf{g}|\mathbf{m}) + \log P(\mathbf{m}) \qquad (1)$$

2.1 Spatial Interaction Model of PC–MRA Images

Generic Markov-Gibbs model of region maps that accounts for only pairwise interactions between each region label and its neighbors has generally an arbitrary interaction structure and arbitrary Gibbs potentials identified from image data. For simplicity, we restrict the interactions to the nearest voxels (26-neighborhood) and assume, by symmetry considerations, that the interactions are independent of relative region orientation, are the same for all classes, and depend only on intra- or inter-region position of each voxel pair (i.e. whether the labels are equal or not). Under these restrictions, the model is similar to the conventional auto-binomial ones and differs only in that the potentials are not related to a predefined function and have analytical estimates. The symmetric label interactions are three-fold: the closest horizontal-vertical-diagonal in the current slice (hvdc), the closest horizontal-vertical-diagonal in the upper slice (hvdu), and the closest horizontal-vertical-diagonal in the lower slice (hvdl). The potentials of each type are bi-valued because only coincidence or difference of the labels are taken into account. Let $\mathbf{V}_a = \{V_a(x,\chi) = V_{a,\text{eq}}$ if $x = \chi$ and $V_a(x,\chi) = V_{a,\text{ne}}$ if $x \neq \chi$: $x, \chi \in \mathbf{X}\}$ denote bi-valued Gibbs potentials describing symmetric pairwise interactions of type $a \in \mathbf{A} = \{\text{hvdc}, \text{hvdu}, \text{hvdl}\}$ between the region labels. Let $\mathbf{N}_{\text{hvdc}} = \{(1,0,0), (0,1,0), (-1,0,0), (0,-1,0)\}$, $\mathbf{N}_{\text{hvdu}} = \{(0,0,1), (-1,-1,1), (-1,1,1), (1,-1,1), (1,1,1)\}$, and $\mathbf{N}_{\text{hvdl}} = \{(0,0,-1), (-1,-1,-1), (-1,1,-1), (1,-1,-1), (1,1,-1)\}$ be subsets of inter-voxel offsets for the 26-neighborhood system. Then the Gibbs probability distribution of region maps is:

$$P(\mathbf{m}) \propto \exp\left(\sum_{(i,j,z) \in \mathbf{R}} \sum_{a \in \mathbf{A}} \sum_{(\xi,\eta,\zeta) \in \mathbf{N}_a} V_a(m_{i,j,z}, m_{i+\xi, j+\eta, z+\zeta})\right) \quad (2)$$

To identify the MGRF model described in Eq. (2), we have to estimate the Gibbs Potentials $\mathbf{V}$. In this paper we introduce a new analytical maximum likelihood estimation for the Gibbs potentials.

$$V_{a,\text{eq}} = \frac{X^2}{X-1}\left(f'_a(\mathbf{m}) - \frac{1}{X}\right) \text{ and } V_{a,\text{ne}} = \frac{X^2}{X-1}\left(f''_a(\mathbf{m}) - 1 + \frac{1}{X}\right) \quad (3)$$

where $f'_a(\mathbf{m})$ and $f''_a(\mathbf{m})$ denote the relative frequency of the equal and non-equal pairs of the labels in all the equivalent voxel pairs $\{((i,j,z), (i+\xi, j+\eta, z+\zeta)) : (i,j,z) \in \mathbf{R}.; (i+\xi, j+\eta, z+\zeta) \in \mathbf{R}; (\xi,\eta,\zeta) \in \mathbf{N}_a\}$, respectively.

2.2 Intensity Model of PC–MRA Images

Let q; $q \in \mathbf{Q} = \{0, 1, \ldots, Q-1\}$, denote the Q-ary gray level. The discrete Gaussian is defined as the probability distribution $\Psi_\theta = (\psi(q|\theta) : q \in \mathbf{Q})$ on $\mathbf{Q}$ such that $\psi(q|\theta) = \Phi_\theta(q+0.5) - \Phi_\theta(q-0.5)$ for $q = 1, \ldots, Q-2$, $\psi(0|\theta) = \Phi_\theta(0.5)$, $\psi(Q-1|\theta) = 1 - \Phi_\theta(Q-1.5)$ where $\Phi_\theta(q)$ is the cumulative Gaussian function with a shorthand notation $\theta = (\mu, \sigma^2)$ for its mean, μ, and variance, σ^2.

We assume the number K of dominant modes, i.e. regions or classes of interest in a given PC–MRA images, is already known. In contrast to a conventional mixture of Gaussians and/or other simple distributions, one per region, we closely approximate the empirical gray level distribution for PC–MRA images with an LCDG having C_p positive and C_n negative components such that $C_p \geq K$:

$$p_{\mathbf{w},\Theta}(q) = \sum_{r=1}^{C_p} w_{p,r} \psi(q|\theta_{p,r}) - \sum_{l=1}^{C_n} w_{n,l} \psi(q|\theta_{n,l}) \quad (4)$$

under the obvious restrictions on the weights $\mathbf{w} = [w_{p,.}, w_{n,.}]$: all the weights are non-negative and

$$\sum_{r=1}^{C_p} w_{p,r} - \sum_{l=1}^{C_n} w_{n,l} = 1 \quad (5)$$

To identify the LCDG-model including the numbers of its positive and negative components, we modify the EM algorithm to deal with the LCDG.

First, the numbers $C_p - K$, C_n and parameters $\mathbf{w}$, $\boldsymbol{\Theta}$ (weights, means, and variances) of the positive and negative Discrete Gaussian (DG) components are estimated with a sequential EM-based initializing algorithm. The goal is to produce a close initial LCDG-approximation of the empirical distribution.

Sequential EM-based Initialization. Sequential EM-based initialization forms an LCDG-approximation of a given empirical marginal gray level distribution using the conventional EM-algorithm [10] adapted to the DGs. At the first stage, the empirical distribution is represented with a mixture of K positive DGs, each dominant mode being roughly approximated with a single DG. At the second stage, deviations of the empirical distribution from the dominant K-component mixture are modeled with other, "subordinate" components of the LCDG. The resulting initial LCDG has K dominant weights, say, $w_{p,1}, \ldots, w_{p,K}$ such that $\sum_{r=1}^{K} w_{p,r} = 1$, and a number of subordinate weights of smaller values such that $\sum_{r=K+1}^{C_p} w_{p,r} - \sum_{l=1}^{C_n} w_{n,l} = 0$.

Modified EM Algorithm for LCDG. Modified EM algorithm for LCDG maximizes the log-likelihood of the empirical data by the model parameters assuming statistically independent signals:

$$L(\mathbf{w}, \boldsymbol{\Theta}) = \sum_{q \in \mathbf{Q}} f(q) \log p_{\mathbf{w}, \boldsymbol{\Theta}}(q) \tag{6}$$

A local maximum of the log-likelihood in Eq. (6) is given with the EM process extending the one in [10] onto alternating signs of the components. Let $p_{\mathbf{w}, \boldsymbol{\Theta}}^{[m]}(q) = \sum_{r=1}^{C_p} w_{p,r}^{[m]} \psi(q|\theta_{p,r}^{[m]}) - \sum_{l=1}^{C_n} w_{n,l}^{[m]} \psi(q|\theta_{n,l}^{[m]})$ denote the current LCDG at iteration m. Relative contributions of each signal $q \in \mathbf{Q}$ to each positive and negative DG at iteration m are specified by the respective conditional weights

$$\pi_p^{[m]}(r|q) = \frac{w_{p,r}^{[m]} \psi(q|\theta_{p,r}^{[m]})}{p_{\mathbf{w}, \boldsymbol{\Theta}}^{[m]}(q)}; \quad \pi_n^{[m]}(l|q) = \frac{w_{n,l}^{[m]} \psi(q|\theta_{n,l}^{[m]})}{p_{\mathbf{w}, \boldsymbol{\Theta}}^{[m]}(q)} \tag{7}$$

such that the following constraints hold:

$$\sum_{r=1}^{C_p} \pi_p^{[m]}(r|q) - \sum_{l=1}^{C_n} \pi_n^{[m]}(l|q) = 1; \; q = 0, \ldots, Q-1 \tag{8}$$

The following two steps iterate until the log-likelihood changes become small:

- **E– step**$^{[m+1]}$: Find the weights of Eq. (7) under the fixed parameters $\mathbf{w}^{[m]}$, $\boldsymbol{\Theta}^{[m]}$ from the previous iteration m, and
- **M– step**$^{[m+1]}$: Find conditional MLEs $\mathbf{w}^{[m+1]}$, $\boldsymbol{\Theta}^{[m+1]}$ by maximizing $L(\mathbf{w}, \boldsymbol{\Theta})$ under the fixed weights of Eq. (7).

Considerations closely similar to those in [10] show this process converges to a local log-likelihood maximum. Let the log-likelihood of Eq. (6) be rewritten in the equivalent form with the constraints of Eq. (8) as unit factors:

$$L(\mathbf{w}^{[m]}, \mathbf{\Theta}^{[m]}) = \sum_{q=0}^{Q} f(q) \left[\sum_{r=1}^{C_\mathrm{p}} \pi_\mathrm{p}^{[m]}(r|q) \log p^{[m]}(q) - \sum_{l=1}^{C_\mathrm{n}} \pi_\mathrm{n}^{[m]}(l|q) \log p^{[m]}(q) \right]$$

Let the terms $\log p^{[m]}(q)$ in the first and second brackets be replaced with the equal terms $\log w_{\mathrm{p},r}^{[m]} + \log \psi(q|\theta_{\mathrm{p},r}^{[m]}) - \log \pi_\mathrm{p}^{[m]}(r|q)$ and $\log w_{\mathrm{n},l}^{[m]} + \log \psi(q|\theta_{\mathrm{n},l}^{[m]}) - \log \pi_\mathrm{n}^{[m]}(l|q)$, respectively, which follow from Eq. (7). At the E-step, the conditional Lagrange maximization of the log-likelihood of Eq. (9) under the Q restrictions of Eq. (8) results just in the weights $\pi_\mathrm{p}^{[m+1]}(r|q)$ and $\pi_\mathrm{n}^{[m+1]}(l|q)$ of Eq. (7) for all $r = 1, \ldots, C_\mathrm{p}$; $l = 1, \ldots, C_\mathrm{n}$ and $q \in \mathbf{Q}$. At the M-step, the DG weights $w_{\mathrm{p},r}^{[m+1]} = \sum_{q \in \mathbf{Q}} f(q) \pi_\mathrm{p}^{[m+1]}(r|q)$ and $w_{\mathrm{n},l}^{[m+1]} = \sum_{q \in \mathbf{Q}} f(q) \pi_\mathrm{n}^{[m+1]}(l|q)$ follow from the conditional Lagrange maximization of the log-likelihood in Eq. (9) under the restriction of Eq. (5) and the fixed conditional weights of Eq. (7). Under these latter, the conventional MLEs of the parameters of each DG stem from maximizing the log-likelihood after each difference of the cumulative Gaussians is replaced with its close approximation with the Gaussian density (below "c" stands for "p" or "n", respectively):

$$\mu_{\mathrm{c},r}^{[m+1]} = \frac{1}{w_{\mathrm{c},r}^{[m+1]}} \sum_{q \in \mathbf{Q}} q \cdot f(q) \pi_\mathrm{c}^{[m+1]}(r|q)$$

$$(\sigma_{\mathrm{c},r}^{[m+1]})^2 = \frac{1}{w_{\mathrm{c},r}^{[m+1]}} \sum_{q \in \mathbf{Q}} \left(q - \mu_{\mathrm{c},i}^{[m+1]} \right)^2 \cdot f(q) \pi_\mathrm{c}^{[m+1]}(r|q)$$

This modified EM-algorithm is valid until the weights $\mathbf{w}$ are strictly positive. The iterations should be terminated when the log-likelihood of Eq. (6) does not change or begins to decrease due to accumulation of rounding errors.

The final mixed LCDG-model $p_C(q)$ is partitioned into the K LCDG-submodels $P_{[k]} = [p(q|k) : q \in \mathbf{Q}]$, one per class $k = 1, \ldots, K$, by associating the subordinate DGs with the dominant terms so that the misclassification rate is minimal.

3 Experimental Results

Experiments were conducted with the PC–MRA images acquired with the Picker 1.5T Edge MRI scanner having spatial resolution of $0.86 \times 0.86 \times 1.0$ mm. The size of each 3D data set is $256 \times 256 \times 123$. The PC–MRA images contain three classes ($K = 3$), namely, darker bones and fat, brain tissues, and brighter blood vessels. A typical PC–MRA slice, its empirical marginal gray level distribution $f(q)$, and the initial 3-component Gaussian dominant mixture $p_3(q)$ are shown in Fig. 1.

Figure 2 presents the final LCDG-model after refining the initial one with the modified EM-algorithm and shows successive changes of the log-likelihood at the refinement iterations. The final LCDG-models of each class are obtained with

Table 1. Minimum ε_n, maximum ε_x, and mean $\bar{\varepsilon}$ segmentation errors, and standard deviations σ of errors on the geometrical 3D PC–MRA phantoms for our (OA) as well as for four other segmentation algorithms using iterative thresholding (IT) [11], gradient based (DMG) [12] or gradient vector flow based (GVF) [13] deformable models, and Chung segmentation approach (C) [8]

	OA	IT	DMG	GVF	C
ε_n,%	**0.07**	3.89	8.9	1.97	0.1
ε_x,%	**1.87**	31.7	19.1	11.1	12.1
$\bar{\varepsilon}$,%	**0.49**	15.7	9.8	4.87	6.2
σ,%	**0.81**	7.01	2.99	1.79	0.93

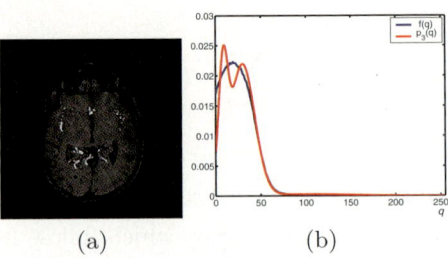

Fig. 1. Typical PC–MRA scan slice (a) and deviations between the empirical distribution $f(q)$ and the dominant 3-component mixture $p_3(q)$ (b)

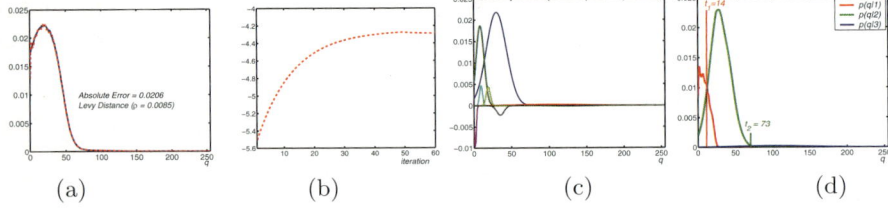

Fig. 2. Final 3-class LCDG-model overlaying the empirical density (a), the log-likelihood dynamics (b) for the refining EM-iterations, the refined model components (c), and the class LCDG-models (d)

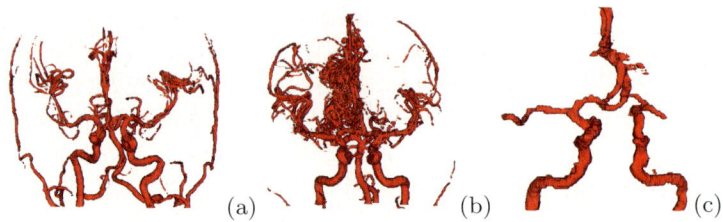

Fig. 3. Segmentation results obtained by the proposed approach

the best separation thresholds $t_1 = 14$ and $t_2 = 73$. The first 47 refining iterations increase the log-likelihood from -5.5 to -4.27. It is clear from Fig. 2(a) that the LCDG helped us to better approximate the tails of the empirical density as well as its main body. Better approximation will lead to good initial segmentation.

The region map obtained first with only the class LCDG-models is further refined using the iterative segmentation algorithm. Changes in the likelihood $L(\mathbf{g}, \mathbf{m})$ become very small after 9 iterations. For this map the initial estimated parameters are $V_{a,eq} = -V_{a,ne} = 1.71$, and the final estimated parameters are $V_{a,eq} = -V_{a,ne} = 2.13$. The final region map produced with these parameters using the Metropolis voxelwise relaxation is shown in Fig. 3(a). More segmentation results are shown in Figs 3(b,c).

4 Validation and Conclusions

It is very difficult to get accurate manually segmented complete vasculare trees to validate our algorithm. To quantitatively evaluate its performance, we created three wooden 3D phantoms in Fig. 4 with geometrical shapes similar to blood vessels. They mimic bifurcations and zero and high curvature existing in any vascular system, and their changing radii simulate both large and small blood vessels. The scanned phantoms were manually segmented to obtain the ground truth. The blood vessel and non-vessel signals for each phantom were generated according to the class distributions $p(q|1), p(q|2)$, and $p(q|3)$ in Fig. 2(d) using the inverse mapping methods. The resulting phantom's histograms are similar to that in Fig. 2(a).

The total segmentation error is evaluated by a percentage of erroneous voxels with respect to the overall number of voxels in the manually segmented 3D phantom. Figure 4 shows the segmentation of the three phantoms using our approach. Table 1 gives error statistics for 440 synthetic slices segmented in the phantoms with proposed approach and compares them to four other known segmentation algorithms. The statistical analysis using a two tailed t-test shows that there is a significant difference ($P < 10^{-4}$) between the error generated by our segmentation approach and the error generated by the other four algorithms that are cited in Table 1 which highlight the advantages of the proposed approach. Figure 4 compares the results of our segmentation approach and the Chung-Noble's segmentation approach, the errors being in terms of the number

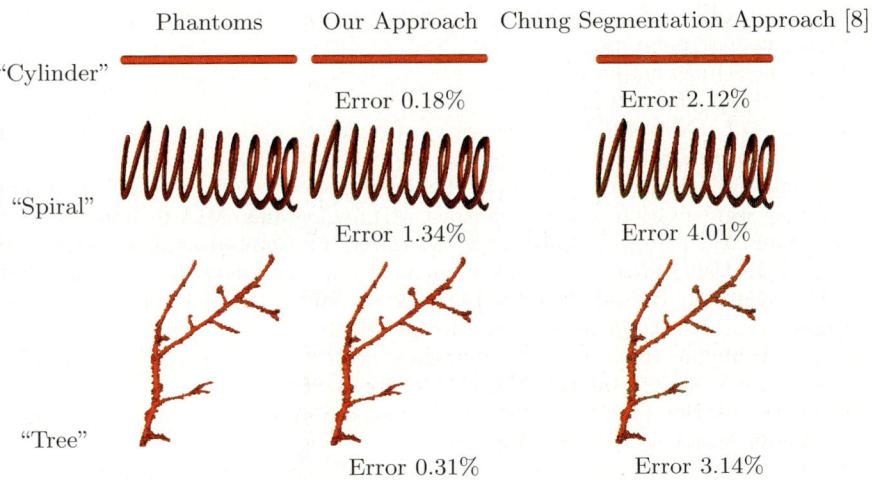

Fig. 4. Segmentation of 3D phantoms. Error shown in green.

of wrong (i.e. missed or extra) voxels relative to the total voxel number in the manually segmented 3D phantoms. In total, our approach produces 0.18-1.34% erroneous voxels comparing to 2.12-4.01% for the Chung-Noble's approach on the synthetic PC-MRA data.

We presented a new stochastic approach to find blood vessels in multi-modal PC–MRA images. The LCDG-model accurately approximates the empirical marginal gray level distribution yielding the high quality segmentation. The accuracy of our approach is validated using a specially designed 3D geometrical phantom. LCDG-model ensures fast convergence of the model refinement with the modified EM algorithm. Also, we introduced a new analytical method for accurate estimation of 3D auto-binomial MGRF model. The proposed approach is not limited only for PC–MRA but also is suitable for segmenting TOF–MRA and CTA medical images. The latter were not included in the paper because of the space limitations, but, the algorithm's code, sample data and segmentation results for the TOF–MRA, PC–MRA, and CTA images will be provided in our web site.

References

1. Caselles, V., Kimmel, R., Sapiro, G.: Geodesic active contours. Int. J. Computer Vision 22, 61–79 (1997)
2. McInerney, T., Terzopoulos, D.: Medical image segmentation using topologically adaptable surface. In: Troccaz, J., Mösges, R., Grimson, W.E.L. (eds.) CVRMed-MRCAS 1997, CVRMed 1997, and MRCAS 1997. LNCS, vol. 1205, pp. 23–32. Springer, Heidelberg (1997)
3. Lorigo, L., Faugeras, O., Grimson, W.E.L., Keriven, R.: Curves: Curve evolution for vessel segmentation. Medical Image Analysis 5, 195–206 (2001)
4. Wink, O., Niessen, W.J., Viergever, M.A.: Fast delineation and visualization of vessels in 3-D angiographic images. IEEE TMI 19, 337–346 (2000)
5. Deschamps, T., Cohen, L.D.: Fast extraction of tubular and tree 3D surfaces with front propoagation methods. In: Proc. 16th ICPR, pp. 731–734 (2002)
6. Lacoste, C., Finet, G., Magnin, I.: Coronary tree extraction from X-ray angiograms using marked point processes. In: Proc. of IEEE International Symposium on Biomedical Imaging: From Nano to Macro (ISBI 2006), Arlington, Virginia, USA, April 6-9, pp. 157–160 (2006)
7. Wilson, D.L., Noble, J.A.: An adaptive segmentation algorithm for time-of-flight MRA data. IEEE Trans. Med. Imaging 18, 938–945 (1999)
8. Chung, A., Noble, J.A., Summers, P.: Fusing speed and phase information for vascular segmentation of phase contrast MR angiograms. MIA 6, 109–128 (2002)
9. Hassouna, M., Farag, A., Hushek, S., Moriarty, T.: Cerebrovascular Segmentation from TOF Using Stochastic Models. Medical Image Analysis 10(1), 2–16 (2006)
10. Schlesinger, M., Hlavac, V.: Ten Lectures on Statistical and Structural Pattern Recognition. Kluwer Academic, Dordrecht (2002)
11. Hu, S., Hoffman, E.A.: Automatic lung segmentation for accurate quantization of volumetric X-ray CT images. IEEE TMI 20, 490–498 (2001)
12. Kass, M., Witkin, A., Terzopoulos, D.: Snakes: Active contour models. Int. J. Computer Vision 1, 321–331 (1987)
13. Xu, C., Prince, J.L.: Snakes, shapes, and gradient vector flow. IEEE TIP 7, 359–369 (1998)

Atlas-Based Improved Prediction of Magnetic Field Inhomogeneity for Distortion Correction of EPI Data

Clare Poynton[1], Mark Jenkinson[2], and William Wells III[1,3]

[1] Computer Science and Artificial Intelligence Lab, MIT, USA
[2] Oxford Centre for Functional Magnetic Resonance Imaging of the Brain (FMRIB), University of Oxford, UK
[3] Brigham and Women's Hospital, Harvard Medical School, USA

Abstract. We describe a method for atlas-based segmentation of structural MRI for calculation of magnetic fieldmaps. CT data sets are used to construct a probabilistic atlas of the head and corresponding MR is used to train a classifier that segments soft tissue, air, and bone. Subject-specific fieldmaps are computed from the segmentations using a perturbation field model. Previous work has shown that distortion in echo-planar images can be corrected using predicted fieldmaps. We obtain results that agree well with acquired fieldmaps: 90% of voxel shifts from predicted fieldmaps show subvoxel disagreement with those computed from acquired fieldmaps. In addition, our fieldmap predictions show statistically significant improvement following inclusion of the atlas.

1 Introduction

Echo-planar imaging (EPI) is the standard pulse sequence employed in functional magnetic resonance imaging (FMRI) and diffusion tensor imaging (DTI) studies due to its high temporal resolution. In order to extract meaningful information from EPI data, scientists and clinicians typically register low resolution EPI data to high resolution anatomical images. A major problem in achieving accurate registration is the inherent distortion of EPI data due to B_0 field inhomogeneity.

Field inhomogeneity results in distortion because the MR image reconstruction assumes a one to one relation between spatial location and the frequency produced by known linear gradient fields. In practice, hardware constraints result in inhomogenities in the main field as high as several hundred parts per million (ppm). This can be corrected to within several ppm using shims [1]. Intrinsic magnetic susceptibility of biological materials causes additional perturbations in the field. In neuroimaging studies, soft tissue and bone have similar susceptibilities of ($\chi_t \approx -9.1 \times 10^{-6}$) [2] and ($\chi_b \approx -11.4 \times 10^{-6}$) [3] respectively, but differ significantly from the susceptibility of air ($\chi_a \approx 0.4 \times 10^{-6}$) [2]. This results in large perturbations around the air-filled sinuses and subsequent distortion of EPI data in the frontal and temporal lobes of the brain.

To correct for this, MR systems contain a set of room-temperature shims that are wound to produce fields based on the first and second order spherical harmonics [1]. Imperfect shimming and higher-order perturbations, however, result in residual subject-specific inhomogeneity, and subsequent distortion of the acquired images. Several techniques have been developed to correct for geometric distortion, the majority of which rely on the acquisition of magnetic fieldmaps [4,5,6]. A fieldmap provides a direct measure of the B_0 inhomogeneity at each point in the image. In EPI, the geometric distortion is a voxel-wise translation restricted predominantly to the phase-encode direction, which can be computed directly from the fieldmap. Fieldmap techniques, however, have several limitations. First, they require additional scan time, which may be difficult to accomodate in clinical settings as well as in DTI studies where many directions need to be acquired in the same session. Second, fieldmaps suffer from low signal-to-noise ratios (SNR) at tissue/air boundaries, which can reduce their reliability in areas where the distortion is most severe. Acquisition of a single fieldmap may also be invalid for unwarping EPI data if there are significant effects due to motion or respiration in the timeseries. Finally, fieldmaps are not available in many retrospective studies.

Given these limitations, there have been several efforts to predict fieldmaps from tissue/air susceptibility distributions of the anatomy using magnetic field models [7,8,2]. Jenkinson et al. showed that the perturbing field can be predicted with high accuracy when CT data of the subject is used to obtain a tissue/air segmentation. Since whole-head CT is rarely available, Koch et al. proposed using registered CT from a reference subject to obtain the tissue/air susceptibility model. Both methods were limited by requiring CT to distinguish air from bone, which have similar intensities in structural MR but significant differences in magnetic susceptibility. Second, these models cannot account for the shim fields present in the scanner that partially compensate for B_0 inhomogeneity during EPI acquisition. Without this additional information, applying the fieldmaps for distortion correction is not possible. In [7] it was shown that tissue/air susceptibility models could be derived from structural MRI by using an intensity-based classifier trained with CT. It was also shown that registration of the EPI and structural MR could be used to search over the unknown shim parameters allowing distortion correction of the EPI that agrees well with results obtained using acquired fieldmaps.

Variability in structural MR acquisitions, however, may limit the efficacy of an intensity-based classifier in cases where the MR intensity properties differ significantly from those of the training data. In [7], CT data sets with MR acquired on the same scanner as the subjects of interest could be used to train the classifier, but this may not be possible in many cases. Limited anatomical information below the brain may also prevent accurate estimation of the perturbing field. Therefore, obtaining more reliable susceptibility models from structural MR is critical for retrospective unwarping of EPI data sets that lack acquired fieldmaps. While previous results predicting fieldmaps from structural MR have shown good agreement with acquired fieldmaps, we hypothesized that improved segmentation methods would result in even greater accuracy.

In this paper we describe a method for using anatomical information from a set of 22 whole-head CT data sets to achieve improved, subject-specific segmentation of structural MR. In this approach a tissue/air atlas is constructed from the CT data to obtain priors on the probability of tissue or air at each location in the anatomy. The corresponding structural MR is used to train a classifier that segments the MR of the subject of interest and this is used as input to a first order perturbation field model to compute a subject-specific fieldmap. The method is evaluated by comparison of predicted fieldmaps and acquired fieldmaps. In addition, the MR classifier can be used to obtain probabilistic bone segmentations from structural MR that show promising agreement with segmented CT.

2 Methods

2.1 Atlas Construction

Automatic segmentation of neuroanatomical structures often relies on the use of probabilistic atlases [9,10,11,12,13]. These atlases are usually constructed by co-registering collections of manual segmentations or other training data. The atlas functions as a spatial prior to represent anatomical variability within a population and compensate for missing information in structural MR images [13]. Although atlas-based methods have typically been applied to the segmentation of brain structures, in this work, we construct a probabilistic tissue/air atlas from 22 CT data sets. By incorporating spatial information into the MR segmentation, we expect improved tissue/air classification in regions where bone is often mislabeled as air.

We obtained 22 datasets consisting of CT and MRI from 3 sources: the publicly available Retrospective Image Registration Evaluation (RIRE) database (17 neurosurgery patients), the Radiology department at Brigham and Women's Hospital (BWH) (4 neurosurgery patients) and the Zubal head phantom (1 subject) [14]. In the RIRE data, each CT image has 27 to 34 slices, 4 mm thick, matrix=512x512, voxel size=0.65x0.65mm. The T1-weighted MRI was acquired on a Siemens SP 1.5 Tesla scanner. MRI for 8 of the 17 subjects has 20 to 26 axial slices, 4 mm thick, no gap, matrix=256x256, voxel size= 1.25x1.25mm, TE/TR=15/650ms. T1-weighted MP-RAGE for the other 9 subjects had TE/TR=4/10ms, matrix=128x256x256 and FOV=160x250x250mm. In the BWH dataset, the CT spanned 36 slices with 512x512 in-plane voxels of size 0.46x0.46x4.8mm. 3D-SPGR MRI of these patients was obtained: slice thickness=1mm, TE/TR=3/8ms, matrix=512x512, voxel size=0.5x0.5x1mm. The Zubal data consists of CT of the head and neck: 1.2mm isotropic voxels spanning 230 slices with 256x256 in-plane voxels, and T1-weighted MRI with 90 slices of thickness 0.2cm, matrix=256x256, and 25.6x25.6cm in-plane resolution.

For each subject, the CT data was registered to its corresponding MR using 6 degrees of freedom (DOF) and mutual information as the cost function. The MR was registered to standard space using the MNI152T1 atlas as the reference, 12 DOF and normalized correlation ratio. These transformations were then applied to the co-registered CT. All registrations were carried out using FLIRT [15,16]. Tissue/air labels were obtained by thresholding the CT data in standard space.

The wide variation in the field of view of the CT data results in highly varying amounts of data at each voxel; in particular only the zubal phantom includes observations in the neck. Probabilistic atlases are frequently constructed by counting the number of occurrences of each tissue class at each voxel and normalizing the result to obtain a probability distribution. In the two class situation, this corresponds to ML estimation of the parameter of a binomial distribution, i.e., if $k \sim \text{Binomial}(n, p)$, then, the ML estimate of p given observed k is $\hat{p} = k/n$.

In the case of only one trial ($n = 1$), or one observation at a given voxel, this will lead to estimates of p that are zero or one, which may be unreasonably certain (i.e. when used as prior probability on tissue class in segmentation, these values would dominate any amount of data in these voxels). One way to avoid this effect, is to put a prior on p; a natural choice is the beta distribution, which is conjugate to the binomial: $p \sim \text{Beta}(\alpha, \beta)$. (The special case of $\alpha = \beta = 1$ corresponds to a flat prior and Laplace's rule of succession). We have chosen to use $\alpha = \beta = \epsilon = 0.05$, and in this case, the posterior expected value of the parameter is $\bar{p} = \frac{k+\epsilon}{n+2\epsilon}$, which avoids, by ϵ, the probability zero and one cases mentioned above. In addition to the tissue/air atlas, a probabilistic atlas of bone was obtained by segmenting bone from CT data and applying the same binomial model and conjugate prior. This was applied to segment bone from MR, which may be useful in other applications such as calculation of attenuation maps for absorption correction in PET or dose calculation in radiotherapy planning.

2.2 Atlas-Based Segmentation

Structural MR was segmented using an MR classifier that incorporates spatially dependent prior information from the probabilistic atlas and MR intensity information (from the subject of interest) to obtain a subject-specific susceptibility model. The classifier was trained using the CT/MR training data described in section 2.1, but applied to segment MR data acquired at a separate site. The accuracy of the segmentations was evaluated by comparing fieldmaps predicted from the atlas-based segmenter to acquired fieldmaps. The fieldmaps were also compared to those predicted using intensity information alone (ie. a spatially constant prior).

We obtained T1-weighted MRI and fieldmaps of 5 subjects previously acquired at Massachusetts General Hospital on a 3T Siemens TimTrio scanner as part of the FBIRN multi-center FMRI study. The MP-RAGE spanned 160 slices, with thickness=1.2mm, matrix=256x256, voxel size=0.86x0.86mm, and TE/TR=2.94/ 2300ms. The gradient echo fieldmaps had 30 slices, thickness=5mm, matrix=64x64, voxel size=3.44x3.44mm, TE1/TE2/TR=3.03/5.49/500ms.

Rigid (6 DOF) registration of the T1 data to the fieldmap magnitude image was carried out using FLIRT [15] so the predicted fieldmaps would be in the same space as the acquired fieldmaps for validation. The MNI152T1 reference image was registered to the fieldmap magnitude image using 12 DOF and the resulting transformation was applied to the atlas-based probability maps.

The prior probabilities of tissue, $P(T \mid X_n)$, and air, $P(T^C \mid X_n)$, at each voxel were obtained from the co-registered atlas. For each of the 22 T1 images in the training data, the MR was scaled according to the parameter that minimized the Kullback-Leibler Distance to the MR of the subject of interest. The data that showed the minimal distance to the subject of interest was used to compute the likelihood terms, $P(I_i \mid T)$ and $P(I_i \mid T^C)$, using tissue/air labels from the corresponding CT. The posterior probability of tissue was computed and applied to segment the MR of the subject of interest. Intensity-based segmentation using spatially stationary priors computed from normalized intensity histograms of the training data was also carried out for comparison to the atlas-based approach.

Bone segmentations were obtained in similar fashion and evaluated using a 'leave-one-out' framework in which one CT was withheld as ground truth and the remaining CT data sets were used to construct the probabilistic bone atlas. A non-linear direct search was performed to solve for the thresholds that maximized the similarity of the estimated bone segmentations to the ground truth segmentation. The similarity was quantified using the dice score, where a value of 0 indicates the volumes have no overlapping voxels and a value of 1 indicates they are exactly the same.

2.3 Fieldmap Estimation

Fieldmaps are predicted from the atlas and intensity-based segmentations using the perturbation field model described in [2]. In this model, a first order perturbation solution of Maxwell's equations is calculated from a tissue/air susceptibility model, where each pixel takes continuous values between 0 (air) and 1 (tissue). For a single voxel, with the B_0 field along z, the predicted field is given by: $F(\mathbf{x}) = \left(\frac{\partial^2 G}{\partial z^2}\right) * (\chi_1 B_z^{(0)})$, where $G(\mathbf{x}) = (4\pi r)^{-1}$, $r = \| \mathbf{x} \| = \sqrt{x^2 + y^2 + z^2}$, $B_z^{(0)}$ is the field strength, and $\chi_1 = 1$ is the susceptibility value of the voxel. Due to the linearity of the perturbing field solution, the total field is given by: $B_z^{(1)}(\mathbf{x}) = \sum_{\mathbf{x}'} \chi_1(\mathbf{x}') F(\mathbf{x} - \mathbf{x}')$ where $\mathbf{x}'$ are the source points (locations of the voxel centers) and $\mathbf{x}$ is the field point where the field is evaluated.

Current field modeling techniques, including the one described in [2], do not account for the shim fields that reduce the B_0 inhomogeneity prior to fieldmap acquisition. Therefore, in order to compare an estimated fieldmap to an acquired one, the shim fields must added to the predicted fieldmaps. This is done by modeling the shim fields using the set of first and second order spherical harmonic basis functions. In addition, a global scaling of the predicted fieldmap must be estimated since the model assumes the magnetic susceptibility throughout the brain, ($\chi_t \approx -9.1 \times 10^{-6}$) [2], is constant, but this may not be accurate near bone interfaces where both partial volume effects and mis-estimation of segmentation values are most likely to occur. Furthermore, the perturbing fieldmaps are calculated assuming a perfectly homogeneous B_0 field, which cannot be achieved in practice due to constraints on the hardware. The fieldmap scaling and shim

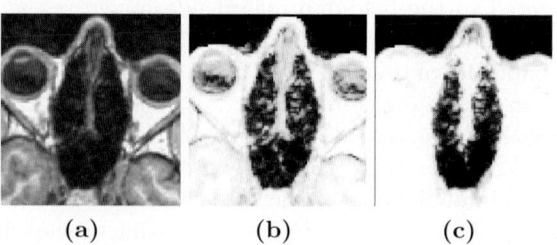

(a) (b) (c)

Fig. 1. Results of the Segmentation. The T1 MR for a representative subject is shown in (a). The tissue probability map computed using the intensity classifier (b) shows misclassification of voxels outside the sinus region where intensities are low in MR. Using the atlas-based classifier significantly reduces these errors while adequately resolving much of the subject-specific sinus anatomy (c).

parameters, θ, can be obtained by least squares fitting to the acquired fieldmap: $\hat{\theta} = \arg\min_{\theta} [\mathbf{B} - \mathbf{A}\theta]^2$ where $\mathbf{A} = \left[\hat{\mathbf{B}}, \mathbf{S_1}, \mathbf{S_2}, ..., \mathbf{S_8}\right]$. The column vectors $\mathbf{B}$, $\hat{\mathbf{B}}$, and $\mathbf{S_i}$, represent the acquired fieldmap, predicted fieldmap, and shim basis functions, respectively. Once these coefficients are known, the predicted fieldmap with shim, $\hat{\mathbf{B}}_\mathbf{s} = \mathbf{A}\hat{\theta}$, can be compared to the acquired fieldmap.

3 Experimental Results

Results of atlas-based segmentation of structural MR is shown in Fig. 1. Fig. 1a shows T1 of the sinus region. Fig. 1b shows the limitations of using the intensity classifier to segment the MR. While it produces reasonable results for many of the voxels in the sinuses, voxels outside this region which are clearly soft tissue or bone are mislabeled with values close to zero. In contrast, using the atlas-based segmenter (as shown in Fig. 1c) achieves similar results for the highly variable subject-specific anatomy within the sinus region, while producing fewer errors in the surrounding area. The intensity and atlas-based segmentations were used as input to the perturbation field model to obtain predicted fieldmaps. The scaling and shim parameters were fit from the acquired fieldmaps as described in section 2.3. The shim fields could then be added to the predicted fieldmaps for comparison to the acquired fieldmaps as shown in Fig. 2. The first column of Fig. 2 shows fieldmaps computed from the intensity-based segmentations, which show significant differences relative to the acquired fieldmaps shown for each subject in column 3. These are especially noticable in areas that have lower signal in MR, such as in the ventricles and major sulci. Fieldmap results from the atlas-based segmentations are shown in the second column of Fig. 2 and show improved agreement with acquired fieldmaps. Quantitative analysis of the absolute error in the B_0 field between these images is given in the table in Fig. 2. Since the bandwidth/pixel for the EPI data acquired in this study is 22.3 Hz, 90% of the voxels in the atlas-based fieldmaps show subvoxel error. The mean of these

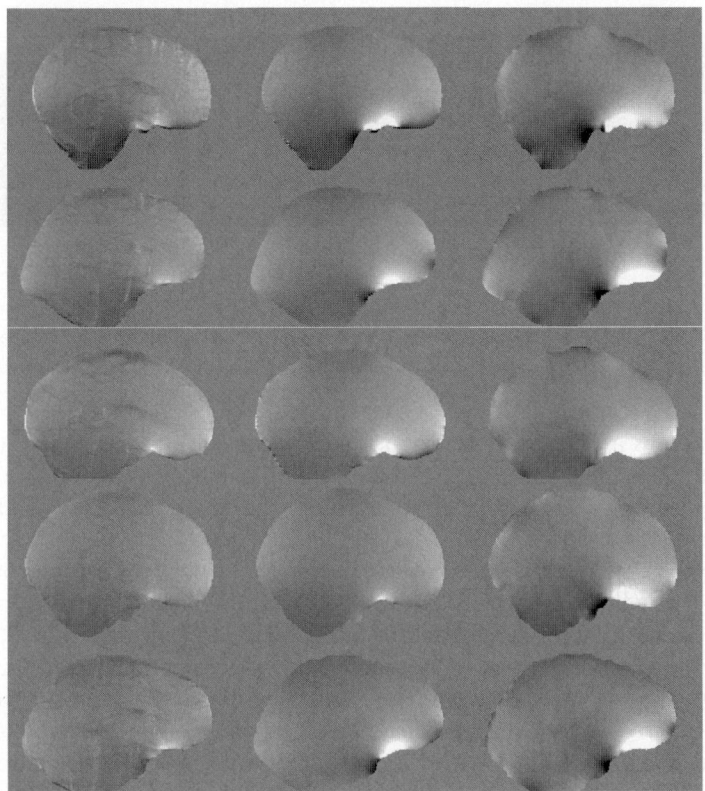

Difference in Field (Hz)	Mean	P80	P85	P90	P95	P99
Subject 1	8.8	12.2	15.0	19.8	31.0	69.1
Subject 2	8.2	11.7	14.2	18.3	27.4	59.8
Subject 3	8.4	12.3	15.1	19.3	27.6	54.6
Subject 4	9.0	12.7	15.7	20.3	30.2	72.6
Subject 5	6.5	8.8	11.0	14.8	22.9	50.1
Koch et al.	12.5	—	—	23.5	—	—
$\mu_{intensity}$	10.0	14.1	17.5	23.2	34.9	74.8
μ_{atlas}	8.2	11.5	14.2	18.5	27.8	61.2
p-values	**0.0080**	0.0087	0.0081	**0.0079**	0.0093	0.0106

Fig. 2. Results of the Fieldmap Estimation. Predicted and acquired fieldmaps for subjects 1-5 are shown in rows 1-5 respectively. Fieldmaps predicted using the intensity classifier (column 1) show significant differences relative to the acquired fieldmaps (column 3), while those computed from the atlas-based segmentation show improved agreement (column 2). The absolute difference between the acquired fieldmaps and the atlas-based fieldmaps are given for each subject in the table above. 90% of voxels show differences that are less than 22.3 Hz, the bandwidth/pixel for the FBIRN EPI data. Results reported by Koch et al. [8] for a single subject are shown, as well as mean statistics across all five subjects for both the intensity classifier and atlas-based classifier. The atlas-based classifier performs better than the Koch and intensity-based methods and the improvement over the intensity method is statistically significant (all p-values < 0.05 for left-sided paired t-test). The scale of the fieldmaps is ± 100 Hz.

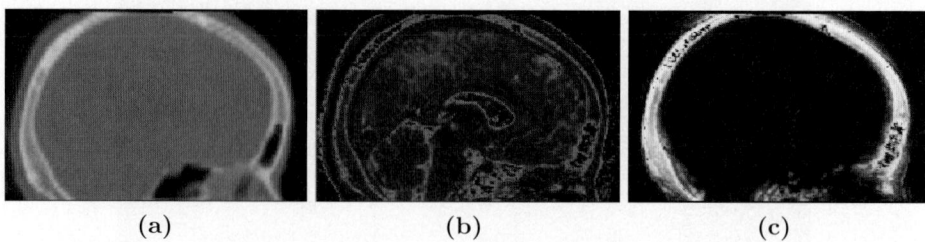

Fig. 3. Results of the Bone Segmentation. Segmentation of bone using the intensity classifier (b) results in significant errors when compared with CT (a), while the atlas-based classifier (c) shows good overall agreement.

statistics across all five subjects is also shown for both the intensity and atlas-based classifiers. The intensity classifier shows a slight improvement over the results reported by Koch et al [8] for a single subject. The atlas-based classifier out performs both the intensity and Koch methods. Paired t-tests comparing the means of the intensity and atlas-based results shows this improvement is statistically significant (all p-values < 0.05). Results of the segmentation of bone from structural MR for a representative subject is shown in Fig. 3. The CT shown in Fig. 3a can be easily thresholded to segment bone from air and soft tissue. Fig. 3b and Fig. 3c show the results of using the intensity and atlas-based classifiers, respectively. While the intensity classifier has some success in segmenting MR into tissue/air classes, it is much less effective in segmenting bone (Fig. 3b). Inspection of the the atlas-based segmentation (Fig. 3c), however, shows good general agreement with the CT, with a dice score of 0.780 for this subject.

Acknowledgments. This research is supported in part by NIH grants: P41RR13218, U54EB005149, U41RR019703, and U24RR021992. Mark Jenkinson was supported by a UK BBSRC David Phillips Fellowship.

References

1. Clare, S., Evans, J., Jezzard, P.: Requirements for room temperature shimming of the human brain. Magn. Reson. Med. 55, 210–214 (2006)
2. Jenkinson, M., Wilson, J.L., Jezzard, P.: Perturbation method for magnetic field calculations of nonconductive objects. Magn. Reson. Med. 52, 471–477 (2004)
3. Hopkins, J.A., Wehrli, F.W.: Magnetic susceptibility measurement of insoluable solids by NMR: magnetic susceptibility of bone. Magn. Reson. Med. 37, 494 (1997)
4. Weisskoff, R.M., Davis, T.L.: Correcting gross distortion on echo planar images. Soc. Magn. Res. Abstr. 11, 4515 (1992)
5. Jezzard, P., Balaban, R.S.: Correction for geometric distortion in echo planar images from b0 field variations. Magn. Reson. Med. 34, 65–73 (1995)
6. Hutton, C., Bork, A., Josephs, O., Deichmann, R., Ashburner, J., Turner, R.: Image distortion correction in FMRI: A quantitative evaluation. Neuroimage 16, 217–240 (2002)

7. Poynton, C., Jenkinson, M., Whalen, S., Golby, A.J., Wells III, W.M.: Fieldmap-free retrospective registration and distortion correction for EPI-based functional imaging. In: Metaxas, D., Axel, L., Fichtinger, G., Székely, G. (eds.) MICCAI 2008, Part II. LNCS, vol. 5242, pp. 271–279. Springer, Heidelberg (2008)
8. Koch, K.M., Papademetris, X., Rothman, D., de Graaf, R.: Rapid calculations of susceptibility-induced magnetostatic field perturbations for in vivo magnetic resonance. Phys. Med. Biol. 51, 6381–6402 (2006)
9. Fischl, B., van der Kouwe, A., Destrieux, C., Halgren, E., Segonne, F., Salat, D., Busa, E., Seidman, L., Goldstein, J., Kennedy, D., Caviness, V., Makris, N., Rosen, B., Dale, A.: Automatically parcellating the human cerebral cortex. Cerebral Cortex 14, 11–22 (2004)
10. Tosun, D., Rettmann, M., Han, X., Tao, X., Xu, C., Resnick, S., Pham, D., Prince, J.: Cortical surface segmentation and mapping. Neuroimage 23, 108–118 (2004)
11. Pohl, K., Bouix, S., Kikinis, R., Grimson, W.: Anatomical guided segmentation with nonstationary tissue class distributions in an expectation-maximization framework. In: ISBI, pp. 81–84 (2004)
12. Heckemann, R.A., Hajnal, J., Aljabar, P., Rueckert, D., Hammers, A.: Automatic anatomical brain MRI segmentation combining label propagation and decision fusion. Neuroimage 33, 115–126 (2006)
13. Zollei, L., Shenton, M., Wells, W., Pohl, K.: The impact of atlas formation methods on atlas-guided brain segmentation. In: MICCAI (2007)
14. Zubal, I.G., Harrell, C.R., Smith, E.O., Rattner, Z., Gindi, G.R., Hoffer, P.B.: Computerized three-dimensional segmented human anatomy. Med. Phys. 21, 299–302 (1994)
15. Jenkinson, M., Smith, S.M.: A global optimisation method for robust affine registration of brain images. Medical Image Analysis 5, 143–156 (2001)
16. Jenkinson, M., Bannister, P., Brady, M., Smith, S.: Improved optimisation for the robust and accurate linear registration and motion correction of brain images. Neuroimage 17(2), 825–841 (2002)

3D Prostate Segmentation in Ultrasound Images Based on Tapered and Deformed Ellipsoids

Seyedeh Sara Mahdavi[1], William J. Morris[2], Ingrid Spadinger[2], Nick Chng[2], Orcun Goksel[1], and Septimiu E. Salcudean[1]

[1] Department of Electrical and Computer Engineering, University of British Columbia, Vancouver, Canada
{saram,orcung,tims}@ece.ubc.ca
[2] Vancouver Cancer Center, British Columbia Cancer Agency, Vancouver, Canada
{jmorris,ispading,nchng}@bccancer.bc.ca

Abstract. Prostate segmentation from trans-rectal transverse B-mode ultrasound images is required for radiation treatment of prostate cancer. Manual segmentation is a time-consuming task, the results of which are dependent on image quality and physicians' experience. This paper introduces a semi-automatic 3D method based on super-ellipsoidal shapes. It produces a 3D segmentation in less than 15 seconds using a warped, tapered ellipsoid fit to the prostate. A study of patient images shows good performance and repeatability. This method is currently in clinical use at the Vancouver Cancer Center where it has become the standard segmentation procedure for low dose-rate brachytherapy treatment.

1 Introduction

Low dose rate (LDR) prostate brachytherapy is a common radiation treatment for early stage prostate cancer. It consists of the permanent implant of 40-100 small radioactive seeds into the prostate with the aim of delivering a sufficiently high radiation dose to the cancerous tissue, while maintaining a tolerable dose to the urethra and rectum. Possible side effects of this procedure include urinary incontinence and erectile dysfunction which are mainly related to inaccurate delivery of the seeds caused by inaccurate visualization of the prostate pre-operatively and intra-operatively.

In a typical pre-operative trans-rectal volume study, a series of 9-14 parallel trans-rectal ultrasound (TRUS) images, from the base to the apex, are collected. These images are then manually segmented to create a 3D model of the prostate, which is used to generate a treatment plan. In typical TRUS images, the prostate is the largest and its boundary is the most discernible in the mid-gland section. Approaching the base and the apex, the boundary almost disappears into the background. Segmentation of these two regions is mainly based on experience and by looking at the mid-portion of the gland, which gives a hint of how far the prostate extends axially. Manual segmentation often requires 5-10 minutes and, in addition to image quality, it greatly relies upon the experience and peculiar habits of the clinician. Therefore, a suitable (semi-)automatic segmentation algorithm can result in less variable contours generated in less time.

Many (semi-)automatic prostate segmentation methods on ultrasound images have been proposed during the last few years [1]. Some methods are based on image enhancement or edge detection techniques such as [2,3,4]. However, methods which rely solely on image information are sensitive to image quality and noise level. Additional information about the shape of the prostate can increase robustness to noise and reduce segmentation time. Deformable models have been widely used for medical image segmentation [5,6,7,8,9] and are generally more successful than the former methods. Fitting ellipses, ellipsoids, super-ellipses, and deformable ellipses or using them for initialization have been relatively attractive approaches for prostate segmentation due to the shape of the gland [10,11,12,13,14].

To the best of our knowledge, there have been no other reports of a 3D (semi) automatic prostate segmentation method reliable enough and fast enough for effective replacement of standard manual segmentation in clinical use. While the extensive study of [12] showed good segmentation results, the method presented is limited to 2D. Previous 3D methods [15,16] are time consuming (> 2 minutes) or require significant user intervention [11]. Our use of an a priori shape allows prostate segmentation in poorly visible regions and therefore can be used in standard clinical practice, thus enabling a more complete validation study than presented with other 3D methods.

In this paper, we propose a method that generates the 3D volume of the prostate based on a combination of the physician's experience, edge detection and prior knowledge of the prostate's shape. The method introduced in [14] has been extended to account for the tapered 3D shape of the prostate. Furthermore, we introduce a novel validation method based on different regions of the gland. This method enables a critical evaluation of prostate segmentation algorithms based on their importance in treatment planning.

2 Methods

2.1 Algorithm

Based on the prostate's shape and considering the effect of the TRUS probe pressure on the gland, we found a warped and tapered ellipsoid with tapering in three axes suitable as the final 3D volume of the prostate. This can be constructed from 2D warped and tapered ellipses generated from each image slice. However, fitting such shapes for each slice can be time-consuming. A solution to this problem is to un-warp and un-taper all images in a pre-processing step that makes the prostate shape approximately ellipsoidal. Un-warping is carried out to remove the posterior concavity of the prostate formed due to TRUS pressure on the gland. Transversal un-tapering is then applied leaving a simple convex ellipse fitting problem for each image. Finally an axially tapered ellipsoid or an 'egg shape' with an elliptical cross-section is fitted to the 2D contours and the results are inversely warped and tapered to match the actual prostate shape. Details of the algorithm are as follows.

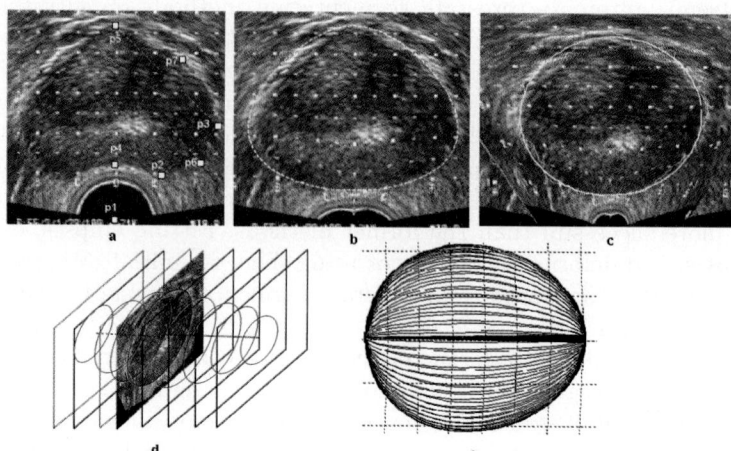

Fig. 1. (a) Initial points, (b) Un-warped mid-gland with initial tapered ellipse fit, (c) Un-tapered, un-warped image with edge detection and ellipse fit, (d) propagation from mid-gland to the remaining slices, (e) tapered ellipsoid

Initialization: The segmentation algorithm is initialized with the user selecting the mid-gland, apex, and base slices. The base and apex are the extreme slices in which the prostate can be seen, superiorly and inferiorly, and the mid-gland slice usually contains the largest and most visible section of the gland. The "slices" used for segmentation throughout the algorithm will be from $base + 1$ to $apex - 1$. On the mid-gland slice, the user selects p_1 the TRUS probe center and six boundary points which are (Fig.1(a)): p_2-lowest posterior lateral, p_3-extreme right, p_4-medial posterior, p_5-medial anterior, p_6 (p_7)- intersection of the mid-perpendicular line between p_2 and p_3 (p_3 and p_5) with the boundary. The aim is to extract the most information from the image while keeping the variability of the initialization low by directing the user to specific regions (superior, lateral, inferior) and using guiding lines.

Un-warping: Based on the selected points, the mid-gland image and initial points are un-warped [13] to reduce the deformation caused by the TRUS probe, using $r_{new} = r - r sin(\theta) exp(-r^2/2\sigma^2)$ where r is the current distance of an image pixel on a radial line starting from the probe center with angle θ ($\theta = 90°$ being the medial line) and r_{new} is the distance of the re-located pixel. According to this sinusoidally weighted Gaussian function, the maximum deformation is achieved when $\theta = 90°$ and is reduced as the distance to the center of the probe increases. The amount of radial stretch is determined by σ which is calculated using the three initial points p_1, p_2, and p_4 for $\theta = 90°$.

Un-tapering: To the un-warped initial points, a tapered ellipse is fitted by solving the following problem using the Levenberg-Marquardt optimization method with the goal of obtaining the parameters $P = (x_0, y_0, a_x, a_y, t_1)$:

$$\min_P \{e^T e \mid e_i = \sqrt{a_x a_y}[(\tfrac{x_i'}{a_x})^2 + (\tfrac{y_i'}{a_y})^2 - 1], \quad i = 1 \ldots N\} \quad (1)$$

$$x_i' = (x_i - x_0)/(\tfrac{t_1}{a_y}(y_i - y_0) + 1), \quad y_i' = (y_i - y_0)$$

with $-1 \leq t_1 \leq 1$ being the tapering parameter ($t_1 = 0$ for ellipse), $[x_0, y_0]$ the center of the shape, a_x and a_y the radii along the x and y axes, and $[x_i, y_i]$ the coordinates of the N boundary points on the mid-gland image. N is determined by the initial points and their reflections about the mid-sagittal plane (Fig.1(b)).

IMMPDA edge detection in mid-gland: The resulting tapered ellipse is used to guide the IMMPDA edge detection algorithm [17] by setting limits on how far from the initial contour the edge detection can search. In order to improve the tapered ellipse fitting, the resulting edge points are once again fed to the Levenberg-Marquardt algorithm. The tapering value of this contour, t_1, is used to 'un-taper' the ultrasound images. We assume that the prostate is most tapered at the mid-gland and the tapering linearly reduces to zero towards the base and the apex. Thus, only one tapering parameter is computed for the entire set of transverse prostate images. Using the negative of the tapering value for each slice, all the images along with the initial points are un-tapered. The combination of un-warping and un-tapering of the images creates images in which the prostate is approximately elliptical in shape, thus simplifying the problem to the convex problem of fitting an ellipse. An ellipse can be fitted to data points by solving a generalized eigenvector problem. Fig.1(c) shows the un-warped and un-tapered mid-gland image along with the IMMPDA edge detection result and final fitted ellipse.

Contour propagation and IMMPDA detection in remaining slices: In order to find the prostate boundary in the rest of the slices, two semi-ellipsoids are first fitted (again using the generalized eigenvector problem): one to the mid-gland contour and the intersection of a line passing the center of the mid-gland contour and parallel to the TRUS with slice $base - 1$, and the second to the mid-gland contour and the intersection of the same line with slice $apex + 1$. The intersection of the two semi-ellipsoids with each of the slices creates initial contours for the delineation of the remaining slices (Fig.1(d)). The IMMPDA edge detection algorithm is applied to each image and the detected edge points are used to fit the final 3D shape. Two semi-ellipsoids instead of one ellipsoid are used because the mid-gland slice is usually closer to the base, thus giving a better initial approximation for the remaining contours.

3D Tapered ellipsoid fit: A tapered ellipsoid is fitted as a final 3D shape to the slice contours obtained (Fig.1(e)). This is no longer a convex problem, and we solve it using the Levenberg-Marquardt algorithm. The following optimization problem is solved in order to find the tapered ellipsoid parameters $P = (x_0, y_0, z_0, a_x, a_y, a_z, t_2, t_3)$:

$$\min_P \{e^T e \mid e_i = \sqrt{a_x a_y a_z}\,[(\tfrac{x_i'}{a_x})^2 + (\tfrac{y_i'}{a_y})^2 + (\tfrac{z_i'}{a_z})^2 - 1], \quad i = 1 \ldots M\} \quad (2)$$

$$x_i' = (x_i - x_0)/(\tfrac{t_2}{a_z}(z_i - z_0) + 1),$$

$$y_i' = (y_i - y_0)/(\tfrac{t_3}{a_z}(z_i - z_0) + 1), \quad z_i' = (z_i - z_0)$$

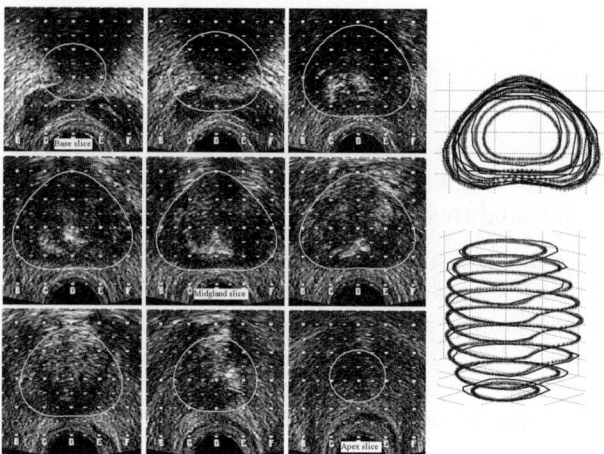

Fig. 2. Final contours on the TRUS B-mode images and the final 3D shape compared with manual segmentation (thin lines)

where a_x, a_y, a_z are the radii along the axes, $[x_0, y_0, z_0]$ is the position of the center of the volume, t_2 and t_3 are respective x and y tapering values in the direction of the ultrasound probe axis and $[x_i, y_i, z_i]$ are the coordinates of M boundary points segmented in the image slices.

The 3D volume fitting is the most time consuming part of the algorithm. To aid the optimization algorithm, an ellipsoid is initially fitted to the data cloud consisting of the ellipse contours of all slices. Since this is a convex problem, the one and only minimum is found almost instantly. The derived center of the ellipsoid and the axes are used along with the two tapering parameters, initially set to 0.05 assuming slight tapering of the prostate towards the apex, as initial values for the optimization algorithm in Eq.2.

Volume re-slicing, tapering and warping: The final volume is sliced, and the resulting contours are inversely tapered and warped. Fig.2 shows the resulting contours in the TRUS B-mode images and a comparison of the final 3D volume generated by the algorithm with the manual contours created by a physician.

2.2 Evaluation

The current algorithm for prostate segmentation is now been used by therapists at the Vancouver Cancer Center, where approximately 300 patients per year are treated. Before treatment planning, radiation oncologists observe and modify the resulting contours, if needed. To evaluate this algorithm we have carried out three comparison studies between 3D shapes generated from: (i) pre- and post-modified semi-automatic contours, (ii) original and repeated pre-modified semi-automatic contours and finally (iii) manually segmented contours and pre-modified semi-automatic contours.

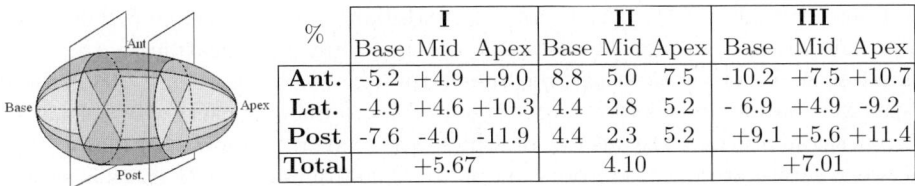

%	I			II			III		
	Base	Mid	Apex	Base	Mid	Apex	Base	Mid	Apex
Ant.	-5.2	+4.9	+9.0	8.8	5.0	7.5	-10.2	+7.5	+10.7
Lat.	-4.9	+4.6	+10.3	4.4	2.8	5.2	- 6.9	+4.9	-9.2
Post	-7.6	-4.0	-11.9	4.4	2.3	5.2	+9.1	+5.6	+11.4
Total	+5.67			4.10			+7.01		

Fig. 3. Percentage of volume errors for each sector. I: pre- *vs.* post modified semi-auto, II: original *vs.* repeated semi-auto, III: semi-auto *vs.* manual.

In all three studies, the 3D prostate shape has been divided into nine sectors (Fig.3). Division in the transverse plane produces three anterior, posterior and lateral regions and axial division results in the apex, base and mid regions. The reason for such a division is to best represent the critical regions involved in the treatment. For example, the boundary of the mid-posterior region should be accurately identified to avoid rectal complications.

For each sector, the percentage of volume error, V_{err}, is calculated. This value is the percentage of the non-overlapping volume of two 3D shapes, as defined in comparison studies (i), (ii) and (iii), to the sum of their volumes. Additionally, the percentage of total volume difference, V_{diff}, is also reported. This is ($V_A - V_B)/V_B \times 100$, with V_A and V_B being the pre- and post-modified (study (i)) and pre-modified and manual volumes (study (iii)), respectively.

Comparison between the pre- and post-modified semi-automatic contours can give a measure of how satisfied the physicians are with the results of the algorithm. This is done on 22 sets of prostate images with an average of 10 images per case. To evaluate the repeatability of the algorithm, 10 of the 22 cases were randomly selected for repeated segmentation. The repeated contours are compared with the pre-modified contours using the same nine-sector analysis.

One can argue that seeing the semi-automatic contours may bias the physician's judgment of where the prostate boundary actually is. To determine the extent to which the a priori shapes generated by the algorithm may cause such bias, 11 cases were segmented both manually (by an expert) and by our algorithm (by a volunteer trained by an expert).

The Mean Absolute Distance (MAD), and Maximum Difference (MAXD) were also calculated for the mid-gland slices in studies (i) and (iii) as measures of the 2D contouring ability of the algorithm. The former(latter) is the average(maximum value) of the absolute radial distance between the two contours to be compared. Finally, a B-mode/MRI volume comparison is carried out.

3 Results

The average normalized volume error for the nine sectors can be seen in the following tables (Fig.3). Column I shows V_{err} between semi-automatic contours and their modified versions for the 22 cases. The positive(negative) signs indicate that the sector is smaller (larger) in the modified version. V_{diff} is 0.61±7.7 (%)

and the average MAD/MAXD for the mid-gland slice is 0.66±0.5/2.06±1.59 (mm) in which 4 of the 22 cases did not need any modification in the mid-gland slice. In order to study the repeatability of the algorithm, 10 of these cases were randomly selected and segmented by a different user two weeks after initial segmentation, the results of which are seen in column II. Finally, V_{err} between semi-automatic contours and manual contours of the 11 cases is shown in column III. In this case, a positive(negative) sign means that the manual sector is smaller (larger). The percentage volume errors are mainly of the order of the pre- and post-modified comparison, which implies that the physician is not significantly biased by the semi-auto contours. V_{diff} is 1.8±5.1 (%) and the MAD/MAXD for the mid-gland slice is 1.25±0.38/3.17±0.73 (mm). Comparison of pre- and post-modified semi-automatic contours with manual MRI contours of 8 patient prostates showed a V_{diff} of 13.1±7.5 (%) between pre-modified and MRI contours. Interestingly, this value is 8.6±5.3 (%) for post-modified and MRI contours (in both cases the MRI volume usually being smaller). This suggests that even the modified contours used for treatment planning create a larger volume than that seen in MRI.

The duration from the moment the initial points are selected until the 3D shape is generated is 14.36±1.39s (max.17s) on a standard PC.

4 Conclusion and Discussion

We have presented a fast algorithm for semi-automatic segmentation of the prostate. The algorithm is presently in clinical use (to date plans for 90 patients were generated) and provides an initial segmentation to radiation oncologists performing brachytherapy. It was shown that only small modifications are required to the initial segmentations, specifically in the mid region of the gland.

It is important to note that the physicians definition of segmentation may not necessarily be what the actual boundaries of the prostate are in B-mode images. Contouring is also affected by how the treatment is planned and carried out. This can be seen in the comparison with MR images which are well known for providing better visibility of the gland. Our results showed that even segmentation results of B-mode images approved for planning have larger volumes than those created from MRI.

A major advantage of this algorithm is that it produces smooth and symmetric contours, in a manner that is physician independent and repeatable. These are suitable for treatment planning and desired by physicians. The algorithm is fast enough to be used in pre-planning. It requires some additional code optimization for intra-operative planning.

Acknowledgments. Financial support from NIH grant R21 CA120232-01 is gratefully acknowledged. The authors would also like to thank the physicians, therapists and staff at the Vancouver Cancer Center who have contributed in this project.

References

1. Noble, J.A., Boukerroui, D.: Ultrasound image segmentation: a survey. IEEE Trans. Med. Imaging 25(8), 987–1010 (2006)
2. Pathak, S.D., Haynor, D.R., Kim, Y.: Edge-guided boundary delineation in prostate ultrasound images. IEEE Trans. Med. Imaging 19(12), 1211–1219 (2000)
3. Boukerroui, D., Baskurt, A., Noble, J., Basset, O.: Segmentation of ultrasound images–multiresolution 2D and 3D algorithm based on global and local statistics. Pattern Recognition Letters 24(4-5), 779–790 (2003)
4. Zaim, A.: An edge-based approach for segmentation of prostate ultrasound images using phase symmetry. In: ISCCSP 2008, pp. 10–13 (2008)
5. Nascimento, J.C., Marques, J.S.: Robust shape tracking with multiple models in ultrasound images. IEEE Trans. Image Process 17(3), 392–406 (2008)
6. Huang, X., Metaxas, D.N.: Metamorphs: deformable shape and appearance models. IEEE Trans. Pattern Anal. Mach. Intell. 30(8), 1444–1459 (2008)
7. Thevenaz, P., Unser, M.: Snakuscules. IEEE Trans. Image Process 17(4), 585–593 (2008)
8. Nanayakkara, N.D., Samarabandu, J., Fenster, A.: Prostate segmentation by feature enhancement using domain knowledge and adaptive region based operations. Phys. Med. Biol. 51(7), 1831–1848 (2006)
9. Hodge, A.C., Fenster, A., Downey, D.B., Ladak, H.M.: Prostate boundary segmentation from ultrasound images using 2D active shape models: optimisation and extension to 3D. Comput. Methods Programs Biomed. 84(2-3), 99–113 (2006)
10. Kachouie, N.N., Fieguth, P., Rahnamayan, S.: An elliptical level set method for automatic TRUS prostate image segmentation. In: Proc. IEEE International Symposium on Signal Processing and Information Technology, pp. 191–196 (2006)
11. Penna, M.A., Dines, K.A., Seip, R., Carlson, R.F., Sanghvi, N.T.: Modeling prostate anatomy from multiple view TRUS images for image-guided HIFU therapy. IEEE Trans. Ultrason Ferroelectr. Freq. Control 54(1), 52–69 (2007)
12. Gong, L., Pathak, S.D., Haynor, D.R., Cho, P.S., Kim, Y.: Parametric shape modeling using deformable superellipses for prostate segmentation. IEEE Trans. Med. Imaging 23(3), 340–349 (2004)
13. Badiei, S., Salcudean, S.E., Varah, J., Morris, W.J.: Prostate segmentation in 2D ultrasound images using image warping and ellipse fitting. Med. Image Comput. Comput. Assist. Interv. Int. Conf. 9(Pt 2), 17–24 (2006)
14. Mahdavi, S., Salcudean, S.E.: 3D prostate segmentation based on ellipsoid fitting, image tapering and warping. In: Conf. Proc. IEEE Eng. Med. Biol. Soc., vol. 1, pp. 2988–2991 (2008)
15. Zhan, Y., Shen, D.: Deformable segmentation of 3-D ultrasound prostate images using statistical texture matching method. IEEE Trans. Med. Imaging 25(3), 256–272 (2006)
16. Tutar, I.B., Pathak, S.D., Gong, L., Cho, P.S., Wallner, K., Kim, Y.: Semiautomatic 3-D prostate segmentation from TRUS images using spherical harmonics. IEEE Trans. Med. Imaging 25(12), 1645–1654 (2006)
17. Abolmaesumi, P., Sirouspour, M.R.: An interacting multiple model probabilistic data association filter for cavity boundary extraction from ultrasound images. IEEE Trans. Med. Imaging 23(6), 772–784 (2004)

An Interactive Geometric Technique for Upper and Lower Teeth Segmentation

Binh Huy Le[1], Zhigang Deng[1,*], James Xia[2], Yu-Bing Chang[2], and Xiaobo Zhou[2,*]

[1] Department of Computer Science, University of Houston, Houston, Texas
[2] The Methodist Hospital Research Institute, Houston, Texas
zdeng@cs.uh.edu, xzhou@tmhs.org

Abstract. Due to the complexity of the dental models in semantics of both shape and form, a fully automated method for the separation of the lower and upper teeth is unsuitable while manual segmentation requires painstakingly user interventions. In this paper, we present a novel interactive method to segment the upper and lower teeth. The process is performed on 3D triangular mesh of the skull and consists of four main steps: reconstruction of 3D model from teeth CT images, curvature estimation, interactive segmentation path planning using the shortest path finding algorithm, and performing actual geometric cut on 3D models using a graph cut algorithm. The accuracy and efficiency of our method were experimentally validated via comparisons with ground truth (manual segmentation) as well as the state of art interactive mesh segmentation algorithms. We show the presented scheme can dramatically save manual effort for users while retaining an acceptable quality (with an averaged 0.29 mm discrepancy from the ideal segmentation).

1 Introduction

Computed tomography (CT) images are commonly used in cranio-maxillofacial (CMF) surgery, orthodontics and dentistry. It is especially true when cone-beam CT (CBCT) scanners are introduced. CBCT scanners have much lower radiation than medical spiral CT scanners while the thickness of each slice is much thinner (0.125mm-0.4mm per slice thickness). CBCT scanners are now extensively used in dental offices to replace the plain cephalometric and panoramic radiographic machines. One of the main interests in CMF surgery and orthodontics is the teeth. In order to quantify the deformity accurately, a CT scan is usually completed when the maxillary (upper) and mandibular (lower) teeth are in centric occlusion (peak and valley on the teeth bite down tightly). This brings us a major problem: *the separation of the maxillary and mandibular teeth.* Due to the irregular 3D geometry of the teeth, they are usually segmented manually by drawing the maxillary and mandibular teeth on each cross-sectional slice. It is time consuming and difficult to segment the peaks of one jaw and the valleys of

---

[*] Corresponding authors.

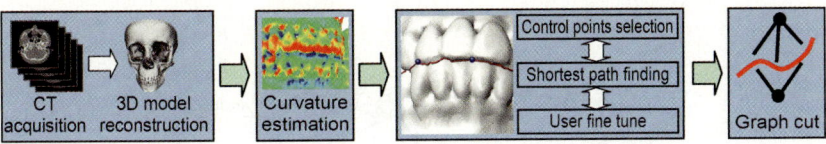

Fig. 1. Schematic view of this interactive approach for the lower and upper teeth segmentation

the opposite jaw on a single slice. It becomes even more difficult if the scatterings (artifacts) are present due to dental restoration and orthodontic braces.

The popularized scheme of current 3D mesh segmentation approaches is to extract and optimize certain application-specific mesh features. One common issue of these automated mesh segmentation approaches is that users cannot control or refine the process if the approaches fail to produce plausible segmentation results on complicated geometric models. Many semi-automatic mesh segmentation algorithms [1,2,3,4,5] were attempted for the purpose of mesh segmentation. Researchers have also developed teeth-specific segmentation techniques to separate individual teeth from a teeth dataset [6,7]. These approaches assume that the upper and lower 3D teeth can be perfectly separated by a plane. Nevertheless, it is nontrivial to extend these methods for the separation of complicated geometrical models such as the maxillary and mandibular teeth in this work.

In this paper, we present a novel interactive technique for segmenting the upper and lower teeth with limited user interventions. First, we reconstruct a 3D triangular mesh model from the acquired teeth CT images. Then, we compute the curvatures of the triangular mesh such that they are more sensitive in the vertical direction than in the horizontal direction. Then, through minimized user interventions such as selecting several control points, we construct a cost function and search for the optimal segmentation path on the mesh. Finally, the graph cut algorithm [8] is employed for handle the remaining isolated sticky parts. Figure 1 shows the schematic view of our approach.

2 Our Approach

2.1 3D Teeth Model Reconstruction

The CT image data of patients' craniofacial skeleton were acquired while the patients were on a centric occlusion. The CT scans were completed using a standard scanning algorithm: a resolution of 512×512 at 0.625-1.25 mm slice thickness, 25cm or lesser field-of-view (FOV), 0° gantry tilt, and 1:1 pitch. Then, we use the open-source OsiriX imaging software (http://www.osirix-viewer.com) to reconstruct their corresponding 3D triangular mesh from the CT images. We remove triangles distant from the teeth to reduce unnecessary computations.

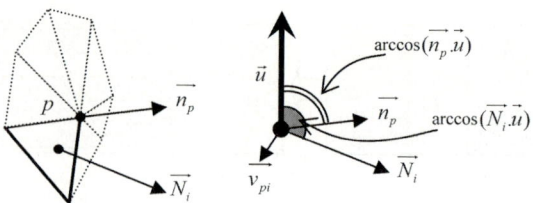

Fig. 2. Illustration of how the curvature of P is computed

2.2 Curvature Estimation

Based on the observation that the upper and lower teeth are expected to be segmented along an approximate horizontal direction, we compute the curvature of each vertex of a 3D teeth model such that it is more sensitive to the vertical direction while less sensitive to other directions. In this process, we use a predefined up vector and then calculate the curvature K_P for each vertex P as the averaged normal vector difference between the normal at the vertex P and the normals of P's neighboring triangles as follows:

$$K_P = \frac{\sum_{i \in nbhd(P)} \left(\arccos(\vec{n_p} \cdot \vec{u}) - \arccos(\vec{N_i} \cdot \vec{u}) \right) \frac{sign(\vec{u} \cdot \vec{v_{pi}})}{|\vec{v_{pi}}|}}{|nbhd(P)|} \quad (1)$$

Here $nbhd(P)$ is the set of P's neighboring triangles, $\vec{n_p}$ is the normal vector of P, $\vec{N_i}$ is the normal vector of a neighboring triangle F_i, $\vec{u}$ is the pre-defined up vector, $\vec{v_{pi}}$ is the vector from P to the centroid of F_i, the sign function $sign(\vec{u} \cdot \vec{v_{pi}})$ determines the vertical direction of $\vec{v_{pi}}$. Eq. 1 incorporates the orientation into the curvature estimation in the following way: angles between normal vectors and the up vector are extracted, then, the sign function is used to determine the concaveness of a neighboring triangle. Finally, we weighted average the estimated curvatures of all neighboring triangles, and the weights are inversely proportional to the distance to the center of the triangle (v_{pi}).

The above estimated curvatures can be used to determine the convex or concave property of the mesh vertices (Figure 2). Vertices with positive curvatures are called convex vertices; otherwise they are concave ones. In this work, we want the segmentation path to travel through the concave area of the mesh by simply thresholding the convex vertices. Note that since the acquired CT slices are in

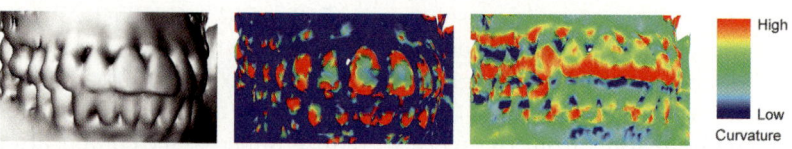

Fig. 3. Original teeth model (left), visualization of Gaussian curvatures (middle) and visualization of the curvatures by our approach (right)

the XY plane, we generally specify the up vector as the Z^+ direction. We also compared our curvature estimation scheme with the widely-used Gaussian curvature estimation algorithm [9]. As shown in Figure 3, the curvatures computed by our approach better separate the concave crevices in the horizontal direction (i.e., potential segmentation path area, shown as blue color in Figure 3) on the 3D teeth model than the Gaussian curvatures [9] where low curvature crevices are distributed everywhere.

2.3 Interactive Segmentation Path Planning

Because the upper and lower teeth are irregularly intertwined each other, an automatic method that fully depends on the curvature guidance would not always produce plausible segmentation. Thus, our approach allows users to select several control points on the model to guide the segmentation planning. Our approach computes an optimal segmentation path that travels through low curvature areas while satisfying the user-specified control points. During this process, users can interactively add or change the control points, and the corresponding segmentation paths will be updated in real-time.

We employ the Dijkstra shortest path algorithm [10] to find the optimal segmentation path between two control points. This algorithm takes two control points as the source and the destination and then minimizes the overall cost. A cost function C between two neighboring vertices i and j is defined as follows:

$$C(i,j) = \frac{d(i,j)}{|K_i| + |K_j|} \tag{2}$$

Where $d(i,j)$ is the Euclidean distance between vertex i and vertex j, K_i and K_j are the computed curvatures for vertices i and j, respectively (Eq. 1).

If the searched shortest path only consists of existing vertices on the 3D model, then it highly depends on the given mesh topology and may not be smooth. To alleviate this problem, many mesh segmentation methods perform a model subdivision (refinement) after an initial cut [5,4,3]. However, due to the lack of user controls on the mesh refinement process, the segmentation path on the refined mesh might measurably deviate from the original computed path, even though it may appear smoother. Mitchell et al. [11] tackle this problem by partitioning an edge into intervals so that the exact segmentation computation can be performed. The computational complexity of this algorithm is $O(n^2 \log n)$

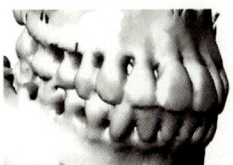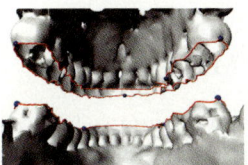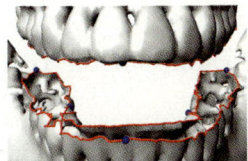

Fig. 4. Results of interactive segmentation path planning (model #1). Selected control points are shown as blue points and the searched segmentation paths are red curves.

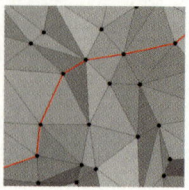 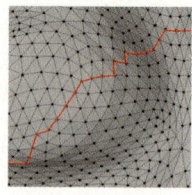 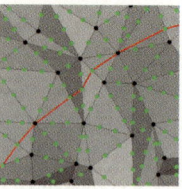

Fig. 5. The searched shortest segmentation path on a mesh without edge-partition (left), on the subdivision mesh (middle), and the mesh with our even edge-partition scheme (right)

in the worst case where n is the number of vertices on the mesh, which is not efficient for practical interactive applications.

In this work, to achieve a trade-off between algorithm efficiency and accuracy, we use a simple while efficient partition strategy that divides an edge into a minimum number of equal intervals and each of them has a user-defined minimum length d_{min}. The curvatures of interval ends are linearly interpolated based on the two end points of the corresponding mesh edge, and we further assume only if two interval-ends belong to the same triangle, then these two points have a cost value; otherwise infinity. The computational complexity of our algorithm is $O(n \log n)$ where n is the number of vertices on the mesh. Figure 4 shows the searched optimal segmentation path from the outside/inside views. Users selected 3 control points in the front side and 2 points inside the mouth. All these control points are illustrated as blue points. In this dataset, there is no gap between the upper and lower teeth, thus our approach can compute a continuous segmentation path surrounding the mesh. Although the distance between two selected control points is relatively large, our algorithm is able to compute a plausible segmentation path with the aid of the estimated curvatures.

We also compared our approach (mesh with even edge-partition) with the original mesh (without edge-partition) and the subdivision mesh. As shown in Figure 5, the shortest path computed from the mesh with even edge-partition is smoother than the other two cases. It is noteworthy that the segmentation path on the subdivision mesh has more vertices than that on the mesh with even edge-partition, which means more computation time. Furthermore, the shortest segmentation path computed from the subdivision mesh is still more rougher than the path on the mesh with our even edge-partition scheme.

2.4 Graph Cut on Teeth Models

After major segmentation paths are computed through the above interactive interface, certain isolated sticky parts may remain to be separated. We automatically segment the remaining sticky parts by applying the graph cut algorithm [8]. This algorithm works on a flow network with multi sources and sinks where nodes are mesh triangles and edges are mesh edges. The sources are triangles on top of the

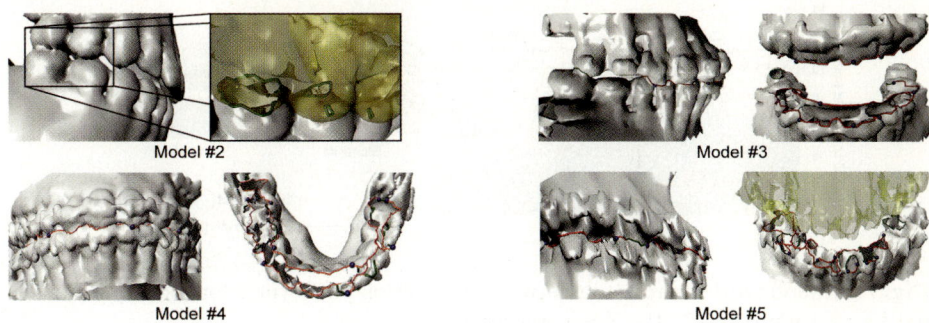

Fig. 6. Segmentation results by our approach: Green curves are the segmentation paths solved by the graph cut, and the semi-transparent yellow region is the upper teeth

mouth and sinks are triangles on the bottom. In this process, if a triangle is intersected with the above searched major segmentation paths (Section 2.3), then the capacities of all the edges of this triangle are set to zero; the capacities of other network edges are set to the length of corresponding mesh edges.

Figure 6 shows the segmentation results after the interactive segmentation path planning and the automated graph cut process are applied to a number of 3D teeth models. Due to the dental braces, many holes as well as rings and loops exist on the models. Despite of their model complexity, the combination of interactive segmentation planning (light red curves) and automated graph cut (bold green curves) is able to plausibly separate the upper and lower teeth. Note that we employ the graph cut not to improve the accuracy but to complete the segmentation, and the interactive segmentation path planning step generates the majority of the cut paths and then the graph cut fills the missing parts in the paths.

3 Results and Evaluation

We performed two experiments including ground truth validation and comparisons between our approach and two of the state of art mesh segmentation algorithms to validate the effectiveness of our approach.

3.1 Ground Truth Validation

In order to quantify the segmentation quality by our approach, we performed the following ground truth validation experiment on two datasets: a single cut (not a loop) from the leftmost to the rightmost of a teeth model, the ground truth segmentation was generated by manually selecting hundreds of segments on the mesh (219 segments for model #1 and 128 segments for model #3), and our semi-automatic approach generated the segmentation path based on several user-specified control points (3 control points for model #1, 5 control points for model #3). We projected these two segmentation paths onto Z-axis to measure their discrepancies, because Z-axis projection maximally shows the trajectory

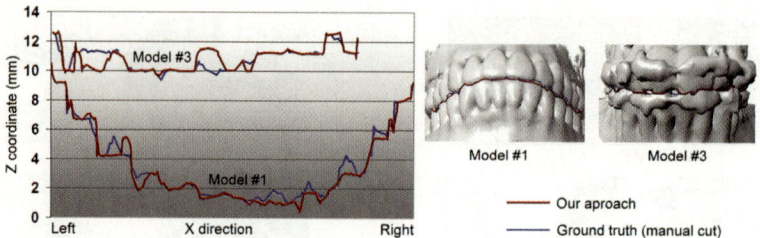

Fig. 7. Ground truth comparison of two segmentation paths (blue for the ground-truth, red for our approach) in the Z-axis projection

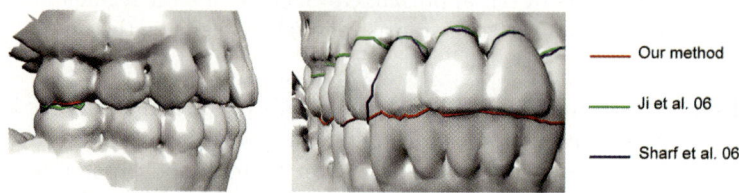

Fig. 8. Segmentation comparison of model #1 between our approach (red) and the other two approaches (blue and green)

difference. Figure 7 shows the Z-coordinates of the two validations. Their maximum errors are 1.57 mm (model #1) and 1.67mm (model #3), and the average errors are 0.28 mm (model #1) and 0.30mm (model #3), respectively.

3.2 Comparisons with State of the Art

We also compared our approach with two state of the art interactive mesh segmentation algorithms [4,5]. Figure 8 shows the comparison results. As shown in this figure, our approach significantly outperformed the other two approaches. Note that the segmentation method proposed by Ji et al. [4] is able to generate smooth segmentation paths due to its refinement algorithm if the teeth only touch in small parts, but it failed to handle this complicated teeth model. In this case, its region growing scheme is uncontrollable with a small number of seeds. Therefore, it requires users to manually select a large number of seeds.

4 Discussion and Conclusions

In this paper we present an effective interactive technique for the upper and lower teeth segmentation. Through numerous experiments on acquired teeth CT datasets, we found that our approach is fast (e.g., tens of times faster than manual approaches) and it required minimized user interventions such as selecting several control points to guide the algorithm process. We also compared our approach with two current interactive mesh segmentation algorithms and found that our approach significantly outperformed them on segmenting complicated teeth models.

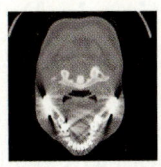 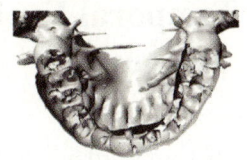 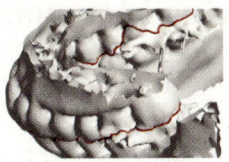

Fig. 9. Metal artifacts on the acquired 2D teeth CT images significantly affect the accuracy of segmentation by our approach

One major limitation of current approach is that when serious artifacts exist in 2D teeth CT images, our approach might fail to produce plausible segmentation results. For example, due to the strong metal artifacts of dental implant in the acquired teeth CT images and thus 3D teeth models, the segmentation accuracy of our approach would be significantly affected (Fig. 9). In the future, we plan to explore effective and automated algorithms to postprocess the acquired 2D teeth CT images and incorporate CT image segmentation with 3D geometric segmentation.

Acknowledgments. This research is supported by a IBIS seed grant (Xiaobo Zhou and Zhigang Deng), and Binh Huy Le is supported by a Fellowship from the Vietnam Education Foundation.

References

1. Gregory, A.D., State, A., Lin, M.C., Manocha, D., Livingston, M.A.: Interactive surface decomposition for polyhedral morphing. The Visual Computer 15(9), 453–470 (1999)
2. Funkhouser, T., Kazhdan, M., Shilane, P., Min, P., Kiefer, W., Tal, A., Rusinkiewicz, S., Dobkin, D.: Modeling by example. ACM Trans. on Graph. 23(3), 652–663 (2004)
3. Lee, Y., Lee, S., Shamir, A., Cohen-Or, D., Seidel, H.P.: Intelligent mesh scissoring using 3d snakes. In: Pacific Conference, pp. 279–287 (2004)
4. Ji, Z., Liu, L., Chen, Z., Wang, G.: Easy mesh cutting. Comput. Graph. Forum 25(3), 283–291 (2006)
5. Sharf, A., Blumenkrants, M., Shamir, A., Cohen-Or, D.: Snappaste: an interactive technique for easy mesh composition. The Visual Computer 22(9-11), 835–844 (2006)
6. Zhao, M., Ma, L., Ta, W., Nie, D.: Interactive tooth segmentation of dental models. In: IEEE EMBC, pp. 654–657 (2005)
7. Gao, H., Chae, O.: Automatic tooth region separation for dental ct images. In: IEEE International Conference on Convergence and Hybrid Information Technology, vol. 1, pp. 654–657 (2005)
8. Boykov, Y., Jolly, M.P.: Interactive graph cuts for optimal boundary and region segmentation of objects in n-d images. In: ICCV 2001, pp. 105–112 (2001)
9. Desbrun, M., Meyer, M., Schroder, P., Barr, A.H.: Discrete differential-geometry operators in nD. Technical report, California Institute of Technology (2000)
10. Dijkstra, E.W.: A note on two problems in connexion with graphs. Numerische Mathematik 1, 269–271 (1959)
11. Mitchell, J.S.B., Mount, D.M., Papadimitriou, C.H.: The discrete geodesic problem. SIAM J. Comput. 16(4), 647–668 (1987)

Enforcing Monotonic Temporal Evolution in Dry Eye Images*

Tamir Yedidya[1], Peter Carr[1], Richard Hartley[1], and Jean-Pierre Guillon[2]

[1] The Australian National University, and National ICT Australia
[2] Faculty of Medicine and Health Sciences, Lions Eye Institute, Australia

Abstract. We address the problem of identifying dry areas in the tear film as part of a diagnostic tool for dry-eye syndrome. The requirement is to identify and measure the growth of the dry regions to provide a time-evolving map of degrees of dryness. We segment dry regions using a multi-label graph-cut algorithm on the 3D spatio-temporal volume of frames from a video sequence. To capture the fact that dryness increases over the time of the sequence, we use a time-asymmetric cost function that enforces a constraint that the dryness of each pixel monotonically increases. We demonstrate how this increases our estimation's reliability and robustness. We tested the method on a set of videos and suggest further research using a similar approach.

1 Introduction

The pre-ocular tear film in humans does not remain stable for long periods of time [1]. When blinking is prevented, the tear film ruptures and dry spots appear over the cornea. This phenomenon is known as Dry Eye Syndrome [2]. The Fluorescein Break Up Time (FBUT) test was designed by Norn [3] to detect dryness. A small amount of fluorescein is instilled in the patient's eye. Then, the tear film is viewed with the help of a yellow filter in front of a slit-lamp (see Fig. 1). A video of the front of the eye is recorded between two consecutive blinks. As time passes after the blink, dark areas form on the iris, indicating the lack of fluorescence and the rupture of the tear film. The degree of blackness of these areas is related to the degree of thinning of the tear film. When a dark area of a certain size first appears on the iris, the time elapsed since the blink is recorded as the Break Up time (BUT). If the eyes are kept open, the area of the break will increase in size and breaks may appear in new areas over the cornea. This is the most commonly used test by clinicians to evaluate dry eyes [4].

In this paper, we present a graph-cut approach for automatic detection of dryness. We transform the video (after alignment) into a spatio-temporal 3D volume, so a relationship between successive images is defined. The 3D image volume is modeled as a 3-dimensional multi-label Markov Random Field (MRF) in which the label assigned to each pixel represents the degree of dryness. A graph-cut approach benefits from lesser sensitivity to spatial noise and misalignment of the eye images. In addition, we introduce the idea of enforcing temporal monotonicity. This reflects the condition that dry

---

* National ICT Australia is funded by the Australian Government's Backing Australia's Ability initiative, in part through the Australia Research Council.

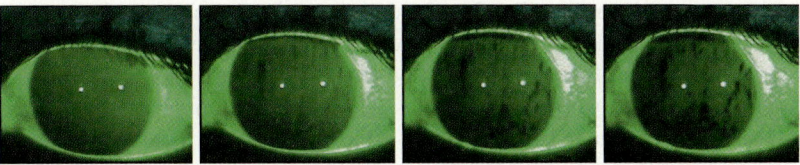

Fig. 1. A sequence of images showing how dryness forms over the iris. The first image is immediately after a blink and then the images are every 4 seconds. The intensity of regions over the iris is related to dryness: the darker the area, the drier it is.

spots on the iris can only become darker (dryer) in temporally successive images as seen in Fig. 1. To enforce the increasing dryness condition, we define asymmetric edge weights in the temporal direction, specifying an infinite (or very large) cost to assigning decreasing labels to a pixel in consecutive frames. The associated energy minimization problem is solved using the alpha expansion algorithm [5].

Previous Work. Assessment of dry-eye was reported by us in [6], but in that work we did not use any sort of spatial or temporal constraints. We compare the new results with our previous method.

There has been some work on 3-dimensional segmentation using graph-cuts. Recently Bokyov et al. [7] described a global N-D graph-cut segmentation approach that can be used to segment the kidney from a 3D MRI. They are interested in identifying three regions of the kidney and conduct three independent binary segmentations sequentially. However, they do not segment all three regions simultaneously using a multi-label approach. Another example for an application that uses 3D volume binary graph-cuts is for the segmentation of brain tumors [8].

Asymmetric cost functions have not seen widespread use. For example, when employed for spatial geometric constraints [9], alpha-expansion was not able to find a good solution. In [10], the authors use an asymmetric cost to segment multiple surfaces in 3D CT images. Even though the surfaces are segmented simultaneously, they use a binary label set (and not a multi-label approach). To our knowledge, asymmetry has not been used before to enforce temporal constraints within volumetric images.

Motivated by the recent report of the international dry eye workshop (DEWS) [2], we apply the monotonic constraint to the dry eye problem. The report notes the lack of gold standard for diagnosis of dry eye and the need for more robust methods.

2 Formulation of the Problem

We formulate our problem as a second-order MRF. In this approach, each variable i must be assigned a label $\mathbf{x}_i$ from the set of labels $\mathcal{L} = \{0, 1, 2, \ldots, \ell\}$. The most probable labeling $\mathbf{x}^\star$ minimizes the associated energy function:

$$E(\mathbf{x}) = \sum_{i \in \mathcal{P}} E_i(x_i) + \sum_{(i,j) \in \mathcal{N}} E_{ij}(x_i, x_j). \quad (1)$$

Here, $\mathcal{P}$ is the set of pixels in the image and $\mathcal{N}$ is the set of pairs of pixels defined over the standard four-connectedness neighborhood.

The unary terms E_i are application dependent, and we employ a dryness measure similar to [6]. The pairwise terms E_{ij} enforce an *a priori* model. In our application, we expect the labels of neighboring pixels to be the same (or at least quite similar). However, large changes are also possible at edges. Therefore, we employ a function based on the truncated linear distance (see Fig. 3(a)), which encourages local smoothness, while limiting the cost of large changes to a threshold T:

$$E_{ij}(x_i, x_j) = \lambda \min(|x_i - x_j|, T). \qquad (2)$$

The alpha-expansion algorithm [5] can minimize functions of the form (2) as they obey the triangle inequality [5,11]. Although an optimal solution is not guaranteed, in practice the method performs quite well.

2.1 3D Graph Construction

Graph-cut minimization is not limited to 2D and is easily extended to 3D applications. The main advantage of a 3D approach to segmenting individual 2D slices is that the relationship between pixels at consecutive slices is considered. Moreover, it allows one to incorporate monotonic constraints (described in the next section) between slices, which would have been impossible otherwise.

Extending the 2D approach to 3D is based on redefining the neighborhood used in the pairwise term. While in the case of MRI segmentation, it is fairly clear what the individual slices are, we offer an approach based on spatial and temporal progression. Even though the image modality is 2D in the case of the FBUT test, it can be perceived as a 3D approach to capture the global relationship between image frames. Denoting image t in a video of length $n + 1$ as I_t, each image is considered as a horizontal slice in the 3D graph (or MRF), creating a graph based on spatial and temporal changes. Therefore slice number 0 in the graph is the image immediately after the blink and slice n is the last image in the sequence. Every other slice is related to the time passed since the blink. The construction of the graph is based on a 6-connectedness neighborhood $\mathcal{N}$, and an example of a 3D MRF showing the 6-connectedness neighborhood is depicted in Fig. 2. Each voxel in the MRF $(x, y, t), t = \{0, \ldots n\}$ is connected to its four immediate neighbors in the same image and to the corresponding pixel (x, y) in the previous and next frames: $(x, y, t - 1)$ and $(x, y, t + 1)$. Another way to look at the neighborhood of a voxel is: $\mathcal{N} = \{left, right, up, down, next, previous\}$. The energy function is still built only from quadratic terms, as each voxel can be seen as being part of a maximum of 6 pairwise cliques. Each voxel is now also dependent on two voxels which are temporally different. This allows the addition of time based constraints. Denoting the set of pixels of frame t by $\mathcal{P}_t$, the new set of pixels is now defined over the whole image sequence: $\mathcal{P} = P_0 \cup \ldots \cup P_n$. The hidden nodes of the MRF are the labels assigned to each voxel from the set $\mathcal{L}$.

2.2 Monotonic Constraint

Multi-label problems usually have an inherent meaning to the ordering of the labels. In the case of the FBUT test, the labels represent the estimated thickness of the tear film. The labeling 0 represents no thinning of the tear film and the final label ℓ corresponds

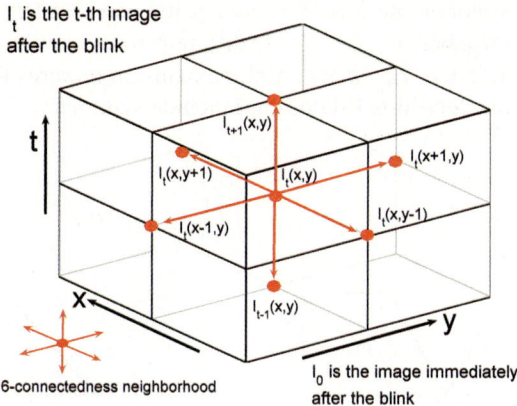

Fig. 2. Explaining the 3D MRF. The x and y axis are the image planes; the t plane is the temporal plane. A pixel $I_t(x,y)$ (or the voxel (x,y,t)) is the pixel (x,y) in the t-th image after the blink. The figure shows the 6-connectedness approach (by the red arrows), where a pixel is connected to its 4 immediate neighbors in the same plane and to two pixels corresponding to the same location at times $t-1$ and $t+1$. Each voxel in the MRF can be assigned any label from the set $\mathcal{L}$.

to a complete absence of fluid, or a break-up of the tear film. Other labels depict the different degrees of thinning of the tear film. Again, we expect the labels to change gradually, so we employ a distance metric for the pairwise cost in the temporal axis:

$$f_{ij}(x_i, x_j) = \gamma |x_i - x_j|. \tag{3}$$

As long as the patient does not blink, the thickness of the tear film can not increase between consecutive images. Formally, the label x_j of a particular pixel at time t_j must be less than the corresponding label x_i of the same pixel at time $t_i = t_j + 1$. We enforce this monotonic dryness condition directly into the pairwise energy term:

$$E_{ij}(x_i, x_j) = \begin{cases} \infty & \text{if } t_i = t_j + 1 \text{ and } x_i < x_j \\ f_{ij}(|x_i - x_j|) & \text{otherwise.} \end{cases} \tag{4}$$

We use the truncated linear term of (2) when i and j are a spatial pair ($t_i = t_j$), and the monotonic function of (4) when they are a temporal pair ($t_i = t_j + 1$).

The monotonic function (4) sets an infinite cost to any labeling **x** where a pair of labels (x_i, x_j) for a particular pixel at times t_j and $t_i = t_j + 1$ decreases — i.e., $x_i < x_j$. Although we associate an infinite cost for violating monotonicity, in general, a finite cost can be employed.

Fig. 3 shows two examples of pairwise functions which can be minimized using alpha-expansion. Part (a) is a cost function based on (2). The maximum penalty for assigning different labels is bounded by T. Part (b) is a cost function based on (4). If the change of labels is negative, the cost is infinity; Otherwise, the penalty is linear and not truncated. When $x_i = x_j$ the function is assigned 0, however it is not mandatory. In our algorithm, we use the first function for spatially neighboring voxels as a large change between labels should happen at edges. The second function is used for temporally neighboring pixels, where changes in labels (dryness) are usually gradual.

The inclusion of a monotonic constraint makes the pairwise terms asymmetric: the cost of changing from label α to β can be different from changing from β to α, or mathematically $E_{ij}(\alpha, \beta) \neq E_{ij}(\beta, \alpha)$. Alpha-expansion requires the cost function to be metric, however this definition [5] does not include symmetry.

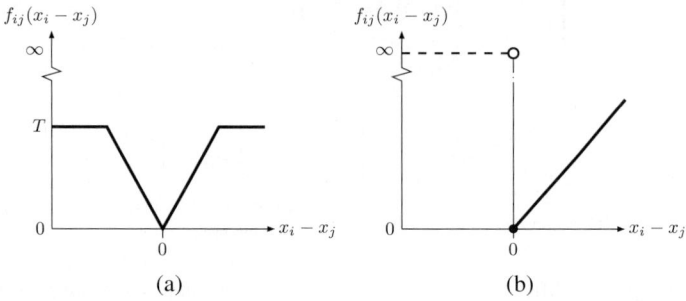

Fig. 3. The spatial (a) and temporal (b) pairwise functions. (a) Neighboring pixels within the same frame are encouraged to have the same label, unless the difference is quite big. In this case, medium and large differences are penalized equally. (b) Temporally, labels must not decrease as time progresses. Moreover, the increase (if any) should not be too large.

3 Application to Detect Dryness

The 2D segmentation approach [6] first detects the iris in each of the video frames. The images are aligned, such that the iris is located roughly at the same location in each image. The segmentation of the dry areas is based on analyzing the aligned video. A cost function examines differences in intensities for each of the pixels in the iris between the first and last images in the video. A dryness image is created, where each pixel is assigned an intensity value which is proportional to its degree of dryness and is denoted by $\tilde{I}(x, y)$. However, the degree of dryness is also computed at each individual slice, and we denote this pixel value by $\tilde{I}(x, y, t)$.

This approach produces good segmentation results and is very fast. Nevertheless, it has a few disadvantages:

1. Small errors in the alignment can completely bias the dryness result for a pixel.
2. The spatial relationships between neighboring pixels in the 2D image are not used.
3. There is no use of the knowledge regarding the temporal change.

3.1 Advantages of the 3D Approach

Given the aligned video created by the 2D segmentation approach, it is possible to incorporate the ideas discussed so far to improve the segmentation results. Instead of looking at individual pixels, and examining every single 2D image for the Break Up Time (BUT), we add the following assumptions:

1. Smoothness constraint - If a pixel becomes dry, it is likely that its neighbors also show a similar degree of dryness.

2. Using temporal knowledge - The video is considered as a 3D volume where each 2D frame is a slice in the 3D image. Segmenting the 3D volume takes into consideration the relationship between the pixel's values at all times.
3. Monotonicity constraint - Temporally, pixels should only become darker, as the amount of fluid in the tear film decreases as time passes. If a pixel becomes brighter it is probably caused by an error in the alignment process or because of shifting of the fluorescein after the blink and not related to the actual dryness.

3.2 Applying the Technique

We show now how the described approach can be easily adopted to the dryness problem. Given the aligned video created in the 2D approach, it is used to create a 3D graph based on temporal changes (see Sec. 2.1). The region of interest in each image is defined as only the pixels belonging to the iris. This region should not be image dependent as after the alignment the iris is resized to the same size at the same location.

The number of labels needed for segmenting dryness depends on the importance of distinguishing between the different degrees of thinning of the tear film. A reasonable choice is to use a set of 9 labels: $\mathcal{L} = \{0, 1, \ldots, 8\}$. This number of labels generally produces suitably precise segmentations of the tear film.

The unary term is defined using the value $\tilde{I}(x, y, t)$ computed in [6] for every pixel for every image $t = \{0, \ldots n\}$. When using a multi-label algorithm, a value has to be assigned for each label $E_i(\mathbf{x}_i), x_i \in \mathcal{L}$. The value $\tilde{I}$ can be associated with the expected label $x_i^\star$ for each pixel. For example, the intensity range of $\tilde{I}$ can be divided into $|\mathcal{L}|$ equally spaced bins, where each bin is associated with a label. The unary term is then defined as a function h proportional to the difference from the expected label:

$$E_i(x_i) = [h(x_i - x_i^\star)]^2. \quad (5)$$

The pairwise term uses linear distance metrics in both the spatial (2) and temporal (4) directions with parameters λ and γ manually tuned to 1. The spatial term is truncated, since large label discontinuities are expected as break-up areas can be local in shape. In the temporal domain, large discontinuities are not expected, so the regular linear distance metric is appropriate. The value of γ is related to the rate of temporally changing labels and can be tuned according to the number of slices in the 3D MRF. The clinical definition of tear film in the FBUT test states that the thickness of the tear film can not increase with time, thus directly encoding a monotonic restriction into (4).

This finalizes the creation of the graph and it is solved using graph-cuts. The labeling for each voxel is its degree of dryness at the time. The labeling of the voxels at time n can be seen as a similar output to the dryness image computed by the 2D approach.

4 Results

To test our method, we used a database of 22 videos with a varying length (4-24 seconds), all having a break of the tear film. Fig. 4(a) shows the result for the sequence in Fig. 1. The brightest areas correspond to areas of maximum thinning. The top slice is the final segmentation result. The t-axis shows the progress of dryness through time.

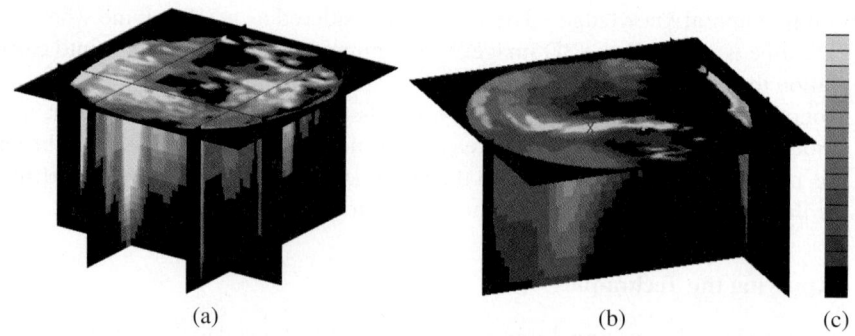

Fig. 4. The top slice shows the final segmentation result. The brighter the colors the more severe the dryness. The t-axis is the temporal axis (not to scale). The 3D view demonstrates how the dryness progresses at specific spatial locations. The monotonic constraint enforces pixels to have non-decreasing intensity. (a) Dryness image of the sequence from Fig. 1 (rotated counterclockwise for clarity). (b) A sequence where the dryness is mainly in the central and superior parts (rotated clockwise). (c) Temporal progress of the voxel highlighted by **x** in (b).

It can be seen how the monotonic constraint enforces the voxels to have only a non-decreasing intensity and that some of the voxels start showing dryness at a later stage but progress faster. Fig. 4(b) shows a similar cut for a different sequence where the dryness mainly develops in the central and superior areas. The area of dryness in the superior part is quite thin, but the smoothness constraint ensures it is a connected area.

In order to show the contribution of the monotonic constraint, we examined the average number of label changes between every two consecutive slices:

$$\mathcal{C} = 1/|\mathcal{P}_i| \sum_{x \in \mathcal{P}_i} \sum_{t=0}^{t=n-1} |x_i^{t+1} - x_i^t|. \tag{6}$$

We denote the label of pixel i at time t by x_i^t. When using the monotonic constraint, the upper bound for $\mathcal{C}$ is defined by the max number of labels: $\mathcal{C} \leq \ell$. Applying (6) to both methods on all 22 videos, we received an average of 0.906 and 0.523 for the 2D approach and 3D approach respectively. Clearly the new approach is much more robust and smooth. We note that in a few videos, most of the image pixels have no thinning of the tear film at all, so the change of labels is focused in a small number of pixels. Therefore, the difference in $\mathcal{C}$ between the approaches is quite meaningful, as in the 2D approach, individual pixels mainly near the eyelids or the iris's borders, had up to 68(!) label changes and a maximum of 8 when using the monotonic 3D approach. Fig. 5(a) shows another segmentation result using our approach. Parts (b) & (c) are temporal cuts, where the y-axis in these images is progression through time. Notice how near the left end side the monotonic constraint creates a smooth transition between labels with no fluctuations while there is a lot of noise in the other approach.

We asked a clinician to measure the BUT in each of the videos. We then automatically computed the BUT using [6] and then using the new method, considering a break of a pixel when it is assigned the highest label in $\mathcal{L}$. The average difference between the clinician's BUT and the approaches was $2.4s$ and $2.34s$ for the old and new method

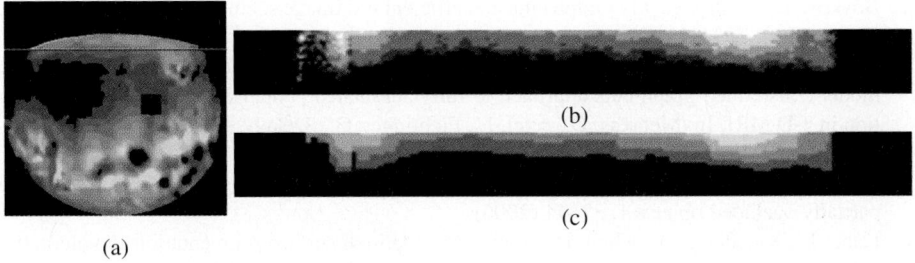

Fig. 5. Example of an x-t cut. (a) Segmentation result using the new approach. An x-t cut (not to scale) at the location of the line in (a) using the (b) 2D approach. (c) 3D approach. The y-axis in (b) & (c) shows temporal progress from bottom to top.

respectively. Considering the high inter-observer variance, these results are on the acceptable range. However, the new method detected small break areas in 2 videos that were not discovered before. This is due to the tendency of our approach to reduce the number of incorrectly segmented pixels. Thus, the result is less sensitive to outliers allowing the use of a lower threshold for computing the BUT (see [6]).

5 Conclusion and Further Research

In this paper, we demonstrated how an asymmetric graph-cuts approach, can be used to segment dryness. The inclusion of a temporally monotonic constraint improves the robustness of the results and reduces the sensitivity to outliers.

The approach presented in this paper can be extended to other medical applications. For instance in segmentation of OCT images of the retina, ordering of the different retinal layers may be enforced using spatially monotonic constraints. In fluoroscopic imaging involving perfusion of contrast agents, temporally monotonic increase and subsequent decrease of intensity may be enforced using an extension of these methods. Finally, spatial relationships and geometric properties such as convexity may be modeled using MRFs with asymmetric edge labels.

References

1. Holly, F.J.: Formation and rupture of the tear film. Exp. Eye Res. 15, 515–525 (1973)
2. Lemp, M.A., Baudouin, C., Dogru, J.B.M., Foulks, G.N., Kinoshita, S., Laibson, P., McCulley, J., Murube, J., Pfugfelder, S.C., Rolando, M., Toda, I.: The definition and classification of dry eye disease: Report of the international dews. The Ocular Surface 5(2) (2007)
3. Norn, M.: Desiccation of the pre corneal film. Acta Ophthal. 47(4), 865–880 (1969)
4. Korb, D., Craig, J., Dought, M., Guillon, J., Smith, G., Tomlinson, A.: The Tear Film, 1st edn. Butterworth Heinemann (2002)
5. Boykov, Y., Veksler, O., Zabih, R.: Fast approximate energy minimization via graph cuts. IEEE Trans. PAMI 23(11), 1222–1239 (2001)
6. Yedidya, T., Hartley, R., Guillon, J.: Automatic detection of pre-ocular tear film break-up sequence in dry eyes. In: DICTA, pp. 442–448 (2008)

7. Boykov, Y., Funka-Lea, G.: Graph cuts and efficient n-d image segmentation. Int. J. Comput. Vision 70(2), 109–131 (2006)
8. Wels, M., Carneiro, G., Aplas, A., Huber, M., Hornegger, J., Comaniciu, D.: A discriminative model-constrained graph cuts approach to fully automated pediatric brain tumor segmentation in 3-D MRI. In: Metaxas, D., Axel, L., Fichtinger, G., Székely, G. (eds.) MICCAI 2008, Part I. LNCS, vol. 5241, pp. 67–75. Springer, Heidelberg (2008)
9. Winn, J., Shotton, J.: The layout consistent random field for recognizing and segmenting partially occluded objects 1, 37–44 (2006)
10. Kang, L., Xiaodong, W., Chen, D., Sonka, M.: Optimal surface segmentation in volumetric images: A graph-theoretic approach. IEEE Trans. on PAMI 28(1) (2006)
11. Kolmogorov, V., Zabih, R.: What energy functions can be minimized via graph cuts? IEEE Trans. PAMI 26(2), 147–159 (2004)

Ultrafast Localization of the Optic Disc Using Dimensionality Reduction of the Search Space

Ahmed Essam Mahfouz and Ahmed S. Fahmy

Center for Informatics Science (CIS), Nile University (NU), Cairo, Egypt

Abstract. Optic Disc (OD) localization is an important pre-processing step that significantly simplifies subsequent segmentation of the OD and other retinal structures. Current OD localization techniques suffer from impractically-high computation times *(few minutes/image)*. In this work, we present an ultrafast technique that requires *less than a second* to localize the OD. The technique is based on reducing the dimensionality of the search space by projecting the 2D image feature space onto two orthogonal (x- and y-) axes. This results in two 1D signals that can be used to determine the x- and y- coordinates of the OD. Image features such as retinal vessels orientation and the OD brightness and shape are used in the current method. Four publicly-available databases, including STARE and DRIVE, were used to evaluate the proposed technique. The OD was successfully located in 330 images out of 340 images (97%) with an average computation time of 0.65 seconds.

1 Introduction

The risk of visual disabilities and blindness due to retinal diseases, whether primary or secondary to other diseases such as diabetes mellitus, could be greatly minimized by early diagnosis. An ophthalmologist needs to examine a large number of retina images to diagnose each patient; therefore, there is a significant need to develop computer-assisted diagnostic (CAD) tools for retina image analysis. The first step in any retina analysis system is to localize the optic disc (OD) [1]. The detected OD location can serve as a seed for OD segmentation, locating other structures such as the fovea [2], classifying left and right eyes in fovea-centered images, and/or a landmark to compensate large translations between retina images before applying any registration algorithm [1]. Although the OD has well defined features, developing fast and robust methods to automatically locate the OD is not an easy task due to retinal pathologies that alter the appearance of the OD significantly.

Several OD localization methods are available in literature. These methods can be classified into two main categories, *appearance-based methods* and *model-based methods* [3]. Appearance-based methods identify the location of the OD as the location of the brightest round object within the retina image. These methods include techniques such as simple threshold, highest average variation, and Principle Component Analysis (PCA) [4]. Although these methods are simple, they fail to correctly localize the OD in diseased retina images where the pathologies have similar properties to the OD.

Model-based methods depend on analyzing the retinal vessels structure. All the currently available techniques segment the retinal vessels as a starting step. These methods incorporate techniques such as geometrical models [1], template matching [5], and convergence of vasculature [6]. Although they have relatively high accuracy, they are computationally very expensive. For example, the geometrical model-based method described in [1] achieves a success rate of 97.5% in STARE database with a computation time of 2 minutes per image. In [2], a new OD localization method based on vasculature convergence has been described. The method achieves an accuracy of 98.77% in STARE database with a computation time of 3.5 minutes per image.

In this work, a novel ultrafast technique for OD localization is proposed. The method is based on converting the search space from a *one 2D space* (image space) to *two 1D spaces* (two 1D signals). The dimensionality reduction of the search space is achieved by projecting certain image features onto two perpendicular axes (horizontal and vertical), resulting in a significant reduction of computation time. Geometric and appearance features of the OD and the vasculature structure have been incorporated into the technique to correctly identify the location of the OD. Evaluation of the proposed method using four publicly available databases showed that it achieves an accuracy of 97% with an average computation time of 0.65 seconds.

2 Theory and Methods

2.1 Dimensionality Reduction and Image Features

Searching for the OD location in a 2D space (image space) renders any localization algorithm highly expensive in terms of computational time. The idea of the proposed method is to significantly enhance the speed of the algorithm by converting the 2D localization problem into two 1D localization problems, i.e. search space dimensionality reduction. This reduction is achieved by projecting certain features of the retina image onto two orthogonal axes (horizontal and vertical). The resulting two 1D signals are then used to determine the horizontal and vertical coordinates of the OD location. The key factor needed for the success of the dimensionality reduction step is to determine the set of features that, when projected on either axes, produce a meaningful signal that can be used to localize the OD. A possible meaningful horizontal/vertical signal is a signal whose maximum value location indicates the horizontal/vertical location of the OD.

In this work, two features are selected to create the two 1D projection signals. The first, and most fundamental, feature is based on the simple observation that the central retinal artery and vein emerge from the OD mainly in the vertical direction and then branch into two main horizontal branches, see fig. 1(a). This retinal vascular structure would suggest that a vertical window (with height equal to image height and a proper width) would always be dominated by vertical edges (vertical vessels) when centered at the OD, location 1 in fig. 1(a). Although the window may contain vertical edges at other locations, e.g. small vascular branches and lesions at location 2 in fig. 1(a), it will always be populated by strong horizontal edges, i.e. the edges of the two main horizontal branches of the retinal vessels. Therefore, the integration of the difference between the vertical and horizontal edges, over a region represented by this window, can be taken as a scoring index of the horizontal location of the OD. The directionality of the retinal vessels is described by the direction of their corresponding edges in the vertical and horizontal edge maps of the retina image. The simple gradient operator [1 0 -1] and its transpose are used to produce the vertical and horizontal edge maps of the retina image, respectively.

The second feature that is used in this work is based on the fact that the OD is usually a bright region. That is, the projection of the intensity values inside the window (which has height and width equal to the OD diameter) has a maximum value at the location of the OD. The following two sections will show the details of projecting these features to reduce the dimensionality of the localization problem.

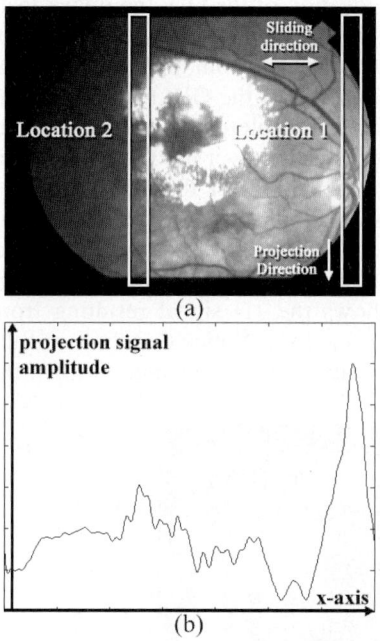

Fig. 1. (a) A retina image, from STARE database, showing the sliding window at two different locations, sliding direction and projection direction. (b) Plot of the 1D signal resulting from projecting the image features onto the horizontal axis ($H_{projection}$).

2.2 Horizontal Localization of the OD

Consider a sliding window whose width and height are equal to double the thickness of a main retinal vessel and the image height, respectively. Let this window scan a retinal image from left to right and project the image features within this window onto a horizontal axis to form a 1D signal. For simplicity, assume that the only image features of interest are the image's horizontal and vertical edges. Fig. 1(a) shows an example of a retina image with the sliding window placed at two different locations (1 & 2). When the window is located over the OD (location 1), it encloses a large number of vertical edges and almost no horizontal edges. Also at location 1, the projection of pixels' intensity within the window returns a minimum value, i.e. the window contains a large number of vessels represented by low intensity pixels. At any other location in the image (location 2), the window may enclose a large number of vertical edges, but it will always contain a large number of horizontal edges (representing the main horizontal branches of the retinal vessels).

Fig. 1(b) shows the 1D signal resulting from projecting the two features described above on the horizontal axis. Notice that the horizontal location of the optic disc is easily identified as the location of the maximum peak of the 1D signal.

2.3 Vertical Localization of the OD

To determine the vertical location of the OD, the image features are projected onto a vertical axis. A vertically sliding window, centered at the pre-determined horizontal location, is defined to scan the image from top to bottom. The height and width of the window are equal to the diameter of the OD. Fig. 2(a) shows an example of a retinal image with the sliding window centered at the pre-determined horizontal location. When the sliding window is located over the OD, it encloses a large number of both vertical and horizontal edges. Also over the OD, the projection of pixels' intensity within the window returns a maximum value (the window contains a maximum number of bright pixels). At any other location along the vertical line defining the pre-determined horizontal location of the OD, the window encloses fewer edges and less bright pixels. Fig. 2(b) shows the 1D signal resulting from projecting the features described above on the vertical axis. Notice that the vertical location of the optic disc is easily identified as the location of the maximum peak of the 1D signal.

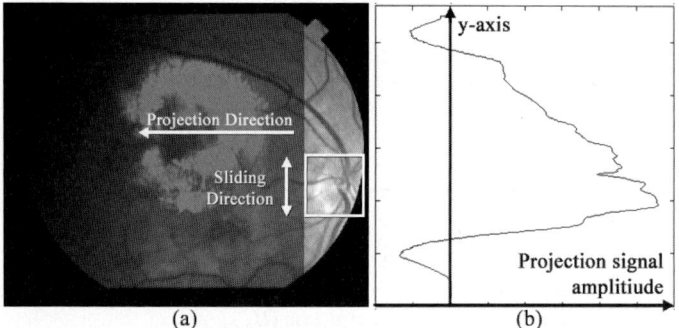

Fig. 2. (a) A retina image, from STARE database, showing the vertically sliding window, sliding direction and projection direction. (b) Plot of the 1D signal resulting from projecting the image features onto the vertical axis ($V_{projection}$).

It is worth noting that the areas outside the camera aperture (circular region) are excluded using a binary mask generated by thresholding the red component of the image based on the method described in [7].

2.4 Algorithm

STEP 1: Get image features
1. Get an image of horizontal edges (E_H) and an image of vertical edges (E_V)
2. Calculate: *EdgeDiff* = $| E_V | - |E_H|$; where $|.|$ *is the absolute operator*
3. Calculate: *EdgeSum* = $|E_H| + |E_V|$

STEP 2: Projection on the horizontal axis
1. Define W_{HRZ} as a rectangular window of size (*image height, 2×main vessel width*) and centered at a horizontal location x.
2. Slide the window W_{HRZ} over the image from left to right and for each x,
   - Calculate: F_{HRZ} = sum of *EdgeDiff* inside the window
   - Calculate: G_{HRZ} = sum of *pixels' intensities* inside the window
   - Calculate: the ratio $H_{projection}(x) = F_{HRZ} / G_{HRZ}$
3. The horizontal location of the optic disc *(cand_H)* is the location of the maximum value in $H_{projection}$

STEP 3: Projection on the vertical axis
1. Define W_{VER} as a rectangular window of size (*OD diameter, OD diameter*) and centered *cand_H*.
2. Slide the window W_{VER} over the image from top to bottom and for each vertical location y,
   - Calculate: F_{VER} = sum of *EdgeSum* inside the window
   - Calculate: G_{VER} = sum of *pixels' intensity* inside the window
   - Calculate the value $V_{projection} = F_{VER} \times G_{VER}$
3. The vertical location of the optic disc *(cand_V)* is the location of the maximum value in $V_{projection}$

2.5 Improving the Technique Robustness

In some cases, the 1D signal resulting from projecting the image features on the horizontal axis ($H_{projection}$) has multiple peaks that are close in their values (not a single prominent peak). These peaks result from various situations: (1) when the small vertical branches of the vessels are represented by strong edges and, at the same time, the OD region in the image is blurred, (2) when the image contains some artifacts. In order to improve the robustness of the proposed technique, a candidate list containing the locations of the two maximum peaks *(cand_H1 & cand_H2)* in $H_{projection}$ is constructed. At each horizontal location, the vertical location is determined as described in section 2.3, which results in two possible candidate locations of the OD.

To determine which one is the correct location of the OD, the geometric properties of the bright regions around these candidates are examined. A basic assumption in this process is that if we center a vertical window at the true location of the OD, it would contain a compact bright region with eccentricity close to unity. The eccentricity is defined as the ratio of the object's major axis length to the object's minor axis length [8] and is used to measure the object's roundness, with the eccentricity of a circle equaling one. The vertical window's size is not critical and can be assumed a rectangle of dimensions: image height × OD diameter. A scoring index is defined for each candidate and is weighed by the eccentricity as follows. The brightest 3.5% pixels within the window are selected. If there is a bright object at the candidate OD location, the eccentricity of this object is calculated and the scoring index of this location, equal to $H_{projection}(cand\_H1)$, is multiplied by the eccentricity of this object. If there is no object present at the candidate location, the eccentricity is set to be 0.1 and the scoring index of this location is multiplied by this eccentricity.

3 Results

Four publicly available databases were used to evaluate the accuracy and the computation time of the proposed technique. The four databases are: (1) STARE database (605 × 700 pixels) [9], (2) DRIVE database (565 × 584 pixels) [10], (3) Standard Diabetic Retinopathy Database 'Calibration Level 0' (DIARETDB0) (1500 × 1152 pixels) [11] and (4) Standard Diabetic Retinopathy Database 'Calibration Level 1' (DIARETDB1) (1500 × 1152 pixels) [11]. Accuracy and computation time results of evaluating the proposed method using these databases are summarized in Table 1. Number of images in each database is also included.

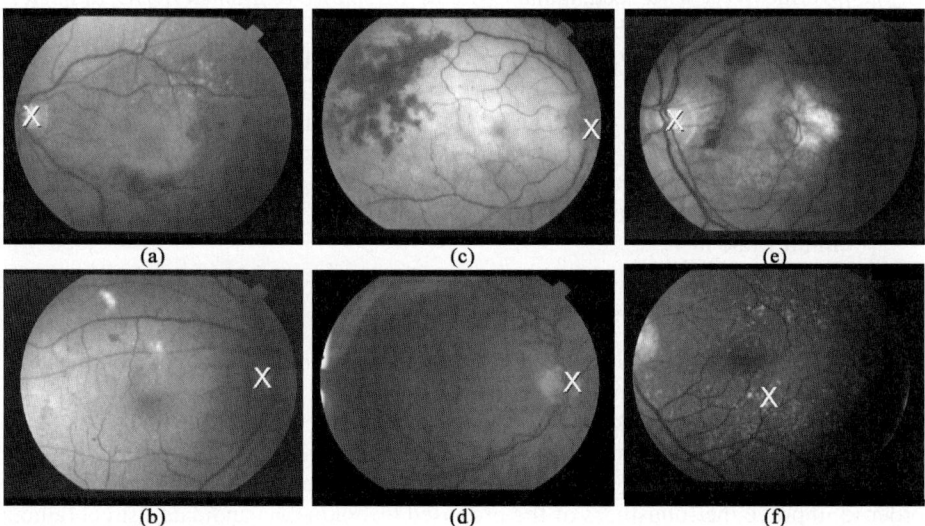

Fig. 3. Success and failure cases in 6 images selected from Stare database. (a) - (e) show successful OD localization samples. (f) shows a sample of failure in OD localization. The white 'X' indicates the location of the OD as detected by the proposed method.

The detected location of the OD is considered correct if it falls within 60 pixels of a manually identified OD center, as proposed by A. Hoover et al. in [6], M. Foracchia et al. in [1] and A. Youssif et al. in [2]. The center of the OD is manually identified as the point from which all the retinal vessels emerge.

The proposed method achieved a total accuracy of 97% when tested using the four databases, i.e. the OD was correctly located in 330 images out of the 340 images tested. The OD was correctly located in 75 images out of STARE's 81 images (92.6%) in 0.46 seconds per image with an average error of 14 pixels and a standard deviation (STD) of 15 pixels. In addition, the OD was correctly located in all the 40 images of DRIVE (100%) taking an average of 0.32 seconds per image with an average error of 11 pixels and a STD of 11 pixels.

Table 1. Accuracy and computation time of the proposed OD localization technique

Database	(1)	(2)	(3)	(4)	Total
Number of Images	81	40	130	89	340
Success	75	40	128	87	330
Accuracy	92.6%	100%	98.5%	97.8%	97%
Computation Time	0.46 sec.	0.32 sec.	0.98 sec.	0.98 sec.	-

4 Discussion

Fig. 3(a)-(e) show samples of successful localization results when applying the proposed method to selected images from STARE database. The technique of vasculature convergence [6] failed to locate the OD correctly in the first three images, while the method in [2] failed to correctly locate the OD in the 4th image. The OD was correctly located in the 4th image by selecting the 2nd peak instead of the first one using the method described in section 2.5. The geometrical model-based technique [1] failed to locate the OD in the 5th image. Fig 3(f) shows an example of an image in which the proposed method failed to locate the OD because it is partially hidden. Both methods described in [1, 6] also failed to locate the OD in this image.

The proposed method reduces the dimensionality of the search space from a 2D space (image space) of order $n \times m$ to two 1D spaces (two 1D signals) of order $n+m$, with n and m being the image dimensions. This dimensionality reduction is achieved through the projection of certain image features onto two orthogonal axes (horizontal and vertical). Two features are selected. The first one is the structure of the retinal vessels. The second feature is the intensity profile of the OD.

In order to increase the accuracy of the proposed method, two candidate locations of the OD are identified and additional scoring of these candidates is done by incorporating the OD geometry (represented by the eccentricity) into the technique. By investigating these two candidate locations instead of one location only, the total accuracy of the technique increased from 93.8% to 97%. As shown in fig. 3, even in the presence of retinal pathologies and/or image artifacts, the selected features were unique to the OD and thus allowed proper localization with relatively high accuracy.

The most computationally demanding operation is convoluting the image with the 3×1 gradient mask used to get the edges. This operation is negligible if compared to the initial step of extracting the retinal vessels, which is required in all model-based techniques. The latter is usually achieved by applying a 2D matched filter (typically 10×15 mask) with several orientations (typically at 12 different angles) [12].

5 Conclusion

A new method for OD localization in retinal fundus images is presented. The method is based on reducing the dimensionality of the search space; that is, decomposing the

2D problem into two 1D problems by projecting certain image features onto two perpendicular axes. The proposed method achieves accurate results in a significantly short computation time relative to currently available techniques.

References

1. Foracchia, M., Grisan, E., Ruggeri, A.: Detection of Optic Disc in Retinal Images by Means of a Geometrical Model of Vessel Structure. IEEE Transaction on Medical Imaging 23(10), 1189–1195 (2004)
2. Youssif, A., Ghalwash, A., Ghoneim, A.: Optic Disc Detection from Normalized digital Fundus Images by means of a Vessels' Direction Matched Filter. IEEE Transaction on Medical Imaging 27(1), 11–18 (2008)
3. Joshi, G.D., Gondle, V., Sivaswamy, J.: Optic Disc Detection Using Topographical Features. In: Proceedings of International EURASIP conf. (BIOSIGNAL), Funchal, Madeira – Portugal (2008)
4. Li, H., Chutatape, O.: Automatic Feature Extraction in Color Retinal Images by a Model Based Approach. IEEE Transaction on Biomedical Engineering 51(2), 246–254 (2004)
5. Lalonde, M., Beaulieu, M., Gagnon, L.: Fast and robust optic disk detection using pyramidal decomposition and Hausdorff-based template matching. IEEE Transaction on Medical Imaging 20(11), 1193–1200 (2001)
6. Hoover, A., Goldbaum, M.: Locating the Optic Nerve in a Retinal Image Using the Fuzzy Convergence of the Blood Vessels. IEEE Transaction on Medical Imaging 22(8), 951–958 (2003)
7. ter Haar, F.: Automatic localization of the optic disc in digital color images of the human retina. M.S. thesis, Utrecht University, Utrecht, The Netherlands (2005)
8. Sonka, M., Hlavac, V., Boyle, R.: Image Processing, Analysis, and Machine Vision. Thomson Learning, USA (2008)
9. STARE project Website Clemson Univ., Clemson, SC,
   http://www.ces.clemson.edu/~ahoover/stare
10. Staal, J.J., Abramoff, M.D., Niemeijer, M., Viergever, M.A., van Ginneken, B.: Ridge based vessel segmentation in color images of the retina. IEEE Transactions on Medical Imaging 23, 501–509 (2004)
11. Kauppi, T., Kalesnykiene, V., Kamarainen, J.K., Lensu, L., Sorri, I., Uusitalo, H., Kälviäinen, H., Pietilä, J.: DIARETDB: Evaluation Database and Methodology for Diabetic Retinopathy, Technical Report
12. Chaudhuri, S., Chatterjee, S., Katz, N., Nelson, M., Goldbaum, M.: Detection of blood vessels in retinal images using two-dimensional matched filters. IEEE Transaction on Medical Imaging 8(3), 263–269 (1989)

Using Frankenstein's Creature Paradigm to Build a Patient Specific Atlas

Olivier Commowick[1], Simon K. Warfield[1], and Grégoire Malandain[2]

[1] CRL, Children's Hospital Boston - Harvard Medical School
Olivier.Commowick@childrens.harvard.edu
[2] INRIA Sophia Antipolis - Asclepios Team, France

Abstract. Conformal radiotherapy planning needs accurate delineations of the critical structures. Atlas-based segmentation has been shown to be very efficient to delineate brain structures. It would therefore be very interesting to develop an atlas for the head and neck region where 7 % of the cancers arise. However, the construction of an atlas in this region is very difficult due to the high variability of the anatomies. This can generate segmentation errors and over-segmented structures in the atlas. To overcome this drawback, we present an alternative method to build a template locally adapted to the patient's anatomy. This is done first by selecting in a database the images that are the most similar to the patient on predefined regions of interest, using on a distance between transformations. The first major contribution is that we do not compute every patient-to-image registration to find the most similar image, but only the registration of the patient towards an average image. This method is therefore computationally very efficient. The second major contribution is a novel method to use the selected images and the predefined regions to build a "Frankenstein's creature" for segmentation. We present a qualitative and quantitative comparison between the proposed method and a classical atlas-based segmentation method. This evaluation is performed on a subset of 58 patients among a database of 105 head and neck CT images and shows a great improvement of the specificity of the results.

1 Introduction

Conformal radiotherapy allows to precisely target the tumor while keeping an acceptable level of irradiation on neighboring critical structures. This however requires to accurately locate the tumor and the organs at risk in order to determine the best characteristics of the irradiation beams. This delineation task is usually done manually and is therefore very long and not reproducible.

To solve this problem, atlas-based segmentation has been shown to produce accurate and automatic segmentations of the brain [1], allowing to take into account easily the relative positions of the structures. The construction of an atlas for other regions such as the head and neck region, where 7 % of the cancers arise, is therefore of great interest [2,3]. Methods have been presented for the construction of an unbiased average model from an image dataset such as [4,5].

We presented in [6] a method to build a symmetric atlas from a database of images manually delineated following the guidelines in [7]. However, anatomical variability is very high in the head and neck region. An average atlas may therefore be very different from the patient, leading to registration discrepancies. Moreover, this variability may cause the mean contours to be too large in the atlas yielding over-segmentations.

To overcome these drawbacks, methods have been presented towards the creation of atlases whose anatomy is adapted to the patient [8,9]. First, Blezek et al. [8] presented an interesting approach to cluster a database into several atlases representing homogeneous sub-populations. However, the selection of the most adequate atlas with respect to a given patient is not addressed. Another method [9] has been introduced to select the most similar images to the patient by comparing a similarity measure between each database image and the patient. This method is however computationally expensive, requiring to register all the database images on the patient. Moreover, a local comparison of the images is more adapted in our case, as our database consists of manually delineated patients who present pathologies that may corrupt a global comparison.

In this paper, we present the development of an atlas locally adapted to the patient to get more precise delineations than with an average atlas. To this end, we first present a new and efficient method to select the most similar images to the patient on predefined regions. Each most similar sample is defined as the one that needs the smallest local deformations to be registered on the patient. These images are then combined into a template image, as an analogy to Frankenstein's creature [10], and used for segmentation.

We first present our approach to select the image that is the most similar to the patient P to delineate on a given region. We then focus on the combination of the local templates selected into one single template for delineation. Finally, we show qualitative and quantitative results on a database of 105 head and neck CT images, showing a great improvement of the specificity of the results.

2 Method

In this section, we present an efficient method to compute a template that is similar to the patient P on predefined regions R_l, based on the following steps:

- Construction of an average atlas M from the database images (pre-computed)
- Non linear registration of the patient P to delineate on M
- Selection of the most similar image $\tilde{I}_l$ for each local region R_l
- Computation of the anatomy $\tilde{M}$ and segmentations from the set of $\tilde{I}_l$

2.1 Selection of the Locally Most Similar Images to a Patient

For each region of interest R_l, we select the most similar image among our database to the patient to delineate. It is defined as the one that is the "less" deformed to be non linearly registered on the patient. We denote by $T_{B \leftarrow A}$ the transformation linking two images A and B, so that B can be resampled on A (i.e.

$A \approx B \circ T_{B \leftarrow A}$). The selection for a given region R_l is then based on a comparison of the non linear transformations $T_{I_j \leftarrow P}$ to bring each image I_j of the database on P, i.e. the most similar image is defined as: $\tilde{I}_l = \arg\min_{I_j} d_{R_l}(I_j, P) = \arg\min_{I_j} d_{R_l}(T_{I_j \leftarrow P}, Id)$, where d_{R_l} will be defined later on. However, this type of comparison is computationally very expensive as it requires to perform all the registrations between P and the images I_j for each patient to segment. To perform an efficient selection, we therefore use an intermediate image: an average atlas M pre-computed from the database using [6].

From the average atlas construction, we obtain for each image I_j an affine transformation $A_{I_j \leftarrow M}$ and a non linear transformation $T_{I_j \leftarrow M}$ bringing it on the average image M. Moreover, when registering P on M, another non linear transformation $T_{P \leftarrow M}$ is computed. The key hypothesis is then to assume that $T_{I_j \leftarrow P}$ can be approximated by $T_{I_j \leftarrow M} \circ T_{P \leftarrow M}^{-1}$. This hypothesis presents many advantages. First, the regions of interest R_l can be defined once and for all on the atlas image M. Moreover, this can be done very easily thanks to the average segmentations available on the atlas. Also, the similarity between P and I_j, $d_{R_l}(T_{I_j \leftarrow P}, Id)$, can be approximated using the following equation:

$$d_{R_l}(T_{I_j \leftarrow M} \circ T_{P \leftarrow M}^{-1}, Id) = \sum_{i \in R_l \circ T_{P \leftarrow M}^{-1}} \| \log(T_{I_j \leftarrow M} \circ T_{P \leftarrow M}^{-1})(i) \| \quad (1)$$

where i corresponds to the voxels of the dense transformation and d_{R_l} is the Log-Euclidean distance on diffeomorphisms [11] between the identity transformation and $T_{I_j \leftarrow M} \circ T_{P \leftarrow M}^{-1}$. Using our hypothesis, we need to perform only one non linear registration between M and P to select the locally most similar images $\tilde{I}_l$ for all regions R_l, therefore reducing drastically the computation time.

2.2 Piecewise Most Similar Atlas Construction

We now focus on the computation of a template for segmentation from the selected images $\tilde{I}_l$ and the regions R_l. This template, similar to the Frankenstein's creature [10], is built by iterating over the following steps to combine the images:

- Registration of the images $\tilde{I}_l$ on the average image at iteration k : $\tilde{M}_k$
- Compute the new average image M_{k+1}, based on the regions $R_{l,k}$
- Compute an average transformation $\bar{T}_k$ from the transformations $T_{\tilde{I}_l \leftarrow \tilde{M}_k}$
- Apply $\bar{T}_k^{-1}$ to M_{k+1} to get the new reference $\tilde{M}_{k+1} = M_{k+1} \circ \bar{T}_k^{-1}$
- Update the regions of interest by applying $\bar{T}_k^{-1}$ to $R_{l,k}$: $R_{l,k+1} = R_{l,k} \circ \bar{T}_k^{-1}$

This algorithm can be seen as an extension of [4] to the construction of an atlas where images have spatially varying weights, depending on the regions R_l. In contrast, Guimond et al. consider implicitly that all images have equal and spatially constant weights ($1/N$ for each image if N images are averaged). The final step is then to associate a set of segmentations to this anatomy. This is done by transforming the manual segmentations of the image $\tilde{I}_l$ present in the region R_l onto $\tilde{M}$, using the transformations obtained in the construction process, and ensuring that no overlap exists between the final structures.

Average Image Computation. To compute M_{k+1} from the images $\tilde{I}_l$ registered on $\tilde{M}_k$, we first need to define the spatial extensions of each region at iteration k : $R_{l,k}$. This will allow to use, on each $R_{l,k}$, only the corresponding $\tilde{I}_l$ and to interpolate between the regions. The weight functions $\bar{w}_{l,k}(x)$ are computed in three steps: locally erode the regions $R_{l,k}$ using the method presented in [12] to ensure a minimal distance between them, compute the inverse of the minimal distance to each $R_{l,k}$: $w_{l,k}(x) = 1/(1 + \alpha \text{dist}(x, R_{l,k}))$, and normalize the $w_{l,k}(x)$: $\bar{w}_{l,k}(x) = w_{l,k}(x) / \sum_{l=1}^{L} w_{l,k}(x)$.

The images $\tilde{I}_l$ are then aligned onto $\tilde{M}_k$, first globally resulting in affine transformations $A_{\tilde{I}_l \leftarrow \tilde{M}_k}$, and then non linearly producing dense transformations $T_{\tilde{I}_l \leftarrow \tilde{M}_k}$. These transformations and the $\bar{w}_{l,k}(x)$ are then used to compute M_{k+1}:

$$M_{k+1}(x) = \sum_{l=1}^{L} \bar{w}_{l,k}(x) \left(\tilde{I}_l \circ A_{\tilde{I}_l \leftarrow \tilde{M}_k} \circ T_{\tilde{I}_l \leftarrow \tilde{M}_k} \right) (x) \qquad (2)$$

Residual Deformation Computation. Similarly to [4], the next step consists in averaging the $T_{\tilde{I}_l \leftarrow \tilde{M}_k}$ into a transformation $\bar{T}_k$ and apply its inverse to M_{k+1} to get the new reference $\tilde{M}_{k+1} = M_{k+1} \circ \bar{T}_k^{-1}$. However, we are averaging transformations using spatially variable weights $\bar{w}_{l,k}(x)$. To take this into account and ensure that $\bar{T}_k$ is a diffeomorphism, we introduce a generalization of the Log-Euclidean (LE) polyaffine transformation to diffeomorphisms, as suggested in [13]. The polydiffeomorphism construction is based on the LE framework for diffeomorphisms [11], allowing to compute operations easily while staying on the manifold of diffeomorphisms. $\bar{T}_k$ is then built by integrating between time 0 : $x(0) = x$ and time 1 : $x(1) = \bar{T}_k(x)$ the following Ordinary Differential Equation (ODE): $\dot{x} = \sum_{l=1}^{N} \bar{w}_{l,k}(x) \log \left(T_{\tilde{I}_l \leftarrow \tilde{M}_k}^{(k)} \right)(x)$. Similarly to the LE polyaffine framework, $\bar{T}_k$ and $\bar{T}_k^{-1}$ are expressed respectively as the exponential of the right hand side of the ODE, and the exponential of its opposite.

3 Evaluation Methodology

To evaluate our method, we have used a database of 105 CT images of patients delineated for head and neck radiotherapy following the guidelines provided in [7]. Segmented structures included 12 structures: lymph nodes II, III and IV, parotids and sub-mandibular glands on each side as well as the spinal cord and the brainstem. On this database, we have repeated a Leave-One-Out approach, each time picking out one patient from the dataset of images. The average atlas is then built from the remaining images. We used this framework to compare two segmentation methods: the average atlas-based segmentation, and the locally most similar image based segmentation. The Frankenstein's creature was built by defining on the average atlas a region of interest for each structure. This gives a total of 12 selected images, combined together into a single composite patient. This image is then registered on the left-out patient to get its segmentation.

The results were then compared to the manual delineations of the left-out patient using two voxel-based overlap measures: sensitivity (rate of true detection of the structure) and specificity (rate of true detection of the background). As they were delineated for radiotherapy, some structures were not available. We have therefore used the Leave-One-Out evaluation on a subset of 58 patients which had 8 or more manual delineations. Finally, the separation between some structures (lymph nodes, brainstem and spinal cord) are made on an arbitrary axial plane, based on possibly moving anatomical landmarks. This may lead to errors in the separations of the automatic segmentations and artificially low quality measures for all methods. We addressed this by evaluating together the brainstem and spinal cord, and by grouping the lymph nodes on each side.

4 Results

4.1 Qualitative Evaluation

We first present in Fig. 1 the visual comparison of the average atlas and locally most similar image for one patient. This example illustrates very well that the average atlas anatomy may be significantly different from the patient after a global registration. This may result in registration discrepancies and in erroneous segmentations. This is particularly visible in the lymph nodes areas (see axes in the images) where the patient is much more corpulent than the atlas. The composite patient is much closer visually to the patient. The deformations between these two images will therefore be easier to recover and this will contribute to minimize the registration errors.

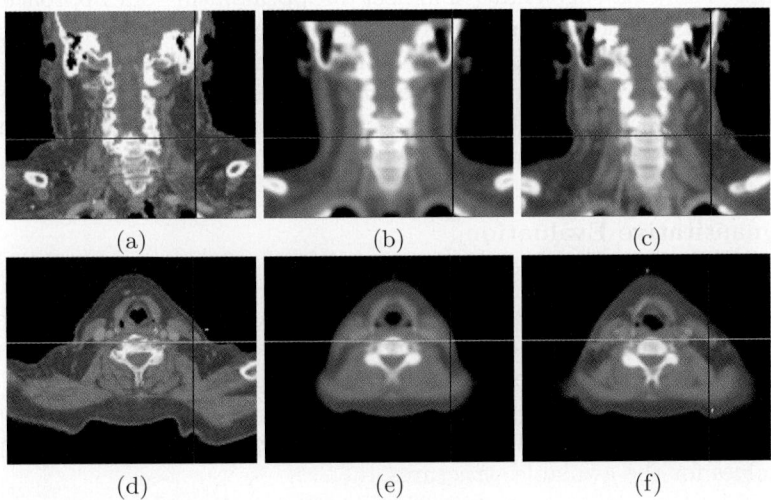

Fig. 1. Example of Computed Piecewise Most Similar Image. Comparison between the patient image (a), (d) ; the average atlas (b), (e) and the locally most similar image (c), (f). All images are globally registered on the patient's image.

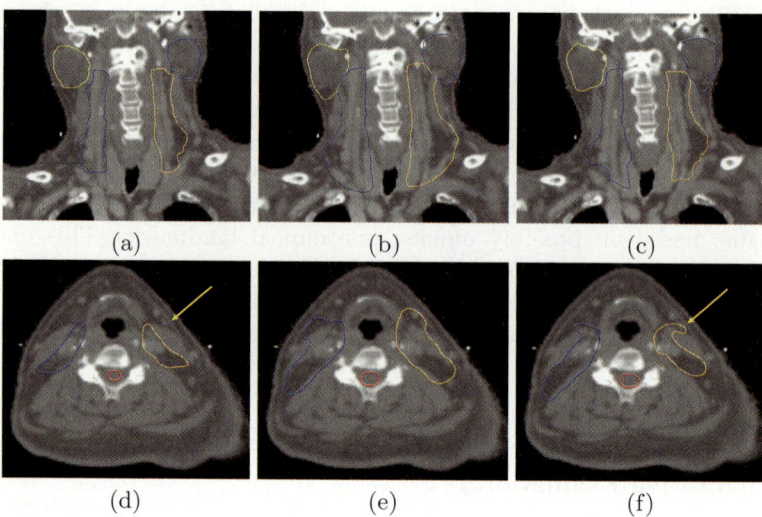

Fig. 2. Qualitative atlas and piecewise most similar image based segmentation results. Comparison between the manual segmentations (a), (d) ; the atlas-based segmentations (b), (e) and the piecewise most similar image segmentations (c), (f).

We then present in Fig. 2 the qualitative evaluation of the segmentation results, using the Leave-One-Out framework. This figure first shows that the atlas-based segmentations (images (b,e)) are overly large when compared to the manual ones. This is due to the inter-expert segmentation variabilities when creating the average segmentations, resulting in overly large segmentations in the atlas itself. This over-segmentation almost disappears using our approach. Only a single manual segmentation is indeed used for each structure, leading to more accurate segmentations, particularly on the lymph nodes areas. Finally, there are still differences in some regions (see arrow in image (f)). These differences are due to the local specificities of the selected manual segmentation, induced by the inter-expert segmentation variability.

4.2 Quantitative Evaluation

We finally present in this section the quantitative evaluation of the results using the Leave-One-Out framework described in section 3. We present in Table 1 the average quantitative results (sensitivity and specificity) computed using the Leave-One-Out framework on 58 patients. We also indicate the number of structures on which each average was performed. The patients in the database were indeed not totally segmented manually and we therefore computed the quantitative values for the available structures.

This table shows an important improvement of the specificity measure in the locally most similar method with respect to classical atlas-based segmentation. This confirms the observations made in the qualitative results as this measure increases as the over-segmentation of the structures with respect to the manual

Table 1. Quantitative Segmentation Results Comparison. Sensitivities (Sens.), specificities (Spec.) and their standard deviations for atlas-based and locally most similar image (Frankenstein) based segmentation (see text).

	Atlas		Frankenstein		Patients
	Sens. ± StD	Spec. ± StD	Sens. ± StD	Spec. ± StD	
Lymph Nodes (L)	0.930 ± 0.051	0.607 ± 0.070	0.692 ± 0.097	0.813 ± 0.072	53
Lymph Nodes (R)	0.923 ± 0.045	0.630 ± 0.078	0.675 ± 0.113	0.832 ± 0.074	46
Spinal Cord	0.938 ± 0.044	0.730 ± 0.065	0.773 ± 0.093	0.867 ± 0.079	47
Left Parotid	0.885 ± 0.072	0.691 ± 0.089	0.700 ± 0.172	0.813 ± 0.074	22
Right Parotid	0.879 ± 0.085	0.703 ± 0.078	0.684 ± 0.107	0.856 ± 0.050	19

segmentations decreases. However, the sensitivity is lower in the locally most similar case. This is mainly due to the inter-expert segmentation variabilities illustrated in Fig. 2. Nevertheless, these results are very promising and show that the locally most similar image allows to obtain an atlas whose anatomy is close to the patient to delineate and to remove the over-segmentation.

5 Conclusion

We have presented a new method to select, up to an affine transformation, the locally most similar images associated to regions of interest predefined on a precomputed average atlas. This is based on the use of a Log-Euclidean distance between transformations obtained through atlas construction and the transformation to register the patient on the atlas. As the atlas is pre-computed, the selection method is very efficient, requiring only one non linear registration. We have then associated to this selection a novel framework to build from these images a composite patient to be used as a template for the patient segmentation.

This method was validated by comparing it to atlas-based segmentation on a subset of 58 CT images among a database of 105 head and neck patients. The segmentations are not over-segmented anymore using our approach. This is seen both on qualitative and quantitative results (specificity). This method has a great interest and could also be applied to many other regions where large variabilities may be seen in the patients anatomies, such as the abdomen region.

We have seen in our experiments that the sensitivity results are corrupted by a large intra- and inter-expert segmentation variability. It is also partially responsible for the overly large segmentations in the average atlas. In the future, we aim at studying further this segmentation variability by computing locally, in the average atlas reference frame, the changes of each delineation, for example using the STAPLE algorithm [14]. This would be of great interest to reduce the variability influence on the segmentation process.

Finally, we will study in the future other selection criterions, such as intensity based comparisons between the images, and compare their performance on the selection of the locally most similar image. We will also study how to combine these different criterions to obtain a very robust selection criterion.

Acknowledgments. This investigation was supported in part by a research grant from CIMIT and by NIH grants R03 CA126466, R01 RR021885, R01 GM074068 and R01 EB008015. This work was undertaken in the framework of the MAESTRO project (IP CE503564) funded by the European Commission.

References

1. Bondiau, P., Malandain, G., Chanalet, S., Marcy, P., Habrand, J., Fauchon, F., Paquis, P., Courdi, A., Commowick, O., Rutten, I., Ayache, N.: Atlas-based automatic segmentation of MR images: validation study on the brainstem in radiotherapy context. Int. J. Radiat. Oncol. Biol. Phys. 61(1), 289–298 (2005)
2. Poon, I., Fischbein, N., Lee, N., Akazawa, P., Xia, P., Quivey, J., Phillips, T.: A population-based atlas and clinical target volume for the head and neck lymph nodes. Int. J. Radiat. Oncol. Biol. Phys. 59(5), 1301–1311 (2004)
3. Zhang, T., Chi, Y., Meldolesi, E., Yan, D.: Automatic delineation of on-line head and neck computed tomography images: Toward on-line adaptive radiotherapy. Int. J. Radiat. Oncol. Biol. Phys. 68(2), 522–530 (2007)
4. Guimond, A., Meunier, J., Thirion, J.: Average brain models: A convergence study. Computer Vision and Image Understanding 77(2), 192–210 (2000)
5. Joshi, S., Davis, B., Jomier, M., Gerig, G.: Unbiased diffeomorphic atlas construction for computational anatomy. Neuroimage 23(Suppl. 1) (2004)
6. Commowick, O., Grégoire, V., Malandain, G.: Atlas-based delineation of lymph node levels in head and neck computed tomography images. Radiotherapy Oncology 87(2), 281–289 (2008)
7. Grégoire, V., Levendag, P., Ang, K.K., Bernier, J., Braaksma, M., Budach, V., Chao, C., Coche, E., Cooper, J.S., Cosnard, G., Eisbruch, A., El-Sayed, S., Emami, B., Grau, C., Hamoir, M., Lee, N., Maingon, P., Muller, K., Reychler, H.: CT-based delineation of lymph node levels and related CTVs in the node-negative neck: DAHANCA, EORTC, GORTEC, NCIC, RTOG consensus guidelines. Radiotherapy Oncology 69(3), 227–236 (2003)
8. Blezek, D.J., Miller, J.V.: Atlas stratification. MedIA 11(5), 443–457 (2007)
9. Aljabar, P., Heckemann, R.A., Hammers, A., Hajnal, J.V., Rueckert, D.: Classifier selection strategies for label fusion using large atlas databases. In: Ayache, N., Ourselin, S., Maeder, A. (eds.) MICCAI 2007, Part I. LNCS, vol. 4791, pp. 523–531. Springer, Heidelberg (2007)
10. Shelley, M.: Frankenstein. Lackington, Hughes, Harding, Mavor and Jones (1818)
11. Arsigny, V., Commowick, O., Pennec, X., Ayache, N.: A log-euclidean framework for statistics on diffeomorphisms. In: Larsen, R., Nielsen, M., Sporring, J. (eds.) MICCAI 2006. LNCS, vol. 4190, pp. 924–931. Springer, Heidelberg (2006)
12. Pitiot, A., Bardinet, E., Thompson, P.M., Malandain, G.: Piecewise affine registration of biological images for volume reconstruction. MedIA 10(3), 465–483 (2006)
13. Arsigny, V.: Processing Data in Lie Groups: An Algebraic Approach. Application to Non-Linear Registration and Diffusion Tensor MRI. PhD, Polytechnique (2006)
14. Warfield, S.K., Zou, K.H., Wells, W.M.: Simultaneous truth and performance level estimation (STAPLE): an algorithm for the validation of image segmentation. IEEE TMI 23(7), 903–921 (2004)

Atlas-Based Automated Segmentation of Spleen and Liver Using Adaptive Enhancement Estimation

Marius George Linguraru, Jesse K. Sandberg, Zhixi Li, John A. Pura,
and Ronald M. Summers

Imaging Biomarkers and Computer-Aided Diagnosis Laboratory, Radiology and Imaging
Sciences, Clinical Center, National Institutes of Health, Bethesda, MD, USA
lingurarum@mail.nih.gov

Abstract. The paper presents the automated segmentation of spleen and liver from contrast-enhanced CT images of normal and hepato/splenomegaly populations. The method used 4 steps: (i) a mean organ model was registered to the patient CT; (ii) the first estimates of the organs were improved by a geodesic active contour; (iii) the contrast enhancements of liver and spleen were estimated to adjust to patient image characteristics, and an adaptive convolution refined the segmentations; (iv) lastly, a normalized probabilistic atlas corrected for shape and location for the precise computation of each organ's volume and height (mid-hepatic liver height and cephalocaudal spleen height). Results from test data demonstrated the method's ability to accurately segment the spleen (RMS error = 1.09mm; DICE/Tanimoto overlaps = 95.2/91) and liver (RMS error = 2.3mm, and DICE/Tanimoto overlaps = 96.2/92.7). The correlations (R^2) with clinical/manual height measurements were 0.97 and 0.93 for the spleen and liver respectively.

1 Introduction

We are working towards using the fully automated segmentation of the spleen and liver as a volumetric diagnostic tool. It had been noted that the 3D shape and size variability of liver and spleen can be an indication of disorders [3,21]. The implementation of a fully automated segmentation allows the radiologist and other health professionals for an easy and convenient access to organ measurements, while avoiding time-consuming manual measurements or biased diagnosis based on 2D projection images [2]. We propose a method to segment the liver/spleen independent of morphological changes due to disease and/or normal anatomical variability.

In clinical practice, the liver size is estimated by height measurements at the mid-hepatic line; similarly, the spleen height is measured as the cephalocaudal height. Liver height, for instance, does not fully characterize the morphology of the liver, such as accounting for an enlarged left lobe. Spleen measurements suffer from similar shortcomings. Alternatively, studies have relied on the liver/spleen volume computed by multiplying the calculated slice area from manual segmentations by the slice thickness. [8].

A variety of automated and interactive methods to segment the liver have been proposed. A technique based on statistical analysis and dimensionality reduction from sparse information models was presented in [5]. In [4] a shape-guided deformable model was introduced using an evolutionary algorithm, but unacceptable segmentations were omitted in the analysis. Most recently, active contours using gradient vector flow were used to address both liver and hepatic tumor segmentation [12], while a hierarchical statistical atlas was employed in [13]. These methods suffer from either heavy manual initialization or present significant segmentation errors.

In 2007, a liver segmentation competition from computed tomography (CT) data was held [6]. Amongst the automated techniques, most notably a combination of shape-constrained statistical deformable models based on a heuristic intensity model had the best performance amongst automated methods [10] with slight under-segmentation of the liver. Region growing was used in [16] with good results, but the technique was sensitive to liver abnormalities. A semantic formulation of knowledge and context was presented in [17], but the segmentation overlap was only 84%.

Despite the abundance of research on liver segmentation, there are few studies focusing on the spleen. However, the segmentation of abdominal multi-organs, including the liver and spleen, has been addressed, but with limited accuracy. In [19,22] a priori probabilistic data were used in combination with measures of relationship and hierarchy between organs and manual landmarks. On a different note, multi-dimensional data from contrast-enhanced CT were employed in [9,11,18], applying variational Bayesian mixture and tissue homogeneity constraints.

We propose a method that involves a combination of appearance, enhancement, and shape and location statistics to segment both the spleen and liver. For the coarse estimation of organs, mean models from an atlas of both liver and spleen are aligned to the patient contrast-enhanced CT image. The estimation is improved by a geodesic active contour. Subsequently, the patient specific contrast-enhancement characteristics are estimated and passed to an adaptive convolution. Only homogenous tissue areas that satisfy the enhancement constraints are labeled as liver/spleen. Lastly, shape and location information from the normalized probabilistic atlas are utilized to provide an accurate representation of each organ's morphology.

2 Methods and Materials

2.1 Data and Statistical Information

192 abdominal CT scans of patients from a mixed population were used; 52 normal livers, 43 normal spleens, 94 splenomegaly (enlarged spleen) and 40 hepatomegaly (enlarged liver) cases. Patients were injected with 130ml of Isovue-300 and images acquired at portal venous phase using fixed delays or bolus-tracking [7]. Data were collected on LightSpeed Ultra and QX/I (GE Healthcare), and Brilliance64 (Philips Healthcare) scanners. Image resolution ranged from 0.62 to 0.82 mm in the axial view with a slice thickness from 1 to 5 mm. The livers and spleens were manually segmented in 14 training and 20 testing CT scans, while their heights (mid-hepatic liver height and cephalocaudal spleen height) were manually measured in all data.

For additional tests, we used 20 more contrast-enhanced CT scans with manual segmentations of the liver downloadable from www.sliver07.isi.uu.nl, addressed as MICCAI data in the paper. These CT data were used for the MICCAI 2007 liver segmentation competition and were acquired in transversal plane with pixel spacing between 0.55 and 0.80 mm and inter-slice distance between 1 and 5 mm. Contrast-enhanced images corresponded to mainly pathological cases and were acquired on a variety of scanners from different manufacturers.

A probabilistic atlas A was constructed from 10 random CT sets (not included in the training or testing data) after manually segmenting the liver and spleen in each image. Organ locations were normalized to an anatomical landmark (xiphoid). A random image from the set was used as reference R and all other images registered to it. We conserved morphological variability by using a size-preserving affine registration. Restricting the degrees of freedom in the transformation (no shear), the organ shape bias from the reference data is minimized. Preserving the size of organs and normalizing their position to that of the xiphoid, we obtain abdominal location normalization with no bias toward the reference size and location. Finally, organs were translated in the atlas to the location of the average normalized centroid.

2.2 Registration and Segmentation

From the construction of A, a mean model $\overline{A}$ was extracted for each organ. Then the patient CT (I) was smoothed with anisotropic diffusion [14] and the result is I_s. First, an affine registration between R and I was performed. The resulting spatial normalization was then applied to both A and $\overline{A}$, which became A_a and $\overline{A}_a$. The affine registration was based on normalized mutual information M [20], where $p(I, \overline{A}_a)$ is the joint probability distribution of images I and $\overline{A}_a$, and $p(I)$ and $p(\overline{A}_a)$ their marginal distributions.

$$M(I_s \mid \overline{A}_a) = \frac{p(I_s) + p(\overline{A}_a)}{p(I_s, \overline{A}_a)}. \tag{1}$$

Next, a more flexible registration of $\overline{A}_a$ was required to compensate for the residual deformation, resulting in $\overline{A}_r$. We employed the non-linear registration algorithm based on B-splines [15]. B-splines allow to locally control the deformation T and a compromise between the similarity provided by M and smoothing S was searched.

$$\arg\min[M(I_s \mid T(I_s)) - S(T)];$$
$$S(T) = \int_{x,y,z} (\partial^2 T)_{x,y,z} dxdydz. \tag{2}$$

To account for possibly missing parts of spleen and liver, a geodesic active contour (GAC) [1] was implemented to correct the organ boundaries based on contrast-enhanced image intensities. To initialize the model, $\overline{A}_r$ was input as zero-level into a GAC I_g. The edge features I_e were computed from the sigmoid of the gradient of I_s. The weights w_1, w_2 and w_3 control respectively the speed c, curvature k and attraction to edges. In our experimental setup, w_1, w_2 and w_3 were set to 1, 0.2 and 1 respectively. Parameters α and β of the image sigmoid were 10 and 8 respectively.

$$I_e = 1 - 1 \bigg/ \left(1 + \exp\left[-\frac{\nabla I_s - (\alpha + \beta)}{3(\alpha - \beta)}\right]\right); \qquad I_{g,t=0} = \overline{A_r};$$

$$\frac{dI_g}{dt} = I_e(w_1 c + w_2 k)|\nabla I_g| + w_3 \nabla I_e \nabla I_g \qquad (3)$$

2.3 Estimation of Enhancement and Shape Correction

A common difficulty in processing contrast-enhanced CT data is the estimation of the optimal time for image acquisition. In practice, fixed delays or bolus-tracking techniques [7] are used to approximate the portal venous phase and can yield a different enhancement and appearance of organs. Hence, variations in an organ's enhancement are common and vary between late-arterial and late-portal venous phases. As both the liver and spleen enhance homogeneously at portal venous phase, we estimated the level of enhancement of these organs to reject volumes that were erroneously captured by the GAC. First, the masks of liver and spleen provided by the GAC segmentation are used to computed the mean (μ_j) and standard deviation (σ_j) of the organs (j=1,2 for liver and spleen). Then outliers are rejected to compute $I_{max}^j = \mu_j + 2\sigma_j$, and $I_{min}^j = \mu_j - 2\sigma_j$ to account for each organ enhancement.

I_{max}^j and I_{min}^j are input to an adaptive erosion filter that is applied to I_g. Thus only regions for which all their voxels in the erosion element E satisfy the intensity criteria are labeled as organs of interest. L represents the labeled image and l_j the labels. L is then dilated to account for the convolution with E. Finally, the normalized A_a (see Section 2.2) is used to correct the shape of the liver/spleen in L. A_a resulted from applying an affine transformation (no shear) to the probabilistic atlas constructed with restricted degrees of freedom (preserving the shape). S is the image of the segmented liver and spleen.

$$L(x,y,z) = \begin{cases} l_j, \text{if} \left(I_{min}^j \leq I_g \circ E \leq I_{max}^j\right); \\ 0, otherwise \end{cases} \qquad S = L \cdot A_a. \qquad (4)$$

The volume overlap (VO) of the automatically segmented livers and spleens with the manual segmentations, and Dice coefficient (DC) were calculated.

$$VO = \frac{V_{manual} \cap V_{CAD}}{V_{manual} + V_{CAD} - (V_{manual} \cap V_{CAD})};$$

$$DC = \frac{2(V_{manual} \cap V_{CAD})}{V_{manual} + V_{CAD}}. \qquad (5)$$

To correlate with clinical evaluations of liver performed by linear measurements of organ height, the mid-hepatic line (MHL) was approximated at the half-distance between the mid-point of the spine and the outer surface of the liver. Then the maximum liver height along the sagittal plane at the location of MHL was computed. The spleen cephalocaudal height was calculated as the Euclidean distance between the top and bottom sagittal slices containing the spleen.

3 Results

Quantitative results from applying our method to the segmentation of liver and spleen are presented in Table 1. We present DC and VO overlaps next to volume estimation error (VER), height estimation error (HER), root mean square error (RMSE) and average surface distance (ASD). Training cases were of low resolution, while test cases of higher resolution: 5mm and 1mm slice thickness respectively. We compared results on training data at incremental steps of the algorithm. Results on testing the algorithm on the MICCAI liver data are also provided in Table 1. The segmentation score was 69, comparable to that of 68 of the competition winner, after using the evaluation tools provided by the competition organizers [6]. Note that our score was obtained on different cases provided by the organizers for training, as we did not have access to the test data used in [6]. Table 1 further presents inter-observer variability for the segmentation of liver and spleen.

Table 1. Statistics for the liver and spleen segmentation results from training and test data. Results at incremental steps of the algorithm are presented for training data: "Atlas"- after non-rigid registration with the probabilistic atlas; 'EE' after enhancement estimation correction; 'Shape' after employing the shape and location correction. Columns present the Dice coefficient (DC), volume overlap (VO), volume estimation error (VER), height estimation error (HER), root mean square error (RMSE) and average surface distance (ASD).

	DC (%)	VO (%)	VER (%)	HER (%)	RMSE (mm)	ASD (mm)
Training Liver 'Atlas'	90.9±3.7	83.6 ± 6	14.9±9.6	12.2±13.2	4.4±2.1	2.6±1.2
Training Liver 'EE"	94.3±1.5	89.3±2.6	3.3±3.7	3.7±3.7	3.8±1.8	1.7±0.8
Training Liver 'Shape'	94.5±0.8	90 ± 1	2 ± 2.1	3.4±3.1	2.9±0.5	1.5±0.3
Test Liver	96.2±0.6	92.7±1.1	2.2±2.1	4.5±6.6	2.3±0.5	1.2±0.2
MICCAI Liver	95.9±0.9	92±1.8	2.9±2.3	4.3±4.6	2.9±1	1.4±0.5
Training Spleen 'Atlas'	87.5±4.8	78±7.5	13.6±10	9.7±9.2	2.9±1.2	1.6±0.7
Training Spleen 'EE"	91±2	83.5±3.3	6.6±5.3	3.5±3.4	2.1±0.5	1±0.2
Training Spleen 'Shape'	90.6±2.1	83±3.5	5.5±4.9	3.5±5.1	2.1±0.6	1.3±0.8
Test Spleen	95.2±1.4	91±2.6	3.3±2.7	1.7±0.7	1.1±0.3	0.7±0.1
Inter-observer Liver	96.4	92.3	1.25	3.9	1.7	0.7
Inter-observer Spleen	96	92.4	2.26	1.67	0.9	0.38

Figure 1 shows a typical example of liver and spleen segmentation from a test case on 2D axial slices of the 3D CT data. Figure 2 illustrates another example of segmentation in 3D along with the segmentation errors between manual and automated segmentation. Finally, automated volumetric and linear 3D measurements were obtained for an additional 168 clinical cases: 19 had normal spleens, 29 had normal livers, while 94 had splenomegaly and 40 cases had hepatomegaly. The height correlations (R^2) between the automatically segmented spleens and livers and the manual linear measurements obtained in clinical practice were 0.97 and 0.93 for spleen and liver respectively, as shown in Figure 3.

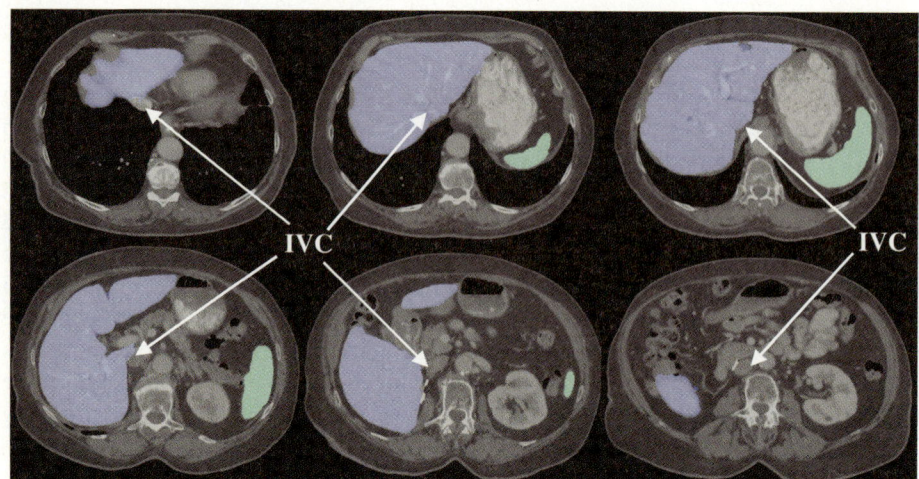

Fig. 1. A typical example of liver (blue) and spleen (green) automatically segmented from a test case on 2D axial views of the 3D CT data. Note the good separation from the heart; parts of the inferior vena cava (IVC) are incorporated in the liver when contrast enhancement is low.

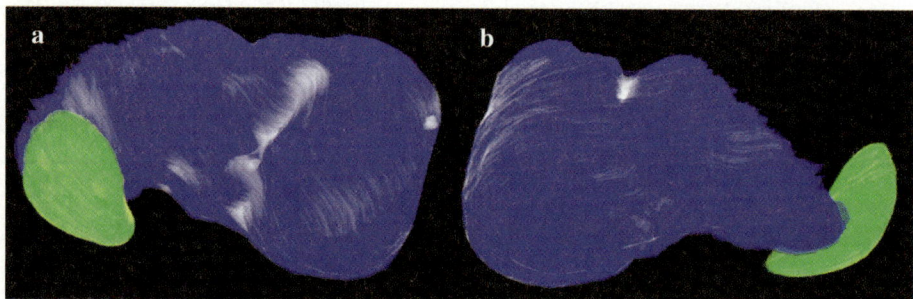

Fig. 2. 3D volume renderings of the segmented liver and spleen; (a) is a posterior view and (b) an anterior view. The liver ground truth is shown in blue with automated segmentation errors overlaid in white; likewise, the spleen ground truth is green and errors are in yellow.

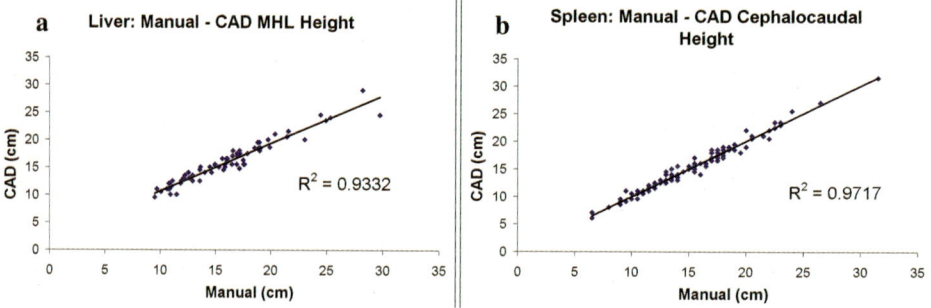

Fig. 3. The correlations (R^2) between automatically generated (CAD) organ height and the manual measurements obtained in clinical practice; (a) shows correlated liver heights at the mid-hepatic line (MHL) from mixed normal and hepatomegaly cases; (b) presents correlated spleen cephalocaudal heights from mixed normal and splenomegaly cases.

4 Discussion

The proposed method involves a combination of appearance, shape and location statistics to automatically segment livers and spleens from clinical contrast-enhanced CT data of mixed populations with normal and abnormal organs. Data from various institutions and scanners were employed. The patient specific contrast-enhancement characteristics were estimated and input into an adaptive convolution that labeled only homogenous tissue areas that satisfy the enhancement constraints of the liver/spleen. Additionally, shape and location information from the normalized probabilistic atlas were utilized to improve the accuracy of the segmentation. Results demonstrated the ability of the technique to segment normal and abnormal spleens with a precision close to the inter-observer variability and errors close to the voxel size.

The method avoided the inclusion of heart volumes in the segmentation of the liver. Although the inferior vena cava was not incorporated in the liver in the majority of cases, parts of the vein may be erroneously segmented in the mid-cephalocaudal liver region, especially when contrast enhancement was low. Also note that the MICCAI data included pathological cases, which made the segmentation of the liver (including the pathologies) more difficult. As expected, segmentation results were more accurate on data with high spatial resolution.

We found that using shape information from a normalized probabilistic atlas changed/improved significantly ($p<0.05$) only the liver volume estimations (see Table 1). This may be explained partly by the small sample of cases used to construct the atlas. But the improvement brought by the adaptive convolution using enhancement estimation and adjusting the parameters to patient specific information was significant for all metrics used in Table 1 ($p<0.04$) in comparison to atlas-based segmentation.

Future work will investigate the use of volumetric measurements to establish more robust diagnosis criteria for the detection of hepato/splenomegaly, and will address additional challenges from a variety of abdominal pathologies. We anticipate to have our method used in routine clinical investigations in the near future.

Acknowledgment. This work was supported by the Intramural Research Program of the National Institutes of Health, Clinical Center.

References

1. Caselles, V., Kimmel, R., Sapiro, G.: Geodesic active contours. International Journal on Computer Vision 22(1), 61–97 (1997)
2. Cools, L., Osteaux, M., Divano, J.L.: Prediction of Splenic volume by a Simple CT Measurement: A Statistical Study. J. Comput. Assist. Tomogr. 7(3), 426–430 (1983)
3. Ellert, J., Kreel, L.: The role of computed tomography in the initial staging and subsequent management of the lymphomas. J. Comput. Assist. Tomogr. 4, 358 (1980)
4. Farraher, S.W., Jara, H., Chang, K.J., Hou, A., Soto, J.A.: Liver and Spleen Volumetry with Quantitative MT Imaging and Dual-Space Clustering Segmentation. Radiology 237(1), 322–328 (2005)
5. Florin, C., Paragios, N., Funka-Lea, G., Williams, J.: Liver segmentation using sparse 3D prior models with optimal data support. Information Processing in Medical Imaging 20, 38–49 (2007)

6. van Ginneken, B., Heimann, T., Styner, M.: 3D Segmentation in the Clinic: A Grand Challenge. In: van Ginneken, B., Heimann, T., Styner, M. (eds.) 3D Segmentation in the Clinic: A Grand Challenge, pp. 7–15 (2007)
7. Goshima, S., Kanematsu, M., Nishibori, H., Kondo, H., Tsuge, Y., Yokoyama, R., Miyoshi, T., Onozuka, M., Shiratori, Y., Moriyama, N., Bae, K.T.: Multi-detector row CT of the kidney: optimizing scan delays for bolus tracking techniques of arterial, corticomedullary, and nephrographic phases. European Journal of Radiology 63(3), 420–426 (2007)
8. Heymsfield, S.B., Fulenwider, T., Nordlinger, B., Barlow, R., Sones, P., Kutner, M.: Accurate measurement of liver, kidney, and spleen volume and mass by computerized axial tomography. Ann. Intern. Med. 90, 185–187 (1979)
9. Hu, X., Shimizu, A., Kobatake, H., Nawano, S.: Independent component analysis of four-phase abdominal CT images. In: Barillot, C., Haynor, D.R., Hellier, P. (eds.) MICCAI 2004. LNCS, vol. 3217, pp. 916–924. Springer, Heidelberg (2004)
10. Kainmueller, D., Lange, T., Lamecker, H.: Shape Constrained Automatic Segmentation of the Liver based on a Heuristic Intensity Model. In: van Ginneken, B., Heimann, T., Styner, M. (eds.) 3D Segmentation in the Clinic: A Grand Challenge, pp. 109–116 (2007)
11. Linguraru, M.G., Summers, R.M.: Multi-Organ Segmentation in 4D Contrast-Enhanced Abdominal CT. In: IEEE Symposium on Biomedical Imaging 2008 (ISBI), pp. 45–48 (2008)
12. Massoptier, L., Casciaro, S.: A New Fully Automatic and Robust Algorithm for Fast Segmentation of Liver Tissue and Tumors from CT Scans. European Radiology 18, 1658–1665 (2008)
13. Okada, T., Shimada, R., Hori, M., Nakamoto, M., Chen, Y.W., Nakamura, H., Sato, Y.: Automated Segmentation of the Liver from 3D CT Images Using Probabilistic Atlas and Multilevel Statistical Shape Model. Academic Radiology 15, 1390–1403 (2008)
14. Perona, P., Malik, J.: Scale-space and Edge Detection using Anisotropic Diffusion. IEEE Trans. on Pattern Analysis and Machine Intelligence (12), 629–639 (1990)
15. Rueckert, D., et al.: Non-rigid registration using free-form deformations: Application to breast MR images. IEEE Transactions on Medical Imaging 18(8), 712–721 (1999)
16. Rusko, L., Bekes, G., Nemeth, G., Fidrich, M.: Fully automatic liver segmentation for contrast-enhanced CT images. In: van Ginneken, B., Heimann, T., Styner, M. (eds.) 3D Segmentation in the Clinic: A Grand Challenge, pp. 143–150 (2007)
17. Schmidt, G., Athelogou, M., Schoenmeyer, R., Korn, R., Binnig, G.: Cognition Network Technology for a Fully Automated 3D Segmentation of Liver. In: van Ginneken, et al. (eds.) 3D Segmentation in the Clinic: A Grand Challenge, pp. 125–133 (2007)
18. Sakashita, M., Kitasaka, T., Mori, K., Suenaga, Y., Nawano, S.: A Method for Extracting Multi-organ from Four-phase Contrasted CT Images based on CT Value Distribution Estimation using EM-algorithm. In: Proceedings of SPIE, vol. 6509, 1C-1-12 (2007)
19. Shimizu, A., Ohno, T., Ikegami, R., Kobatake, H.: Multi-organ Segmentation in Three-dimensional Abdominal CT Images. Int. J. CARS 1, 76–78 (2006)
20. Studholme, C., Hill, D.L.G., Hawkes, D.J.: An overlap invariant entropy measure of 3D medical image alignment. Pattern Recognition 32(1), 71–86 (1999)
21. Tsushima, Y., Endo, K.: Spleen Enlargement in Patients with Nonalcoholic Fatty Liver – Correlation between Degree of Fatty Infiltration in Liver and Size of Spleen. Digestive Diseases and Sciences 45(1), 196–200 (2000)
22. Yao, C., Wada, T., Shimizu, A., Kobatake, H., Nawano, S.: Simultaneous Location Detection of Multi-organ by Atlas-guided Eigen-organ Method in Volumetric Medical Images. Int. J. CARS 1, 42–45 (2006)

A Two-Level Approach Towards Semantic Colon Segmentation: Removing Extra-Colonic Findings

Le Lu[1], Matthias Wolf[1], Jianming Liang[1,2], Murat Dundar[1,3], Jinbo Bi[1], and Marcos Salganicoff[1]

[1] CAD & Knowledge Solutions, Siemens Healthcare, Malvern, PA 19355, USA
[2] Biomedical Informatics Dept., Arizona State University, AZ 85004, USA
[3] Computer Information Science Dept., IUPUI, IN 46202, USA

Abstract. Computer aided detection (CAD) of colonic polyps in computed tomographic colonography has tremendously impacted colorectal cancer diagnosis using 3D medical imaging. It is a prerequisite for all CAD systems to extract the air-distended colon segments from 3D abdomen computed tomography scans. In this paper, we present a two-level statistical approach of first separating colon segments from small intestine, stomach and other extra-colonic parts by classification on a new geometric feature set; then evaluating the overall performance confidence using distance and geometry statistics over patients. The proposed method is fully automatic and validated using both the classification results in the first level and its numerical impacts on false positive reduction of extra-colonic findings in a CAD system. It shows superior performance than the state-of-art knowledge or anatomy based colon segmentation algorithms [1,2,3].

1 Introduction

Colon cancer is the second leading deadly cancer for western population. Early detection and removal of colonic polyps is the critical step which helps to decrease the risk of colon cancer and improve survival. Computed tomographic colonography (CTC) or virtual colonoscopy has been widely used for detecting colorectal neoplasms via 3D computed tomography (CT) abdomen scans of the cleansed and air-distended colon. In the last decade, many computer aided detection and diagnosis systems [4,5,6,7] have been proposed and actively studied to improve the performance and reliability of human radiologists as second readers.

For any CAD system, the first processing is to identify all cleansed and air-distended colon segments, for detecting colonic polyps as next step, in 3D abdomen CT scans. Knowledge or anatomy based colon segmentation algorithms are described in past literature [1,2,3]. A two-step method is proposed, including "anatomy-based extraction" to find and remove non-digestive components, such as outer-air, bones and lung; and "colon-based analysis" to segment out extra-colonic parts (e.g., small bowel and stomach) by region growing from a seed in colon rectum. Removing extra-colonic lumen fragments is our main focus since non-digestive components are more isolated and can often be reliably excluded.

By considering the potential presence of partially or completely collapsed colon regions, multiple colon seeds [1,2] are needed to cover the decent portion of true colon volume. Numerous heuristic rules and thresholding parameters, e.g., when to stop region growing, how many seed points needed and how many slices apart to look for the next seed, are necessary to generate the final results. In [3], a centerline chaining based colon segmentation method is described. However the essential drawbacks of rule-based methods (as above) remains and the colon linking scheme [3] is only valid for well-distended or slightly collapsed colon cases.

In this paper, we present a two-level approach for colon segmentation. First all air segments (after pre-segmentation) are classified as either colon components or extra-colonic parts (small intestine, stomach and others) by statistical modeling on novel geometry feature sets per segment. Then we evaluate the overall segmentation quality using a new colon "daisy-chaining" tracking algorithm integrated with distance and geometry statistics over patients, which handles moderately or poorly distended colon significantly better than previous methods. The proposed method is validated using both the classification results in the first level and its numerical impact on false positive reduction of extra-colonic findings in a CAD system. It shows the superior performance than previous heuristic knowledge or anatomy based colon segmentation algorithms [1,2,3], on a 166 volume dataset. The remainder of this paper is organized as follows. Section 2 gives the details of the materials used and our taken approach. Experimental results and analysis are reported in section 3. Lastly, section 4 concludes the paper and directs future work.

2 Materials and Methods

An accurate segmentation of a specific organ (e.g., colon) is a very crucial part of a CAD system. Only if the organ can be accurately segmented it is possible to perform a reliable and thorough examination of that organ. A case of under-segmentation can lose important parts of an organ which may lead to miss potential lesions whereas an over-segmentation may generate avoidable false positives in areas outside of the organ. Our colon segmentation approach is composed of three steps: intensity-appearance based initial segmentation, independent colon component classification (level 1) and anatomical colon tracking (level 2).

Colon Pre-segmentation: Datasets of 166 prone and supine CT volumes from 92 patients, obtained from four hospitals and scanned using both Siemens and GE machines under different imaging protocols, are used to conduct our study. For pre-segmentation stage, a pixelwise thresholding is first performed on the entire volume based on a predefined air Hounsfield (HU) value (e.g., -800 HU). Pixels are then labeled as foreground (air) and background (non-air). Afterwards, adjacent foreground pixels are merged as fragments or components by running a standard connected component scheme. This step identifies all air-filled regions within the body and can often contain parts other than the colon, such as stomach, lung, small intestine and other random noises. Colon pre-segmentation is a general purpose process and handled similarly by other systems, thought more complicated thresholding and merging rules can be adopted in [1,5].

2.1 Colon Fragment Classification

Annotation & Data: We design and implement a user interface for marking each individual fragment after initial segmentation of potential colon areas. Each segmented component is labeled as one of the five anatomical categories: colon, small intestine, mixed (of colon and small intestine through opened ileo-cecal valve which happens in low frequency), stomach or lung, and noise. Since mixed class contains partial colon volume, both colon and mixed categories are treated as positive class. The rest of the categories are considered negative. It results 165 positive samples and 1665 negative samples in the training dataset of 110 volumes. There are 89 positives and 836 negatives based on a unseen testing dataset with 56 CT scans. Around 40% volumes have collapsed colon segments.

Feature Extraction: The success of colon and non-colon classification relies on discriminative features. In this paper, we explore a set of geometric (+ spatial) features, including volume, length, area, volume-length ratio and area-length ratio. For each potential colon component from pre-segmentation, the volume refers its total volume; the length is an estimation of the length computed by the *shortest-path* algorithm [8]; and the area means its surface area. The volume-length ratio and area-length ratio are the ratios of volume to length and area to length. We denote this as four feature set $\mathcal{F}_4$. Additionally, the normalized centroid position in 3D volume coordinates of each fragment can also be integrated as $\mathcal{F}_7$ where positions are normalized in the range of $[0, 1]$ (i.e., bounded by the extreme positions of initial segmented components).

Classification: Support vector machine (SVM) has been proven as an effective approach for classification. In particular, 1-norm SVM [9] can be used to construct classifiers and select important features simultaneously. The 1-norm SVM determines classifiers by minimizing a regularized training error $\lambda P(\cdot) + \sum_i \xi_i$ where ξ is a hinge loss occurred on the i-th training example and the regularization term $P(\cdot)$ is a 1-norm penalty on the weight vector of the linear classifier. The 1-norm SVM can be formulated as a linear program (LP) which, in general, can be solved efficiently by existing optimization tools. The classification accuracy is cost sensitive to the size or volume measurements of the segmented regions, in the context of colon segmentation task. It is treated as a more severe error if a large segmented volume (i.e., retaining more potential polyp candidates) is misclassified than a small region is missed. Hence we revise 1-norm SVM to associate the hinge loss occurred on each classification instance with a weight, ie. the volume size of the example. At last, we optimize the following problem to construct the classifier $\{w, b\}$

$$\min_{w,b} \lambda ||w||_1 + \sum_i \nu_i \xi_i \\ \text{s.t.} \, y_i(w^T x + b) \geq \xi_i, \quad \xi_i \geq 0. \tag{1}$$

where $x \in \mathcal{F}_4$ or $\mathcal{F}_7$. Given the trained linear classifier, receiver operating characteristic (ROC) curves can be drawn by thresholding the classifier output $(w^T x + b) \geq \tau$ at different operating points τ. The volume fragments classified as positive colon class by setting high detection rate $>= 99\%$ will be used for the next level processing.

2.2 Colon Fragment Tracing

Given the fragments as classified as colon by the previous step, we attempt to provide a global interpretation by incorporating anatomic colon structure and performing a "Daisy-chaining" colon fragments tracing. Algorithm 1 describes the processing details, and Figure 1 shows an illustrative example where a complete colon is composed of five collapsed segments.

```
foreach Colon CT Volume i do
    Identify the rectum R_i and the corresponding component S(R_i);
    Identify the cecum C_i and the corresponding component S(C_i);
    if R_i == true and C_i == true then
        if S(R_i) == S(C_i) then
        |   return component S(R_i) or S(C_i), exit;
        end
        while True do
            Mark the rectum component S(R_i) the first colon fragment;
            Search the component S_j from unidentified colon segments that is
            "closest" (with distance D) to the lastly merged colon fragment;
            if D <= T then
                merge S_j with the already known colon fragments;
                if S_j == S(C_i) then
                |   return all current colon segments, exit;
                end
            end
            if D > T or S_j == false then
            |   return all current colon segments, exit;
            end
        end
    end
end
```

Algorithm 1. Colon "Daisy-chaining" Tracking Algorithm

Rectum and cecum are important landmarks as they describe the course of the entire colon, and they can be reliably located (100% for rectum; $\geq 85\%$ for cecum) via fusing the direct detection of themselves and other more extinctive landmarks on vertebrae and hip bones. In Algorithm 1, if there is no detection of cecum, all cecum relevant checking will be omitted. After colon tracking, a geodesic distance checking between rectum and cecum is used to reject cecum mislocation. The distance threshold T is calibrated using the distance statistics obtained from all valid collapsed colon connections of 110 training volumes. The mean distance is $29.78mm$ with standard deviation as $15.06mm$ and we set $T = 60mm$ for all following evaluations. Other richer descriptive geometry features (e.g., gradient orientations and curvatures on tubular shortest-paths) can be employed and are under study. Overall, $> 92\%$ volumes complete "Daisy-chaining" colon tracking and further remove more false positives. A probabilistic fusing formulation of fragment connectness modeling and verification, other than simple thresholding, can also be investigated in future work.

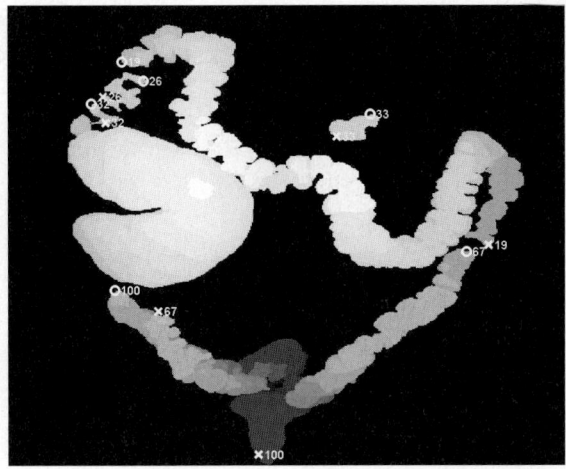

Fig. 1. This shows a colon (as maximum intensity projection image) that is broken into several pieces. The symbols "X" and "O" denote the start and end point of a component. The numbers indicate points belonging to the same component. In this example, the rectum component is #100 and the detected rectum landmark is close to "X100". The cecum component is #32. The complete colon consists of #100, #67, #19, #26, and #32 by our tracking scheme. Component #33 does not belong to the colon.

3 Experimental Results

In this section, we describe both the evaluation of colon segmentation using 1-norm SVM [9] as a single classification issue, and its integration and effectiveness on removing extra-colonic findings (ECR) in a CAD system.

Colon Segmentation Evaluation: We first analyze the performance characteristics of our classification based colon segmentation module. We demonstrate two types of ROC curves using per count or volume (mm^3) as measurement metrics, i.e., how many fragments (or how much volume) are correctly or incorrectly classified, which are plotted in Fig. 3. Our ECR module enables to remove > 90% or higher extra-colonic volumes (mm^3), at the detection rate of 99.5%, for training or testing dataset respectively. In [2], 83.2% ~ 92.8% colon volumes can be semi-automatically segmented or partially segmented. Manual seed placement is required in 16.8% CT scans. [1] detects 98% of the visible colonic walls, and approximately 50% of the extra-colonic components are removed, using 88 volumes. [3] reports sensitivity of 96% for colon volume and it is unclear, to what degree collapsed colons can be handled, in a smaller dataset of total 38 scans. An illustrative example of the MIP (Maximum Intensity Projection) image of a 3D colon volume, before and after ECR colon segmentation, is also shown in Fig. 2.

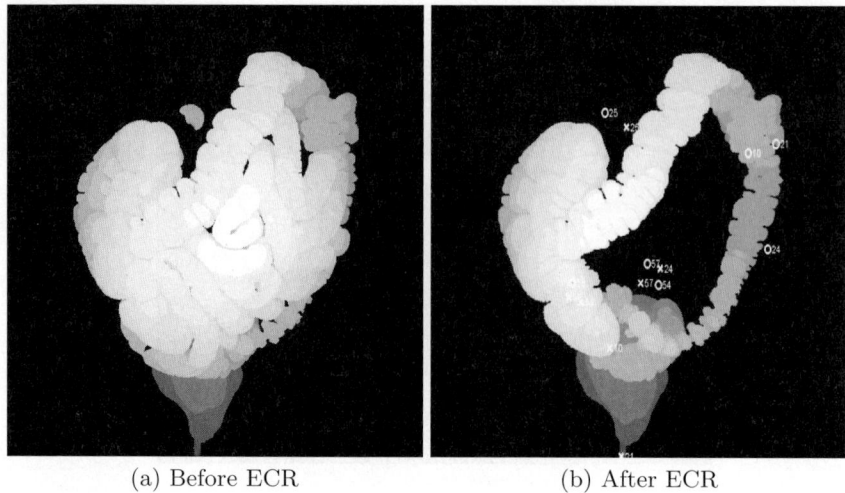

(a) Before ECR (b) After ECR

Fig. 2. An illustrative example of showing the MIP (Maximum Intensity Projection) image of a 3D colon volume before and after ECR colon segmentation

ECR Impacts on CAD False Positive Reduction: We assign each true and false polyp candidate with the classification score $(w^T x + b)$, obtained by the colon fragment which contains itself. The empirical probability density functions (PDF) of positive (true) and negative (false) polyp candidates are plotted for both training and testing CT datasets in Fig. 4. It is clear that the blue peaks around $[0, -5]$ of FP distribution can be removed without significantly affecting the detection rate of true positives in red[1].

In another validation setting, we analyze and manually label 236 total false positive (FP) candidates, as the final outputs of our CAD system, after polyp classification but without applying ECR. 89 of them are verified as extra-colonic FPs and the rest are colonic. Our ECR colon segmentation (as a post-filter module) further removes 80 FP candidates where only 3 of them are actually colonic and 77 are true extra-colonic findings. It results in sensitivity of $77/89 = 86.5\%$ and specificity as $(147-3)/147 = 98\%$, which conforms the high detection rate setting in section 2. For true positive analysis, there is a very minimal but non-zero risk of losing polyps because of ECR colon removing, but we have not seen such cases in our extensive CAD pipeline study (out of 166 volumes used to build ECR). Finally, though our whole colon segmentation subsystem is trained using 110 tagged colon CT scans processed after electronic cleansing, it generalizes well and achieves similar performance on the clean-prep colon cases based on our further study.

---

[1] The kernel density estimation based PDF fitting smooths and slightly skews both distribution curves in Fig. 4. The minimum ECR score for positive polyp candidates is -2.1652. When ECR is used as pre-filtering for our colon CAD system, the total candidate number per volume drops from > 200 to 142, without missing any true polyp candidate.

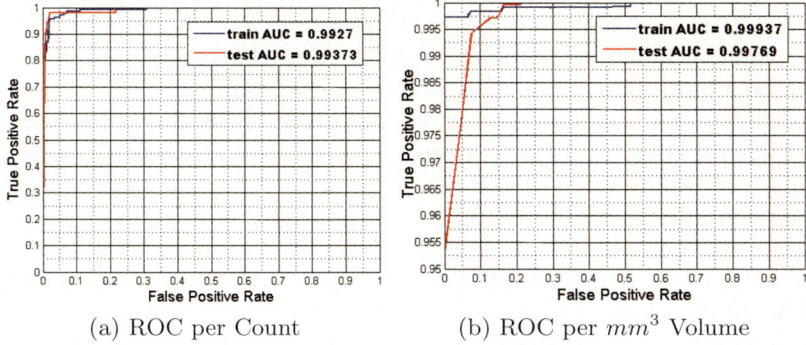

(a) ROC per Count   (b) ROC per mm^3 Volume

Fig. 3. ROC curves for colon fragment (air-filled connected component) classification using norm-1 SVM. (a) is measured as per fragment count, (b) is measured using absolute mm^3 volume. Red curves are for training and blue for testing.

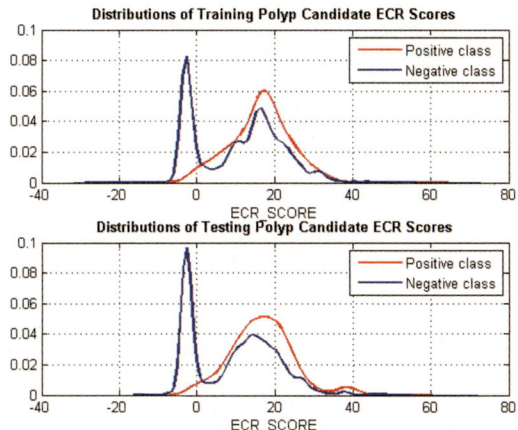

Fig. 4. The plot of ECR scores of positive/negative polyp candidates for both training (Top) and testing (Bottom) CT datasets, as outputs of the linear 1-norm SVM classifier on $\mathcal{F}_4$

4 Discussion

In this paper, we present a fully automatic, statistical based colon segmentation approach. After a generic pre-segmentation, it first classifies all air-filled fragments as binary colon or non-colon classes using continuous 1-norm SVM classifier on newly explored geometric features. Then a colon fragment tracking algorithm is employed to measure the overall colon segmentation confidence using anatomic information. The proposed method is validated using both the classification results on colon segmentation and its numerical impact on false positive reduction of extra-colonic findings in a CAD system. It shows superior performance than previous knowledge or anatomy based colon segmentation work [1,2,3], using different but larger datasets.

The colon segmentation problem benefits from the general statistical models learned from a population, but it can also be considered as a binary testing/decision task of colon or non-colon components per volume case. In future work, the ideal colon classification process should be performed by considering all component information in one volume as a set, to make an optimal binary cut. Pairwise affinity based graph partitioning algorithm [10] can be employed as an alternative solution. Besides exploring more descriptive features for colon structure topology model (as in section 2.2), We also intend to address the model adaptation issue for groupwise or personalized colon segmentation using self-normalized tests [11], which can be capable of applying and adapting the trained model to datasets from different races (e.g., from Caucasian to Asian).

References

1. Näppi, J., MacEneaney, P., Dachman, A., Yoshida, H.: Knowledgeguided automated segmentation of colon for computer-aided detection of polyps in ct colonography. J. Comput. Assist. Tomogr. (2002)
2. Iordanescu, G., Pickhardt, P., Choi, J., Summers, R.: Automated seed placement for colon segmentation in computed tomography colonography. Academic Radiologyg 12, 182–190 (2005)
3. Frimmela, H., Näppi, J., Yoshida, H.: Centerline-based colon segmentation for ct colonographyy. Med. Phys., 2665–2672 (2005)
4. Baker, M., Bogoni, L., et al.: Computer-aided detection of colorectal polyps: Can it improve sensitivity of less-experienced readers? preliminary findings. Radiology 245, 140–149 (2007)
5. Yoshida, H., Näppi, J.: Three-dimensional computer-aided diagnosis scheme for detection of colonic polyps. IEEE Trans. Medical Imaging 20, 1261–1274 (2001)
6. Summers, R., Jerebko, A., et al.: Colonic polyps: Complementary role of computer-aided detection in ct colonography. Radiology 225, 391–399 (2002)
7. Chowdhury, T., Whelan, P., Ghita, O.: A fully automatic cad-ctc system based on curvature analysis for standard and low dose ct data. IEEE Trans. Biomedical Engineering 55, 888–901 (2008)
8. Dijkstra, E.W.: A note on two problems in connections with graphs. Numerische Mathematic 1, 269–271 (1959)
9. Zhu, J., Rosset, S., Hastie, T., Tibshirani, R.: 1-norm support vector machines. In: Neural Information Processing System (2004)
10. Weiss, Y.: Segmentation using eigenvectors: A unifying view. In: Proc. of ICCV, pp. 975–982 (1999)
11. Gangaputra, S., Geman, D.: Self-normalized linear tests. In: Proc. of CVPR, pp. 616–622 (2004)

Segmentation of Lumbar Vertebrae Using Part-Based Graphs and Active Appearance Models*

Martin G. Roberts[1], Tim F. Cootes[1], Elisa Pacheco[1], Teik Oh[1], and Judith E. Adams[1]

School of Imaging Science, University of Manchester, U.K.
martin.roberts@manchester.ac.uk

Abstract. The aim of the work is to provide a fully automatic method of segmenting vertebrae in spinal radiographs. This is of clinical relevance to the diagnosis of osteoporosis by vertebral fracture assessment, and to grading incident fractures in clinical trials. We use a parts based model of small vertebral patches (e.g. corners). Many potential candidates are found in a global search using multi-resolution normalised correlation. The ambiguity in the possible solution is resolved by applying a graphical model of the connections between parts, and applying geometric constraints. The resulting graph optimisation problem is solved using loopy belief propagation.

The minimum cost solution is used to initialise a second phase of active appearance model search. The method is applied to a clinical data set of computed radiography images of lumbar spines. The accuracy of this fully automatic method is assessed by comparing the results to a gold standard of manual annotation by expert radiologists.

1 Introduction

The accurate identification of prevalent vertebral fractures is clinically important in the diagnosis of osteoporosis. However there is no precise definition of exactly what constitutes a vertebral fracture, though a variety of methods of describing such fractures have been developed [1]. These include semi-quantitative methods, requiring some subjective judgement by an expert radiologist; and fully quantitative morphometric methods. The latter require the manual annotation of six (or more) points on each vertebra. The manual marking is time consuming, and such methods are lacking in specificity. More sophisticated classification methods based on statistical models have been reported in [2,3], but these require an accurate segmentation method. Active appearance models [4] (AAM) have been used to segment dual energy X-ray absorptiometry (DXA) images in [5], but the method required a manual initialisation on the centre of each vertebra. Also in clinical practise the use of spinal radiographs is still the gold standard, despite the increasing use of DXA. Radiographs are more challenging as the fan beam

---

* We are thankful to the UK Arthritis Research Council for funding.

used in conventional radiography can lead to parallax errors and apparent scale changes. Some success in automatically locating vertebrae in lumbar radiographs has been reported in [6].

In this work we apply an AAM-based approach similar to [5] to computed radiography images of the lumbar spine. In applications such as large clinical drug trials, it is desirable to eliminate the manual initialisation of the AAM used in [5]. This paper describes a two-phase approach. First a global search is conducted using a set of feature detectors combined with a graph model of their pair-wise geometry. This is then used to initialise a set of AAMs which provide a more detailed segmentation.

A potential problem in the case of the spine is that many vertebrae have a similar appearance. A natural approach is thus to use a parts+geometry model [7,8] as is widely used in the object recognition literature [9]. This work is partly inspired by that of Donner et al.[10], who demonstrate that sparse local models, together with a network of inter-part relationships, can be very useful for locating structures in medical images.

The novelty of the work lies in: a) the combined use of the parts+geometry model with an AAM search, thus providing a fully automatic segmentation method for vertebrae; b) substantial evaluation on a clinical and challenging dataset of spinal radiographs.

2 Methods

2.1 Multi-resolution Patch Models

We first describe the components of the models of parts and geometry used for initial vertebrae location. Given a set of training images in which a particular region has been annotated, we can construct a statistical model of the region. Firstly gross brightness and contrast variation are removed by normalising each pixel using the locally smoothed mean and variance, derived by exponential smoothing with a 50% response radius of 4mm. We then use a simple oriented rectangle, centred on a point, with the axis direction and scales defined by other annotated points (see figure 1).

We search new images using this model by running normalised correlation at a range of positions, orientations and scales in an exhaustive search. To reduce the combinatorial complexity, we perform a multi-resolution search. The coarser resolution models sub-sample smoothed versions of the image, thus covering the same image region with a reduced number of pixels. A fully exhaustive search for local optima is performed only at the coarsest scale to get a set of plausible candidates. Then smaller regions around these candidates are searched, to refine each candidate at the finer resolutions. Only the best candidate is retained when multiple candidate patches overlap. This coarse-to-fine approach usually results in between 10-40 candidates.

We used 6 patches (parts) for each lumbar vertebra: the four corners, a patch on the curved inferior junction of the vertebra with the pedicle; and a wide patch across the spine aligned with the lower pedicle. Note the latter two can

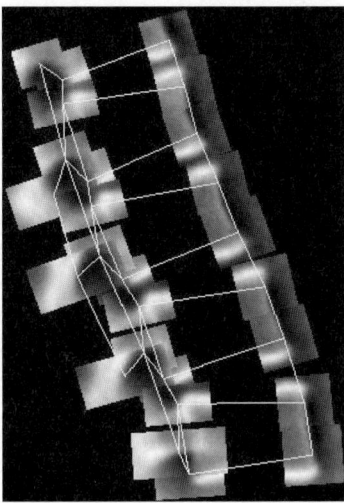

Fig. 1. Mean normalised patches with arc links

overlap somewhat. We chose corner features as they tend to be more distinctive in appearance than other edges. Also the middle of the vertebral endplates tend to have a much more variable appearance due to both parallax tilting (a "bean-can" appearance), and collapse due to fracture. It is doubtful whether normalised correlation of whole vertebral edges would be reliable due to the intrinsic variability of appearance, whereas the corners tend to be more stable in appearance. The curvature of the pedicle join also has a distinctive appearance, and sections of the spine are typically the brightest thing in the image, and so give coarse lateral positional clues.

The node cost of each candidate patch is assigned using a normalised mean absolute deviation from the training set mean patch. For each patch pixel vector $\mathbf{g}$ with mean μ_g and standard deviation σ_g (over the patch), we compute the normalised vector of pixels $\mathbf{v}$, where $\mathbf{v} = \frac{\mathbf{g} - \mu_g}{\max(\sigma_g, \sigma_{min})}$[1].

The mean of each normalised patch is calculated over the training set, to provide a set of patch means $\bar{\mathbf{v}}$. For ease of subscript notation we consider one such patch form. A candidate $\mathbf{v}^{(k)}$ in image j is assigned a cost C_{jk} thus by summing over the absolute deviations from the mean of each of n pixels, with the normalisation factors $\{\hat{\sigma}\}$ evaluated over the training set of N images:

$$C_{jk} = \sum_{i=1}^{n} \frac{|v_{ji}^{(k)} - \bar{v}_i|}{\hat{\sigma}_i} \quad , \hat{\sigma}_i = \frac{1}{N} \sum_{j=1}^{N} |v_{ji} - \bar{v}_i| \qquad (1)$$

Finally the actual cost assigned is further normalised as
$c_{jk} = \frac{C_{jk}}{\alpha}$ where alpha is the standard deviation of $\{C_j\}, j \in \{1 \ldots N\}$ over the training set. Note that this normalisation step ensures that the distribution of

---

[1] Where σ_{min} is a lower-bound, to avoid ill-conditioned behaviour in flat regions.

c (over correctly aligned patches) has approximately unit variance. This ensures a compatible scale for the node and arc costs in the subsequent graph model.

2.2 Geometric Relationships

There are many responses for each part, some of them being duplicated over the similar-looking vertebrae. To resolve the ambiguity, we use a geometric model containing multiple nodes (one per part), together with a model of the pairwise geometrical relationships between them. This is a widely used technique [7,8,10]. We can then use graph algorithms to locate the optimal solution for the combination of feature response candidates and pairwise geometry. The set of vertebral corner and spine features we used form a natural grid with arc set E (see figure 1).

Geometric Constraints. Each candidate response for part r has a central reference point $\mathbf{p}_r$, a scale s_r and an orientation θ_r. The geometric constraints between parts r and q can be represented in the cost function $f_{rq}(\mathbf{p}_r, s_r, \theta_r, \mathbf{p}_q, s_q, \theta_q)$. In general this could be based on a joint probability density function of the parameters.

To allow for the varying scale and orientation between patch candidates, we use similarity transforms. Let the similarity transformation $T(\mathbf{x} : \mathbf{d}, s, \theta)$ apply to $\mathbf{x}$ a scaling of s, a rotation of θ, followed by a translation of $\mathbf{d}$. The corrected relative position of a candidate for patch q is obtained by mapping the position of $\mathbf{p}_q$ into the co-ordinate frame defined by a candidate for r using $\mathbf{t}_{rq} = T^{-1}(\mathbf{p}_q : \mathbf{p}_r, s_r, \theta_r)$.

We compute the 2D mean and variances of the relative position defined by the positional components of $\mathbf{t}_{rq}(\mathbf{p}_q)$ across a training set. We then use the Mahalanabis distance for the cost function f_{rq}. The node cost $c_r(k_r)$ of candidate k_r is obtained as for the $\{c_{jk}\}$ above, but we now drop the image subscript j and use an explicit parts subscript r. The final selection of optimal solution $\tilde{\mathbf{k}}$ from the set of candidate patches $\{P_{rk}\}$ is given by finding the minimum sum of node and arc costs:

$$\tilde{\mathbf{k}} = \operatorname{argmin}_{\mathbf{k}} \left\{ \sum_{r=1}^{R} c_r(k_r) + \sum_{(r,q) \in E} f_{rq}(k_r, k_q) \right\} \qquad (2)$$

We trivially convert this to a maximisation problem and use a loopy belief propagation algorithm [11][2] to solve for the optimal candidate vector $\tilde{\mathbf{k}}$. Note the "loopy" nature of the grid topology means that this is not guaranteed to converge to the true global optimum.

2.3 Data

We obtained anonymised computed radiography (CR) lumbar images from a local hospital, from patients having had spinal radiography over the previous

---
[2] The max-product variant, equivalent to max-sum with log probabilities.

12 months, and with the approval of the local ethics committee. We selected a training subset of 135 images, particularly including those images with evidence of vertebral fracture, to try and ensure a sufficient training of the AAM shape models to cope with fractured cases.

The images were manually annotated using an in-house tool by an experienced radiologist. Each vertebral contour uses 60 points around the vertebral body with 8 further points around the pedicles. The endplate rims were modelled using a quasi-elliptical shape to cope with the dual-edge appearance induced by projective tilting.

2.4 Active Appearance Models

The linked AAM approach of [5] was used to fit a sequence of three AAMs composed of overlapping vertebral triplets covering the spine from L4 up to T12. Note that L5 is not normally used in vertebral fracture assessment as it is very rare for L5 to suffer osteoporotic fracture. The AAM combination algorithm also uses a global shape model of the entire spine, but this is used to guide the initialisation of later sub-models in the fitting sequence (given the earlier sub-model solutions). T12 was included to form the uppermost L1-centred triplet.

As there is little useful information inside the vertebral body we used profile gradient samplers for the AAM texture model, as was used on DXA data [5], with a non-linear renormalisation using a sigmoidal function tuned to the mean absolute gradient. We used a 4-level multi-resolution pyramid search to extend the convergence zone.

3 Experiments

3.1 Feature Detection

A train/test split was performed by picking out 10 images in turn from the CR data. The patch correlators were trained on the remaining CR data, and similarly the means and variances of the relative patch poses were calculated in order to construct relative position functions for the arc costs. The patch correlation followed by graph optimisation was then run on the respective test subsets.

There is a fundamental ambiguity in determining the vertebral levels. This was worsened by the fact that our modelling does not yet include L5, as L5 is not normally assessed for osteoporosis. We therefore cropped the images at 20 mm below L4, which tends to include about half of L5. Because the lumbar images typically include several thoracic vertebrae (e.g. up to T10), we found that the optimal solution is frequently displaced by one vertebal level (i.e. L3 appears to be L4 etc). Even such cases represent a kind of success, as the feature detectors are still locating vertebrae. So we classified each image detection result into three catagories: successful, level-displaced, and unsuccessful. Successful cases require at least 3 lumbar centres to be located within 10mm of the true centre (i.e. about half a vertebral height), so the putative centre is normally inside the

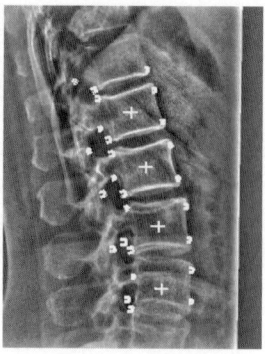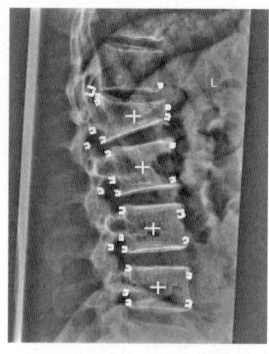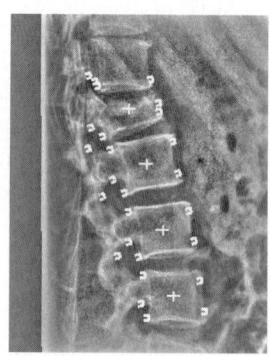

Fig. 2. Successful automatic initialisations. Crosses mark the estimated vertebral centres, other smaller 3-sided markers are drawn around located feature points. Note the L1 wedge fractures in the images ii) and iii).

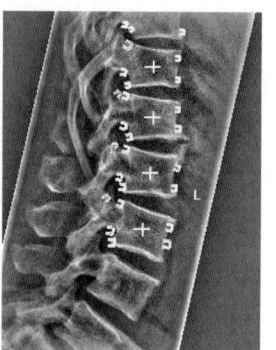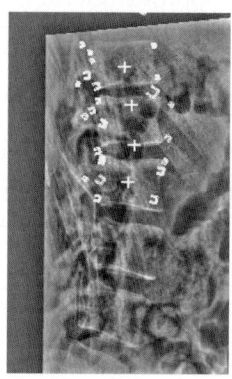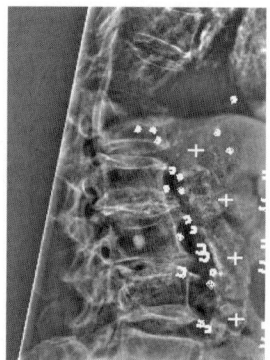

Fig. 3. Unsuccessful automatic initialisations, a)-c) (left first): a) vertebral level displaced upwards by one; b) the middle two vertebra are also compressed into one (edge confusion); c) Completely failure due to scoliosis and anterior calcification

correct vertebra. A level-displaced case is similar but with the levels shifted by one vertebrae; and a failure case is all others. Only successful cases were subject to the secondary stage of AAM search.

3.2 AAM Search

We used a similar train/test cycle of miss-10-out to run the AAM searches. We then took the centre of the 4 lumbar vertebral corner patches and used these vertebral centres to initialise the next phase of AAM search, using a global shape model of T12-L4 (plus vertebral centres). Note that shape constraints are applied in the usual AAM manner, so this initialisation will tend to smooth out outliers. Point-to-line errors were calculated of the converged AAM positions with respect to the gold-standard radiologist manually placed points.

Table 1. Number of Images / (Percentage) for which vertebrae location algorithm succeeds

Successful	Level-Shifted	Failures
98 (73%)	27 (20%)	10 (7%)

Table 2. Search error statistics (point-to-line) for AAM

Vertebra Status	Search Error Statistic				
	Mean (mm)	Median (mm)	75%-ile mm	95%-ile mm	%ge errors >2mm
Normal	0.93	0.53	0.98	1.68	7.3%
Fractured	2.27	1.16	2.44	5.50	30.6%

4 Results

Figure 2 shows three examples of the located features (and vertebral centres), while Figure 3 shows a level-shifted result and two failures.

Table 1 gives the numbers of successful, level-displaced (by one vertebral level), and unsuccessful phase 1 localisations. It can be seen that the ambiguity of vertebral levels is a problem, but only 7% of images result in outright failure. The mean central point error of the successful cases was 3.6mm.

Table 2 gives point-to-line accuracy results from the phase 2 AAM segmentation given the automatic ("successful" only cases) initialisations. These results are decomposed into points within normal or fractured vertebrae. Data are given for the mean, median, 75th and 95th percentiles; and the percentage of point errors in excess of 2mm, which can be viewed as a point failure threshold. The overall mean error was 1.06mm.

5 Discussion and Conclusions

Although there is some degree of failure of the automatic initialisation process, the algorithm sucessfully locates a plausible set of vertebrae in over 90% of cases. The fundamental ambiguity of vertebral levels is a problem (20% level-shifted), but we hope that by more fully modelling L5 and the upper sacrum we will be able to better resolve this ambiguity. We may have to extend the algorithm to include optional thoracic vertebra (e.g. up to T10), and thus deal with potentially missing structure. In some applications it may be possible for the level issue to be resolved by manual pre-cropping of the images. The use of more sophisticated feature representations of the images to reduce spurious feature detections is also under investigation.

Successful cases give adequate accuracy for a secondary phase of detailed AAM segmentation. The overall mean AAM accuracy of 1.06mm is comparable to results on DXA [5], and other methods for lumbar vertebrae (e.g. [6], mean error 1.4mm). Good accuracy is obtained for normal (unfractured) vertebrae, but there is a higher point failure rate and more skewed errors for fractured vertebrae. If severe fractures [3] are excluded, then the mean error over the remaining fractured vertebrae reduces to 1.7mm (median 0.94mm); whereas for severe (grade 3) fractures it is 3.9mm. This deterioration may be partly due to undertraining of the shape models for the more severe fractures, a problem which should be resolved by more training examples.

A parts+geometry model trained on vertebral patches with a grid topology successfully located a sequence of vertebrae in 93% of images. However issues remain over the ambiguity of vertebral level. In successful cases this vertebral detection method provides adequate initialisation for an accurate AAM segmentation, but further AAM training on severe fractures is needed.

References

1. Guermazi, A., Mohr, A., Grigorian, M., Taouli, B., Genant, H.K.: Identification of vertebral fractures in osteoporosis. Seminars in Musculoskeletal Radiology 6(3), 241–252 (2002)
2. de Bruijne, M., Lund, M.T., Tankó, L.B., Pettersen, P.P., Nielsen, M.: Quantitative vertebral morphometry using neighbor-conditional shape models. In: Larsen, R., Nielsen, M., Sporring, J. (eds.) MICCAI 2006. LNCS, vol. 4190, pp. 1–8. Springer, Heidelberg (2006)
3. Roberts, M.G., Cootes, T.F., Pacheco, E.M., Adams, J.E.: Quantitative vertebral fracture detection on DXA images using shape and appearance models. Academic Radiology 14, 1166–1178 (2007)
4. Cootes, T.F., Edwards, G.J., Taylor, C.J.: Active appearance models. IEEE Transactions on Pattern Analysis and Machine Intelligence 23, 681–685 (2001)
5. Roberts, M.G., Cootes, T.F., Adams, J.E.: Vertebral morphometry: semi-automatic determination of detailed shape from DXA images using active appearance models. Investigative Radiology 41(12), 849–859 (2006)
6. de Bruijne, M., Nielsen, M.: Image segmentation by shape particle filtering. In: International Conference on Pattern Recognition, pp. 722–725. IEEE Computer Society Press, Los Alamitos (2004)
7. Fergus, R., Perona, P., Zisserman, A.: A visual category filter for google images. In: Pajdla, T., Matas, J(G.) (eds.) ECCV 2004. LNCS, vol. 3021, pp. 242–256. Springer, Heidelberg (2004)
8. Felzenszwalb, P., Huttenlocher, D.: Pictorial structures for object recognition. Int. Journal of Computer Vision 61(1), 55–79 (2005)
9. Ponce, J., Hebert, M., Schmid, C., Zisserman, A. (eds.): Towards Category-Level Object Recognition. Springer, Heidelberg (2006)
10. Donner, R., Micusik, B., Langs, G., Bischof, H.: Sparse MRF appearance models for fast anatomical structure localisation. In: Proc. British Machine Vision Conference, vol. 2, pp. 1080–1089 (2007)
11. Weiss, Y., Freeman, W.: On the optimality of solutions of the max-product belief propagation algorithm in arbitrary graphs. IEEE Trans. Inf. Theory 47, 736–744 (2001)

---

[3] i.e. grade 3 fractures in the Genant system [1], suffering over 40% height loss.

Utero-Fetal Unit and Pregnant Woman Modeling Using a Computer Graphics Approach for Dosimetry Studies

Jérémie Anquez, Tamy Boubekeur, Lazar Bibin, Elsa Angelini, and Isabelle Bloch

Telecom ParisTech, CNRS UMR 5141 LTCI, Paris, France

Abstract. Potential sanitary effects related to electromagnetic fields exposure raise public concerns, especially for fetuses during pregnancy. Human fetus exposure can only be assessed through simulated dosimetry studies, performed on anthropomorphic models of pregnant women. In this paper, we propose a new methodology to generate a set of detailed utero-fetal unit (UFU) 3D models during the first and third trimesters of pregnancy, based on segmented 3D ultrasound and MRI data. UFU models are built using recent geometry processing methods derived from mesh-based computer graphics techniques and embedded in a synthetic woman body. Nine pregnant woman models have been generated using this approach and validated by obstetricians, for anatomical accuracy and representativeness.

1 Introduction

Several organizations and institutes like the World Health Organization or the Mobile Manufacturers Forum, have pointed out the need for studies of interactions between electromagnetic fields and biological tissues. For this purpose, experiments performed *in vivo* on animals and *in vitro* at the cellular level are complemented by simulated dosimetry studies. These studies require rasterized computational body models in order to simulate the electromagnetic field and derive the energy absorption at each point of the model.

With the advent of fast whole body acquisition imaging protocols, voxel-based models are nowadays built using segmented medical data acquired on volunteers. Numerous adult and children voxel-based models are available [1], which have enabled extensive dosimetric studies. In 2006, the World Health Organization designated studies aiming at assessing fetal exposure during pregnancy as a new priority. Since gathering whole body medical data on a pregnant woman is unethical, hybrid models were built by merging stylized models with organs built with surface equations, voxel-based models and/or synthetic models from the computer graphics community. Only few works modeled pregnant women at different stages of pregnancy. However, detail and realism of the UFU models remained limited in these models, and did not allow precise fetal exposure assessment. Stylized models were used in [2], which are inherently simplified anatomical representations.

A detailed set of models of pregnant women was already proposed in [3], but was limited by the fact that the fetus models contained a realistic but coarse skeleton extracted from a CT scan, scaled and combined with different synthetic envelopes not generated from medical data. Moreover, only a limited set of fetal tissues were distinguished (including soft tissues, skeleton, brain). The set of models proposed in [4] was the only one built using medical images, but UFU models at different gestational ages were obtained by scaling a single model extracted from MRI data obtained at 35 weeks of amenorrhea (WA). This transformation seems inappropriate as fetal limbs and organs do not develop at the same moment nor grow linearly. Therefore, there is still a need for more complex models.

In this paper, we propose to fill this gap by building a set of pregnant woman models, embedding detailed and realistic UFU models. Realism is ensured by the use of medical images, obtained with two modalities used in routine pregnancy follow up: 3D ultrasound (3DUS) during the first trimester and magnetic resonance imaging (MRI) during the second and third trimesters. Detailed segmentations, validated by expert physicians, are then processed using several point-based graphics tools, in particular the MLS operator, which have recently emerged as efficient and robust techniques in digital geometry processing. We introduce their use in medical imaging by meshing smooth surfaces sampled from medical volume data. This mesh representation preserves smoothness during the discretization of the UFU anatomy on the Cartesian grid used for dosimetric simulations, which is crucial as surface singularities induce bias in the simulation results. UFU models are merged with a synthetic woman model, overlapping the maternal bulk extracted from the images and under control of obstetricians.

The originality of this work is three-fold: an emerging problematic is addressed; an extensive database of images acquired with state-of-the-art modalities used in obstetrics has been gathered (Section 2); recent geometry processing methods derived from mesh-based computer graphics techniques are used to provide a smooth representation of the UFU anatomical structures (Section 3). Preliminary results and future works are presented in Section 4.

2 Images Database and Utero-Fetal Unit Segmentation

3DUS Image Data. With the collaboration of obstetricians from the Port-Royal and Beaujon hospitals (Paris, France), we obtained eighteen 3DUS images between 8 and 14 WA. These images have a submillimetric and isotropic resolution (typically $0.6 \times 0.6 \times 0.6$ mm^3) and contain the whole UFU. First, voxels are classified into two classes, the amniotic fluid on the one hand, and the fetal and maternal tissues on the other hand. This is performed using the method described in [5], where statistical distributions of voxel intensities within each class are exploited in a deformable model segmentation framework. Then, the fetus is manually disconnected from the uterine wall and from the umbilical cord. Finally, the placenta and the endometrium are identified.

MRI Image Data. In collaboration with pediatric radiologists from the Cochin-St Vincent de Paul hospital (Paris, France), a database of twenty-two routine

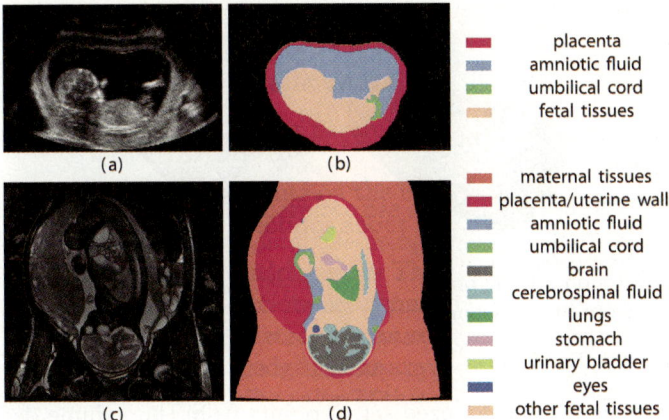

Fig. 1. 3DUS (a) and MRI (c) images at 13 and 34 WA, with corresponding segmentation results (b) and (d)

MRI exams has been gathered, of fetuses between 26 and 35 WA. Images were acquired using the Balanced Steady State Free Precession sequence, which enables to acquire volumes encompassing the UFU in less than thirty seconds. Thus, images free from fetal motion related artifacts can be obtained, guaranteeing three dimensional consistency of the UFU anatomical structures. Moreover, intensities in fluids are strikingly higher than in fetal soft tissues and high contrasts enable easy delineation of the fetus and its anatomy [6]. The typical images resolution is $1 \times 1 \times 4$ mm^3. First, maternal tissues, uterine wall, placenta, amniotic fluid, umbilical cord and fetus are segmented using semi-automatic segmentation tools. Then, fetal anatomy is refined by segmenting the brain, cerebrospinal fluid, spine, eyes, lungs, heart, stomach and urinary bladder. The overall segmentation is time consuming and automated approaches are currently being developed. Accurate results have already been obtained for eyes, brain [7], cerebrospinal fluid and spine automated segmentation. Typical 3DUS and MRI data images are shown in Figure 1, together with the corresponding segmentation results, which were individually validated by obstetricians.

3 Utero-Fetal Unit and Pregnant Woman Modeling

3.1 Surface Reconstruction

For dosimetry studies, Finite Difference Time Domain method is frequently used for numerical simulations on a spatial grid, with labeled anthropomorphic models which need to be smooth to avoid simulation bias on singularities. Naive direct meshing approaches generate "steps" effects (see Figure 2) in the surface models, especially when MRI images with anisotropic resolution are considered. In this section, we describe a method for generating a high quality triangle mesh from a presegmented volume of interest (see Figure 2). We adopt a generic approach

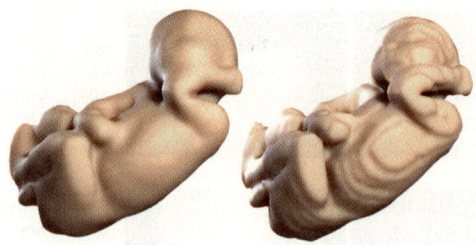

Fig. 2. Illustration on a fetus body of the proposed surface reconstruction (left) versus direct meshing from image segmentation (right)

by first extracting an unorganized set of points from the volume data and then generating a mesh by sampling a smooth surface which approximates this point set. The entire process is performed in a few seconds.

The mesh reconstruction algorithm is composed of three main steps, detailed below (see Figure 3 for an illustration). With this algorithm, a mesh of arbitrary resolution can be extracted from an arbitrary sparse point set. Consequently, the system allows producing dense enough surface sampling to enable both accurate subsequent deformations of the objects and robust rasterization within the original volume domain. **Point-Normal Sampling.** In addition to the position $\mathbf{p}_i$ of a point sample, the algorithm requires a surface normal estimate $\mathbf{n}_i$ at this point, in order to generate a mesh $\mathcal{M}$ from the point-normal sampling $\mathcal{P}^N = \{\{\mathbf{p}_0, \mathbf{n}_0\}, ... \{\mathbf{p}_m, \mathbf{n}_m\}\}$. We compute an approximate normal vector at each point by using a *Principal Component Analysis* [8] in 3D space. More precisely, the normal is given as $\mathbf{u}_i$, the eigen vector associated with the smallest eigen value of the covariance matrix of the k-nearest-neighborhood of $\mathbf{p}_i$. In practice, the anisotropic nature of the original sampling induces a rather large value for k, usually $k \in [50, 120]$, and we use a kD-Tree data structure [9] to efficiently compute the k-neighborhood queries.

In our case, the sign of the normal can be resolved using additional information available from the volume data: the vector $\mathbf{a}_i$, from the surface point $\mathbf{p}_i$ to the corresponding point on a dilated volume boundary, always points from the surface to the outside of the object. Thus, we get

$$\mathbf{n}_i = \frac{\overline{\mathbf{n}_i}}{||\overline{\mathbf{n}_i}||} \text{ with } \overline{\mathbf{n}_i} = \begin{cases} \mathbf{u}_i & \text{if } \mathbf{u}_i \cdot \mathbf{a}_i > 0 \\ -\mathbf{u}_i & \text{otherwise} \end{cases}.$$

Note that $\mathbf{n}_i$ is only an estimate, with a smoothness controlled by k. To increase the quality of this estimate for later stages of the reconstruction pipeline, the normals are re-estimated after each major processing step in this algorithm.

MLS Operator. The Moving Least Square (or MLS) projection operator [10,11] is a scattered data approximation method intensively used in geometry processing. We make use of it for both filtering and meshing steps, as it provides a simple and powerful tool for the sparse sampling $\mathcal{P}^N$ extracted from volume data. We

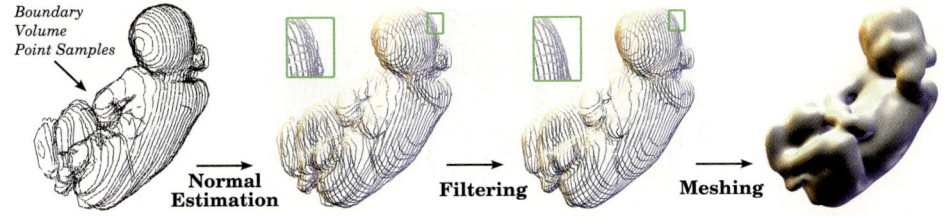

Fig. 3. Illustration on a fetus body of the reconstruction pipeline

consider a variation of a recent simplification of the MLS operator [12]. Let consider $\mathbf{q} \in \mathbb{R}^3$. The MLS operator is defined as:

$$MLS^{\mathcal{P}^N} : \mathbb{R}^3 \to \mathbb{R}^3, \mathbf{q} \to \Pi^\infty(\mathbf{q})$$

It is based on the orthogonal projection $\Pi(\mathbf{q})$ of $\mathbf{q}$ onto a weighted least square plane $H_\mathbf{q} = \{c(\mathbf{q}), n(\mathbf{q})\}$: $\Pi(\mathbf{q}) = \mathbf{q} - <\mathbf{q} - c(\mathbf{q}).n(\mathbf{q})> n(\mathbf{q})$ where

$$c(\mathbf{q}) = \frac{\sum_i \omega(\|\mathbf{q}-\mathbf{p_i}\|)\mathbf{p_i}}{\sum_i \omega(\|\mathbf{q}-\mathbf{p_i}\|)} \text{ and } n(\mathbf{q}) = \frac{\sum_i \omega(\|\mathbf{q}-\mathbf{p_i}\|)\mathbf{n_i}}{\|\sum_i \omega(\|\mathbf{q}-\mathbf{p_i}\|)\mathbf{n_i}\|}$$

define a weighted combination over a local neighborhood of surface point samples near $\mathbf{q}$ with $\{\mathbf{p}_i, \mathbf{n}_i\} \in \mathcal{P}^N$. For efficiency reasons, we use Wendland's [13] compactly supported, piecewise polynomial function as the weighting kernel:

$$\omega(t) = \begin{cases} (1-\frac{t}{h})^4(\frac{4t}{h}+1) & \text{if } 0 \le t \le h \\ 0 & \text{if } t > h \end{cases},$$

where h controls the size of the support (i.e. smoothness). By applying iteratively this projection procedure, we define $\Pi^{i+1}(\mathbf{q}) = \Pi(\Pi^i(\mathbf{q}))$ and generate a sequence of points $\{\mathbf{q}, \Pi(\mathbf{q}), ..., \Pi^i(\mathbf{q}), ...\}$ which — considering $\mathbf{q}$ in the vicinity of $\mathcal{P}^N$ [14] — converges toward a stationary point $\Pi^\infty(\mathbf{q})$. The set of points in $\mathbb{R}^3$ which are stationary by this MLS projection of $\mathcal{P}^N$ is called the *point set surface* (or PSS) [15] of $\mathcal{P}^N$. This procedure converges very quickly in the vicinity of $\mathcal{P}^N$. In practice, we bound the number of iterations to 5 and the precision to a user-defined value, i.e. $\|\Pi^{i+1}(\mathbf{q}) - \Pi^i(\mathbf{q})\| < \epsilon$. Note that $\omega(t)$ has a compact support, which allows us to consider only a small and local set of neighbors in $\mathcal{P}^N$. Again, a kD-Tree is used to query them in logarithmic time. **Filtering.** The manual segmentation may often lead to inaccurate volume boundary and unwanted samples in $\mathcal{P}^N$. Consequently, we need to filter $\mathcal{P}^N$ prior to the mesh generation stage. In practice, this filtering boils down to smooth $\mathcal{P}^N$ and remove its *outliers*, which are samples located far away from the estimated surface. The former can be addressed by applying the MLS projection on every sample of $\mathcal{P}^N$, using h to control the low-pass filtering effect (i.e. $\mathcal{P}^N$ is projected onto the PSS it defines). We address the later problem using an iterative classification inspired from the method of Bradley et al. [16]: we compute the *Plane Fit Criterion* proposed by Weyrich et al. [17], remove the detected outliers and restart with a

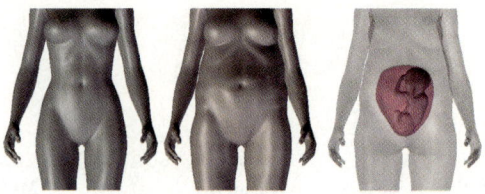

Fig. 4. Pregnant woman modeling: original trunk of the synthetic woman (left), deformed trunk (center) and final model (right)

quadratically decreasing bound until a user-defined threshold. Our experiments show that the number of iterations can be fixed to 3. **Mesh Generation.** We finally generate the mesh $\mathcal{M}$ from $\mathcal{P}^N$ using two distinct approaches:

- in most cases, we use the implicit form of the PSS:

$$f^{\mathcal{P}^N} : \mathbb{R}^3 \to \mathbb{R}, \mathbf{q} \to n(\mathbf{q})^\top (\mathbf{q} - c(\mathbf{q}))$$

to define a scalar field with zero set — $f^{\mathcal{P}^N}(\mathbf{q}) = 0$ — corresponding to a smooth surface approximating $\mathcal{P}^N$. We contour it by feeding the *extended marching cube* algorithm [18] with $f^{\mathcal{P}^N}$ (i.e., $f^{\mathcal{P}^N}$ is evaluated at marching cube grid vertices).
- in some cases, exhibiting large missing surface regions in the sampling obtained from volume data, we use the *Poisson Reconstruction* algorithm, as proposed by Kazhdan et al. [19]. We use their code, publicly available.

As a result, we obtain a triangle mesh $\mathcal{M}$ sampling at arbitrary precision (controlled by the marching cube grid size) a smooth surface defined from the input boundary samples extracted from volume data. Surface meshes for all segmented objects in Figure 1 have been generated with our method. These mesh models can then be used for further interactive skinning, deformation and visualization.

3.2 Pregnant Woman Modeling

No segmented woman model is freely available and an approach similar to [4] has been adopted. Pregnant women models are built by inserting UFU models into a synthetic woman model, Victoria, distributed by DAZ studio (www.daz3d.com). UFU models generated using ultrasound data are registered rigidly into Victoria. Those models correspond to early pregnancy stages. Consequently, Victoria's body is not altered, as the abdominal morphology of a pregnant woman is not modified at such stages by the growing UFU, given its small volume.

However, a different insertion process has to be considered when models generated from MRI data are inserted (see Figure 4). First, UFU and the maternal bulk models are positioned by rigidly registering the pubis. Then, a realistic inclination is defined. Finally, Victoria's thigh and trunk are morphed using free form deformations to fit the maternal bulk. The final pregnant woman model is obtained by removing the maternal bulk. Positioning and morphing operations were supervised by experienced obstetricians.

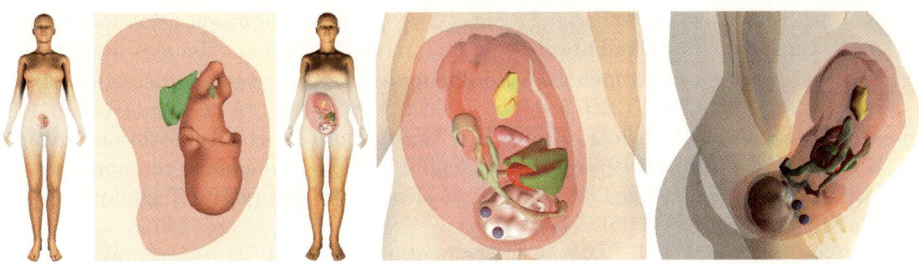

Fig. 5. Pregnant women models at 13 WA (left two images) and 35 WA (right three images), generated using US3D and MRI data, respectively

4 Preliminary Results and Future Works

Nine pregnant woman models have been generated using the method presented in this paper: four from 3DUS images (8, 9, 10 and 13 WA) and five from MRI images (30, 32, 32, 33 and 35 WA). Models at 13 and 35 WA are shown in Figure 5. All models were anatomically validated by obstetricians and pediatric physicians, and will be shared with other researchers in a near future. Preliminary dosimetry studies on models derived from MRI have been performed and results show that fetal position and morphology have a direct influence on fetal exposure [20], demonstrating the importance of considering multiple models with similar gestational ages.

Future works include the computation of additional models, especially for the second pregnancy trimester. During this period, 3DUS cannot be used due to limited field of view and MRI images quality is often altered by fetal motion related artifacts. However, an artifact free MRI volume was recently obtained at 26 WA and the corresponding model is currently under construction. A fetus model has also been articulated, to be morphed into different anatomical position. This enables the study of the posing influence on dosimetry. Finally, this model can be used as a tool for segmentation. Indeed, registering this model on fetal landmark points (e.g. joints cartilage) in a new image dataset to initialize a graphcut segmentation provided promising results in preliminary experiments for the fetal envelope segmentation.

Acknowledgments. This work has been partially founded by a grant from the Fondation Santé et Radiofréquences and by Orange Labs. The authors thank all the radiologists and obstetricians involved in the models building process.

References

1. Caon, M.: Voxel-based computational models of real human anatomy: a review. Radiation and Environmental Biophysics 42(4), 229–235 (2004)
2. Dimbylow, P.: Development of pregnant female, hybrid voxel-mathematical models and their application to the dosimetry of applied magnetic and electric fields at 50 Hz. Physics in Medicine and Biology 51(10), 2383–2394 (2006)

3. Xu, X., Taranenko, V., Zhang, J., Shi, C.: A boundary-representation method for designing whole-body radiation dosimetry models: pregnant females at the ends of three gestational periods–RPI-P3,-P6 and-P9. Physics in Medicine and Biology 52(23), 7023–7044 (2007)
4. Wu, D., Shamsi, S., Chen, J., Kainz, W.: Evaluations of specific absorption rate and temperature increase within pregnant female models in magnetic resonance imaging birdcage coils. IEEE Transactions on Microwave Theory and Techniques 54(12 Part 2), 4472–4478 (2006)
5. Anquez, J., Angelini, E., Bloch, I.: Segmentation of fetal 3D ultrasound based on statistical prior and deformable model. In: ISBI, pp. 17–20 (2008)
6. Anquez, J., Angelini, E., Bloch, I., Merzoug, V., Bellaiche-Millischer, A., Adamsbaum, C.: Interest of the Steady State Free Precession (SSFP) sequence for 3D modeling of the whole fetus. In: EMBS, pp. 771–774 (2007)
7. Anquez, J., Angelini, E., Bloch, I.: Automatic segmentation of head structures on fetal MRI. In: ISBI (2009)
8. Hoppe, H., DeRose, T., Duchamp, T., McDonald, J., Stuetzle, W.: Surface reconstruction from unorganized points. In: ACM SIGGRAPH (1995)
9. Bentley, J.L.: Multidimensional binary search trees used for associative searching. Communications of the ACM 18(9), 509–517 (1975)
10. Levin, D.: The approximation power of moving least-squares. Mathematics of Computation 67(224), 1517–1531 (1998)
11. Levin, D.: Mesh-independent surface interpolation. Geometric Modeling for Scientific Visualization 3 (2003)
12. Alexa, M., Gross, M., Pauly, M., Pfister, H., Stamminger, M., Zwicker, M.: Point-based computer graphics. In: ACM SIGGRAPH Course Notes (2004)
13. Wendland, H.: Piecewise polynomial, positive definite and compactly supported radial functions of minimal degree. Advances in Computational Mathematics 4(4), 389–396 (1995)
14. Amenta, N., Kil, Y.J.: Defining point-set surfaces. In: ACM SIGGRAPH, pp. 264–270 (2004)
15. Alexa, M., Behr, J., Cohen-Or, D., Fleishman, S., Levin, D., Silva, C.T.: Point set surfaces. In: Vis, pp. 21–29 (2001)
16. Bradley, D., Boubekeur, T., Heidrich, W.: Accurate multi-view reconstruction using robust binocular stereo and surface meshing. In: CVPR, pp. 1–8 (2008)
17. Weyrich, T., Pauly, M., Keiser, R., Heinzle, S., Scandella, S., Gross, M.: Post-processing of scanned 3d surface data. In: PBG, pp. 85–94 (2004)
18. Kobbelt, L., Botsch, M., Schwanecke, U., Seidel, H.P.: Feature sensitive surface extraction from volume data. In: ACM SIGGRAPH, pp. 57–66 (2001)
19. Kazhdan, M., Bolitho, M., Hoppe, H.: Poisson surface reconstruction. In: SGP, pp. 61–70 (2006)
20. Bibin, L., Anquez, J., Hadjem, A., Angelini, E.D., Wiart, J., Bloch, I.: Dosimetry studies on a fetus model combining medical image information and synthetic woman body. In: WC (2009)

Cross Modality Deformable Segmentation Using Hierarchical Clustering and Learning

Yiqiang Zhan, Maneesh Dewan, and Xiang Sean Zhou

CAD R&D, Siemens Healthcare, Malvern, PA USA

Abstract. Segmentation of anatomical objects is always a fundamental task for various clinical applications. Although many automatic segmentation methods have been designed to segment specific anatomical objects in a given imaging modality, a more generic solution that is directly applicable to different imaging modalities and different *deformable surfaces* is desired, if attainable. In this paper, we propose such a framework, which learns from examples the *spatially adaptive appearance* and *shape* of a 3D surface (either open or closed). The application to a new object/surface in a new modality requires *only* the annotation of training examples. Key contributions of our method include: (1) an automatic clustering and learning algorithm to capture the spatial distribution of appearance similarities/variations on the 3D surface. More specifically, the model vertices are hierarchically clustered into a set of anatomical primitives (sub-surfaces) using both geometric and appearance features. The appearance characteristics of each learned anatomical primitive are then captured through a cascaded boosting learning method. (2) To effectively incorporate non-Gaussian shape priors, we cluster the training shapes in order to build multiple statistical shape models. (3) To our best knowledge, this is the first time the same segmentation algorithm has been directly employed in two very diverse applications: a. Liver segmentation (closed surface) in PET-CT, in which CT has very low-resolution and low-contrast; b. Distal femur (condyle) surface (open surface) segmentation in MRI.

1 Introduction

In recent decades, automatic/semi-automatic algorithms for the delineation of anatomical structures has become more and more important in assisting and automating specific radiological tasks. Hence, it is not surprising that there have been multitude of algorithms developed in recent years, each tailored towards a particular anatomical structure and imaging modality, typically with a few key parameters to tweak for the algorithm to work. In spite of the availability of all these algorithms [1][2][3][4], generally, it is not easy to make these algorithms to work on another structure/organ and/or imaging modality.

To that end, in this paper, we propose a learning-based hierarchical deformable model to segment various organs (or structures) from different medical imaging modalities. Compared to the existing methods in the "deformable model" family, our method has three hallmarks. *First*, the boundary appearance is hierarchically modeled and learned in a spatially adaptive way. More specifically, the vertices of the deformable model are hierarchically clustered based on both the geometric and appearance similarity. Boundary characteristics of each cluster is then captured by training a boundary detector using a cascade boosting method, finally providing a hierarchically learned model for deformation. *Second*, shape priors are modeled by multiple statistical shape models built upon clustered shape instances. Since each cluster of shape instances represents one of the distribution modes in the shape space, multiple statistical shape models are able to provide more "specific" refinement to the deformable model. *Third*, and finally we demonstrate the efficacy of our algorithm (without changing any parameters), on two different anatomical structures (liver and distal end of femur) in two contrasting imaging modalities (PET-CT and MR).

2 Related Work

Deformable model is a vigorously studied model-based approach in the area of medical image segmentation. The widely recognized potency of deformable models comes from their ability to segment anatomic structures by exploiting constraints derived from the image data (bottom-up) together with prior knowledge about these structures (top-down). The deformation process is usually formulated as an optimization problem whose objective function consists of external (image) term and internal (shape) term. While internal energy is designed to preserve the geometric characteristics of the organ under study, the external energy is defined to move the model toward organ boundaries. Traditional external energy term usually comes from edge information [5], e.g.,

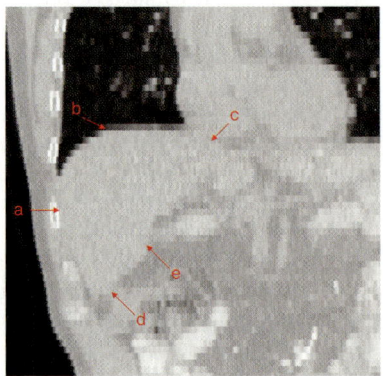

Fig. 1. An example of liver CT images. Arrows *a-e* point to boundaries between liver and rib, lung, heart, abdomen and colon that show heterogenous appearance.

image gradient. In recent years, more effort has been invested on the integration of other image features, e.g., local regional information [1][2] and texture models [3]. By combining different image features as the external energy, deformable model achieves tremendous success in various clinical practices. However, as these external energy terms are usually designed for specific imaging modality and organ, they lack scalability to different medical imaging modalities. Machine learning technologies have opened the door for a more generic external energy design. By using learning-based methods, boundary characteristics can be learned from training data [6][7]. In other words, the "design" of external energy becomes data driven and extensible to different imaging modalities. A potential problem is that the boundary characteristics of organs can seldom be learned by a single classifier due to heterogenous characteristics along organ boundaries (c.f. Fig 1). To address this problem, a "divide-and-conquer" strategy is desired. More specifically, the deformable model should be decomposed into a set of sub-surfaces with relatively similar boundary characteristics.

Moreover, by hierarchically decomposing the deformable model into a set of deformation units, the speed and the robustness of segmentation can be highly improved [8]. However, the hierarchical structure was designed heuristically in [8]. Hence, a more principled way to generate the hierarchical structure, as presented in this work, would be highly desirable.

3 Method

3.1 Overview

In our study, we aim to develop a deformable model that is extensible to different imaging modalities. To achieve this purpose, we propose a learning-based hierarchical model, which is purely data-driven. Given a set of manually segmented training data, the hierarchical structure of the deformable model is constructed through an iterative clustering and feature selection method. As shown in Fig. 3, every node of the hierarchical structure represents a sub-surface of the deformable model. For each primitive sub-surface, i.e., leaf nodes in the hierarchical tree, a boundary detector is learned using a cascade boosting method. The ensemble of these learned boundary detectors actually capture the appearance characteristics of a specific organ in a specific imaging modality. Their responses guide the deformable model to the desired organ boundary. In addition to the hierarchical model and the boundary detectors, a set of statistical shape models are built upon clustered shape instances in the learning stage. These shape priors will be used to constrain the deformable model at run-time. The diagram of our method is shown in Fig 2.

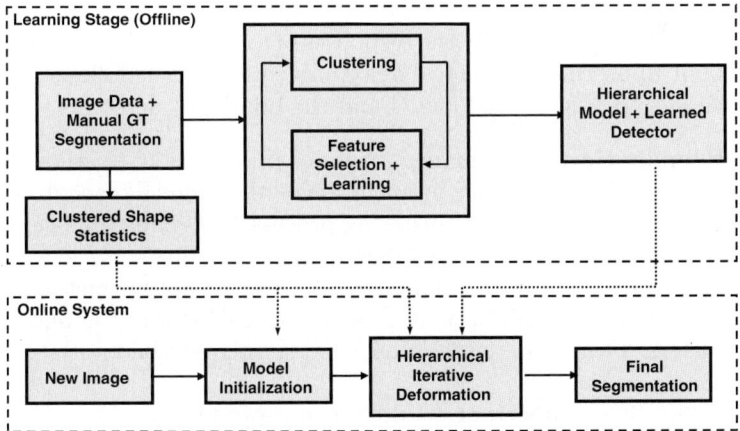

Fig. 2. Flowchart of the learning-based hierarchical model showing both the offline learning and the online testing system

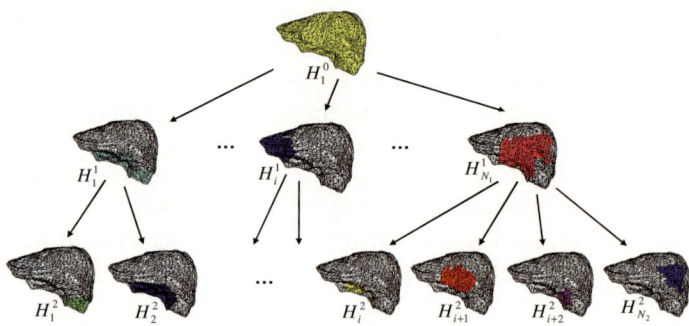

Fig. 3. Hierarchical structure of the deformable model. Color patches depict the sub-surfaces (H_i^j) at jth hierarchical level comprised of vertices in the ith cluster.

Model Description. Our deformable model is represented by a triangle mesh: $S \equiv (V, T)$, where $V = \{v_i | i = 1, \ldots, N\}$ denotes the vertices of the surface and $T = \{t_j | j = 1, \ldots, M\}$ denotes the triangles defined by vertices. Mathematically, the segmentation problem is formulated as the minimization of an energy function defined as:

$$E(S) = E_{ext}(S) + E_{int}(S) = \sum_{i=1}^{N} E_{ext}(v_i) + E_{int}(S) \qquad (1)$$

where E_{ext} and E_{int} are the image (external) energy term and shape (internal) energy term. A hierarchical deformation strategy is employed to solve this high dimensional optimization problem (Refer [6] for details). Due to page limits, we will focus on the energy terms in the remainder of this paper.

3.2 Hierarchical Model with Learning-Based Boundary Detectors

Our external energy is defined by the responses of a set (or ensemble) of boundary detectors built upon the hierarchical deformable model. The following steps are used to generate the hierarchial model and the boundary detectors.

Affinity Propagation Clustering. "Affinity propagation" method [9] is employed to cluster vertices. Affinity propagation method models each data point as a node in a network. During the clustering process, real-valued messages are recursively exchanged between data points until a high quality set of exemplars and corresponding clusters emerge. Compared to other clustering methods, affinity propagation considers each data point as a potential cluster center and gradually generate clusters. Therefore, the solution is not sensitive to bad initialization and hard decision.

In our study, it is important to design an appropriate similarity between vertices since it determines the clustering results of affinity propagation. We put two constraints on the clustered vertices. First, to facilitate the characterization of heterogenous boundary, vertices in the same cluster should have relatively similar image features. Second, the hierarchical deformable model requires the vertices within a cluster to be proximal to each other on the surface. In this way, the cluster center can be treated as a "driving vertex" and drive its neighborhood in the deformation process. To achieve these two purposes, the similarity between vertices is defined as follows.

$$s(v_i, v_j) = 1 - (1/K) \sum_{k=1}^{K} [\alpha G(v_i^k, v_j^k) + (1-\alpha) C(\mathcal{F}(v_i^k), \mathcal{F}(v_j^k))] \quad (2)$$

Here, K is the number of training subjects, v_i^k denotes the ith vertex of the kth subject. $G(v_i^k, v_j^k)$ denotes the geodesic distance between v_i^k and v_j^k. $C(\mathcal{F}(v_i^k), \mathcal{F}(v_j^k))$ denotes the Euclidean distance between image feature vectors calculated at v_i^k and v_j^k.

Iterative Feature Selection/Clustering. To construct the hierarchical structure of the deformable model, vertices are recursively clustered. Assume H_i^j is the ith cluster at the jth hierarchical level, vertices belonging to H_i^j are further clustered to a set of sub-clusters $\{H_k^{j+1}, k = 1, \ldots, N_i\}$:

$$H_i^j = \bigcup_{k=i_1}^{i_{N_i}} H_k^{j+1} \text{ and } \bigcap_{k=i_1}^{i_{N_i}} H_k^{j+1} = \emptyset \quad (3)$$

The remaining problem is the selection of appropriate $\mathcal{F}(.)$ in Eq. 2. This is actually an "egg-and-chicken" problem. On one hand, to achieve the desired clusters, we need to know the distinctive feature sets for boundary description. On the other hand, distinctive features for local boundary can be obtained only after we have the vertices cluster. To address this problem, we propose an iterative clustering and feature selection method.

For the first level of cluster, we use intensity profile along normal of the vertices as $\mathcal{F}(.)$. After that, assume $H_i^j = \{v_l\}$, we use *Adaboost* method to select the features that are most powerful to distinguish $\{v_l\}$ from the points along their normal directions, both inside and outside of the surface. The selected feature set are used as $\mathcal{F}(.)$ in Eq. 2 to further cluster $\{v_l\}$ to a set of sub-clusters $\{H_k^{j+1}, k = i_1, \ldots, i_{N_i}\}$. Feature selection and clustering are iteratively executed until boundary characteristics within a cluster becomes learnable.

Learn Boundary Detectors. For each primitive cluster, i.e., the leaf node of the hierarchical tree, a boundary detector is learned to characterize local boundary. In principle, we follow the idea of [10] to use an extensively redundant feature pool and a cascade *Adaboost* method to learn a boundary detector. Given an image I, $\mathfrak{F}(\mathbf{x}; I)$ denotes the redundant feature vector of $\mathbf{x}$. (In practice, we use 2D, 3D or 4D Haar-like features depends on the dimensionality of different image modalities.) In run-time system, each learned classifier generates a boundary probability map $P(\mathbf{x}|I)$. Hence, the external energy term in Eq. 1 is defined as:

$$E_{ext}(v_i) = 1 - P(v_i|I) = 1 - C_{\hbar_{v_i}}(\mathfrak{F}(v_i; I)) \quad (4)$$

where $\hbar_{v_i}$ is the cluster index of v_i and $C_{\hbar_.}$ defines the corresponding classifier.

3.3 Multiple Statistical Atlas Built on Clustered Shape Instances

In the well-known active shape model [11], shape prior is modeled by a statistical model built upon the whole population of shape instances. However, the assumption that the shape instances follow a mono-Gaussian distribution in the shape space might not always hold for some organs. An effective solution is to build sub-population models [12]. Inspired by this idea, we build multiple shape models upon clustered shape instances. Given a set of training shapes, they are firstly clustered according to pair-wise shape similarity, which is defined by the Euclidean distance between shape vectors. A set of statistical models are then built on each clusters, respectively. In the run time, the deformable model is constrained by the most similar statistical shape model. More specifically, the deformed model is mapped to the eigen-spaces of each shape cluster, respectively. The shape statistical model that gives the most compact description is selected to refine the deformed model. Hence, the internal energy of Eq. 1 is formulated as:

$$E_{int}(S) = 1 - \max_i e^{(-S-S_i)^T \Xi_i (-S-S_i)} \qquad (5)$$

where S_i and Ξ_i denote the average shape and the covariance matrix of the ith shape cluster, respectively.

4 Results

Liver segmentation in wholebody PET-CT. Wholebody PET-CT provides fused morphological and functional information, which benefits cancer diagnosis and therapy evaluation. As the standardized uptake value of liver is usually higher than surrounding tissues, it is desired to segment liver from PET-CT for an organ-specific PET-CT interpretation. In this study, the learning-based hierarchial model was trained by 20 wholebody PET-CT scans with manually delineated liver surfaces. (To jointly exploit CT-PET information, 4D Haar-like filters are used for feature extractor.[13]) As shown in Fig. 4, the generated model has two hierarchical levels with 8 and 25 vertices clusters, respectively. The automatic segmentation results on 30 testing dataset (PET: $5 \times 5 \times 5mm$; CT: $1.3 \times 1.3 \times 5mm$) are compared with manually delineated organ surfaces (see Fig. 5). Accuracy measurements include median distance between surfaces, average distance between surfaces, volume difference and volume overlap difference. In Table 1, we compare our proposed

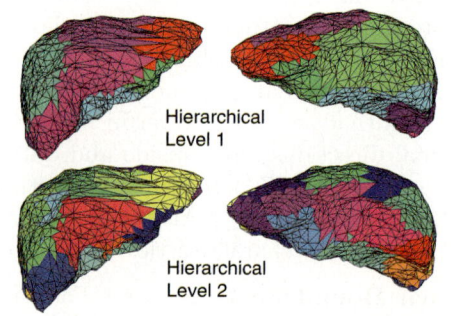

Fig. 4. 3D rendering of the hierarchical structure of a liver model. Color patches denote the vertices belonging to the same cluster. Left: Anterior View. Right: Posterior view.

Table 1. Quantitative comparison of learning based methods on PET-CT liver segmentation

	Med Surf. Dist.(voxel)	Avg Surf. Dist (voxel)	Vol. Diff. (%)	Overlap Diff. (%)
Method1	0.84	1.01	3.13	7.61
Method2	1.27	1.61	5.16	12.1

method (*Method1*) with *Method2*, which is a learning-based deformable model with *heuristically* designed hierarchical structure. More specifically, in *Method2* the hierarchical structure is determined by clustering neighboring vertices, based only on geodesic information[1]. Therefore, the spatially clustered vertices in *Method2* might have larger appearance variation, which is difficult to learn. Hence, *Method2* shows inferior performance.

Distal femur condyle surface segmentation in MR T1 image. The morphological shape and geometry of the condyle surface is not only important for understanding the kinematic function of the knee, but also has clinical significance in areas of total knee arthroplasty and anterior cruciate ligament reconstruction [14]. The automatic segmentation of condyle surface is useful to knee disease diagnosis and therapy planning. We apply the same method on the segmentation of distal femur MR T1 images. As shown in Fig. 5, the automatic segmentation is very close to manual segmentation. Tested on 21 knee MR images (T1, $1.953 \times 1.953 \times 2mm$), the average distance between manually the automatically delineated surfaces is **1.87**mm (in sub-voxel precision).[2]

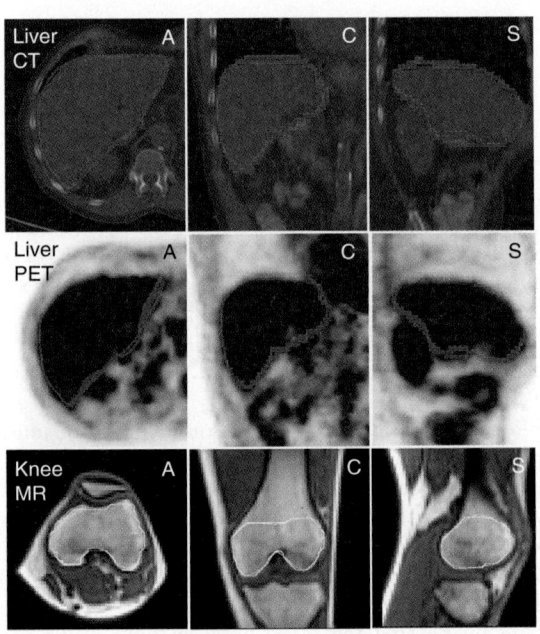

Fig. 5. Comparison of manual and automatic segmentation. Blue/yellow and red/blue contours denote the automatic and manual segmentation, respectively.

---

[1] Note that *Method2* only differs from *Method1* in the way their hierarchical structures are built.

[2] As the distal femur surface is an open surface, we cannot provide the volume error in this experiment.

Importantly, for both liver PET-CT and femur distal surface segmentation, we use exactly same parameters. The accurate results shows that our method is transparent to different imaging modalities and different organs.

5 Conclusion

In this paper, we proposed a learning-based hierarchical deformable model for automatically segmenting anatomic structures across different imaging modalities. The boundary appearance of the anatomical structure is hierarchically modeled through an iterative clustering and learning framework. In addition, the non-gaussian shape variations of these anatomical structures are modeled through multiple statistical shape models, built upon clustered shape instances. The algorithm does not require tweaking of any parameters and the only input required by the algorithm is the image data along with the corresponding annotations. Experimental results on two different structures (liver and distal femur) demonstrated the potential of this method in dealing with segmentation problems in contrasting image modalities.

References

1. Vese, L., Chan, T.F.: A multiphase level set framework for image segmentation using the mumford and shah model. International Journal of Computer Vision 50(3), 271–293 (2002)
2. Ronfard, R.: Region-based strategies for active contour models. International Journal of Computer Vision 13(2), 229–251 (1994)
3. Huang, X., Metaxas, D., Chen, T.: Metamorphs: Deformable shape and texture models. In: CVPR 2004, pp. 496–503 (2004)
4. Pham, D.L., Xu, C., Prince, J.L.: Current methods in medical image segmentation. Annual Review of Biomedical Engineering 2, 315–338 (2000)
5. Xu, C., Prince, J.L.: Snakes, shapes, and gradient vector flow. IEEE Transactions on Image Processing 7(3), 359–369 (1998)
6. Zhan, Y., Shen, D.: Deformable segmentation of 3-d ultrasound prostate images using statistical texture matching method. IEEE TMI 25, 256–272 (2006)
7. Zheng, Y., Barbu, A., et al.: Four-chamber heart modeling and automatic segmentation for 3-d cardiac ct volumes using marginal space learning and steerable features. IEEE Transactions on Medical Imaging 27(11), 1668–1681 (2008)
8. Shen, D., Davatzikos, C.: An adaptive-focus deformable model using statistical and geometric information. IEEE PAMI 22(8), 906–913 (2000)
9. Frey, B.J., Dueck, D.: Clustering by passing messages between data points. Science 315, 972–976 (2007)
10. Viola, P., Jones, M.J.: Robust real-time face detection. International Journal of Computer Vision 57, 137–154 (2004)
11. Cootes, T., Taylor, C.J., Cooper, D.H., Graham, J.: Active shape models-their training and application. CVIU 61(1), 38–59 (1995)

12. Shi, Y., Shen, D.: Hierarchical shape statistical model for segmentation of lung fields in chest radiographs. In: Metaxas, D., Axel, L., Fichtinger, G., Székely, G. (eds.) MICCAI 2008, Part I. LNCS, vol. 5241, pp. 417–424. Springer, Heidelberg (2008)
13. Zhan, Y., Peng, Z., Zhou, X.: Towards organ-specific pet-ct interpretation: generic organ segmentation using joint pet-ct information. In: MICCAI 2008 Workshop on Analysis of Functional Medical Images (2008)
14. Eckhoff, D.G., Bach, J.M., et al.: Three-dimensional morphology and kinematics of the distal part of the femur viewed in virtual reality. Journal of Bone and Joint Surgery 85, 97–104 (2003)

3D Multi-branch Tubular Surface and Centerline Extraction with 4D Iterative Key Points

Hua Li[1], Anthony Yezzi[2], and Laurent Cohen[3]

[1] Department of Radiology, Mayo Clinic College of Medicine, Rochester, MN 55905, USA
[2] School of ECE, Georgia Institute of Technology, Atlanta, GA 30332, USA
[3] CEREMADE, CNRS UMR 7534, University Paris-Dauphine, 75775 Paris Cedex, France

Abstract. An innovative 3D multi-branch tubular structure and centerline extraction method is proposed in this paper. In contrast to classical minimal path techniques that can only detect a single curve between two pre-defined initial points, this method propagates outward from only one initial seed point to detect 3D multi-branch tubular surfaces and centerlines simultaneously. First, instead of only representing the trajectory of a tubular structure as a 3D curve, the surface of the entire structure is represented as a 4D curve along which every point represents a 3D sphere inside the tubular structure. Then, from any given sphere inside the tubular structure, a novel 4D iterative key point searching scheme is applied, in which the minimal action map and the Euclidean length map are calculated with a 4D freezing fast marching evolution. A set of 4D key points is obtained during the front propagation process. Finally, by sliding back from each key point to the previous one via the minimal action map until all the key points are visited, we are able to fully obtain global minimizing multi-branch tubular surfaces. An additional immediate benefit of this method is a natural notion of a multi-branch tube's "central curve" by taking only the first three spatial coordinates of the detected 4D multi-branch curve. Experimental results on 2D/3D medical vascular images illustrate the benefits of this method.

1 Introduction

Image segmentation is often the first task for solving problems in the fields of image processing and computer vision. In medical imaging, the extraction of vascular objects such as coronary arteries and retinal blood vessels, has attracted the attention of more and more researchers [1, 2]. Numerous segmentation methods have been proposed that depend upon organ structures, imaging modalities, application domains, user-interaction requirements, and so on [3].

Centerline extraction methods have been proposed to extract only the centerline (or skeleton) of a tubular object, thereby requiring further processing to obtain the 3D surface or shape. By assuming a centerline corresponded to a minimal cost path, some methods have been designed based on path finding procedures [4, 5, 6, 7, 8, 9, 10]. Specially, Deschamps and Cohen [11] simplified the problem of generating centerlines into the problem of finding minimal paths [12] by utilizing fast marching schemes [13]. The minimal path approach [12] has several advantages such as finding global minimizers, fast computation, ease of implementation, and powerful incorporation of user input.

Unfortunately, despite these numerous advantages, traditional minimal path techniques exhibit some disadvantages both in general and in the particular application of vessel segmentation [14]. First, follow-up vessel boundary extraction is by no means straight forward, even in 2D where the longitudinal cross-sectional boundary of a vessel is completely described by two curves on either side of the detected trajectory. Second, the detected interior trajectory does not always yield remain central to the vessel. Third, in 3D (just as in 2D), traditional purely spatial minimal path techniques can be used only for curve extraction, whereas vessels and other tubular structures, despite sharing some characteristics with curves, are in fact surfaces. Finally, only a single branch can be detected for each pair of initializing seed points. Multiple initialization pairs would be required in order to detect multi-branch structures.

As an improvement, Li and Yezzi [14] proposed a 4D minimal path technique to extract full 3D tubular surfaces and their centerlines simultaneously. They represented the surface of a tubular structure as the envelope of a one-parameter family (curve) of spheres with different centers (three coordinates) and different radii (fourth coordinate). So the *3D surface* extraction problem is translated into the problem of finding a *4D curve* which encodes this family of 3D spheres. As such, the tubular surface and its centerline can be detected simultaneously in this one-dimension-higher 4D space. However, in their method, the user input is still a pair of initial points (or spheres), and thus only a single branch can be detected for each pair of initializations. This disadvantage significantly limits its application to most vessels which have complex branching topologies such as the coronary arteries and abdominal aorta.

In this paper, we propose an innovative 3D *multi-branch* tubular structure and centerline extraction method with all the merits of minimal path techniques while further limiting the required user-interaction to a single initial point. By modeling the surface as a 4D trajectory as in [14], a set of branching 3D tubular surfaces and their centerlines are simultaneously detected with a guarantee that the centerline curves also connect at branch points. By starting with a single 4D point (i.e. a single sphere inside the 3D vessel or other tubular structure) a novel scheme is applied to find a set of 4D iterative key points along an optimal 4D path which is free to branch whenever it is energetically favorable. Then, by sliding back from each key point to the previous one along the minimal action map until all the key points are visited, we obtain the final global minimizing multi-branch 4D trajectory from which we may directly construct the branching tubular 3D surface along with its 3D "central curve", both of which are guaranteed to exhibit the exact same branching topology. Experimental results on 2D/3D medical vascular images illustrate the benefits of this method.

2 Multi-branch Tubular Structure Extraction

When only a single initial starting point is provided by the user, detecting an optimal branching trajectory using minimal cost path searching schemes is dependent upon finding one or more appropriate destination points on the desired path. Furthermore, in order to detect multi-branch structures, at least one destination point along each individual branch should be found. We may then slide back from each destination point toward the starting point to obtain the multi-branch tubular structure. Here, we propose a 4D key point searching scheme to carry out these tasks.

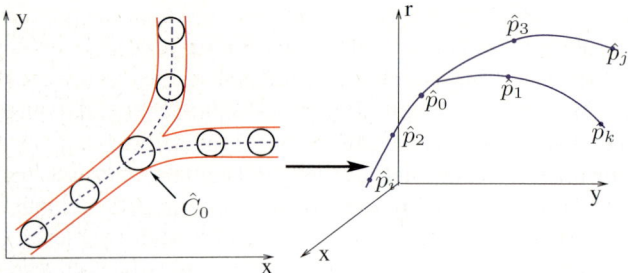

Fig. 1. The entire multi-branch structure extraction is reduced to finding structures between all adjacent key point pairs. The 4D path length D between each key point pair is equal to d_{step}. For easier visualization, the same concept is illustrated here using circles instead of spheres.

2.1 4D Key Point Searching Scheme

Motivated by the 4D minimal path technique [14], we first represent the entire vessel as a 4D curve, where each 4D point represents a 3D sphere (three coordinates for the center point and one for the radius). The *3D surface* extraction problem is translated into the problem of finding a *4D curve* which encodes this family of 3D spheres.

For detecting multi-branch tubular structures, the new 4D iterative key point searching scheme is proposed and illustrated in Fig. 1. The energy minimization model is

$$E(\hat{C}) = \int_{\Omega} \{\omega + P(\hat{C}(c(s), r(s)))\} ds = \int_{\Omega} \widetilde{P}(\hat{C}) ds, \qquad (1)$$

where s represents the arc-length parameter over an interval Ω, $c(s)$ represents the location of a point in the original image domain Ω_I either in $\mathbb{R}^2$ $[c(s) = (x(s), y(s))]$ or in $\mathbb{R}^3$ $[c(s) = (x(s), y(s), z(s))]$, $r(s) \in [0, r_{max}]$ represents the radius of a circle/sphere centered at $c(s)$ (r_{max} is the largest allowed thickness of the vessel to be captured), $\hat{C}(c(s), r(s)) \in \Omega_I$ represents a multi-branch "path" composed by a family of circles/spheres in Ω_I, $E(\hat{C})$ represents the energy which is the integral of $\widetilde{P}$ along $\hat{C}(c(s), r(s))$, P is the potential that enhances the boundary of the vascular tree, ω is a real positive constant, and $\widetilde{P} = P + w$. We call $\Omega_{I_r} = \Omega_I \times [0, r_{max}]$.

Alternatively, as shown in Fig. 1, energy E along the entire structure can be treated as the summation of energy E_k along a path $\hat{C}_k$ between every two adjacent key points $\hat{p}_{k_0}$ (as the starting point) and $\hat{p}_k$ (as the ending point),

$$E(\hat{C}) = \sum_{k=1}^{N} E_k(\hat{C}_k) = \sum_{k=1}^{N} (\int_{\Omega} \widetilde{P}_k(\hat{C}_k) ds). \qquad (2)$$

where P_k may be different for finding different minimal cost path C_k. It is well known that an appropriate $\widetilde{P}_k$ with lower values near the optimal path will cause fronts starting from the initial point $\hat{p}_{k_0}$ to propagate faster along the desired minimal path. Here we define an additional item: the distance step d_{step}. We choose the first reached point at which a front starting from the initial point $\hat{p}_0$ travels d_{step}, and we labeled it as key point $\hat{p}_1$. We then trace back the optimal minimal path between it and $\hat{p}_0$. The next key point $\hat{p}_2$ will be the first reached point at which a front, starting simultaneously from $\hat{p}_0$ and $\hat{p}_1$, travels the distance d_{step}. This will become the destination point for the minimal path segment $\hat{C}_2$. Repeating this process, the new key point $\hat{p}_k$ is always the first reached point at which a front, starting simultaneously from points $\hat{p}_0$ to $\hat{p}_{(k-1)}$, travels the distance d_{step}. In this way, the front may propagate to different branches of the tubular structure, and key points along different branches may be obtained. The process stops when no new key point can be found, which is guaranteed by freezing fast marching schemes and will be discussed later.

To find each minimal path segment $\hat{C}_k$ (minimizing the energy E_k) between key point pairs $\hat{p}_{k_0}$ and $\hat{p}_k$ (the starting point $\hat{p}_{k_0}$ may be any one of the points $\hat{p}_0$ to $\hat{p}_{(k-1)}$), the 4D minimal path technique [14] is applied. At any 4D point $\hat{p} \in \Omega_{I_r}$, we define the minimal action map $U_k(\hat{p})$ as the minimal energy integrated along any possible path between the starting point $\hat{p}_{k_0}$ and the point $\hat{p}$,

$$U_k(\hat{p}) = \inf_{A_{\hat{p}_{k_0},\hat{p}}} \{\int_\Omega \widetilde{P}_k(\hat{C}(c(s), r(s))) ds\} = \inf_{A_{\hat{p}_{k_0},\hat{p}}} \{E_k(\hat{C})\}, \quad (3)$$

where $A_{\hat{p}_{k_0},\hat{p}}$ is defined as the set of all paths between $\hat{p}_{k_0}$ and $\hat{p}$. So, from the ending point $\hat{p}_k$, the minimal path between $\hat{p}_{k_0}$ and $\hat{p}_k$ can be deduced by calculating $U_k(\hat{p}_k)$ and then sliding back from $\hat{p}_k$ along the action map U_k to $\hat{p}_{k_0}$ via gradient descent. $U_k(\hat{p})$ can be computed by solving the Eikonal equation,

$$||\nabla U_k|| = \widetilde{P}_k(\hat{p}) \quad \text{with} \quad U_k(\hat{p}_{k_0}) = 0, \quad \hat{p} \in \Omega_{I_r}, \quad (4)$$

using the fast marching algorithm [13]. 3D (or 4D) fast marching schemes are utilized to solve the Eikonal equations and calculate the action maps for 2D (or 3D) spheres respectively. The 3D vessel structure is then obtained as the envelope of the family of spheres traversed along this 4D curve. Also because all the spheres on the detected minimal path are tangential to the boundary of the tubular structure, the union of their center points describes the central path (medial axis) of the tubular structure.

In order to find appropriate key points and also reduce the computational cost, we would like to limit the front propagation within the long tubular structure. A freezing fast marching method proposed in [15] is utilized to stop the propagation of these fronts when they reach the structure boundary. Obviously, we would like to freeze points at the "tail" of the front, especially when it reaches the actual boundary of tubular shape, and keep the points at the "head" of the front propagating further. To be able to distinguish points at the "head" from those at the "tail", the path lengths $D_k(\hat{p})$ from the starting point $\hat{p}_{k_0}$ to any other point $\hat{p}$ should be computed. $D_k(\hat{p})$ is the Euclidean distance traveled by the front from the starting point $\hat{p}_{k_0}$ to any other point $\hat{p}$. When $D_k(\hat{p})$ is smaller than the current maximum path length d_{max} (initial $d_{max} = 0$),

$$D_k(\hat{p}) < max((d_{max} - \widetilde{d}), 0) \quad with \quad \widetilde{d} > 0, \quad (5)$$

point $\hat{p}$ is frozen by setting the speed to 0, where $\widetilde{d}$ is a pre-defined threshold value. Eq. 5 ensures that no point is frozen till one point on the front has traveled at least the Euclidean distance $\widetilde{d}$, which enables the front to stay inside the long and thin structure.

The distance threshold $\tilde{d}$ is a parameter which should be larger than the expected maximum branch segment of the object, otherwise the algorithm will wrongly freeze points prematurely within incomplete branches. An appropriate $\tilde{d}$ should be chosen based on different image qualities, vessel structures, noise levels, and so on. Instead of calculating D_k after extracting the minimal path according to gradient descent, we may solve D_k locally using the same neighbors involved for solving U_k in Eq. 4,

$$\begin{cases} ||\nabla U_k|| = \tilde{P}_k & \text{with} \quad U(\hat{p}_{k_0}) = 0 \\ ||\nabla D_k|| = 1 & \text{with} \quad D(\hat{p}_{k_0}) = 0. \end{cases} \quad (6)$$

Second, since key point $\hat{p}_k, k \in \{1, ..., N\}$ is the first reached point at which a front, starting simultaneously from multiple points $\hat{p}_0$ to $\hat{p}_{(k-1)}$, travels the distance d_{step}, the optimal minimal cost path $\hat{C}_k$ should connect $\hat{p}_k$ to the appropriate previous key point $\hat{p}_{k_0}, k_0 \in \{0, ..., (k-1)\}$. Here we separate the back tracking process into each new key point searching step to avoid false connections. Each time when we obtain a new key point $\hat{p}_k$, we slide back right away from $\hat{p}_k$ according to the gradient descent on the minimal action map until reaching any point in the group of points $\hat{p}_0$ to $\hat{p}_{(k-1)}$ and obtaining the minimal path $\hat{C}_k$. Parameter d_{step} also defines the accuracy and computational cost of the method. If it is big, it decreases the computational cost of tracking the connectivity of the fronts. However, it misses branches shorter than d_{step}.

Furthermore, if the detected tubular structure only has one branch, the 4D iterative process can be simplified to the following process. First, an initial point $\hat{p}_0$ should be chosen at the end of the tubular structure in order to detect the whole structure. Similarly, if the front starting from $\hat{p}_0$ will travel at least the distance $N \times d_{step}$, the first reached points when the front travels the distance $n \times d_{step}, n \in \{1, ..., N\}$ are chosen as the labeled key points $\hat{p}_n$. The 4D minimal path between the initial point $\hat{p}_0$ and the last iterative key point $\hat{p}_N$ can be easily deduced by sliding back from point $\hat{p}_N$ to its previous point $\hat{p}_{(N-1)}$ along the action map via gradient descent until reaching the initial point $\hat{p}_0$. For single branch detection, we may use this simplified process with an initial point located at one end of the tubular structure.

2.2 Potentials

The potential $\tilde{P}_k$ is designed as a measurement which incorporates the full set of image values within the sphere surrounding the corresponding image point. Any sphere sp in the image domain Ω_I is defined as a point $\hat{p}$ in Ω_{I_r}, $sp = (p, r)$, where p is the center point and r is the radius. The entire sphere should lie inside the desired object and be as big as possible (so that it is tangential to the object boundary). Such spheres should exhibit lower values of $\tilde{P}_k$ compared to smaller spheres which lie inside the desired object or to any sphere which lies outside (fully or partially) the desired object.

For any image point p with gray value $I(p)$ in an image I, we define the mean intensity value $\mu(sp)$ and variance $\sigma^2(sp)$ for the sphere $sp = (p, r)$ as

$$\mu(sp) = \frac{\int_{B(p,r)} I(\tilde{p}) d\tilde{p}}{\int_{B(p,r)} d\tilde{p}}, \quad \sigma^2(sp) = \frac{\int_{B(p,r)} (I(\tilde{p}) - \mu(sp))^2 d\tilde{p}}{\int_{B(p,r)} d\tilde{p}}, \quad (7)$$

where $B(p, r)$ represents the ball of radius r centered at p. We propose an example potential

$$\widetilde{P}_k(\hat{p}) = \widetilde{P}_k(sp) = 1/(w + \lambda_1(|\mu(sp_2) - \mu(sp)|^2) + \lambda_2(|\sigma^2(sp_2) - \sigma^2(sp)|^2)), \quad (8)$$

where $\mu(sp_2)$ and $\sigma^2(sp_2)$ represent the mean and the variance for the sphere $sp_2 = (p, 2r)$, ω is a real positive constant to control the smoothness of the obtained path, λ_1 and λ_2 are two real positive weights for the mean difference and variance difference between the detected sphere and a bigger sphere which has the same center point but twice the radius. These parameters should be selected based on the size and interior information of detected vessels, image noise levels, etc.

The potential shown in Eq. 8 considers the mean and variance differences between the detected sphere and the bigger sphere which shares the same center point with the detected sphere but has a bigger radius. It is irrelevant to k. If a sphere's radius is larger or smaller than the width of the tubular structure, the mean and variance differences between this sphere and the bigger sphere will decrease, and the related potential $\widetilde{P}_k$ will increase. This potential gives smallest values on spheres when they are exactly with center on centerline and the radii are as half as the width of the detected vessel. Also, this *region based* potential does not consider the difference between the current sphere and the starting sphere which therefore helps to avoid accumulation of detection errors along the fast gradient descent.

3 Experimental Results and Analysis

In this section, we demonstrate our approach on various 2D and 3D real images. For each test, users need to specify the center location and radius of the starting point, the potential, and the largest allowed radius of the tubular object. Users also need to specify the parameters d_{max}, $\widetilde{d}$, and d_{step} for the 4D freezing fast marching scheme. Furthermore, all the results shown in this paper were processed on the original image data (i.e. no pre-processing steps were applied beforehand).

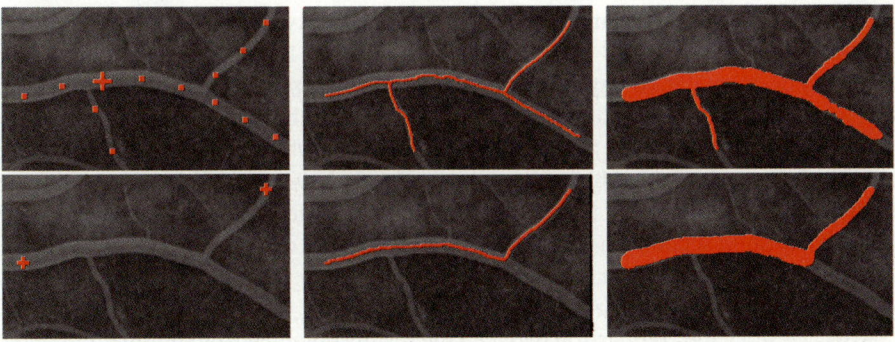

Fig. 2. Vessel segmentation for an angiogram 2D projection image based on the proposed method (upper row) versus the 4D minimal path method [14] (lower row). The initial point is shown with the red cross. Panels from left to right show the initial point and the detected iterative key points, the detected multi-branch centerlines, and the detected vessel surfaces.

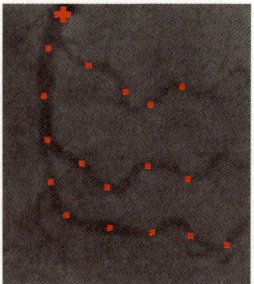 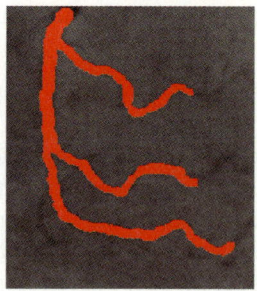

Fig. 3. Segmentation results via the proposed method on another 2D projection angiogram image. Panels from left to right show the initial point and the detected iterative key points and the detected vessel surfaces.

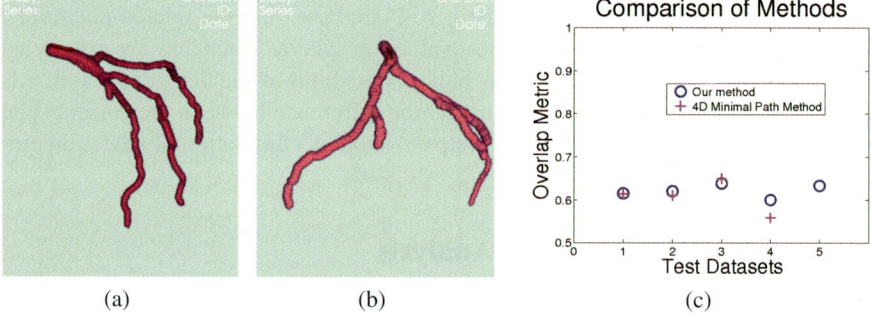

Fig. 4. 3D segmentation results shown for two out of five real 3D CTA data sets, plus comparisons for all five sets between the proposed method versus the 4D minimal path method [14] in terms of overlap with an expert's manual segmentations

Be begin in Fig. 2 with a 2D segmentation result for a noisy 2D projection angiogram image. We set $r_{max} = 15$, $r_{initial} = 9$, $d_{max} = 0$, $\tilde{d} = 100$, and $d_{step} = 50$ for the test. The initial point is located in the middle of the vessel structure. The potential is defined by Eq. 8 with $\omega = 10$, $\lambda_1 = 10$, and $\lambda_2 = 10$. The result shows that by utilizing our 4D iterative key point scheme, multiple branches can be detected only with one initial point. For comparison, we also present the segmentation result on the same image based on the 4D minimal path method [14] which requires two input points instead of one and is incapable of branching. Fig. 3 shows an additional segmentation result with our algorithm on another 2D MRA projection image. In Fig. 4, we test the iterative key point scheme on two 3D CTA datasets of the coronary artery. The potential is defined by Eq. 8 with $\omega = 10$, $\lambda_1 = 10$, and $\lambda_2 = 10$. In these two tests, the initial points are located at the top of the left coronary artery.

Also, we show the comparison between the results obtained from our method (which required only one initial seed point per experiment) and the 4D minimal path method in [14] (which required 5 initial seed points per experiment in order to separately detect each branch). The comparison was done via overlap with manually aquired segmentations for the five 3D clinical CTA coronary datasets. No preprocessing was applied to the date for any of these experiments. Overlap Metric, $OM = 2 \cdot \frac{N_B \cap N_R}{N_B + N_R}$, is applied to evaluate the detection accuracy, in which N_R and N_B are the number of reference ground truth voxels and the number of the detected voxels. For this comparison, we cropped a small region in which the vessel structures were detected by both our method and 4D minimal path method. The comparison illustrates that the proposed method can receive better results as the 4D minimal path technique with far less initial input demanded from the user.

4 Conclusions

In this paper, we proposed an innovative approach to extract multi-branch tubular structures using minimal user input. First, a novel 4D iterative key point searching method is proposed and utilized to detect multi-branch tubular structures with only one initial point. In contrast to standard minimal path techniques which require two initial points and can only detect one single branch between them, this new approach may propagate a tubular surface from only an initial seed point and detect 3D multi-branch surfaces and their centerlines simultaneously. Second, the freezing fast marching method is extended to 4D to reduce the computational cost of the iterative key point search. Finally, the designed potential, which is recalculated each time that a new key point is obtained, can avoid the path difference accumulation along a long tubular structure. It is a novel design and can be implemented easily in the iterative key point searching procedure.

References

1. Frangi, A., Niessen, W., Hoogeveen, R., van Walsum, T., Viergever, M.: Model-based Quantitation of 3D Magnetic Resonance Angiographic Images. IEEE Transactions on Medical Imaging 18(10), 946–956 (1999)
2. Duncan, J., Ayache, N.: Medical Image Analysis: Progress over Two Decades and the Challenges Ahead. IEEE Transactions on Pattern Analysis and Machine Intelligence 22(1), 85–105 (2000)
3. Kirbas, C., Quek, F.: A Review of Vessel Extraction Techniques and Algorithms. ACM Computing Surveys (CSUR) 36(2), 81–121 (2004)
4. Sato, Y., Nakajima, S., Shiraga, N., Atsumi, H., Yoshida, S., Koller, T., Gerig, G., Kikinis, R.: Three-dimensional Multi-scale Line Filter for Segmentation and Visualization of Curvilinear Structures in Medical Images. Medical Image Analysis 2(2), 143–168 (1998)
5. Lorigo, L., Faugeras, O., Grimson, W., Keriven, R., Kikinis, R., Nabavi, A., Westin, C.: CURVES: Curve Evolution for Vessel Segmentation. Medical Image Analysis 5(3), 195–206 (2001)
6. Aylward, S., Bullitt, E.: Initialization, Noise, Singularities, and Scale in Height Ridge Traversal for Tubular Object Centerline Extraction. IEEE Transactions on Medical Imaging 21(2), 61–75 (2002)
7. Wink, O., Niessen, W., Viergever, M.: Multiscale Vessel Tracking. IEEE Transactions on Medical Imaging 23(1), 130–133 (2004)
8. Chung, A., Noble, A., Summers, P.: Vascular Segmentation of Phase Contrast Magnetic Resonance Angiograms Based on Statistical Mixture Modeling and Local Phase Coherence. IEEE Transactions on Medical Imaging 23(12), 1490–1507 (2004)

9. Bouix, S., Siddiqi, K., Tannenbaum, A.: Flux Driven Automatic Centerline Extraction. Medical Image Analysis 9(3), 209–221 (2005)
10. Yan, P., Kassim, A.: Segmentation of Volumetric MRA Images by Using Capillary Active Contour. Medical Image Analysis 10(3), 317–329 (2006)
11. Deschamps, T., Cohen, L.: Fast Extraction of Minimal Paths in 3D Images and Applications to Virtual Endoscopy. Medical Image Analysis 5(4), 281–299 (2001)
12. Cohen, L., Kimmel, R.: Global Minimum for Active Contour Models: A Minimal Path Approach. In: IEEE International Conference on CVPR (CVPR 1996), pp. 666–673 (1996)
13. Sethian, J.: Fast Marching Methods. SIAM Review 41(2), 199–235 (1999)
14. Li, H., Yezzi, A.: Vessels as 4D Curves: Global Minimal 4D Paths to Extract 3D Tubular Surfaces and Centerlines. IEEE Transactions on Medical Imaging 26(9), 1213–1223 (2007)
15. Cohen, L., Deschamps, T.: Segmentation of 3D Tubular Objects with Adaptive Front Propagation and Minimal Tree Extraction for 3D Medical Imaging. Computer Methods in Biomechanics and Biomedical Engineering 10(4), 289–305 (2007)

Multimodal Prior Appearance Models Based on Regional Clustering of Intensity Profiles

François Chung and Hervé Delingette

Asclepios Research Team, INRIA Sophia-Antipolis, France
francois.chung@inria.fr

Abstract. Model-based image segmentation requires prior information about the appearance of a structure in the image. Instead of relying on Principal Component Analysis such as in Statistical Appearance Models, we propose a method based on a regional clustering of intensity profiles that does not rely on an accurate pointwise registration. Our method is built upon the Expectation-Maximization algorithm with regularized covariance matrices and includes spatial regularization. The number of appearance regions is determined by a novel model order selection criterion. The prior is described on a reference mesh where each vertex has a probability to belong to several intensity profile classes.

1 Introduction

Intensity profiles were among the first image representations used to describe appearance for segmentation purposes. Cootes used intensity profiles to build Statistical Appearance Models [1]. They are sampled in training images and both mean profile and its principal modes of variation are extracted for each landmark. Intensity and gradient profiles were used to optimize image forces of deformable models [2]. The idea was to better discriminate organ contours in images by comparing intensity profiles, using two generic models and checking the similarity variation with the normalized cross-correlation. A thorough study on intensity profiles can be found in [3].

Several issues may be raised with statistical appearance methods based on Principal Component Analysis (PCA). First, they require an accurate pointwise registration as the statistical analysis of appearance is performed at each point. Defining homologous points for 3D structures is difficult and therefore registering those points accurately is still considered challenging. A second limitation common to most appearance models (*e.g.* Active Appearance Models) is that they are *monomodal*, *i.e.* they rely on the hypothesis that the probability density function is well described by a single Gaussian distribution. This hypothesis is often violated by the presence of pathologies but also by the fact that shape is not necessarily correlated with appearance (see for instance livers of Fig. 2 where top regions corresponding to the lungs vary in size). Instead of having one mode with large covariance, it is preferable for image segmentation or image detection purposes to have several modes with lower covariance.

In this paper, we describe how to build a Multimodal Prior Appearance Model from a training set of P meshes. Intensity profile classes are estimated for each mesh and not for each point (*i.e.* without the need for any registration). Registration between subjects is only used to estimate the posterior probabilities on a reference mesh. Furthermore, the proposed method is fully automated and one single threshold $\mathcal{J}$ controls the number of classes. Finally, we introduce new regularization strategies of covariance matrices in the Expectation-Maximization algorithm (EM) and the *OSI* index to determine the optimal number of classes.

2 Building Multimodal Prior Appearance Models

2.1 Principles

In Fig. 1, we overview our automated method to create a Multimodal Prior Appearance Model. The input is a set of P meshes $\mathcal{M}_p$ corresponding to the segmentation of the same structure in different images. The meshes may have different number of vertices, or even different topologies. At each vertex i of $\mathcal{M}_p$, we extract M regularly sampled intensities to build an intensity profile of dimension M along the normal direction, noted $\mathbf{x}_i^p$. This profile can extend inward, outward or both sides, depending on the application. Note that intensity profiles act as feature vectors that could be replaced by any other local or global features such as isophote curvature, texture descriptors, oriented filters, etc. Changing the feature vector would only change the regularization of the covariance matrices (section 2.2).

For each mesh, we propose to automatically cluster the profiles using an EM classification. The number of classes, a hyperparameter, is selected in an automatic fashion through a model order selection based on a new criterion (section 2.3). Classification is improved by performing spatial regularization of the posterior probabilities (section 2.4). The creation of the prior is done in two steps. First, all intensity profile classes from the P subjects are compared and classes corresponding to the same tissues are possibly merged. Finally, all P meshes are registered to the same reference mesh $\mathcal{M}^\star$ and a unique prior model is created. Each vertex i of $\mathcal{M}^\star$ is given a probability $\tilde{\gamma}_i^m$ to belong to a reference class m (section 2.5).

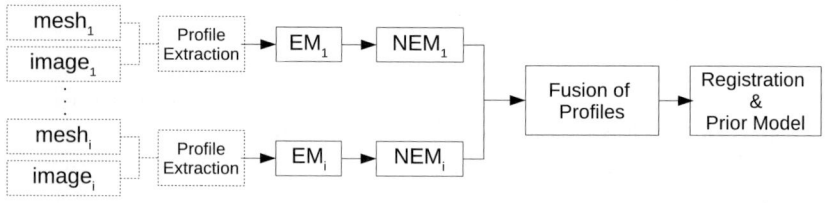

Fig. 1. Proposed pipeline for Multimodal Prior Appearance Model construction

2.2 EM Classification of Intensity Profiles

The classification for a given mesh $\mathcal{M}_p$ is formulated in the context of a probability density estimation using Gaussian Mixture Models. The approach is semi-parametric because the number of classes $\mathcal{K}_p$ is an unknown parameter. In the remainder, intensity profile class is denoted by *mode* and we write μ_k^p, Σ_k^p, π_k^p and $^p\gamma_i^k$ for the mean, covariance matrix, mixing coefficient and posterior probabilities of class k from mesh $\mathcal{M}_p$.

Initialization. EM is initialized with the Fuzzy C-Means algorithm (FCM). After convergence, FCM cluster centers and data membership values are used to initialize the EM mode means μ_k^p, posterior probabilities $^p\gamma_i^k$, mixing coefficients π_k^p and covariance matrices Σ_k^p. FCM are themselves initialized with random cluster centers.

Coping with Missing Data. Since segmented structures may be close to the image boundaries, profiles are likely to be incomplete. In order to use those incomplete profiles in the classification, a valid dimension range $M_i \leq M$ is determined for each profile i. In the E-step, the term $\exp((\mathbf{x}_i^p)^T (\Sigma_k^p)^{-1} (\mathbf{x}_i^p))$ is only computed for the valid dimension range and multiplied by M/M_i. In the M-step, the mode means and covariance matrices are normalized by the total number of valid values for each index u of the profile ($1 \leq u \leq M$). FCM have also been extended in similar fashion to cope with incomplete data.

Covariance Matrix Regularization. The EM log-likelihood maximization may lead to local maxima or degeneracy. For profiles of dimension M (typically $M \approx 10$), degeneracy of covariance matrices Σ_k^p may occur due to the coarse sampling (typically $N \approx 4000$) of this high dimensional space. We propose 3 distinct methods to regularize Σ_k^p based on a regularization parameter h ($0 \leq h \leq 1$). The first one is based on *Spectral Regularization*. The covariance matrix is diagonalized $\Sigma_k^p = \mathbf{P}\mathbf{\Lambda}\mathbf{P}^T$ and the h lowest eigenvalues are set to 1% of the highest eigenvalue, thus leading to a new diagonal matrix $\hat{\mathbf{\Lambda}}_h$. The inverse is then computed as $^h(\Sigma_k^p)^{-1} = \mathbf{P}\hat{\mathbf{\Lambda}}_h^{-1}\mathbf{P}^T$. This can be seen as performing PCA and filtering the matrix by discarding high frequencies. In a second approach, *Diagonal Regularization*, the covariance matrix is regularized towards a diagonal matrix controlled by parameter h. The u, v element of matrix $^h\Sigma_k^p$: $^h(\Sigma_k^p)_{u,v} = (1-h)(\Sigma_k^p)_{u,v} + h\, \delta_{u,v}\, (\Sigma_k^p)_{u,v}$ ($\delta_{u,v}$ is the Kronecker symbol). The higher h, the more diagonal dominant the covariance matrix. This approach has been used in climate modeling to cope with missing

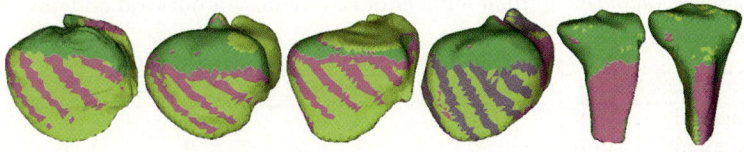

Fig. 2. EM classification of outward profiles performed on 4 livers and 2 tibias

values [4]. The last approach, *Constant Regularization*, regularizes the covariance matrix towards a constant matrix $\mathbf{Id}\ tr(\boldsymbol{\Sigma}_k^p)/M$ controlled by parameter h : $^h(\boldsymbol{\Sigma}_k^p) = (1-h)\ (\boldsymbol{\Sigma}_k^p) + h\ \mathbf{Id}\ tr(\boldsymbol{\Sigma}_k^p)/M$. With a high value of h, the covariance matrix converges towards a diagonal matrix with the same variance. The choice of a covariance matrix regularization method depends on the nature of the data. We have tested the three methods on profiles and we found that *Diagonal* or *Constant Regularization* method with $h = 0.9$ leads to the most intuitive classification results.

2.3 Model Order Selection

The objective of model order selection is to find the number of modes that best represents the data without any under or overfitting. To this end, we propose to estimate a criterion measuring the quality of EM classification for a given number of modes $\mathcal{K}$. We then keep the number of modes $\mathcal{K}_{opt}$ that maximizes (or minimizes) that criterion. Several criteria based on information theory have been proposed in the literature such as the Akaike Information Criterion (AIC) and the second-order AIC (AIC_c). The often preferred EM criterion is the Bayesian Information Criterion (BIC) [5]. We also investigated FCM criteria such as cluster validity indices [6] and the Fuzzy Vector Quantization [7].

In addition, we propose a new non parametric model order selection criterion called *Overlap Separation Index* (OSI) inspired by Kim *et al.* [6]. This criterion is solely based on the posterior probabilities $^p\gamma_i^k$ and penalizes the overlap between modes while encouraging their separation. More precisely, the criterion is computed as $OSI = \frac{C_1}{C_2}$. The first term C_1 sums the amount of overlap $2\ ^p\gamma_i^s/(^p\gamma_i^r + ^p\gamma_i^s)$ between the best two modes r and s for profile i (*i.e.* modes with the highest $^p\gamma_i^k$). The second term C_2 is the minimum separation between any pair of modes. The separation between pair of modes r and s is computed as the sum of $2\ ^p\gamma_i^s/(^p\gamma_i^r + ^p\gamma_i^s)$ for all profile i being classified to mode r and $2\ ^p\gamma_i^r/(^p\gamma_i^r + ^p\gamma_i^s)$ for all profile i being classified to mode s.

Table 1 shows the performance of the different model order selection criteria with varying regularization methods (spectral method has been discarded here). The number of modes being tested varies between 2 and 10, which takes around 15 minutes for a mesh with few thousand points. For outward profiles, the expected number of modes is at least 3 (air, bones, soft tissue) while for inward profiles 2 modes are expected (parenchyma and non-parenchyma). Based on Table 1 and further analysis on 6 other liver meshes, we found that *OSI* criterion

Table 1. Selection of the optimal number of EM modes for outward and inward profiles

Regularization	h	Outward profiles					Inward profiles				
		OSI	FVQ	AIC	AIC_c	BIC	OSI	FVQ	AIC	AIC_c	BIC
Diagonal	0.9	4	2	3	3	2	2	2	4	4	2
Diagonal	1.0	3	2	3	3	2	2	2	4	4	2
Constant	0.9	4	2	5	5	2	2	2	6	6	2
Constant	1.0	3	2	3	3	2	2	2	5	5	2

gave the most consistent results with a limited sensitivity to regularization methods and h parameter.

2.4 Spatial Regularization

EM does not take into account the neighborhood information of profiles. This leads to non smooth posterior probability maps $^p\gamma_i^k$, which impairs the fusion of appearance regions. To account for the connectivity between profiles, we use the Neighborhood EM algorithm (NEM) [8] since it nicely extends EM and leads to efficient computation (compared to Markov Random Field). NEM is an alternate optimization of the L functional :

$$\mathcal{L}(^p\gamma_i^k, \pi_k^p, \mu_k^p, \Sigma_k^p) = L(^p\gamma_i^k, \pi_k^p, \mu_k^p, \Sigma_k^p) + \beta \sum_{k=1}^{K}\sum_{i=1}^{N}\sum_{j=1}^{N} {}^p\gamma_i^k \, {}^p\gamma_j^k \, v_{ij} \quad (1)$$

$$L(^p\gamma_i^k, \pi_k^p, \mu_k^p, \Sigma_k^p) = \sum_{k=1}^{K}\sum_{i=1}^{N} {}^p\gamma_i^k \, \log(\pi_k^p G(\mathbf{x}_i^p|\mu_k^p, \Sigma_k^p)) - \sum_{k=1}^{K}\sum_{i=1}^{N} {}^p\gamma_i^k \log(^p\gamma_i^k)$$

where $G(\mathbf{x}_i^p|\mu_k^p, \Sigma_k^p))$ is the Gaussian probability density function.

The former term L leads to the classical EM [9] while the latter is a spatial regularization term controlled by β. The neighborhood parameter v_{ij} sets the amount of smoothing and is non-zero only if profile i is neighbor to profile j. $\mathcal{L}$ functional is minimized with an alternate optimization leading to a modified E-step where the posterior probabilities are iteratively estimated until a fixed point value is reached [8]. In our setup, profiles are extracted from 2-simplex meshes for which each vertex has only 3 neighbors [10]. Thus, v_{ij} has only three non-zero values, which substantially speeds-up the computation. In practice, less than 5 iterations are necessary to obtain stable posterior probabilities.

As neighborhood parameter v_{ij}, we choose the correlation coefficient between neighboring profiles i and j. With this choice, the spatial regularization of posterior probabilities is stronger between similar neighboring profiles, similarly to anisotropic diffusion in image processing. This prevents the blurring of tissue modes that would have occurred with a constant v_{ij} value.

The choice of the β parameter is an important issue and we set this parameter automatically by using an heuristic proposed by Dang [11]. It consists in using

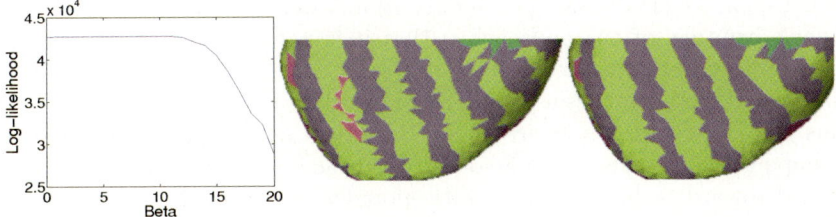

Fig. 3. $\mathcal{L}$ w.r.t β (left), liver before (middle) and after (right) NEM regularization

NEM with increasing values of β, and then detecting the β value above which the log-likelihood $\mathcal{L}$ sharply decreases (see left of Fig. 3). Indeed, too much spatial regularization leads to a significantly worse profile classification captured by the $\mathcal{L}$ functional. The proposed approach is a fully automatic way to spatially regularize posterior probabilities.

2.5 Fusion of Modes from P Meshes

The objective of this section is to merge the modes from the profile classification performed on P meshes into a single Multimodal Prior Appearance Model. This is done in two steps. The first step consists in comparing and merging the appearance regions extracted on the same structure for P different subjects. Profiles of each mesh $\mathcal{M}_p$ have been classified and lead to $\mathcal{K}_p$ modes ($\mathcal{K}_p$ may vary among meshes, e.g. due to the occurrence of pathologies). In order to have a meaningful comparison, an intensity normalization is required (e.g. to cope with the different nature or settings of the imaging systems). This may be done by histogram normalization or many other approaches proposed in the literature. With CT images, we found best not to perform any normalization.

In order to merge similar regions, we measure the similarity between any pair of modes $(\mu_k^p, \Sigma_k^p), (\mu_l^q, \Sigma_l^q)$ for $p \neq q$ by using the Jaccard index (ratio of the intersection of two sets over their union) of the region spanned by the mean and standard deviation $\mu_k^p \pm \sqrt{\sigma_k^p}$ where σ_k^p is the diagonal of the covariance matrix (see Fig. 4). A threshold $\mathcal{J}$ between 0 and 1 is used to decide whether two modes k and l are equivalent. Thus, we create a graph where nodes represent the modes and arcs link the modes found to be equivalent. The number of connected components of this graph is the number of independent modes $\mathcal{K}$. For connected components with only one node (i.e. without equivalence), modes are directly included in the prior with a new index m. For connected components having r equivalent nodes, we compute the mean of the new mode as the weighted sum of profile means μ_r^p with the weight $\sum_i^p \gamma_i^r$ while covariance matrices are recomputed. This computation leads to $\mathcal{K}$ independent modes $(\tilde{\mu}_m, \tilde{\Sigma}_m)$ and an equivalence table $\eta(p, m)$ establishing the new index m of mode k.

An alternative to this first step could be to perform an EM classification of all profiles for all P subjects with model order selection to find the optimal number of modes. This approach would lead to a more time consuming task, which would need to be performed each time a new dataset is added. Instead, we prefer to achieve a separate clustering of each dataset followed by a merging of all modes. Another advantage of our approach is that it is not biased by the variation of mesh resolution between datasets.

The second step provides a geometric embedding for the independent modes. To this end, we register non-rigidly all P meshes $\mathcal{M}^p$ towards the same reference shape with a coarse-to-fine deformable surface approach where each mesh is registered towards a binary image with globally-constrained deformations [10]. After defining a reference mesh $\mathcal{M}^\star$ on the reference shape, each posterior probability $^p\gamma_i^k$ is resampled on $\mathcal{M}^\star$ using a closest point approach. Finally, for each

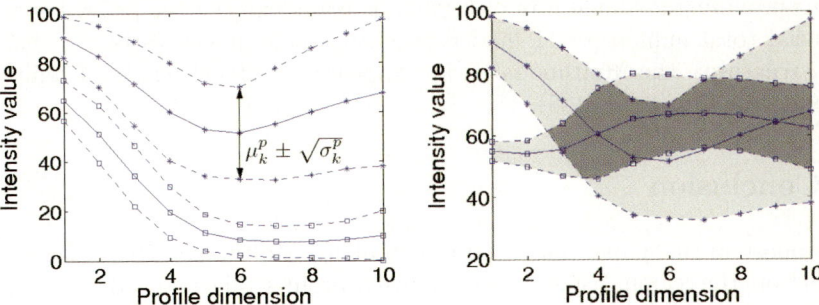

Fig. 4. Left: μ_k^p (solid lines) and $\sqrt{\sigma_k^p}$ (dashed lines) of 2 modes (asterisk and square) after EM classification of profiles (σ_k^p is the diagonal of $\boldsymbol{\Sigma}_k^p$). Right: Similarity between pairs of modes defined as the ratio of the intersection (dark gray) over the union (light gray) of their variance surface.

vertex i of $\mathcal{M}^\star$, we compute the posterior probability $\tilde{\gamma}_i^m$ by summing and normalizing the posterior probabilities associated to each mode : $\tilde{\gamma}_i^{\eta(p,m)} += {}^p\gamma_i^m$. In practice, this approach leads to sparse probabilities where only a few modes have non-zero posterior probabilities (as opposed to performing an E-step based on the mode means and covariances).

3 Results

We tested our method on 7 livers segmented from CT images and 4 tibias (cropped at knee level) segmented from MR images (see Fig. 2). For both structures, outward profiles (10 samples extracted every mm) were generated from meshes with $\approx$ 4000 vertices. As said before, EM classification using *Diagonal* or *Constant Regularization* with $h = 0.9$ leads to the most intuitive results. The optimal number of modes were estimated with the *OSI* criterion. NEM was launched $\approx$ 10 times to find the optimal β (see left of Fig. 3). For the livers, an initial total number of 24 modes leads to 14 new modes after the merging of profiles with $\mathcal{J} = 0.6$. With a lower $\mathcal{J} = 0.5$, the number of modes goes down to

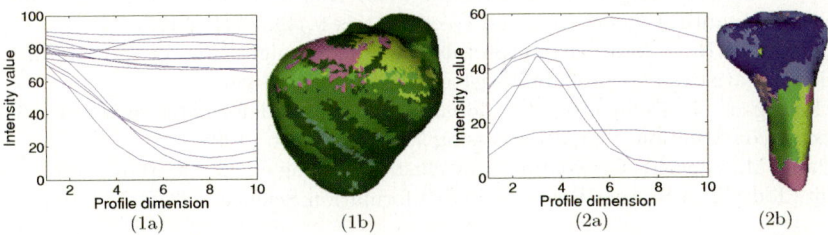

Fig. 5. Multimodal Prior Appearance Model for the livers (1) and tibias (2). For both structures, plot of the new mode means (a) and the new classification (b).

6, thus providing a simple way to taylor the complexity of the prior. For tibias, an initial total number of 11 modes leads to 6 new modes with $\mathcal{J} = 0.5$. For both structures, the Multimodal Prior Appearance Model has been built from these new modes (see Fig. 5).

4 Conclusion

We propose in this paper a method that builds a Multimodal Prior Appearance Model from the regional clustering of intensity profiles. The main advantage of our approach is that modes are built without requiring an accurate pointwise registration. Another advantage is that a meaningful prior may be built with very few datasets (in fact one dataset suffices), which makes it well suited for a bootstrapping strategy. Furthermore, the prior is multimodal therefore able to cope with large variation of appearances including pathologies. We have also introduced the *OSI* index and included spatial anisotropic regularization of EM classification. Future work will focus on the use of this prior in image segmentation.

Acknowledgments. This work is supported by the EU Marie Curie project 3D Anatomical Human (MRTN-CT-2006-035763).

References

1. Cootes, T., Taylor, C.: Using grey-level models to improve active shape model search. In: Proceedings of ICPRE, vol. 1, pp. 63–67 (1994)
2. Gilles, B.: Anatomical and kinematical modelling of the musculoskeletal system from MRI. Phd Thesis, University of Geneva (August 2007)
3. Heimann, T.: Statistical Shape Models for 3D Medical Image Segmentation. VDM Verlag Dr. Muller Aktiengesellschaft & Co., KG (2009)
4. Schneider, T.: Analysis of incomplete climate data. J. Clim. 14(5), 853–871 (2001)
5. Schwarz, G.: Estimating the dimension of a model. Ann. Stat. 6(2), 461–464 (1978)
6. Kim, D.W., Lee, K.H., Lee, D.: On cluster validity index for estimation of the optimal number of fuzzy clusters. Pattern Recognition 37, 2009–2025 (2004)
7. Saha, S., Bandyopadhyay, S.: A new cluster validity index based on fuzzy granulation-degranulation criterion. In: 15th ADCOM 2007, pp. 353–358 (2007)
8. Ambroise, C., Dang, M., Govaert, G.: Clustering of spatial data by the em algorithm. Quantitative Geology and Geostatistics 9, 493–504 (1997)
9. Hathaway, R.J.: Another interpretation of the em algorithm for mixture distributions. Statistics and probability letters 4(2), 53–56 (1986)
10. Montagnat, J., Delingette, H.: Globally constrained deformable models for 3D object reconstruction. Signal Processing 71(2), 173–186 (1998)
11. Dang, M., Govaert, G.: Spatial fuzzy clustering using em and markov random fields. Int. Journal of System Research and Information Science, 183–202 (1998)

3D Medical Image Segmentation by Multiple-Surface Active Volume Models

Tian Shen and Xiaolei Huang

Department of Computer Science and Engineering,
Lehigh University, Bethlehem, PA 18015, USA

Abstract. In this paper, we propose Multiple-Surface Active Volume Models (MSAVM) to extract 3D objects from volumetric medical images. Being able to incorporate spatial constraints among multiple objects, MSAVM is more robust and accurate than the original Active Volume Models [1]. The main novelty in MSAVM is that it has two surface-distance based functions to adaptively adjust the weights of contribution from the image-based region information and from spatial constraints among multiple interacting surfaces. These two functions help MSAVM not only overcome local minima but also avoid leakage. Because of the implicit representation of AVM, the spatial information can be calculated based on the model's signed distance transform map with very low extra computational cost. The MSAVM thus has the efficiency of the original 3D AVM but produces more accurate results. 3D segmentation results, validation and comparison are presented for experiments on volumetric medical images.

1 Introduction

Object boundary extraction is an important task in medical image analysis. A large variety of 2D algorithms have been proposed over the last few decades. 3D volumetric medical images are usually analyzed as a sequence of 2D image slices [2] due to concerns over the exponential increase in computational cost in 3D.

PDE-based segmentation methods became popular after Kass et al. proposed the Snakes [3]. Because local image gradient constraints in Snakes make the model sensitive to initialization and noise, Xu et al. proposed Gradient Vector Flow(GVF) [4], which increases the attraction range of the original Snakes. Region analysis strategies [2] have also been incorporated in PDE-based models to improve robustness to noise. Another class of deformable models is level set based geometric models [5]. This approach evolves the model based on the theory of curve evolution, with speed function specifically designed to incorporate image gradient information. Because level set models are topologically free and can be easily used in any dimension, they are widely used in tubular structure and 3D cortex segmentation tasks.

In noisy medical images, statistical modeling approaches such as ASM [6] and AAM [7] are adopted by adding constraints learned offline. Integrating high-level prior knowledge, these models deform in ways constrained by the training data and thus are often more robust in image interpretation. However, training data collection and landmark annotation are laborious in building statistical models, especially in 3D.

In many medical image applications, we are interested in extracting boundaries of several surfaces that are coupled in such a way that their relative positions are known and the distances between them are within a specific range. Clearly, integrating this high-level spatial constraint into the segmentation model will further improve accuracy and robustness. A 2D method [8] segments left ventricular Epi- and Endocardial borders using coupled active contours but needs a precise manual initialization. In 3D, Zeng et al. [9] incorporated spatial constraints about gray matter and white matter into the level set framework which greatly improved cortex segmentation accuracy. In [10], a graph-theoretic approach detects multiple interacting surfaces by transforming the problem into computing a minimum s-t cut. Deformation of multiple surfaces in [11] has intersurface proximity constraints which allow each surface to guide other surfaces into place. All of the three 3D methods [9,10,11] require manually specifying the expected thickness between surfaces as model-based constraint.

Active volume models (AVM) were recently proposed [1] to segment 3D objects directly from volumetric medical image dataset. Compared with active contours and ASM/AAM, the AVM is a "self-contained" generative object model that does not require off-line training. In this paper, we propose the Multiple-Surface AVMs to segment coupled medical objects simultaneously. Instead of setting up a fixed distance constraint during initialization, multiple-surface AVMs dynamically update the distance constraint between the interacting surfaces based on current model surfaces' spatial inter-relations. Integrating the distance constraint strategy with other energy terms based on image gradient and region information, 3D MSAVMs are more robust to initial positions and yield more accurate segmentation results.

2 Methodology

2.1 Review of 3D AVM and Boundary Prediction Module

An AVM is a deformable solid that minimizes internal and external energy. The internal constraint ensures the model has smooth boundary surface. The external constraints come from image data, prior, and/or user-defined features. Different from most of deformable models, one of the novel features of AVM is its unsupervised adaptive object boundary prediction scheme. The model alternates between two operations: deform according to the current object boundary prediction, and predict according to current appearance statistics of the model. Next we introduce the 3D AVM model representation and its boundary prediction module.

3D AVM [1] adopts a polyhedron mesh as the model representation which places vertices regularly on the model. More specifically, a 3D AVM is considered as an elastic solid and defined as a finite element triangulation Λ, which can be tetrahedron, octahedron or icosahedron. Using the finite element method (FEM), the internal energy function can be written compactly as:

$$E_{int} = \frac{1}{2} \int_\Lambda (\mathbf{B}\mathbf{v})^T D(\mathbf{B}\mathbf{v}) d\Lambda \qquad (1)$$

where $\mathbf{B}$ is the differential operator for the model vertices $\mathbf{v}$ and D is the stress matrix (or constitutive matrix).

External constraints from any sources can be accounted by probabilistic integration. Suppose we have n independent constraints from image information. Each constraint corresponds to a probabilistic boundary prediction module, and it generates a confidence-rated probability map to indicate the likelihood of a pixel being +1 (*object* class), or -1 (*non_object* class). The feature used in the kth constraint is f_k, $L(\mathbf{x})$ denotes the label of a pixel $\mathbf{x}$. AVM combines the multiple independent modules and applies the Bayes rule to evaluate the final confidence rate:

$$Pr(L(\mathbf{x})|f_1, f_2, ..., f_n) = (Pr(f_1, f_2, ..., f_n|L(\mathbf{x}))Pr(L(\mathbf{x}))/(Pr(f_1, f_2, ..., f_n)) \\ \propto Pr(f_1|L(\mathbf{x}))Pr(f_2|L(\mathbf{x}))...Pr(f_n|L(\mathbf{x}))Pr(L(\mathbf{x})) \qquad (2)$$

For each independent module, the probability $Pr(f_k|L(\mathbf{x}))$ is estimated based on the AVM's current statistics about feature f_k as well as the overall feature statistics in the image [1]. Once the posterior probabilities $Pr(L(\mathbf{x})|f_1, f_2, ..., f_n)$ are estimated, we apply the Bayesian decision rule to obtain a binary map P_B whose foreground represents the Region of Interest(ROI). That is, $P_B(\mathbf{x}) = 1$ (object pixel) if $Pr(L(\mathbf{x}) = +1|f_1, f_2, ..., f_n) \geq Pr(L(\mathbf{x}) = -1|f_1, f_2, ..., f_n)$, , and $P_B(\mathbf{x}) = 0$ otherwise. Let signed distance transform of the ROI shape be Φ_R. Combining Φ_R and Φ_M, a region-based external energy term is defined as:

$$E_R = \int_\Lambda E_R(\mathbf{v}) d\Lambda = \int_\Lambda \Phi_M(\mathbf{v}) \Phi_R(\mathbf{v}) d\Lambda \qquad (3)$$

The multiplicative term provides two-way balloon forces that deform the model toward the predicted ROI boundary.

The external energy of AVM also consists of a gradient term $E_g = -|\nabla I|^2$. Putting together internal and external energy terms, the overall energy function for AVM is defined as:

$$E = E_{int} + E_{ext} = E_{int} + (E_g + k_{reg} \cdot E_R) \qquad (4)$$

where k_{reg} is a constant that balances the contributions of the gradient term and the region term.

2.2 Multiple-Surface Active Volume Models

Due to limitations in medical imaging techniques, in some regions of an image, there may not be enough information (e.g. contrast) that can be derived from the image to clearly distinguish an object boundary or surface. Therefore, a single surface based deformable model may stop at local minima or leak to converge to an outer boundary. When spatial constraints between multiple surfaces are available, such information can help deform all interacting surfaces simultaneously with better accuracy, in a multiple surface based model framework.

The Multiple-Surface AVM we propose is initialized as several AVMs inside an outer AVM. Let i, j be the surface indices, the mean Euclidean distance value of the ith surface, M_i, from other surfaces is defined as:

$$\overline{dist}_i = \frac{\int_\Lambda dist_v d\Lambda}{\int_\Lambda d\Lambda}, \text{ where } dist_v = \{d|d = min(|\Phi_{M_j}(\mathbf{v})|), \forall j, j \neq i\} \quad (5)$$

Φ_{M_j} is the signed distance transform of the jth surface, M_j.

To deform the multiple surfaces simultaneously with adaptive spatial constraints, we construct two distance-related Gaussian Mixtures (GM) functions to modulate the external force at each vertex. For a vertex v on the ith surface, its minimum distance value to all other surfaces $dist_v$ can be calculated based on Eq. (5). Then the GM distance functions at this vertex are defined in Eq. 6 and illustrated in Figure 1.

$$\begin{aligned} g_D(dist_v) &= (1+\alpha) - e^{-(dist_v - \overline{dist}_i)^2 / 2\sigma_1^2} - \alpha e^{-(dist_v - \overline{dist}_i)^2 / 2\sigma_2^2} \\ g_R(dist_v) &= e^{-(dist_v - \overline{dist}_i)^2 / 2\sigma_1^2} + \alpha e^{-(dist_v - \overline{dist}_i)^2 / 2\sigma_2^2} \end{aligned} \quad (6)$$

where $\alpha \in (0,1)$ is the GM weighting parameter, σ_1 and σ_2 ($\sigma_1 < \sigma_2$) are the standard deviations of the two Gaussians.

Then the overall energy function of MSAVM is defined as:

$$E = E_{int} + \int_\Lambda (E_g(\mathbf{v}) + g_R(dist_v) \cdot E_R(\mathbf{v}) + g_D(dist_v) \cdot E_{dist_v}) \quad (7)$$

where $E_{dist_v} = dist_v$ is the energy term enforcing the distance constraint.

According to $g_R(dist_v)$ and $g_D(dist_v)$ (Fig. 1(a-b)), if $dist_v$ is close to the surface's mean distance (from other surfaces), $\overline{dist}_i$, then the region term $E_R(\mathbf{v})$ makes more contribution toward the surface's local deformation near v; conversely, if $dist_v$ is far away from $\overline{dist}_i$, which means the local surface near the vertex may be stuck at local minima or have a leakage, the distance constraint, E_{dist_v}, is given more power to deform the surface and guide it into place.

Different from the distance constraint function in [9], which only works well in the case of brain segmentation since the cortical layer has a nearly constant thickness, MSAVM adopts the above $g_R(dist)$ and $g_D(dist)$ functions to adaptively balance the contributions of region term and spatial constraint term. MSAVM thus has broader applications. It not only can be used for brain segmentation, but also has very good performance in extracting ventricles from heart and lungs from the thorax even though distances between these coupled ventricular surfaces vary greatly. Figure 1c and 1d show two segmentation results by distance-color (DC) mapping the spatial distance information into color space.

Instead of setting the spatial constraint manually or empirically, we update $\overline{dist}$ based on the spatial relationship among current model surfaces. After getting $\overline{dist}$, we shift $g_R(dist)$ and $g_D(dist)$ functions accordingly to make sure

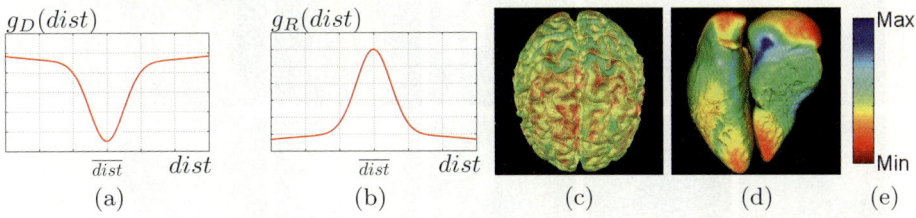

Fig. 1. (a)(b) Functions to balance the contributions of region term and spatial constraint term, (c)DC mapping of brain gray matter segmentation; the range for distance between Gray and white matters is 2∼15 voxels, (d)DC mapping of heart segmentation; the distance range is 2∼25 voxels, (e)the color bar used to map the spatial information.

the new $\overline{dist}$ still corresponds to the extrema of these functions. This unsupervised learning strategy, both for multiple surface spatial constraint and for region appearance statistics, allows MSAVM to have flexible initialization and fast convergence.

2.3 The Model's Deformation

Minimization of the MSAVM's energy function can be achieved by solving several independent linear systems. For the ith surface,

$$A_{3D} \cdot V_i = L_{V_i}; \qquad (8)$$

where A_{3D} is the stiffness matrix derived from Eq. 1. V_i is the vector of vertices on the ith surface. L_{V_i} is the corresponding external force vector. Using the finite differences method [12], we adopt the following steps to deform the MSAVM to match the desired object surfaces.

1. Initialize the MSAVM, stiffness matrix A_{3D} and $\overline{dist}$ for each surface.
2. For each surface, compute Φ_M based on the current model; predict R and compute Φ_R; and update $\overline{dist}$ based on Eq. (5) and shift $g_R(dist_v)$ and $g_D(dist_v)$ according to $\overline{dist}$.
3. Deform MSAVM according to Eq. 8.
4. Adaptively decrease the degree of surface stiffness/smoothness.
5. Repeat steps 2-4 until convergence.

3 Experimental Results

We applied MSAVM to segmenting various organ surfaces in volumetric medical images. First, we put the model into a thorax CT stack to segment the lungs. The model was initialized as one outer ellipsoid around the thorax and two inside ellipsoids whose long axes are perpendicular to the axial image plane. Figure 2 shows the 3D DC mapping images during deformation. A 2D coronal projection view is also included in 2f to show the initial model and converged result.

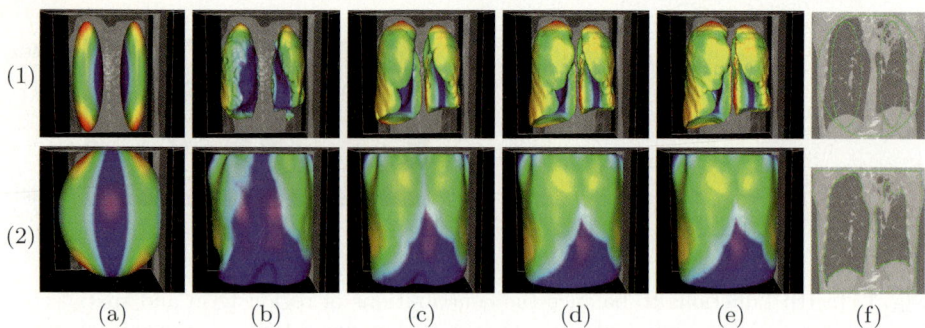

Fig. 2. DC mapping of lung surfaces segmentation using MSAVM, the distance range is 3-45 voxels. (1)(a)-(e)deformation progress of inner surfaces, (2)(a)-(e)outer surface; (a)Initial model after (b)3, (c)9, (d)21, (e)26(converged result) iterations; (1)(f)initial model in a 2D slice, (2)(f)converged result in a 2D slice.

Then we experimented with the model on segmenting heart surfaces in a cardiac CT stack. The MSAVM model is initialized as three ellipsoids: one for epicardial surface of the myocardium, one for endocardial surface of the left ventrile, and a third one for endocardial surface of the right ventricle. Some boundary condition is also specified so that the model does not deform beyond the top and bottom slices. Figure 3 and Figure 4 show the deformation steps of the heart from two 3D viewpoints. 2D sagittal and coronal projection views are also provided in Figure 3f and Figure 4f. Due to intensity inhomogeneity caused by papillary muscles inside the left ventricle, it would be difficult for a single surface deformable model to reach the desired boundary without supervised learning priors. However, deforming according to the on-line predicted object boundary with spatial constraints, MSAVM can overcome the inhomogeneity problem and extract accurately the multiple cardiac surfaces.

Table 1 shows the running times and quantitative evaluation of *sensitivity* (P), *specificity* (Q) and *dice similarity coefficient* (DSC) on a PC workstation with Intel Duo Core 3GHz E6850 processor. Compared with the 3D AVM

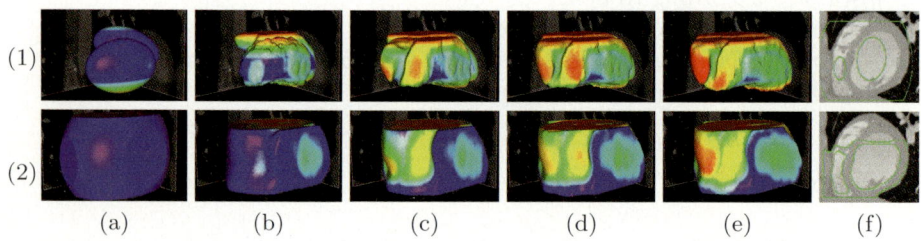

Fig. 3. DC mapping of heart segmentation using MSAVM viewed from the right, the distance range is 2-25 voxels, (1)(a)-(e)deformation progress of inner surfaces, (2)(a)-(e)DC mapping for outer surface; (a)Initial model after (b)3, (c)9, (d)21, (e)27(converged result) iterations; (1)(f)initial model in a 2D slice, (2)(f)converged result in a 2D slice

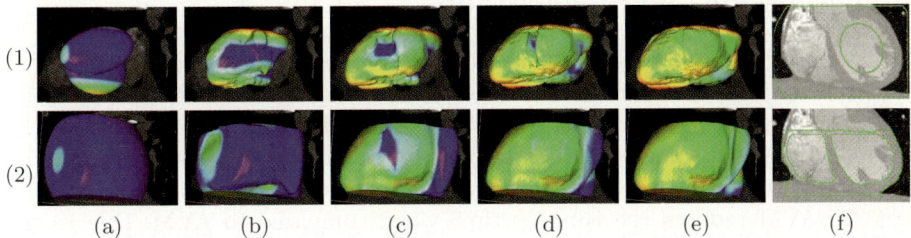

Fig. 4. DC mapping of heart segmentation using MSAVM viewed from the left, the distance range is 2-25 voxels, (1)(a)-(e)deformation progress of inner surfaces, (2)(a)-(e)outer surface; (a)Initial model after (b)3, (c)9, (d)21, (e)27(converged result) iterations; (1)(f)initial model in a 2D slice, (2)(f)converged result in a 2D slice

Table 1. Quantitative evaluation and performance comparison

	MSAVM					3D AVM				
	P	Q	DSC	Iterations	Time	P	Q	DSC	Iterations	Time
Lung in Fig. 2	95.5	99.8	96.2	26	870s	92.3	99.8	94.6	33	1000s
Heart in Fig. 3	92.0	99.0	92.2	27	1535s	90.7	98.9	91.1	39	2023s

without spatial constraint, MSAVM improved segmentation results in all the cases. Even though MSAVM needs extra time to calculate the spatial distances among surfaces, it has faster convergence so MSAVM is actually faster than 3D AVM.

To demonstrate the MSAVM more clearly, we put a set of 2D axial projection slices from a case of 3D heart segmentation in Figure 5, and compare them with the converged result of original 3D AVM using the same initialization in Figure 5f. Due to intensity inhomogeneity inside the inner surfaces and obscure boundary of the outer surface, original 3D AVM either leaks to the outer-most (e.g. outer surface) or stops at local minima (e.g. left ventricle). However, deforming under the spatial constraints, MSAVM can avoid such leakage and overcome the local minima to find the desired object boundary.

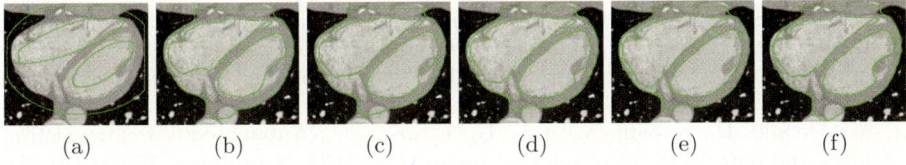

Fig. 5. Heart segmentation progress in a 2D slice projection. (a)Initial MSAVM, after (b)9, (c)15, (d)21, (e)29(converged result) iterations, (f)converged result of three separate AVMs after 36 iterations.

4 Discussions and Conclusion

In this paper, we proposed Multiple-Surface Active Volume Models to segment 3D objects in volumetric medical images. Combining high-level spatial information with predicted ROI region, MSAVM achieves better performance than the original 3D AVM. Because of the implicit representation of AVM, the spatial distance constraints can be obtained with very low extra computational cost. In fact, MSAVM reduces the running time when compared to AVM. Due to the local smoothness of simplex-mesh, it is still hard for the model to reach some tip locations (e.g., top-right tip of the right ventricle in figure 5). As future work we plan to address this problem by reparameterizing the model near tips since vertices in these areas tend to be sparser than those distributed on the main body.

References

1. Shen, T., Li, H., Qian, Z., Huang, X.: Active volume models for 3d medical image segmentation. In: IEEE Conference on Computer Vision and Pattern Recognition, CVPR 2009, pp. 1–8 (2009)
2. Shen, T., Zhu, Y., Huang, X., Huang, J., Metaxas, D., Axel, L.: Active volume models with probabilistic object boundary prediction module. In: Metaxas, D., Axel, L., Fichtinger, G., Székely, G. (eds.) MICCAI 2008, Part I. LNCS, vol. 5241, pp. 331–341. Springer, Heidelberg (2008)
3. Kass, M., Witkin, A., Terzopoulos, D.: Snakes: Active contour models. Int'l Journal on Computer Vision 1, 321–331 (1987)
4. Xu, C., Prince, J.: Snakes, shapes and gradient vector flow. IEEE Trans. on Image Processing 7, 359–369 (1998)
5. Malladi, R., Sethian, J., Vemuri, B.: Shape modeling with front propagation: A level set approach. IEEE Trans. on Pattern Analysis and Machine Intelligence 17(2), 158–175 (1995)
6. Cootes, T., Taylor, C., Cooper, D., Graham, J.: Active shape model - their training and application. Computer Vision and Image Understanding 61, 38–59 (1995)
7. Cootes, T., Edwards, G., Taylar, C.: Active appearance models. In: Proc. of European Conf. on Computer Vision, vol. 2, pp. 484–498 (1998)
8. Spreeuwers, L., Breeuwer, M.: Detection of left ventricular epi- and endocardial borders using coupled active contours. Computer Assisted Radiology and Surgery, 1147–1152 (2003)
9. Zeng, X., Staib, L., Schultz, R., Duncan, J.: Segmentation and measurement of the cortex from 3-d MR images using coupled-surfaces propagation. IEEE Transactions on Medical Imaging 18, 927–937 (1999)
10. Li, K., Wu, X., Chen, D., Sonka, M.: Optimal surface segmentation in volumetric images-a graph-theoretic approach. IEEE Transactions on Pattern Analysis and Machine Intelligence 28(1), 119–134 (2006)
11. MacDonald, D., Kabani, N., Avis, D., Evans, A.C.: Automated 3-d extraction of inner and outer surfaces of cerebral cortex from MRI. NeuroImage 12(3), 340–356 (2000)
12. Cohen, L., Cohen, I.: Finite-element methods for active contour models and balloons for 2-D and 3-D images. IEEE Trans. on Pattern Analysis and Machine Intelligence 15, 1131–1147 (1993)

Model Completion via Deformation Cloning Based on an Explicit Global Deformation Model*

Qiong Han[1], Stephen E. Strup[2], Melody C. Carswell[1], Duncan Clarke[1], and Williams B. Seales[1]

[1] Center for Visualization and Virtual Environments, University of Kentucky, USA
[2] Division of Urology, Department of Surgery, University of Kentucky, USA
qhan@engr.uky.edu

Abstract. Our main focus is the registration and visualization of a pre-built 3D model from preoperative images to the camera view of a minimally invasive surgery (MIS). Accurate estimation of soft-tissue deformations is key to the success of such a registration. This paper proposes an explicit statistical model to represent global non-rigid deformations. The deformation model built from a reference object is cloned to a target object to guide the registration of the pre-built model, which completes the deformed target object when only a part of the object is naturally visible in the camera view. The registered target model is then used to estimate deformations of its substructures. Our method requires a small number of landmarks to be reconstructed from the camera view. The registration is driven by a small set of parameters, making it suitable for real-time visualization.

1 Introduction

The distinct advantage of minimally invasive surgery (MIS) is that it induces less trauma to patients. Preoperative images reveal important substructures of target objects, which are unfortunately not visible under a laparoscopic camera view. Incorporating preoperative images into MIS is thus focused by many researchers. Among different approaches, reconstructing 3D points from a camera video sequence and registering a pre-built 3D model to the reconstructed 3D points has the strength of converting the 3D-to-2D registration to a 3D-to-3D registration.

Devernay et al. proposed a 5 step method for augmented reality of cardiac MIS [1]. [2] uses stereo images to reconstruct dense depth cues of surgical scenes. [3] fused stereo depth cues with monocular depth cues based on surface shading. Stereo based methods in general require repeatable tracking of a large number of feature points in order to reconstruct a dense set of surface points. Structure from motion (SFM) method is also adapted to MIS, and Hu et al. used a Competitive

---

* We thank the Medical Image Display & Analysis Group (MIDAG) at UNC-Chapel Hill for providing the kidney data and source codes. This work was done with support from U.S. Army grant W81XWH-06-1-0761.

Evolutionary Agent-based (CEA) method to deal with the missing data problem in SFM [4].

Statistical models of deformations and motions have also been proposed. In [5], a statistical deformation model is built from simulated finite element model (FEM) deformations of the prostate. However, proper tissue property parameters are difficult to determine for FEM simulations. [6] explicitly included material properties in their FEM simulations and built a statistical motion model to guide the deformation estimation of the prostate. [7] proposed an explicit 1D motion model to represent and compensate the motion of the mitral valve annulus.

Our driving clinical applications are laparoscopic cryoablation and laparoscopic partial nephrectomy on small renal tumors. 3D visualization of a kidney and its tumor is expected to increase the positioning accuracy of the tumor. Furthermore, surgical plans based on the same preoperative scans, from which the 3D model is built, can be visualized in real time to improve the precision of needle insertion for cryoablation or of incision site and depth for partial nephrectomy. The challenge is that there are always non-rigid intra-object deformations between the kidney in the CT scans and the kidney during an MIS. This paper proposes an explicit global deformation model, which is statistically built from a reference object and its deformed shapes. Furthermore, training data to learn a deformation model is sometimes difficult to acquire. Therefore, we propose to *clone* a learned deformation model to a new target object to guide the registration of the target object into the camera view, based on a small number of landmarks reconstructed from a camera video sequence.

Next section details our proposed method by its main steps. Section 3 describes the evaluation of the proposed method and shows the results. Section 4 concludes the paper with discussions.

2 Method

Our method takes a 5-step process shown as follows and detailed in the following subsections.

1. Build a statistical deformation model from a reference object and its deformed shapes;
2. Build a 3D model of a target object from the pre-operative computed-tomography (CT) scans;
3. Capture a video sequence of the exposed target object with a calibrated laparoscopic camera, and reconstruct 3D landmarks of the target object using the SFM method;
4. Clone the statistical deformation model to the target object model to register the target model to the reconstructed 3D landmarks;
5. Apply the deformation of the registered target object to its substructures.

2.1 A Statistical Deformation Model

The *discrete m-rep* [8] is chosen as the shape model because of its unique property of modeling and parameterizing both the surface and the interior volume of an object. A discrete m-rep $\mathbf{M}$ consists of a quad-mesh of n_M medial atoms $\{\mathbf{m}_i, i = 1, 2, ..., n_M\}$. Each internal atom $\mathbf{m}_i$ has a hub position $\mathbf{p}_i$, two spokes $\mathbf{S}_i^{+1,-1}$ with a radius r_i and direction $\mathbf{U}_i^{+1,-1}$. Atoms at the edge of the quad-mesh are treated differently. For simplicity, all medial atoms are considered the same in this paper.

To learn a statistical deformation model based on m-reps, a series of deformed shapes of a reference object are captured either by a set of CT scans or by a series 3D reconstructed meshes. This paper uses the latter. An m-rep is fitted to each mesh to form a training set of m-reps. Principal geodesic analysis (PGA) [9] is applied to the training set of m-reps to form a statistical deformation model, given as a Frechét mean $\overline{\mathbf{M}}$, the first n_{PGA} principal geodesic directions $\mathbf{v}_j, j = 1, 2, ..., n_{PGA}$, representing more than 95% of the total deformation variations, and the corresponding variances λ_j of the principal geodesic directions.

Now given a set of principal geodesic components $c_j \in \mathbb{R}, j = 1, 2, ..., n_{PGA}$, a deformed reference object $\mathbf{M}_{PGA}$ can be reconstructed from $\overline{\mathbf{M}}$ and a tangent vector $\sum_{j=1}^{n_{PGA}} c_j \mathbf{v}_j$ via the *exponential map* [9]. The deformation between $\mathbf{M}_{PGA}$ and $\overline{\mathbf{M}}$ can be represented by the *residue* between the two m-reps [10], which is defined as the set of residues between all corresponding atom pairs $(\mathbf{m}_{PGA,i}, \overline{\mathbf{m}}_i)$.

Each medial atom is an element of a Riemannian symmetric space $\mathcal{G} = \mathbb{R}^3 \times \mathbb{R}^+ \times \mathcal{S}^2 \times \mathcal{S}^2$. The following operator defines the difference between a pair of atoms $(\mathbf{m}_{PGA,i}, \overline{\mathbf{m}}_i)$:

$$\mathbf{m}_{PGA,i} \ominus \overline{\mathbf{m}}_i = (\mathbf{p}_{PGA,i} - \overline{\mathbf{p}}_i, \frac{r_{PGA,i}}{r_i}, \mathbf{R}_{\mathbf{S}_{PGA,i}^{+1}}(\overline{\mathbf{S}}_i^{+1}), \mathbf{R}_{\mathbf{S}_{PGA,i}^{-1}}(\overline{\mathbf{S}}_i^{-1})) \quad (1)$$

where for any $\mathbf{w} = (w_1, w_2, w_3) \in \mathcal{S}^2$, $\mathbf{R}_\mathbf{w} \in \mathcal{SO}(3)$ is the rotation around the axis passing the origin $(0, 0, 0)$ and $(w_2, -w_1, 0)$ with the rotation angle being the geodesic distance between a chosen point $\mathbf{p}_0 = (0, 0, 1)$ and $\mathbf{w}$ on the unit sphere. Let $\Delta \mathbf{m}_i = \mathbf{m}_{PGA,i} \ominus \overline{\mathbf{m}}_i$. $\Delta \mathbf{m}_i$ is also an element of $\mathcal{G}$, and it is called the residue of $\mathbf{m}_{PGA,i}$ to $\overline{\mathbf{m}}_i$, which records the deformation of $\mathbf{m}_{PGA,i}$ relative to $\overline{\mathbf{m}}_i$'s coordinates.

The residue, i.e., the deformation, between a pair of atoms can then be cloned to a new atom via an operator $\oplus$:

$$\mathbf{m}_i \oplus \Delta \mathbf{m}_i = (\mathbf{p}_i + \Delta \mathbf{p}_i, r_i \Delta r_i, \mathbf{R}_{\mathbf{S}_i^{+1}}^{-1}(\Delta \mathbf{S}_i^{+1}), \mathbf{R}_{\mathbf{S}_i^{-1}}^{-1}(\Delta \mathbf{S}_i^{-1})) \quad (2)$$

where $\mathbf{R}_\mathbf{w}^{-1} \in \mathcal{SO}(3)$ is the inverse rotation of $\mathbf{R}_\mathbf{w}$.

Based on operators $\ominus$ and $\oplus$, the residue $\Delta \mathbf{M}$ between two m-reps $\mathbf{M}_{PGA}$ and $\overline{\mathbf{M}}$ and the deformation cloning of $\Delta \mathbf{M}$ to a target m-rep $\mathbf{M}_t$ are defined as follows:

$$\Delta \mathbf{M} = \mathbf{M}_{PGA} \ominus \overline{\mathbf{M}} = \{\Delta \mathbf{m}_i, i = 1, 2, ..., n_M\}, \quad (3)$$
$$\mathbf{M}_{deformed,t} = \mathbf{M}_t \oplus \Delta \mathbf{M} = \{\mathbf{m}_{t,i} \oplus \Delta \mathbf{m}_i, i = 1, 2, ..., n_M\}. \quad (4)$$

$\Delta \mathbf{M}$ is the explicit statistical deformation model learned from the reference object, which is a function of the principal geodesic components $\{c_j\}$.

2.2 A Pre-built 3D Model for the Target Object

The 3D m-rep model $\mathbf{M}_t$ is built from a manual segmentation of pre-operative CT scans of the target object by experts, and an m-rep is fitted into the segmentation using the binary fitting method described in [11]. An automatic segmentation tool will be highly desirable for this step.

2.3 Reconstruction of 3D Landmarks

Using the structure from motion (SFM) method, a dense set of object surface points $\mathbf{L}_{all} = \{\mathbf{l}_k, k = 1, 2, ..., N_{L_{all}}\}$ are reconstructed from a laparoscopic video sequence of the target object. A small subset of $\mathbf{L}_{all}$ are identified as a set of 6 to 9 anatomical landmarks $\mathbf{L} = \{\mathbf{l}_k, k = 1, 2, ..., n_L\}$. At the same time, an initial correspondence is established between the set of landmarks $\mathbf{L}$ and a set of surface points on the m-rep $\mathbf{M}_t$. This correspondence will, however, be automatically updated in the registration step whenever necessary, via the iterative closest point (ICP) method [12].

In order to get a robust reconstruction of the landmarks, fiducial markers can be used because of the small size of the landmark set. Although this step is not the main focus of this paper, the accuracy of the 3D reconstruction is crucial to the consequent steps. The effect of reconstruction errors on the registration step are evaluated in section 3.

2.4 Model Registration via Deformation Cloning

By cloning $\Delta \mathbf{M}$ to a target m-rep $\mathbf{M}_t$, we transfer the deformation learned from the reference object to the target object. As a result, we have a specific deformation model for the target object. An alignment step is required to properly clone a deformation to the target object. The alignment is described first, followed by a full description of the registration step.

Alignment step: in order to properly apply a deformation residue $\Delta \mathbf{M}(\{c_j\})$ to $\mathbf{M}_t$, $\mathbf{M}_t$ must be aligned to the mean reference object $\overline{\mathbf{M}}$ via a similarity transformation $\mathbf{T}_{sim} = \{\mathbf{p}_{sim} \in \mathbb{R}^3, r_{sim} \in \mathbb{R}^+, \mathbf{R}_{sim} \in \mathcal{SO}(3)\}$: $\mathbf{T}_{sim} = \arg\min_{\mathbf{T}} dis^2_{geodesic}(\mathbf{T}(\mathbf{M}_t), \overline{\mathbf{M}})$, where $dis^2_{geodesic}(\mathbf{M}_1, \mathbf{M}_2)$ is the squared geodesic distance between two m-reps $\mathbf{M}_1$ and $\mathbf{M}_2$ [9].

Let $\mathbf{M}_t^{aligned} = \mathbf{T}_{sim}(\mathbf{M}_t)$. A deformed target object with cloned deformation $\Delta \mathbf{M}$ is defined as $\mathbf{M}_{deformed,t} = \mathbf{M}_t^{aligned} \oplus \frac{\Delta \mathbf{M}}{r_{sim}}$, where r_{sim} is the scaling factor in $\mathbf{T}_{sim}$, and where $\frac{\Delta \mathbf{M}}{r_{sim}} = \{\frac{\Delta \mathbf{m}_i}{r_{sim}}\}$. $\frac{\Delta \mathbf{m}_i}{r_{sim}}$ means each $\Delta \mathbf{p}_i \in \mathbf{m}_i$ is replaced by $\frac{\Delta \mathbf{p}_i}{r_{sim}}$ because the translation component in an m-rep atom deformation is scale-dependent, but the scaling and rotational components are scale-independent.

$\mathbf{M}_{deformed,t}$ is then registered (fitted) to the set of reconstructed landmarks $\mathbf{L} = \{\mathbf{l}_k, k = 1, 2, ..., n_L\}$. For each $\mathbf{l}_k$, there is a corresponding surface point $\mathbf{f}_k$ on the implied surface of $\mathbf{M}_t$. The fitting is implemented by minimizing an objective function:

$$\mathbf{M}'_t = \arg\min_{\mathbf{T}_{rigid}, \mathbf{M}_{deformed,t}} F(\mathbf{T}_{rigid}(\mathbf{M}_{deformed,t}(\{c_j, j = 1, 2, ..., n_{PGA}\}))) \quad (5)$$

where $F(\mathbf{M}'_t)$ has three components as $F(\mathbf{M}'_t) = t_1 F_{fit}(\mathbf{M}'_t) + t_2 F_{maha}(\mathbf{M}'_t) + (1 - t_1 - t_2) F_{leg}(\mathbf{M}'_t)$, with t_1, t_2, and $t_1 + t_2 \in (0, 1)$ as two tuning parameters: $F_{fit} = \Sigma_{k=1}^{n_L} (\frac{dis(\mathbf{f}_k(\mathbf{M}'_t), \mathbf{l}_k)}{r_{mean}})^2$ measures the fitting quality of the model to the set of landmarks by the Euclidean distance function dis and the geometric mean of the radii of all medial atoms r_{mean}; $F_{maha} = \Sigma_{i=1}^{n_{PGA}} (\frac{c_j}{\lambda_j})^2$ is the squared Mahalanobis distance between the current m-rep $\mathbf{M}'_t$ and the m-rep $\mathbf{M}_t^{aligned}$ without deformations, penalizing big deformations of $\mathbf{M}'_t$; $F_{leg} = \Sigma_{i=1} n_M f_{leg}(\mathbf{m}'_{t,i})$, where $\mathbf{m}'_{t,i}$ is a medial atom in $\mathbf{M}'_t$, and where f_{leg} is the illegality penalty term defined by equation (12) in [11]. This component penalizes shape illegalities, such as creasing or folding.

The overall algorithm is shown as follows:

1. Initialize $\{c_j\}$ to $\{0\}$, and calculate an initial alignment $\mathbf{T}_{rigid}$ to minimize $F(\mathbf{M}_t^{aligned})$;
2. Optimize $F(\mathbf{M}'_t)$ over $\{c_j\}$ and $\mathbf{T}_{rigid}$ via the conjugate gradient method until the objective function converges. Because of the compactness of the deformation model, n_{PGA} is usually smaller than 5, and the optimization usually converges within 30-40 sub-steps;
3. If $F_{fit}(\mathbf{M}'_t)$ is bigger than an empirically set threshold ε, an iteration of ICP is used to re-establish the correspondence between $\mathbf{M}'_t$ and the landmark set $\mathbf{L}$, and go back to step 2.

Step 3 is often not necessary if the initial correspondence between the small set of reconstructed landmarks L and the target m-rep is good. For majority of the testing cases, to be shown in next section, one iteration of the optimization of the objective function $F(\mathbf{M}'_t)$ is sufficient. However, by updating an initial correspondence that is of poor quality, the overall algorithm is more robust to correspondence errors.

2.5 Deformation Propagation to Substructures

The target models before and after the registration are used to imply a deformation field for the interior and the adjacent exterior volume of the target object. The deformation field is propagated to the substructure volume, voxel by voxel. Because of the enforced legality of the deformed $\mathbf{M}'$ by the component F_{leg}, the volumetric legalities of both the models, before and after the registration, are guaranteed. Therefore, the implied deformation field is guaranteed to be legal. Next section evaluates the proposed method.

3 Result

In order to evaluate the proposed method, a set of kidney models with synthetic deformations is generated. Synthetic data provide the ground truth to better evaluate our method. Also, the impact of reconstruction errors by the SFM method is studied. One set of *in vivo* data is also used to test our method.

The rationale of using synthetic deformations is that the types of deformations a kidney undergoes during an MIS can be well described and modeled by experienced surgeons so it is a reasonable approximation to population deformations. However, our method can be applied to dynamic CT or range data sets to learn arguably more realistic organ deformations.

3.1 Generating Synthetic Testing Data

There are two parts of data generations:

- Generation of the statistical deformation models: 20 kidney m-reps $\mathbf{M}_{kid,i}$, $i \in [1, 20]$ from different patients are used. A series of simulated deformations are applied to each kidney m-rep. Each kidney m-rep and its deformed shapes are used to build a statistical deformation model $\Delta \mathbf{M}_{kid,i}(\{c_j\})$ of the reference m-rep $\overline{\mathbf{M}}_{kid,i}$. Each statistical deformation model is then used to guide the registration of all the other 19 kidneys. In total there are 20×19 registration results. A tumor m-rep is also added to each kidney m-rep.
- Generation of video sequences for SFM reconstructions: a diffeomorphic deformation, independent from the deformations used to generate the statistical deformation models, is applied to the m-rep implied surface meshes of the kidney and tumor.

  A kidney texture image, stitched from an *in vivo* video, is used as the texture for each deformed kidney mesh $\mathbf{Mesh}_{kid,i}$. Using the parameters of a calibrated Stryker laparoscope, a series of 15 images $\mathbf{I}_i$ are generated at the resolution of 640×480 to cover about half of each kidney surface, assuming no deformations among these image frames. A set of 100 surface points are randomly selected as the ground truth reconstructed surface points $\mathbf{L}_{truth,all,i}$. 6 to 9 landmarks of anatomical significance are selected from each mesh as the set $\mathbf{L}_{truth,i}$. Initial correspondence between $\mathbf{L}_{truth,i}$ and the m-rep $\mathbf{M}_i$ is also automatically established.

3.2 Experimental Results from Synthetic Data

Guided by the statistical deformation model learned from the reference kidney $\mathbf{M}_i \in [1, 20]$, each m-rep $\mathbf{M}_j, j \neq i$ was registered into its video sequence $\mathbf{I}_j$ to acquire the registered m-rep $\mathbf{M}'_{i,j}$. Each $\mathbf{M}'_{j,i}$ was compared to the ground truth landmark points $\mathbf{L}_{truth,j}$ to calculate the average point-to-point distance (APD), and $\mathbf{M}'_{j,i}$ was also compared to each ground truth mesh $\mathbf{Mesh}_{kid,j}$ to calculate the average surface distance (ASD) Each $\mathbf{M}'_{j,i}$ was then used to estimate and apply propagation deformations to its tumor model. The deformed tumor model was compared to the ground truth tumor mesh $\mathbf{Mesh}_{tumor,j}$ to calculate the ASD. A deformation model and 3 testing kidney models are shown in figure 1.

All the experiments were conducted with different levels of Gaussian noise added to the reconstructed surface points $\mathbf{L}_{all,j}$: the standard deviations are 1, 3, and 5 voxels. The size of 1 voxel is approximately $0.78mm$. The average experimental results are shown in table 1. The deformation propagation errors of the tumor are

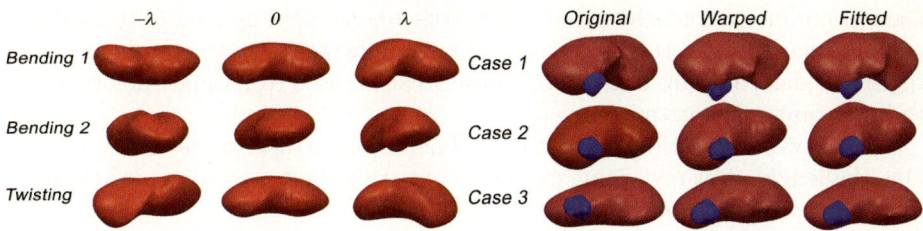

Fig. 1. Left: 3 main modes of a deformation model: each row shows one mode from $-\lambda$, 0, to λ; Right: 3 testing kidney m-reps, from left to right: the original target kidney m-rep $\mathbf{M}_i$ (in red), the ground truth surface mesh of the kidney and tumor (in blue) reconstructed from warped object volume, and the registered m-rep $\mathbf{M}'$ with the deformation applied to its attached tumor model

Table 1. All units are in voxels, with the size of $0.78mm$, except the number of iterations

STD of Noise	Kidney Avg. APD	Kidney Avg. ASD	Tumor Avg. ASD	Avg. Number of Iterations	Kidney Avg. ASD Without ICP
1	0.57 ± 0.88	0.75 ± 0.65	1.38 ± 0.69	1.36 ± 0.53	1.14 ± 0.78
3	2.24 ± 1.35	2.59 ± 0.95	3.25 ± 1.06	3.00 ± 0.87	3.76 ± 2.03
5	3.27 ± 1.45	3.41 ± 1.30	4.19 ± 1.41	5.81 ± 1.54	6.82 ± 3.44

bigger than the registration errors of kidneys, which is expected. As the noise level for the reconstruction error increases, the registration errors increase too, but at a slower pace. At a lower noise level, most registrations only require 1 iteration of optimization. However, the ICP step is necessary to keep the registration robust as the noise increases. The last column shows that the registration results deteriorate rapidly without the ICP to correct a poor initial correspondence.

3.3 Results from a Set of *in vivo* Data

A CT scan of $1mm \times 1mm \times 3mm$ was used to build the initial m-rep model for the target kidney. Because of the lack of enough training data, the deformation model built from the synthetic data was used to guide the registration of the m-rep to the video sequence. There is no ground truth surface mesh available. A dense set of 200 surface points were reconstructed from the video sequence and were used in the registration. The average distance between the surface points to the implied boundary surface of the registered m-rep is $2.65mm$.

4 Discussion

Our method has the advantages as follows: the registration via deformation cloning uses a statistical deformation model learned from often very limited training data, and the registration completes the deformed target object; only a small number of reconstructed landmarks are required as long as a good correspondence between the landmark set and the target model is established; the registered deformations of the target object can be used to estimate deformations to important substructures.

We are working on live animal experiments to further validate our method. One challenging but rewarding extension of our method is to combine and apply multiple deformation models to a new target object.

References

1. Devernay, F., Mourgues, F., Coste-Maniere, F.: Towards endoscopic augmented reality for robotically assisted minimally invasive cardiac surgery. In: Proceedings of the International Workshop on Medical Imaging and Augmented Reality (MIAR 2001), pp. 16–20 (2001)
2. Lau, W., Ramey, N., Corso, J., Thakor, N., Hager, G.: Stereo-based endoscopic tracking of cardiac surface deformation. In: Barillot, C., Haynor, D.R., Hellier, P. (eds.) MICCAI 2004. LNCS, vol. 3217, pp. 494–501. Springer, Heidelberg (2004)
3. Lo, B.P., Scarzanella, M.V., Stoyanov, D., Yang, G.Z.: Belief propagation for depth cue fusion in minimally invasive surgery. In: Metaxas, D., Axel, L., Fichtinger, G., Székely, G. (eds.) MICCAI 2008, Part II. LNCS, vol. 5242, pp. 104–112. Springer, Heidelberg (2008)
4. Hu, M., Edwards, P., Figl, M., Hawkes, D.J.: 3D reconstruction of internal organ surfaces for minimal invasive surgery. In: Ayache, N., Ourselin, S., Maeder, A. (eds.) MICCAI 2007, Part I. LNCS, vol. 4791, pp. 68–77. Springer, Heidelberg (2007)
5. Mohamed, A., Davatzikos, C., Taylor, R.: A combined statistical and biomechanical model for estimation of intra-operative prostate deformation. In: Dohi, T., Kikinis, R. (eds.) MICCAI 2002. LNCS, vol. 2489, pp. 452–460. Springer, Heidelberg (2002)
6. Hu, Y., Morgan, D., Ahmed, H.U., Pends, D., Sahu, M., Allen, C., Emberton, M., Hawkes, D., Barratt, D.: A statistical motion model based on biomechanical simulations for data fusion during image-guided prostate interventions. In: Metaxas, D., Axel, L., Fichtinger, G., Székely, G. (eds.) MICCAI 2008, Part I. LNCS, vol. 5241, pp. 737–744. Springer, Heidelberg (2008)
7. Yuen, S.G., Kesner, S.B., Vasilyev, N.V., Nido, P.J.D., Howe, R.D.: 3D ultrasound-guided motion compensation system for beating heart mitral valve repair. In: Metaxas, D., Axel, L., Fichtinger, G., Székely, G. (eds.) MICCAI 2008, Part I. LNCS, vol. 5241, pp. 711–719. Springer, Heidelberg (2008)
8. Pizer, S.M., Fletcher, T., Fridman, Y., Fritsch, D.S., Gash, A.G., Glotzer, J.M., Joshi, S., Thall, A., Tracton, G., Yushkevich, P., Chaney, E.L.: Deformable m-reps for 3d medical image segmentation. International Journal of Computer Vision - Special UNC-MIDAG issue 55(2), 85–106 (2003)
9. Fletcher, P.T., Lu, C., Pizer, S.M., Joshi, S.: Principal geodesic analysis for the nonlinear study of shape. Transactions on Medical Imaging (TMI) 23(8), 995–1005 (2004)
10. Lu, C., Pizer, S.M., Joshi, S., Jeong, J.Y.: Statistical multi-object shape models. IJCV 75(3), 387–404 (2007)
11. Han, Q., Merck, D., Levy, J., Villarruel, C., Damon, J.N., Chaney, E.L., Pizer, S.M.: Geometrically proper models in statistical training. In: Karssemeijer, N., Lelieveldt, B. (eds.) IPMI 2007. LNCS, vol. 4584, pp. 751–762. Springer, Heidelberg (2007)
12. Besl, P., Mckay, N.: A method for registration of 3-d shapes. IEEE TPAMI 14(2), 239–256 (1992)

Supervised Nonparametric Image Parcellation

Mert R. Sabuncu[1], B.T. Thomas Yeo[1], Koen Van Leemput[1,2,3],
Bruce Fischl[1,2], and Polina Golland[1]

[1] Computer Science and Artificial Intelligence Lab, MIT
[2] Department of Radiology, Harvard Medical School
[3] Dept. of Information and Computer Science, Helsinki University of Technology

Abstract. Segmentation of medical images is commonly formulated as a supervised learning problem, where manually labeled training data are summarized using a parametric atlas. Summarizing the data alleviates the computational burden at the expense of possibly losing valuable information on inter-subject variability. This paper presents a novel framework for Supervised Nonparametric Image Parcellation (SNIP). SNIP models the intensity and label images as samples of a joint distribution estimated from the training data in a non-parametric fashion. By capitalizing on recently developed fast and robust pairwise image alignment tools, SNIP employs the *entire* training data to segment a new image via Expectation Maximization. The use of multiple registrations increases robustness to occasional registration failures. We report experiments on 39 volumetric brain MRI scans with manual labels for the white matter, cortex and subcortical structures. SNIP yields better segmentation than state-of-the-art algorithms in multiple regions of interest.

1 Introduction

Image segmentation in medical imaging aims to partition images into various regions of interest (ROIs), such as anatomical structures. Except in cases where the ROIs are distinguishable based on intensity information alone, prior information is typically needed in the form of manually labeled data. A common approach is to summarize the training data with a parametric model, usually referred to as an *atlas* [1,2,3,4,5]. Atlases aid segmentation by introducing a global coordinate system that restricts the number of possible structures occurring at a particular position and may encode the appearance of anatomical structures.

Atlas-based segmentation relies on the alignment of a new image to the atlas coordinate frame. Conventional methods utilize off-the-shelf inter-subject registration tools as pre-processing before segmentation [6,7,3]. Because the quality of registration can be improved with better segmentation and vice versa, several approaches have been proposed to unify the two problems [8,4,5].

An alternative strategy is to employ the entire training data set. Such an approach can exploit recently-developed fast and accurate, pairwise nonlinear registration algorithms, e.g. [9,10]. The label fusion (propagation) method [11,12] transfers the labels of training images to a test image after pairwise registration.

The segmentation labels of the test image are then estimated via majority voting. This method yields improved segmentation, since errors in the registration procedures are averaged out. A recent extension of label fusion [11] uses a subset of the training data, consisting of the subjects most similar to the test subject. Yet, segmentation is still performed via majority voting, where each relevant training subject has the same weight. Isgum et al. propose an ad-hoc method that uses local and soft weighting within the label-fusion framework [13].

In this paper, we develop a supervised nonparametric image parcellation (SNIP) framework conceptually similar to label fusion [12] and its extensions [11,13]. In contrast to these methods, we adopt a Bayesian approach, where segmentation is inferred via the Maximum A Posteriori (MAP) principle and the joint label and intensity image distribution is estimated in a nonparametric fashion. The transformations between the test image and each training image are modeled as nuisance random variables and marginalized using standard Bayesian approximations. Marginalization accounts for the uncertainty in registration, commonly ignored in the literature (see [14,15] for notable exceptions). The resulting optimization is efficiently solved using Expectation Maximization. Unlike [12], the similarity between a warped training image and test image plays an important role: more similar training images are weighted more in segmentation.

The soft weighting of training subjects was recently used for shape regression [16], where the weights were a function of age difference between the subjects. The proposed SNIP framework is also related to STAPLE [17], which fuses multiple segmentations of a single subject. In contrast, SNIP handles multiple subjects and accounts for inter-subject registration.

We report experiments on 39 brain MRI scans that have corresponding manual labels, including the cortex, white matter, and sub-cortical structures. We demonstrate that SNIP compares favorably to state-of-the-art segmentation algorithms in multiple regions of interest.

2 Theory

Let $\{I_i\}$ be N training images with corresponding label maps $\{L_i\}$, $i = 1, \ldots, N$. We assume the label maps take discrete values that indicate the label identity at each spatial location. Let $I : \Omega \mapsto \mathbb{R}$ denote a new, previously unseen test image defined on a discrete grid $\Omega \subset \mathbb{R}^3$. One common approach to estimate its label map $\hat{L}$ is via MAP estimation:

$$\hat{L} = \underset{L}{\operatorname{argmax}}\, p(L|I, \{L_i, I_i\}) = \underset{L}{\operatorname{argmax}}\, p(L, I|\{L_i, I_i\}), \qquad (1)$$

where $p(L, I|\{L_i, I_i\})$ denotes the joint probability of the label map L and image I given the training data. Rather than using a parametric model for $p(L, I|\{L_i, I_i\})$, we employ a non-parametric estimate:

$$p(L, I|\{L_i, I_i\}) = \frac{1}{N} \sum_{i=1}^{N} p(L, I|L_i, I_i). \qquad (2)$$

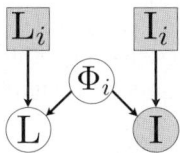

Fig. 1. Generative model for (L, I) given the template (L_i, I_i). Φ_i is the mapping from the image coordinates to the template coordinates. Squares indicate non-random parameters, while circles indicate random variables. Shaded variables are observed.

Eq. (2) can be viewed as a kernel density (Parzen window) estimate of the underlying distribution, or equivalently, a mixture distribution. $p(L, I|L_i, I_i)$ is the probability of (L, I), given that the new subject was generated from training subject i. Let $\Phi_i : \Omega \mapsto \mathbb{R}^3$ denote the unknown transformation that maps a test image grid point to a location in the training image i. Fig. 1 illustrates the generative model for $p(L, I|L_i, I_i)$, which assumes that the image I and label L are conditionally independent if the transformation Φ_i is observed. This yields:

$$\begin{aligned} p(L, I|L_i, I_i) &= p(I|L_i, I_i)p(L|I, L_i, I_i) \\ &= p(I|I_i) \int_{\Phi_i} p(L|\Phi_i, L_i, I_i)p(\Phi_i|I, L_i, I_i)d\Phi_i \\ &\approx p(I|I_i) \int_{\Phi_i} p(L|\Phi_i, L_i, I_i)\delta(\Phi_i - \Phi_i^*)d\Phi_i \\ &= p(I|I_i)p(L|\Phi_i^*, L_i), \end{aligned} \quad (3)$$

where we used the standard mode approximation for the integral and

$$\Phi_i^* \triangleq \underset{\Phi}{\operatorname{argmax}}\, p(\Phi_i|I, L_i, I_i) = \underset{\Phi}{\operatorname{argmax}}\, p(I|\Phi, I_i)p(\Phi), \quad (4)$$

is the most likely transformation between test image I and training image I_i. Substituting Eqs. (2) and (3) into Eq. (1) yields

$$\hat{L} = \underset{L}{\operatorname{argmax}} \sum_{i=1}^{N} p(I|I_i)p(L|\Phi_i^*, L_i). \quad (5)$$

The objective function in Eq. (5) can be viewed as a mixture distribution, where the label likelihood terms $p(L|\Phi_i^*, L_i)$ are the mixture components and the image likelihood terms $p(I|I_i)$ – which encode the similarity between the test image I and training image I_i – are the mixing coefficients. This optimization problem can be solved efficiently using Expectation Maximization (EM). In the next section, we instantiate the model and present the corresponding EM algorithm.

3 Model Instantiation

In our current implementation, we assume the image likelihood is a spatially independent Gaussian with a stationary variance σ^2:

$$p(I|I_i, \Phi_i) = \prod_{x \in \Omega} \frac{1}{\sqrt{2\pi\sigma^2}} \exp\left[-\frac{1}{2\sigma^2}\left(I(x) - I_i(\Phi_i(x))\right)^2\right]. \tag{6}$$

We model the label likelihoods as a product of independent multinomials:

$$p(L|L_i, \Phi_i) = \prod_{x \in \Omega} \pi_{L_i}(L(x); \Phi_i(x)), \tag{7}$$

where $\pi_{L_i}(l; \Phi_i(x))$ encodes the probability of observing label l at grid location $x \in \Omega$ of the test image, given that the test image is generated by training image i and Φ_i is the mapping from the coordinates of the image to those of the training image i. We compute $\pi_{L_i}(\cdot; \Phi_i(x))$ by applying the transformation Φ_i to the vector image $\pi_{L_i}(\cdot; x)$ where each voxel is assigned a length-$\mathcal{L}$ probability vector, with one indicating the manual label, and zero elsewhere. Non-grid values are obtained via trilinear interpolation.

Using the one-parameter subgroup of diffeomorphism, we parameterize a warp Φ with a smooth, stationary velocity field $v : \mathbb{R}^3 \mapsto \mathbb{R}^3$ via an ODE [9]: $\frac{\partial \Phi(x,t)}{\partial t} = v(\Phi(x,t))$ and initial condition $\Phi(x, 0) = x$. The deformation $\Phi(x) = \exp(v)(x)$ can be computed efficiently using scaling and squaring and inverted by using the negative of the velocity field: $\Phi^{-1} = \exp(-v)$ [18].

We impose an elastic-like regularization on the stationary velocity field:

$$p(\Phi = \exp(v)) = \frac{1}{Z_\lambda} \exp\left[-\lambda \sum_{y \in \Omega} \sum_{j,k=1,2,3} \left(\frac{\partial^2}{\partial x_j^2} v_k(x)\bigg|_{x=y}\right)^2\right], \tag{8}$$

where $\lambda > 0$ is the warp stiffness parameter, Z_λ is a partition function that depends only on λ, and sub-scripts denote coordinates (dimensions). A higher warp stiffness parameter yields more rigid warps.

3.1 Efficient Pairwise Registration

To evaluate the joint probability in Eq. (3), we need to compute Φ_i^* defined in Eq. (4). Using Eqs. (6) and (8), we can rewrite Eq. (4) as

$$\hat{v}^i = \underset{v}{\operatorname{argmin}} \sum_{y \in \Omega} \left[(I(y) - I_i(\exp(v)(y)))^2 + 2\lambda\sigma^2 \sum_{j,k=1,2,3} \left(\frac{\partial^2}{\partial x_j^2} v_k(x)\bigg|_{x=y}\right)^2\right], \tag{9}$$

where $\Phi_i^* = \exp(\hat{v}^i)$. To solve Eq. (9), we use the bidirectional log-domain Demons framework [10], which decouples the optimization of the first and second terms by introducing an auxiliary transformation. The update warp is first computed using the Gauss-Newton method. The regularization is achieved by smoothing the updated warp parameters. The smoothing kernel corresponding to Eq. (8) can be approximated with a Gaussian: $K(x) \propto \exp(-\alpha \sum_{i=1,2,3} x_i^2)$, where $\alpha = \frac{\gamma}{8\lambda\sigma^2}$ and $\gamma > 0$ controls the step size of the Gauss-Newton step.

3.2 The Image Likelihood

The image likelihood $p(I|I_i)$ is needed to evaluate the joint probability in Eq. (3). We expand $p(I|I_i)$ using the generative model in Fig. 1 and approximate the resulting integral using Laplace's method [19]:

$$p(I|I_i) = \int_\Phi p(I|\Phi, I_i) p(\Phi) d\Phi \approx p(I|\Phi_i^*, I_i) p(\Phi_i^*) \sqrt{(2\pi)^{3|\Omega|}/\det H}, \qquad (10)$$

where Φ_i^* is defined in Eq. (4) and computed in the previous section. det denotes matrix determinant, H is the Hessian matrix with entries $-\frac{\partial^2 \log[p(I|\Phi, I_i)p(\Phi)]}{\partial v_j(x) \partial v_k(y)}|_{\Phi = \Phi_i^*}$, for all $x, y \in \Omega \subset \mathbb{R}^3$ and $j, k = \{1, 2, 3\}$, and $|\Omega|$ is the number of voxels.

We approximate the determinant of the Hessian by ignoring the second derivative terms and interactions between neighboring voxels, cf.[15]:

$$\det H \propto \prod_{x \in \Omega} \det \left(\nabla I_i(\exp(v)(x))(\nabla I_i(\exp(v)(x)))^T + \frac{9}{2}\lambda\sigma^2 \mathrm{Id}_{3\times 3} \right), \qquad (11)$$

where $\nabla I_i(\exp(v)(x))$ is the 3×1 gradient of the warped training image I_i and $\mathrm{Id}_{3\times 3}$ is the 3×3 identity matrix.

3.3 Segmentation via EM

With our model instantiation, the solution of Eq. (5) cannot be found in closed form, since a mixture of factorized distributions is not factorized. Yet, an efficient solution to this MAP formulation can be obtained via Expectation Maximization (EM). The derivation of the EM algorithm is straightforward. Here, we present a summary. The E-step updates the weights associated with each training image:

$$m_i^{(n)} \propto p(I|I_i) \prod_{x \in \Omega} \pi_{L_i}(\hat{L}^{(n-1)}(x); \Phi_i^*(x)), \qquad (12)$$

where $\hat{L}^{(n-1)}(x)$ is the segmentation estimate of the test image from the previous iteration and the weights sum to 1, $\sum_i m_i^{(n)} = 1$. The M-step updates the segmentation estimate through the following maximization:

$$\hat{L}^{(n)}(x) = \underset{L(x)}{\mathrm{argmax}} \sum_{i=1}^{N} m_i^{(n)} \log\left(\pi_{L_i}(L(x); \Phi_i^*(x)) \right). \qquad (13)$$

The M-step in Eq. (13) performs an independent optimization at each voxel $x \in \Omega$. Each of these optimizations simply entails determining the mode of a length $\mathcal{L}$ vector, where $\mathcal{L}$ is the number of labels. The EM algorithm is initialized with $m_i^{(1)} \propto p(I|I_i)$ and iterates between Equations (13) and (12), until convergence.

4 Experiments

We validate SNIP with 39 T1-weighted brain MRI scans of dimensions $256 \times 256 \times 256$, 1mm isotropic. Each MRI was manually delineated by an expert anatomist into left and right White Matter (WM), Cerebral Cortex (CT), Lateral Ventricle (LV), Hippocampus (HP), Thalamus (TH), Caudate (CA), Putamen (PU), Pallidum (PA) and Amygdala (AM). We use volume overlap with manual labels, as measured by the Dice score [20], to quantify segmentation quality. The Dice score ranges from 0 to 1, with higher values indicating improved segmentation.

4.1 Setting Parameters through Training

SNIP has three independent parameters: (a) the image intensity variance σ^2 in Eq. (6), (b) the warp stiffness parameter λ in Eq. (8), and (c) the step size γ in the registration algorithm in Section 3.1. In particular, the registration component of SNIP is completely determined by γ and $\alpha = \frac{\gamma}{8\lambda\sigma^2}$, while the segmentation component is determined by σ^2 and λ.

Nine subjects were used to determine the optimal values of these parameters. First, 20 random pairs of these nine subjects were registered for a range of values of γ and α. Registration quality was assessed by the amount of pairwise label overlap and used to select the optimal (γ^*, α^*) pair.

We used the optimal (γ^*, α^*) pair to register all 72 ordered pairs of the 9 training subjects. We performed nine leave-one-out segmentations using these alignments with different pairs of σ^2 and λ that satisfy the relationship $\lambda \sigma^2 = \frac{\gamma^*}{8\lambda^*}$. The pair that yielded the best segmentation results was deemed optimal and used in validation on the remaining 30 subjects.

4.2 Benchmarks

First, we consider our implementation of the Label Fusion algorithm [12]. We use the pairwise registrations obtained with (γ^*, α^*) to transfer the labels to the training subject via nearest-neighbor interpolation. Segmentation is then computed through majority voting at each voxel. In the second benchmark, we use the label probability maps, where each training image voxel has a length-$\mathcal{L}$ vector, with one for the entry corresponding to the manual label, and zero otherwise. Segmentation for each voxel is determined to be the label corresponding to the mode of the label probability obtained by averaging the warped label probability maps, computed using the pairwise registrations and trilinear interpolation. We call this method Probabilistic Label Fusion.

4.3 Results

We report results for the 30 subjects not included in the group used for setting the algorithm parameters γ, σ, α. For each test subject, we treat the remaining subjects as training data. We note that the results from the two hemispheres are very similar and report results averaged across two hemispheres.

Fig. 2 shows box-plots of Dice scores for the two benchmarks and SNIP. These results indicate that SNIP outperforms the two benchmarks in all structures,

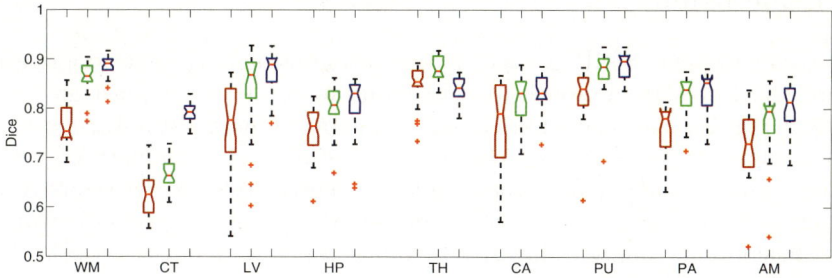

Fig. 2. Boxplots of Dice scores for Label Fusion (red), Probabilistic Label Fusion (green) and SNIP (blue). Medians are indicated by horizontal bars. Boxes indicate the lower and upper quartiles and vertical lines extend to 1.5 inter-quartile spacing.

Table 1. Comparison with FreeSurfer [1] and FreeSurfer Atlas Renormalization [2]

	HP	TH	CA	PU	PA	AM
SNIP	0.81 ± 0.07	0.84 ± 0.03	0.84 ± 0.04	0.89 ± 0.03	0.83 ± 0.04	0.80 ± 0.05
FS [1]	0.79 ± 0.09	0.88 ± 0.02	0.79 ± 0.10	0.81 ± 0.07	0.71 ± 0.09	0.71 ± 0.12
FSAR [2]	0.82 ± 0.04	0.88 ± 0.02	0.84 ± 0.05	0.85 ± 0.04	0.76 ± 0.06	0.75 ± 0.07

except the thalamus. The improvement is particularly significant in the White Matter, Cortex, Lateral Ventricle and Hippocampus. Between the two benchmarks, the performance of Probabilistic Label Fusion is consistently higher than that of Label Fusion. We note, however, that the results we report for SNIP are in the same ball-park as the ones reported for Label Fusion [12], and thus higher than what we achieve with our Label Fusion implementation. This might be due to differences in the data and/or registration algorithm. Specifically, normalized mutual information (NMI) was used as the registration cost function in [12]. Entropy-based measures such as NMI are known to yield more robust alignment results. We leave a careful analysis of this issue and an extension of SNIP that utilizes entropy-based similarity measures to future work.

Segmentation results for six subcortical structures were reported by two other state-of-the art atlas-based segmentation methods: FreeSurfer (FS) [1] and the FreeSurfer Atlas Renormalization (FSAR) technique [2]. Table 1 lists the average and s.t.d. of the dice scores reported in [1,2]. These results suggest that SNIP's performance is better for 3 ROIs (PU, PA, AM), equivalent for two ROIs (CA, HP) and worse for one ROI (TH).

The computational complexity of SNIP grows linearly with the number of training subjects. With the 39 training images we tested on, the segmentation procedure of each test subject took about 30 hours of CPU time on a modern computer. This run-time can be significantly reduced by solving the registrations in parallel. In comparison, Freesurfer took 10 hours and our Label Fusion implementation took 24 hours. Managing large training datasets within the SNIP framework is an important open question that we leave to future research.

5 Conclusion

This paper presents SNIP, a novel segmentation framework that adopts a nonparametric Bayesian approach to segmentation. By leveraging fast and robust nonrigid registration algorithms, SNIP exploits the entire training set, rather than a summary of it. In contrast to Label Fusion [12], similarities between the test image and training images play a central role in the segmentation. Our experiments indicate that SNIP promises to improve the performance of Label Fusion and compares favorably against other state-of-the-art atlas based segmentation methods in several regions of interest. One particularly promising future direction is to incorporate an entropy-based similarity measure into the computation of the image likelihood and pairwise registrations.

Acknowledgments. Support for this research is provided in part by: NAMIC (NIH NIBIB NAMIC U54-EB005149), the NAC (NIH NCRR NAC P41-RR13218), the mBIRN (NIH NCRR mBIRN U24-RR021382), the NIH NINDS R01-NS051826 grant, the NSF CAREER 0642971 grant, NCRR (P41-RR14075, R01 RR16594-01A1), the NIBIB (R01 EB001550, R01EB006758), the NINDS (R01 NS052585-01), the MIND Institute, and the Autism & Dyslexia Project funded by the Ellison Medical Foundation. B.T. Thomas Yeo is funded by the A*STAR,Singapore.

References

1. Fischl, B., Salat, D., van der Kouwe, A., Makris, N., Segonne, F., Quinn, B., Dale, A.: Sequence-independent segmentation of magnetic resonance images. Neuroimage 23, 69–84 (2004)
2. Han, X., Fischl, B.: Atlas renormalization for improved brain MR image segmentation across scanner platforms. IEEE TMI 26(4), 479–486 (2007)
3. Mazziotta, J., Toga, A., Evans, A., Fox, P., Lancaster, J.: A probabilistic atlas of the human brain: Theory and rationale for its development: The international consortium for brain mapping (ICBM). Neuroimage 2(2), 89–101 (1995)
4. Pohl, K., Fisher, J., Grimson, W., Kikinis, R., Wells, W.: A bayesian model for joint segmentation and registration. Neuroimage 31, 228–239 (2006)
5. Yeo, B., Sabuncu, M., Desikan, R., Fischl, B., Golland, P.: Effects of registration regularization and atlas sharpness on segmentation accuracy. Medical Image Analysis 12(5), 603–615 (2008)
6. Guimond, A., Meunier, F., Thirion, J.: Average brain models: A convergence study. Computer Vision and Image Understanding 77(2), 192–210 (2000)
7. Joshi, S., Davis, B., Jomier, M., Gerig, G.: Unbiased diffeomorphism atlas construction for computational anatomy. Neuroimage 23, 151–160 (2004)
8. Ashburner, J., Friston, K.: Unified segmentation. Neuroimage 26, 839–851 (2005)
9. Vercauteren, T., Pennec, X., Perchant, A., Ayache, N.: Symmetric log-domain diffeomorphic registration: A demons-based approach. In: Metaxas, D., Axel, L., Fichtinger, G., Székely, G. (eds.) MICCAI 2008, Part I. LNCS, vol. 5241, pp. 754–761. Springer, Heidelberg (2008)
10. Sabuncu, M., Yeo, B., Vercauteren, T., Leemput, K.V., Golland, P.: Asymmetric image template registration. In: Yang, G.-Z., et al. (eds.) MICCAI 2009, Part I. LNCS, vol. 5761, pp. 565–573. Springer, Heidelberg (2009)

11. Aljabar, P., Heckemann, R.A., Hammers, A., Hajnal, J.V., Rueckert, D.: Classifier selection strategies for label fusion using large atlas databases. In: Ayache, N., Ourselin, S., Maeder, A. (eds.) MICCAI 2007, Part I. LNCS, vol. 4791, pp. 523–531. Springer, Heidelberg (2007)
12. Heckemann, R., Hajnal, J., Aljabar, P., Rueckert, D., Hammers, A.: Automatic anatomical brain MRI segmentation combining label propagation and decision fusion. Neuroimage 33(1), 115–126 (2006)
13. Isgum, I., Staring, M., Rutten, A., Prokop, M., Viergever, M., van Ginneken, B.: Multi-atlas-based segmentation with local decision fusion-application to cardiac and aortic segmentation in CT scans. TM (in press, 2009)
14. Allassonniere, S., Kuhn, E., Trouve, A.: Construction of Bayesian deformable models via stochastic approximation algorithm: a convergence study. arXiv.org (2009)
15. Van Leemput, K.: Probabilistic brain atlas encoding using bayesian inference. In: Larsen, R., Nielsen, M., Sporring, J. (eds.) MICCAI 2006. LNCS, vol. 4190, pp. 704–711. Springer, Heidelberg (2006)
16. Davis, B., Fletcher, P., Bullitt, E., Joshi, S.: Population shape regression from random design data. In: Proc. of ICCV, pp. 1–7 (2007)
17. Warfield, S., Zou, K., Wells, W.: Simultaneous truth and performance level estimation (STAPLE): an algorithm for validation of image segmentation. TMI 23(7), 903–921 (2004)
18. Arsigny, V., Commowick, O., Pennec, X., Ayache, N.: A log-euclidean framework for statistics on diffeomorphisms. In: Larsen, R., Nielsen, M., Sporring, J. (eds.) MICCAI 2006. LNCS, vol. 4190, pp. 924–931. Springer, Heidelberg (2006)
19. MacKay, D.: Information Theory, Pattern Recognition and Neural Networks (2003)
20. Dice, L.: Measures of the amount of ecologic association between species. Ecology 26(3), 297–302 (1945)

Thermal Vision for Sleep Apnea Monitoring

Jin Fei[1], Ioannis Pavlidis[1], and Jayasimha Murthy[2]

[1] Computational Physiology Lab,
University of Houston, Houston, TX, USA
jin.fei@gmail.com, ipavlidis@uh.edu
[2] Division of Pulmonary, Critical Care and Sleep Medicine,
University of Texas Health Science Center, Houston, TX USA
Jayasimha.Murthy@uth.tmc.edu

Abstract. The present paper proposes a novel methodology to monitor sleep apnea through thermal imaging. First, the nostril region is segmented and it is tracked over time via a network of cooperating probabilistic trackers. Then, the mean thermal signal of the nostril region, carrying the breathing information, is analyzed through wavelet decomposition. The experimental set included 22 subjects (12 men and 10 women). The sleep-disordered incidents were detected by both thermal and standard polysomnographic methodologies. The high accuracy confirms the validity of the proposed approach, and brings non-obtrusive clinical monitoring of sleep disorders within reach.

1 Introduction

Sleep apnea is a respiratory disorder in which the breath stops repetitively during sleep. It can occur hundreds of times during a single night and each breath pause takes more than ten seconds. Sleep apnea is a common disorder and its prevalence can be as high as 30% among middle aged adults. It is associated with the development of high blood pressure and other cardiovascular diseases, and may lead to metabolic, organic, central nervous system, and endocrine ailments [1]. Therefore, there is a strong need for unobtrusive breathing measurement methods, where lengthy sleep studies with the minimum amount of discomfort are required.

Various contact modalities have been developed to assess the likelihood of apnea that capitalize on different aspects of the breathing phenomenon. Polysomnography (PSG) is the most reliable diagnostic method for the detection of sleep apnea syndrome. It is a multi-channel wired signal acquisition system which typically records ECG, nasal airflow, abdominal and thoracic movements, and blood oxygen saturation SpO_2. The sensor probes and cables are uncomfortable for a patient under monitoring. They may interfere with the usual sleep pattern of the patient and influence the results of the test.

Human breathing consists of expiration and inspiration phases. The expired air has higher temperature than the inspired air due to heat exchange in the lungs and respiratory passageways [2]. This thermal nature of breath around the nostril area creates an opportunity for a thermal measurement. Thermal infrared imaging is a passive contact-free modality. The sensing element itself can be viewed as a 2D array of contact-free thermistors, and therefore has a principle of operation similar to the nasal thermistor probe in PSG.

In this paper, we introduce a novel thermal imaging method to detect sleep apnea in the clinical sleep lab. It is based on automatic tracking/localization of the nasal region and wavelet analysis. The sleep apnea events were automatically detected from the onset of higher energy at lower frequency wavelets. In Section 2, we describe the tracking and localization algorithms as well as the wavelet-based detection method. We discuss the experimental setup in Section 3.1 and present the experimental results in Section 3.2. Section 4 concludes the paper.

2 Methodology

To measure the breathing function in thermal video we need to track the motion of subject, localize the measurement region, and analyze the extracted signal. We address each of these issues in detail in the following subsections.

2.1 Tracking

We chose the coalitional tracking algorithm [3] to track facial tissue during breath measurements. It optimizes multi-tracker interaction via game theory. The coalitional tracking method was developed to address the conflicting goals of generality and accuracy that arise in the context of thermo-physiological measurements on the face. Thermal imaging is functional imaging that depicts an evolving physiological process. The dynamic nature of thermal imaging poses a modeling challenge to tracking. Particle filter trackers [4] overcome this challenge because they are general and adapt well to changes. The accuracy of these trackers peaks when the real estate they cover is neither too large nor too small. By optimizing the behavior of a spatially distributed cluster of particle filter trackers (coalition), one gains in accuracy without sacrificing adaptability.

We use a coalition grid composed of four particle filter trackers. The grid outline is drawn interactively by a click and drag operation on the first frame.

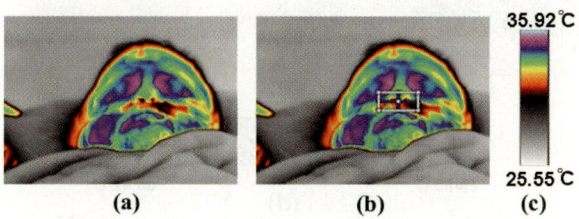

Fig. 1. (a) Thermal snapshot of a subject's face. (b) Initialization of coalitional tracker (TROI). (c) Thermal color map.

It encompasses comfortably the nostril region without any stricter specification. The grid outline constitutes the Tracking Region of Interest (TROI) - see white rectangle in Figure 1. The localization algorithm (see Section 2.2) operates within TROI and determines more rigorously the nostril region of measurement.

2.2 Localization

The source of thermal signal is the nostrils where we select the Measurement Region of Interest (MROI) for breathing. This region features both spatial and temporal variances. First, the shape of the nostril region is different for different individuals. Thermal imaging is a functional imaging modality that records the changing image physiology. In the case of breathing, thermal imagery registers the temperature fluctuation between the inspiration and expiration phases. This, however, increases the segmentation difficulty, as the shape of nostrils varies temporally due to the varying thermal signature of inspiration and expiration.

Figure 2 shows how within TROI the nostrils are separated from the rest of the facial tissue due to colder boundaries formed by cartilage. This feature can help to localize MROI. The contrast at the boundary of the nose is quite strong not only in thermal imagery but also in visual imagery, for different reasons. The nose is a distinct 3D feature in an otherwise 2D facial surface and forms strong edges at the seams. Due to similar nose boundary properties, we can leverage some of the work performed in the visual spectrum for thermal imaging purposes. Specifically, Brunelli and Poggio [5] showed that the horizontal gradients are useful in detecting the left and right visual boundaries of nose, whereas vertical gradients can detect the nose base. Kotropoulos and Pitas [6] demonstrated that the vertical and horizontal projection profiles of human nose are obtained by summing-up visual pixel intensities row-wise and column-wise, respectively. We have used elements of these approaches transplanted in the thermal infrared domain.

Let $I(x,y)$ be the original thermal image and $E_X(x,y)$ and $E_Y(x,y)$ be the edge images after applying the Sobel edge detectors. We perform integral

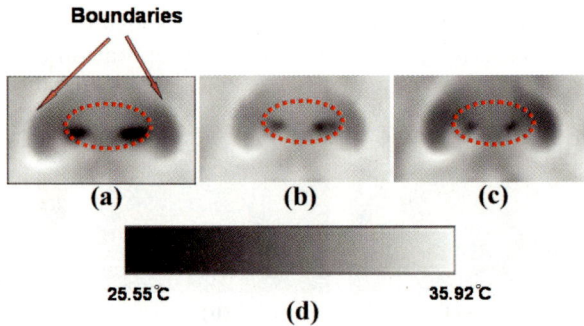

Fig. 2. Temporal variance of nostril region in thermal imagery during breathing. (a) Inspiration phase. (b) Transition phase. (c) Expiration phase. (d) Thermal color map.

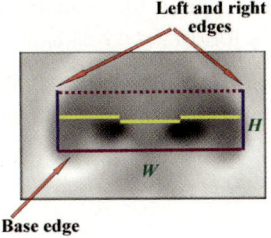

Fig. 3. MROI based on mean nose edges and anthropometric estimates

projections on the edge images to extract the outer edges of nostrils. The vertical and horizontal integral projections are:

$$P_v(x) = \sum_{y=y_1}^{y_m} E_X(x,y), \tag{1}$$

$$P_h(y) = \sum_{x=x_1}^{x_n} E_Y(x,y). \tag{2}$$

The left- and right-most peaks of $P_v(x)$ yield the left and right outer nostril edges correspondingly. The maximum of $P_h(y)$ yields the base edge.

The MROI selection varies from frame to frame. Some projections are weak and the locations vary as well. We use a time window of $4-5\ sec$ to compute the mean vertical and horizontal projections. Such window is representative of the full spatio-temporal evolution, as it covers both expiration and inspiration phases.

Based on anthropometric knowledge [7], the distance between left and right alares is about 30 mm and the distance between subnasale and columella is about 10 mm. Therefore, we estimate the nostril's height H as one third of its base edge segment W, which is delineated by the left and right outer nostril edges. Thus, we construct the MROI $W \times H$ (see Figure 3). We compute the mean temperature within MROI in every frame. This produces a quasi-periodic thermal signal along the timeline, which is indicative of the breathing function.

2.3 Wavelet Analysis

We perform wavelet analysis on the imaged thermal signal to detect the incidents of sleep apnea. Wavelet is the appropriate analysis tool as breathing is a non-stationary process.

The thermal video sampling rate fluctuates. A constant sampling rate is necessary for optimal results in wavelet decomposition. We choose the re-sampling rate of the thermal signal as 10 fps.

We normalize and perform wavelet analysis on sliding segments (windows) of the re-sampled thermal signal. As the sliding window travels along the evolving timeline of the re-sampled and normalized signal, we compute a series of wavelet energy coefficients. This renders apnea incident detection real time. The details of each algorithmic step are as follows:

Normalization. We define as $S(t)$, $t \in \{0, \cdots, N\}$, the re-sampled breathing signal. We normalize the signal amplitude as follows:

$$S'(t) = \frac{S(t) - \mu}{\sigma}, \qquad (3)$$

where μ and σ are the mean and standard deviation of $S(t)$ respectively. The normalization transforms signal $S(t)$ to $S'(t)$ with mean $\mu' = 0$ and standard deviation $\sigma' = 1$.

Wavelet Transform. We perform Continuous Wavelet Transformation (CWT) on the resampled and normalized thermal signal:

$$\Psi_{S'}^{\psi}(\tau, s) = \frac{1}{\sqrt{|s|}} \int S'(t) \psi(\frac{t-\tau}{s}) dt, \qquad (4)$$

where ψ is the 'mother wavelet', τ represents the translation parameter, while s denotes the scale at which the signal is examined. We use the Mexican Hat (MH) as the mother wavelet.

Wavelet Energy. CWT allows analysis at all scales, hence, facilitating the extraction of the signal component of interest (i.e., breathing and apnea). We assume that the wavelet energy at scale s_i corresponding to the wavelet coefficients $WT_i(t)$ is:

$$P_i = \sum |WT_i(t)|^2. \qquad (5)$$

We define P_n and P_o the wavelet energies of normal and obstructive breathing respectively. In normal breathing, P_n is larger than P_o. However, P_o increases at low frequency (higher scale) during sleep apnea incidents. Hence, we choose to monitor P_o for detection of sleep apnea events.

3 Experiments

3.1 Experimental Setup

The center-piece of the imaging system we used in our experiments is a FLIR SC6000 Mid-Wave Infra-Red (MWIR) camera with an Indium Antimonite (InSb) detector operating in the range $3-5$ μm [8]. The camera has a focal plane array (FPA) with maximum resolution of 640×512 pixels. The sensitivity is $0.025°$ C. The camera is outfitted with a MWIR 100 mm lens $f/2.3$, $Si:Ge$, bayonet mount from FLIR Systems [8]. The MWIR camera was calibrated with a two-point calibration at $28°$ C and $38°$ C, which are the end points of a typical temperature distribution on a human face.

The experiments took place in a climate controlled room according to an approved protocol by the Institutional Review Board of the University of Texas

Health Science Center. Subjects, lying in a comfortable bed, were positioned 10 ft away from the imaging system. The subjects were fitted with standard polysomnography (PSG) to ground-truth the imaging measurements. We recorded approximately one-hour long thermal clips (and the corresponding PSG signals) for each of the twenty-two subjects (twelve men, ten women). The age range was 24 to 66 years and the Body Mass Index (BMI) 19.71 to 45.57 kg/m^2. The control group included twelve subjects who had no history of obstructive sleep apnea. The pathological group had ten subjects with clinical diagnosis of obstructive sleep apnea. The ground-truth apnea events were detected by clinical specialists and reviewed by clinical doctors.

3.2 Results

The thermal signal produced in the vicinity of the nasal area is detectable when subjects are at sleep and can be recovered in pristine form with the help of the tracker. The interweaved inspiration and expiration phases produce periodic breathing signals. Figure 4 depicts a breathing signal from a patient suffering from obstructive sleep apnea. We report the presence of apnea (events) in 30 sec epochs, following established standards for clinical diagnosis. The computerized method features redundant epochs that overlap consecutive epochs by a half epoch. Therefore, we can detect the apnea event in $Epoch_{i+3}$, in the example shown in Figure 4. This event may be missed if only the consecutive epochs $Epoch_{i+2}$ and $Epoch_{i+4}$ are considered.

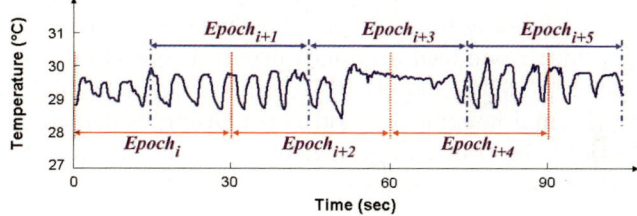

Fig. 4. Analysis of thermal breathing signals with overlapped epochs

We compute the wavelet energy from the thermal breathing curves. Apnea incidents are detected when P_o drops at the frequency of 6 cpm. In Figure 5, the spikes represent the epochs with apnea incidents. The wavelet energy threshold corresponding to the chosen P_o threshold is 2000 - it is computed from the simulated signal (similar to $Epoch_{i+3}$ in Figure 4).

Professional sleep medicine specialists manually scored the sleep events from PSG. Physicians certified in the specialty of Sleep Medicine reviewed scoring of apneas and finalized the interpretation of PSG. the apnea reports. The detected apnea events based on the computerized method are nearly the same as in the clinical report. The main difference is that the scoring process has been automated.

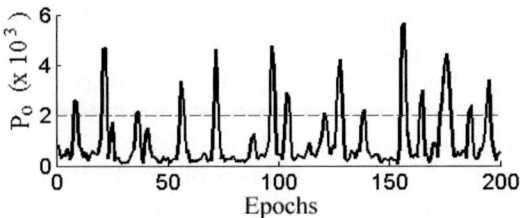

Fig. 5. Energy P_o for all the epochs

Table 1. Performance

Group	PSG Event	TP	TN	FP	FN	Accuracy	Precision	Recall
Control	22	19	2553	92	3	96.44	86.36	96.52
Pathological	145	132	1337	123	13	91.53	91.03	91.58
Overall	167	151	3890	215	16	94.59	90.42	94.76

We evaluated the measurement accuracy with three performance indicators: Accuracy, precision, and recall. Table 1 compares the results of true positive (TP), true negative (TN), false positive (FP), and false negative (FN) from both the control and pathological groups. Overall, the doctors reported 167 apnea events from PSG - 151 of these were detected by thermal imaging. There were 16 'false negative' cases. Most inconsistencies arose from 'false positive'. Such faults mainly resulted from tracking failures, when the tracker was misdirected to the background and away from the periodic effect of breathing. This resulted in a flat signal, which resembled an apnea event. The accuracy, precision, and recall were 94.59%, 90.42%, and 94.76%, respectively. The high performance proves that the thermal imaging method is promising in detecting incidents of sleep apnea. Besides the contact-free benefits, thermal imaging analysis could also assist in automating the diagnosis of sleep apnea.

4 Discussion and Conclusion

The current mean edge localization algorithm has been designed to deal with front views only. When the subject is on lateral posture (subject #3 and #21), we need to manually select the MROI. A pose estimation enhancement may fix this problem in the future. In case where both the nasal and oral areas are blocked by the blanket no measurement is feasible. Fortunately, such incidents happen rarely and do no last very long.

In general, the imaging method accurately recorded incidents of sleep apnea concomitantly with the standard detection instrument. Where the imaging method really shines is the highly automated and totally unobtrusive nature of its operation and the potential for improved post-processing, following the development of improved algorithms. By contrast, the subject needs to be outfitted with obtrusive sensors and cables in traditional PSG. The discomfort caused by such a monitoring method may interfere with the sleep routine of the subject, thus, biasing the experiment. This imaging method may be especially beneficial in pediatric patients or in patients with facial trauma.

In this paper, for the first time we have described a new methodology based on passive imaging to detect sleep apnea in clinical studies. The present method can automatically localize the nasal region. After applying Wavelet Transform, the method detects sleep apnea events based on the onset of high energy at low frequency wavelets. The sensing system can operate as a computer peripheral, which opens the way for home-based sleep monitoring in the future.

Acknowledgments. This material is based upon work supported by the National Institutes of Health Clinical and Translational Sciences Award (UL1RR024148; PI: Frank C. Arnett, M.D.) at the University of Texas Health Science Center, a research contract by the Defense Academy for Credibility Assessment, and National Science Foundation Awards (IIS-0812526, CNS-0521527, and IIS-0414754) - PI: Ioannis Pavlidis, Ph.D. - at the University of Houston. Any opinions, findings, and conclusions or recommendations expressed in this material are those of the authors and do not necessarily reflect the views of the funding agencies.

References

1. Pack, A.: Centennial review: advances in sleep-disordered breathing. Am. J. Respir. Crit. Care Med. 173, 7–15 (2006)
2. Zhang, Y.: Quantitative measurement of radiation properties for opaque and semi-transparent greybodies. Infrared Physics 30(2), 149–153 (1990)
3. Dowdall, J., Pavlidis, I., Tsiamyrtzis, P.: Coalitional tracking. Computer Vision and Image Understanding 106(2-3), 205–219 (2007)
4. Isard, M., Blake, A.: Condensation-conditional density propagation for visual tracking. International Journal of Computer Vision 29(1), 5–28 (1998)
5. Brunelli, R., Poggio, T.: Face recognition: Features versus templates. IEEE Transactions on Pattern Analysis and Machine Intelligence 15(10), 1042–1052 (1993)
6. Kotropoulos, C., Pitas, I.: Rule-based face detection in frontal views. In: IEEE International Conference on Acoustics, Speech, and Signal Processing, Munich, Germany, April 21-24, vol. 4, pp. 2537–2540 (1997)
7. Farkas, L.G.: Anthropometry of the Head and Face in Medicine. Elsevier, New York (1981)
8. FLIR Systems (2007), http://www.flir.com

Tissue Tracking in Thermo-physiological Imagery through Spatio-temporal Smoothing

Yan Zhou[1], Panagiotis Tsiamyrtzis[2], and Ioannis T. Pavlidis[1]

[1] Department of Computer Science, University of Houston, Houston, TX 77024, USA
[2] Department of Statistics, Athens University, Athens 10434, Greece
{yzhou9,ipavlidis}@uh.edu, pt@aueb.gr

Abstract. Accurate tracking of facial tissue in thermal infrared imaging is challenging because it is affected not only by positional but also physiological (functional) changes. This article presents a particle filter tracker driven by a probabilistic template function with both spatial and temporal smoothing components, which is capable of adapting to abrupt positional and physiological changes. The method was tested on tracking facial regions of subjects under varying physiological and environmental conditions in 12 thermal clips. It demonstrated robustness and accuracy, outperforming other strategies. This new method promises improved performance in a host of biomedical applications that involve physiological measurements on the face, like unobtrusive sleep studies.

1 Introduction

In the last few years, facial tracking in the thermal infrared spectrum received increasing attention. Initially, applications in surveillance and face recognition were the driving force, where thermal imaging has the distinct advantage of being impervious to lighting conditions [1][2]. Later, physiological variables, like vital signs, proved measurable in this modality [3][4][5][6], which gave rise to applications in Human-Computer Interaction [7], Medicine [8], and Psychology [9]. The degree of success of such measurements depends on a tracking method that can reliably follow the tissue of interest over time. For example, in sleep studies, if the tracker momentarily loses the nasal region of interest (see Figure 1), the generated breathing signal is far from accurate, which affects the ensuing analysis. Thus, the specification of a facial tracker in thermal infrared needs to be quite stringent.

The proposed method uses a particle-filter tracker, which is driven by a template-based objective function. The choice has to do with the peculiarities of thermal imaging and the needs of the targeted applications. Model-based tracking [10] is not very appealing in facial thermal imaging, because the modality images function not structure. Consequently, one is difficult to construct reliable shape-driven models.

To give an example and drive the point home, imagine that a tracker constructed out of deformable models is assigned to track the nose of a subject in thermal infrared imagery. Under normal conditions, the nose is colder than the surrounding tissue due to convection from nasal air flow. This translates to a

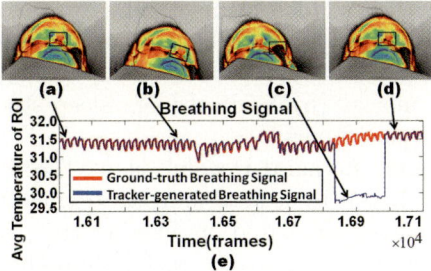

Fig. 1. (a) The initial frame with the rectangular ROI centered on the nostrils. (b) & (d) When the tracker works well, the generated breathing signal is good. (c) When the tracker loses the ROI, the generated breathing signal is far from accurate. (e) Tracker-generated compared with ground-truth breathing signal.

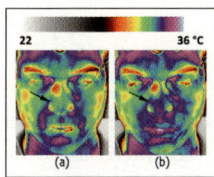

Fig. 2. Nose (a) in shape (b) out of shape

characteristic thermal shape similar to the one appearing in visual (structural) images (see Figure 2 (a)). At some point, an irritant reaches the subject's nostrils, there is an allergic reaction that blocks air flow in the nostrils and breathing continues mainly through the mouth. Because there is no air flow convection anymore, the temperature over the nasal tissue rises and the nostrils blend with the surrounding tissue in the imagery (see Figure 2 (b)). The nose is functionally 'gone' and so its characteristic thermal signature. In such cases where stochastic physiological changes affect thermal emission, a model tracker may encounter significant difficulties. Also, many of the targeted applications are in medicine and HCI. This necessitates a computationally 'light' tracker for real-time performance and with no training requirements, as the scenario variability is overwhelming.

Particle filtering is a general mechanism, free of strong modeling, which can accommodate very efficiently the predict-update loop. Assume that the update operation in this loop is realized through a template algorithm, capable of dealing with changes due to motion and thermal emission. The combination can potentially produce a fast, flexible, and accurate tracker, fullfiling the specifications of the application domain.

1.1 Previous Work

The literature in particle-filter tracking and templates is vast and well-known. This section focuses on a few representative methods that have been used as comparative yardsticks in the experimental part. It is by no means an exhaustive literature account.

In [11], Jepson at al. proposed a statistical appearance template, which weighted pixels with stable behavior heavier than pixels with less stable one. Appearance modeling is a powerful template mechanism, but has two weak points:

It does not cope well with sudden change and saturates after a long tracking period (needs re-starting). Both are problematic in the context of thermal facial imaging because: (a) Physiology can produce abrupt changes (e.g., perspiration) and the head sudden moves. (b) Medical (e.g., sleep studies) or psychological observations sometimes last hours.

In the thermal imaging domain, Dowdall et al. [12] proposed a network of particle-filter trackers driven by a deterministic template function. Each template pixel was updated or not, based on whether the respective difference exceeded or not a predetermined threshold. Such a Zero-One approach (i.e., either do not or do update a pixel) could not handle well abrupt orientation and/or physiology changes. It was also plagued by the drifting problem, due to its rigid nature.

The present paper describes a particle filter tracking method driven by a novel probabilistic template mechanism. This mechanism is based on the Matte algorithm, which was originally developed for segmentation purposes [13]. To the best of our knowledge, it is the first time that it is adopted for tracking purposes. The strong point of Matte for the problem at hand is that is based on pixel dependence (spatial smoothness). Indeed, there is spatial smoothness in thermophysiological imagery of the face. Muscular areas are relatively homogeneous and so are vascular areas. This is in contrast to the pixel independence assumption of appearance modeling, which is not realistic here. The authors have also introduced a temporal smoothness assumption, by modifying the Matte formula accordingly. This assumption holds true for appropriately small time windows and reduces oscillation.

The rest of the paper is organized as follows: Section 2 describes the methodology. In section 3, the experimental results demonstrate the relative advantage of the method with respect to other plausible approaches. Finally, section 4 concludes the paper.

2 Methodology

The particle filter tracker features 80 particles and performs a single iteration per frame. It is driven by a semi-stochastic optimization method. Initially, the method selects the most stable and unstable pixels in the ROI. These pixels constitute the seeds for the Matte computation step. The criteria for extracting maximally stable and unstable pixels are met, when pixel-wise intensity differences of the current frame from the template exceed predetermined thresholds. We used $\lambda_1 = 5$ and $\lambda_2 = 20$ as threshold values. Sensitivity analysis proved that the method is not very sensitive to these thresholds as far as the values do not get very close.

To compute the Matte of the current ROI, one assumes that the intensity of each pixel is a convex combination of a stable and an unstable map:

$$I_i = \alpha_i S_i + (1 - \alpha_i) U_i \tag{1}$$

where, I_i is the intensity of the ith pixel of the current ROI, α_i is the Matte value of the ith pixel and S, U refer to the stable and unstable maps respectively. The parameters on the right hand side of Eq. (1) are unknown and the goal is to solve for α_i. The composite Eq. (1) is similar to the one appearing in [13] and various methods to solve for α_i have been proposed. In the present paper, the authors introduce a novel cost function with both spatial and temporal smoothing terms:

$$\alpha_{i,t} = \arg\min_{a,b} \sum_{j \in I}(\sum_{i \in \omega_j}(\alpha_{i,t} - a_j I_i - b_j)^2 \\ + \epsilon a_j^2 + (\alpha_{i,t} - \alpha_{i,t-1})^2) \quad (2)$$

where, $a_j = 1/(S_j - U_j)$, $b_j = U_j/(S_j - U_j)$, ω is a small image window (usually 3×3), and ϵ is a small constant used for numerical stability.

The more unstable the pixels are, the more aggressive updating they need. The estimated Matte values indicate the necessary degree of updating for each pixel. More precisely, the pixel of the updated template at time t, will arise as a weighted sum of the previous template $T_i^{(t-1)}$, which was estimated at time $t-1$, and the ROI pixel $I_i^{(t)}$ from the current frame at time t; the weight α_i is being determined by the Matte value:

$$T_i^{(t)} = \alpha_i T_i^{(t-1)} + (1-\alpha_i)I_i^{(t)}. \quad (3)$$

One can deduce from Eq. (3) that for a stable seed the template value will not change (since $\alpha_i = 1$), while for an unstable seed the template value will update to the corresponding pixel in the current ROI (since $\alpha_i = 0$). Given the computed Matte, the new template will not only update the unstable seeds and reserve the stable seeds, but will also proportionally update their surrounding pixels based on the Matte values.

3 Experimental Results

For the purpose of testing the Spatio-Temporal Matte (STM) template update method in the context of particle filter tracking, the authors used 12 thermal clips from 11 subjects. The clips were generated as part of a clinical study on breathing [8] and a stress study related to lie detection [9], per the approval of the appropriate institutional review boards; they were kindly released to the authors. The set included clips that had at minimum $\sim 6,500$ and at maximum $\sim 49,500$ frames. The targeted facial areas included the nostrils, where vital physiological function is resident, or the periorbital, supraorbital, or maxillary where sympathetic activation is manifested.

The STM particle filter tracker is compared with the Zero-One particle filter tracker reported in [12] and the OAM template tracker reported in [11]. The Zero-One method uses a deterministic objective function to drive a particle-filter tracking loop. OAM is a probabilistic template tracker, but without spatial and temporal smoothness assumptions. Thus, they offer complementary opportunities to compare the effectiveness of STM's three main features: probabilistic nature, spatial smoothness, and temporal smoothness.

The trackers optimize three state variables, which serve as ROI descriptors. These are (x, y) for translation and ϕ for rotation on the image plane. The templates in all three trackers are formed out of normalized thermal values. All three tracking methods achieved real-time(>25fps) performance on a PentiumIV 4-core computer, with 4G memory. The particle filter tracker of the Zero-One method featured identical parameterization with that of STM. For every subject, all three trackers were tasked to track a selected facial tissue (ROI) from the exact same initial frame.

3.1 Qualitative Results

In thermal image tracking of the face, there are two major factors that affect the tracker's performance: Subject's motion and physiological changes. The first one alters the ROI location, while the second affects the spatial distribution of pixel values within the ROI. The data set features subjects that were experiencing small/large changes in the position and/or the physiology of the ROI. Based on the above, the following grouping was adopted: (1) Scenario 1: Large positional and small physiological changes. (2) Senario2: Small positional and large physiological changes. (3) Scenario 3: Large positional and large physiological changes.

Figure 3(a) shows a case representative of the first scenario. The video clip shows a subject that has abruptly turned his head, producing large positional change. Large positional change should not be interpreted here as in a surveillance context, where a person walks around. In a biometric or biomedical context, such as this, ROI motion is caused by head rotation. Although, in world coordinates this motion may be a few centimeters, in image plane coordinates spans almost the length of the image plane because the face covers the entire field of view. Even more important, the accuracy requirements are very strict, as a positional error of just a couple of pixels may invalidate the biomedical measurements. As the figure shows, STM copes well with the abrupt appearance changes due to motion. OAM adapts to the change at frame # 7868, but fails

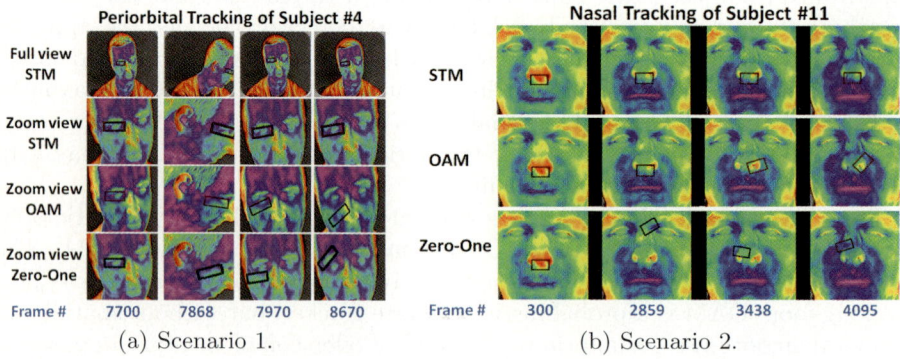

Fig. 3. Tracking examples from scenarios 1 and 2

when the subject snaps back his head at frame # 7970. The Zero-One method cannot adapt to change and fails outright at # frame 7868.

Figure 3(b) shows a case representative of the second scenario. The subject was under stress during a critical interview. As a result his physiology changed dramatically after 2 min into the process. STM copes well with the thermo-physiological change. OAM adapts to the physiological change at frame # 2859, but saturates after a few more thousands of frames and has already stalled at frame # 4095. The Zero-One method fails altogether.

3.2 Quantitative Results

To quantify how well each tracker performed, one needs to have the ground-truth location of the ROI and compare the tracker's ROI with the ground-truth ROI through the timeline. In medical imaging, the ground-truth data are usually obtained by manually segmenting the ROI in each frame. But with thousands of frames in the data set, manual ground-truthing was not practical. Instead, each of the three trackers were used to generate tracking results. The results were examined and where each tracker appeared to have failed, it was manually repositioned and tracking was initiated again from that point onward, to correct the error. At the end, ground-truth trackers were formed as the means of the individual corrected trackers.

Tracking performance correlates to the Euclidean distance and angular difference between the ground-truth ROI and the ROI that each of the three competing strategies produces. The closer these are, the better.

The 12 clips of the data set, when partitioned according to the three scenarios given above, they provide 7, 2, and 3 clips per scenario respectively. Figure 4(a) shows a graphical representation of the distribution of translational (Euclidean) errors for all subjects categorized by scenario. As the plot indicates, the STM approach outperformed the other two template update strategies in all scenarios. The OAM method has distinct difficulty with large combined positional-physiological changes, while the Zero-One with large positional changes. Figure 4(b) shows a graphical representation of the distribution of rotational errors for all

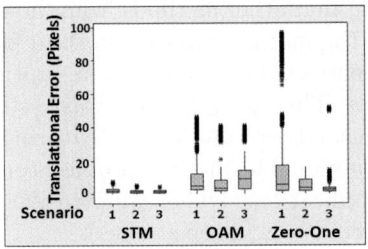
(a) Positional Box-Plot.

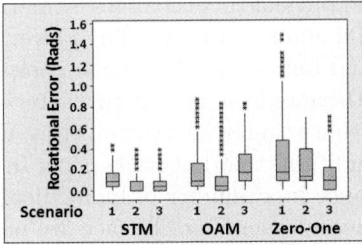
(b) Rotational Box-Plot.

Fig. 4. The box-plots of the positional and rotational error distributions for all three methods and subjects categorized by scenario

subjects categorized by scenario. STM still outperforms the others across the spectrum, but the relative error magnitude increased with respect to the translational error.

3.3 Benefit of Temporal Smoothing

To specify the beneficial effect of temporal smoothing, a simulation was run where a thermal nasal region was translated only in the x direction, while the y direction and angle of rotation ϕ were kept constant. The region featured semi-periodic fluctuation in temperature akin to the effect of breathing. This region was tracked first with a particle filter tracker driven by the classical Matte formula with spatial smoothing only. Then, it was tracked with the same particle filter tracker but driven by STM, that is, the modified Matte formula with both spatial and temporal smoothing. The trajectory results in Figure 5 demonstrate the fault oscillation introduced in the y and rotational dimensions by the classical Matte method.

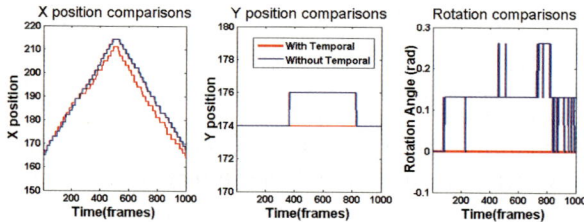

Fig. 5. Comparative trajectory results of Matte vs STM for controlled simulation experiment

4 Conclusions

This paper presents a new probabilistic template update method that when drives a particle filter tracker is capable of producing sophisticated tracking behavior in thermal facial imaging. Specifically, the method can cope with both large positional and physiological changes, something that other methods from the thermal or visual domain fail to do. The power of the method appears to stem from the spatial and temporal smoothness components of the template that capture well natural thermophysiological characteristics. The new approach was tested on a data set consisting of 12 thermal clips, thousands of frames each, featuring a variety of conditions that naturally occur in practice. The method promises improved performance in a number of biomedical applications, where unobtrusive physiological measurements on the face are preferred (e.g., sleep studies).

Acknowledgments. This material is based upon work supported by the National Science Foundation (NSF) under Grant No. #IIS-0812526, entitled "Do Nintendo Surgeons Defy Stress," and a research contract from the Defense

Academy for Credibility Assessmenr (DACA). Any opinions, findings, and conclusions or recommendations expressed in this material are those of the authors and do not necessarily reflect the views of the funding agencies.

References

1. Eveland, C., Socolinsky, D., Wolff, L.: Tracking human faces in infrared video. Image and Vision Computing 21, 579–590 (2003)
2. Kong, S., Heo, J., Abidi, B., Paik, J., Abidi, M.: Recent advances in visual and infrared face recognition - A review. Computer Vision and Image Understanding 97, 103–135 (2005)
3. Sun, N., Garbey, M., Merla, A., Pavlidis, I.: Imaging the cardiovascular pulse. In: Proceedings of the IEEE Computer Society Conference on Computer Vision and Pattern Recognition, San Diego, California, vol. 2, pp. 416–421 (2005)
4. Sun, N., Pavlidis, I., Garbey, M., Fei, J.: Harvesting the thermal cardiac pulse signal. In: Larsen, R., Nielsen, M., Sporring, J. (eds.) MICCAI 2006. LNCS, vol. 4191, pp. 569–576. Springer, Heidelberg (2006)
5. Murthy, R., Pavlidis, I.: Noncontact measurement of breathing function. IEEE Engineering in Medicine and Biology Magazine 25(3), 57–67 (2006)
6. Chekmenev, S., Farag, A., Essock, E.: Thermal imaging of the superficial temporal artery: An arterial pulse recovery model. In: Proceedings of the 2007 IEEE Conference on Computer Vision and Pattern Recognition, Minneapolis, Minnesota, June 17-22 (2007)
7. Pavlidis, I., Dowdall, J., Sun, N., Puri, C., Fei, J., Garbey, M.: Interacting with human physiology. Computer Vision and Image Understanding 108(1-2), 150–170 (2007)
8. Murthy, J., Faiz, S., Fei, J., Pavlidis, I., Abeulhagia, A., Castriota, R.: Remote infrared imaging: A novel non-contact method to monitor airflow during polysomnography. In: Chest Meeting Abstracts, Chicago, Illinois, October 20-25, vol. 132, p. 464 (2007)
9. Tsiamyrtzis, P., Dowdall, J., Shastri, D., Pavlidis, I., Frank, M., Ekman, P.: Imaging facial physiology for the detection of deceit. International Journal of Computer Vision 71(2), 197–214 (2006)
10. Faser, B., Luettin, J.: Automatic facial expression analysis: A survey. Pattern Recognition 36(1), 259–275 (2003)
11. Jepson, A., Fleet, D., El-Maraghi, T.: Robust online appearance models for visual tracking. IEEE Transactions of Pattern Analysis and Machine Intelligence 25(10), 415–422 (2003)
12. Dowdall, J., Pavlidis, I., Tsiamyrtzis, P.: Coalitional tracking. Computer Vision and Image Understanding 106(2-3), 205–219 (2007)
13. Levin, A., Lischinski, D., Weiss, Y.: A closed form solution to natural image matting. IEEE Transactions on Pattern Analysis and Machine Intelligence 30(2), 228–242 (2008)

Depth Data Improves Skin Lesion Segmentation

Xiang Li[1], Ben Aldridge[2], Lucia Ballerini[1], Robert Fisher[1], and Jonathan Rees[2]

[1] School of Informatics, University of Edinburgh, UK
x.li-29@sms.ed.ac.uk, lucia.ballerini@ed.ac.uk, rbf@inf.ed.ac.uk
[2] Dermatology, University of Edinburgh, UK
ben.aldridge@ed.ac.uk, jonathanlrees@mac.com

Abstract. This paper shows that adding 3D depth information to RGB colour images improves segmentation of pigmented and non-pigmented skin lesion. A region-based active contour segmentation approach using a statistical model based on the level-set framework is presented. We consider what kinds of properties (e.g., colour, depth, texture) are most discriminative. The experiments show that our proposed method integrating chromatic and geometric information produces segmentation results for pigmented lesions close to dermatologists and more consistent and accurate results for non-pigmented lesions.

1 Introduction

Segmentation is the first step of computer-based skin lesion diagnosis and its importance is twofold. First, the lesion boundary provides important information for accurate diagnosis. Second, the extraction of other clinical features critically depends on the accuracy of the boundary [1]. Due to reasons such as low contrast between the lesion and its background, artifact inference, etc., segmentation is a very challenging task. In recent years, many methods have been proposed for lesion boundary detection. Classic algorithms such as histogram thresholding, region-growing, k-means are widely used to segment lesions into homogeneous regions based on their intensity values. Xu et al. [2] introduced a semi-automatic method based on thresholding. Experiment results showed an average error that was about the same as that obtained by experts. Iyatomi et al. [3] proposed a dermatologist-like lesion region extraction algorithm that combined both pixel-based and region-based methods and introduced a region-growing approach which aimed to bring the extraction results closer to those determined by dermatologists. More recently, optimization based segmentation methods, especially active contours, have been applied to segment lesion images and have become more popular as they can produce decent results [4,5]. Tang presented a skin cancer segmentation algorithm using a multi-directional gradient vector flow snake [6]. The performance of their algorithm is close to human segmentation. Yuan et al. [7] proposed a novel multi-modal skin lesion segmentation method based on region fusion and narrow band energy graph partitioning. Comparisons showed that their method outperformed the state of the art methods with a mean error rate of 12.41% for XLM (oil immersion and cross-polarizaion mode of epiluminescence microscopy (ELM)) images and 12.28% for TLM (side-transillumination mode of ELM) images. They only used intensity features and an extension to incorporate colour and texture features was considered as future work. Unfortunately, most of these methods are developed for dermoscopy images and focus on pigmented melanocytic lesions (e.g., distinguishing melanoma from benign naevi). They are not suitable for the non-pigmented lesions, including two other important skin cancers **BCC** (Basal Cell Carcinoma) and **SCC** (Squamous Cell Carcinoma) for which early and correct diagnosis is also of great importance. They are included in our work.

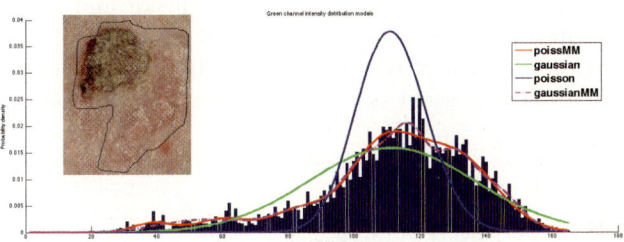

Fig. 1. The univariate density models of the lesion region on the green channel. The top-left shows the corresponding lesion - a **SCC** with dried exudate (The lesion region is identified with the black curve).

In this paper, we present a region-based active contour segmentation approach and apply it to both pigmented and non-pigmented lesion data including 2D conventional colour data and 3D topological (depth) data, which correlates strongly with human visual assessment of lesion surface appearance. The skin lesion data in this research is collected with a non-contact instantaneous dense stereophotometry system (equipped with ring flash for consistent lighting and a Macbeth colour chart), which outputs both dense 3D point cloud data and 1:1 aligned colour images [8]. An example of the image data is shown in Fig. 1 and Fig. 2(e)

For the level-set formulation of active contour segmentation, partitioning a given image is achieved by minimizing appropriate energy functions. Partial differential equations are used to drive the contours, which are implicitly represented as the (zero) level line of some embedding function, to evolve in the direction of a negative energy gradient [9]. Chan et al. proposed a region-based segmentation model using the Mumford-Shah functional [10]. Our method is inspired by another region-based level set segmentation using Bayesian inference [9]. It partitions the image domain by progressively fitting statistical models to the properties in each of a set of regions. The probabilistic formulation of the segmentation problem considers segmentation as a process of finding an optimal partition $P(\Omega)$ of the image domain by maximizing the *a posteriori* probability $p(P(\Omega)|I)$ for a given image I, integrating a regularity constraint.

2 Method

For active contour segmentation, an initial contour is needed as a first step of segmentation. We use a semi-automatic strategy, in which the initial contour is drawn roughly by hand. The level-set segmentation framework is used to refine this initial contour according to the regional information of the lesions.

For binary segmentation, the level-set formulation [9] is expressed as

$$E(\phi) = \int_{\phi \in \Omega} -H(\phi) \log p_1(f) - (1 - H(\phi)) \log p_2(f) + \nu |\nabla H(\phi)| d\phi. \quad (1)$$

$H(\phi)$ denotes the heaviside step function, p_1/p_2 are the pdfs inside/outside the contour. The first two terms in (1) model the areas inside and outside the contour while the last term represents the length of the separating contour. Considering the associated Euler-Lagrange equation for ϕ, the minimization of the energy functional by a gradient descent of the embedding function ϕ is [11]:

$$\frac{\partial \phi}{\partial t} = -\frac{\partial E(\phi)}{\partial \phi} = \delta(\phi) \left(\nu div(\frac{\nabla \phi}{|\nabla \phi|}) + \log \frac{p_2(f(x))}{p_1(f(x))} \right). \quad (2)$$

$\delta(\phi)$ has value 1 at the lesion boundary and 0 elsewhere.

In the following, the two questions concerning the above function are addressed: 1) how to chose a probabilistic model to fit the density distribution of properties and 2) which features or properties $f(x)$ should be used.

2.1 Distributions

Parametric density functions $p(f(x)|\theta)$ are used to model distributions. For a particular choice of parametric density, parameters θ modeling the distribution depend on the associated regions and update with the evolution of the contour.

Gaussian Mixture Model Extension. Lesion regions usually do not have a homogeneous content, especially for **BCC** and **SCC** (this is also the case for the background normal skin region because of hairs and skin markings). Hence, the density distribution of a property may have multiple peaks. This implies that the commonly used single multivariate Gaussian or Poisson model might not fit the data well. A multivariate Gaussian mixture model developed using an expectation-maximization(EM) algorithm was the final selected representation, shown in Fig. 1. The initial cluster parameters of components are determined by k-means algorithm. The number of the clusters are determined by optimization which chooses the largest average silhouette of the data (typically $K = 2$ to 3 for lesion region and $K = 1$ to 2 for skin region). The final evolution equation is

$$\frac{\partial \phi}{\partial t} = \delta(\phi) \left(\nu div(\frac{\nabla \phi}{|\nabla \phi|}) + \log \frac{p_{mixSkin}(f(x)|\mu_1, \Sigma_1, \ldots, \mu_K, \Sigma_K)}{p_{mixLesion}(f(x)|\mu_1, \Sigma_1, \ldots, \mu_K, \Sigma_K)} \right). \quad (3)$$

2.2 Image Properties

One central question is which properties characterize lesions and distinguish them from the background skin?

Colour. Colour is the most direct and critical property for dermatologists to assess and diagnose skin lesions, but which colour space or colour elements should be used? Here, the colour representation of lesions combines the results from different channels of different colour spaces. It includes 1) the Saturation of HSV, 2) $a*$ of CIE_Lab, 3) the normalized blue of RGB as lesions are often more prominent in this channel [1] and 4) the Hue of HSV. Hence, each image position is associated with a colour-valued feature vector, as $f(x) = (I_{saturation}, I_{a*}, I_{blue}, I_{hue})^T$. As shown in Fig. 2, the lesion area, especially the right part which is similar to surrounding skin is enhanced compared with the conventional RGB representation.

Relative depth. Lesion surface appearance attributes can be grouped into two major categories - chromatic and geometric attributes. The former has been extensively used. Little research has been done on geometric (or depth) properties to lesion segmentation. Our stereo imaging system obtains depth information as well as colour. We extract the relative depth I_{depth} between the current pixel and a quadric surface fitted to the background [8] to account for local surface shape, shown in Fig. 2(e). The texture of the depth data is also used.

Texture. Texture is an important property for lesion diagnosis, since it differs among different lesion types, as well as different locations of skin (e.g., lesion and healthy skin). We assign a local texture signature to each image location. A well known local representation is the gradient structure tensor which has good properties for texture discrimination and is widely used to represent texture [9]. It is a matrix of first partial derivatives. For an intensity image, the structure tensor is expressed as $J = \begin{pmatrix} I_{x1}^2 & I_{x1}I_{x2} \\ I_{x1}I_{x2} & I_{x2}^2 \end{pmatrix}$. The associated texture properties at each image location can be represented as $f(x) = (J_1, J_2, J_3) = \left(\frac{I_{x1}^2}{|\nabla I|}, \frac{2I_{x1}I_{x2}}{|\nabla I|}, \frac{I_{x2}^2}{|\nabla I|} \right)^T$. The first derivatives (I_{x1} and I_{x2}) of an image are not rotationally invariant. To compensate, we adopted the steerable Gaussian filter proposed in [12] to calculate the directional derivative I_{x1} oriented at angle α with respect to the x-axis and I_{x2} at degree $\alpha + 90°$. α starts at $0°$ degrees and increases by $15°$ until $90°$. The texture property at each image location is the average. Next, we sum the tensors of the individual channels. An adaptive anisotropic diffusion method is applied to smooth homogeneous regions while inhibiting diffusion in highly textured regions: $\frac{\partial J}{\partial t} = div[c(|\nabla J|)\nabla J], J(t=0) = J_0$.

We adopted the diffusion conductance proposed by Perona and Malik [13] as $c(x) = \exp\left(-\frac{x^2}{P^2}\right)$. c varies as a function of the texture properties. It is small where the gradient of the property image is large, resulting in lower diffusion near the textured locations like boundaries [14]. Two modifications are applied to improve the performance of the diffusion filter. First, the property image is smoothed by a Gaussian filter with parameter σ decreasing at each iterations. Second, we compute P adaptively as a function of time - higher at beginning and lower gradually. The time duration for the evolution of the diffusion function is determined experimentally as 20 iterations. The diffused structure tensor images

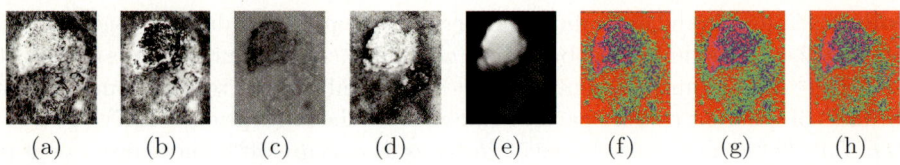

(a) (b) (c) (d) (e) (f) (g) (h)

Fig. 2. Colour properties of the lesion in Fig 1. (a) Saturation, (b) $a*$, (c) Blue, (d) Hue, (e) Stretched depth, (f)-(h)colour coded tensor elements $\frac{I_{x1}^2}{|\nabla I|}$, $\frac{2I_{x1}I_{x2}}{|\nabla I|}$ and $\frac{I_{x2}^2}{|\nabla I|}$.

are given in Fig. 2 (f), (g), (h). The textural difference can be seen between the lesion and its surrounding skin. The final property vector with colour, depth and texture properties is

$$f(x) = \left(I_{saturation}, I_{a*}, I_{blue}, I_{hue}, I_{depth}, \sum_{i=1}^{M} \frac{I_{ix1}^2}{|\nabla I_i|}, \sum_{i=1}^{M} \frac{I_{ix1}I_{ix2}}{|\nabla I_i|}, \sum_{i=1}^{M} \frac{I_{ix2}^2}{|\nabla I_i|} \right)^T, \quad (4)$$

where M is the number of colour and depth images. Here, M = 5.

3 Results

To reduce the influence of artifacts like hair and intrinsic cutaneous features (e.g., blood vessels, skin lines), image smoothing using 5×5 mean filtering is applied. After segmentation, post processing included hole filling, small segment deletion and local region growing.

The 20 test images used in our comparison are randomly selected from our lesion data-base, including 2 **SCC**, 4 **ML** (Melanocytic nevus), 7 **BCC**, 1 **AK** (Actinic Keratosis) and 6 **SK** (Seborrhoeic Keratosis). Seven of them are pigmented

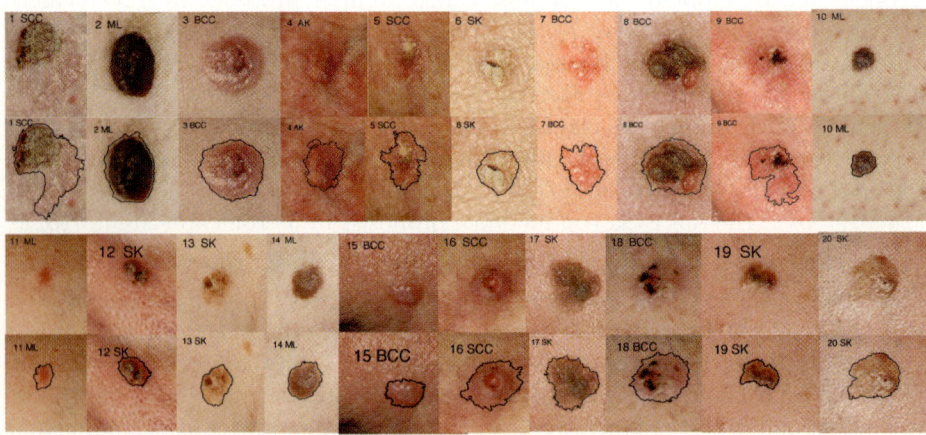

Fig. 3. The 20 test images and our segmentation results

lesions; while the other 13 are non-pigmented. These images are shown in Fig. 3 along with our segmentation results and corresponding lesion types. Manual segmentations given by 8 dermatologists from the Dermatology department of Edinburgh University are used for performance evaluation. A standard tumour area (**STA**) is defined as the region selected by four or more dermatologists.

The standard deviation (**SD**) of the area of manual segmentations is calculated for each lesion image and the value is normalized by the corresponding **STA**. There are big variations between dermatologists. The average **SD** over our 20 test images is 20.69%. There is more variation in clinical opinion of lesion boundaries for non-pigmented lesions (**SD** = 24.09%) than pigmented ones (**SD** = 9.74%).

To evaluate computer-based segmentations, we used the popular segmentation evaluation criteria XOR measure (or Error rate) defined as:

$$XOR = \frac{Area(AB \bigoplus MB)}{Area(AB + MB)} \times 100\%, \qquad (5)$$

where AB and MB are the binary images obtained by computer and the reference segmentation (**STA**), respectively. $\bigoplus$ denotes exclusive-OR and gives the pixels for which AB and MB disagree; + means union.

Based on this quantitative metric, we performed a comparison study of our method using different properties and the results are summarized as:

1. Our colour combination performed the best (average error rate of 11.14%) compared to the commonly used CIE_Lab colour space (11.71%).
2. Integrating colour and depth information reduces the error rate from 11.14% to 10.74%. Similarly, the colour structure tensor results are reduced from 10.80% to 9.68% by being extended with depth as shown in Fig. 4.

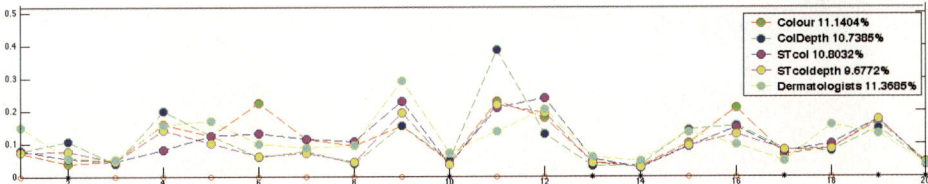

Fig. 4. Segmentation comparison. The associated lesions are shown in Fig. 3. Red ○ identifies non-pigmented lesions, black ∗ identifies pigmented lesions. Colour uses components 1-4 of $f(x)$, ColDepth uses 1-5, STcol uses 1-4, 6-8, STcoldepth uses 1-8.

We compared our method to both manual segmentations and a popular segmentation method [10] using the Mumford-Shah functional (**MS** method). The results are summarized in Table 1. The error rate of individual dermatologists and its variation is calculated. Our method produces very close segmentation to the dermatologists on pigmented lesions and more consistent segmentations on most non-pigmented lesions. This improvement can be explained as the integration of depth information which cannot be visualized by dermatologists from 2D

Table 1. Average segmentation error rates and their standard deviations

Error Rate %(XOR)	Dermatologists	MS [10]	Our method
Overall	11.37(8.22)	15.42(8.67)	9.68(5.90)
Pigmented	6.39(3.09)	10.46(7.9)	6.8(5.08)
Non-pigmented	14.05(6.13)	18.10(8.11)	11.23(5.89)

colour images as well as complicated texture associated with depth information. Fig. 5 shows contours obtained using different segmentation methods of several non-pigmented lesions (e.g., case 6, where the error rate improves significantly by integration depth and texture information, see Fig. 4).

It is hard to directly compare our approach to other algorithms because most other algorithms are designed for 1) other input modalities (e.g., dermoscopy) and 2) only melanocytic lesions. We did evaluate the Skin Cancer Segmentation software package [2], which is based on colour differences between the lesion and the surrounding skin and the thresholding algorithm (here called the DT method). Of our 20 test images, 12 failed totally, because the lesions did not have significant pigmentation. We only compared the segmentation performance on the remaining 8. Some results are shown in Fig. 5. (We tried to obtain the best performance by tuning of the DT method's 6 parameters.) Over the 8 usable lesions, our method provides a smaller average error rate (5.50% versus 12.46%) and for some cases, the error rate difference is significant (7.43% versus 34.75% in Fig. 5 (a)).

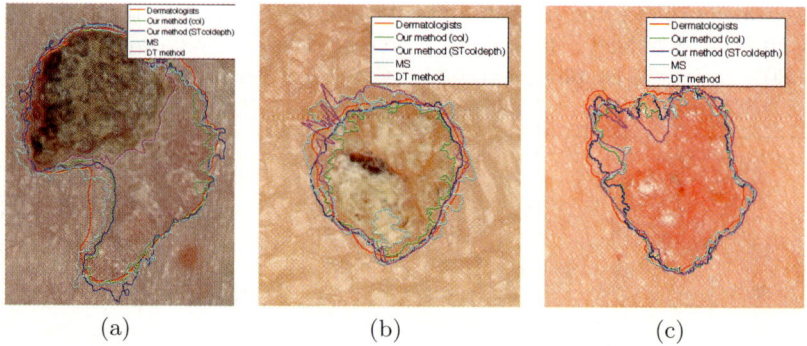

Fig. 5. The contours (cases 1, 6, 7 in Fig. 4) obtained by the dermatologists, MS [10], DT [2] methods and our methods based on colour (col) or colour and depth structure tensor (STcoldepth) properties

4 Conclusion and Further Work

A region-based probabilistic segmentation formulation using a statistical model within the level-set framework is applied to isolate lesions from their background. A multivariate gaussian mixture model is considered to be the best way to model the density distribution of properties. Upon comparison, we conclude that both depth and texture properties help to improve the segmentation result by reducing error rate from 15.42%±8.67% to 9.68%±5.90%. Our method integrating colour, depth and texture information produces the best results compared to those by the MS method [10], the DT method [2] and dermatologists.

There are several potential improvements and follow-up work to be considered: 1) In addition to the structure tensor, other texture features should be considered. 2) Better colour representation of lesion images is needed as well as better preprocessing to reduce the influence of artifacts such as specular reflections. 3) We have not implemented weight selection between different kinds of properties (i.e., colour, depth and texture) and just treat them equally.

References

1. Celebi, M.E., Iyatomi, H., Schaefer, G., Stoecker, W.V.: Lesion border detection in dermoscopy images. Comp. Medical Imaging and Graphics 33, 148–153 (2009)
2. Xu, L., Jackowski, M., Goshtasby, A., Roseman, D., Bines, S., Yu, C., Dhawan, A., Huntley, A.: Segmentation of skin cancer images. Image and Vision Computing 17(1), 65–74 (1999)
3. Iyatomi, H., Oka, H., Saito, M., Miyaka, A., Kimoto, M., Yamagami, J.: Quantitative assessment of tumour area extraction from dermoscopy images and evaluation of the computer-based methods for automatic melanoma diagnostic system. Melanoma Research 16(2), 183–190 (2006)
4. Chung, D.H., Sapiro, G.: Segmenting skin lesions with partial-differential-equations-bassed image processing algorithms. IEEE Transactions on Medical Imaging 19(7), 763–767 (2000)
5. Erkol, B., Moss, R., Stanley, R., Stoecker, W., Hvatum, E.: Automatic lesion boundary detection in dermoscopy images using gradient vector flow snakes. Skin Research and Technology 11(17-26) (2005)
6. Tang, J.: A multi-direction GVF snake for the segmentation of skin cancer images. Pattern Recognition 42, 1172–1179 (2009)
7. Yuan, X., Situ, N., Zouridakis, G.: A narrow band graph partitioning method for skin lesion segmentation. Pattern Recognition 42, 1017–1028 (2009)
8. McDonagh, S.: Skin cancer surface shape based classification. Thesis, School of Informatics, University of Edinburgh (2008)
9. Cremers, D., Rousson, M., Deriche, R.: Reviews of statistical approaches to level set segmentation: integrating color, texture, motion and shape. International Journal of Computer Vision 72(2), 195–215 (2007)
10. Chan, T.F., Vese, L.A.: Active contours without edges. IEEE Transactions in Image Processing 10(2), 266–277 (2001)
11. Bertelli, L., Sumengen, B., Manjunath, B.S., Gibou, F.: A variational framework for multiregion pairwise-similarity-based image segmentation. IEEE Transactions on Pattern Analysis and Machine Intelligence 30(8), 1400–1415 (2008)
12. Freeman, W.T., Adelson, E.H.: The design and use of steerable filters. IEEE Transactions on Pattern Analysis and Machine Intelligence 13(9), 891–906 (1991)
13. Perona, P., Malik, J.: Scale-space and edge detection using anisotropic diffusion. IEEE Trans. on Pattern Analysis and Machine Intell. 12(7), 629–639 (1990)
14. Weeratunga, S.K., Kamath, C.: Pde-based non-linear diffusion techniques for denoising scientific and industrial images: an empirical study. In: Image Processing: Algorithms and Systems Conference, SPIE, vol. 4667, pp. 279–290 (2002)

A Fully Automatic Random Walker Segmentation for Skin Lesions in a Supervised Setting

Paul Wighton[1,2,3], Maryam Sadeghi[1,3], Tim K. Lee[1,2,3], and M. Stella Atkins[1]

[1] School of Computing Science, Simon Fraser University, Canada
pwighton@sfu.ca
[2] Department of Dermatology and Skin Science, University of British Columbia and Vancouver Coastal Health Research Institute, Canada
[3] Cancer Control Research Program and Cancer Imaging Department, BC Cancer Research Centre, Canada

Abstract. We present a method for automatically segmenting skin lesions by initializing the random walker algorithm with seed points whose properties, such as colour and texture, have been learnt via a training set. We leverage the speed and robustness of the random walker algorithm and augment it into a fully automatic method by using supervised statistical pattern recognition techniques. We validate our results by comparing the resulting segmentations to the manual segmentations of an expert over 120 cases, including 100 cases which are categorized as difficult (i.e.: low contrast, heavily occluded, etc.). We achieve an F-measure of 0.95 when segmenting easy cases, and an F-measure of 0.85 when segmenting difficult cases.

1 Introduction

The segmentation of skin lesions is a crucial step in the process of automatically diagnosing melanoma. Inaccurate segmentations will affect all downstream processes such as feature extraction, feature selection and even the final diagnosis. Accurate segmentations are especially crucial for features that measure properties of the lesion border. Additionally, a recent study found that all commercially available automated systems evaluated had difficulty segmenting when the contrast between the lesion and skin was low[1]. We seek to improve skin lesion segmentations by employing supervised techniques to automatically initialize the random walker (RW) algorithm[2], which has been shown useful for interactive segmentations where boundaries are not clearly defined.

2 Previous Work

2.1 Skin Lesion Segmentation

The closest related work in skin lesion segmentation is by Celebi et. al.[3]. They reduce a dermoscopic image to 20 distinct colour groups, and assign labels to pixels based on the group to which they belong. They then define a metric, the *J-value*, which measures the spatial separation or isolation of each group. The *J-value* is derived from the separability criterion used by Fisher in Linear Discriminant Analysis[4]. Next, they define a localized *J-value* for a specific pixel by computing the metric over a neighbourhood around the pixel. By varying the neighbourhood size, they create several of these *J-images*. Multiscale methods are used to combine the images into a final segmentation. By creating a class map via color reduction, and employing various neighbourhood sizes they are incorporating, on some levels, textural information into their segmentation. In a follow-up study [5] Celebi et. al. apply their segmentation method to a set of dermoscopic images. Images are excluded if 1) the entire lesion is not visible, 2) the image contains too much occluding hair or 3) there is insufficient contrast between the lesion and surrounding skin. In total, 596 images are segmented, 32 of which are deemed to be unsatisfactory.

As will be seen in section 3, our method employs two of these concepts from [3]: the use of textural information in segmentation and the use of Fisher's separability criterion. Our application of these concepts, however, is substantially different.

2.2 Random Walker

The RW algorithm[2] is a general purpose, interactive, multi-label segmentation technique where a user labels the image with 'seed points' which denote the ground truth label for that pixel. Then, for an arbitrary pixel, the probability of a random walker reaching a seed of a specific label (before reaching seeds of any other label) is computed. However, the RW algorithm is sensitive to the exact placement of seeds and to the number of seeds placed[6]. While the RW algorithm is fast, intuitive and robust, it has been determined that a large number of seed points (up to 50% of the image) is required to reproduce a segmentation with only minor differences[6].

We have adopted the RW method described above into a novel framework, to automatically segment skin lesions from dermoscopic images.

3 Method

In this paper we present an approach to leverage the advantages of RW for automatic skin lesion segmentation. We initialize the RW algorithm automatically with seed points generated by 'learning' (by means of a training set) the difference between the properties of 'skin lesion pixels' and 'healthy skin pixels'.

3.1 Supervised Probabilistic Segmentation

We begin with a set of 120 expertly segmented dermoscopic images taken from atlases[7][8]. Each pixel is assigned either the label 'inside' (l_1) or 'outside' (l_2)

based on the ground truth segmentation. In this stage we aim to learn the difference between these two groups. Images are converted to L*a*b* space, and each channel is filtered with a set of Gaussian and Laplacian of Gaussian filters. Let m denote the number of filters employed. Pixels are then represented as a $1 \times 3m$ vector since each filter is applied to each of the 3 image channels. Linear Discriminant Analysis (LDA)[4] is then used to determine the linear combination of filters that best discriminate 'inside' and 'outside' pixels. LDA is similar to Principal Component Analysis (PCA), but where PCA is an *unsupervised* technique that reduces dimensionality while maintaining variance, LDA is a *supervised* technique that reduces dimensionality while maintaining class separability. This is achieved through an eigenvalue decomposition of an $3m \times 3m$ scatter matrix, which represents the separability of the classes with respect to each filter. Since this is a 2-class problem, we consider only the principle eigenvector. This eigenvector results in a linear combination of the filtersets for each image channel. Since the filterset employed is a series of low-pass (Gaussian) and high-pass (Laplacian of Gaussian) filters, the resulting 'eigenfilters' can be interpreted as either a high, low, or multiple-band-pass filters. We are therefore not only learning the colour difference between these two groups of pixels, but also the difference in the spatial variation of colours. This process is illustrated in Figure 1.

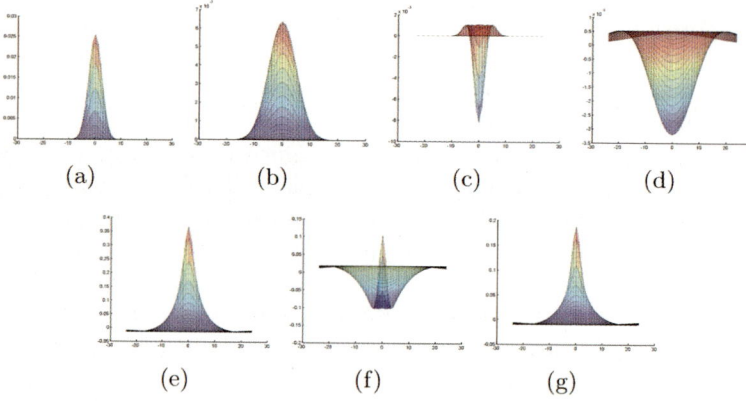

Fig. 1. Learning the difference between pixels inside and outside the segmentation. a)-d): Some filters from the filterset applied to each channel of each image. The filterset consists of Gaussian filters (a,b) and Laplacian of Gaussian filters (c,d) and the 'eigenfilters' as a result of LDA for the L*, a* and b* channels respectively (e,f,g).

Next, the response of the pixel groups ('inside' and 'outside') along this eigenvector are modeled as Gaussian distributions

$$P(p|l_i) = \frac{1}{\sigma\sqrt{2\pi}} \exp\left(-\frac{(x-\mu)^2}{2\sigma^2}\right) \qquad (1)$$

We create probability maps for unseen images by filtering the image with the resulting eigenfilters from LDA, and for each pixel p, assigning it a normalized probability that the pixel is inside the lesion

$$P = \frac{P(p|l_1)}{P(p|l_1) + P(p|l_2)} \quad (2)$$

The creation of a probability map is illustrated in Figure 2

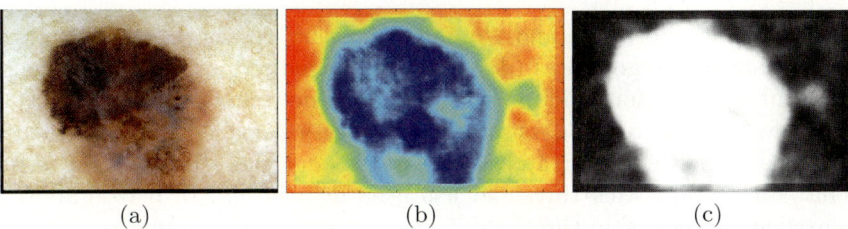

(a)   (b)   (c)

Fig. 2. The creation of a supervised probabilistic segmentation. a) The original dermoscopic image b) The image's response to the 'eigenfilter' from Figure 1 c) The resulting probability map by applying equation 2. Note the high response to the photodamaged skin to the right of the lesion. This is due to the fact that this pattern (known as a *pigment network*) usually occurs within lesions.

3.2 Initializing the Random Walker Algorithm

The original RW algorithm is an interactive segmentation which requires the user to place seed points. In our proposed automatic RW approach, there is no user interaction and the object and the background seeds are automatically determined from the probability map generated in section 3.1. To generate seed points, two thresholds must be determined. Let T_S represent the skin threshold and T_L represent the lesion threshold. Once these thresholds are determined, an arbitrary number of seeds can be automatically generated as long as the thresholding constraints are satisfied. Let $P(p)$ represent the probability a pixel p is a part of the lesion, as determined by equation 2. A pixel is a candidate for a background seed if $P(p) < T_S$. Similarly, a pixel is a candidate for an object seed if $P(p) > T_L$.

To determine T_S and T_L, we analyze the histogram of the probability map (shown in Figure 3(b),(f)). We fit a Gaussian Mixture Model to the histogram and extract the dominant Gaussians that represent the skin and lesion[9]. Let μ_S and μ_L represent the means of the 'skin' and 'lesion' Gaussians respectively. Similarly, let σ_S and σ_L represent the variances. Thresholds are then determined by:

$$T_S = \mu_S + 3\sigma_S \quad (3)$$

$$T_L = \mu_L - 3\sigma_L \quad (4)$$

Now, let $F(x)$ represent the cumulative histogram of the probability map. We then define two metrics α_H and β_H, using the subscript H ('histogram') to differentiate from the β parameter of the RW algorithm:

$$\alpha_H = \frac{F(T_L) - F(T_S)}{F(T_S)} \quad (5)$$

$$\beta_H = \frac{F(T_L) - F(T_S)}{F(1) - F(T_L)} \quad (6)$$

Low values for both α_H and β_H imply an easy to segment, high contrast image, as shown in Figure 3(a)-(d). The area shaded red in Figure 3(b) denotes the amount of pixels for which a label cannot be determined with certainty.

If however, either α_H, β_H or both are above a certain threshold, then the contrast between the lesion and skin is poor, and the segmentation is more difficult. Empirically, this threshold has been defined as 2.0. If α is above 2.0 then we define a new skin threshold T'_S as the median of the uncertainty range (the range between T_S and T_L). Similarly, if β is above 2.0 we define T'_L as the median of the uncertainty range. If both α and β are above 2.0, we take the larger value to determine which threshold to shift. This threshold adaptation is illustrated in Figure 3(e)-(h). Initially α_H and β_H are computed in Figure 3(e). The amount of uncertain pixels is large (grey and red shaded are) which is reflected in the high value $\beta_H = 7.88$. Since $\beta_H > 2.00$, we define $T'_L = 0.42$, which reduces the uncertain region (red) considerably.

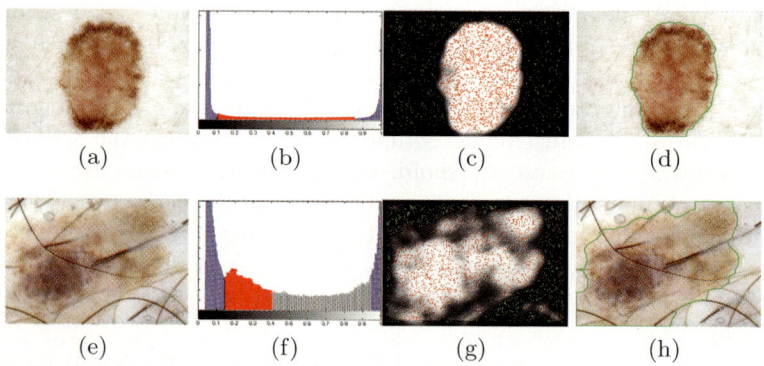

Fig. 3. Automatically initializing the RW algorithm. First row: A high contrast, easy to segment image. a) The initial image. b) The histogram of the image's probability map as generated by section 3.1. The blue area denotes candidate seed pixels ($\alpha_H = 1.27, \beta_H = 1.74, T_S = 0.10, T_L = 0.85$). c) Seed pixels randomly selected. d) The resulting segmentation. Second row: A difficult low-contrast lesion with occluding hair. The original parameters ($\alpha_H = 0.77, \beta_H = 7.88, T_S = 0.18, T_L = 0.97$) indicate its difficulty since, $\beta_H > 2.0$. T'_L is therefore set to 0.42 (reducing the uncertainty area to the red shaded region).

After determining the thresholds for the skin (T_S or T'_S) and the lesion (T_L or T'_L) pixels, seed points can now be chosen according to these thresholding constraints. We randomly choose 3% of pixels as seeds. Since spatial filtering methods are inaccurate near image borders (as can be seen in Figure 2(b) we impose an additional constraint and do not consider pixels in proximity to the image border as seed point candidates.

After placing seeds in the areas of high certainty, RW segments the image. RW gracefully handles the uncertain area in the probability map along the lesion border. We initialize the RW graph edge weights using a Gaussian function of the image intensity as Grady does[2]. The Gaussian width in this function, which we denote as β_{RW}, is a free parameter that determines the degree to which two intensities are considered similar. Throughout this paper, this parameter has been fixed at 30. Finally, after applying the RW algorithm, the segmentations undergo morphological post-processing to fill holes and break isthmuses.

4 Results

We tested our method on a dataset of images taken from [7] and [8]. We begin by selecting 100 images that pose a challenge to segmentation methods, and call this imageset 'challenging'. These represent images that are often excluded from other studies[3]. An image is considered challenging if one or more of the following conditions is met: 1) the contrast between the skin and lesion is low, 2) there is significant occlusion by either oil or hair, 3) the entire lesion is not visible, 4) the lesion contains variegated colours or 5) the lesion border is not clearly defined. Next, we select 20 images that do not meet any of the above conditions, and call this imageset 'simple'. We merge these two imagesets, calling the resulting imageset 'whole'. Finally, we create an imageset to measure the intraobserver agreement of our expert. We randomly select 10 images from the 'challenging' imageset. These images undergo a random rotation of 90, 180 or 270 degrees, and some are randomly inverted along the X and/or Y axes. This is done to reduce the likelihood that the dermatologist would recognize the duplicate image while performing the segmentation task. We call this imageset 'intra'.

Probability maps for all images are generated as described in section 3.1 using ten-fold cross validation. Seeds are placed automatically as described in section 3.2. The results are summarized in Table 1. We also compare our results to the Otsu thresholding method[10] and measure the intra-observer variability of the expert. Segmentations obtained from our modified random walker algorithm, the Otsu method and the dermatologist are denoted as 'MRW', 'Otsu' and 'Derm' respectively. For all comparisons we compute precision, recall, F-measure[11], and border error[12].

As can be seen in Table 1, while the Otsu method consistently achieves a higher precision, its recall is much worse. This implies that the Otsu method consistently underestimates the lesion border, labeling many pixels as 'skin' that ought to be labeled as 'lesion'. When examining the more comprehensive metrics such as F-measure or border error, it is apparent that our modified random

Table 1. Comparing the results of our modified random walker segmentation algorithm (MRW) to that of Otsu's thresholding method[10] (Otsu), and a dermatologist's manual segmentation which acts as ground truth (Derm). Comparisons are performed over simple and challenging imagesets taken from [7] and [8]. See Section 4 for a description of these imagesets.

Comparison	Imageset	n	Precision	Recall	F-measure	Mean BE	Std BE
MRW vs. Derm	simple	20	0.96	0.95	0.95	0.079	0.024
MRW vs. Derm	challenging	100	0.83	0.90	0.85	0.31	0.19
MRW vs. Derm	whole	120	0.87	0.92	0.88	0.24	0.18
Otsu vs. Derm	simple	20	0.99	0.86	0.91	0.15	0.083
Otsu vs. Derm	challenging	100	0.88	0.68	0.71	0.44	0.40
Otsu vs. Derm	whole	120	0.91	0.74	0.78	0.34	0.36
Derm vs. Derm	intra	10	0.95	0.91	0.93	0.085	0.036

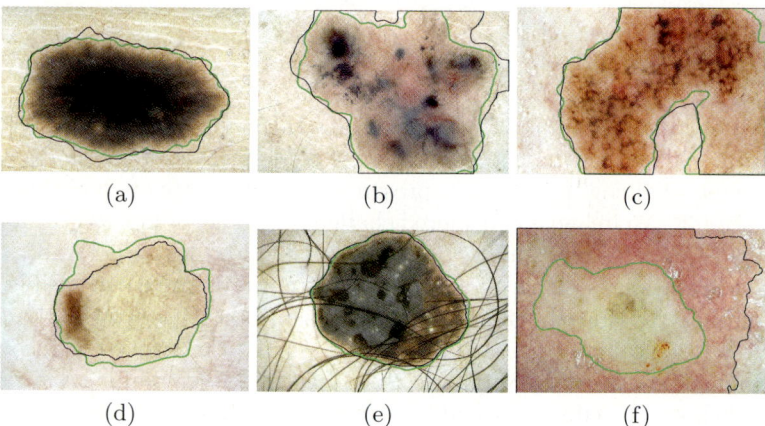

Fig. 4. Sample segmentation results for our method (denoted in black) compared to ground truth (denoted in green). a) A typical, easy to segment lesion. b) A lesion with variegated colours. c) An example of the entire lesion not being visible. Also, the lesion border is unclear in the bottom right hand side. d) A low contrast lesion. e) A lesion occluded significantly by hair. f) A difficult case where our method fails.

walker outperforms Otsu's method. The poorer F-measure and border error results for the Otsu method on the challenging imagest indicates its degree of difficulty. This is also born out by the results of the intra-observer agreement of the expert dermatologist on the 'intra' imageset.

Figure 4 shows sample results of the segmentations obtained from our method (denoted in black) as well as the ground truth segmentation (denoted in green) for a variety of lesions, including several difficult lesions.

5 Conclusion

We have developed a fully automatic method for segmenting unseen skin lesions by leveraging knowledge extracted from expert ground truth, and the random walker algorithm. Our method uses colour as well as texture to perform the segmentation and adapts itself to handle difficult, low-contrast images. Clinically, this is the first step towards an automated skin lesion diagnosis system. Future work will refine the method, and validate it on a larger dataset.

Acknowledgments. This research was funded by NSERC, CIHR and MITACS. The authors would also like to thank their collaborators Dr. Harvey Lui, Dr. David McLean and Dr. Bernardita Ortiz-Policarpio for their guidance and segmentations.

References

1. Braun, R.P., Rabinovitz, H.S., Oliviero, M., Kopf, A.W., Saurat, J.H.: Can automated dermoscopy image analysis instruments provide added benefit for the dermatologist? British Journal of Dermatology 157(5), 926–933 (2007)
2. Grady, L.: Random walks for image segmentation. IEEE Transactions on Pattern Analysis and Machine Intelligence 28(11), 1768–1783 (2006)
3. Celebi, M., Aslandogan, et al.: Unsupervised border detection in dermoscopy images. Skin Research and Technology 13(4), 454–462 (2007)
4. Fitzpatrick, J.M., Sonka, M.: Handbook of Medical Imaging, Volume 2. Medical Image Processing and Analysis (SPIE Press Monograph Vol. PM80). 1s edn. SPIE– The International Society for Optical Engineering (June 2000)
5. Celebi, M.E., Kingravi, H.A., Uddin, B., Iyatomi, H., Aslandogan, Y.A., Stoecker, W.V., Moss, R.H.: A methodological approach to the classification of dermoscopy images. Computerized Medical Imaging and Graphics, 362–373 (2007)
6. Grady, L., Schiwietz, T., Aharon, S., Munchen, T.U.: Random walks for interactive organ segmentation in two and three dimensions: Implementation and validation. In: Duncan, J.S., Gerig, G. (eds.) MICCAI 2005. LNCS, vol. 3750, pp. 773–780. Springer, Heidelberg (2005)
7. Argenziano, G., Soyer, H., et al.: Interactive Atlas of Dermoscopy (Book and CD-ROM). Edra medical publishing and new media (2000)
8. Soyer, H., Argenziano, G., et al.: Dermoscopy of Pigmented Skin Lesions. An Atlas based on the Consesnsus Net Meeting on Dermoscopy. Edra medical publishing and new media (2000)
9. Huang, Z., Chau, K.: A new image thresholding method based on Gaussian mixture model. Applied Mathematics and Computation 205(2), 899–907 (2008)
10. Otsu, N.: A threshold selection method from gray-level histograms. IEEE Transactions on Systems, Man and Cybernetics 9(1), 62–66 (1979)
11. Makhoul, J., Kubala, F., Schwartz, R., Weischedel, R.: Performance measures for information extraction. In: Broadcast News Workshop 1999, p. 249 (1999)
12. Hance, G., Umbaugh, S., Moss, R., Stoecker, W.: Unsupervised color image segmentation: with application to skin tumor borders. IEEE Engineering in Medicine and Biology Magazine 15(1), 104–111 (1996)

Author Index

Abbott, Jake J. I-540
Abd-Elmoniem, Khaled Z. II-331
Abolmaesumi, Purang I-75, I-803, II-795
Abou El-Ghar, Mohamed II-682, II-943
Abugharbieh, Rafeef II-474, II-490
Adams, Judith E. II-1017
Aganj, Iman II-423
Aguet, François II-625
Ahmed, Hashim Uddin I-787
Aickelin, Uwe I-984
Aja-Fernández, Santiago I-919, I-951, II-415
Akselrod-Ballin, Ayelet I-632
Al-Ahmad, Amin I-9
Alberola-López, Carlos I-156
Albrecht, Thomas II-1
Aldridge, Ben II-1100
Alexander, Daniel C. I-329
Allain, Baptiste I-491
Allard, Jérémie I-198
Allen, Clare I-787
Alvino, Christopher II-34
Amunts, Katrin II-795
An, Hongyu II-232
Ananthanarayanan, Rajagopal I-861
Andersson, Mats I-1000
Angelini, Elsa D. I-222, II-1025
Anquez, Jérémie II-1025
Anwander, Alfred I-886
Arai, Andrew II-741
Arbel, Tal II-109
Argibay-Quiñones, Daniel I-903
Armspach, Jean-Paul I-959, II-566
Arnold, Douglas L. II-584, II-601
Arzhaeva, Yulia II-724
Ashraf, Haseem II-699
Assemlal, Haz-Edine II-406
Atasoy, Selen I-499
Athanasiou, Thanos I-410
Atkins, M. Stella II-1108
Auzias, Guillaume I-730
Avedissian, Christina II-506
Avramescu, Taina II-316

Awate, Suyash P. II-141, II-200, II-852
Ayache, Nicholas I-214, I-297

Baillet, Sylvain I-730
Bainbridge, Daniel I-516
Balicki, Marcin I-108
Ballerini, Lucia II-1100
Barenstz, Jelle O. II-836
Barillot, Christian II-584
Barkovich, A. James I-289
Barmpoutis, Angelos I-640
Barratt, Dean I-787
Barrot Cortés, Emilia II-275
Barysheva, Marina I-845, I-967, II-498, II-506
Basser, Peter J. I-181
Baumann, Michael I-67
Bazin, Pierre-Louis I-943
Becher, Harald II-893
Beg, Mirza Faisal I-713, II-549
Bello, Fernando I-34
Ben Ayed, Ismail II-373, II-901
Bergeles, Christos I-540
Bernhardt, Boris I-214
Beširević, Armin II-356
Beymer, David I-648
Bhotika, Rahul I-239
Bi, Jinbo II-1009
Bibin, Lazar II-1025
Biesdorf, Andreas I-607
Bijnens, Bart H. I-140, II-759
Biros, George II-257, II-885
Bischof, Horst II-860
Blake, Andrew II-558
Blanc, Julie I-214
Blanc, Rémi II-84
Bloch, Isabelle I-222, II-1025
Blumberg, Hilary P. II-18
Bock, Davi I-632
Boctor, Emad I-507
Boesecke, Robert I-402
Boettger, Thomas I-828
Bogovic, John I-943
Boisgontier, Hervé I-959

Boissonnat, Jean-Daniel II-283
Boisvert, Jonathan I-803
Boltcheva, Dobrina II-283
Boselie, Toon I-524
Bossa, Matías Nicolás II-240
Boubekeur, Tamy II-1025
Boudjemline, Younes I-214
Bouix, Sylvain I-345
Brady, Michael II-398
Breteler, Monique M.B. I-853
Brodlie, Ken W. II-43
Brooks, Rupert I-51
Brost, Alexander I-394
Brückner, Marcel I-386
Brun, Caroline C. II-498, I-967
Brun, Luc II-406
Buatti, John II-827
Buechert, Martin II-665
Buhmann, Joachim M. II-633
Bullitt, Elizabeth I-321
Bulpitt, Andy J. II-43
Bunyak, Filiz II-617
Burdette, Everette C. I-59

Caan, Matthan I-869
Cahill, Nathan D. I-574
Cairncross, J. Gregory II-522
Camus, Estelle I-9
Cao, Kunlin I-739
Capuano, Ermanno I-369
Cárdenes, Rubén I-903
Cardoso, M. Christina II-617
Cardoso, Manuel Jorge II-441
Carlier, Stéphane II-776
Carneiro, Gustavo II-575
Carney, Paul R. I-190
Carr, Peter II-976
Carswell, Melody C. II-1067
Casula, Roberto I-34
Cates, Joshua II-167
Cavallaro, Alexander I-255
Cecchi, Guillermo A. I-1018
Chagin, Vadim II-617
Chan, Kap Luk II-803
Chan, Tony F. I-337, I-133
Chandran, Sharat I-230
Chang, Yu-Bing II-968
Chappell, Michael A. II-514
Chefdhotel, Christophe II-741

Chen, Albert Y. II-715
Chen, Elvis I-803
Chen, Mei I-100
Chen, Terrence II-877
Chen, Ting I-43
Chen, Yasheng II-232
Cheng, Guang I-190
Cheng, Jian I-911
Chiang, Ming-Chang I-967, II-506
Chiba, Toshio I-83
Chiu, Ing-Sh II-266
Chng, Nick II-960
Chong, Jaron II-373, II-901
Chou, Yi-Yu I-967, II-498
Christensen, Gary E. I-739, II-795
Chuang, Ming II-100
Chung, Albert C.S. I-696, II-59
Chung, François II-1051
Chung, Moo K. II-158, II-549
Ciompi, Francesco II-869
Ciuciu, Philippe I-975
Clark, Chris A. II-150
Clark, James I-410
Clarke, Colin I-516
Clarke, Duncan II-1067
Clarkson, Matthew J. II-441
Clarysse, Patrick II-365
Clayden, Jonathan D. II-150
Cobzas, Dana II-531
Cohen, Laurent II-1042
Collins, D. Louis II-109, II-584, II-592, II-601
Colliot, Olivier I-730
Comaniciu, Dorin I-17, I-116, I-255, II-575, II-767, II-877
Combès, Benoît II-175
Commowick, Olivier II-993
Connelly, Kim II-750
Cook, Richard I-491
Cootes, Tim F. II-1017
Corso, Jason II-715
Cotin, Stéphane I-198, II-291, I-377
Coukos, George I-230
Coupé, Pierrick II-601
Couton, Mathieu II-300
Criminisi, Antonio II-558

D'Haese, Pierre-François I-557
Daanen, Vincent I-67
Dahnke, Robert II-125

Dai, Wei II-133
Dalton, Kim M. II-158
Darzi, Ara I-410
Das, Sandhitsu R. II-141
Dassopoulos, Themos I-582
Datar, Manasi II-167
Davatzikos, Christos I-680, II-257
Davidson, Richard J. II-158
Dawant, Benoit M. I-557
De, Suvranu II-348
de Boer, Renske I-853
de Bruijne, Marleen II-51, II-699
De Craene, Mathieu I-140, II-759
de Groot, Marius I-853
Deguchi, Daisuke II-707
de Hoop, Bartjan I-263
Deinzer, Frank I-386, I-590
de Jong, Pim A. II-724
de Korte, Chris L. II-927
Delingette, Hervé I-214, II-1051
del Nido, Pedro J. I-26
Delorme, Sébastien I-51
Deng, Zhigang II-968
Denzler, Joachim I-386
Dequidt, Jeremie I-377
Deriche, Rachid I-911
De Robles, Paula II-522
Descoteaux, Maxime I-886, II-482
Deux, Jean-François I-672
Devlin, Steven I-75
Dewan, Maneesh II-715, II-1033
de Zubicaray, Greig I. I-845, I-967, II-498, II-506
Diallo, Mamadou I-9, I-828
Díaz, Alejandro II-690
Dick, Alexander II-750
Ding, Kai I-739
Dinov, Ivo II-208
Dione, Donald P. I-688
Doblaré Castellano, Manuel II-275
Dobrucki, Lawrence W. I-688
Dohi, Takeyoshi I-83, I-418, I-451
Dojat, Michel II-540
Donner, René II-860
Dougherty, Robert F. I-861
Drabycz, Sylvia II-522
Dubuisson, Florian I-475
Duchateau, Nicolas II-759
Duncan, James S. I-206
Dundar, Murat II-1009

Duong, Christophe I-9
Duriez, Christian I-377, II-291
Durrleman, Stanley I-214, I-297

Ebrahimi, Mehran I-811
Edenbrandt, Lars I-664
Edwards, Philip J. I-34
Eggers, Georg I-402
Ehrhardt, Jan I-755
Eklund, Anders I-1000
El-Baz, Ayman I-281, II-682, II-943
Elhawary, Haytham I-837
Elson, Daniel I-483
Emberton, Mark I-787
Engelbrecht, Rainer I-467
Eom, Jaesung II-348
Ernst, Floris II-356
Ersoy, Ilker II-617
Essafi, Salma II-919
Estépar, Raúl San José II-690
Euler, Ekkehard I-173

Fahmy, Ahmed S. II-985
Fahrig, Rebecca I-9
Falk, Robert II-682, II-943
Fang, Le I-198
Faraco, Carlos I-313
Fei, Jin II-1084
Feldman, Michael D. I-230
Fernández-Nofrerías, Eduard II-869
Feulner, Johannes I-255
Feußner, Hubertus I-459, I-467
Fichtinger, Gabor I-59, I-803
Figl, Michael I-34
Fillard, Pierre I-886, I-927
Fischl, Bruce I-598, II-1075
Fisher, Robert II-1100
Fleming, Ioana I-507
Fletcher, P. Thomas II-167
Fleuret, François II-625
Floros, Xenofon II-633
Fonteijn, Hubert I-329
Forbes, Florence II-540
Foroughi, Pezhman I-507
Fox, Nick C. II-441
Frangi, Alejandro F. I-140, II-759
Fua, Pascal II-625
Fuchs, Thomas J. II-633
Funka-Lea, Gareth I-222, II-34

Gangl, Alfred   I-247
García-Lorenzo, Daniel   II-584
Garg, Rahul   I-1018
Gaser, Christian   II-125
Gedamu, Elias   II-601
Gee, James C.   II-141, II-200, II-466, II-852
Gehlbach, Peter   I-108
Gelas, Arnaud   II-641
Geng, Xiujuan   II-795
Georgescu, Bogdan   I-17, II-767
Gerber, Samuel   I-305
Gerig, Guido   I-297, I-321, II-167
Ghosh, Aurobrata   I-911
Giannarou, Stamatia   I-483, I-499
Gibson, Eli   I-713
Gill, Sean   I-803
Gilmore, John   II-232
Gimel'farb, Georgy   I-281, II-682, II-943
Ginel Cañamaque, Ángel   II-275
Girgis, Hani   I-582
Glaunès, Joan   I-730
Glenn, Orit A.   I-289
Glocker, Ben   I-499, I-672
Goh, Alvina   I-877
Goksel, Orcun   II-248, II-960
Golland, Polina   I-272, I-565, I-598, I-1009, II-1075
Gong, Ren Hui   I-75
González Ballester, Miguel A.   II-275
González, Germán   II-625
Goodlett, Casey   I-321
Gouaillard, Alexandre   II-641
Gouttard, Sylvain   I-321, II-167
Grady, Leo   II-910
Grau, Vicente   II-893
Grimbergen, Cornelis   I-869
Grisoni, Laurent   II-291
Grossman, Murray   II-852
Gruionu, Gabriel   II-316
Gruionu, Lucian Gheorghe   II-316
Gu, Xianfeng   II-133
Guébert, Christophe   II-291
Guehring, Jens   II-741, II-910
Guevara, Pamela   I-935
Guillon, Jean-Pierre   II-976
Guo, Lei   I-313, II-184, II-458
Gurmeric, Serhan   II-776
Gutiérrez Boronat, Javier   I-459

Habas, Piotr A.   I-289
Hadjidemetriou, Stathis   II-665
Häfner, Michael   I-247
Hager, Gregory D.   I-91, I-426, I-435, I-507, I-582
Hall, Matt G.   I-329
Hämäläinen, Matti   I-1009
Hamarneh, Ghassan   II-649
Hambrock, Thomas   II-836
Hamm, Jihun   I-680
Han, Jae-Ho   I-108
Han, Qiong   II-1067
Handa, James   I-108
Handels, Heinz   I-755
Harel, Noam   II-423
Hartley, Richard   II-976
Hartov, Alexander   I-795, II-308
Hasegawa, Yosihnori   II-707
Hata, Nobuhiko   I-1, I-837
Hawkes, David J.   I-34, I-491, I-574, I-787
Heining, Sandro Michael   I-173
Heitz, Fabrice   I-959, II-566
Hennig, Juergen   II-665
Heredia, David   II-682, II-943
Herrero Jover, Javier   II-275
Hervé, Pierre-Yves   I-984
Hietala, Jarmo   II-216
Hinrichs, Chris   II-786
Ho, Harvey   II-323
Ho, Hon Pong   II-18
Hoffman, Eric A.   I-739
Hogeweg, Laurens   II-724
Höller, Kurt   I-459, I-467
Horiuchi, Tetsuya   I-451
Hornegger, Joachim   I-17, I-132, I-255, I-394, I-459, I-467, I-549, II-26, II-575, II-767, II-819
Houle, Helene   II-767
Howe, Robert D.   I-26
Hu, Mingxing   I-34, I-491
Hu, Yipeng   I-787
Huang, Albert   II-474
Huang, Wei   II-803
Huang, Xiaolei   II-673, II-1059
Huber, Martin   I-17, II-575
Huisman, Henkjan J.   II-836, II-927
Hunter, Peter   II-323
Hurtig, Mark   I-75

Ibrahim, Joseph G.   II-192
Idier, Jérôme   I-975
Iliescu, Nicolae   II-316
Inoue, Jiro   I-75
Ionasec, Razvan Ioan   I-17, II-767
Iordachita, Iulian   I-108
Irfanoglu, Mustafa Okan   I-181
Iseki, Hiroshi   I-443
Isguder, Gozde Gul   II-776
Ishii, Masaru   I-91
Ishikawa, Hiroshi   I-100
Islam, Ali   II-373, II-901
Itoh, Kazuko   I-443
Iwano, Shingo   II-707

Jacques, Robert   II-100
Jacques, Steven L.   II-657
Jäger, Florian   II-819
Jagersand, Martin   II-531
Jahanshad, Neda   II-498
Jahn, Jasper   I-459
Jain, Ameet K.   I-59
Janka, Rolf   II-819
Janowczyk, Andrew   I-230
Jayender, Jagadeesan   I-1
Jenkinson, Mark   I-705, II-951
Jezzard, Peter   II-514
Ji, Songbai   I-795, II-308
Ji, Yongnan   I-984
Jiang, Di   I-51
Jiang, Tianzi   I-911
John, Matthias   I-9
Johnson, Sterling   II-786
Johnsrude, Ingrid S.   II-795
Joldes, Grand Roman   II-300
Jolly, Marie-Pierre   II-910
Joshi, Sarang   I-305

Kabus, Sven   I-747
Kadir, Timor   I-771, II-34
Kadoury, Samuel   II-92
Kagiyama, Yoshiyuki   I-532
Kainmueller, Dagmar   II-76
Kaiser, Hans-Jürgen   I-607
Kakadiaris, Ioannis A.   II-885
Kane, Gavin   I-402
Kang, Jin   I-108
Kao, Chris   I-557
Kapusta, Livia   II-927
Kauffmann, Claude   I-475

Kazhdan, Michael   II-100
Keil, Andreas   II-389
Keller, Merlin   II-450
Kellman, Peter   II-741
Keriven, Renaud   II-482
Kerrien, Erwan   I-377
Khamene, Ali   I-9, I-828, II-381
Khan, Ali R.   I-713, II-549
Khudanpur, Sanjeev   I-426
Kier, Christian   II-935
Kikinis, Ron   II-690
Kim, Kio   I-289
Kim, Peter T.   II-158
Kim, Sung   I-43
Kindlmann, Gordon   I-345
King, Martin D.   II-150
Kirchberg, Klaus J.   II-68
Kitasaka, Takayuki   II-707
Kleemann, Markus   II-356
Klein, Stefan   I-369, I-853
Klinder, Tobias   I-747
Knösche, T.R.   I-886
Knutsson, Hans   I-1000
Koay, Cheng Guan   I-181
Kobayashi, Kazuto   I-532
Koch, Christoph   II-356
Kohlberger, Timo   II-34
Komodakis, Nikos   I-672
Konrad, Peter E.   I-557
Krishnan, Arun   II-715
Kumar, Rajesh   I-582
Kumar, Vedant   II-943
Kunz, Manuela   I-75
Kurhanewicz, John   II-844
Kutter, Oliver   I-763
Kwitt, Roland   I-247
Kwok, Ka-Wai   I-410
Kybic, Jan   II-365

Labat, Christian   I-59
Lahrech, Abdelkabir   I-148
Lamecker, Hans   II-76
Langs, Georg   II-860, II-919
Lara Rodríguez, Laura   II-275
Lauritsch, Günter   II-68, I-132, II-389
Lavielle, Marc   II-450
Law, Max W.K.   II-59
Le, Binh Huy   II-968
Lecoeur, Jeremy   II-584
Lee, Agatha D.   I-967, II-498

Lee, Junghoon   I-59
Lee, Tim K.   II-1108
Leemans, Alexander   I-853
Legg, Philip A.   I-616
Lenglet, Christophe   I-877, II-423
Leow, Alex D.   I-845
Leow, Wee Kheng   II-266
Leporé, Natasha   I-967, II-498
Lerotic, Mirna   I-410
Lesage, David   I-222
Levner, Ilya   II-522
Li, Chao   I-165
Li, Fuhai   II-609
Li, Gang   I-313, II-184, II-458
Li, Hao   II-266
Li, Hongsheng   II-673
Li, Hua   II-1042
Li, Huiqi   II-803
Li, Kaiming   I-313
Li, Rui   I-557
Li, Shuo   II-373, II-901
Li, Xiang   II-1100
Li, Yang   I-624
Li, Zhixi   II-1001
Liang, Jianming   II-1009
Liao, Hongen   I-83, I-418, I-451
Liao, Rui   I-394
Liao, Shu   I-696
Licht, Daniel   II-200
Lieberman, Jeffrey   II-192
Lim, Joo Hwee   II-803
Lin, Ching-Long   I-739
Lin, Fa-Hsuan   I-1009
Lin, Henry   I-426
Lin, Weili   I-321, I-721, II-192, II-232
Lin, Zhuohua   I-443
Ling, Haibin   I-116
Linguraru, Marius George   II-1001
Linte, Cristian A.   I-361
Liu, Fenghong   II-308
Liu, Huafeng   II-732
Liu, Jiang   II-803
Liu, Tianming   I-313, II-184, II-458
Liu, Xiaofeng   II-331
Liu, Yunlong   II-827
Lo, Pechin   II-51, II-699
Lollis, S. Scott   II-308
Lopata, Richard G.P.   II-927
López Villalobos, José Luís   II-275
Lorenz, Christine H.   II-741

Lorenz, Cristian   I-747
Lovat, Laurence B.   I-491
Lu, Le   II-715, II-1009
Lu, Yingli   II-750
Lurz, Philipp   I-214
Lüthi, Marcel   II-1
Lythgoe, Mark F.   I-329

Ma, Songde   I-198
Machiraju, Raghu   I-181
Madabhushi, Anant   I-230, II-844
Madsen, Sarah K.   I-967
Mahdavi, Seyedeh Sara   II-339, II-960
Mahfouz, Ahmed Essam   II-985
Makrogiannis, Sokratis   I-239
Malandain, Grégoire   II-993
Malcolm, James G.   I-894
Mallinson, Gordon   II-323
Mangin, Jean-François   I-730, I-927, I-935, II-117
Manjón, José V.   II-601
Mansi, Tommaso   I-214
Marchal, Maud   II-291
Mareci, Thomas H.   I-190
Mariano-Goulart, Denis   I-148
Marmulla, Rüdiger   I-402
Marshall, David   I-616
Martín-Fernández, Marcos   I-156, I-903
Martín-Fernández, Miguel Ángel   I-156
Martel, Anne L.   I-811
Martens, Volker   II-356
Masamune, Ken   I-83, I-418, I-451
Mateus, Diana   I-499
Mauri, Josepa   II-869
McGregor, Robert H.P.   I-124
McKeown, Martin J.   II-490
McLaughlin, Robert A.   II-657
McLennan, Andrew   II-398
McMahon, Katie L.   I-845, I-967, II-498, II-506
McNutt, Todd   II-100
Megason, Sean   II-641
Meining, Alexander   I-499
Melhem, Elias R.   II-141
Melvær, Eivind Lyche   I-771
Mendizabal-Ruiz, E. Gerardo   II-885
Menke, Ricarda A.   I-705
Mertins, Alfred   II-935
Metaxas, Dimitris   I-43
Metz, Coert T.   I-369

Meyer-Wiethe, Karsten II-935
Michaud, Gregory F. I-1
Milko, Sergiy I-771
Miller, James V. I-239
Miller, Karol II-300
Miller, Stephen I-313
Mirota, Daniel I-91
Mitchell, Ross II-522
Mithraratne, Kumar II-323
Mizutani, Masahiro I-451
Moch, Holger II-633
Modat, Marc II-441
Modha, Dharmendra S. I-861
Moore, John I-361, I-516
Mora, Vincent I-51
Moradi, Mehdi II-339
Morgan, James E. I-616
Mori, Kensaku II-707
Mori, Masaki II-707
Morosan, Patricia II-795
Morra, Jonathan H. II-432
Morris, William J. II-339, II-960
Morrison, Paul R. I-837
Mosaliganti, Kishore II-641
Mosayebi, Parisa II-531
Motomura, Noboru I-451
Motreff, Pascal I-475
Mountney, Peter I-483
Mousavi, Parvin I-803
Mozer, Pierre I-67
Mühling, Joachim I-402
Mullin, Gerard I-582
Muñoz-Moreno, Emma I-903
Muralidhar, Krishnamurthy I-124
Murphy, Keelin I-747
Murtha, Albert II-531
Murthy, Jayasimha II-1084
Mylonas, George P. I-353, I-410

Nakamoto, Masahiko I-532
Natori, Hiroshi II-707
Navab, Nassir I-173, I-499, I-763, I-779, II-389, II-767
Neefjes, Lisan A. I-369
Neimat, Joseph S. I-557
Nelson, Bradley J. I-540
Ng, Bernard II-490
Nichols, Thomas E. I-992
Nie, Jingxin I-313, II-184, II-458
Nielles-Vallespin, Sonia II-741

Nielsen, Mads II-699
Niessen, Wiro J. I-369, I-853
Nillesen, Maartje M. II-927
Noble, J. Alison I-574, II-893
Noblet, Vincent I-959, II-566
Noche, Ramil II-641

Obholzer, Nikolaus II-641
Oguro, Sota I-837
Oh, Teik II-1017
Ohlsson, Henrik I-1000
Ohlsson, Mattias I-664
Okada, Toshiyuki I-532, II-811
Okell, Thomas W. II-514
Olmos, Salvador II-240
Ostermeier, Martin I-116, II-877
Ota, Shunsuke II-707
Otomaru, Itaru I-532
Ou, Wanmei I-1009
Ourselin, Sebastien I-491, II-441

Pace, Danielle I-516
Pacheco, Elisa II-1017
Pajevic, Sinisa I-181
Palaniappan, Kannappan II-617
Pallavaram, Srivatsan I-557
Pan, Chunhong I-198
Panagiotaki, Eleftheria I-329
Papademetris, Xenophon I-206, I-688, II-18
Paragios, Nikos I-672, II-92, II-919
Pastrama, Stefan II-316
Patel, Rajni V. I-1
Paulsen, Keith D. I-795, II-308
Pavlidis, Ioannis T. II-1084, II-1092
Péchaud, Mickaël II-482
Pedersen, Jesper Johannes Holst II-51
Pendsé, Doug I-787
Penne, Jochen I-459, I-467, I-549
Pennec, Xavier I-214, I-297
Penney, Graeme P. I-34
Pérez, Frederic II-275
Pérez del Palomar, Amaya II-275
Perrin, Douglas P. I-26
Perrot, Matthieu I-730, II-117, II-450
Peters, Terry M. I-361, I-516
Petersen, Dirk II-356
Petrović, Aleksandar I-705
Pfefferbaum, Adolf II-224
Pham, Dzung L. I-943

Pichora, David   I-803
Pitiot, Alain   I-984
Platel, Bram   I-524
Pluim, Josien P.W.   I-263, I-747
Poupon, Cyril   I-886, I-927, I-935
Poynton, Clare   II-951
Pozo, Jose M.   I-140
Prastawa, Marcel   I-321
Price, Anthony   I-329
Prima, Sylvain   II-175
Prince, Jerry L.   I-59, I-943, II-331
Prokop, Mathias   I-263
Pruessner, Jens C.   II-592
Prümmer, Marcus   I-132
Prummer, Simone   I-116, II-877
Pujol, Oriol   II-869
Punithakumar, Kumaradevan   II-373, II-901
Pura, John A.   II-1001

Raczkowsky, Jörg   I-402
Radau, Perry   II-750
Radeva, Petia   II-869
Raij, Tommi   I-1009
Rainey, Sabrina   II-682
Rajagopal, Gunaretnam   I-43
Rajan, Purnima   I-582
Rajpoot, Kashif   II-893
Rangarajan, Anand   I-648
Rao, A. Ravishankar   I-1018
Rathi, Yogesh   I-894
Rechsteiner, Markus P.   II-633
Reed, Galen   II-844
Rees, Jonathan   II-1100
Reich, Daniel   I-943
Reichardt, Wilfried   II-665
Reid, R. Clay   I-632
Reiley, Carol E.   I-426, I-435
Reinartz, Rianne   I-524
Reinhardt, Joseph M.   I-739
Remple, Michael S.   I-557
Renard, Félix   I-959
Reyes, Mauricio   II-84
Ricco, Susanna   I-100
Rico, Agnès   I-148
Ridgway, Gerard R.   II-441
Rietzel, Eike   I-828
Riklin Raviv, Tammy   I-272
Risser, Laurent   I-975
Rivaz, Hassan   I-507

Rivière, Denis   I-935, II-117
Robbins, Peter   II-657
Roberts, David W.   I-795, II-308
Roberts, Martin G.   II-1017
Robles, Montserrat   II-601
Roca, Pauline   I-935
Roche, Alexis   II-450
Rodríguez Panadero, Francisco   II-275
Rohkohl, Christopher   I-132, I-549
Rohlfing, Torsten   II-224
Rohr, Karl   I-607
Roldan, Gloria   II-522
Rosen, Mark   II-844
Rosin, Paul L.   I-616
Ross, Ian   II-373
Ross, James C.   II-690
Rousseau, François   I-289, II-566
Rueckert, Daniel   I-34, II-466
Rumbach, Lucien   I-959, II-566
Rydell, Joakim   I-1000

Sabuncu, Mert R.   I-565, I-598, II-1075
Sadeghi, Maryam   II-1108
Sage, Caroline   I-869
Sahu, Mahua   I-787
Salcudean, Septimiu E.   II-248, II-339, II-960
Salganicoff, Marcos   II-715, II-1009
Salimi-Khorshidi, Gholamreza   I-992
Sampson, David D.   II-657
Samset, Eigil   I-771
Sandberg, Jesse K.   II-1001
Sands, Gregory   II-323
Sapiro, Guillermo   II-423
Sarrut, David   II-365
Sarry, Laurent   I-475
Sarunic, Marinko   II-649
Sasaki, Tomoya   I-443
Sasaroli, Dimitra   I-230
Sato, Yoshinobu   I-532, II-811
Saunders, Christobel   II-657
Savadjiev, Peter   I-345
Schaap, Michiel   I-369
Schaller, Christian   I-549
Scheinost, Dustin   I-688
Scherrer, Benoit   II-540
Schlichting, Stefan   II-356
Schmauss, Bernhard   I-467
Schmid, Holger   II-323
Schmidt-Richberg, Alexander   I-755

Schneider, Armin   I-459, I-467
Schrauder, Thomas   I-467
Schultz, Carl   I-369
Schuman, Joel   I-100
Schwab, Siegfried   II-819
Schweikard, Achim   II-356
Scolaro, Loretta   II-657
Seales, Williams B.   II-1067
Seidel, Günter   II-935
Seifert, Sascha   I-255
Seiler, Christof   II-84
Seim, Heiko   II-76
Sermesant, Maxime   I-214
Serruys, Patrick W.   I-369
Seshamani, Sharmishtaa   I-582
Sessa, Salvatore   I-443
Shaffer, Teresa   II-682
Shamaei, Kamran   I-540
Sharma, Swati   II-566
Shen, Dinggang   I-656, I-721, II-232
Shen, Tian   II-673, II-1059
Shenton, Martha E.   I-345, I-894
Sherbondy, Anthony J.   I-861
Shi, Chengyu   II-348
Shi, Pengcheng   II-732
Shi, Xiaoyan   II-192
Shi, Yonggang   II-208
Shotton, Jamie   II-558
Shyn, Paul B.   I-837
Silva, Etel   II-759
Silverman, Edwin K.   II-690
Silverman, Stuart G.   I-837
Simari, Patricio   II-100
Singh, Rajendra   I-230
Singh, Vikas   II-158, II-786
Sinusas, Albert J.   I-206, I-688
Siow, Bernard   I-329
Sitges, Marta   II-759
Sjöstrand, Karl   I-664
Skinner Jr., John   I-239
Slosman, Daniel O.   II-34
Smith, Benjamin   II-649
Smith, Mark   II-827
Smith, Stephen M.   I-705, I-992
Song, Danny Y.   I-59
Song, Qi   II-827
Song, Yi   II-43
Sonka, Milan   II-827
Sørensen, Lauge   II-699
Sotiras, Aristeidis   I-672

Soza, Grzegorz   II-26
Spadinger, Ingrid   II-960
Spinas, Giatgen   II-633
Sporring, Jon   II-51, II-699
Staib, Lawrence H.   II-18
Stewart, James   I-75
Stippich, Christoph   I-607
Stoyanov, Danail   I-353
Strauss, Olivier   I-148
Strobel, Norbert   I-394
Strup, Stephen E.   II-1067
Studholme, Colin   I-289
Stürmer, Michael   I-467, I-549
Styner, Martin   II-192
Suenaga, Yasuhito   II-707
Sugano, Nobuhiko   I-532, II-811
Suh, Jung W.   I-688
Sullivan, Edith V.   II-224
Summers, Ronald M.   II-9, II-1001
Sun, Loi Wah   I-410
Sun, Ying   I-165
Sun, Zhong Yi   II-117
Sunaert, Stefan   I-869
Sundar, Hari   II-257, II-381
Suzuki, Takashi   I-443
Syeda-Mahmood, Tanveer   I-648
Szczerba, Dominik   I-124
Székely, Gábor   I-124, II-84
Szmigielski, Cezary   II-893

Tada, Yukio   I-532, II-811
Tahmasebi, Amir M.   II-795
Takabatake, Hirotsugu   II-707
Takamoto, Shinichi   I-451
Takanishi, Atsuo   I-443
Takao, Masaki   I-532, II-811
Tam, Roger   II-474
Tao, Yimo   II-715
Tasdizen, Tolga   I-305
Tatli, Servet   I-837
Taylor, Andrew M.   I-17, I-214
Taylor, Russell H.   I-91, II-100, I-108
Telle, Benoît   I-148
ter Haar Romeny, Bart   I-524
Thijssen, Johan M.   II-927
Thompson, Paul M.   I-337, I-845, I-877, I-967, II-133, II-432, II-498, II-506
Tiwari, Pallavi   II-844
Toews, Matthew   II-109

Toga, Arthur W.   I-337, I-845, I-967, II-133, II-208, II-432, II-498, II-506
Tohka, Jussi   II-216
Trabelsi, Olfa   II-275
Traub, Joerg   I-173
Tristán-Vega, Antonio   I-919, I-951, II-415
Troccaz, Jocelyne   I-67
Trouvé, Alain   I-297, I-730
Tschumperlé, David   II-406
Tsiamyrtzis, Panagiotis   II-1092
Tsin, Yanghai   II-68
Tsukihara, Hiroyuki   I-451
Tu, Zhuowen   II-432
Tucholka, Alan   II-117
Tuncali, Kemal   I-837

Ugurbil, Kamil   II-423
Uhl, Andreas   I-247
Unal, Gozde   II-776
Unser, Michael   II-625
Uzunbaş, M. Gökhan   II-34

Vandemeulebroucke, Jef   II-365
van der Graaf, Maaike   I-869
van der Lugt, Aad   I-853
van Geuns, Robert Jan   I-369
van Ginneken, Bram   I-263, I-747, II-724
Van Leemput, Koen   I-272, I-565, II-1075
van Mameren, Henk   I-524
van Rikxoort, Eva M.   I-263
van Santbrink, Henk   I-524
van Vliet, Lucas   I-869
van Walsum, Theo   I-369
Varadarajan, Balakrishnan   I-426
Vasilyev, Nikolay V.   I-26
Vass, Melissa   I-239
Vavylonis, Dimitrios   II-673
Vécsei, Andreas   I-247
Vemuri, Baba C.   I-190, I-640, I-648
Vercauteren, Tom   I-565
Verma, Ragini   I-624, I-680
Vernooij, Meike W.   I-853
Vetter, Thomas   II-1
Vidal, René   I-877
Viergever, Max A.   I-263, II-724
Villa-Uriol, Maria-Cruz   I-140
Vincent, Thomas   I-975
Visentini-Scarzanella, Marco   I-353

Vitanovski, Dime   I-17
Vogel, Jakob   II-389
Voigt, Ingmar   I-214, II-767
von Elverfeldt, Dominik   II-665
Vos, Frans   I-869
Vos, Pieter C.   II-836

Wachinger, Christian   I-779
Wacker, Matthias   I-590
Waldman, Stephen D.   I-75
Wandell, Brian A.   I-861
Wang, Fei   I-648
Wang, Fei   II-18
Wang, Hanzi   I-91
Wang, Lejing   I-173
Wang, Linwei   II-732
Wang, Peng   II-877
Wang, Qian   I-656
Wang, Yalin   I-337, II-133
Wang, Yang   II-767
Warfield, Simon K.   I-632, II-300, II-993
Washko, George R.   II-690
Wedlake, Chris   I-361, I-516
Wei, Yiyi   I-198
Weidert, Simon   I-173
Wein, Wolfgang   I-9, I-763
Wells III, William M.   II-109, I-272, II-951
Wels, Michael   II-575
Wen, Xu   II-339
Werner, Rene   I-755
Westin, Carl-Fredrik   I-345, II-415, II-690, I-919
Whitaker, Ross   I-305, II-167
Wighton, Paul   II-1108
Wildenauer, Horst   II-860
Wiles, Andrew D.   I-361, I-516
Wimmer, Andreas   II-26
Wittek, Adam   II-300
Wittenberg, Thomas   I-459
Wolf, Matthias   II-1009
Wollstein, Gadi   I-100
Wong, Ken C.L.   II-732
Wong, Stephen T.C.   II-609
Wong, Tien Yin   II-803
Woo, John H.   II-141
Woolrich, Mark W.   II-514
Wörn, Heinz   I-402
Wörz, Stefan   I-607
Wrba, Friedrich   I-247

Wright, Graham II-750
Wright, Margaret J. I-845, I-967, II-498, II-506
Wu, Binbin II-100
Wu, Guorong I-656, I-721
Wu, Xiaodong II-827

Xia, James II-968
Xu, Chenyang I-9, II-68, II-381
Xu, Guofan II-786
Xu, Xie George II-348
Xuan, Jianhua II-715
Xue, Hui II-741, II-910

Yacoub, Essa II-423
Yamanaka, Noriaki I-83
Yamashita, Hiromasa I-83, I-418, I-451
Yang, Guang-Zhong I-353, I-410, I-483, I-499
Yao, Jianhua II-9
Yap, Pew-Thian I-656, I-721
Yatziv, Liron II-381
Yau, Shing-Tung II-133
Yazdanpanah, Azadeh II-649
Yedidya, Tamir II-976
Yeo, B.T. Thomas I-565, I-598, II-1075
Yezzi, Anthony II-1042
Yi, Zhao II-558
Yin, Youbing I-739
Yip, Michael C. I-26
Ynnerman, Anders I-1000
Yo, Ting-Shuo I-886
Yokota, Futoshi II-811
Yotter, Rachel Aine II-125
Yue, Ning I-43

Yuen, Shelten G. I-26
Yushkevich, Paul A. II-141, II-200, II-466
Yvinec, Mariette II-283

Zachow, Stefan II-76
Zacur, Ernesto II-240
Zecca, Massimiliano I-443
Zellars, Richard I-507
Zhan, Liang I-845
Zhan, Yiqiang II-1033
Zhang, Chong I-140
Zhang, Heye II-732
Zhang, Hui II-141, II-466
Zhang, Tuo II-184
Zhang, Wei I-116
Zhao, Hong II-609
Zhao, Lu II-216
Zhao, Qun I-313
Zheng, Guoyan I-820
Zheng, Yefeng II-575
Zheng, Yuanjie II-852
Zhou, Jinghao I-43
Zhou, Kevin Shaohua I-116, I-255
Zhou, Xiang Sean II-1033
Zhou, Xiaobo II-609, II-968
Zhou, Yan II-1092
Zhu, Hongtu I-721, II-192, II-232
Zhu, Siwei I-845
Zhu, Ying II-877
Zhu, Yun I-206
Zikic, Darko I-828
Zinser, Max II-76
Zuehlsdorff, Sven II-741
Zuo, Siyang I-418

Printing: Mercedes-Druck, Berlin
Binding: Stein+Lehmann, Berlin